REA'S TEST PREP FOR TODAY'S PRE-MED STUDENT

Your R_X for the MCAT® CBT

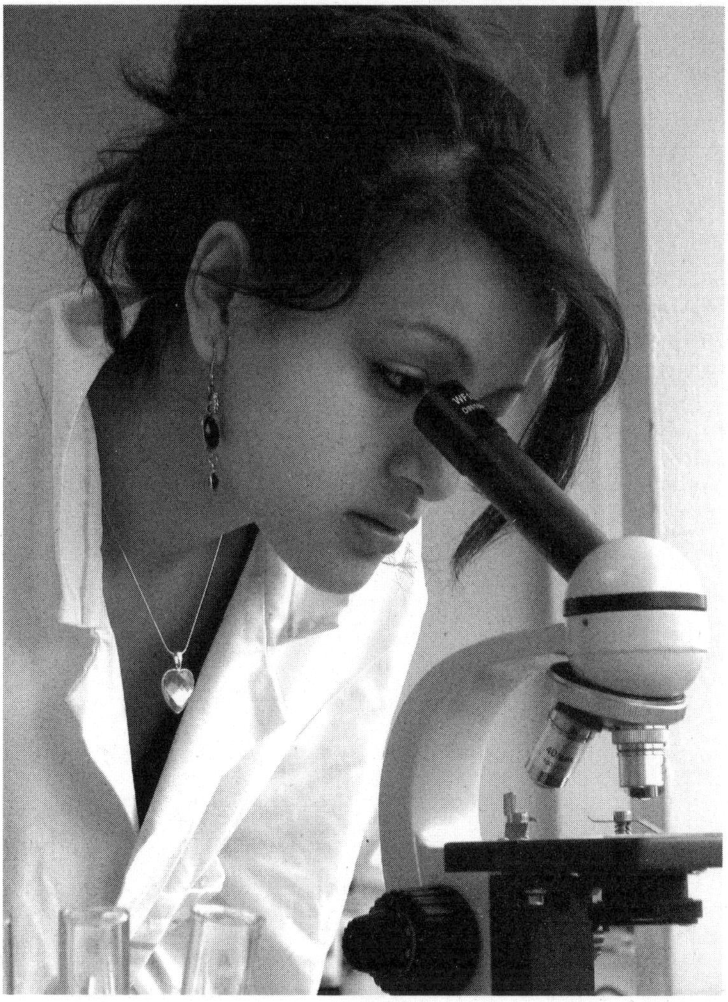

Susan D. Van Arnum, Ph.D.

TestWare® Edition

Research & Education Association
Visit our website: www.rea.com

Research & Education Association
61 Ethel Road West
Piscataway, New Jersey 08854
E-mail: info@rea.com

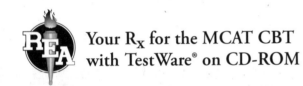

Your R_X for the MCAT CBT with TestWare® on CD-ROM

Printed in the United States of America

Library of Congress Control Number 2009940782

ISBN-13: 978-0-7386-0387-2
ISBN-10: 0-7386-0387-2

L09-0101

TABLE OF CONTENTS

FOREWORD

Welcome medical school candidates! By purchasing this comprehensive test prep, you have begun preparing for the Medical College Admission Test (MCAT), one of several criteria used to assess potential candidates for medical school admission.

Why study for the MCAT?

The MCAT, administered by the Association of American Medical Colleges, is required for admission to almost all medical schools in the United States and many medical schools in Canada and 14 other countries. Over 70,000 applicants take the test each year, and test results (along with your undergraduate academic courses and personal interviews) are used by the admissions committee to assemble the next entering medical school class. While the MCAT is not the only criterion used to determine medical school admission, it *is* a significant one, and your performance on the test is an important component of your overall presentation to the admissions committee.

What does the MCAT measure?

At its most basic, practicing medicine involves the ability to apply knowledge to solve, or to help patients manage, health-related problems. The physician must identify the health issue, assess severity, determine whether acute or chronic, and then develop a plan, along with the patient, to manage the issue. These steps are labeled assessment, diagnosis, and treatment.

The MCAT assesses your knowledge base in the physical and biological sciences, and your ability to apply that knowledge to solve problems. The Verbal Reasoning section assesses Reading Comprehension because reading and absorbing information from textbooks and journals is critical to keeping abreast of changes in medical treatment and procedures. The Writing Sample measures your ability to communicate via the written word. Communicating your findings and opinions on patients to colleagues and ancillary medical personnel is a skill used daily in medical practice. As you can see, the MCAT measures your proficiency in areas a physician uses to manage patient care. The test itself consists of three multiple-choice sections and a writing section.

How can this test prep help me pass the MCAT?

At REA, we have been preparing test preps for the academic arena for 50 years. Our newly revised MCAT review has been completely updated and is designed to reflect the scope, difficulty level, and overall feel of the latest computerized MCAT test series. We have included reviews of mathematics, physics, the biological sciences, chemistry and organic chemistry, as well as Verbal Reasoning, plus we have provided several opportunities for you to practice the Writing Sample. The reviews contain questions and explanations as well as sample tests. We have also included suggestions on how to use the reviews to prepare, how to score your sample tests, and we offer helpful test-taking strategies. Knowing what to expect is key to scoring well on any standardized test, and our test prep will help you succeed on the MCAT and get one step closer toward medical school admission.

Best wishes as you move into the next stage of your professional career!

Sussan K. Sutphen, MD

About the Author

Susan D. Van Arnum, Ph.D., is a process research and development chemist. She has approximately fifteen years of experience in the fine chemical and pharmaceutical industries in drug development and manufacturing. She holds undergraduate degrees in chemistry and biology and has a Ph.D. in physical organic chemistry from Rutgers University in New Brunswick, New Jersey. She has published research articles on green chemistry, photochemistry and heterocyclic synthesis. In addition, she was a contributor to the *Kirk-Othmer Encyclopedia of Chemical Technology* and the *Journal of Chemical Education*. Dr. Van Arnum is a member of the American Chemical Society.

About the Technical Editor

Sussan K. Sutphen, M.D., graduated from the Medical College of Wisconsin in Milwaukee, Wisc., in 1982 and completed her emergency medicine residency in 1986. She served 3 years in the U.S. Public Health Service and as a result of that experience practiced primarily in small rural community hospitals in Indiana and Georgia. She switched to Occupational Medicine in 2002. She also has an M.A. in professional writing from Kennesaw State University and is a medical writer and editor. She has had continuing medical education articles published on Medscape, a website for healthcare professionals.

About Research & Education Association

Founded in 1959, Research & Education Association (REA) is dedicated to publishing the finest and most effective educational materials—including software, study guides, and test preps—for students in middle school, high school, college, gradute school, and beyond.

REA's Test Preparation series includes books and software for all academic levels in almost all disciplines. REA publishes test preps for students who have not yet entered high school, as well as high school students preparing to enter college. Students from countries around the world seeking to attend college in the United States will find the assistance they need in REA's publications. For college students seeking advanced degrees, REA publishes test preps for many major graduate school admission examinations in a wide variety of disciplines, including engineering, law, and medicine. Students at every level, in every field, with every ambition can find what they are looking for among REA's publications.

REA's publications and educational materials are highly regarded and continually receive an unprecedented amount of praise from professionals, instructors, librarians, parents, and students. Our authors are as diverse as the subject matter represented in the books we publish. They are well known in their respective disciplines and serve on the faculties of prestigious high schools, colleges, and universities throughout the United States and Canada.

Today, REA's wide-ranging catalog is a leading resource for teachers, students, and professionals.

We invite you to visit us at *www.rea.com* to find out how "REA is making the world smarter."

Contributor Acknowledgments

In addition to our author and editor, we wish to thank our entire team of contributors, including: Joseph A. Alvarez, M.A.; Pauline Beard, Ph.D.; Robert Chasnov, Ph.D.; Anita P. Davis, Ed.D.; Larry A. Geismann, Ph.D.; Gary F. Greif, Ph.D.; Timothy M. Hagle, J.D., Ph.D.; Marie Hankins, Ph.D.; Thomas C. Kennedy, Ph.D.; James S. Malek, Ph.D.; Mary Rengo Murnik, Ph.D.; Jack C. Norma, Ph.D.; William R. Oliver, Ph.D.; John G. Robinson, Ph.D.; Garret Ward Sheldon, Ph.D.; William L. Stone, Ph.D.; Barbara A. D. Swyhart, Ph.D.; Gail D. Thomas, M.S.; William C. Uhland, M.S.; William F. Wacholtz, Ph.D.; Chalres M. Wynn, Ph.D; Kurt Vandervoort; Linda Gregory; Brian Dinkelmeyer; Tamara Trout; Aruoriwo Oboh, M.D.; Susan Arvay; Jason Biegel; Aaron Bram; Eric Hollekim; Andrew McIntosh; Paul Olson; Nicholas Paraskevopoulos; Kimberly Parke; Andrew Parks; Muhammad Qureshi; Alexandra Sonshine; Cindy Coe Taylor, Ph.D.; Jeanine Todaro; John Tsinetakes; and Albert Zaretskie.

REA Acknowledgments

We thank Larry B. Kling, Vice President, Editorial, for his overall direction; Pam Weston, Vice President, Publishing, for setting the quality standards for production integrity; Michael Reynolds, Managing Editor, for project management; Macmillan Publishing Solutions for designing and typesetting the book; and Christine Saul, Senior Graphic Artist, for designing the cover.

MCAT Study Schedule

Week	Activity
1	Read Chapter 1, "Preparing for the MCAT," and study our introduction to the MCAT on the following pages. Be sure you understand the format of the MCAT and know exactly what is tested on the exam. Now would be a good time to plan your study schedule. When and where will you study? How will you balance your daily responsibilities with your studying schedule? Decide when and where you study best, and get ready to take on the MCAT!
2	Start your study routine by taking the MCAT Practice Test 1 on CD to determine your strengths and weaknesses. Make sure you give yourself at least 5 hours (preferably on a weekend, or at another convenient time) to take the exam. You will need to concentrate, so take the practice test at a time and place where you will not be disturbed. When you take the test, try to do your best, even on sections where you may not know the answer. After you have finished the test, record your scores for each section. This will help you track your progress as you study and highlight areas in which you need improvement. For example, if you answered several questions in the Physical Sciences Section incorrectly, you should carefully study the Physics and Chemistry review chapters to improve your skills in those areas. Later in the week, study the detailed explanations of answers for the questions you answered incorrectly. In the cases where you erred, find out why. Take notes and pay attention to sections where you missed a lot of questions. You will need to spend more time reviewing the related material.
3	Make a firm commitment to study for *at least* two hours a day, every day for the next few weeks. It may seem hard to find time in your busy schedule, but remember: the more you study, the better prepared you will be for the MCAT. This week, study the Mathematics Review (Chapter 2). Take your time and carefully review all the theories and formulas. Try to solve the practice problems included throughout the chapter, and make sure you understand the solutions.
4	Study the Physics Review (Chapter 3). We've provided Problem-Solving Tips to help you better understand the material and successfully solve the practice problems. If Physics isn't your strongest area, consider breaking the chapter into sections and review a few topics at a time. Practice and review areas in which you feel you need improvement.

(continued)

MCAT Study Schedule *(continued from previous page)*

Week	Activity
5	Keep working your way through the review chapters and sample problems. Your hard work is paying off! This week, study the Biology Review (Chapter 4). Don't become overwhelmed at the size and scope of the chapter. You have an entire week to work through the various sections and practice problems. Take your time and focus on one or two subjects at each study session. Once you've grasped the material in one area, you can make your way through the rest of the chapter.
6	Congratulations! You've reached the halfway point! Success is just around the corner, but keep going, there's more work to be done. Now it's time to study Chemistry and Organic Chemistry (Chapters 5 and 6). Make sure you understand all the formulas and equations included in the reviews. If any section seems confusing, or if you find yourself in need of clarification on a subject, you may want to consult your chemistry textbook or ask a classmate or professor for additional help. Test what you've learned by trying to solve the practice problems on your own, and note any areas in which you need improvement. Give yourself a break and do something fun – after you've finished studying for the week.
7	It's time to take Practice Test 3. You've been studying for weeks, and now is a good time to test what you've learned. After taking the exam, record your score and measure your progress. How much have you improved since you took Practice Test 1? Go back and study the detailed explanations of answers to any questions you answered incorrectly. You may want to revisit the sections (or chapters) in which you need extra reinforcement.
8	Practice makes perfect! Start off Week 8 by focusing on the Writing Sample and Verbal Reasoning Reviews (Chapters 7 and 8). Make sure you understand what is being tested in these sections, and take note of the suggested techniques for writing essays in chapter 7. Now is a good time to review any supplemental materials (such as a writing handbook) that will aid you in writing clearer, better-focused essays. Try writing a few practice essays on your own and ask a coworker, spouse, or friend to give you feedback.
9	This week, set aside a few hours to take the MCAT "for real." By now you should be familiar with the format of the exam, so take Practice Test 2 on CD. Take your time and think about each question as you answer it. Time yourself, or ask a spouse or friend to let you know when "time's up." Score your practice test and see how well you did!
10	This week, before you take Practice Test 4, review any questions you answered incorrectly on the previous practice tests. Study the detailed explanations of answers and make sure you understand why you answered the question wrong, so you can improve your test-taking skills. When you're ready, take Practice Test 4. Your score should improve with each practice exam.
11	Now you're ready for Practice Test 5. Allow yourself at least 5 hours to take the test. Focus, remember what you've learned, and answer every question to the best of your ability. After you've completed the test, review all the answer explanations for the questions you answered incorrectly.
12	You have just about reached your goal! After a day or two of additional study to reinforce any areas of weakness, take Practice Test 6. Use the rest of your time to restudy any topics in which you need improvement and review the answer explanations for the questions you answered incorrectly. You may want to re-read the review chapters or work on the practice questions to help you boost your skills. If time permits, why not retake Practice Test 1 for additional practice? After you've completed the exam, compare your two scores and see how far you've come in just a matter of weeks!

Congratulations! You've worked hard and you're ready for the MCAT!

MCAT

MEDICAL COLLEGE ADMISSION TEST

Preparing for the MCAT

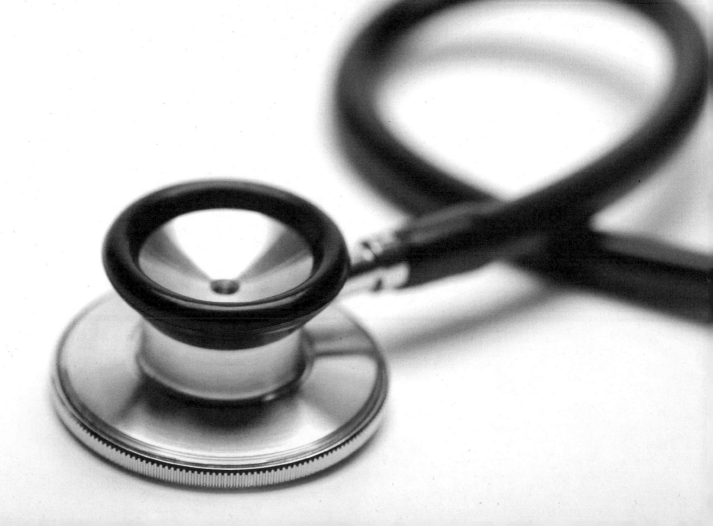

CHAPTER 1

PREPARING FOR THE MCAT

HOW YOU CAN ACHIEVE A TOP MCAT SCORE

By reviewing and studying the material in this book, you can achieve a top score on the Medical College Admission Test (MCAT). This book has been designed to thoroughly prepare you for the MCAT by providing you with six full-length exams that accurately reflect the MCAT in both the level of difficulty and nature of the questions. The exams provided are based on the current computerized format of the MCAT and include every type of question you may encounter during the actual examination.

Following each exam is an answer key, complete with detailed explanations and solutions designed to clarify the material. Our objective is to provide you with not only answers but also explanations of why one answer is more acceptable than another. Our topical reviews will take you through the very material you're most likely to encounter on the MCAT. By completing all six practice exams and studying the explanations that follow, you can discover your strengths and weaknesses. Then you can concentrate on the sections of the exam that give you the most difficulty. Our reviews cover each topic on the test: chemistry, biology, physics, and mathematics. You'll also find powerful tips on writing the essays and completing the Verbal Reasoning section. The reviews themselves are interspersed with drills to raise your comfort level.

Two of the practice tests in this book and software package are included in two formats: in printed form in this book, and in TestWare® format on the enclosed CD. **We recommend that you begin your preparation by first taking the practice exams on your computer.** The software provides timed conditions, automatic scoring, and scoring information that makes it easier to target your strengths and weaknesses.

Also included on the CD is REA's Visual Medical Reference Library. We provide 22 full-color charts that clearly present human anatomy. These charts will be of great help with your MCAT studies and beyond.

ABOUT THE MCAT

The MCAT is required by virtually all American medical schools and is a top criterion for admission. The test is also given internationally in 15 other countries, including Canada and China. Every year, more than 70,000 medical school applicants to submit MCAT results, along with other undergraduate records, as part of the highly competitive medical school admissions process.

Each medical school has a formula for evaluating your application, and different schools attach different weight to your MCAT scores. As a general rule, however, MCAT scores are equally as important as your overall grade-point average and interview performance. In a word, you *must* achieve a high MCAT score to have a reasonable chance for admission. And, of course, the MCAT's importance is heightened if you are applying to a highly competitive medical school.

The MCAT is administered by the Association of American Medical Colleges several times from late January to early September. You should choose the test date appropriate to the application requirements of the medical school(s) of your choice. However, medical school admissions advisors generally suggest that you take the MCAT in the spring before the year you plan to begin your studies. Spring test dates are preferable because test results will be ready in time for early processing of your medical school application. In addition, if you perform poorly on the MCAT administered in the spring, you will have an opportunity to retake the test in the summer. Scores for the late-summer administration of the MCAT are available in time to meet most application deadlines.

The only way to register for the MCAT is online. You will be able to access the Web registration site approximately 120 days before each test date. Candidates are urged to register early, at least 60 days before the test date. Registrations are processed in the order received, so submitting your registration early increases your chance to get tested at your first-choice test center. The regular registration deadline is 14 calendar days before the test date. Accommodations are possible for certain disabilities, in accordance with the Americans with Disabilities Act. If you are disabled, you must submit documentation with your MCAT registration, and you will receive written notification regarding your request and specific instructions pertaining to the accommodation.

About five weeks before each test date, the MCAT Program Office begins mailing appointment times, admission tickets, and identification (ID) cards. If you do not receive your confirmation e-mail, admission ticket, and ID card within a reasonable time after registration, call the MCAT Program Office. The admission ticket will show the exact address of the test center and the date and time of your test. Keep it in a safe place and remember to bring it to the test.

If you have any further questions, ask your academic supervisor, or contact:

MCAT Program Office
Association of American Medical Colleges
Section for Applicant Assessment Services
2450 N Street, NW
Washington, DC 20037-1127
Phone: (202) 828-0690
FAX: (202) 828-4799
Web site: *www.aamc.org*
E-mail: mcat@aamc.org

FORMAT OF THE MCAT

In addition to testing your basic scientific knowledge in the fields of biology, chemistry, and physics, the MCAT will test your problem-solving, critical thinking, and writing skills. The exam appointment, which lasts 5 hours 20 minutes, is composed of four basic sections, each containing brief passages that outline a situation. Following the passages are multiple-choice questions, which are designed to test your knowledge and various skills that the Association of American Medical Colleges has determined are prerequisites for medical school and the practice of medicine.

Physical Sciences (70 minutes)

This section consists of 52 physics and general chemistry questions.

Verbal Reasoning (60 minutes)

This section consists of 40 reading comprehension questions based on nine passages.

Writing Sample (30 minutes each essay)

This section consists of two separate essays on assigned topics.

Biological Sciences (70 minutes)

This section consists of 52 general biology and organic chemistry questions.

Survey (10 minutes)

Total Content Time: 4 hours and 20 minutes

Test Section	Number of Questions	Minutes per Section	Minutes per Break Period
Tutorial	—	10	10 (optional)
Nondisclosure Agreement	—	5	—
Physical Sciences	52	70	10 (optional)
Verbal Reasoning	40	60	10 (optional)
Writing Sample	2 essays	20	10 (optional)
Biological Sciences	52	70	—
Void Question	—	10	—
Survey	—	10	—
Total Testing Time: 5 hours and 20 minutes			

Testing is by appointment, beginning at 8:00 a.m., 12:00 p.m., or 2:00 p.m. local time on the test date. The overall length of the appointment time is 5 hours 20 minutes; however, it may be shorter if you choose not to take all the breaks. Individuals work at their own pace, and breaks are optional. All examinees must sign the nondisclosure agreement.

REVIEW SECTIONS

- The **Mathematics Review** sharpens the necessary skills required for the science sections of the MCAT by reviewing the key areas of math you'll need to master before taking the exam.
- The **Physics Review** covers all the topics that constitute the general physics half of the Physical Sciences test section.
- The **Biology Review** covers all the topics that constitute the general biology half of the Biological Sciences section of the MCAT.
- The **Chemistry Review** presents all the topics that constitute the general chemistry half of the Physical Sciences test section.
- The **Organic Chemistry Review** presents all the topics that constitute the organic chemistry half of the Biological Sciences test section.
- The **Writing Sample Review** provides pointers on completing the Writing Sample section of the MCAT. It also discusses ways to gear your writing skills and organize your thoughts in a limited amount of time.
- The **Verbal Reasoning Review** introduces all the skills that will help you succeed in that section of the MCAT.

THE TEST SECTIONS

As discussed earlier, the MCAT contains four sections: Physical Sciences, Verbal Reasoning, Writing Sample, and Biological Sciences. The following outline explains these sections in detail and contains helpful hints for selecting the correct answer.

Physical Sciences

The Physical Sciences section is based on several short passages, each outlining a situation. You must interpret, analyze, and apply the provided information as you answer the questions. This section requires you to do the following:

- Understand and apply basic concepts
- Balance simple chemical equations
- Solve general physics problems

All the questions asked will be at the level of first-year college material. You will not need advanced or special knowledge to answer these questions.

Suggested Techniques for Answering Physical Sciences Questions

- Read each passage thoroughly.
- Be sure you understand what each question is asking.
- Take notes on scratch paper.
- Don't try to work out the problems in your head.
- If you don't know the answer to a question, try to make an educated guess.

Verbal Reasoning

The Verbal Reasoning section includes questions testing your comprehension, evaluation, and application and incorporation of information of nine reading passages. Each passage is approximately 500 to 600 words in length and followed by 5 to 10 questions. The questions do not ask about detailed facts from the passage but include material that requires you to do the following:

- Understand the theme of a passage
- Determine and evaluate the important points of an argument
- Draw inferences from facts and reach conclusions

You can answer all the questions solely on the basis of information provided in the passages and do not need any medical or special knowledge. The passages for this section are drawn from many disciplines, including the social sciences, humanities, and philosophy.

Suggested Techniques for Answering Verbal Reasoning Questions

- Read the passage for content. Be sure you understand the words and statements in it.
- Skim some of the questions first before reading the passage. This may help you focus on the important points in the passage.
- Try not to spend too much time deciphering the meaning of words and statements on first reading the passage. You may find it helpful to go over specific parts of the passage later, after reading each question.
- While reading the passage, look specifically for inferences and the mood or tone of the passage. Such things may hint at the type of questions that might be asked.
- The main idea or theme of a passage is usually in the first and/or last sentences.
- Opinion pieces are the core of the MCAT Verbal Reasoning section. Observe how the author's opinion differs from the general opinion surrounding the issue.
- You should remember that correct choices usually paraphrase the information from the passages. This is especially true of inferential questions.

- Choices that repeat the material from a passage word-for-word are usually used as a lure to steer you into choosing the wrong answer.

Note that each multiple-choice section includes experimental items that do not count toward your score.

Writing Sample

The Writing Sample section requires you to write two essays on assigned topics. You are given a short statement or quote to analyze. You must then write a logical and concise essay, addressing all the required writing tasks in the time allotted. You are not required to have prior knowledge of medicine to write your essays because topics on medicine are not assigned. However, you are expected to do the following:

- Review and understand the topic statement or quotation
- Formulate a clear position
- Support your position eloquently and effectively
- Use correct grammar and vocabulary

Suggested techniques on writing the essays are given in Chapter 7.

Biological Sciences

The Biological Sciences section is based on several short passages, each outlining a situation. You must be able to interpret, analyze, and apply the information provided. In this section, you are required to do the following:

- Understand and apply basic concepts
- Answer general biology questions
- Solve organic chemistry problems

All questions are at the level of first-year college material. You are not required to possess prior or advanced knowledge to answer these questions.

Suggested Techniques for Answering Biological Sciences Questions

- Read each passage thoroughly.
- Be sure you understand what each question is asking.
- Skim some of the questions before reading each passage.

MCAT SCORING

Your MCAT test score is composed of four individual scores — one for each section of the test. All the multiple-choice sections of your MCAT are first given a raw score. Your raw score for a particular section is determined by totaling the number of correct answers for that section. Then your raw score is converted into a scaled score, with 1 the lowest and 15 the highest. This conversion is necessary to account for differences in the difficulty of test questions. Even though some test forms are slightly more difficult or slightly easier than others, a scaled score represents the same level of skill mastery in every test form used. Each writing sample is scored by two readers using a six-point scale. These scores are added up and converted to an alphabetical scale for score reporting, from J to T for the lowest to highest scores, respectively. You can expect to receive your official scores approximately 30 days after you take the test, and the scores are available through the Testing History System (THx) at the MCAT Web site.

Depending on your level of confidence, you should take an MCAT practice test either before or after reading the applicable review section in this book. The MCAT practice tests presented here provide the best barometer of your strengths and weaknesses.

SCORING YOUR PRACTICE TESTS

1. Use the answer key after each test to check your answers.
2. Use the space below to mark your raw score.
3. Use the Score Conversion Chart to convert your raw scores into scaled scores.

Total Number of Correct Answers (Raw Score)	
Verbal Reasoning Section	______________________
Physical Sciences Section	______________________
Biological Sciences Section	______________________

Use the following table to convert your raw score to a scaled score. Remember that the conversion value of raw scores to scaled scores will vary slightly from year to year and from practice test to practice test to compensate for different levels of question difficulty.

Your estimated percentile rank indicates your rank in comparison to other students who have taken the exam. For example, if your Verbal Reasoning raw score is 35 (correct answers), then according to the table your percentile rank is between 78 and 90, indicating that you achieved a higher score than 78–90% of all MCAT examinees.

Score Conversion Chart

Verbal Reasoning			Physical Sciences			Biological Sciences		
Estimated Rank	Raw Score	Scaled Score	Estimated Rank	Raw Score	Scaled Score	Estimated Rank	Raw Score	Scaled Score
15	38–40	93–99	15	49–52	96–99	15	49–52	98–99
14	35–37	78–90	14	45–48	90–95	14	46–48	92–97
13	31–34	63–75	13	41–44	82–89	13	43–45	83–90
12	28–30	48–60	12	37–40	73–81	12	40–42	73–81
11	25–27	36–46	11	33–36	62–71	11	36–39	61–71
10	22–24	25–33	10	29–32	50–59	10	33–35	49–59
9	19–21	16–23	9	25–28	39–47	9	28–32	37–47
8	16–18	9–14	8	21–24	25–35	8	24–27	26–35
7	14–15	4–7	7	17–20	14–23	7	20–23	16–24
6	11–13	3–4	6	13–16	5–12	6	17–19	7–14
5	9–10	2–3	5	11–12	4–5	5	14–16	2–6
4	7–8	2	4	8–9	3–4	4	11–13	2
3	5–6	1	3	6–7	2–3	3	8–10	1
2	3–4	1	2	4–5	1–2	2	5–7	1

SCORING THE WRITING SAMPLES

Your MCAT writing samples are graded on a scale of 1 to 6, with 1 being "poor" and 6 "excellent." Each writing sample is graded independently by two readers. The raw score assigned to your essays is a combination of four evaluations: two for your first essay and two for your second essay. If there is a discrepancy of more than one point between the two readers, a third reader evaluates your essay and assigns a final score.

After the initial scoring, the evaluations for both of your essays are added together and assigned a letter grade on a scale from J to T, with J the lowest score and T the highest. Your scores for the writing samples are also reported to the medical schools to which you are applying. Each medical school receives a written explanation describing the meaning of each letter grade, your percentile ranking, and score distributions.

Here are the scoring criteria for evaluating your MCAT writing samples:

Writing Sample Point Values

1	The essay shows very poor spelling and punctuation. The essay may not answer the assigned topic. The structure and writing of the essay may make it difficult to understand.
2	The essay contains major structural and/or grammatical errors. The analysis of the essay topic may be incorrect or incomplete. One or more of the required writing assignments may be executed incompletely or incorrectly.
3	The essay indicates that the writer's basic skills are adequate, but errors are noticeable. The essay may be disorganized or poorly planned. One or more of the required writing assignments may be addressed only on a superficial level.
4	The essay is well organized, with only minor digressions from the topic. Points are logical and clearly written but should have been developed in greater depth. All required writing assignments have been addressed but one or more required more development.
5	The essay addresses all required writing assignments clearly and thoroughly. The essay's points are concise and well organized. Grammar and punctuation in the essay are correct.
6	The essay thoroughly addresses the required writing assignments in depth. The essay's points are clear and well organized. The grammar and punctuation of the essay are excellent.

MCAT TEST-TAKING STRATEGIES

How to Beat the Clock

Every second counts when you are taking the MCAT, so you should use your testing time as efficiently as possible. Because the MCAT is composed of questions that vary in degree of difficulty, you should answer first the questions you feel are easy, saving the difficult ones for last. Also, you should not spend a great deal of time working out a single difficult question when you could be solving the questions that are easier to answer. Although you should work quickly, do not rush through the exam because this will cause you to answer the questions with less accuracy. Pace yourself and work steadily.

Make every effort to maintain your concentration during the test. Don't waste time watching the proctor or looking around the room. This only saps valuable minutes that you'll regret having lost as you approach the end of the exam.

Guessing Strategy

If you are uncertain of a question, guess at the answer rather than not answer it at all. You will not be penalized for answering incorrectly because wrong answers are not counted. This means you should never have an unanswered question on the answer screen. Even if you do not have time to guess at an answer, be sure to fill in every space on the answer screen. Because you are not assessed a penalty for a wrong answer, you receive credit for any questions you answer correctly by luck. Remember, your chances of selecting the correct answer are automatically improved if you do not leave the question blank.

Try to make an educated guess if you don't know the answer. However, if time is short and you cannot make educated guesses, don't simply guess at random. Choose one letter and fill in all your guesses with that letter. This has been statistically proven to be one-and-a-half times as effective as blind guessing.

Other Must-Do Strategies

As you work on the test, make sure your answers correspond with the numbers and letters on the answer screen. You do not want your answer to be marked incorrect simply because you selected the wrong circle.

Don't hesitate to use scratch paper. You should not try to solve difficult problems or questions in your head. Taking the actual exam is a high-pressure situation, and you may become confused. Using scratch paper enables you to see your work on paper and makes the problem easier to solve.

If you are completely uncertain of a question, skip it at first. Mark the question on scratch paper so you can go back to it later. This allows you to go on to questions about which you are certain. Then, if time allows, go back and try to make educated guesses for the questions you skipped.

THE DAY OF THE TEST

Try to get a good night's rest and get up early on the test day. Have a good breakfast because a growling stomach could distract you and other candidates. Arrive at the testing center at least 30 minutes before your scheduled appointment time. Dress in layers; the test center typically is comfortable only for the proctor. Arrive early at the test center because no one is admitted after the test has begun.

You must take the following with you to the test center: your admission ticket or other MCAT Program Office authorization; your completed MCAT ID card; a valid government-issued identification that contains both your photo and your signature (e.g., a driver's license or passport). The test center provides scratch paper, ear covers, and pencils.

Phones, pagers, cameras, watches, and aids of any kind are prohibited in the test center. A timer is visible on your testing monitor. Eating, drinking, and smoking are not allowed in the testing room. Lockers are provided for personal items. If you remove a sweater or jacket in the testing room, you must place it in the locker. Time does not stop while you are away from your test station.

When you arrive at the test center, a supervisor asks you for your personal identification and MCAT paperwork. On making a positive identification, the supervisor assigns you a seat. Testing centers may contain up to 16 workstations. Follow all instructions given by the proctor because failure to do so may result in the cancellation of your scores. The test center administrator captures your identification electronically, including your fingerprints and photograph. This process simplifies your reentry to the exam after breaks.

When you have finished the test, go home and sleep for a day or so. You've earned it.

Good luck on the MCAT!

MCAT

MEDICAL COLLEGE ADMISSION TEST

Mathematics Review

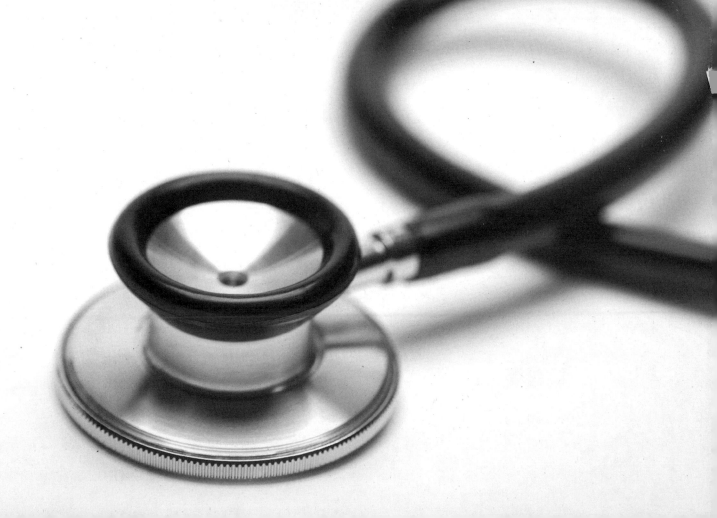

GENERAL CONSIDERATIONS

Calculators are not allowed on the MCAT. In addition to knowledge of mathematical transformations and expressions, it is important to know the numerical value of certain mathematical quantities. Skill in mental math — that is, reducing the complexity of mathematical expressions without the use of paper and pencil — will save time. As an MCAT test taker, you should be familiar with the decimal values and percentage values of common fractions. For example, $\frac{1}{8}$ equals 0.125 or 12.5%; $\frac{6}{8}$ equals $\frac{3}{4}$, 0.75, or 75%. You should also know the second and third powers of the numbers 1 through 10; and you should memorize that the numerical value for the square root of 2 is 1.414 and the numerical value for the square root of 3 is 1.732. Instantaneous recognition of these expressions will save time on the MCAT.

In an effort to save time and avoid long division and multiplication, you should round fractional quantities on a regular basis. It is unlikely that the difference between two answers on the MCAT will be that one answer was rounded and the other was not. With the time you save, you can make sure that you properly set up the problem, the units cancel, and your arithmetic is correct.

I. ARITHMETIC

1. INTEGERS AND REAL NUMBERS

Most of the numbers used in algebra belong to a set called the real numbers, or reals. This set can be represented graphically by the real number line.

On a number line like that shown here, a point can be fixed and labeled with the number 0. In a similar manner, any point on the line can be labeled with one of the real numbers, depending on its position relative to 0. Numbers to the right of zero are positive, and numbers to the left are negative. Value increases from left to right, so that if *a* is to the right of *b*, it is said to be greater than *b*.

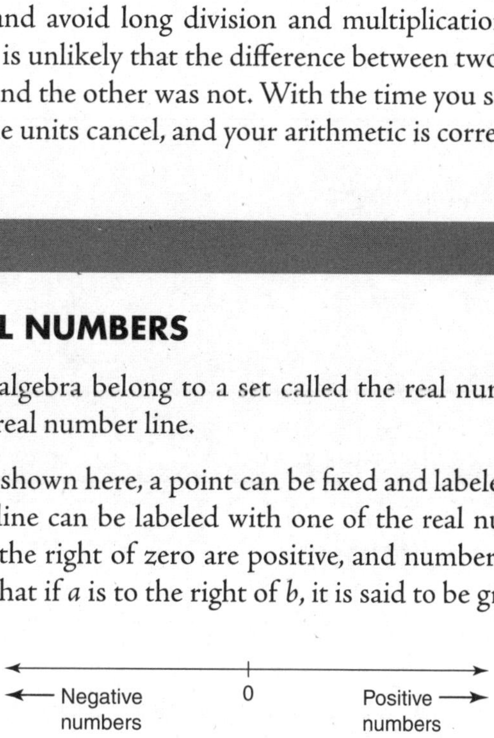

The number line can be divided into equal segments and the points of division labeled with real numbers. For example, the point two lengths to the left of zero is −2, and the point three lengths to the right of zero is +3 (the + sign is usually assumed, so +3 is written simply as 3). The number line now looks like this:

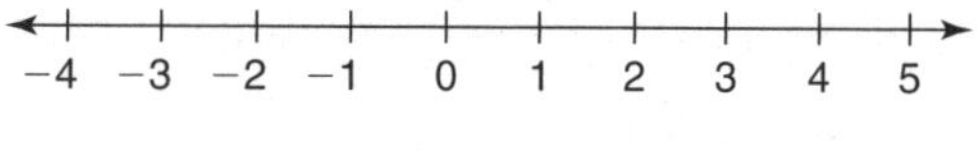

These boundary points represent the subset of the reals known as the integers. The set of integers is made up of the positive and negative whole numbers: $\{\ldots -4, -3, -2, -1, 0, 1, 2, 3, 4, \ldots\}$. Following are some subsets of integers:

Natural numbers or positive numbers — the set of integers starting with 1 and increasing: $N = \{1, 2, 3, 4, \ldots\}$.

Whole numbers — the set of integers starting with 0 and increasing: $W = \{0, 1, 2, 3, \ldots\}$.

Negative numbers — the set of integers starting with −1 and decreasing: $Z = \{-1, -2, -3 \ldots\}$.

Prime numbers — the set of positive integers greater than 1 that are divisible only by 1 and themselves: $\{2, 3, 5, 7, 11, \ldots\}$.

Even integers — the set of integers divisible by 2: $\{\ldots, -4, -2, 0, 2, 4, 6, \ldots\}$.

Odd integers — the set of integers not divisible by 2: $\{\ldots, -3, -1, 1, 3, 5, 7, \ldots\}$.

Problem

Classify each of the following numbers into as many different sets as possible; for example, real number, integer, and so on.

A. 0 B. 9 C. $\sqrt{6}$

D. $\frac{1}{2}$ E. $\frac{2}{3}$ F. 1.5

Solution

A. Zero is a real number and an integer.
B. 9 is a real number, a natural number, and an integer.
C. $\sqrt{6}$ is a real number.
D. $\frac{1}{2}$ is a real number.
E. $\frac{2}{3}$ is a real number.
F. 1.5 is a real number and a decimal.

2. RATIOS AND PROPORTIONS

The ratio of two numbers x and y, written $x{:}y$, is the fraction x/y where $y \neq 0$. A proportion is an equality of two ratios.

Given a proportion $a{:}b = c{:}d$, a and d are called the extremes, b and c are called the means, and d is called the fourth proportional to a, b, and c. If the two means are equal, as in the proportion $a{:}b = b{:}c$, then c is called the third proportional to a and b.

Fundamental Properties of Proportions

If $a{:}b = c{:}d$, then:

1. $ad = bc$, the product of the means is equal to the product of the extremes. For example, if

$$4{:}8 = 9{:}x, \text{ then}$$
$$4x = 72 \text{ and } x = 18$$

2. $a{:}b = c{:}d$. Following from property 1, $ad = bc$, either pair can be made the means and the other pair the extremes.

   In this case, $a{:}b = c{:}d$, bc are the means, and ad are the extremes.

3. $b{:}a = d{:}c$, inversion.
4. $(a + b){:}b = (c + d){:}d$, addition.
5. $(a - b){:}b = (c - d){:}d$, subtraction.

Problem

Write the following ratios reduced to simplest form.

A. 12 inches to 2 feet

B. 15 minutes to 2 hours

C. 1100 yards to 1 mile

D. $(x^3 + x^2 - 6x) : (x^3 - 4x^2 + 4x)$

Solution

A. Convert the quantities being compared to the same units. Convert 2 feet to inches.
12 inches to 24 inches = 12:24 = 1:2

B. Convert 2 hours to minutes.
15 minutes to 120 minutes = 15:120 = 1:8

C. Convert 1 mile to yards.
1,100 yards to 1,760 yards = 1,100:1,760 = 5:8

D. Factor each polynomial separately

$$\frac{x^3 + x^2 - 6x}{x^3 - 4x^2 + 4x} = \frac{x(x^2 + x - 6)}{x(x^2 - 4x + 4)} = \frac{x(x-2)(x+3)}{x(x-2)(x-2)}$$

Cancel equivalent terms

$$\frac{x+3}{x-2} \text{ or } (x+3) : (x-2)$$

Problem

Find the fourth proportional to 2, 5, and 6.

Solution

Set up the proportion:

$2{:}5 = 6{:}x$

By definition, x is the fourth proportional:

$2x = 30,$

$x = 15.$

Problem

Find the third proportional to 9 and 5.

Solution

Set up the proportion:

$9{:}5 = 5{:}x$

By definition, x is the third proportional:

$9x = 25$

$$x = 2\frac{7}{9}.$$

Problem

Find the mean proportional between 4 and 16.

Solution

Set up the proportion:

$4:x = x:16$

x is the mean proportional, solve for x:

$x^2 = 64$

$x = \pm 8$

Problem

Find the value of x in the proportion:

$(x + 2):(2x - 8) = 5:(x - 5)$

Solution

Using property 1, $ad = bc$:

$(x + 2)(x - 5) = 5(2x - 8)$

Multiply out both sides:

$x^2 - 3x - 10 = 10x - 40$

$x^2 - 13x + 30 = 0$

$(x - 3)(x - 10) = 0$

$x = +3, x = +10$

Problem

If $9x = 4y$, find the ratio of $x:y$.

Solution

Using property 2, $a:b = c:d$, either pair can be made the means and the other pair the extremes. Choosing $9x$ as the extremes, you will have $x:y = 4:9$.

Problem

Solve the proportion $\frac{x+1}{4} = \frac{15}{12}$.

Solution

Cross multiply to determine x; that is, multiply the numerator of the first fraction by the denominator of the second, and equate this to the product of the numerator of the second and the denominator of the first.

$(x + 1)\,12 = 4 \cdot 15$

$12x + 12 = 60$

$x = 4.$

3. PERCENTAGES

A percentage is a number out of 100. A percentage can be defined by fractions with a denominator of 100. Decimals can also represent a percentage. For instance,

$$56\% = 0.56 \text{ or } \frac{56}{100}.$$

Problem

Compute the value of the following:

A. 90% of 400

B. 180% of 400

C. 50% of 500

D. 200% of 4

Solution

The symbol % means "per hundred"; therefore, $5\% = \frac{5}{100}$.

A. $90\% \text{ of } 400 = \frac{90}{100} \times \frac{400}{1} = 90 \times 4 = 360$

B. $180\% \text{ of } 400 = \frac{180}{100} \times \frac{400}{1} = 180 \times 4 = 720$

C. $50\% \text{ of } 500 = \frac{50}{100} \times \frac{500}{1} = 50 \times 5 = 250$

D. $200\% \text{ of } 4 = \frac{200}{100} \times \frac{4}{1} = 2 \times 4 = 8$

Problem

What percentage of

A. 100 is 99.5?

B. 200 is 4?

Solution

A. $99.5 = x \times 100$

$99.5 = 100x$

$99.5 = x,$

but this is the value of x per hundred. Therefore,

$x = 99.5\%.$

B. $4 = x \times 200$

$4 = 200x$

$0.02 = x.$

Again this must be changed to a percentage, so

$x = 2\%.$

4. RECIPROCALS

The reciprocal of a number x is the fraction $\frac{1}{x}$, where x can be any real number.

Problem

Find the reciprocal of each of the following numbers and express them as decimals.

A. 5

B. $\frac{4}{9}$

C. $2\frac{4}{5}$

D. 4.25

Solution

A. The reciprocal of 5 is $\frac{1}{5}$. In decimal notation, $\frac{1}{5} = 0.2$.

B. The reciprocal of $\frac{4}{9}$ is

$$\frac{1}{\frac{4}{9}} = 1 + \frac{4}{9} = 1 \times \frac{9}{4} = \frac{9}{4} = 2.25.$$

C. First, express $2\frac{4}{5}$ as a fraction: $2\frac{4}{5} = \frac{14}{5}$. The reciprocal of $\frac{14}{5}$ is

$$\frac{1}{\frac{14}{5}} = 1 + \frac{14}{5} = 1 \times \frac{5}{14} = \frac{5}{14} = 0.357.$$

D. First, express 4.25 as a fraction: $4\frac{1}{4} = \frac{17}{4}$ The reciprocal of $\frac{17}{4}$ is

$$\frac{1}{\frac{17}{4}} = 1 + \frac{17}{4} = 1 \times \frac{4}{17} = \frac{4}{17} = 0.235.$$

II. SCIENTIFIC CALCULATIONS

1. EXPONENTS

Given the expression $a_n = b$, in which a, n, and b are real numbers, a is called the base and n is called the exponent or power. For example, in 3^2, 3 is the base and 2 is the exponent.

Given the expression $x^n = y$, in which n is a positive integer and x and y are real numbers, x is said to be the nth root of y, written

$$x = \sqrt[n]{y} = \frac{1}{y^n}.$$

A. Positive Integral Exponent

If n is a positive integer, then a^n represents the product of n factors, each of which is a.

B. Negative Integral Exponent

If n is a positive integer,

$$a^{-n} = \frac{1}{a^n} \quad a \neq 0.$$

Therefore,

$$2^{-4} = \frac{1}{2^4} = \frac{1}{16}.$$

C. Positive Fractional Exponent

$$a^{\frac{m}{n}} = \sqrt[n]{a^m},$$

where m and n are positive integers. For example,

$$4^{\frac{3}{2}} = \sqrt[2]{4^3} = \sqrt{64} = 8.$$

D. Negative Fractional Exponent

$$a^{\frac{m}{n}} = \frac{1}{a^{\frac{m}{n}}}.$$

For example,

$$27^{\frac{2}{3}} = \frac{1}{27^{\frac{2}{3}}} = \frac{1}{\sqrt[3]{27^2}} = \frac{1}{\sqrt[3]{729}} = \frac{1}{9}.$$

E. Zero Exponent

$$a^0 = 1, a \neq 0$$

F. General Laws of Exponents

A. $a^p a^q = a^{p+q}$

B. $(a^p)^q = a^{pq}$

C. $\dfrac{a^p}{a^q} = a^{p-q}, a \neq 0$

D. $(ab)^p = a^p b^p$

E. $\left(\dfrac{a}{b}\right)^p = \dfrac{a^p}{b^p}, b \neq 0$

Problem

Simplify the following expressions:

A. -3^{-2} B. $(-3)^{-2}$ C. $\dfrac{-3}{4^{-1}}$

Solution

A. Here the exponent applies only to 3. Thus,

$$x^{-y} = \frac{1}{x^y}, -3^{-2} = -(3^{-2}) = -\frac{1}{3^2} = -\frac{1}{9}.$$

B. In this case the exponent applies to the negative base. Thus,

$$(-3)^2 = -\frac{1}{(-3)^2} = \frac{1}{(-3)(-3)} = \frac{1}{9}.$$

C. $> \frac{-3}{4^{-1}} = \frac{-3}{\left(\frac{1}{4}\right)^1} = \frac{-3}{\frac{(1^1)}{(4^1)}} = -\frac{3}{\frac{1}{4}}.$

Division by a fraction is equivalent to multiplication by that fraction's reciprocal. Thus,

$$\frac{-3}{\frac{1}{4}} = -3 \times \frac{4}{1} = -12$$

and

$$\frac{-3}{4^{-1}} = -12.$$

Problem

Find the indicated roots:

A. $\sqrt[5]{32}$

B. $\pm\sqrt[4]{625}$

C. $\sqrt[3]{-125}$

D. $\sqrt[4]{-16}$

Solution

The following two laws of exponents can be used to solve these problems:

$$(1)\ \left(\sqrt[n]{a}\right)^n = \left(a^{\frac{1}{n}}\right) = a^1 = a \text{ and } (2)\ \left(\sqrt[n]{a}\right)^n = \sqrt[n]{a^n}$$

A. $\sqrt[5]{32} = \sqrt[5]{2^5} = \left(\sqrt[5]{2}\right)^5 = 2.$

This result is true because $(2)^5 = 32$; that is, $2 \times 2 \times 2 \times 2 \times 2 = 32$.

B. $\sqrt[4]{625} = \sqrt[4]{5^4} = \left(\sqrt[4]{5}\right)^4 = 5.$

This result is true because $(5)^4 = 625$; that is, $5 \times 5 \times 5 \times 5 = 625$.

$$-\sqrt[4]{625} = -\left(\sqrt[4]{5^4}\right) = \left[\left(\sqrt[4]{5}\right)\right]^4 = -[5] = -5.$$

This result is true because $(-5)^4 = 625$, that is, $(-5) \times (-5) \times (-5) \times (-5) = 625$.

C. $\sqrt[3]{-125} = \sqrt[3]{(-5)^3} = \left(\sqrt[3]{-5}\right)^3 = -5.$

This result is true because $(-5)^3 = -125$, that is, $(-5) \times (-5) \times (-5) = -125$.

D. There is no solution to $\sqrt[4]{-16}$ because any number raised to the fourth power is a positive number; that is, $N^4 = (N) \times (N) \times (N) \times (N)$ = a positive number, not a negative number.

2. LOGARITHMS

The logarithm of a number N is the power a to which the base b must be raised to get the number N. The exponent a must be positive.

A. Exponential Form

$b^a = N$

B. Logarithmic Form

$\log_b N = a$

Problem

Express $2^6 = 64$ in logarithmic form.

Solution

Find the base b, exponent a, and number N. Place in the form

$\log_b N = a.$

Base: $b = 2$

Number: $N = 64$

Exponent: $a = 6$

Therefore, the logarithmic form is $\log_2 64 = 6$.

Problem

Express $3^{-4} = \frac{1}{81}$ in logarithmic form.

Solution

Base: $b = 3$

Number: $N = \frac{1}{81}$

Exponent: $a = -4$

Place in the form $\log_b N = a$:

$$\log_3 \frac{1}{81} = -4$$

Problem

Express $\log_5 625 = 4$ in exponential form.

Solution

Base: $b = 5$

Number: $N = 625$

Exponent: $a = 4$

Place in the form $b^a = N$:

$$5^4 = 625.$$

Problem

Express $\log_{16} \frac{1}{32} = -\frac{5}{4}$ in exponential form.

Solution

Base: $b = 16$

Number: $N = \frac{1}{32}$

Exponent: $a = -\frac{5}{4}$

Place in form $b^a = N$:

$$16^{-\frac{5}{4}} = \frac{1}{32}$$

Problem

Find the value of x in the following equation:

$$\log_{128} 16 = x$$

Solution

First, find the base, exponent, and number:

Base: $b = 128$

Exponent: $a = x$

Number: $N = 16$

Place in exponential form $b^a = N$:

$$128^x = 16$$

Find a common base between the numbers. In this case, the base is 2:

$$(2^7)^x = 2^4$$

Equate the exponents:

$$7x = 4$$

$$x = \frac{4}{7}$$

C. Properties of Logarithms

A. $\log_a MN = \log_a M + \log_a N$

B. $\log_a \dfrac{M}{N} = \log_a M - \log_a N$

C. $\log_a M^k = k \log_a M$

Problem

Express $\log_a \dfrac{\sqrt[3]{17}}{\sqrt{10}}$ in terms of logarithms of prime numbers.

Solution

Use property B:

$$\log_a \frac{\sqrt[3]{17}}{\sqrt{10}} = \log_a \sqrt[3]{17} - \log_a \sqrt{10}$$

Express radicals as exponents:

$$\log_a (17)^{\frac{1}{3}} - \log_a (10)^{\frac{1}{2}}$$

Express the number 10 as prime numbers:

$$\log_a (17)^{\frac{1}{3}} - \log_a (5 \times 2)^{\frac{1}{2}}$$

Use property A:

$$\log_a (17)^{\frac{1}{3}} - \left(\log_a 5^{\frac{1}{2}} + \log_a 2^{\frac{1}{2}}\right)$$

Use property C:

$$\frac{1}{3}\log_a 17 - \frac{1}{2}\log_a 5 - \frac{1}{2}\log_a 2$$

D. Logarithms with Base 10

Any positive number except 1 can be used as the base, but for computational purposes, it is convenient to use 10 as the base. When the base is omitted, base 10 is assumed.

The logarithms of numbers that are integral powers of 10 are very easy to find. For example,

$$\log 1 = 0, \log 10 = 1, \log 100 = 2, \log 1000 = 3, \log 0.1 = -1, \text{ and } \log 0.01 = -2.$$

For some general number that is not a power of 10, the logarithm has a whole-number (integer) part called the characteristic, and a decimal part called the mantissa. For example,

$$2580 = 10^{3.4116} \text{ or } \log 2580 = 3.4116,$$

so the characteristic is 3 and the mantissa is .4116.

E. Natural Logarithms

For scientific and mathematical purposes, sometimes another base is used instead of base 10. This base is denoted by e, where $e = 2.71828$. The logarithm with base e is called the natural logarithm.

To find out the natural logarithm, it is convenient to use the following formula:

$$\log_e x = \log_e 10 \cdot \log_{10} x = 2.303 \log_{10} x.$$

3. SCIENTIFIC NOTATION

To simplify the expression of very large or very small numbers, scientific notation is used.

A real number expressed in scientific notation is written as a product of a real number n and an integral power of 10; the value of n is $1 \leq n < 10$.

Problem

Express the distance between the earth and the moon, 236,121 miles, in scientific notation.

Solution

First, find the n between 1 and 10:

$n = 2.3$

Then move the decimal point five places to the right to get 236,121. Each movement to the right represents a multiplication by 10. Therefore, 5 places equals a multiplication by 10^5.

Expressed in scientific notation:

$$236{,}121 = 2.3 \times 10^5 \text{ miles}$$

Problem

Express the wavelength of the new Ka band police radar, 0.011 m, in scientific notation.

Solution

The number n between 1 and 10 is 1.1. The decimal must now be moved 2 places to the left. Two places to the left equals a multiplication of 10^{-2}.

Expressed in scientific notation:

$$0.011 = 1.1 \times 10^{-2} \text{ m}$$

Problem

Convert the number 6.38×10^6 to ordinary decimal notation.

Solution

Multiplication by 10^6 is equivalent to moving the decimal point six places to the right. Therefore, $6.38 \times 10^6 = 6,380,000$.

4. METRIC UNITS

The international system of units (abbreviated SI), commonly known as the metric system, is divided into three classes: base units, supplementary units, and derived units. The list of all the units is very long, so Table 1 lists the basic units used most often.

TABLE 1. Basic Metric Units

Quantity	Unit	Symbol
Length	Meter	m
Mass	Kilogram	kg
Time	Second	s
Angle	Radian	rad
Temperature	Celsius	C
Volume	Liter	L

A. Prefixes

Prefixes are used to form the multiple and submultiple of the SI units. Table 2 lists the prefixes most commonly used.

TABLE 2. Metric Prefixes

Multiplication Factor	Prefix	Abbreviation
10^9	Giga	G
10^6	Mega	M
10^3	Kilo	k
10^2	Hecto	h
10^1	Deka	da
10^{-1}	Deci	d
10^{-2}	Centi	c
10^{-3}	Milli	m
10^{-6}	Micro	µ
10^{-9}	Nano	n

B. Conversion Factors

Table 3 lists the multiplying factors necessary to convert from one unit of measure to another, and to convert back to the original unit, for the basic metric units listed in Table 1.

TABLE 3. Conversion Factors

To Convert	Into	Multiply by	To Convert Back, Multiply by
Meters	Feet	3.28	30.48×10^{-2}
Meters	Inches	39.37	2.54×10^{-2}
Meters	Miles	6.212×10^{-4}	1609.35
Meters	Yards	1.094	0.9144
Kilograms	Pounds	2.205	0.4536
Radians	Degrees	57.27	1.746×10^{-2}
Kelvin	Fahrenheit	1.8 K – 459.67	(°F + 459.67)/1.8
Kelvin	Celsius	K – 273.1 = °C	°C + 273.1 = K
Liters	Gallons (U.S.)	0.2642	3.785
Liters	Pints (U.S. fluid)	2.113	0.4732

III. ALGEBRA AND TRIGONOMETRY

1. SIMPLIFYING ALGEBRAIC EXPRESSIONS

The following concepts are important to factoring or simplifying algebraic expressions.

The factors of an algebraic expression consist of two or more algebraic expressions that, when multiplied together, produce the given algebraic expression.

Some important formulas useful for the factoring of algebraic expressions are listed below.

$$a(c + d) = ac + ad$$
$$(a + b)(a - b) = a^2 - b^2$$
$$(a + b)(a + b) = (a + b)^2 = a^2 + 2ab + b^2$$
$$(a - b)(a - b) = (a - b)^2 = a^2 - 2ab + b^2$$
$$(x + a)(x + b) = x^2 + (a + b)x + ab$$
$$(ax + b)(cx + d) = acx^2 + (ad + bc)x + bd$$
$$(a + b)(c + d) = ac + bc + ad + bd$$
$$(a + b)(a + b)(a + b) = (a + b)^3 = a^3 + 3a^2b + 3ab^2 + b^3$$
$$(a - b)(a - b)(a - b) = (a - b)^3 = a^3 - 3a^2b + 3ab^2 - b^3$$
$$(a - b)(a^2 + ab + b^2) = a^3 - b^3$$
$$(a + b)(a^2 - ab + b^2) = a^3 + b^3$$
$$(a + b + c)^2 = a^2 + b^2 + c^2 + 2ab + 2ac + 2bc$$
$$(a - b)(a^2 + ab + b^2) = a^3 - b^3$$
$$(a - b)(a^3 + a^2b + ab^2 + b^3) = a^4 - b^4$$

$(a-b)(a^4+a^3b+a^2b^2+ab^3+b^4)=a^5-b^5$

$(a-b)(a^5+a^4b+a^3b^2+a^2b^3+ab^4+b^5)=a^6-b^6$

$(a-b)(a^{n-1}+a^{n-2}b+a^{n-3}b^2+\ldots+ab^{n-2}+b^{n-1})=a^n-b^n$, where n is any positive integer $(1, 2, 3, 4, \ldots)$.

$(a+b)(a^{n-1}-a^{n-2}b+a^{n-3}b^2-\ldots-ab^{n-2}+b^{n-1})=a^n+b^n$, where n is any positive odd integer $(1, 3, 5, 7, \ldots)$.

The procedure for factoring an algebraic expression completely is as follows:

Step 1: Find the greatest common factor, if there is one. Then examine each factor remaining for greatest common factors.

Step 2: Continue factoring the factors obtained in step 1 until all factors other than monomial factors are prime.

For example, here is how to factor $4-16x^2$:

$4-16x^2=4(1-4x^2)=4(1+2x)(1-2x)$

Problem

Express each of the following as a single term.

A. $3x^2+2x^2-4x^2$

B. $5axy^2-7axy^2-3xy^2$

Solution

A. Factor x^2 in the expression.

$3x^2+2x^2-4x^2=(3+2-4)x^2=1x^2=x^2.$

B. Factor xy^2 in the expression and then factor a.

$$\begin{aligned}5axy^2-7axy^2-3xy^2&=(5a-7a-3)xy^2\\&=[(5-7)a-3]xy^2\\&=(-2a-3)xy^2.\end{aligned}$$

Problem

Simplify $\dfrac{\frac{1}{x-1}-\frac{1}{x-2}}{\frac{1}{x-2}-\frac{1}{x-3}}$.

Solution

Simplify the expression in the numerator by using the following addition rule:

$$\frac{a}{b}+\frac{c}{d}=\frac{ad+bc}{bd}$$

Notice that bd is the least common denominator, or LCD. Using the addition rule gives

$$\frac{x-2-(x-1)}{(x-1)(x-2)}=\frac{-1}{(x-1)(x-2)}$$

in the numerator.

Repeating this procedure for the expression in the denominator

$$\frac{x-3-(x-2)}{(x-2)(x-3)} = \frac{-1}{(x-2)(x-3)}$$

results in

$$\frac{\dfrac{-1}{(x-1)(x-2)}}{\dfrac{-1}{(x-2)(x-3)}},$$

which is simplified by inverting the fraction in the denominator, multiplying it by the numerator, and canceling like terms:

$$\frac{-1}{(x-1)(x-2)} \cdot \frac{(x-2(x-3))}{-1} = \frac{x-3}{x-1}.$$

2. EQUATIONS

An equation is defined as a statement of equality of two separate expressions.

Equations with the same solutions are said to be equivalent equations.

A. Replacing an expression of an equation by an equivalent expression results in an equation equivalent to the original one. Consider the equation

$$3x + y + x + 2y = 15.$$

The commutative and distributive laws can be applied to the left side of the equation to get

$$3x + y + x + 2y = 4x + 3y.$$

Because these are equivalent, the expression in the original equation can be replaced with the simpler form to get

$$4x + 3y = 15.$$

B. The addition or subtraction of the same expression on both sides of an equation results in an equation equivalent to the original one. For example, given the equation

$$y + 6 = 10,$$

(-6) can be added to both sides

$$y + 6 + (-6) = 10 + (-6)$$

to get $y + 0 = 10 - 6 \rightarrow y = 4$. So $y + 6 = 10$ is equivalent to $y = 4$.

C. The multiplication or division on both sides of an equation by the same expression results in an equivalent equation to the original. For example,

$$3x = 6 \rightarrow \frac{3x}{3} = \frac{6}{3} \rightarrow x = 2.$$

Therefore, $3x = 6$ is equivalent to $x = 2$.

D. If both members of an equation are raised to the same power, then the resultant equation is equivalent to the original equation. For example,

$$a = x^2y,\ (a)^2 = (x^2y)^2, \text{ and } a^2 = x^4y^2.$$

This applies to negative and fractional powers as well. For example,

$$x^2 = 3y^4.$$

If both members are raised to the -2 power, the result is

$$(x^{-2})^{-2} = (3y^4)^{-2}$$

$$\frac{1}{(x^2)^2} = \frac{1}{(3y^4)^2}$$

$$\frac{1}{x^4} = \frac{1}{9y^8}$$

If both members are raised to the $\frac{1}{2}$ power, which is the same as taking the square root, the result is

$$(x^2)^{\frac{1}{2}} = (3y^4)^{\frac{1}{2}}$$

$$x = \sqrt{3y^2}$$

E. The reciprocal of both members of an equation is equivalent to the original equation.
Note: The reciprocal of zero is undefined.

$$\frac{2x+y}{z} = \frac{5}{2} \quad \frac{z}{2x+y} = \frac{2}{5}$$

Problem

Solve, justifying each step: $3x - 8 = 7x + 8$.

Solution

$$3x - 8 = 7x + 8$$

Add 8 to both members: $3x - 8 + 8 = 7x + 8 + 8$

Apply the additive inverse property: $3x + 0 = 7x + 16$

Apply the additive identity property: $3x = 7x + 16$

Add $(-7x)$ to both members: $3x - 7x = 7x + 16 - 7x$

Commute: $-4x = 7x - 7x + 16$

Apply the additive inverse property: $-4x = 0 + 16$

Apply the additive identity property: $-4x = 16$

Divide both sides by -4: $\frac{-4x}{-4} = \frac{16}{-4}$

$$x = -4$$

Check: Replace x with -4 in the original equation:

$$3x - 8 = 7x + 8$$

$$3(-4) - 8 = 7(-4) + 8$$

$$-12 - 8 = -28 + 8$$

$$-20 = -20$$

A. Linear Equations

A linear equation with one unknown is one that can be put into the form $ax + b = 0$, where a and b are constants, $a \neq 0$.

To solve a linear equation means to transform it into the form $x = \frac{-b}{a}$.

A. If the equation has unknowns on both sides of the equality, it is convenient to put similar terms on the same sides. For example,

$$\begin{aligned}
4x + 3 &= 2x + 9 \\
4x + 3 - 2x &= 2x + 9 - 2x \\
(4x - 2x) + 3 &= (2x - 2x) + 9 \\
2x + 3 &= 0 + 9 \\
2x + 3 - 3 &= 0 + 9 - 3 \\
2x &= 6 \\
\frac{2x}{2} &= \frac{6}{2} \\
x &= 3.
\end{aligned}$$

B. If the equation appears in fractional form, it is necessary to transform it using cross multiplication. Then the same procedure as in step A is repeated.

$$\frac{3x+4}{3} \times \frac{7x+2}{5}$$

Using cross-multiplication results in

$$3(7x + 2) = 5(3x + 4).$$

This is equivalent to

$$21x + 6 = 15x + 20,$$

which can be solved as in step A:

$$\begin{aligned}
21x + 6 &= 15x + 20 \\
21x - 15x + 6 &= 15x - 15x + 20 \\
6x + 6 - 6 &= 20 - 6 \\
6x &= 14 \\
x &= \frac{14}{6} \\
x &= \frac{7}{3}
\end{aligned}$$

C. If there are radicals in the equation, it is necessary to square both sides and then perform step A:

$$\begin{aligned}
\left(\sqrt{3x+1}\right) &= 5 \\
\left(\sqrt{3x+1}\right)^2 &= 52 \\
3x + 1 &= 25 \\
3x + 1 - 1 &= 25 - 1 \\
3x &= 24 \\
x &= \frac{24}{3} \\
x &= 8
\end{aligned}$$

Problem

Solve the equation $2(x + 3) = (3x + 5) - (x - 5)$.

Solution

Transform the given equation to an equivalent equation in which the solution set is easily recognized:

$2(x + 3) = 3x + 5 - (x - 5)$

Distribute: $2x + 6 = 3x + 5 - x + 5$

Combine terms: $2x + 6 = 2x + 10$

Subtract $2x$ from both sides: $6 = 10$

Because $6 = 10$ is not a true statement, there is no real number that will make the original equation true. The equation is inconsistent, and the solution set is Φ, the empty set.

Problem

Solve the equation $2\left(\frac{2}{3y} + 5\right) + 2(y + 5) = 130$.

Solution

The procedure for solving this equation is as follows:

Distribute: $\frac{4}{3y} + 10 + 2y + 10 = 130$

Combine like terms: $\frac{4}{3y} + 2y + 20 = 130,$

Subtract 20 from both sides: $\frac{4}{3y} + 2y = 110,$

Convert $2y$ into a fraction with denominator: $\frac{4}{3y} + \frac{6}{3y} = 110$

Combine like terms: $\frac{10}{3y} = 110,$

Divide by $\frac{10}{3}$: $y = 110 \times \frac{3}{10} = 33$,

Check: Replace y by 33 in the original equation:

$2(2/3(33) + 5) + (2(33 + 5) = 130$

$2(22 + 5) + 2(38) = 130$

$2(27) + 76 = 130$

$54 + 76 = 130$

$130 = 130$

Therefore, the solution to the given equation is $y = 33$.

B. Two Linear Equations

Equations of the form $ax + by = c$, where a, b, c are constants and $a, b \neq 0$, are called linear equations with two unknown variables.

There are three ways to solve systems of linear equations in two variables.

Method 1: Addition or subtraction — If necessary, multiply the equations by numbers that will make the coefficients of one unknown in the resulting equations numerically equal. If the signs of equal coefficients are the same, subtract the equation; otherwise, add. The result is one equation with one unknown. Solve the equation and substitute the value into the other equations to find the unknown that was first eliminated.

Method 2: Substitution — Find the value of one unknown in terms of the other. Substitute that value in the other equation and solve.

Method 3: Graphing — Graph both equations. The point of intersection of the drawn lines is a simultaneous solution for the equations, and its coordinates correspond to the answer that would be found analytically.

If the lines are parallel, they have no simultaneous solution.

Dependent equations are equations that represent the same line; therefore, every point on the line of a dependent equation represents a solution. Because there is an infinite number of points, there is an infinite number of simultaneous solutions. For example,

$$2x + y = 8$$
$$4x + 2y = 16.$$

These equations are dependent, they represent the same line, and all points that satisfy either of the equations are solutions of the system.

A system of linear equations is consistent if there is only one solution for the system. A system of linear equations is inconsistent if it does not have any solutions.

Example of a consistent system — Find the point of intersection of the graphs of the equations

$$x + y = 3, \text{ and}$$
$$3x - 2y = 14.$$

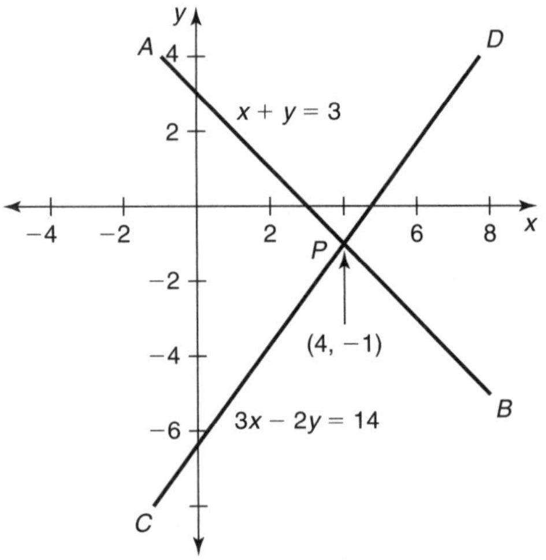

To solve these linear equations, solve for y in terms of x. The equations will be in the form $y = mx + b$, where m is the slope and b is the intercept on the y-axis.

$x + y = 3$
Subtract x from both sides: $y = 3 - x$
Subtract $3x$ from both sides: $3x - 2y = 14$
Divide by -2: $-2y = 14 - 3x$

$$y = -7 + 3/2x$$

The graphs of the linear functions $y = 3 - x$ and $y - 7 + \frac{3}{2x}$ can be determined by plotting only two points. For example, for $y = 3 - x$, if $x = 0$, then $y = 3$; and if $x = 1$, then $y = 2$. The two points on this first line are $(0, 3)$ and $(1, 2)$. For $y - 7 + \frac{3}{2x}$, let $x = 0$, then $y = -7$. Let $x = 1$, then $y = -5\frac{1}{2}$.

The two points on this second line are $(0, -7)$ and $\left(1, -5\frac{1}{2}\right)$.

To find the point of intersection P of

$$x + y = 3 \text{ and } 3x - 2y = 14,$$

solve them algebraically. Multiply the first equation by 2. Add the two equations to eliminate the variable y:

$$\begin{array}{r} 2x + 2y = 6 \\ 3x - 2y = 14 \\ \hline 5x = 20 \end{array}$$

Solve for x to obtain $x = 4$. Substitute that into $y = 3 - x$ to get $y = 3 - 4 = -1$. P is $(4, -1)$. AB is the graph of the first equation, and CD is the graph of the second equation. The point of intersection P of the two graphs is the only point on both lines. The coordinates of P satisfy both equations and represent the desired solution to the problem. From the graph, P seems to be the point $(4, -1)$. These coordinates satisfy both equations and thus are the exact coordinates of the point of intersection of the two lines.

To show that $(4, -1)$ satisfies both equations, substitute that point into both equations.

$$\begin{array}{rr} x + y = 3 & 3x - 2y = 14 \\ 4 + (-1) = 3 & 3(4) - 2(-1) = 14 \\ 4 - 1 = 3 & 12 + 2 = 14 \\ 3 = 3 & 14 = 14 \end{array}$$

Example of an inconsistent system — Solve the equations $2x + 3y = 6$ and $4x + 6y = 7$ simultaneously.

There are two equations in two unknowns:

$$2x + 3y = 6 \qquad (1)$$

and

$$x + 6y = 7 \qquad (2)$$

There are several methods to solve this problem. Try multiplying each equation by a different number so that when the two equations are added, one of the variables drops out:

Multiply equation (1) by 2: $4x + 6y = 12$ (3)
Multiply equation (2) by -1: $-4x - 6y = -7$ (4)
Add equations (3) and (4): $0 = 5$

That is a peculiar result!

Actually, what this shows is that, if there were a simultaneous solution to the given equations, then 0 would equal 5. But the conclusion is impossible; therefore, there can be no simultaneous solution to these two equations and thus no point satisfying both.

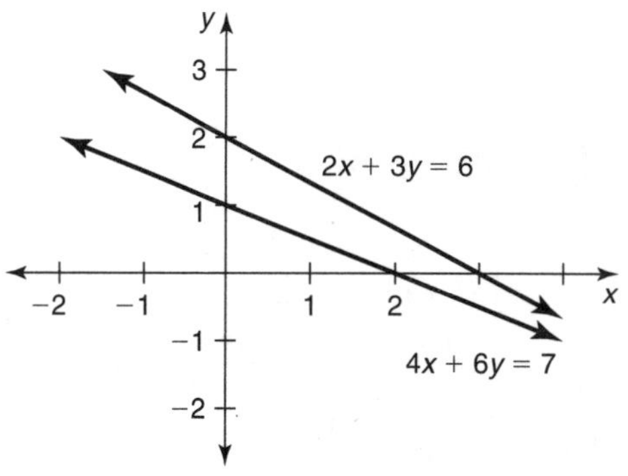

The straight lines that are the graphs of these equations must be parallel if they never intersect. But they are not identical, which can be seen from the graph of these equations (see the accompanying diagram).

Example of a dependent system — Solve the equations $2x + 3y = 6$ and $y = -\left(\frac{2x}{3}\right) + 2$ simultaneously.

There are two equations in two unknowns:

$$2x + 3y = 6 \qquad (1)$$

and

$$y = -\left(\frac{2x}{3}\right) + 2 \qquad (2)$$

There are several methods of solution for this problem. Because equation (2) already gives an expression for y, the method of substitution can be used. Substituting $-\left(\frac{2x}{3}\right) + 2$ for y in the first equation results in the following:

$$2x + 3\left(\frac{-2x}{2}\right) + 2 = 6$$

Distribute: $2x - 2x + 6 = 6$

$$6 = 6$$

Apparently, this method leads nowhere! The result $6 = 6$ is true but indicates no solution. Actually, this shows that no matter what real number x is, if y is determined by the second equation, then the first equation will always be satisfied.

The reason for this peculiarity may be seen by taking a closer look at the equation $y = -\left(\frac{2x}{3}\right) + 2$. It is equivalent to $3y = -2x + 6$, or $2x + 3y = 6$.

In other words, the two equations are equivalent. Any pair of values of x and y that satisfies one satisfies the other.

It is hardly necessary to verify that, in this case, the graphs of the given equations are identical lines, and that there are an infinite number of simultaneous solutions of these equations.

A system of three linear equations in three unknowns is solved by eliminating one unknown from any two of the three equations and solving them. After finding two unknowns, substitute them in any of the equations to find the third unknown.

Problem

Solve the system

$$2x + 3y - 4z = -8 \qquad (1)$$
$$x + y - 2z = -5 \qquad (2)$$
$$7x - 2y + 5z = 4 \qquad (3)$$

Solution

No variable can be eliminated from two pairs of equations by a single multiplication. However, both x and z may be eliminated from equations (1) and (2) by multiplying equation (2) by -2. Then

$$2x + 3y - 4z = -8 \quad (1)$$
$$-2x - 2y + 4z = 10 \quad (4)$$

By addition, $y = 2$. Although now either x or z can be eliminated from another pair of equations, it is more convenient to substitute $y = 2$ in equations (2) and (3) to get two equations in two variables. Thus, making the substitution $y = 2$ in equations (2) and (3) results in

$$x - 2z = -7 \qquad (5)$$
$$7x + 5z = 8. \qquad (6)$$

Multiply equation (5) by 5 and multiply equation (6) by 2 and add the two new equations. Then $x = -1$. Substitute x in either equation (5) or (6) to find z.

The solution of the system is $x = -1$, $y = 2$, and $z = 3$. Check by substitution.

A system of equations, like the following, that has all constant terms $b_1, b_2, \ldots, b_n$ equal to zero is said to be a homogeneous system:

$$\begin{cases} a_{11}x_1 + a_{12}x_2 + a_{1n}x_m = b_1 \\ a_{21}x_1 + a_{22}x_2 + a_{2n}x_m = b_2 \\ \vdots \quad \vdots \quad \vdots \quad \vdots \\ a_{n1}x_1 + a_{n2}x_2 + \cdots + a_{mn}x_m = b_n \end{cases}$$

A homogeneous system always has at least one solution, called the trivial solution, which is $x_1 = 0$, $x_2 = 0, \ldots, x_m = 0$.

For any given homogeneous system of equations in which the number of variables is greater than or equal to the number of equations, there are nontrivial solutions.

Two systems of linear equations are said to be equivalent if and only if they have the same solution set.

Problem

Solve for x and y.

$$x + 2y = 8 \qquad (1)$$
$$3x + 4y = 20 \qquad (2)$$

Solution

Solve equation (1) for x in terms of y:

$$x = 8 - 2y \qquad (3)$$

Substitute $(8 - 2y)$ for x in equation (2):

$$3(8 - 2y) + 4y = 20 \qquad (4)$$

Solve equation (4) for y as follows:

Distribute: $24 - 6y + 4y = 20$

Combine like terms: $24 - 2y = 20$

Subtract 24 from both sides: $24 - 24 - 2y = 20 - 24$

$$-2y = -4$$

Divide both sides by -2: $y = 2$

Substitute 2 for y in equation (1):

$$x + 2(2) = 8$$
$$x = 4$$

Thus, the solution is $x = 4, y = 2$.

Check: Substitute $x = 4, y = 2$ in equations (1) and (2):

$$4 + 2(2) = 8$$
$$8 = 8$$
$$3(4) + 4(2) = 20$$
$$20 = 20$$

Problem

Solve algebraically:

$$4x + 2y = -1 \qquad (1)$$
$$5x - 3y = 7 \qquad (2)$$

Solution

Arbitrarily choose to eliminate x first.

Multiply equation (1) by 5: $20x + 10y = -5$ (3)
Multiply equation (2) by 4: $20x - 12y = 28$ (4)
Subtract equation (3) from equation (4): $22y = -33$ (5)

Divide equation (5) by 22: $y = -\frac{33}{22} = -\frac{3}{2}$

To find x, substitute $y = -\frac{3}{2}$ in either of the original equations. Using equation (1) results in

$4x + 2\left(-\frac{3}{2}\right) = -1, 4x - 3 = -1,\ 4x = 2,\ x = \frac{1}{2}.$

The solution $\left(\frac{1}{2}, -\frac{3}{2}\right)$ should be checked in both equations of the given system.

Replacing $\left(\frac{1}{2}, \frac{3}{2}\right)$ in equation (1):

$$4x + 2y = -1$$
$$4\left(\frac{1}{2}\right) + 2\left(-\frac{3}{2}\right) = -1$$
$$4/2 - 3 = -1$$
$$2 - 3 = -1$$
$$-1 = -1$$

Replacing $\left(\frac{1}{2}, -\frac{3}{2}\right)$ in equation (2):

$$5x - 3y = 7$$
$$5\left(\tfrac{1}{2}\right) - 3\left(-\tfrac{3}{2}\right) = 7$$
$$\tfrac{5}{2} + \tfrac{9}{2} = 7$$
$$\tfrac{14}{2} = 7$$
$$7 = 7$$

Instead of eliminating x from the two given equations, it is possible to eliminate y by multiplying equation (1) by 3, multiplying equation (2) by 2, and then adding the two derived equations.

C. Quadratic Equations

A second-degree equation in x of the type $ax^2 + bx + c = 0$, where $a \neq 0$ and a, b, and c are real numbers, is called a quadratic equation.

To solve a quadratic equation is to find values of x that satisfy $ax^2 + bx + c = 0$. These values of x are called solutions, or roots, of the equation.

A quadratic equation has a maximum of two roots. Methods of solving quadratic equations include the following

Method 1: Direct solution — Given $x^2 - 9 = 0$, the solution can be found directly by isolating the variable x:

$x^2 = 9$
$x = \pm 3.$

Method 2: Factoring — Given a quadratic equation $ax^2 + bx + c = 0$, where $a, b, c \neq 0$, to *factor* means to express it as the product $a(x - r_1)(x - r_2) = 0$, where r_1 and r_2 are the two roots.

Following are some helpful hints:

$r_1 + r_2 = -\frac{b}{a}$.

$r_1 r_2 = \frac{c}{a}$.

For example, consider the equation $x^2 - 5x + 4 = 0$. Because $r_1 + r_2 = -\frac{b}{a} = \frac{-(-5)}{1} = 5$, possible solutions to that equation are (3, 2), (4, 1), and (5, 0). Because $r_1 r_2 = \frac{c}{a} = \frac{4}{1} = 4$, this equation is satisfied only by the second pair, so $r_1 = 4$, $r_2 = 1$, and the factored form is $(x - 4)(x - 1) = 0$.

If the coefficient of x^2 is not 1, it is necessary to divide the equation by this coefficient and then factor. For example, consider the equation $2x^2 - 12x + 16 = 0$. Dividing by 2 gives

$$x^2 - 6x + 8 = 0.$$

Because $r_1 + r_2 = -\frac{b}{a} = 6$, the possible solutions are (6, 0), (5, 1), (4, 2), (3, 3). Because $r_1 r_2 = 8$, the only possible answer is (4, 2), and the expression $x^2 - 6x + 8 = 0$ can be factored as $(x - 4)(x - 2)$.

Method 3: Using the quadratic equation — For the equation in the form, $ax^2 + bx + c$, the solution to x is given by the quadratic equation, which states that

$$x = \frac{-b \pm \sqrt{b^2 - 4ac}}{2a}$$

Problem

Solve the equation $x^2 + 8x + 15 = 0$.

Solution

This equation is in the form of the quadratic equation, where $a = 1$, $b = 8$, *and* $c = 15$. Substituting into the quadratic equation gives

$$x = \frac{-8 \pm \sqrt{8^2 - 4(1)(15)}}{2(1)},$$

which simplifies to

$$x = \frac{-8 \pm 2}{2}$$

Note that $x = -5$ OR $x = -3$. This does not mean that $x = -5$ AND $x = -3$. Also, check that both these numbers do actually satisfy the given equations and thus are solutions.

Check: Replacing x by (-5) in the original equation:

$$\begin{aligned} x^2 + 8x + 15 &= 0 \\ (-5)^2 + 8(-5) + 15 &= 0 \\ 25 - 40 + 15 &= 0 \\ -15 + 15 &= 0 \\ 0 &= 0 \end{aligned}$$

Replacing x by (-3) in the original equation:

$$\begin{aligned} x^2 + 8x + 15 &= 0 \\ (-3)^2 + 8(-3) + 15 &= 0 \\ 9 - 24 + 15 &= 0 \\ -15 + 15 &= 0 \\ 0 &= 0 \end{aligned}$$

Problem

Solve the following equations by factoring.

A. $2x^2 + 3x = 0$

B. $y^2 - 2y - 3 = y - 3$

C. $z^2 - 2z - 3 = 0$

D. $2m^2 - 11m - 6 = 0$

Solution

A. $2x^2 + 3x = 0$. Factoring out the common factor of x from the left side of the given equation,

$$x(2x + 3) = 0.$$

Whenever a product $ab = 0$, where a and b are any two numbers, either $a = 0$ or $b = 0$. Then, either

$x = 0$ or $2x + 3 = 0$

$2x = -3$

$x = -\frac{3}{2}$

Hence, the solution set to the original equation $2x^2 + 3x = 0$ is $\left\{-\frac{3}{2}, 0\right\}$

B. $y^2 - 2y - 3 = y - 3$. Subtract $(y - 3)$ from both sides of the given equation:

$$y^2 - 2y - 3 - (y - 3) = y - 3 - (y - 3)$$
$$y^2 - 2y - 3 - y + 3 = y - 3 - y + 3$$
$$y^2 - 3y = 0.$$

Factor out a common factor of y from the left side of this equation:

$$y(y - 3) = 0.$$

Thus, $y = 0$ or $y - 3 = 0, y = 3$. Therefore, the solution set to the original equation $y^2 - 2y - 3 = y - 3$ is $\{0,3\}$.

C. $z^2 - 2z - 3 = 0.$

Factor the original equation into a product of two polynomials:

$$z^2 - 2z - 3 = (z - 3)(z + 1) = 0$$

Hence, $z - 3 = 0$ or $z + 1 = 0$; and $z = 3$ or $z = -1$.

Therefore, the solution set to the original equation $z^2 - 2z - 3 = 0$ is: $\{-1, 3\}$.

D. $2m^2 - 11m - 6 = 0.$

Factor the original equation into a product of two polynomials:

$$2m^2 - 11m - 6 \quad = \quad (2m + 1)(m - 6) = 0$$

Thus, $2m + 1 = 0$ or $m - 6 = 0$

$$2m = -1 \quad m = 6$$
$$m = -\frac{1}{2}$$

Therefore, the solution set to the original equation $2m^2 - 11m - 6 = 0$ is $\{-\frac{1}{2}, 6\}$.

3. FUNCTIONS

Constant — A symbol that represents one particular number during a discussion. For example, numbers 5, -3, π, and $2\frac{6}{7}$ are constants.

Variable — A symbol to which may be assigned any of several numbers during the course of a discussion.

Function — If two variables, x and y, are so related that to each permissible value of x, there corresponds one or more values of a second variable, then y is called a function of x. In the formulation, x is called the independent variable, while y is called the dependent variable. In order to express the fact that y is a function of x, the symbol used is $y = f(x)$.

Problem

If $f(x) = x^2 + 3x - 7$, then find $f(2)$.

Solution

$f(2)$ indicates that 2 is to be substituted for x.

$$f(2) = 2^2 + 3.2 - 7 = 4 + 6 - 7 = 3$$

Problem

If $f(x) = x^3 + 2x - 6$, then find

A. $f(-1)$. B. $f(0)$. C. $f(1/a)$.

Solution

$f(x) = x^3 + 2x - 6$

A. $f(-1)$ means that $x = -1$ is substituted into $f(x)$.

$$f(-1) = (-1)^3 + 2(-1) - 6$$
$$= -1 - 2 - 6$$
$$= -9$$

B. $f(0)$ substitute in $x = 0$

$$f(0) = (0)3 + 2(0) - 6$$
$$= 0 + 0 - 6$$
$$= -6$$

C. $$f\left(\frac{1}{a}\right) = \left(\frac{1}{a}\right)^3 + 2\left(\frac{1}{a}\right) - 6$$
$$= \frac{1}{a^3} + \frac{2}{a} - 6$$
$$= \frac{1}{a^3} + \frac{2a^2}{a^3} - \frac{6a^3}{a^3} \text{ get common denominator}$$
$$= \frac{1 + 2a^2 - 6a^3}{a^3}$$

Problem

If $f(x) = x^2 - 3x + 9$, then find

A. $f(y + 1)$. B. $f(a + b)$.

Solution

$f(x) = x^2 - 3x + 9$

A. $f(y + 1)$ means that $x = y + 1$ is substituted into $f(x)$

$$f(y + 1) = (y + 1)^2 - 3(y + 1) + 9$$

Expand terms: $= y^2 + 2y + 1 - 3y - 3 + 9$

Add like terms: $= y^2 - y + 7$

B. $f(a + b)$ substitute in $x = a + b$

$$f(a + b) = (a + b)2 - 3(a + b) + 9$$

Expand terms: $= a^2 + 2ab + b2 - 3a - 3b + 9$

4. GRAPHS

The graph shown on the next page is called the Cartesian coordinate plane. The graph consists of a pair of perpendicular lines called coordinate axes. The vertical axis is the y-axis and the horizontal axis is the x-axis. The point of intersection of these two axes is called the origin; it is the zero point of both axes.

Further, points to the right of the origin on the x-axis and above the origin on the y-axis represent positive real numbers. Points to the left of the origin on the x-axis or below the origin on the y-axis represent negative real numbers.

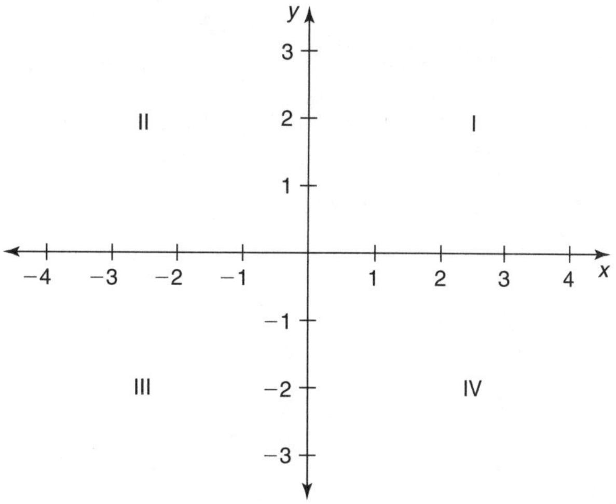

The four regions cut off by the coordinate axes are called, in counterclockwise direction from the top right, the first, second, third and fourth quadrant. The first quadrant contains all points with two positive coordinates.

In the following graph, two points are identified by the ordered pair (x, y) of numbers. The x-coordinate is the first number and the y-coordinate is the second number. In this case, point A has the coordinates $(4, 2)$, and the coordinates of point B are $(-3, -5)$.

The number indicating how many units a point is to the right or to the left of the y-axis is called the abscissa. In the case of point A, the abscissa is 4, while for point B the abscissa is -3.

The number indicating how many units a point is above or below the x-axis is called the ordinate. The ordinate for point A is 2, while for point B, the ordinate is -5.

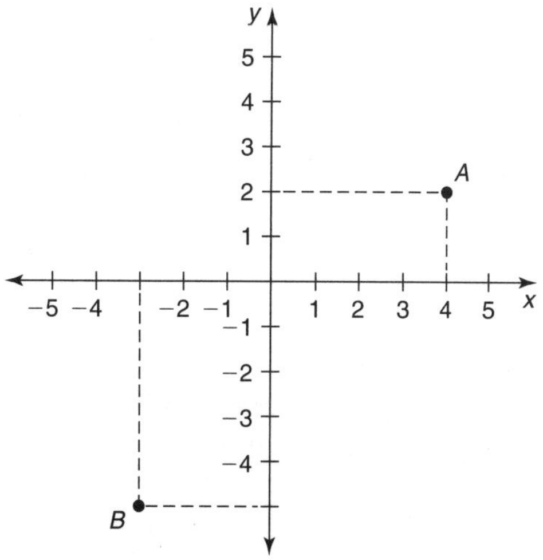

A. Graph of a Function

The graph of a function $y = f(x)$ consists of all the points whose coordinates satisfy the relationship $y = f(x)$.

Problem

Plot the graph of $4x - 2y = 10$.

Solution

Creating the graph requires a set of ordered pairs (x, y).

Determine the pairs by first solving the equation for y and substituting appropriate values for x:

$$4x - 2y = 10$$
$$2y = 4x - 10$$
$$y = 2x - 5$$

Then form a table by substituting values for x:

x	−2	−1	0	1	2	3
y	−9	−7	−5	−3	−1	1

Plot the points of ordered pairs:

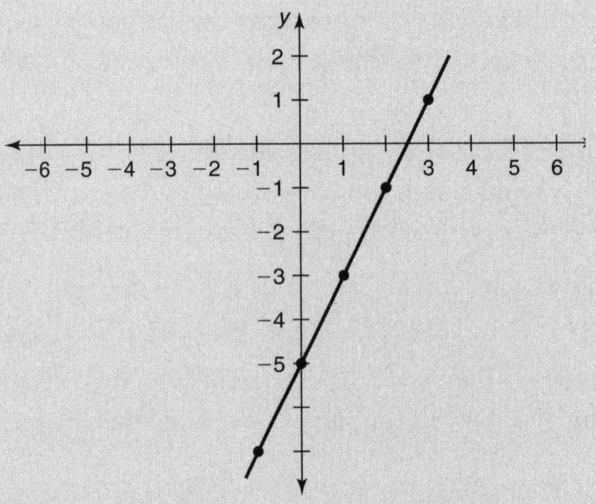

Recognize the similarities and differences in the following graph of three straight lines, which are in the general form $y = mx + b$, where m is the slope of the line and b is the y-intercept:

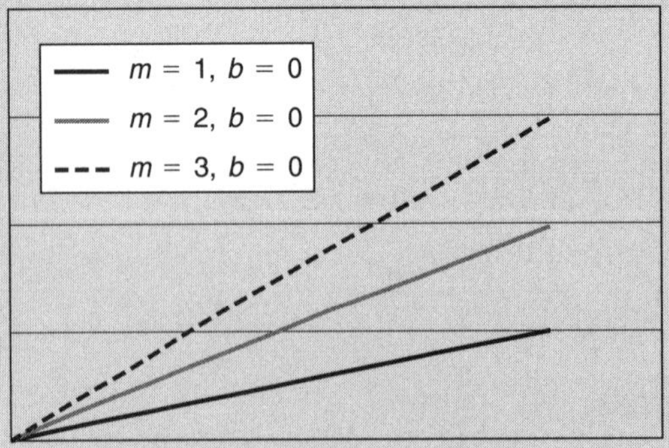

In the following graph, the lines are offset by one positive unit, because the y-intercept = 1:

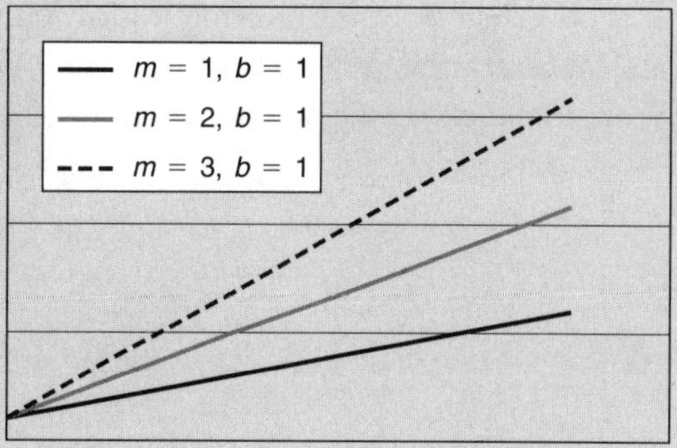

Here the line is offset by two negative units:

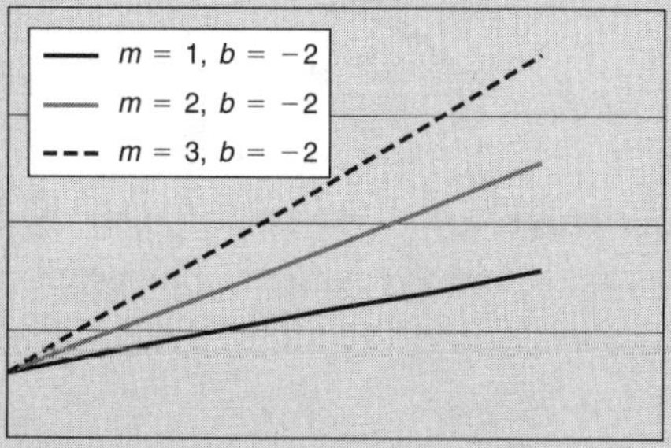

For a straight line with a negative slope, the value of y decreases as x increases, as shown here:

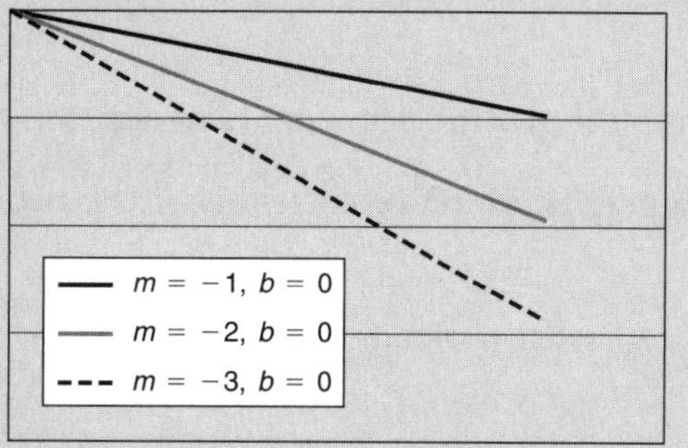

A straight line means that y is linearly related to x. Two important graphical relationships to recognize are the power equation and the reciprocal relationship.

Figure 1

$y = x^n$

Figure 2

$y = x^n + b$

Figure 3

$$y = \frac{1}{x^n}$$

Figure 4

$$y = \frac{1}{x^n} + b$$

In the latter graph, y is approaching b, and in the former graph, y is approaching zero.

Problem

An inhibitor is a substance that can influence the rate of an enzymatic reaction. The structures of the inhibitor and the enzyme influences how the rate of the enzymatic reaction will be affected. In Figure 1, Graph A represents a plot of substrate concentration versus rate of reaction without an inhibitor. Graphs B and C represent plots of substrate concentration versus rate of reaction with an inhibitor present.

FIGURE 1

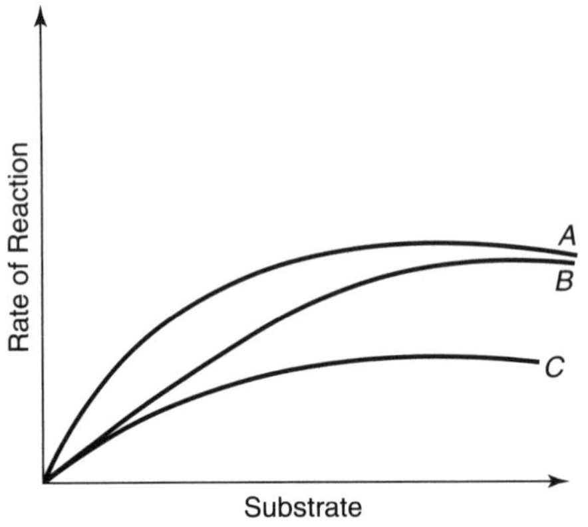

Question — Which graph represents a system in which the same rate of reaction will be achieved at high substrate concentration as the system represented by graph A?

Answer — Graph B.

Question — In the absence of the substrate, is there enzymatic activity in these systems?

Answer — No, the *y*-intercept for all graphs is zero.

Question — Which graph represents a system in which the maximum rate is the smallest value?

Answer — Graph C.

Question — Which graph shows the dependence of reaction rate on enzyme concentration?

Answer — None. The graphs are representations of the dependence of reaction rate on substrate concentration.

The graphs in Figure 2 represent a system in which consecutive chemical reactions can occur.

B -> C -> A

FIGURE 2

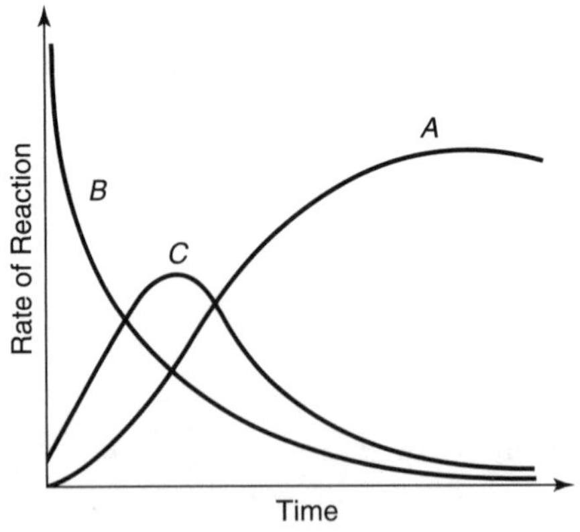

Question — At 60 minutes, what species is in greatest concentration?

Answer — Species A because it is the product of the reaction.

Question — At 10 minutes, what species is in the greatest concentration?

Answer — Species B because it is the starting material.

Question — At what time does species C reach its maximum concentration?

Answer — At approximately 25 minutes, species C reaches a maximum concentration.

B. Scales

Three kinds of scales are usually used for plotting functions:

1. **Arithmetic** — when the abscissa is x and the ordinate is y. This kind of scale is the most commonly used.
2. **Semilog** — when either the abscissa is log x and the ordinate is y, or when the abscissa is x and the ordinate is log y. This type of scale is used when either x is larger than y, or vice versa.
3. **Log-log** — when the abscissa is log x and the ordinate is log y. This type of scale is used when both x and y are large numbers.

5. DISTANCE

For any two points A and B with coordinates (X_A, Y_A) and (X_B, Y_B), respectively, the distance between A and B is represented by

$$AB = \sqrt{(X_A - X_B)^2 + (Y_A - Y_B{}^2)}\ .$$

This is commonly known as the distance formula or the Pythagorean theorem.

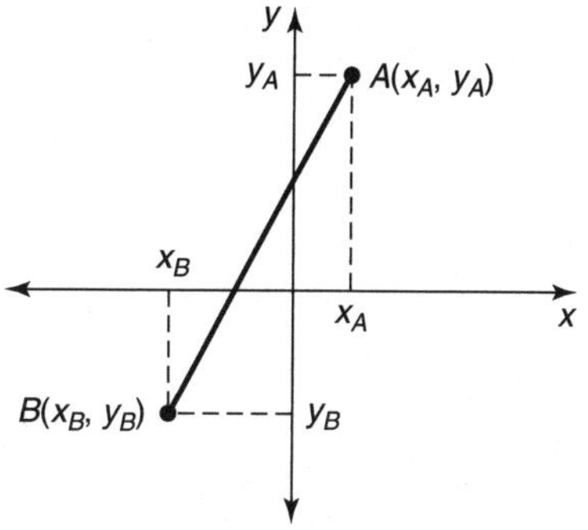

Problem

Find the distance between points $A(1, 3)$ and $B(5, 3)$.

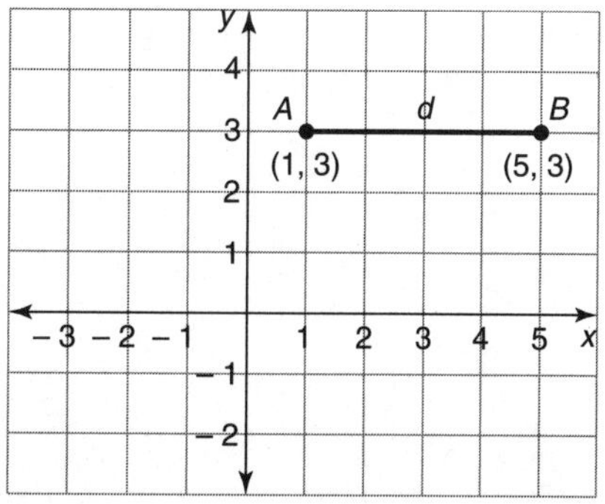

Solution

In this case, where the ordinate of both points is the same, the distance between the two points is given by the absolute value of the difference between the two abscissas. In fact, this case reduces to merely counting boxes, as the figure shows.

Let, x_1 = abscissa of A y_1 = ordinate of A

x_2 = abscissa of B y_1 = ordinate of B

d = the distance

Therefore, $d = |x_1 - x_2|$. By substitution, $d = |1-5| = |-4| = 4$. This answer can also be obtained by applying the general formula for distance between two points.

$$d = \sqrt{(x_1 - x_2)^2 + (y_1 - y_2)^2}$$

By substitution,

$$d = \sqrt{(1-5)^2 + (3-3)^2} = \sqrt{(-4)^2 + (0)^2} = \sqrt{16} = 4.$$

Thus, the distance is 4.

6. SLOPE OF A STRAIGHT LINE

The slope of a straight line containing two points (x_1, y_1) and (x_2, y_2) is given by

$$slope = m = \frac{y_2 - y_1}{x_2 - x_1}.$$

Horizontal lines have a slope of zero, and the slope of vertical lines is undefined. Parallel lines have equal slopes, and perpendicular lines have slopes that are negative reciprocals.

Problem

Find the slope of the straight line that contains points A and B. Also determine the slope of the perpendicular line.

A. $A(-1, 2), B(-2, -1)$

B. $A(1, 0), B(0, 1)$

C. $A(-1, 0), B(1, 0)$

Solution

A. Treat the coordinates of A as $A(x_1, y_1)$ and of B as $B(x_2, y_2)$. Then,

$$m = \frac{y_2 - y_1}{x_2 - x_1} = \frac{-1-2}{-2-(-1)} = \frac{-3}{-2+1} = \frac{-3}{-1} = 3.$$

The slope of the perpendicular line is the negative reciprocal of m, which is $-\frac{1}{3}$.

B. $m = \frac{1-0}{0-1} = \frac{1}{-1} = -1$

The slope of the perpendicular line $= -\frac{1}{m} = 1$.

C. $m = \dfrac{0-0}{1-(-1)} = \dfrac{0}{1+1} = \dfrac{0}{2} = 0$

Because m is 0, this line is a horizontal line, and the line perpendicular to that line is a vertical line whose slope is undefined.

7. TRIGONOMETRIC RATIOS

The following definitions of trigonometric ratios are based on the right triangle ΔABC shown here.

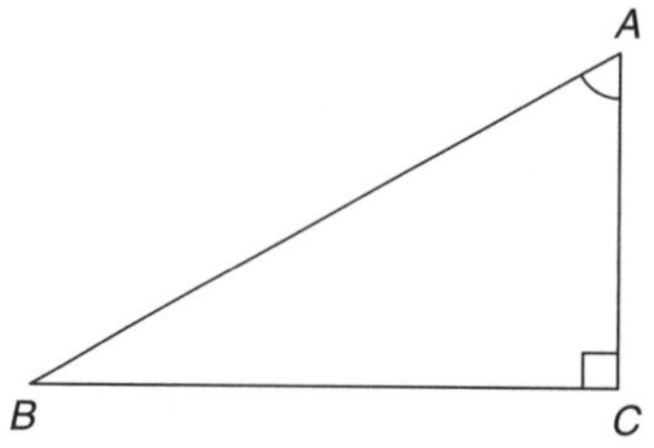

Definition 1:

$$\sin A = \frac{BC}{AB} = \frac{\text{measure of side opposite } \angle A}{\text{measure of hypotenuse}}$$

Definition 2:

$$\cos A = \frac{AC}{AB} = \frac{\text{measure of side adjacent } \angle A}{\text{measure of hypotenuse}}$$

Definition 3:

$$\tan A = \frac{BC}{AC} = \frac{\text{measure of side opposite } \angle A}{\text{measure of side adjacent to } \angle A}$$

Definition 4:

$$\cot A = \frac{AC}{BC} = \frac{\text{measure of side adjacent } \angle A}{\text{measure of side opposite } \angle A}$$

$$\sec A = \frac{AB}{AC} = \frac{\text{measure of hypotenuse}}{\text{measure of side adjacent to } \angle A}$$

$$\csc A = \frac{AB}{BC} = \frac{\text{measure of hypotenuse}}{\text{measure of side opposite to } \angle A}$$

Table 4 gives the values of sine, cosine, tangent, and cotangent for some special angles.

TABLE 4. Value of Common Trigonometric Functions

α	**Sin** α	**Cos** α	**Tan** α	**Cot** α
0°	0	1	0	∞
$\frac{\pi^R}{6} = 30°$	$\frac{1}{2}$	$\frac{\sqrt{3}}{2}$	$\frac{1}{\sqrt{3}}$	$\sqrt{3}$
$\frac{\pi^R}{4} = 45°$	$\frac{1}{\sqrt{2}}$	$\frac{1}{\sqrt{2}}$	1	1

(Continued)

TABLE 4. *Continued*

α	Sin α	Cos α	Tan α	Cot α
$\frac{\pi^R}{3} = 60°$	$\frac{\sqrt{3}}{2}$	$\frac{1}{2}$	$\sqrt{3}$	$\frac{1}{\sqrt{3}}$
$\frac{\pi^R}{2} = 90°$	1	0	∞	0

8. PYTHAGOREAN THEOREM

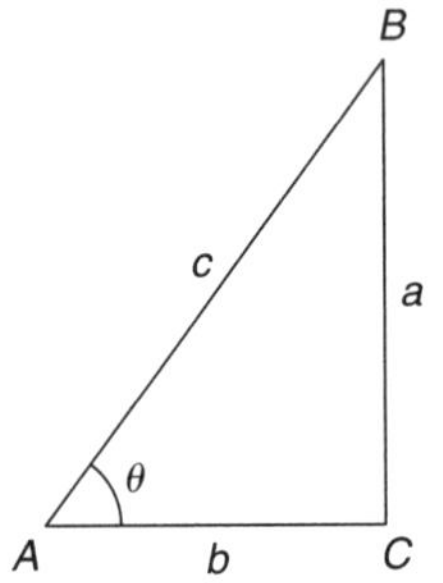

In the right triangle *ABC* shown here, C is the length of the hypotenuse, and *a* and *b* are the lengths of the other two sides. The Pythagorean theorem says that

$$c^2 = a^2 + b^2.$$

Problem

For the right triangle shown above, $\sin\theta = \frac{4}{5}$. Find

A. $\cos\theta$

B. $\tan\theta$

Solution

By definition,

$$\sin\theta = \frac{a}{c} = \frac{4}{5}.$$

Therefore, $a = 4$ and $c = 5$. Applying the Pythagorean theorem,

$$b^2 = c^2 - a^2 = 5^2 - 4^2 = 25 - 16 = 9$$
$$\text{or } b = \sqrt{9} = 3.$$

A. Therefore, $\cos\theta = \frac{b}{c} = \frac{3}{5}$.

B. $\tan\theta = \frac{a}{b} = \frac{4}{3}$.

The relationships between the sides of a right triangle can be determined using Table 4. For example if $\theta = 30$, then

$$\sin\theta = \frac{a}{c} = \frac{1}{2}.$$

This implies that $2a = c$. So for a right triangle with $\theta = 30$, the length of the hypotenuse is twice the length of *a*. Similarly, if $\theta = 45°$, then

$$\tan\theta 45 = \frac{a}{b} = 1,$$

which implies $a = b$. If = 60°, then

$$\cos\theta = \frac{b}{c} = \frac{1}{2},$$

which implies that $2b = c$.

9. INVERSE TRIGONOMETRIC FUNCTIONS

If the values of some trigonometric functions are known, based on the definitions presented in the previous section, then the corresponding angles can be determined by taking the inverse trigonometric function. A unique value is assigned to each inverse trigonometric function in each quadrant. Usually, when the trigonometric function of some angle A is given, and nothing more is specified, it is assumed that angle A is in the first quadrant. In other words, it is assumed that angle A is between 0° and 90°. However, in general, an infinite number of angles correspond to the same trigonometric values.

Here are the trigonometric functions and their inverses:

If $y = \sin x$, then $x = \sin^{-1} y = \text{Arcsin } y$

$y = \cos x$, $x = \cos^{-1} y = \text{Arccos } y$

$y = \tan x$, $x = \tan^{-1} y = \text{Arctan } y$.

The others are written the same way.

Problem

For the triangle ABC shown here, find all the remaining sides and the angles.

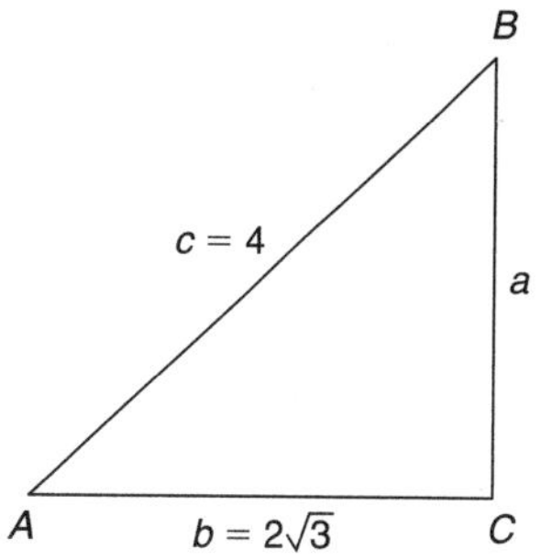

Solution

Because $b = 2\sqrt{3}$ and $c = 4$, applying the Pythagorean theorem gives

$$a^2 = c^2 - b^2$$
$$= 4^2 - (2\sqrt{3})^2 = 16 - 12 = 4$$
$$\text{or } a = \sqrt{4} = 2$$

To find angle A:

$$\sin A = \frac{a}{c} = \frac{2}{4} = \frac{1}{2}$$

$$\text{or } A = \sin^{-1}\left(\frac{1}{2}\right)$$

Table 4 shows that the angle whose sin is $\frac{1}{2}$ is a 30° angle.

The sum of all the angles in a triangle is 180; therefore, when $A = 30°$ and $C = 90°$, it follows that $B = 60°$.

IV. VECTORS AND SCALARS

A vector is a quantity that has both magnitude and direction, such as displacement, velocity, force, acceleration, momentum, electric field strength, and magnetic field strength.

A scalar is a quantity that has magnitude but no direction, such as mass, length, time, density, energy, temperature, etc.

1. ADDITION AND SUBTRACTION OF VECTORS: GEOMETRIC METHODS

A. Vector Addition

Triangle Method (Head-to-Tail Method)

The following two steps constitute the triangle method of vector addition:

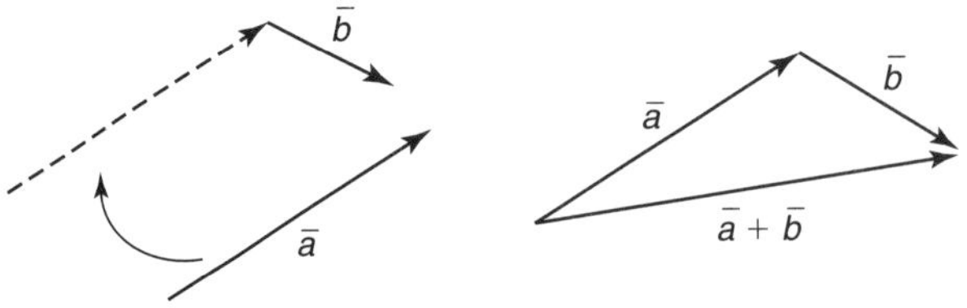

(i) Attach the head of $\bar{a}$ to the tail of $\bar{b}$. (ii) By connecting the head of $\bar{a}$ to the tail of $\bar{b}$, the vector $\bar{a} + \bar{b}$ is defined.

Parallelogram Method (Tail-to-Tail Method)

The following two steps describe the parallelogram method of vector addition:

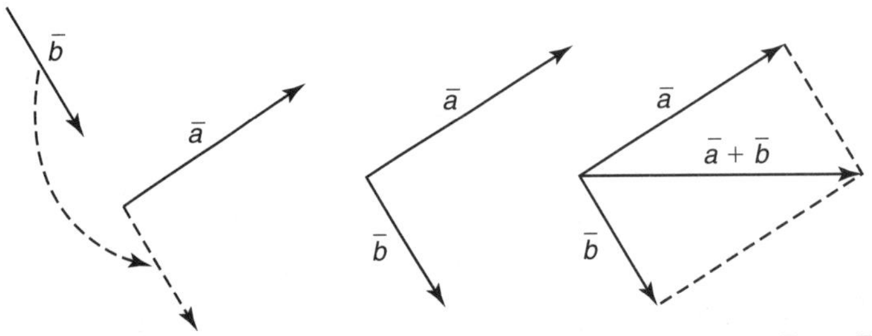

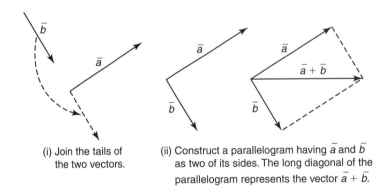

(i) Join the tails of the two vectors. (ii) Construct a parallelogram having $\bar{a}$ and $\bar{b}$ as two of its sides. The long diagonal of the parallelogram represents the vector $\bar{a} + \bar{b}$.

B. Vector Subtraction

The subtraction of a vector is defined as the addition of the corresponding negative vector. Therefore, the vector $\mathbf{P} - \mathbf{F}$ is obtained by adding the vector $(-\mathbf{F})$ to the vector $\mathbf{P}$, or $\mathbf{P} + (-\mathbf{F})$.

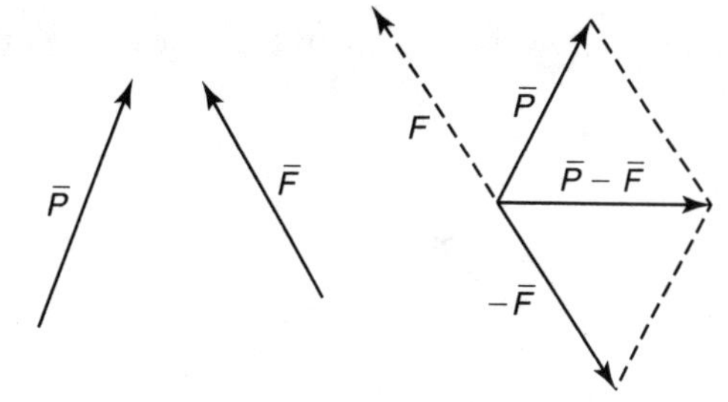

$\bar{P} - \bar{F} = \bar{P} + (-\bar{F})$

C. Multiplication of a Vector by a Scalar

The product of vector **a** and scalar k, written as $k\mathbf{a}$, is a new vector whose magnitude is k times the magnitude of **a**. If k is positive, the new vector has the same direction as **a**; if k is negative, the new vector has a direction opposite that of **a**.

The following rules also hold:

$k(\mathbf{a} + \mathbf{b}) = k\mathbf{a} + k\mathbf{b}$

$k(a - \mathbf{b}) = k\mathbf{a} - k\mathbf{b}$

Problem

A bicyclist is moving northward at 30 mph, and a wind of 40 mph is blowing directly from the east. What is the apparent magnitude and direction of the wind experienced by the bicyclist?

Solution

Construct the two vectors representing the motion of the bicyclist and the wind as follows:

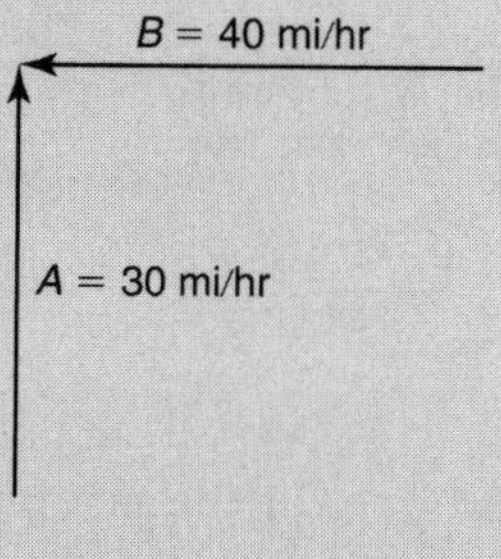

The effective magnitude and direction of the wind is the vector **B** − **A**. Applying the triangle rule for vector subtraction, add **B** and −**A**. The following diagram shows the resultant vector:

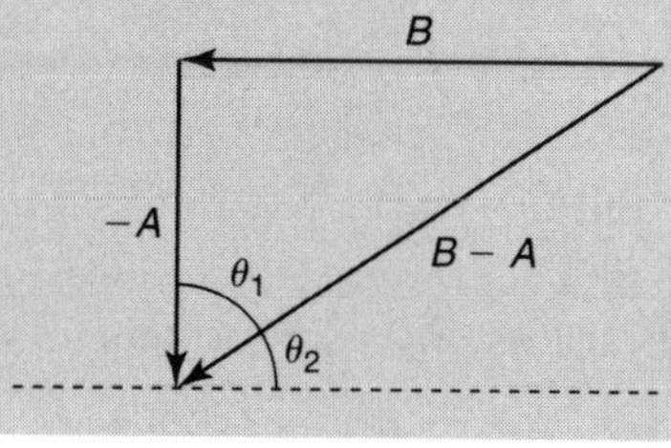

Applying the Pythagorean theorem, the magnitude of **B** − **A** is found:

$$|B - A|^2 = |B|^2 + |A|^2$$

$$= 40^2 + 30^2 = 2500$$

or $$|B - A|^2 = 50$$

To find the direction, apply the trigonometric ratios:

$$\sin \theta_1 = \frac{\text{magnitude of B}}{\text{magnitude of B} - \text{A}} = \frac{40}{50} = \frac{4}{5}$$

$$\theta_1 = \sin^{-1} \frac{4}{5} = 53°$$

$$\theta_2 = 90° - 53° = 37°$$

2. COMPONENTS OF A VECTOR

Formation of Vector Components on the Positive *x*- and *y*-Axes

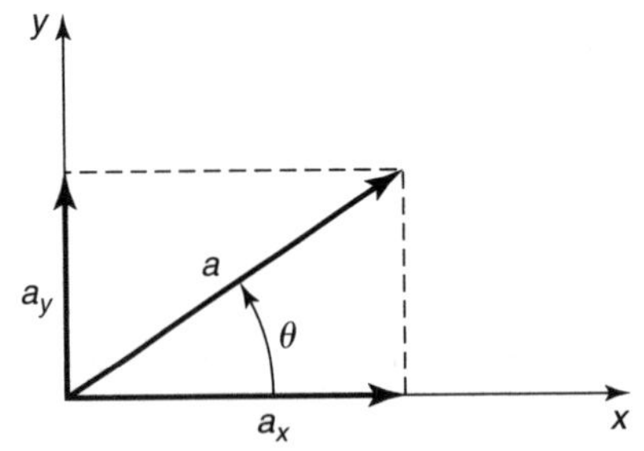

a_x and a_y are the components of a vector **a**. The angle θ is measured counterclockwise from the positive x-axis. The components are formed by drawing perpendicular lines to the chosen axes.

A. The components of a vector are given by

$A_x = A \cos \theta$
$A_y = A \sin \theta.$

A component is equal to the product of the magnitude of vector **A** and cosine of the angle between the positive axis and the vector.

B. The magnitude can be expressed in terms of the components.

$$A = \sqrt{A_x^2 + A_y^2}$$

For the angle θ,

$$\tan \theta = \frac{A_y}{A_x}$$

C. A vector **F** can be written in terms of its components *Fx* and *Fy*

$$\mathbf{F} = \mathbf{i}Fx + \mathbf{j}Fy$$

where **i** and **j** represent perpendicular unit vectors (magnitude = 1) along the *x*-axis and *y*-axis.

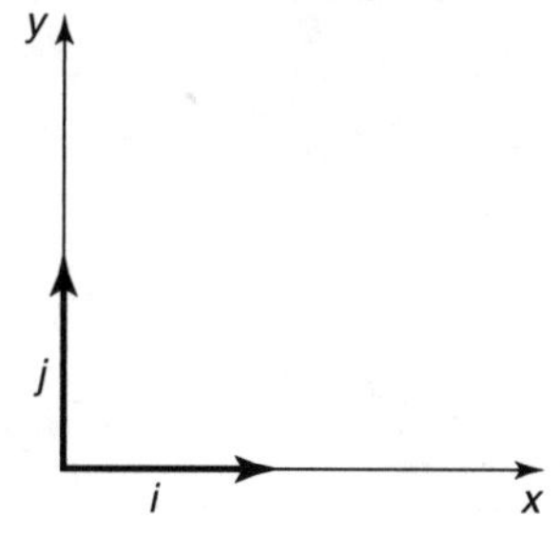

(a) The unit vectors **i** and **j** of the two-dimensional rectangular coordinate system

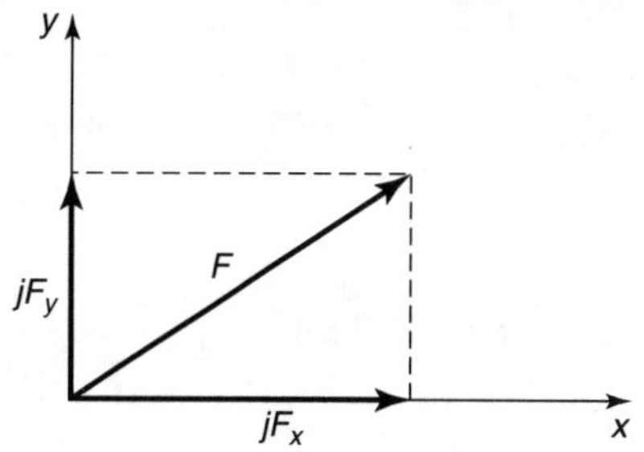

(b) The components of F_x and F_y

A unit vector in the direction of a vector **a** is given by

$$\mathbf{u} = \frac{\mathbf{a}}{|\mathbf{a}|} = \frac{\mathbf{a}}{a} = \left(\frac{a_x}{a}\mathrm{i} + \frac{a_y}{a}\mathrm{j}\right).$$

3. ADDING VECTORS ANALYTICALLY

Analytical addition involves adding the components of the individual vectors to produce the sum, expressed in terms of its components.

To find **a** + **b** = **c** analytically:

1. Resolve **a** in terms of its components:

$$\mathbf{a} = \mathbf{i}a_x + \mathbf{j}a_y$$

2. Resolve **b** in terms of its components:

$$\mathbf{b} = \mathbf{i}b_x + \mathbf{j}b_y$$

3. The components of **c** equal the sum of the corresponding components of **a** and **b**:

$$\mathbf{c} = \mathbf{i}(a_x + b_x) + \mathbf{j}(a_y + b_y)$$

and

$$\mathbf{c} = \mathbf{i}c_x + \mathbf{j}c_y$$

and the magnitude

$$|c| = \sqrt{c_x^2 + c_y^2}$$

with θ given by

$$\tan\theta = \frac{c_y}{c_x}$$

Problem

An airplane would be flying in a direction 30° northeast at 200 mph if it were not for a wind of 50 mph blowing from south to north. What is the velocity of the airplane with respect to the ground?

Solution

As shown in the figure, the air velocity of the plane resolves into its components V_x and V_y.

$$Vx = 200 \quad \cos 30° = 173 \text{ mph}$$
$$V_y = 200 \quad \sin 30° = 100 \text{ mph}$$

Combine the y components to obtain the total velocity in the y-direction, which is

$$100 \text{ mph} + 50 \text{ mph} = 150 \text{ mph}.$$

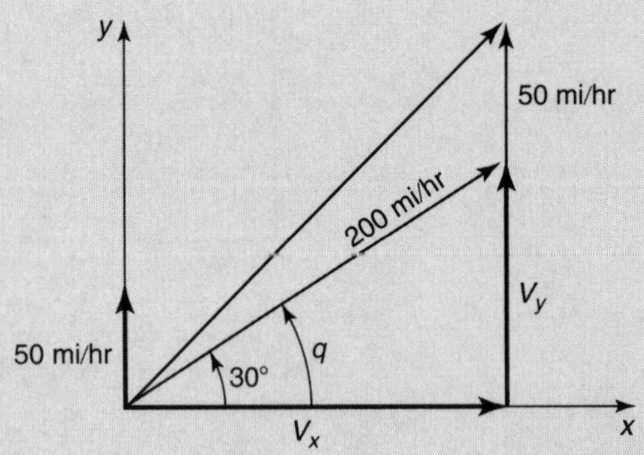

The only velocity component in the x-direction, Vx, is 173 mph. Hence the magnitude of the resultant velocity is

$$V = \sqrt{(150)^2 + (173)^2} = 230 \text{ min}/hr$$

The resultant velocity is in a direction that makes an angle q with the positive x-direction, where

$$\tan \theta = \frac{150}{173} \text{ or } \theta = \tan^{-1} \frac{150}{173} = 41°.$$

V. PROBABILITY AND STATISTICS

1. PROBABILITY

Let e denote an event that can happen in k ways out of a total of n possible ways. All n ways are equally likely. The probability of event e occurring is defined as

$$p = pr\{e\} = \frac{k}{n}.$$

The probability of e occurring is called its success. The probability of failure (nonoccurrence) of the event is denoted by q and defined as

$$q = pr\{not\ e\} = \frac{n-k}{n} = 1 - \frac{k}{n} = 1 - p$$

Thus, $p + q = 1$. The event "not e" is denoted by $\tilde{e}$ or ~e.

For example, a toss of a coin will produce one of two possible outcomes: heads or tails. Let e be the event that tails will turn up in a single toss of a coin. Then,

$$p = \frac{1}{1+1} = \frac{1}{2}$$

In another example, event e occurs when the number 5 or 6 turns up in a single toss of a die. A single toss of a die has six equally likely outcomes:

$$\{1, 2, 3, 4, 5, 6\}$$

Thus, $n = 6$. The event e can occur in two ways:

$$p = pr\{e\} = \frac{2}{6} = \frac{1}{3}$$

The probability of failure of e is

$$q = pr\{\sim e\} = 1 - \frac{1}{3} = \frac{2}{3}.$$

For any event e,

$$0 \le pr\{e\} \le 1$$

If the event cannot occur, its probability is 0. If the event must occur, its probability is 1.

The definition of the odds is as follows: Let p be the probability that an event will occur. The odds in favor of its occurrence are $p{:}q$ and the odds against it are $q{:}p$.

For instance, to determine the probability that at least one tail appears in two tosses of a coin, let h denote heads and t tails. The possible outcomes of two tosses are

$$(h, h), (h, t)\ (t, h), (t, t).$$

Three cases are favorable. Thus,

$$p = \frac{3}{4}.$$

In another example, suppose event e occurs when the sum 8 appears in a single toss of a pair of dice. There are $6 \times 6 = 36$ outcomes:

$$(1, 1), (2, 1), (3, 1), \ldots, (6, 6).$$

The sum 8 appears in five cases:

$$(2, 6), (6, 2), (3, 5), (5, 3), (4, 4)$$

Then,

$$p\{e\} = \frac{5}{36}$$

The concept of probability is based on the concept of random experiment. A random experiment is an experiment with more than one possible outcome, conducted such that it is not known in advance which outcome will occur. The set of possible outcomes is denoted by a capital letter — say, X. Usually, each outcome is either a number (a toss of a die) or something to which a number can be assigned (heads = 1, tails = 0 for a toss of a coin).

2. MEAN, MEDIAN, AND MODE

A. MEAN

The mean is the arithmetic average. That is, the sum of the variables divided by the number of variables is the mean. For example,

$$\frac{4 + 3 + 8}{3} = 5.$$

Problem

Find the mean salary for four company employees whose hourly wages are \$5, \$8, \$12, and \$15.

Solution

The mean salary is the average:

$$\frac{\$5+\$8+\$12+\$15}{4}=\frac{\$40}{4}=\$10\,/\,\text{hr}$$

Problem

Find the mean length of five fish with lengths of 7.5 in, 7.75 in, 8.5 in, 8.5 in, and 8.25 in.

Solution

The mean length is the average length:

$$\frac{7.5+7.75+8.5+8.5+8.25}{5}=\frac{40.5}{5}=8.1\text{ in}$$

B. Median

The median is the middle value of a set of an odd number of values. Therefore, the number of values larger than the median is equal to the number of values smaller than the median. In a set with an even number of values, the average of the two middle values is the median. For example,

The median of (2, 3, 5, 8, 9) is 5.

The median of (2, 3, 5, 9, 10, 11) is $\frac{5+9}{2}=7$.

C. Mode

The mode is the most frequently occurring value in the set of values. For example, the mode of the set composed of 4, 5, 8, 3, 8, 2 is 8.

Problem

For this series of observations find the mean, median, and mode.

500, 600, 800, 800, 900, 900, 900, 900, 900, 1000, 1100

Solution

The mean is the value obtained by adding all the measurements and dividing by the number of measurements:

$$\frac{500+600+800+800+900+900+900+900+1000+1100}{11}$$

$$=\frac{9300}{11}=845.45$$

The median is the observation in the middle. There are 11 numbers, so the median of this set of numbers is the sixth, 900.

The mode is the observation that appears most frequently, which is also 900 because it appears five times in the set.

All three of these numbers are measures of central tendency. They describe the "middle" or "center" of the data.

Problem

Nine rats run through a maze. The time each rat took to traverse the maze is recorded as follows:

1 min., 2.5 min., 3 min., 1.5 min., 2 min., 1.25 min., 1 min., 9 min., 30 min.

Which of the three measures of central tendency would be the most appropriate in this case?

Solution

Calculate the three measures of central tendency and then compare them to determine which would be the most appropriate in describing these data.

The mean is the sum of observations divided by the number of observations. In this case,

$$\frac{1 = 2.5 + 3 + 1.5 + 2 + 1.25 + 1. + .9 + 30}{9} = \frac{43.15}{9} = 4.79.$$

The median is the middle number in any array of observations from lowest to highest.

0.9, 1.0, 1.0, 1.25, 1.5, 2.0, 2.5, 3.0, 30.0

The median is the fifth observation in this array, which is 1.5. There are four observations larger than 1.5 and four observations smaller than 1.5.

The mode is the most frequently occurring observation in the sample. In this data set, the mode is 1.0.

Mean = 4.79
Median = 1.5
Mode = 1.0

The mean is not appropriate here. Only one rat took more than 4.79 minutes to run the maze, and that rat took 30 minutes. Thus, the mean has been distorted by one large observation.

The median or mode best describes this data set and would be more appropriate to use.

3. STANDARD DEVIATION

The standard deviation is a measure of the dispersion of data with respect to its mean or average value. By definition, the standard deviation of a set $x_1, x_2, \ldots, x_n$ of n numbers is defined by

$$s = \sqrt{\frac{\sum_{i=1}^{n}\left(x_i - \overline{x}\right)^2}{n-1}}$$

where $\overline{x}$ is the mean of $x_1, x_2, \ldots, x_n$.

If some number x_i in the data set occurs f_i times, then f_i is called the frequency of the number x_i. The formula for the standard deviation holds when the frequency of each number is 1. When the frequency of some or all of the numbers is greater than 1, the data is called grouped data. For grouped data, the modified formula is used for the standard deviation. Let the frequencies of the numbers $x_1, x_2, \ldots, x_n$ be $f_1, f_2, \ldots, f_n$, respectively; then

$$s = \sqrt{\frac{\sum_{i=1}^{n} \left(x_i - \overline{x}\right)^2}{\sum_{i=1}^{n} f_i}}.$$

The variance of a set of numbers is the square of the standard deviation.

Simplified formulas exist for finding the standard deviation. These are

$$s = \sqrt{\frac{\sum_{i=1}^{n} x_i^2}{n} - \left(\frac{\sum_{i=1}^{n} x_i}{n}\right)^2}$$

and, for grouped data,

$$s = \sqrt{\frac{\sum_{i=1}^{n} f_i x_i^2}{\sum_{i=1}^{n} f_i} - \left(\frac{\sum_{i=1}^{n} f_i x_i}{\sum_{i=1}^{n} f_i}\right)^2}.$$

Problem

Find the standard deviation of the numbers 3, 5, 6, 8, 13, 21.

Solution

$$\sum_{i=1}^{n} x_i^2 = 3^2 + 5^2 + 6^2 + 8^2 + 13^2 + 21^2 = 744$$

$$\sum_{i=1}^{n} x_i = 56$$

$$S = \sqrt{\frac{744}{6} - \left(\frac{56}{6}\right)^2} = 6.07$$

Problem

The height of 100 students was measured and recorded. Find the standard deviation for the data shown here:

Height (inches)	Class Mark (x)	x²	Frequency (f)	fx²	fx
60–62	61	3,721	7	26,047	427
63–65	64	4,096	21	86,016	1,344
66–68	67	4,489	37	166,093	2,479
69–71	70	4,900	26	127,400	1,820
72–74	73	5,329	9	47,961	657

Solution

Apply the formula

$$s = \sqrt{\frac{\sum fx^2}{\sum f} - \left(\frac{\sum fx}{\sum f}\right)^2}.$$

Sum the data in the appropriate columns

$\Sigma f = 100 \qquad \Sigma fx^2 = 453{,}517 \qquad \Sigma f = 6{,}727$

and substitute into the equation:

$s = \sqrt{4.535 - 4.525} = 3.16$

4. CORRELATION COEFFICIENT

The correlation coefficient is a measure of the relationship between two sets of data. The most commonly used relationship is the linear relationship. The corresponding correlation coefficient r for two sets of data $\{x_1, x_2, \ldots, x_n\}$ and $\{y_1, y_2, \ldots, y_n\}$ is given by

$$r = \frac{\sum_{i=1}^{n}\left(x_i - \bar{x}\right)\left(y_i - \bar{y}\right)}{\sqrt{\sum_{i=1}^{n}\left(x_i - \bar{x}\right)^2\left(\sum_{i=1}^{n}\left(y_i - \bar{y}\right)^2\right)}}$$

where $\bar{x}$ is the mean of $\{x_1, x_2, \ldots, x_n\}$ and is the mean of $\{y_1, y_2, \ldots, y_n\}$.

The value of the correlation coefficient is always between -1 and 1. Negative values show that the two data sets are "opposite" each other. This is one type of correlation. Thus, if $r = -1$, it means that the two sets of data are strongly negatively correlated. If $r = 0$, no correlation exists or the data sets are independent of each other. Positive values show that two data sets are "similar" to each other. If $r = 1$, the two data sets are almost similar.

Problem

Compute the correlation coefficient for the following sets of data:

x	y	$x_i - \bar{x}$	$y_i - \bar{y}$	$(x_i - \bar{x})(y_i - \bar{y})$	$(x_i - \bar{x})^2$	$(y_i - \bar{y})^2$
9.2	9.6	2.41	1.16	2.80	5.81	1.35
9.7	8.6	2.91	0.16	0.47	8.47	0.03
8.1	11.2	1.31	2.76	3.62	1.72	7.62
5.5	8.7	−1.29	0.26	−0.34	1.66	0.07
7.7	10.2	0.91	1.76	1.60	0.83	3.10
5.6	8.4	−1.19	−.04	0.05	1.42	0.0016
5.7	4.4	−1.09	−4.04	4.40	1.19	16.32
5.4	7.6	−1.39	−0.84	1.17	1.93	0.71
2.3	10.1	−4.49	1.66	−7.45	20.16	2.76
8.7	5.6	1.91	−2.84	−5.42	3.65	8.07

Solution

Apply the following formula:

$$r = \frac{\sum_{i=1}^{n} \left(x_i - \bar{x}\right)\left(y_i - \bar{y}\right)}{\sqrt{\sum_{i=1}^{n} \left(x_i - \bar{x}\right)^2 \left(\sum_{i=1}^{n} \left(y_i - \bar{y}\right)^2\right)}}$$

Take the averages of x and y:

$$\bar{x} = 6.79,\ \bar{y} = 8.44$$

Perform the necessary summations:

$$\sum_{i=1}^{n} (xi - \bar{x})(yi - \bar{y}) = 0.90$$

$$\sum_{i=1}^{n} (xi - \bar{x})^2 = 46.84$$

$$\sum_{i=1}^{n}(yi - \overline{y})^2 = 40.03$$

Substitute totals into formula:

$$r = \frac{0.90}{\sqrt{(46.84)(40.03)}} = \frac{.90}{43.30} = 0.02$$

Because r is close to 0, the data sets x and y are very weakly related to each other.

MCAT

MEDICAL COLLEGE ADMISSION TEST

Physics Review

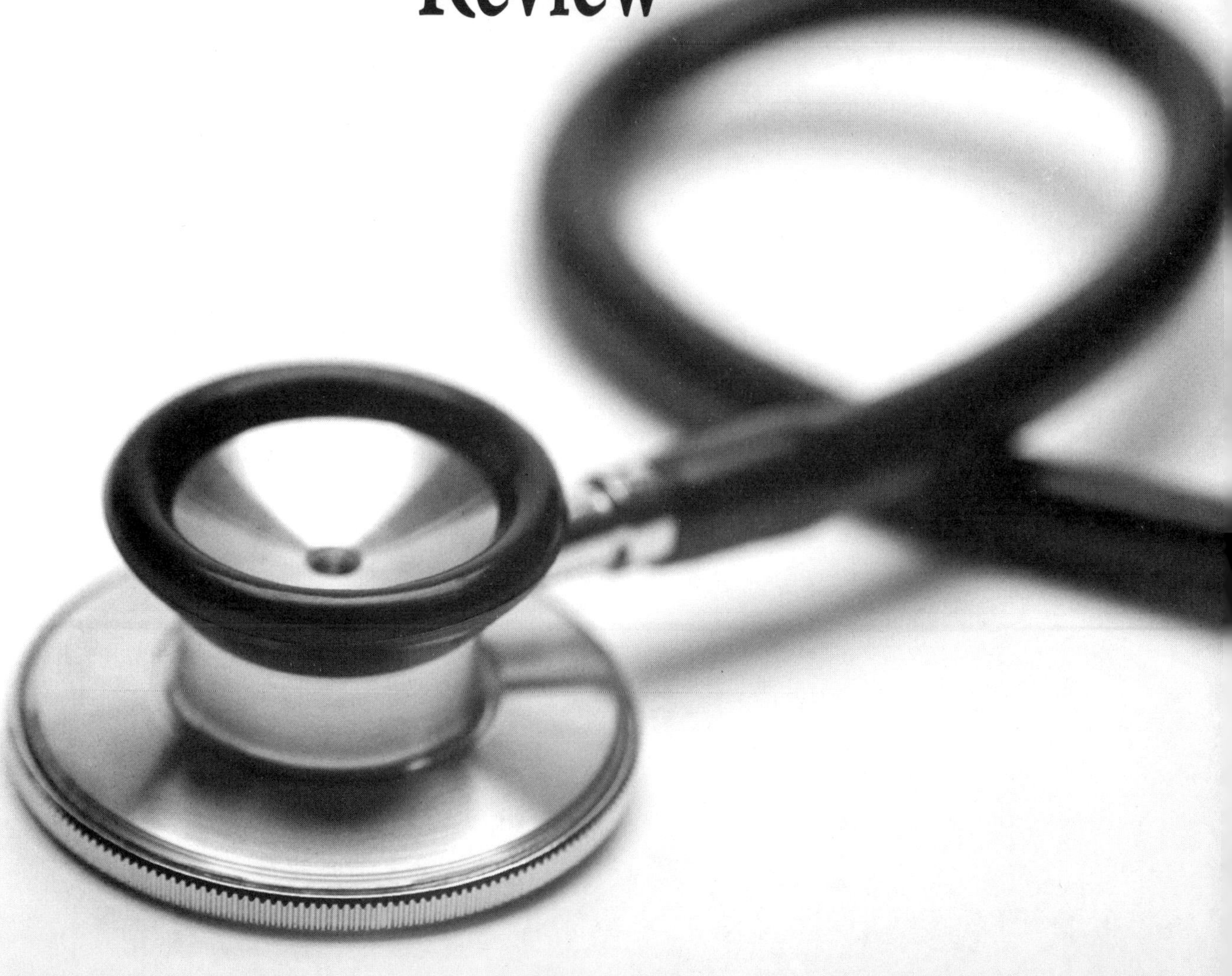

PROBLEM-SOLVING TIPS

1. Make a sketch of the problem showing dimensions, forces, and angles.
2. Focus only on the body or bodies to which the question refers.
3. Recall a formula that uses the variables for which you have the values. Do this carefully because these formulas may be used for other problems.
4. Check that all quantities are in the correct units and that the units cancel. The only units that should remain are the units for the answer. This check verifies that you have recalled the correct formula and used it properly.
5. Substitute the values and calculate the answer.

I. TRANSLATIONAL MOTION

Motion may be defined as a continuous change of position. Motion is critical for all living things. Mechanics deals with the relationships among motion, force, and matter. The branch of mechanics related to motion is called kinematics.

1. DIMENSIONS AND UNITS

Conversion Factors

1 mile = 5,280 ft acceleration of gravity (g) = 9.8 m/sec^2 = 10 m/sec^2
1 ft = 0.305 m = 32.2 ft/sec^2
1 in = 0.54 cm
(See Appendix A for more dimensions and units.)

2. VECTORS AND SCALARS

A. Basic Definitions of Vectors and Scalars

A vector is a quantity that has both magnitude and direction. Some typical vector quantities are displacement, velocity, force, acceleration, momentum, electric field strength, and magnetic field strength.

A scalar is a quantity that has magnitude but no direction. Some typical scalar quantities are mass, length, time, density, energy, and temperature.

B. Addition of Vectors (a + b): Geometric Methods

Triangle Method (Head-to-Tail Method)

The following two steps constitute the triangle method of vector addition:

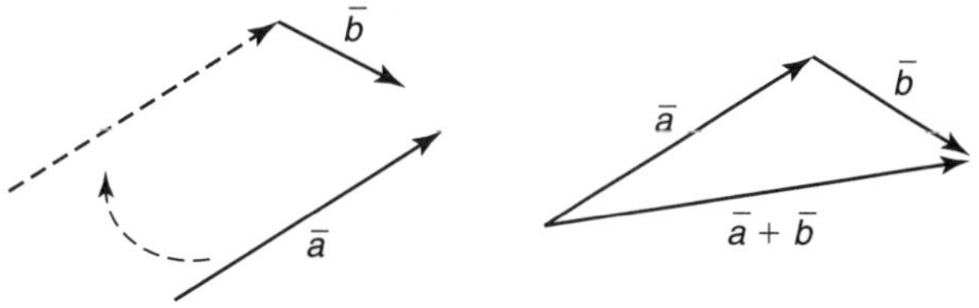

(i) Attach the head of $\bar{a}$ to the tail of $\bar{b}$. (ii) By connecting the head of $\bar{a}$ to the tail of $\bar{b}$, the vector $\bar{a} + \bar{b}$ is defined.

Parallelogram Method (Tail-to-Tail Method)

The following two steps constitute the parallelogram method of vector addition:

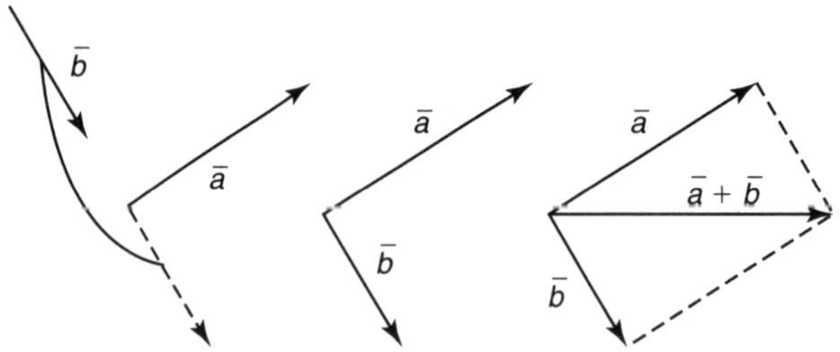

(i) Join the tails of the two vectors.

(ii) Construct a parallelogram having $\bar{a}$ and $\bar{b}$ as two of its sides. The long diagonal of the parallelogram represents the vector $\bar{a} + \bar{b}$.

C. Subtraction of Vectors

The subtraction of a vector is defined as the addition of the corresponding negative vector. Therefore, the vector **P** − **F** is obtained by adding the vector (−**F**) to the vector **P** — that is, **P** + (− **F**), as shown in the following figure:

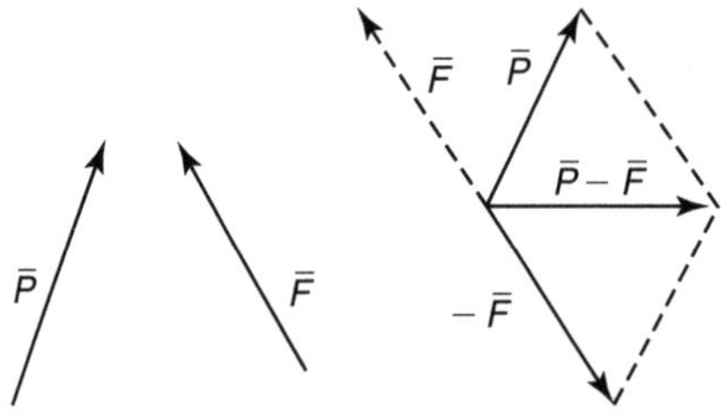

$\bar{P} - \bar{F} = \bar{P} + (-\bar{F})$

D. Components of a Vector

The following figure illustrates the formation of vector components on the positive *x*- and *y*-axes:

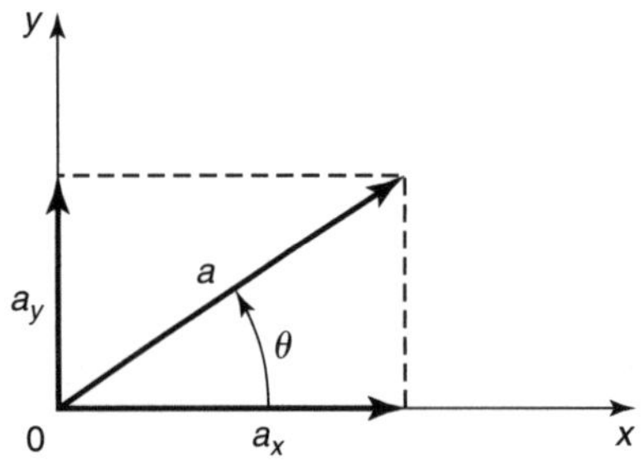

a_x and a_y are the components of vector **a**. The angle θ is measured counterclockwise from the positive *x*-axis. The components are formed by drawing perpendicular lines to the chosen axes.

The components of a vector are as follows:

$A_x = A \cos \theta$

$A_y = A \sin \theta.$

A component is equal to the product of the magnitude of vector A and the cosine of the angle between the positive axis and the vector.

The magnitude can be expressed in terms of the components:

$$A = \sqrt{A_x^2 + A_y^2}$$

For the angle θ,

$$Tan\theta = \frac{A_y}{A_x}$$

Problem

Two hikers set off in an eastward direction. Hiker 1 travels 3 km, while hiker 2 travels six times the distance covered by hiker 1. What is the displacement of hiker 2?

Solution

From the information given, the displacement vector is directed eastward. The magnitude of the displacement vector for hiker 2 is six times the magnitude of the displacement vector for hiker 1. Therefore, its magnitude is

$$6 \times (3 \text{ km}) = 18 \text{ km}$$

Problem

Two wires are attached to a corner fence post, with the wires making an angle of 90° with each other. If each wire pulls on the post with a force of 50 pounds, what is the resultant force acting on the post? See Figure 1.

FIGURE 1

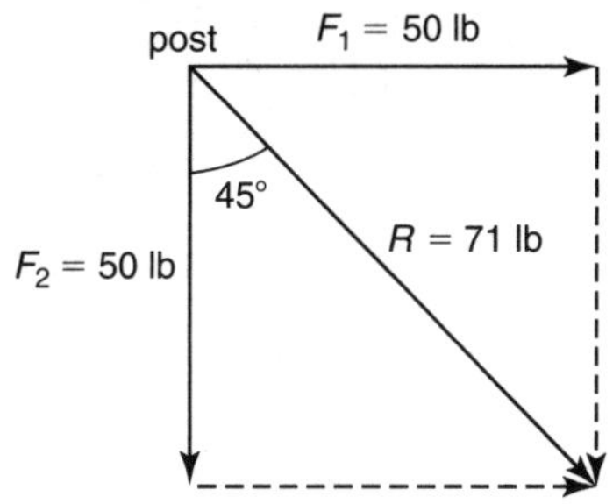

Solution

Complete the parallelogram, as shown by the dashed lines in the figure. Measure R and scale it to find it is equal to about 71 pounds. The angle of the resultant is 45° from either of the component vectors.

Use the fact that the component vectors are at right angles to each other to write

$$R^2 = 50^2 + 50^2.$$

Therefore, $R = 71$ pounds at approximately 45° to each wire.

3. UNIFORMLY ACCELERATED MOTION

Consider the special case of constant or uniform acceleration **a** equal to the constant rate of change in velocity/time. In one dimension, the statement is that a = constant, and the acceleration–time curve is given by Figure 2. The average acceleration is

$$\langle \mathbf{a} \rangle = \Delta\mathbf{v}/\Delta t = (\mathbf{v} - \mathbf{v}_0)/(t - 0).$$

The meaning of this physics problem-solving technique is that the area under the acceleration–time curve is the change in velocity (the shaded area in Figure 2).

FIGURE 2

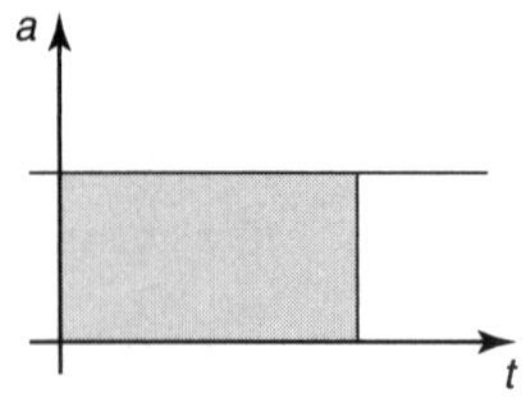

In one dimension, the first equation for motion is

$$v = v_0 + at.$$

Therefore, if the changes in velocity and the time are known, the acceleration can be found. This means that the slope of the velocity–time curve is the acceleration. See Figure 3.

FIGURE 3

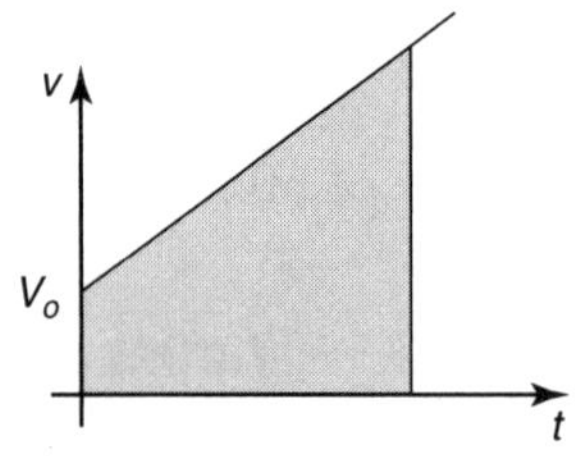

Now, the definition of velocity is $\mathbf{v}$ = rate of change in direction/time. The average velocity is

$$<\mathbf{v}> = \Delta\mathbf{r}/\Delta t = (\mathbf{r} - \mathbf{r}_0)/(t - 0).$$

Therefore, if the distance covered and the time taken are known, the average velocity can be found. For the special case of uniform acceleration only,

$$<\mathbf{v}> = (\mathbf{v} + \mathbf{v}_0)/2,$$

as would be expected for an average value.

In one dimension, the second important equation is

$$x = x_0 + v_0t + 1/2at^2.$$

Figure 4 shows the position–time curve. Note that the slope of the position–time curve at any time is the instantaneous velocity.

FIGURE 4

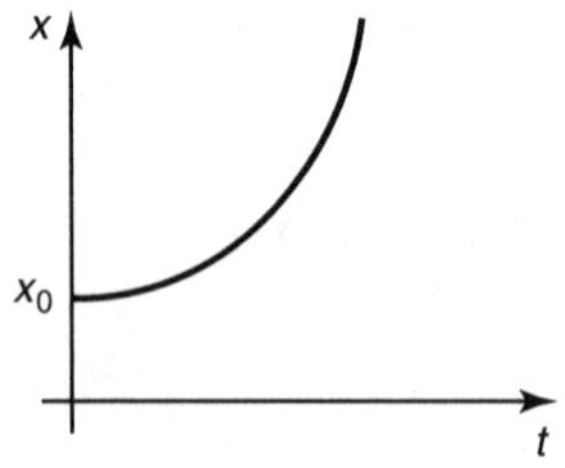

A third important formula is obtained by solving for the time

$$t = (v - v_0)/a$$

and substituting into

$$x - x_0 = <v>t$$

to get

$$v^2 = v_0^{\,2} + 2a(x - x_0).$$

This formula is useful if the time is not part of the given information in the problem.

Problem

An airplane lands on a carrier deck at 150 mph and is brought to a stop uniformly, by an arresting device, in 500 ft. Find the acceleration and the time required to stop.

Solution

Convert units to ft/sec:

$$v_0 = (150mi\ /\ hr) \times \left(\frac{5280\ ft/hr}{3600\ hr/\sec}\right) = 220\,ft\ /\ \sec.$$

Because there is a constant deceleration,

$$2as = v_1^{\,2} - v_0^{\,2}$$

$$2a(500\,ft) = 0 - (220\,ft/\sec)^2$$

$$a = \frac{-(220/ft/\sec)^2}{2(500\,ft)} = -48.4\,ft/\sec^2$$

Solve for t using the following formula:

$$v_1 = v_0 + at$$

$$v_1 = v_0 + at$$

$$t = \frac{v_1 - v_0}{a} = \frac{0 - 220\,ft\ /\ \sec}{-48.4\,ft\ /\ \sec^2} = 4.55\ \sec.$$

Problem

A body moves from rest with constant acceleration of 6 m/sec^2. Find the following:

A. The instantaneous speed at the end of 5 seconds

B. The average speed for the 5-second interval

C. The distance covered in 5 seconds from rest

Solution

A. Instantaneous speed $= v_0 + at$

$$= 0 + 6\ \text{m/sec}^2 \times 5\ \text{sec}$$

$$= 30\ \text{m/sec}$$

B. Average speed $= \frac{1}{2}(v_0 + v)$

$= \frac{1}{2}(0 + 30)$ m/sec

$= 15$ m/sec

C. Distance $= v_0 t + \frac{1}{2}at^2$

$= 0 + \frac{1}{2}(6 \text{ m/sec}^2)(5\text{sec})^2$

$= 75$ m

$=$ Average speed $\times$ Time

$= 15$ m/sec $\times$ 5 sec

$= 75$ m

Problem

A sled starting from rest slides down an inclined plane with uniform acceleration and travels 9 m in 3 sec. In what time from rest will it acquire a velocity of 24 m/sec down the plane?

Solution

Time $= (v - v_0)/a$

$v_0 = 0$ and $v = 24$ m/sec

Because $v_0 = 0$, distance $= \frac{1}{2}at^2$

$$a = \frac{2 \times \text{distance}}{t^2}$$

$$a = \frac{2 \times (9 \text{ m})}{(3 \text{ sec})^2}$$

$= 2$ m/sec^2

time $= v/a$

$= (24 \text{ m/sec})/(2 \text{ m/sec}^2)$

$= 12$ sec

4. FREELY FALLING BODIES

Free fall in one dimension is a special case of constant acceleration translational kinematics. If the direction downward is taken as negative, then

$$a = -g = -9.8 \text{ m/sec}^2,$$

and the first two formulas become

$$v = v_0 - gt \text{ and } y = y_0 + v_0 t - \frac{1}{2}gt^2.$$

The displacement–time curve is thus a parabola. If an object is projected upward with a positive initial velocity, the time to reach the apex, where $v = 0$, is just $t = v_0/g$.

Problem

A boy leaning over a railway bridge 49 ft high sees a train approaching with uniform speed and attempts to drop a stone down the funnel. He releases the stone when the engine is 80 ft away from the bridge and sees the stone hit the ground 3 ft in front of the engine. What is the speed of the train?

Solution

Apply the equation applicable to uniform acceleration:

$$x - x_0 = v_0 t + \frac{1}{2}at^2.$$

From the dropping of the stone 49 ft from rest under the action of gravity, the time t the stone is in motion can be found. The initial velocity of the stone v_0 is zero. The distance the stone travels is

$$x + x_0 = 49 \text{ ft}.$$

Therefore,

$$49 \text{ ft} = 0 + \left(\frac{1}{2}\right)(32 \text{ ft/sec}^2)\,(t^2)$$

$$\therefore t = \sqrt{\frac{2 \times 49\,ft}{32\,ft/s^2}} = \frac{7}{4}s.$$

In the $\frac{7}{4}$ seconds it takes the stone to drop, the engine has moved with uniform speed u a distance of (80 − 3) ft.

$$\therefore u = \frac{d}{t} = \frac{77\,ft}{\frac{7}{4}} = 44\,ft/sec = 30mi$$

Problem

A bomb is dropped from a balloon that is 875 feet above the ground and is ascending at 40 ft/sec. Find the maximum height reached.

Solution

The origin is at the point that the bomb was released and is equal to 875 feet above the ground. The upward initial velocity is positive at 40 ft/sec. The acceleration due to gravity is −32 ft/sec^2. At the highest point, the velocity is equal to zero.

$$v^2 = v_0^{\,2} + 2as$$

$$0 = (40 \text{ ft/sec})^2 + 2(-32 \text{ ft/sec}^2) \times \text{Distance}$$

$$-1{,}600 \text{ ft}^2/\text{sec}^2 = -64 \text{ ft/sec}^2 \times \text{Distance}$$

$$\text{Distance} = 25 \text{ ft}$$

$$\text{Maximum height} = 875 \text{ ft} + 25 \text{ ft} = 900 \text{ ft}$$

5. PROJECTILES

Projectile motion in two dimensions follows from keeping track of the components in the first two kinematic formulas:

$$v_y = v_{0y} - gt \text{ and } y = y_0 + v_0 yt - \frac{1}{2}gt^2$$

$$v_x = v_{0x} = \text{constant and } x = x_0 + v_{0x}t.$$

The y-versus-x curve may be shown to be parabolic. Note that because velocity is a vector,

$$v_{0x} = v_0 \cos\theta \text{ and } v_{0y} = v_0 \sin\theta,$$

where θ is the initial angle of projection, as shown in Figure 5. The time to reach the apex of the path is again $t = v_{0y}/g$, and the height may be found by substituting into the $y = y(t)$ equation. Also, the range is found by substituting $t_R = 2t$ into the equation $x = x_0 + v_x t$.

FIGURE 5

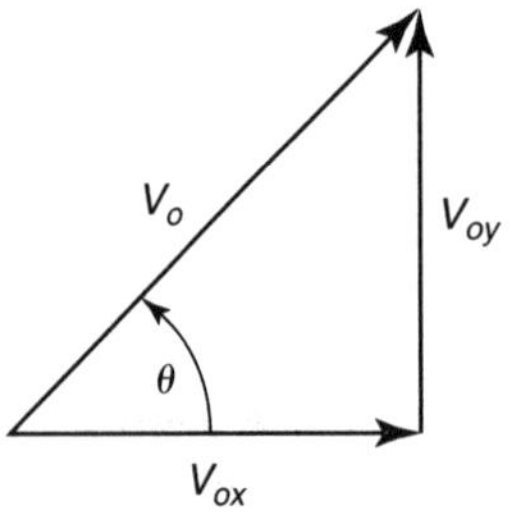

Problem

A ball is thrown with an initial velocity v_0 of 160 ft/sec, directed at an angle θ_0 of 53 with the ground.

A. Find the x- and y-components of v_0.

B. Find the position of the ball and the magnitude and direction of its velocity when $t = 2$ seconds.

C. At the highest point of the ball's path, what is the ball's altitude (h), and how much time has elapsed?

D. What is the ball's range d? See Figure 6.

FIGURE 6

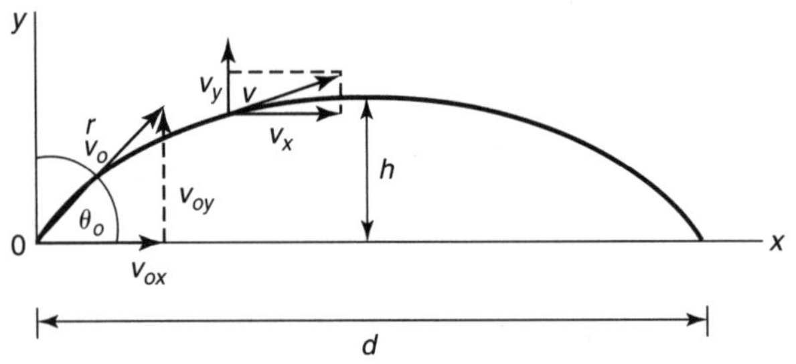

Solution

A. Using the figure,

$$v_{ox} = v_o\cos\theta_o;\ v_{ox} = v_o\sin\theta_o.$$

Therefore,

$v_{ox} = 160ft/\text{sec}.\cos 53° = 160ft/\text{sec}\ \frac{3}{5} = 96ft/\text{sec}$

$v_{oy} = 160ft/\text{sec}.\sin 53° = 160ft/\text{sec}\ \frac{4}{5} = 128ft/\text{sec}$

B. The acceleration due to gravity is constant. Further, there is no force acting on the projectile in the x-direction; its acceleration in this direction is therefore zero. Thus,

$a_x(t) = 0$	$a_x(t) = -g$
$v_x(t) = v_{ox}$	$v_x(t) = v_{oy} - gt$
$x(t) = x_o + v_{ox}t$	$y(t) = y_o t + v_{oy}t - \frac{1}{2}gt^2$

Here, x_0 and y_0 are the initial coordinates of the projectile, and v_{0x} and v_{0y} are the initial x- and y-components of the ball's velocity. Taking the origin (0) as shown in the figure, at $t = 2$ seconds,

$v_x = 96$ ft/sec

$x = (96 \text{ ft/sec})(2 \text{ sec}) = 192$ ft

$v_y = 128 \text{ ft/sec} - (32 \text{ ft/sec}^2)(2 \text{ sec}) = 64$ ft/sec

$y = (128 \text{ ft/sec})(2 \text{ sec}) - \left(\frac{1}{2}\right)(32 \text{ ft/sec}^2)(4 \text{ sec}^2)$

$y = 256 \text{ ft} - 64 \text{ ft} = 192$ ft.

The magnitude of the ball's velocity is

$v = (v_x^2 + v_y^2)^{1/2}$

$v = ((64 \text{ ft/sec})^2 + (96 \text{ ft/sec})^2)^{1/2}$

$v = 115.4$ ft/sec.

The direction of the velocity relative to the x-axis is

$$\tan\theta = \frac{v_y}{v_x} = \frac{64}{96} = \frac{2}{3}$$

$\theta = 34°$

C. At the highest point of the path, the ball has no vertical velocity. Then, by the kinematics equations,

$v_y = 0 = v_o - gt$

$v_y = 0 = v_o - gt$

$$t = \frac{v_{oy} - 0}{g} = \frac{128\,ft/\text{sec}}{32\,ft/\text{sec}^2} = 4\text{ sec.}$$

It takes 4 seconds for the ball to reach its maximum height. It has traveled a vertical distance of

$y_{\max} = v_{oy}t - \frac{1}{2}gt^2$

$= (128 \text{ ft/sec})(4 \text{ sec}) - \frac{1}{2}(32 \text{ ft/sec}^2)(4 \text{ sec})^2$

$= 512 \text{ ft} - 256 \text{ ft} = 256$ ft.

D. It takes the ball as much time to fall as it does to rise. Therefore, the entire trajectory requires 8 seconds. By the kinematics equations, its horizontal position at the end of its trajectory can be found:

$$x(t) = v_{0x}t = 96 \text{ ft/sec} \cdot 8 \text{ sec} = 768 \text{ ft}.$$

II. FORCE, MOTION, AND GRAVITATION

Force can be defined as an external entity that causes a change in the motion of a body. A force can also be defined as a push or pull. This chapter deals with the relationship between force and motion. Forces are vectors and have both magnitude and direction.

1. NEWTON'S FIRST LAW

In the absence of any applied force, a body either remains at rest or moves uniformly in a straight line.

For a given body, the ratio of the magnitude of the force to that of the acceleration is a constant and is called its mass:

$$m = \frac{F}{a} = \text{constant (for a given body)}.$$

The unit of mass is the kilogram (kg).

The weight of a body is the gravitational force exerted on the body by the earth and is given by the product of the mass and the gravitational acceleration.

$$W = mg$$

The unit of weight is the newton (N).

Problem

Consider a weight hanging from the ceiling by a vertical cord, as shown in Figure 7. If the weight weighs 20 N, what is the tension in the cord?

Solution

FIGURE 7

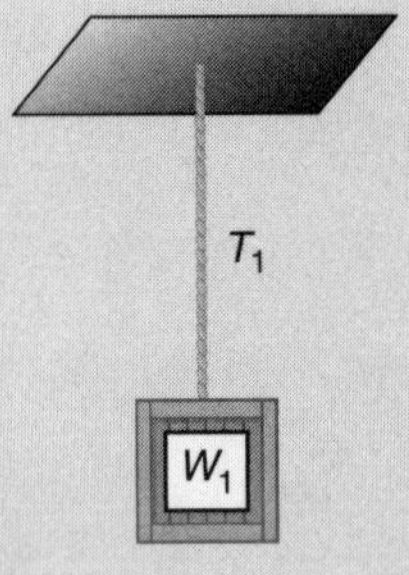

From the equilibrium condition, $F_y = 0$

$$F_y = T_1 - w_1 = 0$$
$$T_1 = w_1$$
$$T_1 = 20 \text{ N}$$

2. NEWTON'S SECOND LAW

If the force **F** acting on a particle of mass m is different from zero, the particle will have an acceleration **a**. The direction of the acceleration will be in the same direction as the force, as shown in the following equation:

$$\mathbf{F} = m\mathbf{a}$$

Problem

A 10-ton engine pulls a 50-ton train on a level track and gives it an acceleration of 4 ft/sec². What acceleration would the engine give to a 20-ton train when exerting the same force?

Solution

When pulling a 50-ton train, the force moved a weight w_1 of (10 + 50) tons = 60 tons. When pulling a 20-ton train, the force moved a weight w_2 of (10 + 20) tons = 30 tons.

$$F = a_1 m_1$$

$$F = a_2 m_2$$

$$a_2 = \frac{a_1 m_1}{m_2}$$

$$m_1 = w_1/g$$

$$m_2 = w_2/g$$

$$a_2 = \frac{a_1 w_1/g}{w_2/g}$$

$$= \frac{a_1 w_1}{w_2}$$

$$= \frac{(4\text{ ft/sec}^2)(60\text{ tons})}{30\text{ tons}}$$

$$= 8\text{ ft/sec}^2$$

Problem

A 2,000-kg truck is speeding at 88 m/sec. Determine the retarding force of the brakes required to stop it in 220 m on a level road.

Solution

$$F = ma$$

$$(2{,}000\text{ kg})\ (a)$$

$$v_t^2 = v_o^2 + 2as$$

$$v_t^2 - v_o^2 = 2as$$

When the brakes are applied, v_t is equal to 0.

$$(0\text{ m/sec})^2 - (88\text{ m/sec})^2 = 2\ a\ 220\text{ ft}$$

$$F = 2{,}000\text{ kg} \times 17.6\text{ m/sec}^2$$

$$= 352{,}000\text{ N}$$

Problem

A 2-kg mass hangs at the end of a rope, as shown in Figure 8. Find the tension T in the rope if the acceleration is 10 m/sec^2 upward.

FIGURE 8

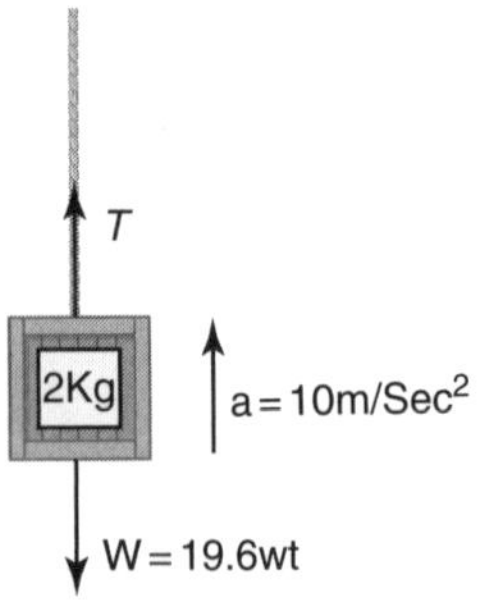

Solution

The weight of the 2 kg mass is $w = mg$

$= 2 \text{ kg} \times 9.8 \text{ m/sec}^2$
$= 19.6 \text{ N}$

When the acceleration is upward, the net force is directed upward.

Unbalanced force upward = Mass × Upward acceleration

$T - 19.6 \text{ N} = 2 \text{ kg} \times 10 \text{ m/sec}^2$
$= 39.6 \text{ N}$

Problem

Neglecting friction, a cord is passed over a pulley with a 7-kg mass at one end and a 9-kg mass at the other end. Determine the tension in the cord.

Solution

The unbalanced force on the entire system equals the mass times the acceleration of the system:

$(9 \times 9.8 - 7 \times 9.8) \text{ N} = (9 + 7) \text{ kg} \times a$

$a = 1.22 \text{ m/sec}^2$

The unbalanced force downward on the 9-kg mass equals the mass times the downward acceleration:

$9(9.8) \text{ N} - T = 9 \text{ kg} \times 1.22 \text{ m/sec}^2$

$T = 77.1 \text{ N}$

3. NEWTON'S THIRD LAW

For every action, there is a corresponding *equal* and opposing reaction.

$F_A = -F_B$

Problem

A car on a country road in Maryland passes over an old-fashioned hump-backed bridge. The center of gravity of the car follows the arc of a circle of radius 88 ft. Assuming that the car has a weight of 2 tons, find the force exerted by the car on the road at the highest point of the bridge if the car is traveling at 30 mph. At what speed will the car lose contact with the road? See Figure 9.

FIGURE 9

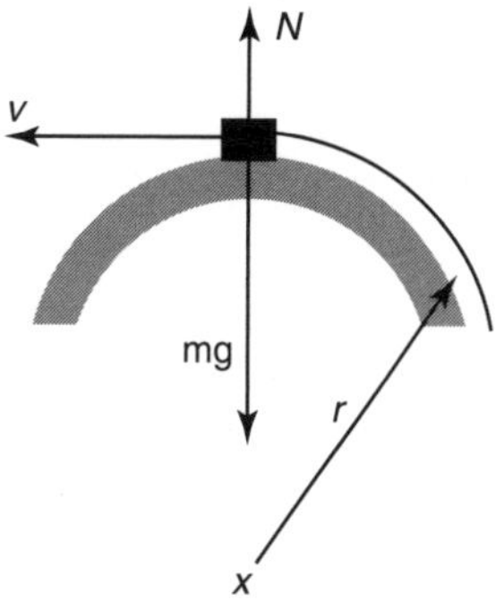

Solution

The forces acting on the car at the highest point of the bridge are its weight $W = m\mathbf{g}$ downward and the normal force **N** exerted by the bridge upward. These cannot be equal because a net downward force must provide the acceleration necessary to keep the car traveling in a circle. Thus, by Newton's second law:

$$mg - N = m\left(\frac{v^2}{r}\right),$$

$$N = m\left(g - \frac{v^2}{r}\right) = \frac{W}{g}\left(g - \frac{v^2}{r}\right) = W\left(1 - \frac{v^2}{rg}\right)$$

where W is the height of the car.

Here $v = 30$ mph $= 44$ ft/sec.

$$N = 2 \text{ tons}\left(1 - \frac{44^2\, ft^2/s^2}{88 \times 32\, ft/s^2}\right)$$

$$= 2\left(1 - \frac{11}{16}\right) ton = \frac{5}{8} ton$$

But action and reaction are equal and opposite. Thus, if the road exerts a force of 5/8 ton on the car, the car exerts the same force on the road.

The car loses contact with the road when $N = 0$ — that is, when $v^2 = rg$. Thus, the speed required is

$$v = \sqrt{rg} = \sqrt{88\, ft \times 32\, \text{ft/s}^2} = 16\sqrt{11}\, ft/s$$

$$= 53.1 \text{ ft/sec} = 36 \text{ mph}$$

4. NEWTON'S LAW OF GRAVITATION

Between every two objects in the universe, there exists an attractive force of gravitation that is proportional to the masses of the objects and inversely proportional to the distance squared between them.

$$F = \frac{Gm_1m_2}{r^2}$$

$$G = 6.7 \times 10^{-11} \frac{Nm^2}{kg^2}$$

Problem

At what distance from the center of the earth does the acceleration due to gravity have one half of the value that it has on the surface of the earth?

Solution

Newton's second law implies that $W = mg$. W is the weight of an object of mass m (that is, the gravitational force of attraction between the earth and the object), and g is the acceleration due to gravity. Then, by Newton's law of universal gravitation,

$$W = \frac{GM_em}{R^2} = mg$$

where R is the distance of the object of mass m from the center of the earth, and M_e is the mass of the earth. Therefore,

$$g(R) = \frac{GM_e}{R^2} \text{ at the surface of the earth, and}$$

$$g(R_e) = \frac{GM_2}{R_e^{\,2}}.$$

But the problem requires finding $g(R) = \frac{1}{2}g(R_e)$. Therefore,

$$\frac{GM_e}{R^2} = \frac{1}{2}\frac{GM_e}{R_e^{\,2}}$$

$$R^2 = 2R_e^{\,2}$$

$$R = \sqrt{2}R_e$$

$$= 1.414 \times 6.38 \times 10^6\text{m} = 9.02 \times 10^6\text{m}$$

The acceleration due to gravity is reduced to one-half of its usual value at a distance of 9.02×10^6 meters from the center of the earth. This is equivalent to a height of 2.64×10^6 meters or 1640 miles above the surface of the earth.

5. UNIFORM CIRCULAR MOTION, CENTRIPETAL FORCE

The force acting on a body of mass m undergoing uniform circular motion is the centripetal force, given by

$$F = ma = m\frac{v^2}{r}$$

A body of mass m is traveling in uniform circular motion. The body is pulled toward the center of the circle of radius r with a force.

$F = \frac{mv^2}{r}$. See Figure 10.

FIGURE 10

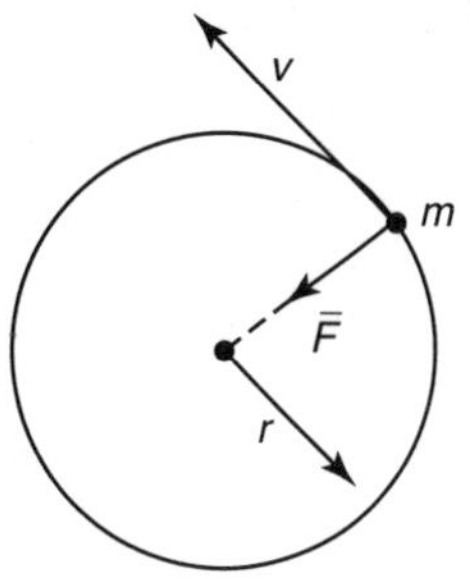

Here, v is the magnitude of velocity, which is constant, and r is the radius of the circle.

Problem

A 3-lb body is tied to the end of a cord and is whirled in a horizontal circle of radius 5 feet at 4 revolutions per second. What is the linear speed of the body?

Solution

$$\begin{aligned} \text{Velocity} &= 2\pi r \times \text{Angular speed} \\ &= 2\pi \times 5 \times 4 \\ &= 40\pi \text{ ft/sec} \\ &\sim 126 \text{ ft/sec} \end{aligned}$$

6. FRICTION

For impending motion,

Frictional force $= F_s = \mu_s N$

where μ_s = Coefficient of static friction and N = Normal force.

For a body already in motion,

$$F_k = \mu_k N,$$

where μ_k = Coefficient of kinetic friction.

Problem

See Figure 11. If the coefficient of sliding friction for steel on ice is 0.05, what force is required to keep a man weighing 150 pounds moving at constant speed along the ice?

FIGURE 11

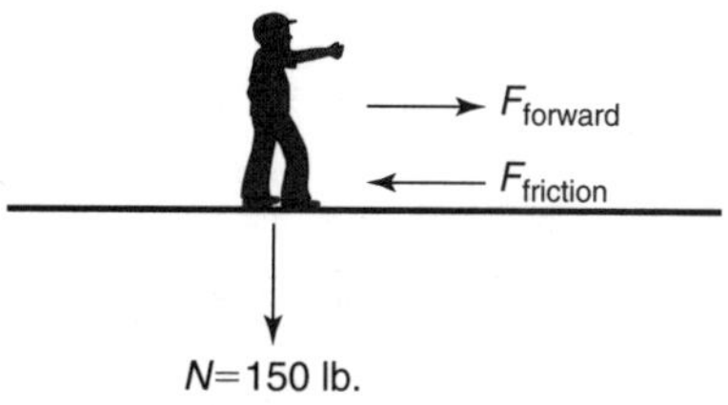

Solution

To keep the man moving at constant velocity, the force of friction tending to retard his motion must be opposed by an equal but opposite force. See Figure 11.

The force of friction is given by:

$$F = \mu_{kinetic} N$$

By Newton's third law

$$F_{\text{forward}} = F_{\text{friction}}.$$

Therefore,

$F_{\text{forward}} = \mu_{kinetic} N$
$F_{\text{forward}} = (.05)\,(150 \text{ lb}) = 7.5 \text{ lb}.$

7. INCLINED PLANES

The key to solving incline problems is to resolve all the forces acting on the object to their components along and perpendicular to the plane.

Problem

What is the acceleration of a block on a frictionless plane inclined at an angle q with the horizontal? See Figure 12.

FIGURE 12

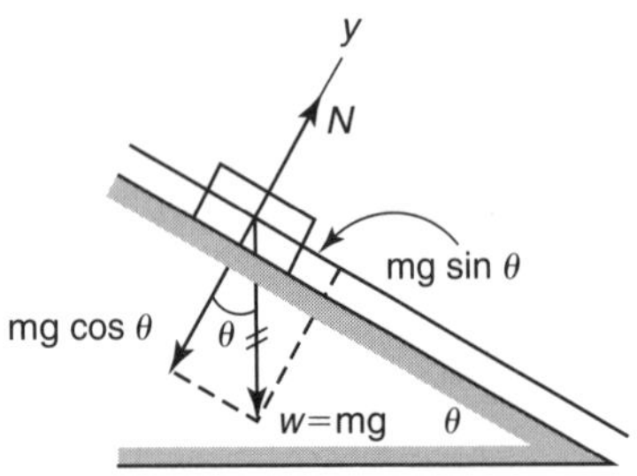

Solution

To find the acceleration *a* of the block, calculate the net force *F* on the block and relate that to its acceleration via Newton's second law, $F = ma$. (Here *m* is the mass of the block.)

The only forces acting on the block are its weight *mg* and the normal force *N* exerted by the plane. See Figure 12. Take axes parallel and perpendicular to the surface of the plane and resolve the weight into *x*- and *y*-components. Then

$$\Sigma F_y = N - mg \cos \theta,$$
$$\Sigma F_x = mg \sin \theta.$$

The acceleration is in the *y* direction, and $a_y = 0$ because the block does not accelerate off the surface of the inclined plane. The equation $\Sigma F_y = ma_y$ reveals that $N = mg \cos \theta$. The equation $\Sigma F_x = ma_x$, where a_x is the acceleration of the block in the *x* direction, reveals that

$mg \sin \theta = ma_x$
$a_x = g \sin \theta.$

The mass does not appear in the final result, which means that any block, regardless of its mass, will slide on a frictionless inclined plane with an acceleration down the plane of $g \sin \theta$. (Note that the velocity is not necessarily down the plane.)

8. PULLEY SYSTEMS

Remember that the tension at all points along a rope in a pulley system is the same.

Problem

For the block and tackle shown in Figure 13:

A. Find the displacement ratio.

B. What force F must be exerted on the free end of the rope to lift a 200-lb load?

FIGURE 13

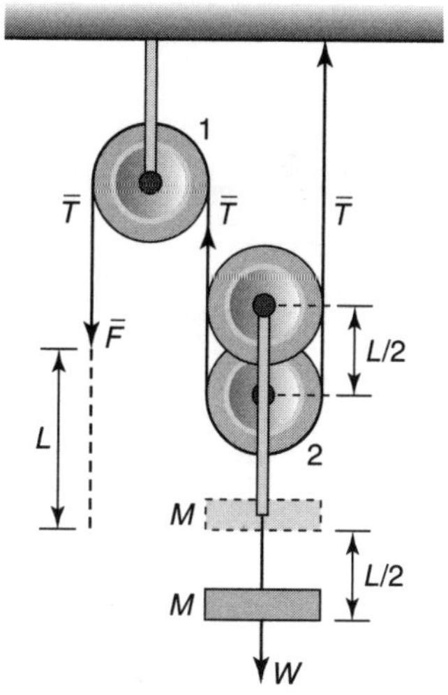

Solution

A. When F pulls down the rope by an amount L, pulley 2 moves up by ½L (as shown in Figure 13) because the shortening of the rope is shared by the two segments of rope that hold the pulley. Therefore, the ratio of the displacement of load to the displacement of rope is

$$\frac{\frac{1}{2}L}{L} = \frac{1}{2}.$$

B. The figure shows that the load is held up by a force $2T$, where T is the tension in the rope. Therefore, to lift the load, the minimum tension should satisfy

$$W = 2T$$
$$T = \frac{1}{2}W$$

where W is the weight of the load.

F is equal to T as long as the rope does not break because the stress in the rope is caused by the action of F. Thus,

$$F = T = \frac{W}{2}$$
$$= \frac{200lb}{2} = 100lb$$

III. EQUILIBRIUM AND MOMENTUM

1. EQUILIBRIUM

A. Translational Equilibrium

Fundamental to physics is the concept of force. Intuitively, force is the push or pull acting on some object. Newton's laws provide for a more precise definition of force. Newton's first law states that an object at rest remains at rest and an object in motion remains in motion with constant velocity in the absence of external forces. Newton's second law is the basis of dynamics, but one consequence of it is that the weight force of any mass is $W = mg$, where g is gravitational acceleration (9.8 m/sec^2 near the surface of the earth).

Other than weight, several important forces are tension (the force in a string or cable); the normal force N acting perpendicular to a surface; the force of static friction, which is

$$F_S \leqslant \mu_S N$$

the force of kinetic friction, which is

$$F_k = \mu_k N;$$

and a pivot or reaction force R acting at an angle θ with respect to the surface. For example, when standing on the floor, you exert a force of magnitude W on the floor, and the floor responds by exerting a force $N = R$ on you. The reaction force of the floor prevents you from falling through the floor.

To solve a statics (or any) physics problem, first write down the information in terms of numbers and symbols. Then draw a figure showing the relevant objects and angles. Next, choose points in the system and draw free-body diagrams for those points. For example, in Figure 14, two important free-body diagrams are shown for the case of a mass suspended by a cord from a ceiling.

FIGURE 14

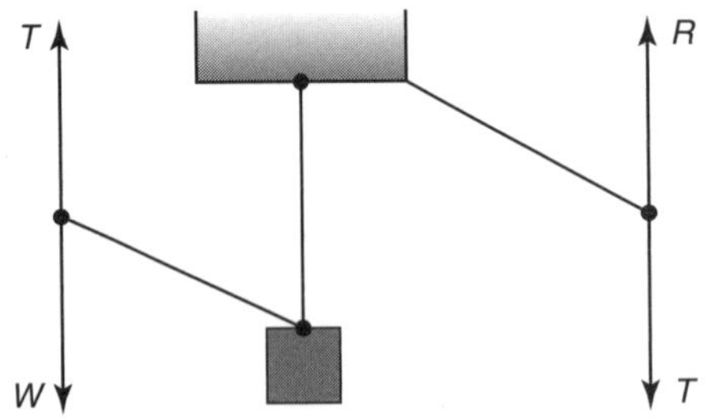

In statics, the next step is to apply the two conditions of equilibrium. The first condition is that the sum of the forces in each direction is zero:

$$\Sigma \mathbf{F} = 0.$$

The equilibrium is said to be static if the velocity also equals zero:

$$\mathbf{v} = 0.$$

For example, in Figure 14, choosing the positive direction as down results in

$$\Sigma F_y = W - T = 0 \text{ and } T - R = 0.$$

Therefore, $T = W$ and $R = T$; the weight determines both the tension in the string and the reaction force of the ceiling. In Figure 15, a force F pushes an object of mass m on a flat but rough surface with coefficient of static friction μ_s and coefficient of kinetic friction μ_k. Resolving F into its x- and y-components reveals that

$$F_x = F \cos \theta \text{ and } F_y = F \sin \theta.$$

FIGURE 15

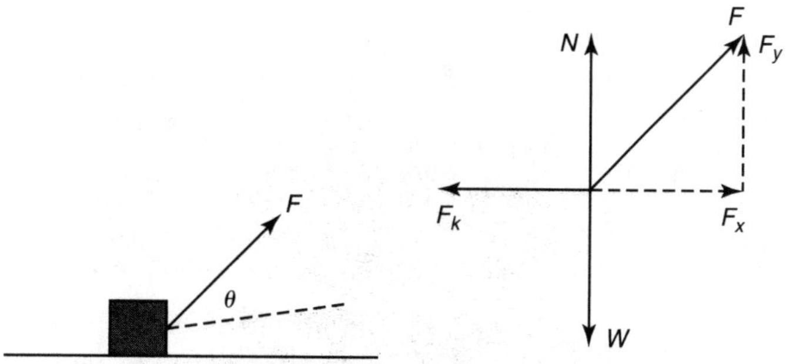

Static equilibrium in the y-direction gives

$$\Sigma F_y = F_y + N - W = 0 \text{ or } N = mg - F \sin \theta,$$

which can be used to find the normal force. Note that the normal force is not always equal to mg. If the object starts at rest, it will begin to move when

$$\Sigma F_x = F_x - F_s = 0 \text{ or } F \cos \theta = \mu_s N.$$

If the object is moving at constant velocity, then

$$\Sigma F_x = F_x - F_k = 0 \text{ or } \mu_k N = F \cos \theta.$$

Problem

A 200-lb man hangs from the middle of a tightly stretched rope so that the angle between the rope and the horizontal direction is 5°, as shown in Figure 16. Calculate the tension in the rope, as illustrated in Figure 17.

FIGURE 16

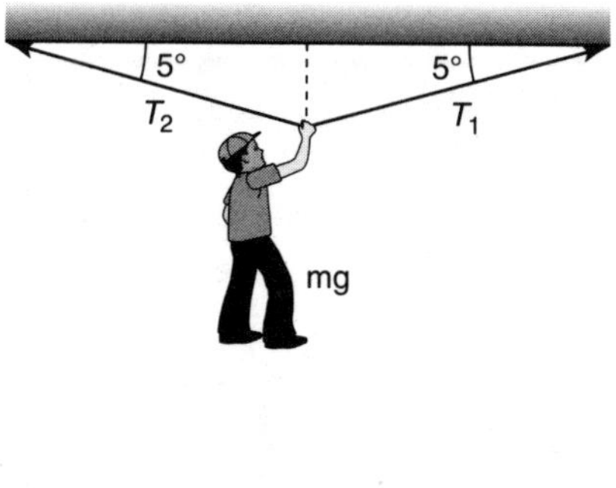

FIGURE 17

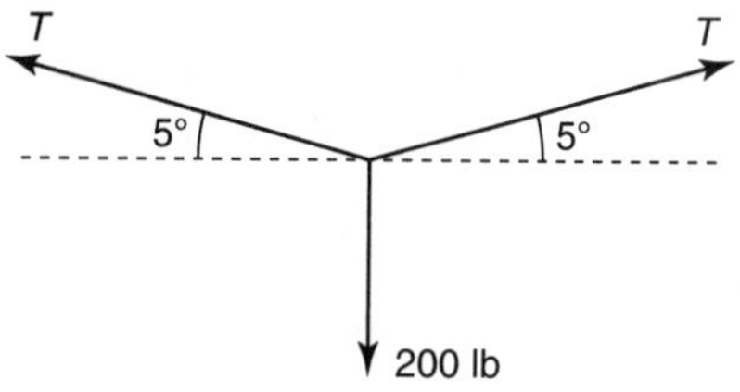

Solution

Because the two sections of the rope are symmetrical with respect to the man, the tensions in them must have the same magnitude (Figure 17). This can be arrived at by summing the forces in the horizontal direction and setting them equal to zero because the system is in equilibrium. Then

$$\Sigma F_x = T_1 \cos 5° - T_2 \cos 5° = 0$$

and $T_1 - T_2 - T$

Considering the forces in the vertical direction,

$$\Sigma F_y = T \sin 5° + T \sin 5° - 200 \text{ lb} = 0$$

$$200 \text{ lb} = 2T \sin 5° = 2T(0.0871)$$

$$T = \frac{(200)}{(2)(0.0871)} = 1150 \text{ 1bs.}$$

Note the significant force that can be exerted on objects at either end of the rope by this arrangement. The tension in the rope is more than five times the weight of the man. Had the angle been as small as 1°, the tension would have been

$$T = \frac{200}{2 \sin 1°\cdot} = \frac{200}{(2)().0174)} = 5730 \text{ lbs}$$

This technique for exerting a large force would be useful only to move something a very small distance because any motion of one end of the rope would change the small angle considerably, and the tension would decrease accordingly.

B. Rotational Equilibrium

The second condition, that of rotational equilibrium, is that the sum of all torques is zero:

$$\Sigma \mathbf{t} = 0$$

where the torque

$$\mathbf{t} = \mathbf{r} \times \mathbf{F}$$

is a cross product. Note that position vector **r** where the force acts and the force **F** must be drawn with a common origin to find the angle θ between them; then the right-hand rule is used to find the direction of the torque. Figure 18 shows a standard boom problem, where the boom has a weight $B = m_b g$ and the person has weight $W = mg$. The first equilibrium gives

$$\Sigma F_x = R_x - T_x = 0 \text{ thus } R_x = T \cos \theta.$$

FIGURE 18

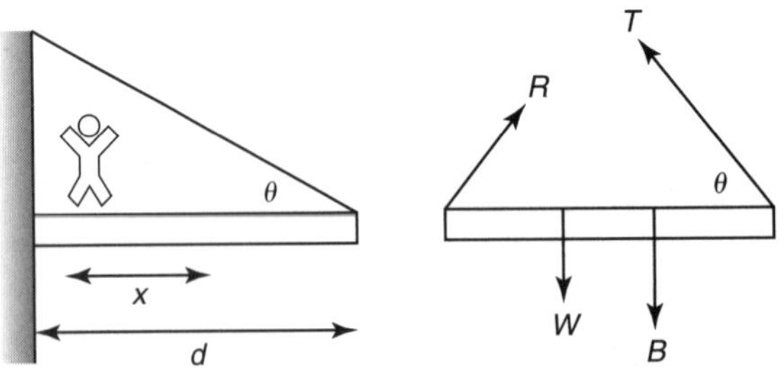

Also,

$$\Sigma F_y = R_y + T_y - W - B = 0 \text{ or } R_y = W + B - T \sin \theta.$$

If R and T are unknown, they cannot be found from these two equations alone. Thus, choose the point where the boom contacts the wall as the origin for calculating torques. Rotational equilibrium then implies that

$$\begin{aligned}\Sigma t &= \Sigma rF \sin \theta \\ &= (0)(R) - xW \sin 90 - d/2\, B \sin 90 + dT \sin(180 - \theta) \\ &= 0,\end{aligned}$$

or solving for the tension:

$$T = (xW + bD/2) / (d \sin \theta).$$

The positive and negative directions come from the right-hand rule. The angles come from moving the position vector such that it and the force have a common origin. See Figure 19.

FIGURE 19

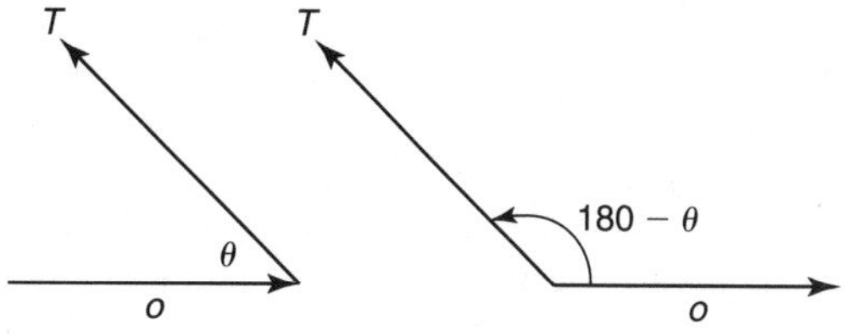

The concept of rotational equilibrium can also be used to locate the center of gravity or gravitational center of a system of objects. This is just the pivot point where the system balances, as in a child's seesaw. More important, the center of gravity often coincides with the center of mass of an object, where

$$r_{cm} = \Sigma m\mathbf{r} / \Sigma m.$$

In the boom problem (see Figure 18), the weight of the boom was assumed to have acted at the center of the mass of the boom $\frac{d}{2}$.

Problem

What scale readings would you predict when a uniform 120-lb plank 6.0 ft long is placed on two balances, as shown in Figure 20, with 1.0 ft extending beyond the left support and 2.0 ft extending beyond the right support?

FIGURE 20

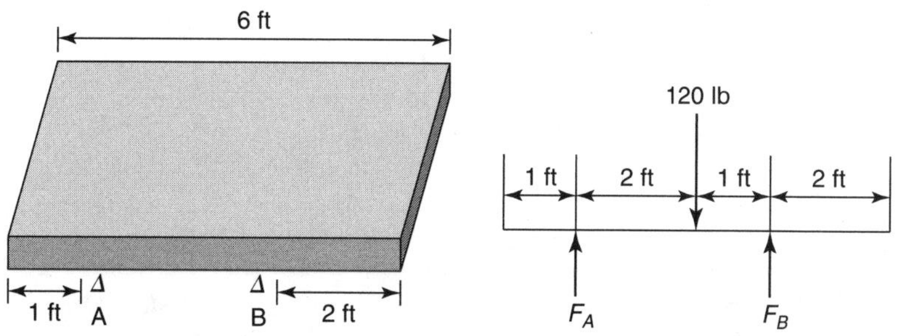

(A) Beam with Supports (B) Diagram of Forces

Solution

From the first condition for equilibrium, the forces upward must equal the forces downward:

$$F_A + F_B - 120 \text{ lb} = 0$$

The plank is uniform, meaning that the center of mass is at the center of the beam, 3 ft from each end. This is the point at which the 120-lb gravitational force can be considered to act.

Torque about a point is defined as the tendency of a force to cause rotation about the point. The magnitude of the torque is given by the product of the magnitude of the force and the perpendicular distance of the line of action of the force (the line along which the force acts) from the point of rotation. The direction of the torque can be found using the right-hand rule. Place the fingers of the right hand in the direction of the distance vector. Rotate the distance vector into the direction of the force vector. If this rotation is in the clockwise direction, the torque is negative. For counterclockwise rotation, the torque is positive. For equilibrium, the sum of all the torques about any point in the body must equal zero.

To apply this second condition for equilibrium, write torques about an axis through A, noting that the center of mass of the plank is 2.0 ft from A:

$$-120 \text{ lb} \times 2.0 \text{ ft} + F_B (3.0) \text{ ft} = 0 \text{ or } F_B = 80 \text{ lb}$$

Substitution of 80 lb for F_B in the first equation gives $F_A = 40$ lb. Alternatively, write a second torque equation, this time about an axis through B:

$$+120 \text{ lb} \times 1.0 \text{ ft} - F_A (3.0 \text{ ft}) = 0 \text{ or } F_A = 40 \text{ lb}$$

2. MOMENTUM

A. Conservation of Linear Momentum

Recall that the momentum of an object is given by

$$\mathbf{p} = m\mathbf{v}.$$

Because momentum is a vector, it is important to keep track of the components when calculating it. The law of conservation of momentum states that the total momentum of a system of particles is conserved in the absence of external forces:

$$\Sigma \mathbf{p}_0 = \Sigma \mathbf{p}$$

Consider the problem of Figure 21. One object of mass m_1 and speed v_1 is about to collide with another of mass m_2 at rest. This is the initial situation. Then the two objects collide or interact via internal forces. The final situation is shown in Figure 22: the first mass moves off with velocity (v'_1, θ) and the second mass with velocity $(v'_2, -\phi)$. From Figure 21, conservation of momentum in the x-direction gives

$$m_1 v_1 = m_1 v'_1 \cos \theta + m_2 v'_2 \cos \theta.$$

Similarly, in the y-direction,

$$0 = m_1 v'_1 \sin \theta - m_2 v'_2 \sin.$$

FIGURE 21

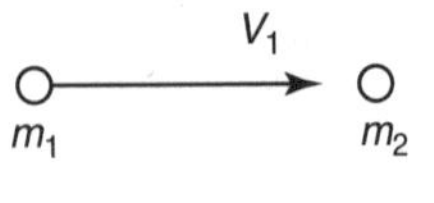

FIGURE 22

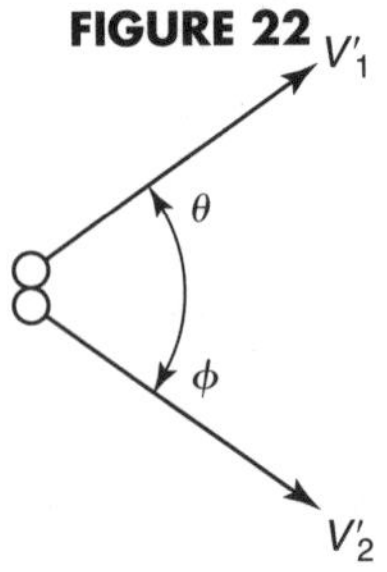

B. Elastic and Inelastic Collisions

If the collision is elastic, then the kinetic energy also is conserved:

$$\Sigma K_0E = \Sigma KE$$

This means

$$\frac{1}{2} m_1 v_1^{\,2} = \frac{1}{2} \; m_1 v_1^{\,2} + \frac{1}{2} m_2 v_2^{\,2}$$

Thus, if v_1 is known, v_2' (for example) can be found in terms of v'_1. The momentum conservation equations then become two equations in two unknowns.

If the collision is inelastic, then the loss of kinetic energy is given by

$$\Delta KE \quad KE \quad K_0E$$
$$= \frac{1}{2} \; m_1 v_1^{\,2} + \frac{1}{2} m_2 v_2^{\,2} - \frac{1}{2} \; m_1 v_1^{\,2} - \frac{1}{2} \; m_2 v_2^{\,2}$$

Problem

A cue ball traveling at a speed of 3 m/sec collides with a stationary billiard ball and imparts a speed of 1.8 m/sec to the billiard ball, as shown in Figure 23. If the billiard ball moves in the same direction as the oncoming cue ball, what is the velocity of the cue ball after the collision? Assume that both balls have the same mass.

FIGURE 23

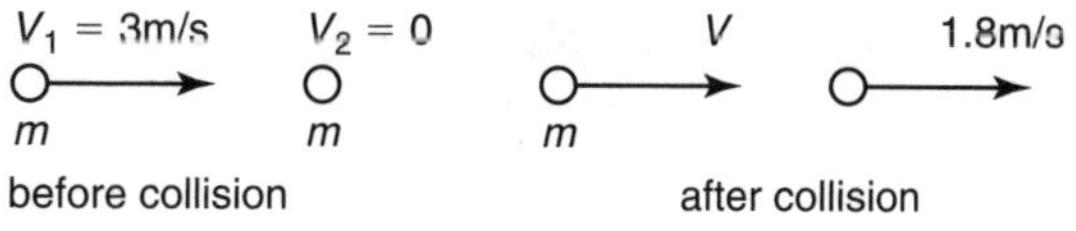

Solution

Linear momentum must be conserved in this isolated, two-particle system. Thus, the initial momentum of the system must equal the system's final momentum. Because the collision is one-dimensional, drop the vector nature of momentum and write

$$P_f = P_i$$
$$mv + m\,(1.8\text{ m/sec}) = m\,(3\text{ m/sec}) + m(0\text{ m/sec})$$
$$m(v + 1.8\text{ m/sec}) = m\,(3\text{ m/sec})$$
$$v + 1.8\text{ m/sec} = 3\text{ m/sec}$$
$$v = 1.2\text{ m/sec}$$

C. Impulse

The impulse momentum theorem follows from Newton's second law:

$$F = \Delta p \,/\, \Delta t$$

Therefore, the impulse is

$$I = \Delta p = Ft$$

Problem

A 100-kg man jumps into a swimming pool from a height of 5 m. It takes 0.4 seconds for the water to reduce his velocity to zero. What average force did the water exert on the man?

Solution

The man's initial velocity (before jumping) is zero. Therefore, as he strikes the water, his velocity v is

$$v^2 = v_0^2 + 2gh,$$

which reduces to $v^2 = 2gh$. Thus,

$$v = \sqrt{2gh} = \sqrt{2 \times (9.8m/s^2) \times 5m}$$
$$= 10\text{m/s}$$

Therefore, the man's momentum on striking the water was

$$p_1 = mv$$
$$= (100 \text{ kg}) \times (10 \text{ m/sec})$$
$$= 1000 \text{ kg-m/sec}$$

The final momentum was $p_2 = 0$, so that the average force was

$$F = \frac{\Delta p}{\Delta t} = \frac{p_2 \quad p_1}{\Delta t}$$
$$= \frac{0\text{-}1000 \text{ kg m/s}^2}{0.4 \text{ sec}}$$
$$= 2500 \text{ N}$$

The negative sign means that the retarding force was directed opposite to the downward velocity of the man.

Problem

Two inelastic masses move in opposite directions toward each other. Their respective masses are 16 and 4 grams with velocities of 30 and 50 cm/sec. If they are stuck together on collision, find the resulting velocity of the combined balls.

Solution

Because of the law of conservation of momentum, the momentum of the system before impact is equal to the momentum of the system after impact.

$$(16 \text{ g} \times 30 \text{ cm/sec}) - (4 \text{ g} \times 50 \text{ m/sec}) = (16 + 4) \text{ g} \times \text{Velocity}$$
$$\text{Velocity} = 14 \text{ cm/sec}$$

IV. WORK AND ENERGY

1. WORK

Work is given by the product of force and displacement; if force and displacement are in the same direction, work is simply force times the distance. In general, the calculation is

$$Fd \cos \theta,$$

as illustrated in Figure 24. Work can also be negative; for example, frictional work is energy dissipative and in the simplest case given by $-\mu_k Nx$.

$W = (F \cos \theta)d$

FIGURE 24

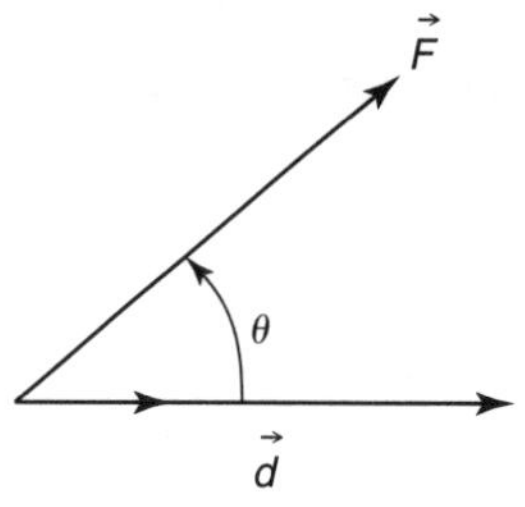

Any unit of work is equal to a unit of force times a unit of length. One newton-meter (N-m) is equal to one joule (J).

Problem

A block of mass of 5 kg is lifted 2 meters in 3 seconds. Compute the work done.

Solution

Weight of block $= m \times g$

$= 5 \text{ kg} \times 9.8 \text{ m/sec}^2$

$= 49 \text{ N}$

Work = Force × distance moved in the direction of the force

$= 49 \text{ N} \times 2 \text{ meters}$

$= 98 \text{ J}$

Problem

A wagon is drawn a distance of 10 meters across level ground, as shown in Figure 25. The pull of the rope is 100 N, and the angle between the rope and the ground is 30°. Find the work done.

FIGURE 25

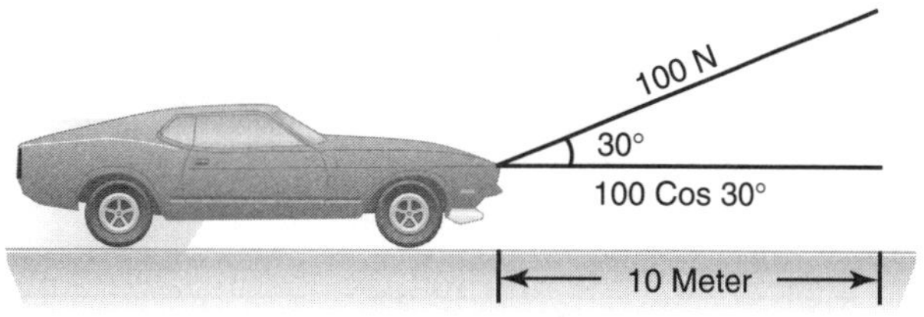

Solution

Work = Component force parallel to displacement × Displacement

$= 100 \cos 30° \times 10 \text{ m}$

$= 866 \text{ N}$

2. KINETIC AND POTENTIAL ENERGY

Kinetic energy is energy of motion and for a single particle given by

$$\text{KE} = \frac{1}{2}mv^2 = p^2/2m.$$

Therefore, if the speed, momentum, and mass are known, the kinetic energy can be calculated numerically. Consider the kinematics of a single particle subject to acceleration:

$$v^2 = v_0{}^2 + 2a(x - x_0).$$

Multiplying this equation by $\frac{1}{2}m$ gives

$$W = \Delta T = T - T_{0,}$$

which is the work energy theorem: work done on an object changes the kinetic energy of that object.

The concept of work leads immediately to the idea of potential, or stored, energy:

$$PE = Fs$$

For the gravitational force, in moving an object up, the force and the displacement point in opposite directions; therefore, the potential energy is just mgh near the surface of the earth.

For every conservative force, a potential energy can be defined. If a spring is compressed or stretched a distance x from equilibrium, according to Hooke's law, the potential energy is $\frac{1}{2}kx^2$. Thus, calculating potential energy can be a matter of simply plugging numbers into formulas. Alternatively, the calculation may have to use the fact that potential energy can be transformed. For example, a mass can fall and compress a spring transforming the gravitational potential energy mgh into compressional potential energy $\frac{1}{2}kx^2$.

Problem

Air consists of a mixture of gas molecules that are constantly moving. Compute the kinetic energy KE of a molecule that is moving with a speed of 500 m/sec. Assume that the mass of this particle is 4.6×10^{-26} kg.

Solution

The mass of the gas molecule, $m = 4.6 \times 10^{-26}$ kg, and its speed $v = 5 \times 10^2$ m/sec, are the known observables. Using the equation $K_E = \frac{1}{2}mv^2$:

$$KE = \left(\frac{1}{2}\right)(4.6 \times 10^{-26}\ \text{kg})(5.0 \times 10^2\ \text{m/sec})^2$$
$$= 5.75 \times 10^{-21}\ \text{J}.$$

Problem

How much work is required to raise a 100-g block to a height of 200 cm and simultaneously give it a velocity of 300 cm/sec?

Solution

The work done is the sum of the potential energy,

$$PE = mgh,$$

and the kinetic energy,

$$
\begin{aligned}
KE &= 1/2\, mv^2 \\
PE &= mgh \\
&= (100\text{ g}) \times (980\text{ cm/sec}^2) \times (200\text{ cm}) \\
&= 1.96 \times 10^7\text{ g-cm}^2/\text{sec}^2 \\
&= 1.96 \times 10^7\text{ ergs} \\
KE &= \frac{1}{2}\, mv^2 \\
&= \frac{1}{2} \times (100\text{ g}) \times (300\text{ cm/sec})^2 \\
&= 4.5 \times 10^6\text{ g-cm}^2/\text{sec}^2 \\
W &= PE + KE \\
&= 1.96 \times 10^7\text{ ergs} + 0.45 \times 10^7\text{ ergs} \\
&= 2.41 \times 10^7\text{ ergs} \\
&= 2.41\text{ J}
\end{aligned}
$$

3. CONSERVATION OF ENERGY

The law of conservation of mechanical energy states that total mechanical energy

$$E = KE + PE$$

is conserved:

$$\Sigma E_0 = \Sigma E.$$

For a single particle, that means

$$\Delta KE = -\ PE.$$

For the mass on a spring system shown in Figure 26, that means

$$\frac{1}{2}\, kA^2 = \frac{1}{2}\, mv^2 + \frac{1}{2}\, kx^2$$

for any value of the displacement x. For example, as a mass on a spring moves from $x = A$ to $x = 0$ to $x = -A$, the potential energy $\frac{1}{2}kx^2$ is transformed into kinetic energy:

$$KE = \frac{1}{2}\, mv^2$$

and then back again into stored energy. A good method of attack in solving energy problems is to draw two pictures, one showing the initial situation (e.g., mass on spring stretched to $x = A$) and the other showing the final situation (e.g., mass on spring at $x = 0$).

FIGURE 26

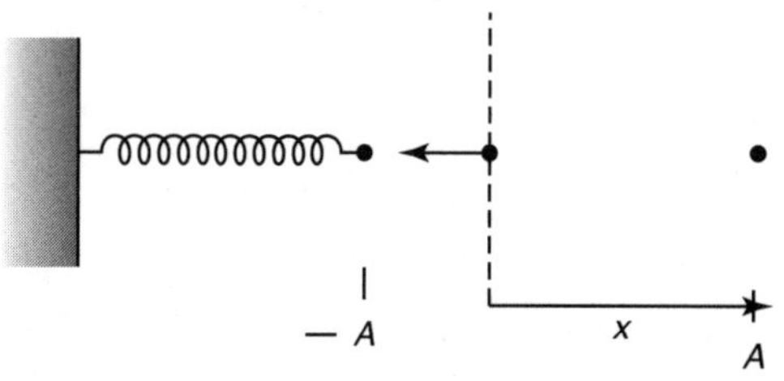

For an object projected upward, as show in Figure 27, this principle can be used to find the height because

$$\frac{1}{2}mv_0^{\ 2} = mgh + \frac{1}{2}mv_{0x}^{\ 2}, \text{ or } \frac{1}{2}mv_{0y}^{\ 2} = mgh.$$

FIGURE 27

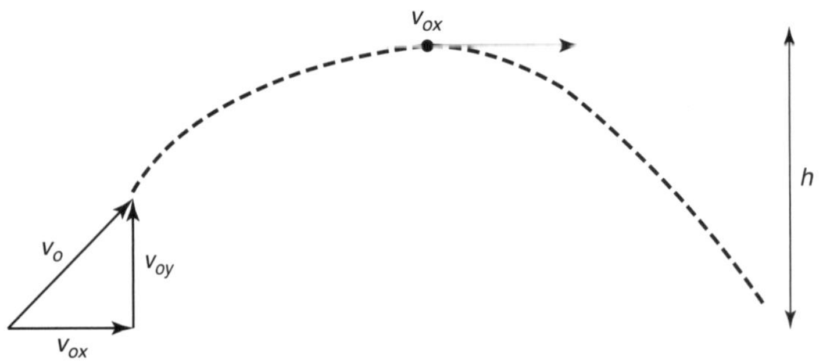

Note that the energy problem-solving method gives the same answer as that for kinematics:

$$h = \frac{v_{0y}^{\ 2}}{2g}.$$

For distances in between $y = 0$ and $y = h$, for an object projected straight upward ($\theta = 90°$),

$$\frac{1}{2}mv^2 + mgy = mgh.$$

If friction is involved in a problem, the fact that some energy is lost or goes into frictional heat must be considered. For example, in sliding down the incline depicted in Figure 28, the law of conservation of energy must be written as

$$mgh = mgy + \frac{1}{2}mv^2 + \mu_k N_x$$

and the usual dynamics approach is used to find N.

FIGURE 28

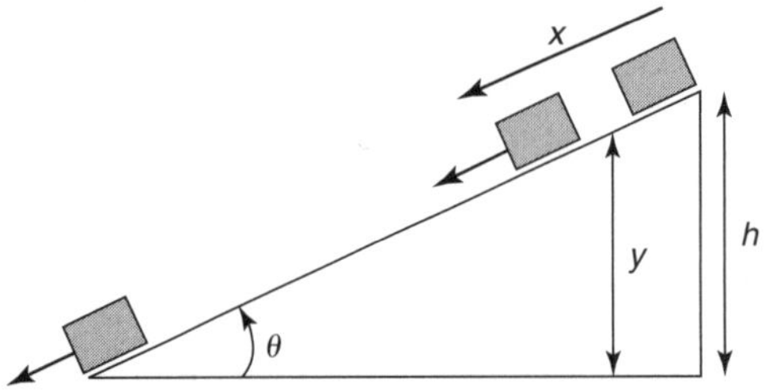

Problem

A 1-kg block slides down a rough inclined plane whose height is 1 m. At the bottom, the block has a velocity of 4 m/sec. Is energy conserved?

Solution

Energy will be conserved if the kinetic energy gained by the block is equal to the potential energy lost. At top:

$$\begin{aligned} PE &= mgh \\ &= (1\text{ kg}) \times (9.8\text{ m/sec}^2) \times (1\text{ m}) \\ &= 9.8\text{ J}. \end{aligned}$$

At bottom:

$$KE = \frac{1}{2} mv^2$$
$$= \frac{1}{2} \times (1\ \text{kg}) \times (4\ \text{m/sec})^2$$
$$= 8\ \text{J}.$$

Apparently, energy is not conserved. Evidently, a certain amount of energy (1.8 J) has been expended in overcoming the friction between the block and the rough plane. This amount of energy appears as thermal energy and could be detected by measuring the temperature rise in the block and the plane after the slide is completed.

Problem

A 5-kg body falls freely through a height of 3 m. Find its kinetic energy when it hits the ground. What was its potential energy?

Solution

$$KE = \tfrac{1}{2} mv^2$$
$$= \tfrac{1}{2} 5v^2$$

After falling 3 meters

$$v^2 = 2 \times g \times h$$
$$= 2 \times 9.8\ \text{m/sec}^2 \times 3\ \text{m}$$
$$= 58.8\ \text{m}^2/\text{sec}^2$$
$$KE = \tfrac{1}{2} 5\text{kg} \times 58.8\ \text{m}^2/\text{sec}^2$$
$$= 147\ \text{J}$$
$$PE = m \times g \times h$$
$$= 5\ \text{kg} \times 9.8\text{m/sec}^2 \times 3\ \text{m}$$
$$= 147\ \text{J}$$

By applying the law of conservation of energy, a quicker answer for the kinetic energy can be obtained by calculating the potential energy.

4. POWER

Power is the work done per unit of time:

$$\frac{\Delta W}{\Delta t}$$

In the simplest case, the work can be found by simply multiplying power by time. For translational motion, power is

$$P = F \times v.$$

Power companies calculate people's electric bills according to kilowatt-hours of energy used, or 10^3 W $\times$ 3600 sec = 3.6 $\times$ 10^6 J, or 3.6 megajoules.

Problem

A constant horizontal force of 10 N is required to drag an object across a rough surface at a constant speed of 5 m/sec. What power is being expended? How much work would be done in 30 min?

Solution

Power is the rate of doing work:

$$P = \frac{\Delta W}{\Delta t} = \frac{F\Delta s}{\Delta t}$$

(Note that in this problem, the work reduces to the force multiplied by the distance the object is moved.) But $\Delta s/\Delta t$ is just the velocity. Therefore,

$$\begin{aligned} P &= Fv \\ &= (10\text{ N}) \times (5\text{ m/sec}) \\ &= 50\text{ J/sec} \\ &= 50\text{ W} \\ W &= Pt \\ &= (50\text{ W}) \times (\tfrac{1}{2}\text{ hr}) \\ &= 25\text{ W-hr.} \end{aligned}$$

The work, of course, is done against the force of sliding friction.

V. WAVE CHARACTERISTICS AND PERIODIC MOTION

1. WAVE CHARACTERISTICS

A wave is considered to be a disturbance that propagates through some material medium or space. There are two classifications of waves. Waves that travel through a material medium are called mechanical waves. Waves that carry the various forms of light are electromagnetic waves, and they travel at the speed of light through a vacuum.

A. Transverse and Longitudinal Motion

Both mechanical and electromagnetic waves can travel by means of a transverse wave. Transverse waves cause matter to move in a direction perpendicular to the direction of wave propagation. Figure 29 shows four points along a wave medium. As the wave travels to the right, the matter within the medium moves up, and then the matter moves down as the wave passes. Thus, the wave is transverse.

FIGURE 29

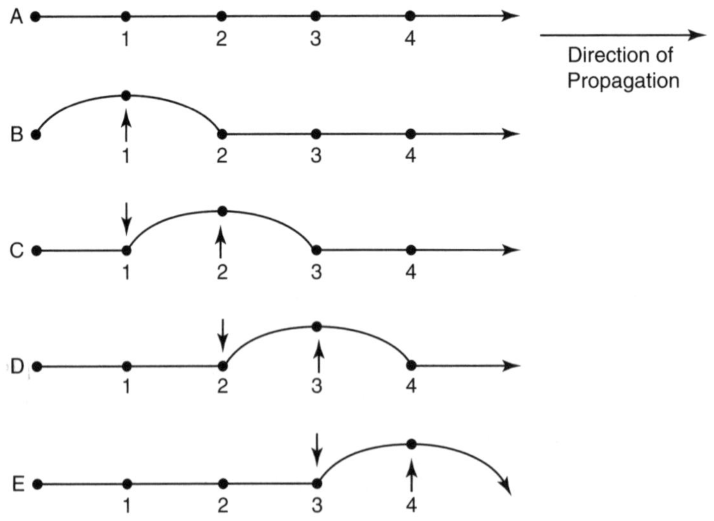

A second type of mechanical wave is the longitudinal, or compression, wave. Longitudinal waves cause material in the medium to move parallel to wave propagation. Figure 30 shows a compression wave pulse through a coil spring. When released, the compressed area attempts to spread out, which will compress the coils to their right. This process continues throughout the length of the spring.

FIGURE 30

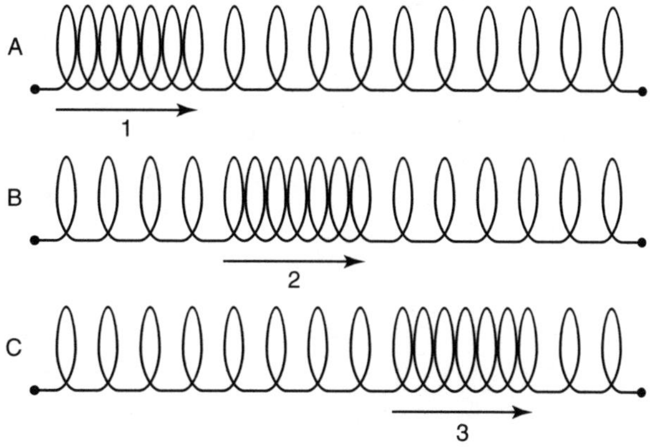

Sound waves are the best example of compression waves. The shock from a sound compresses the air near the source, which sends a compression wave through the air in all directions. You hear the sound when the compression shock hits your eardrum.

B. Wavelength, Frequency, and Velocity

If a source that creates a wave does so repeatedly at equal time intervals, then a periodic wave will result. Figure 31 shows a periodic transverse wave with equal disturbances over equal time periods.

FIGURE 31

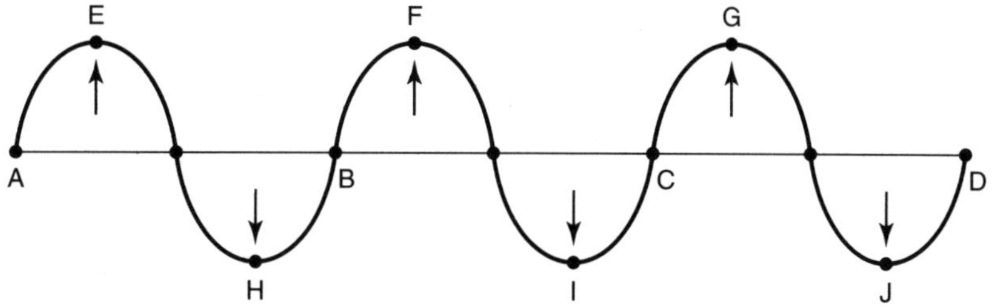

The figure shows three complete waves, each with an upper displacement crest and a lower displacement trough. The distance from a point on one wave to the same point on the next wave is called one wavelength. For the wave in Figure 31, the wavelength, λ (lambda), could be measured from A to B, one crest and one trough; from E to F, crest to crest; or from H to I, trough to trough.

A wave that travels through one crest and one trough has completed one cycle. The number of waves that pass a given point in a specified time interval is the wave frequency. Frequency, f, is measured in cycles per second, or hertz (Hz). The period T for a wave is the time for one complete wave to pass a reference point. Finally, a wave that moves in a given direction must have velocity in that direction. Wavelength, frequency, period, and velocity all relate to each other. Figure 32 shows two waves traveling one meter from x to y. Each wave can travel from x to y in 1 second.

FIGURE 32

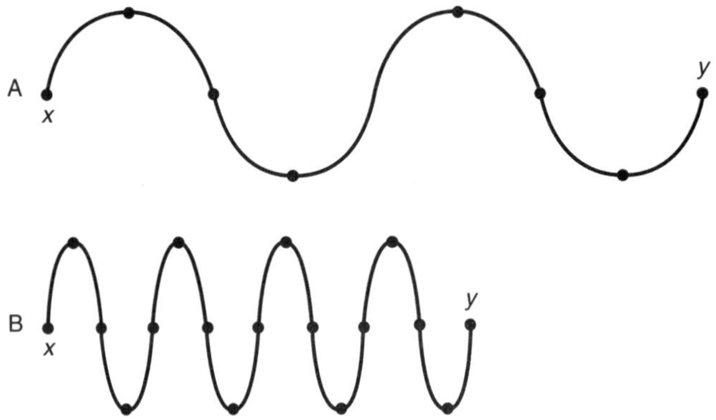

For wave A, two complete waves will pass point Y in one second, which gives a frequency equal to 2 Hz. For wave B, four waves pass y in one second, which gives a frequency of 4 Hz. Because the waves are traveling 2 per second in A, the period for wave A is ½ second. In B, waves pass 4 per second, and the period is $\frac{1}{4}$ second. Notice that the frequency and period are reciprocals. Thus,

$$f = \frac{1}{T} \text{ and } T = \frac{1}{f}$$

Because each wave travels a distance λ in time T,

$$v = \frac{\lambda}{T}.$$

Substituting for $\frac{1}{T}$ gives

$$v = \frac{\lambda}{T} = \left(\frac{1}{T}\right)(\lambda) = f\lambda$$

$$v = f\lambda$$

This final equation is true for all periodic waves, transverse or longitudinal, regardless of medium material.

Problem

The wave shown in Figure 33 is represented by the equation

$$y = 0.20 \sin 0.40\pi (x - 60t),$$

where all distances are measured in centimeters and time in seconds. Determine the following characteristics of the wave:

A. Amplitude
B. Wavelength
C. Speed
D. Frequency

E. Displacement at $x = 5.5$ cm and $t = 0.020$ sec

FIGURE 33

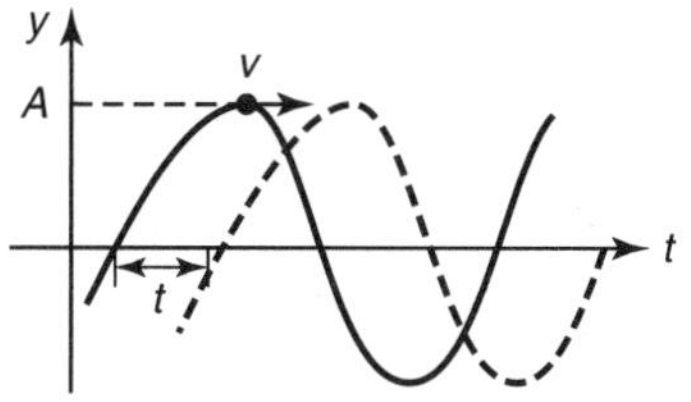

Solution

The displacement y of the medium due to wave motion at a position x at a time t is

$$y = A \sin \frac{2\pi}{\lambda}(x - vt).$$

where A is the amplitude, λ is the wavelength, and v is the velocity with which the wave is traveling along the x-axis. Compare this equation with the expression given in the question:

A. $A = 0.20$ cm

B. $\frac{2\pi}{\lambda} = 0.40\pi \qquad \lambda = \frac{2}{0.40} cm = 5.0cm$

C. $v = 60$ cm/sec

D. $f = \frac{v}{\lambda} = \frac{60cm / \sec}{5.0cm} = 12 / \sec$

E. $y = (0.20 \text{ cm}) \sin [0.40\pi(5.5 - 60 \times 0.020)]$
$= (0.20 \text{ cm}) \sin [0.40\ \pi(5.5 - 1.2)]$
$= (0.20 \text{ cm}) \sin (0.40 \times 4.3\ \pi)$
$= (0.20 \text{ cm}) \sin 1.72\pi$
$= (0.20 \text{ cm}) (-0.77) = -0.15 \text{ cm}$

C. Superposition of Waves, Interference, and Phase

Superposition is the algebraic summing of the amplitudes of two traveling waves when they pass through each other. The waves then travel on past each other unchanged. If the sum of the two waves is greater than the amplitudes of each individual wave, then the waves are said to constructively interfere. Destructive interference occurs if the algebraic sum of the waves is less than the amplitude of each individual wave.

For two waves traveling in the same direction at the same speed, superposition will also occur. The waves in this case will not pass each other, but the effects of constructive or destructive interference will be seen for as long as the two waves are traveling at the same speed. The amount of interference will depend on the *phase* difference between the two waves. For example, in Figure 34 the two waves with equal wavelength traveling at the same speed are in phase because the maximum points at the crests of both waves line up. Two waves in phase have a phase difference f of zero between them and constructively interfere to produce a resultant wave.

FIGURE 34

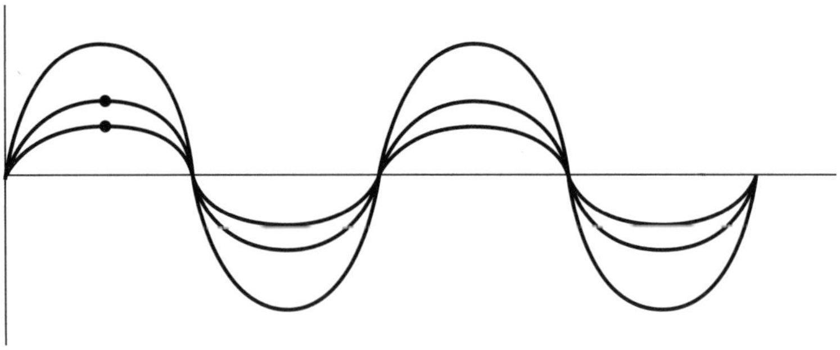

When a phase difference of Ø = 180° occurs, the waves will destructively interfere. In fact, waves with equal amplitudes will completely cancel each other out, as shown in Figure 35.

FIGURE 35

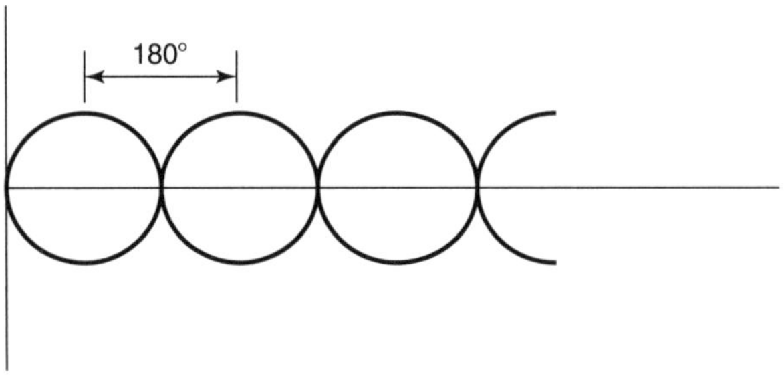

Phase differences between Ø = 0° and = 180° will form a resultant wave that is the algebraic sum of the two original waves because at some points the waves may constructively interfere and at other points the waves may destructively interfere.

D. Beats

If two waves do not have the same wavelength (frequency) but their frequencies are very close, the waves will continuously constructively and destructively interfere. As a result, a wave with a beat frequency

$$f_{beat}\,|f_1 - f_2|$$

will be formed.

Problem

When two tuning forks are sounded simultaneously, a beat note of 5 cycles per second is heard. If one of the forks has a known frequency of 256 cycles per second, and if a small piece of adhesive tape fastened to this fork reduces the beat note to 3 cycles per second, what is the frequency of the other fork?

Solution

This problem involves the phenomenon of beats. When two similar waves are superimposed, the beat frequency represents the numerical difference in their frequencies. Thus, for the case in question,

$$n = (256 \pm 5) \text{ cycles/sec}$$

where n represents the unknown frequency.

It appears that n has two possible values: 251 or 261. When the standard fork is loaded with the tape, its frequency will decrease. Because the beat frequency is then reduced to 3 cycles per second, the unknown frequency must be less than, not more than, 256. Thus, $n = 251$.

2. PERIODIC MOTION

A. Hooke's Law

$$F_s = -kx$$

where F_s is the force produced by the spring along its length, x is the displacement of the spring, and k is the spring's constant. The force of the spring is always opposite to the direction of displacement; therefore, a negative sign is included in the formula.

Problem

A weight is hung from a spring, and the spring stretches 0.5 m. Determine the period of vibration of the spring if it is pulled a little and then released.

Solution

$$T = 2\pi\sqrt{\frac{m}{k}} = 2\pi\sqrt{\frac{w/g}{k}} = 2\pi\sqrt{\frac{w}{gk}}$$

$$k = \frac{\text{upward restoring force}}{\text{downward displacment produced by the stretching forc}} = \frac{\text{w}}{0.5\text{t}}$$

$$\text{T} = 2\pi\sqrt{\frac{\text{kg}}{2\text{kg/m} \times 9.8\ \text{m/s}^2}} = 1.42\ \text{sec}$$

B. Simple Harmonic Motion

Equations of Motion: Variables for Simple Harmonic Motion

The period of motion is

$$T = \frac{2\pi}{\omega} = 2\pi\sqrt{\frac{m}{k}} \rightarrow \textit{units : Seconds}.$$

The frequency of motion is

$$f = \frac{1}{T} = \frac{\omega}{2\pi} = \frac{1}{2\pi}\sqrt{\frac{k}{m}} \rightarrow \text{units} : \frac{1}{\text{seconds}}.$$

The angular frequency of motion is

$$\omega = 2\pi f = \frac{2\pi}{T} = \sqrt{\frac{k}{m}} \rightarrow \text{units} : \frac{\text{Rads}}{\text{sec}}$$

Simple harmonic oscillation is depicted in Figure 36.

FIGURE 36

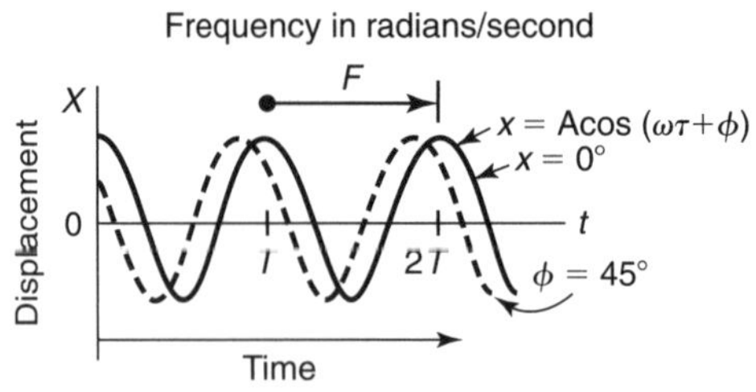

Differential Equations of Motion

Displacement:

$$\mathbf{x} = A \cos(\omega t + \phi)$$

Velocity:

$$\frac{dx}{dt} = v = -\omega \sin(\omega t + \phi)$$

Problem

One end of a fingernail file is clamped in a vise, and the other end is given a to-and-fro vibration. The motion of the free end is approximately simple harmonic motion. If the frequency is 10 vibrations per second and the amplitude is 4 millimeters, what is the velocity when the displacement of the free end is 2 millimeters?

Solution

The problem states that the motion is nearly simple harmonic motion. Therefore, the displacement of the file is

$x = A \sin(\omega t + a)$, (1)

where A is the amplitude, α is a constant, and ω is the angular frequency of the vibration. If f is the frequency of the motion

$$\omega = 2\pi f.$$

The velocity of the end of the file is, differentiating equation (1),

$v = A\,\omega \cos(\omega t + \alpha)$ (2)

At the position $x = 2$ mm, using equation (1) gives

$$2 \text{ mm} = 4 \text{ mm} \sin(\omega t + \alpha)$$

$$\sin(\omega t + \alpha) = \frac{1}{2}$$

where $(\omega t + \alpha) = 30^\circ$.

Therefore, using equation (2),

$v = A\,\omega \cos(30^\circ)$

$v = A\,(2\pi f) \cos(30^\circ)$

$v = (4 \text{ mm})\,(6.28)\,(10 \text{ per sec})$

$$v = \left(\frac{40\text{mm}}{\text{sec}}\right)(6.28)(0.866) = 218\text{mm}/sec$$

C. Pendulum Motion

FIGURE 37

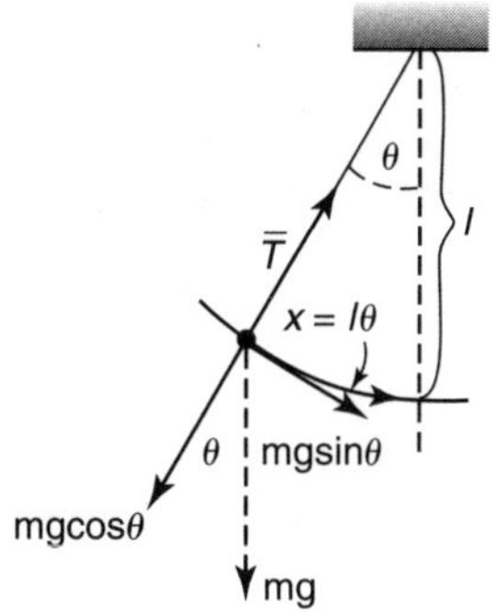

Force, F:

$$F = -mg\theta = \frac{-mg}{L}x$$

Period T:

$$T = 2\pi\sqrt{\frac{L}{g}}$$

Problem

A pendulum makes 90 vibrations in 1 minute. Determine the period and frequency.

Solution

$$T = \frac{\text{Elapsed time}}{\text{Vibrations made}}$$
$$= \frac{60 \text{ sec}}{90}$$
$$= 0.67 \text{ sec}$$
$$f = \frac{\text{Vibrations made}}{\text{Elapsed time}}$$
$$= \frac{90}{60 \text{ sec}}$$
$$= 1.5 \text{ sec}^{-1}$$

Problem

Compute the acceleration due to gravity at a place where a simple pendulum, 150 cm long, makes 100 vibrations in 246 seconds.

Solution

$$T = \frac{(246 \text{ sec})}{100} = 2.46 \text{ sec}$$

$$T = 2\pi(l/g)^{0.5}$$

$$T^2 = 4\pi^2 l/g$$

$$g = \frac{4\pi^2 \times l}{T^2}$$

$$= \frac{4\pi^2 \times 1.50\text{ m}}{(2.46\text{ sec})^2}$$

$$= 9.79\text{ m/sec}^2$$

VI. SOUND

1. PRODUCTION OF SOUND

Sound waves are treated exactly like other waves, with frequency and wavelength related by

$$v = f \times \lambda.$$

Sound waves, however, are mechanical waves. They are longitudinal waves corresponding to the compression and rarefaction (expansion) of the medium in which the waves are traveling.

Problem

What is the wavelength of the sound wave emitted by a standard tuning fork of 440 cycles per second?

Solution

Given that velocity (v), frequency (f), and wavelength (λ) of sound are related by $v = f \times \lambda$, and assuming the velocity of sound to be 34,000 cm/sec, or approximately 1,100 ft/sec, then

$$\lambda = \frac{v}{f} = \frac{1100\,ft}{440} = 2.5\,ft \text{ (approx.)}$$

Problem

What is the frequency of a 2-cm sound wave in seawater? The velocity of sound in seawater is $v = 1.53 \times 10^5$ cm/sec.

Solution

The 2 cm is the wavelength l of the sound wave. The frequency is given by

$$f = \frac{v}{\lambda}$$

$$= \frac{1.53 \times 10^5\text{ cm / sec}}{2\text{ cm}}$$

$$= 7.6 \times 10^4\text{ Hz} = 76\text{ kHz}$$

which is an ultrasonic wave (that is, above the human audible range). A 2-cm sound wave in air would be audible.

2. RELATIVE SPEED OF SOUND IN SOLIDS, LIQUIDS, AND GASES

A. Wave Speed in a Fluid

$$v = \sqrt{\frac{B}{\rho}}$$

v = Speed of sound in a fluid
B = Modulus of elasticity
ρ = Density of medium

B. Wave Speed in a Solid

To determine the speed of a wave traveling in a solid, the value of B is replaced by a parameter appropriate to the particular situation. For a wave traveling along a taut rope, B is replaced by the tension, T.

C. Wave Speed in a Gas

$$vg = \sqrt{\frac{\gamma p}{\rho}}$$

v_g = Speed of sound in a gas
γ = Ratio of specific heats for a gas
p = Undisturbed pressure
ρ = Density of medium

3. INTENSITY OF SOUND

A. Average Intensity (I)

$$I = \frac{1}{2}\frac{P_m{}^2}{\sqrt{B\rho}}$$

P_m = Pressure amplitude
B = Bulk modulus of elasticity
ρ = Density of medium

B. Loudness

Loudness of sound is measured in decibels and defined as

$$\text{Loudness} = 10 \log \frac{I}{I_0}$$

where $I_0 = 10^{-12}\,\text{Wb/m}^2$, which is the lowest sound a human ear can hear.

In contrast, a very loud stereo system can crank out 100 decibels (dB), which corresponds to an intensity $I = 10^{-2}\,\text{Wb/m}^2$. An intensity of 1 Wb/m^2 or 120 dB is at the threshold of pain for the human ear.

4. DOPPLER EFFECT

One interesting idea regarding wave velocity is the Doppler effect. This effect refers to a wave that originates from a source traveling with some velocity. In essence, the source velocity appears to be added to or subtracted from the wave velocity. The Doppler effect is best explained by examining sound waves.

The frequency of a sound wave determines a characteristic known as pitch. Interpreting pitch is how the human ear distinguishes among frequencies. The higher the frequency, the higher the pitch. If the source of sound is in motion relative to the listener, the Doppler effect occurs and the pitch heard is not the true pitch of the wave. Figure 38 shows the Doppler effect. Remember that sound travels by compression waves, but for this diagram they are shown as transverse.

FIGURE 38

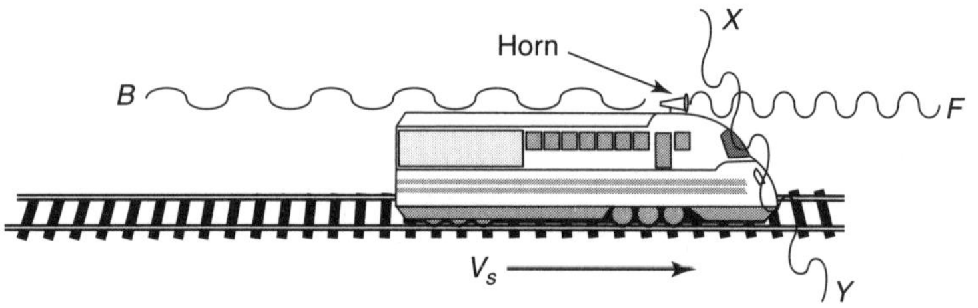

The listeners at positions X and Y hear the wave perpendicular to the motion of the train. These waves are unaffected by the motion of the source, and the true pitch is heard. Listener F hears a wave that is traveling the same direction as the source. As the source approaches, the frequency heard increases and the pitch is higher. Listener B hears the opposite effect. Because the sound is moving opposite the source, the frequency heard decreases and the pitch is lower.

To describe the Doppler effect more analytically, let v_s be the velocity of the source and v_0 that of the observer. Then the frequency observed by the observer is

$$f' = f(v \pm v_0) / (v \pm v_s).$$

For example, in the situation shown in Figure 39, $v_s = 0$ and the observer is moving away from the source, so the expectation is that $\lambda' > \lambda$ or $f' < f$. More precisely,

$$f'' = f(v - v_0)/v.$$

In the situation of Figure 40, where $v_0 = 0$ and the source is moving toward the observer, $\lambda' < \lambda$ and therefore $f' > f$. More precisely,

$$f'' = fv/(v - v_s).$$

FIGURE 39

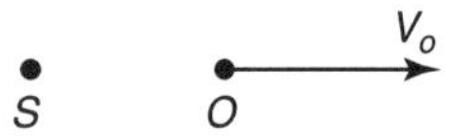

FIGURE 40

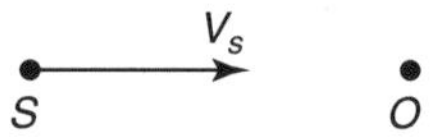

Problem

A researcher notices that the frequency of a note emitted by an automobile horn appears to drop from 284 cycles•sec^{-1} to 266 cycles•sec^{-1} as the automobile passes him. From this observation, he is able to calculate the speed of the car, knowing that the speed of sound in air is 1,100 ft•sec^{-1}. What value does he obtain for the speed?

Solution

This is an example of the Doppler effect. When there is no movement of the surrounding medium, the relationship between the frequency as heard by a moving observer and that emitted by a moving source is

$$\frac{f_L}{u \pm v_L} = \frac{f_s}{u \mp v_s}$$

where f_L is the frequency heard by the listener, f_s the frequency emitted by the moving source, v_L the velocity of the listener, v_s the velocity of the source, and u the velocity of sound (= 1,100 ft•sec^{-1}). The upper signs (+ left side of equation, − right side) correspond to the source and observer moving along the line joining the two and approaching each other, and the lower signs (− left, + right) correspond to source and observer receding from one another.

In this case, the frequencies heard by the stationary listener ($v_L = 0$) are

$$f_L = uf_s/(u \mp v_s)$$

As the automobile approaches the observer, he records a frequency of 284 cycles•sec^{-1}, and as the automobile moves away from him, he records 266 cycles•sec^{-1}. Thus

$$284\ s^{-1} = \frac{uf_s}{u - v_s} \qquad (1)$$

and

$$266\ s^{-1} = \frac{uf_s}{u + v_s} \qquad (2)$$

Dividing equation (1) by equation (2):

$$\frac{u + v_s}{u - v_s} = \frac{284}{266}$$

$$266(u + v_s) = 284(u - v_s)$$

or

$$\frac{v_s}{u} = \frac{18}{550}.$$

$$\therefore v_s = \frac{18}{550} \times 1100\,ft \cdot s^{-1} = 36\,ft \cdot s^{-1}$$

$$= 36\,ft \cdot s^{-1} \times \frac{1mile}{5280\,ft} \times \frac{60s}{1\min} \times \frac{60\min}{1hr} = 24.5mph$$

5. RESONANCE IN PIPES AND STRINGS, AND HARMONICS

As mentioned in the last section, a traveling wave moving to the right and one moving to the left may interfere to produce standing waves of amplitude A. For a string of length L, the usual condition is $L = n\lambda/2$, where n = 1, 2, and 3 waveforms, as in Figure 41. The points where $y = \pm A$ are called antinodes, and the points where $y = 0$ are termed nodes. Thus, n is the number of antinodes.

The situation in a pipe closed at both ends is exactly the same, $L = n\lambda/2$, except it is pressure or sound waves interfering. For a pipe open at both ends, $L = n\lambda/2$ also applies (as in Figure 42). Finally for a pipe open at one end and closed at the other, you could draw the waveforms and see that $L = n\lambda/4$, where n = 1,3,5, and so on.

Because $f = v/\lambda$, the frequencies are

$$f_n = nv/2L = nf_1$$

where f_1 is called the fundamental frequency or the first harmonic. The term *harmonic* is used here because a harmonic series or quantized equation exists. Similarly, f_2 and f_3 are the second and third harmonics.

FIGURE 41

FIGURE 42

Problem

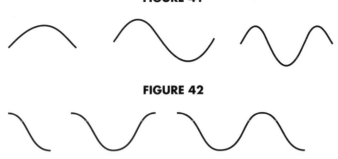

The average person can hear sounds varying in frequency from 20 to 20,000 vibrations per second. Determine the wavelength in each case. The speed of sound is 340 m/sec.

Solution

$$\frac{v}{f} = \lambda$$

$$\frac{340 \text{ m/sec}}{20 \text{ sec}} = 17 \text{ m}$$

$$\frac{340 \text{ m/sec}}{20,000 \text{ sec}} = 0.017 \text{ m} = 1.7 \text{ cm}$$

See Biology Review, Hearing, page 200.

Problem

A rod 200 cm long is clamped 50 cm from one end and set into longitudinal vibrations, as shown in Figure 43. The lowest frequency produced by the rod is 3,000 vibrations per second. What is the speed of sound in the rod?

FIGURE 43

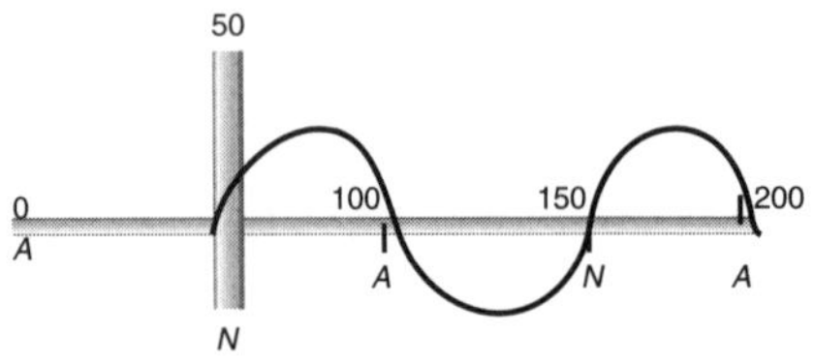

Solution

There is a node on the clamp and an antinode at each end.

Wavelength $\lambda = 2 \times$ Distance between nodes

$= 2 \times 100$ cm

$= 200$ cm

$$v = f\lambda = \frac{3,000}{\text{sec}} \times 2.00 \text{ m}$$

$$= 6,000 \text{ m/sec}$$

Problem

Determine the shortest length of closed pipe and of open pipe that will resonate in air at 0°C with a fork of frequency 160 ft/sec. The speed of sound equals 1,087 ft/sec.

Solution

Wavelength of sound $\lambda = v/f$

$$= \frac{1,100 \text{ ft/sec}}{160 \text{ ft/sec}}$$

$$= 6.8 \text{ ft}$$

Shortest piece of closed pipe $= \frac{1}{4}\lambda$

$$= \frac{1}{4}(6.8 \text{ ft})$$

$$= 1.7 \text{ ft}$$

Shortest piece of open pipe $= \frac{1}{2}\lambda$

$$= \frac{1}{2}(6.8 \text{ ft})$$

$$= 3.4 \text{ ft}$$

VII. FLUIDS AND SOLIDS

1. FLUIDS

A. Density and Specific Gravity

Density (ρ) is the ratio of mass over volume. Specific gravity (s) is the ratio of the density of a substance to that of a reference substance:

$$\rho = M/V$$

$$s = \rho/\rho_{ref}$$

The most commonly used reference density is that of water at a standard temperature (4.0°C), 1 gram per cubic centimeter.

Problem

The specific weight of water at ordinary pressure and temperature is 62.4 lb/ft^3 (9.81 kN/m^3). The specific gravity of mercury is 13.55. Compute the density of water and the specific weight and density of mercury.

Solution

Density ρ and specific weight γ of a fluid are related as follows:

$$\rho = \frac{\gamma}{g} \text{ or } \gamma = \rho g$$

Specific gravity s of a liquid is the ratio of its density to that of pure water at a standard temperature. Therefore,

$$\rho_{water} = \frac{\gamma_{water}}{g} = \frac{62.4 \text{ lb/ft}^3}{32.2 \text{ ft / s}^2} = 1.94 \text{slugs/ft}^3$$

$$= \frac{9.81 kN \text{ / m}^3}{9.81 \text{ m/s}^2} = 1.00 Mg \text{ / m}^3 = 1.00 g \text{ / cm}^3$$

$\gamma_{mercury} = s_{mercury}\, \gamma_{water} = 13.55\,(62.4) = 846\ \text{lb/ft}^3$

$13.55\,(9.81) = 133\ \text{kN/m}^3$

$\rho_{mercury} = s_{mercury}\, \rho_{water} = 13.55\,(1.94) = 26.3\ \text{slugs/ft}^3$

$13.55\,(1.00) = 13.55\ \text{Mg/m}^3$

B. Archimedes' Principle

Archimedes' principle describes the effects of buoyancy. The mass of a floating object equals the mass of the fluid displaced. Also, the upward force of an immersed object equals the volume displaced times the difference between the weight of fluid displaced and that of the object.

Problem

To determine their density, drops of blood are placed in a mixture of xylene of density 0.867 g?m^{-3} and bromobenzene of density 1.497 g?cm^{-3}, the mixture being altered until the drops do not rise or sink. The mixture then contains 72% of xylene and 28% of bromobenzene by volume. What is the density of the blood?

Solution

Using the definition of density,

$$\text{Density} = \frac{\text{Mass}}{\text{Volume}},$$

every 72 cm^3 of xylene has a mass of

$$72\ \text{cm}^3 \times 0.867\ \text{g}\cdot\text{cm}^{-3} = 62.424\ \text{g},$$

and every 28 cm^3 of bromobenzene has a mass of

$$28\ \text{cm}^3 \times 1.497\ \text{gm}\cdot\text{cm}^{-3} = 41.916\ \text{g}.$$

Thus, 100 cm^3 of the mixture has a mass of

$$(62.424 + 41.916)\ \text{g} = 104.340\ \text{g}.$$

Thus, the density of the mixture is 1.0434 g·cm^{-3}.

However, blood neither rises nor sinks in this mixture, showing that the blood has no net force acting on it. Thus, the weight of any drop of blood is exactly equal to the upthrust acting on it. By Archimedes' principle, the upthrust is the weight of an equal volume of mixture. Therefore, the blood and the mixture have the same densities, and the density of blood is 1.0434 g·cm^{-3}.

See Biology Review, Properties of Water, page 135.

Problem

Icebergs are of glacial origin and consist of freshwater. The specific gravity of ice is 0.92. What fraction of an iceberg will be submerged when floating in seawater? The specific gravity of seawater is 1.03.

Solution

Because the ice floats, the weight of displaced liquid (mxg) equals the weight of ice (W). If v_t is the total volume and V_s is the submerged volume, then

$$W = mxg$$

$$9.8 \text{ m/sec}^2 \times V_t = 1.03 \times 9.8 \text{ m/sec}^2 \times V_s$$

$$\frac{V_s}{V_t} = 0.92/1.03 = 0.893$$

C. Hydrostatic Pressure

Pressure = Force per unit area

$$= \frac{\text{Force } F \text{ acting perpendicular to an area}}{\text{Area } A \text{ over which the force is distributed}}$$

$$P = \frac{F}{A}$$

The pressure in a column of fluid of height h and density ρ is

$$P = h\rho g$$

Hydrostatic pressure is the pressure exerted at the bottom of a column of fluid divided by the area of the base. It is equal to the pressure at the top of the column plus the force exerted by the fluid:

$$P = P_0 + \frac{w}{A} = P_0 + pgh \; (V = A \times h)$$

Problem

Find the pressure at the bottom of a vessel 76 cm deep when the vessel is filled with water and with mercury. The density of mercury is 13.6 g/cm^3.

Solution

With water as the fluid,

$$P = h\rho g$$
$$= 0.76 \text{ m} \times 1{,}000 \text{ kg/m}^2 \times 9.8 \text{ m/sec}^2$$
$$= 7.5 \times 10^3 \text{ N/m}^2$$

With mercury as the fluid,

$$P = h\rho\rho g$$
$$= 0.76 \text{ m} \times (13.6 \times 1{,}000 \text{ kg/m}^2) \times 9.8 \text{ m/sec}^2$$
$$= 1.0 \times 10^5 \text{ N/m}^2$$

D. Bernoulli Equation

The Bernoulli equation is a simplified form of the mechanical energy equation used when changes in the kinetic and potential energies of a fluid are to be determined. It relates changes in pressure, height, and velocity.

$$p_1 + \frac{1}{2}\rho v_1{}^2 + \rho g y_1 = p_2 + \frac{1}{2}\rho v_2{}^2 + \rho g y_2{}^2 = \text{constant}$$

Problem

An open tank containing water has an orifice located near the bottom of the tank, as shown in Figure 44. Demonstrate that, for ideal flow, the discharge velocity at the orifice is $\sqrt{2gh}$. Assume steady flow.

FIGURE 44

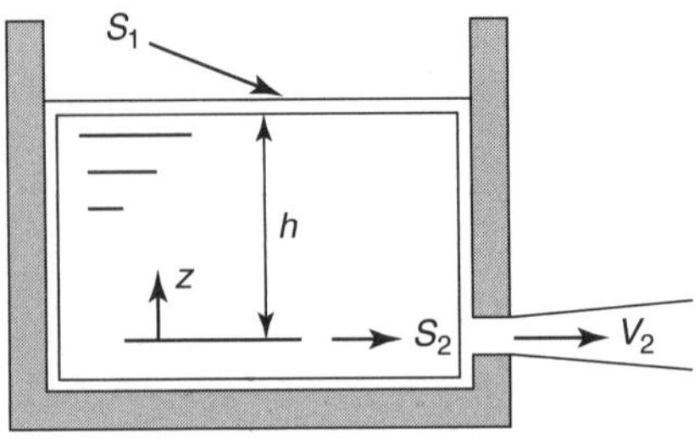

Solution

Consider the control volume shown in Figure 44. Apply the Bernoulli equation to sections s_1 and s_2.

$$\frac{p_1}{\rho} + \frac{v_1^2}{2g_c} + \frac{gz_1}{g_c} = \frac{p_2}{\rho} + \frac{v_2^2}{2g_c} + \frac{gz^2}{g_c} \quad (1)$$

Experiments indicate that the pressure at any section open to the atmosphere can be taken to be at atmospheric pressure. Therefore,

$$p_1 = p_2 = p_{atm}.$$

Using the continuity equation,

$$v_1A_1 = v_2A_2 \quad (2)$$

and the fact that $A_1 >> A_2$, leads to $v_1 << v_2$. Thus, v_1 can be neglected. Under these circumstances, equation (1) reduces to

$$\frac{v_2^2}{2g} = z_1 - z_2 = h.$$

or

$$v_2 = \sqrt{2gh}$$

E. Pascal's Principle

When the pressure on any part of a confined fluid (liquid or gas) is changed, the pressure on every other part of the fluid is changed by the same amount.

Problem

In a hydraulic press, the large piston has a cross-sectional area $A_1 = 200\ \text{in}^2$, and the small piston has a cross-sectional area $A_2 = 5\ \text{in}^2$. If a force F_2 of 25 lb is applied to the small piston, find the force F_1 on the large piston.

Solution

FIGURE 45

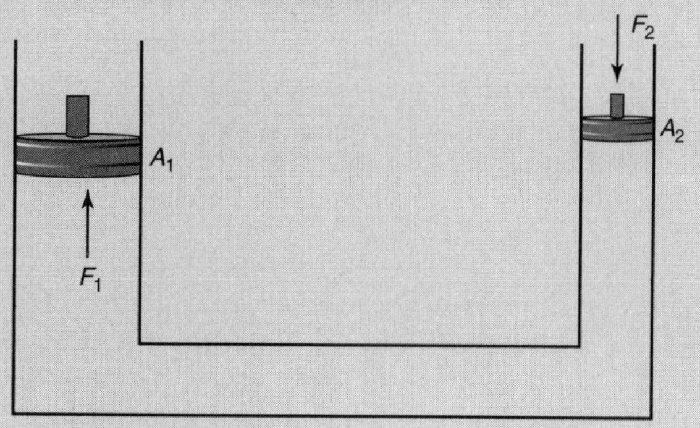

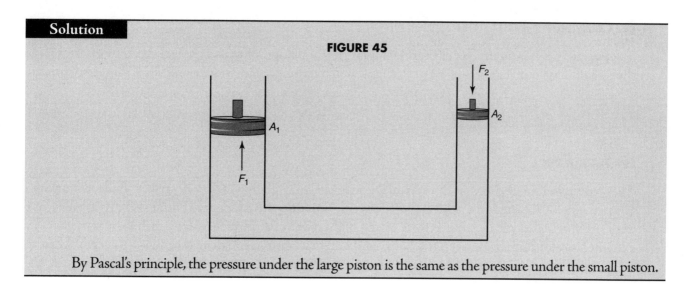

By Pascal's principle, the pressure under the large piston is the same as the pressure under the small piston.

F. Viscosity

Viscosity (η) of a fluid relates the force required to produce motion in a fluid. The units are force times time divided by area:

$$F = \eta \frac{Av}{L}$$

A = Area of liquid over which force is applied
L = Transverse dimension
v = Velocity

Problem

The space between two parallel plates 1.5 cm apart is filled with an oil of viscosity η of 0.050 kg/m sec. A thin 30 × 60 cm rectangular plate is pulled through the oil 0.50 cm from one plate and 1.00 cm from the other. What force is needed to pull the plate at 0.40 m/sec?

FIGURE 46

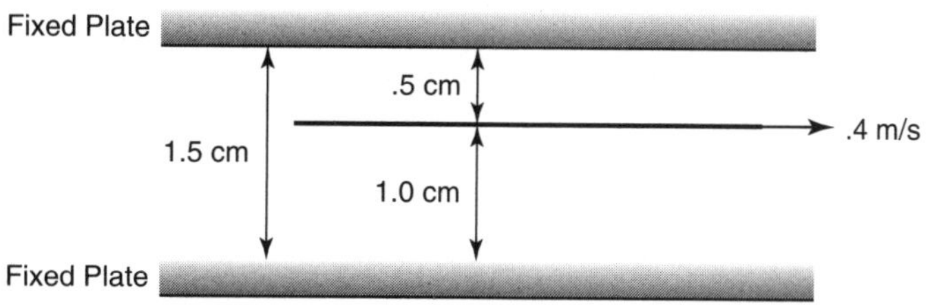

Solution

The total force overcomes the viscous shear over both the upper and the lower surface of the moving plate as indicated in Figure 46. Thus,

$$\begin{aligned} F_{total} &= F_{upper} + F_{lower} \\ &= \text{(Upper shear stress) (Area)} + \text{(Lower shear stress) (Area)} \\ &= \eta(V/h_{upper})(A) + \eta(V/h_{lower})(A) \\ &= (0.050)(0.40/0.005)(0.180) + (0.050)(0.40/0.010)(0.180) \\ &= 0.72 + 0.36 \\ &= 1.08\ \text{N} \end{aligned}$$

G. Continuity Equation

The equation of continuity states that the rate of accumulation of mass equals the rate of mass in minus the rate of mass out. Taken over a fixed volume and assuming steady state conditions, this simplifies to

$$(pAv)_{in} = (pAv)_{out}$$

where v = Velocity of the fluid.

H. Turbulence

There are two flow regimes in the typical Newtonian fluid. Laminar flow describes fluids as flowing in layers over one another. In a typical pipe flow, the boundary (the pipe wall) fluid velocity is taken to be zero. At the center of the pipe, flow is at the highest velocity. Flow becomes turbulent at higher flow rates because of mixing between the layers and eddy currents. Turbulent flow tends to occur when the Reynolds number exceeds 2,100. The dimensionless Reynolds number is the diameter times the bulk flow times the density divided by the viscosity.

$$N_r = \frac{rvD}{h}$$

r = Density of fluid
v = Average velocity
D = Diameter of pipe
h = Coefficient of viscosity

I. Surface Tension

The attractive forces between molecules pull them closer to each other to form more stable, lower-energy forms — similar to the way atoms combine to form molecules to decrease their energy. These molecular attractions will cause the molecules to form shapes with the lowest possible energy. For a liquid, this shape is a sphere, which is why water droplets always have a spherical shape. At the surface of a glass of water, the molecules are not bound on all sides like the water molecules below them, so they try to reduce the surface area as much as possible. Surface tension decreases with increasing temperature and changes depending on the gas in contact with the surface.

Surface tension is a cause of capillarity — the creeping up of water on the inside of a filled test tube. In the case of water, the attraction of the water to the glass is greater than the surface tension, and a concave meniscus forms in the tube. For mercury, the attraction between Hg molecules is greater than the attraction of Hg to the glass so the mercury forms a convex meniscus. The convex shape keeps all the mercury molecules as close to each other as possible.

2. SOLIDS

A. Elastic Properties

When the stress on a solid object is linearly proportional to the strain of the object, this stress–strain relationship is governed by Hooke's law:

$\sigma = E\varepsilon$
$\sigma \equiv$ Axial stress
$\varepsilon \equiv$ Axial strain
E = Modulus of elasticity

A little beyond the point where stress is linearly proportional to strain, the elastic deformation limit occurs. Further stress applied beyond this limit will result in a permanent or plastic deformation of the solid object.

VIII. ELECTROSTATICS AND ELECTROMAGNETISM

1. ELECTROSTATICS

A. Coulomb's Law

Electrostatics is the study of discrete or continuous systems of electric charge at rest. Electric charge comes in two varieties: positive and negative, the MKS unit being the coulomb. Like charges repel one another, and unlike charges attract each other (see Figure 47). Fundamental to electricity is Coulomb's law, which states that between every two charges, there exists an electric force given by

$$\mathbf{F} = \frac{k_e q_1 q_2}{r^2 \mathbf{r}}$$

where $k_e = 9.0 \times \frac{10^9 \text{ N-m}^2}{\text{C}^2}$ is the MKS coulomb force constant. If using the CGS system of units, $k_e = 1$ exactly, and the charge is measured in electrostatic units (esu). If more than one charge is in the vicinity, then the sum of the vector forces from all the nearby charges equals the resultant force (see the "Vectors and Scalars" section of this review); this is called the principle of superposition.

FIGURE 47

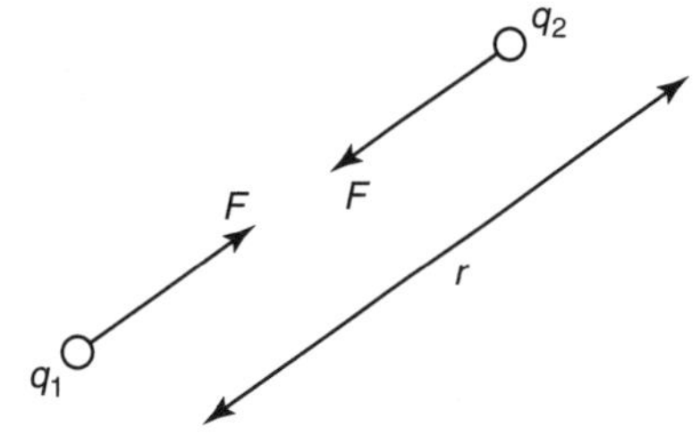

Problem

Calculate the resultant force on the charge q_3 in Figure 48.

FIGURE 48

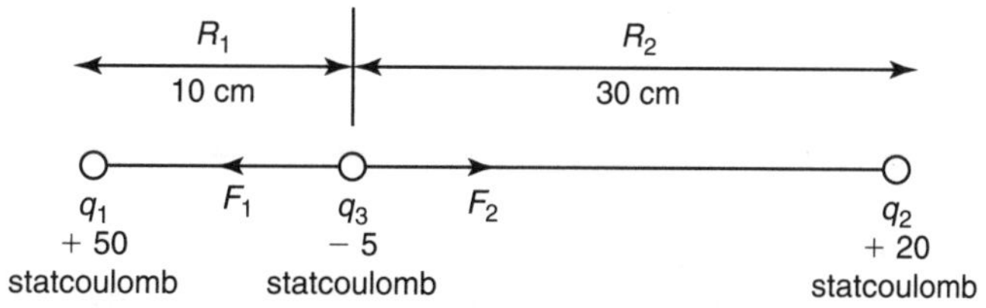

Solution

The force exerted by q_1 on q_3 is

$$F_1 = \frac{q_1 q_2}{R_1^{\,2}}$$
$$= \frac{(50(-5))}{(10)^2} = -2.5 \text{ dyne}.$$

The negative sign denotes an attractive force. The force exerted on q_3 by q_2 is

$$F_1 = \frac{q_1 q_2}{R_1^{\,2}}$$
$$= \frac{(20(-5))}{(10)^2} = -\frac{-100}{900}$$
$$= -0.111 \text{ dyne}$$

Because q_2 is positive and q_3 is negative, this force is attractive and is directed to the right toward q_2.

The resultant force on q_3 is

$$F_r = F_1 - F_2 = -2.5 - (-0.111)$$

and is directed to the left.

B. Charge on Conductors and Insulators

A better understanding of electrostatics requires examining how an object first obtained a charge. Nearly everything in nature is electrically neutral, meaning that everything contains an equal amount of positive and negative charges. However, if an additional charge is added to a normally neutral object by touching the object with a charged rod, the neutral object will then have an extra positive or negative charge. This is known as charging by contact. All extra charges, now on the previously neutral object, are of the same type (all positive or negative). Each charge of the same type will repel one another; therefore, they will spread out, as much as they can, throughout the object. That is why charge can be removed from an object by grounding it to the earth. The earth is very large, allowing the charges to leave the small charged object and spread far from each other, making the object neutral again.

Problem

Show how two metal balls mounted on insulating glass stands may be electrostatically charged with equal amounts but opposite sign charges.

Solution

The two metal balls are assumed to be initially uncharged and touching each other. (Any charge on them may first be removed by touching them to the earth, providing a path for the charge on the spheres to move to the ground.) A charged piece of amber is brought near one of the balls (B) as shown in Figure 49.

FIGURE 49

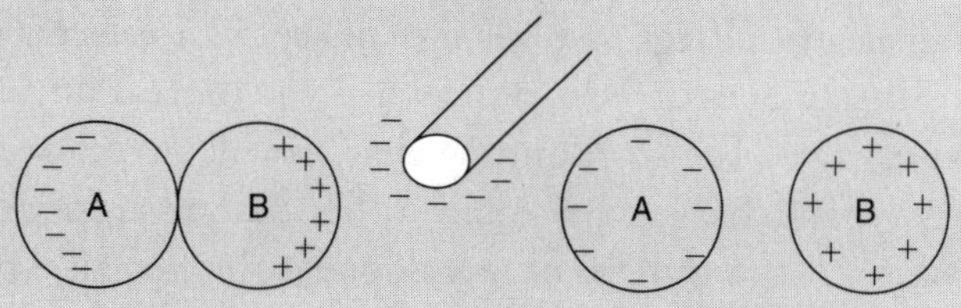

Figure (A) Figure (B)

The negative charge of the amber will repel the electrons in the metal and cause them to move to the far side of *A*, leaving *B* charged positively. If the balls are now separated, *A* retains a negative charge and *B* has an equal amount of positive charge. This method of charging is called charging by induction because it was not necessary to touch the objects being electrified with a charged object (the amber). The charge distribution is induced by the electrical forces associated with the excess electrons present on the surface of the amber.

C. Electric Field

The electric field acting on a charge is defined as the electric force acting on that charge divided by the magnitude of the charge. Therefore, for a single point charge, the electric field is given by

$$\vec{E} = k_e q/r^2\hat{r}.$$

The electric field at a point in space due to a system of point charges can also be found using superposition, summing up the electric fields of the individual point charge. Positive charges are sources of electric field and negative charges are sinks (see Figure 50), which means that electric field vectors point away from positive charges ($+\hat{r}$ direction) and toward negative charges ($-\hat{r}$ direction). Electric field lines are found by connecting electric field vectors, as shown in Figure 51.

FIGURE 50

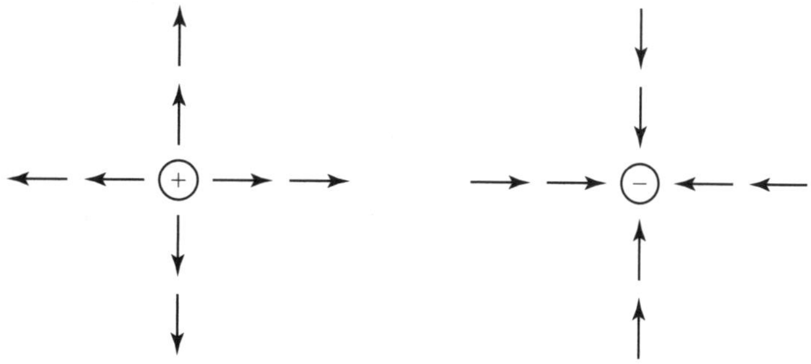

FIGURE 51

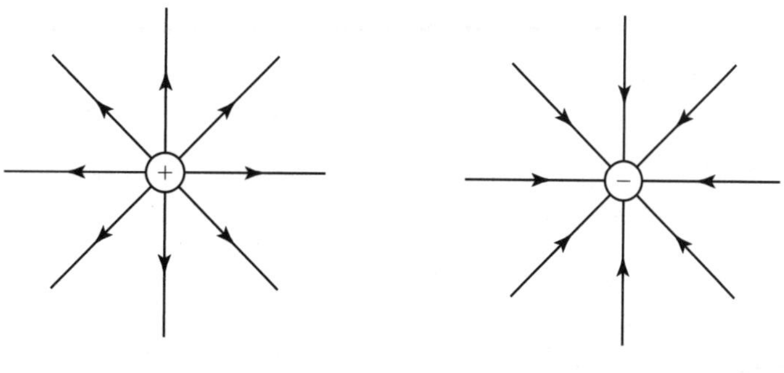

D. Potential Difference

Studying the effect of an electric charge involves the concept of an electrical potential, also known as voltage. Electric potential is the amount of work done when you move a single charge, let's call it a test charge, near an area with other charges. The surrounding charges will attract or repel the test charge. Therefore, work must be done to move the charge while all the other charges are acting on it. If the test charge moves from position *A* to position *B*, the amount of work done is the electrical potential:

$$V = \frac{W}{Q}$$

Using the electric field, the potential difference is

$$V = V_a - V_b = -E_d,$$

where *E* is a constant electric field and *d* is the distance from *B* to *A*.

2. MAGNETICS

A. Magnetic Fields

Magnetics is familiar to all of us from the childhood magnet, which has north and south poles. The magnetic field lines extend from the north pole to the south pole, as shown in Figure 52. Like poles repel one another, and unlike poles attract one another. A magnetic field is produced by the motion of electric charges. Thus, in addition to the electric field, a magnetic field will also be created around a moving electron.

FIGURE 52

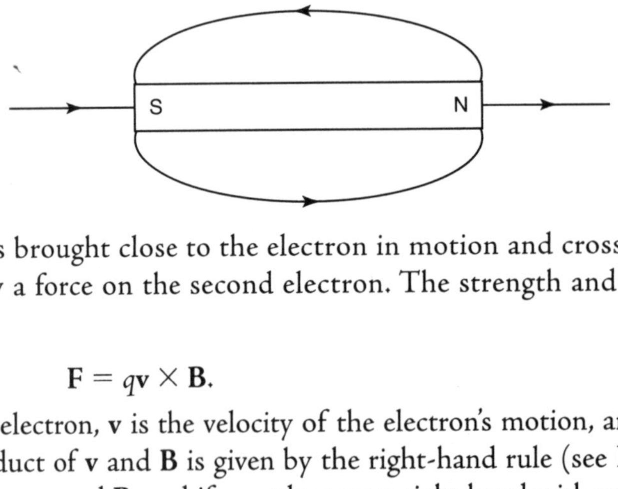

If another electron is brought close to the electron in motion and crosses its magnetic field, the magnetic field will apply a force on the second electron. The strength and direction of this force is given by

$$\mathbf{F} = q\mathbf{v} \times \mathbf{B}.$$

F is the force on the electron, **v** is the velocity of the electron's motion, and **B** is the magnetic field produced. The cross product of **v** and **B** is given by the right-hand rule (see Figure 53). If the vector **v** is moved counterclockwise toward **B,** and if you place your right hand with your fingers curled counterclockwise, the force will be in the direction your thumb is pointing. Remember, the force is related by a cross product, so if an electron is traveling parallel to the magnetic field, no magnetic force will act on it. For a direction other than parallel to the field, the perpendicular component of the velocity will determine the strength of the force. However, regardless of the electron's motion, an electric force will always occur between two electrons.

FIGURE 53

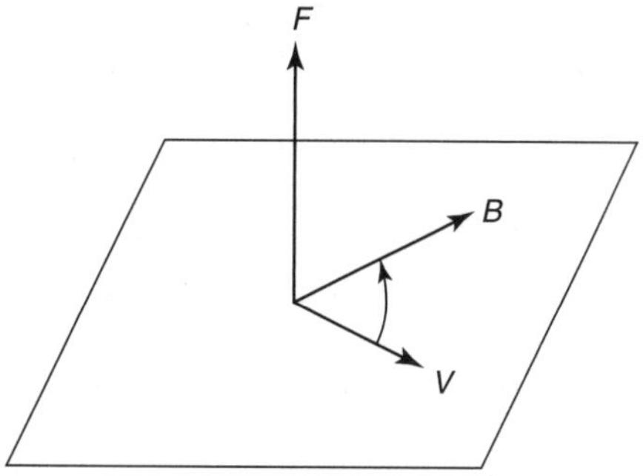

When dealing with problems involving both electric and magnetic forces, the two forces can be calculated separately. Then their influence on another object can be added together. A wire carrying current will also produce a magnetic field because it has a flow of electrons passing through it. To find the magnetic field around the wire, use the formula

$$B = \frac{\mu I}{2\pi r}.$$

The direction of the magnetic field is again given by the right-hand rule. If you hold the wire with your right hand and make sure your thumb is pointing in the direction of the current, your fingers will curl around the wire in the direction of the magnetic field.

Problem

The current from a DC supply is carried to an instrument by two long parallel wires 10 cm apart. What is the magnetic flux density midway between the wires when the current carried is 100 A?

Solution

The magnetic field due to each wire in the diagram at the point midway between them will be into the paper. This may be seen by use of the right-hand rule. If the thumb of your right hand points in the direction of current through the wire, then your fingers will curl in the direction of the magnetic field (or magnetic flux density) created by the current. Application of this rule to both current-carrying wires indicates that the field of each is into the page (see Figure 54). The effects due to the wires are therefore additive at that point and the total effect is twice the effect of either alone.

FIGURE 54

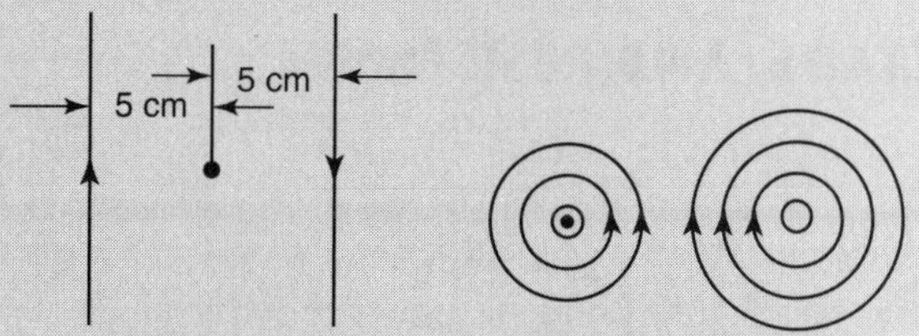

Figure (A): Side View   Figure (B): Top View

Thus, midway between the wires, the magnetic field due to one wire is

$$B = \frac{u_0}{2\pi}\frac{I}{r}$$

where the permeability is

$$\mu_0 = 4\pi \times 10^{-7}\,\text{N-A}^{-2}.$$

I is the current through the wire, and *r* is the distance from the point being considered to the wire. Thus,

$$\text{B} = 2\times10^{-7}\ \text{N-A}^2 \times \frac{100\ \text{A}}{0.05\ \text{m}} = 4\times10^{-4}\ \text{Wb/m}^{-2}$$

The magnetic field due to both wires is then

$$B_T = 2B = 8 \times 10^{-4}\,\text{Wb/m}^{-2}.$$

B. Electromagnetic Spectrum

FIGURE 55

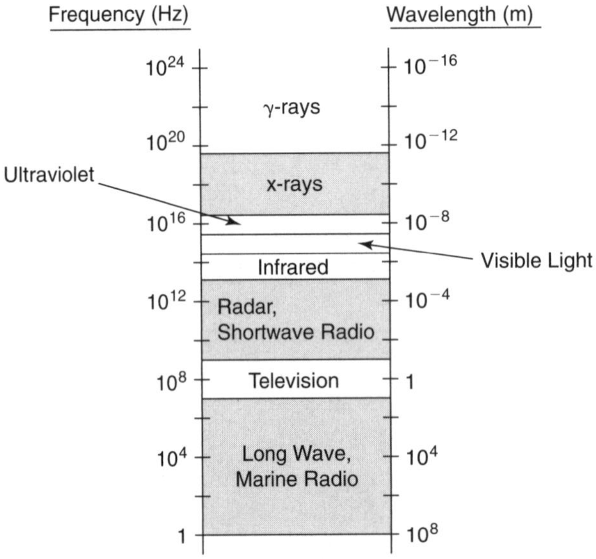

IX. ELECTRIC CIRCUITS

1. CURRENT, VOLTAGE, AND RESISTANCE

A. Current

A current *I* of electricity exists in a conductor whenever electric charge *Q* is being transferred from one point to another point to another point in that conduction.

$$\text{i(Current)} = \frac{\text{q (charge transferred)}}{\text{t (time taken to transfer this charge)}}$$

$$\text{I (amperes)} = \frac{\text{q(coulombs)}}{\text{t (seconds)}}$$

B. Resistance

The basic element of all electric circuits is resistance because all elements in a circuit have some resistance. However, modern technology has found some devices, called superconductors, that have zero resistance. Because use of superconductors is still under development, resistance is still a factor. Resistance is the slowing down of the flow of energy throughout a circuit.

C. Ohm's Law

Current I is the motion of charge through a conductor. A conductor has a current of 1 ampere (amp) when a charge of 1 coulomb per second flows through it. Voltage V is the force or potential that pushes charge through the circuit. For most material, resistance R is the ratio of $\frac{V}{I}$, which is a constant. This is Ohm's law:

$$R = \frac{V}{I} \text{ or } V = IR.$$

For example, a 10-ohm resistor requires 10 volts across it for a current of 1 ampere to flow.

Problem

A car battery supplies a current I of 50 amp to the starter motor. How much charge passes through the starter in 30 seconds?

Solution

Current I is defined as the net amount of charge Q passing a point per unit of time T. Therefore,

$$Q = IT = (50 \text{ amp})\ (30 \text{ sec}) = 1{,}500 \text{ C}.$$

Problem

Find the current through the filament of a light bulb with a resistance of 240 ohms when a voltage of 120 volts is applied to the lamp.

Solution

To find the current, use Ohm's law in the form

$$I = \frac{V}{R}$$

$$V = 120 \text{ volts}$$

$$R = 240 \text{ ohms}$$

$$I = \frac{120}{240} = 0.5 \text{ ampere}$$

Problem

The voltage across the terminals of a resistor is 6.0 volts, and an ammeter connected as in Figure 56 reads 1.5 amp.

A. What is the resistance of the resistor?

B. What would the current be if the potential difference were raised to 8.0 volts?

FIGURE 56

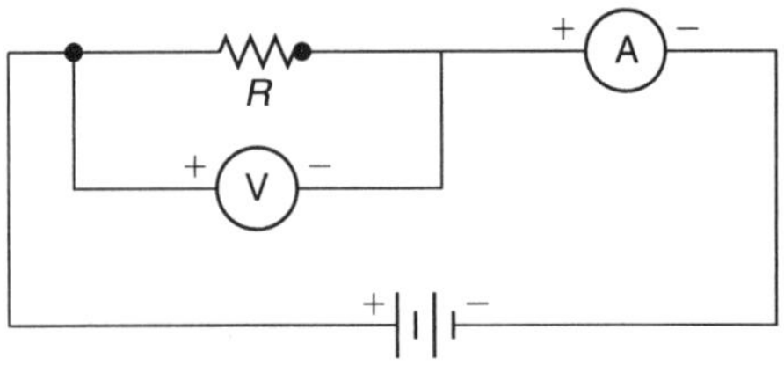

Solution

A. $R = \dfrac{V}{I} = \dfrac{6.0 \text{ volts}}{1.5 \text{ amp}} = 4.0 \text{ ohms}$

B. $I = \dfrac{V}{R} = \dfrac{8.0 \text{ volts}}{4.0 \text{ ohms}} = 2.0 \text{ amps}$

Part A of this solution used the definition of resistance, but part B used Ohm's law — that is, the fact that R is constant.

2. RESISTORS

The value of a resistor is determined by its physical dimensions and a characteristic of the material called resistivity. For a conducting wire, the resistance is given by

$$R = \frac{\rho L}{A},$$

where L is the wire length and A is its cross-sectional area. The resistance is temperature dependent because the resistivity varies with temperature:

$$\Delta R = \alpha R \Delta T$$

This variation is known for different materials and is given by the factor a, the temperature coefficient of resistance.

Problem

What is the resistance of a piece of nichrome wire 225 cm long with a cross-sectional area of 0.015 cm^2? The resistivity (r) for nichrome is 100×10^{-6} ohm-cm.

Solution

To solve this problem, use the relation

$R = \rho \underline{L/A}$
where R = Resistance
ρ = Resistivity
L = Wire length
A = Cross-sectional area

This basic relationship states that resistance is directly proportional to resistivity and length and inversely proportional to cross-sectional area. In the case of a wire, that means resistance depends on the nature of the substance (which appears in the equation as resistivity) and that resistance increases as the wire gets longer and decreases as the wire gets thicker.

The resistivity ρ for nichrome is 100×10^{-6} ohm-cm. The length is 225 cm, and the area is 0.015 cm^2. Thus,

$$R = \frac{10^{-4}\ \text{ohm-cm} \times 225\ \text{cm}}{0.015\ \text{cm}^2} = 1.5\ \text{ohm}.$$

3. PARALLEL-PLATE CAPACITORS

FIGURE 57

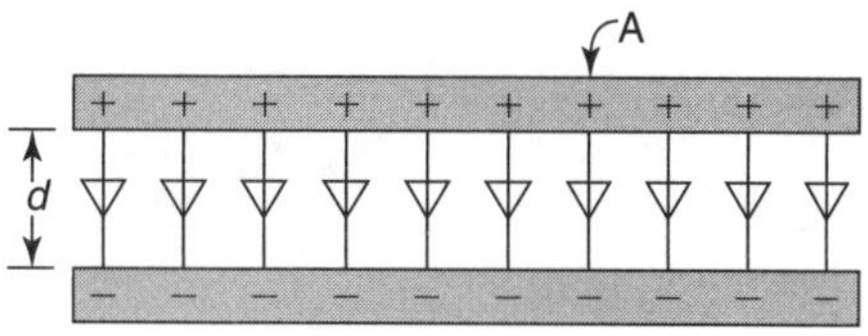

Parallel-plate capacitor

$$C = \frac{Q}{V} = \frac{\epsilon_0 A}{d} \rightarrow \text{units: } \frac{\text{coulomb}}{\text{volt}} = \text{farad}$$

C = Capacitance
Q = Electric charge
V = Electric potential
ε_0 = Permittivity constant
A = Cross-sectional area of plates
d = Distance between plate surfaces

Problem

A given conductor has a potential of 200 volts when charged with 6×10^{-9} coulomb. What is the capacitance of the capacitor formed by the conductor and its surroundings?

Solution

$$\text{Capacitance } C = \frac{\text{charge } Q}{\text{potential } V} = \frac{6 \times 10^{-9}\ \text{coulomb}}{200\ \text{volts}} = 3 \times 10^{-11}\ \text{farad}$$

4. KIRCHHOFF'S VOLTAGE AND CURRENT LAWS FOR A CIRCUIT

The voltage and currents in a circuit can be explained by Kirchhoff's laws. Kirchhoff's voltage law states that the sum of all the voltage drops around a closed loop must equal zero. Thus, for the voltages in Figure 58,

$$V_1 + V_2 + V_3 + V_4 = 0.$$

Kirchhoff's current law states that the sum of all the currents into a node, a point where three or more circuit elements are connected, must equal zero. Therefore, for the circuit of Figure 59,

$$I_1 + I_2 + I_3 = 0.$$

FIGURE 58

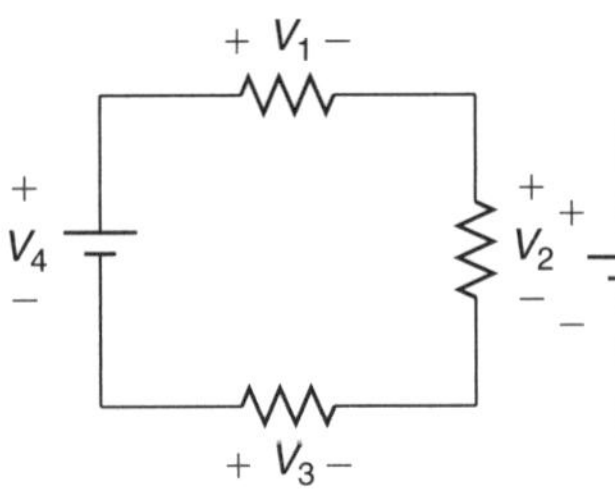

Figure 59

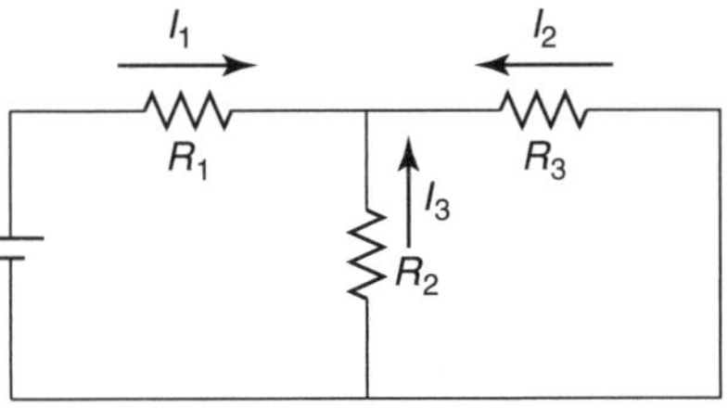

Problem

Two capacitors of capacitance $c_1 = 200$ microfarads (μF) and $c_2 = 600\ \mu$ F are connected in parallel and then charged to a potential of 120 volts. Determine the charge (Q) on each capacitor.

Solution

$Q_1 = c_1$ volts $= 200 \times 10^{-12}$ farads $\times$ 120 v $= 2.4 \times 10^{-8}$ coulombs
$Q_2 = c_2$ volts $= 600 \times 10^{-12}$ farads $\times$ 120 volts $= 7.2 \times 10^{-8}$ coulombs

5. SERIES AND PARALLEL CONNECTIONS

Electric circuits or parts of electric circuits involving series resistances can be simplified by using the fact that series resistances add up:

$$R_T = \Sigma R_i$$

For example, the resistances of the three resistors depicted in Figure 59 can be replaced by one resistor:

$$R_T = R_1 + R_2 + R_3$$

Parallel resistors (R_p) in a circuit, such as R_2 and R_3 in Figure 59, add with the reciprocal rule:

$$1/R_p = \frac{1}{R_2} + \frac{1}{R_3}$$

Thus, the total resistance R_T across the battery in Figure 59 is

$$R_T = R_1 + R_p = R_1 + \frac{R_2 + R_3}{R_2 R_3}$$

Problem

Find the equivalent resistor R and the equivalent capacitor C as shown in Figure 60, where μ F is equivalent to 10^{-6} farad.

Solution

First, examine the resistors. Note that the 2-ohm (Ω) and 6-Ω resistors are in series and can be replaced by a single resistance of $6 + 2 = 8\ \Omega$. Now the 8-Ω and 4-Ω resistors are in parallel. Combine them to get a single resistance R given by

$$\frac{1}{R} = \frac{1}{8} + \frac{1}{4}$$

FIGURE 60

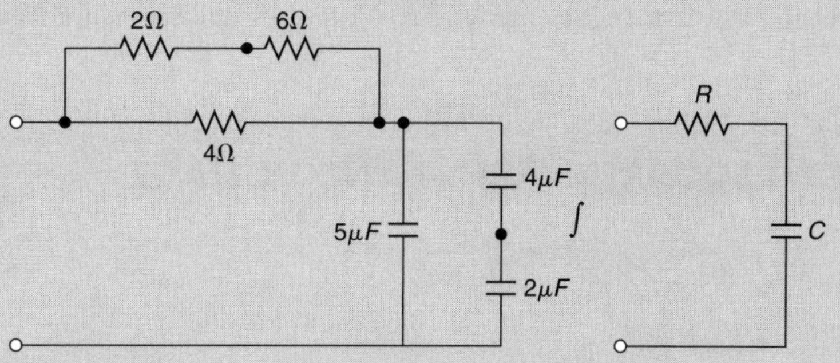

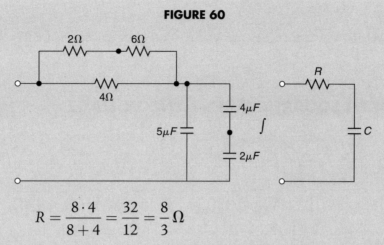

$$R = \frac{8 \cdot 4}{8+4} = \frac{32}{12} = \frac{8}{3}\,\Omega$$

For the capacitors, the 2-μF and 4-μF capacitors are in series, and they can be combined to give a capacitor

$$\frac{2 \cdot 4}{2+4}\mu F \text{ or } \frac{4}{3}\mu F.$$

This will be in parallel with a 5μF capacitor. Therefore,

$$C = 5 + \frac{4}{3} = \frac{19}{3}\mu F.$$

Note that the rule for capacitors is different. Capacitors in series add like resistors in parallel by the reciprocal rule, and capacitors in parallel add like resistors in series.

Problem

Each of five cells has an EMF of 2 volts and internal resistance of 0.6 ohm. What current will they supply to an external resistance of 17 ohm when they are (a) connected in series and (b) connected in parallel?

Solution

a. $\text{Current} = \dfrac{\text{Total EMF}}{\text{Total resistance}}$

$= \dfrac{5 \times 2 \text{ volts}}{(5 \times .6 + 17) \text{ ohm}}$

$= 0.5 \text{ amp}$

b. $\text{Current} = \dfrac{\text{Total EMF}}{\text{Total resistance}}$

$= \dfrac{2 \text{ volts}}{(0.6/5 = 17) \text{ ohm}}$

$= 0.117 \text{ amp}$

6. POWER

To find the power used by a circuit element, the voltage across that element is multiplied by the current through it, or $P = VI$, where P is the power in watts.

7. ROOT MEAN SQUARE CURRENT AND VOLTAGE

To compare the energy an AC signal can deliver to a circuit with the energy a DC signal delivers, an effective or root mean square (RMS) value of current and voltage is used.

$$I_{rms} = \frac{I_m}{\sqrt{2}}$$

$$V_{rms} = \frac{V_m}{\sqrt{2}}$$

I_m = Peak current value (maximum amplitude)
V_m = Peak voltage value

X. LIGHT AND GEOMETRIC OPTICS

1. REFRACTION, REFRACTIVE INDEX, SNELL'S LAW

Recall that light propagates at the following speed in a vacuum.

$$c = f \times \lambda$$

or speed in a medium of index of refraction n:

$$v = \frac{c}{n}$$

Usually, the propagation of light is also represented as a ray moving in a straight line. Many problems in optics use the fact that, for a ray of light, the angle of incidence is equal to the angle of reflection from a mirrored surface. Therefore, the first part of solving an optics problem is to draw an accurate ray diagram.

To solve problems involving the propagation of light from one medium (or index of refraction n_i) to another (or index of refraction n_r), Snell's law is used (see Figure 61). Snell's law states that

$$n_i \sin \theta_i = n_r \sin \theta_r.$$

Therefore, given any three of the four variables, one can solve for the other. Note that for a vacuum or near vacuum (sometimes a good approximation for air), the index of refraction is 1.

FIGURE 61

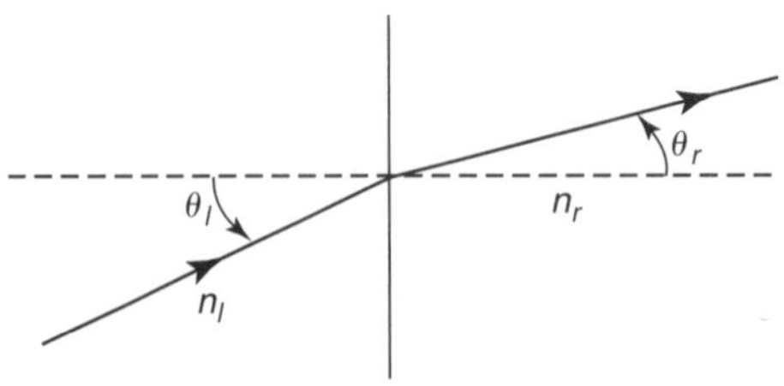

Problem

How fast does light travel in glass of refractive index 1.5?

Solution

By definition, the refractive index n is the ratio of the velocity of light in a vacuum (3.00×10^{10} cm/sec) to the velocity of light in the medium in question. Therefore,

$$n = \frac{3 \times 10^{10} \text{cm/ s}}{v} = 1.5$$

and

$$v = \frac{3 \times 10^{10} \text{ cm/s}}{1.5}$$
$$= 2.00 \times 10^{10} \text{ cm/sec}$$

2. TOTAL INTERNAL REFLECTION

Figure 62 shows that it is conceivable to have an angle of refraction of 90°. When that happens, the angle of incidence is called the critical angle θ_c, given by $\sin \theta_c = \frac{n_r}{n_1}$. An angle of incidence greater than the critical angle indicates total internal reflection: light cannot escape from the first medium. This principle is used to transmit pulses of light in fiber optic communication.

For critical angle θ_c,

$$\sin \theta_c = \frac{n_2}{n_1}, \frac{n_2}{n_1} < 1.$$

FIGURE 62

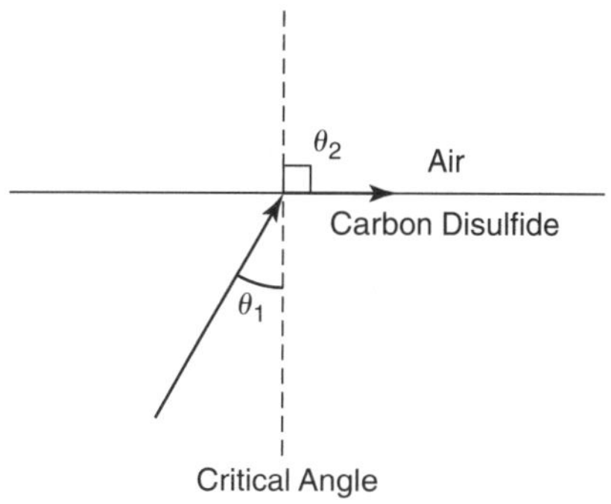

Problem

What is the critical angle between carbon disulfide and air?

Solution

Carbon disulfide is a more optically dense material than air. Therefore, as a beam of light passes from carbon disulfide to air, the angle of refraction is larger than the angle of incidence. There is an angle of incidence smaller than 90° for which the angle of refraction is equal to 90°, meaning that the beam of light emerges parallel to the boundary between the two mediums. This angle of incidence is called the critical angle. If the angle of incidence is greater than this value, the light will not escape from the carbon disulfide. It will be reflected back into the carbon disulfide, following the regular law of reflection. Solving for the critical angle θ_1, let θ_2 be 90°. The index of refraction for carbon disulfide is 1.643 and for air it is 1.00. Using Snell's law,

$$n_1 \sin \theta_1 = n_2 \sin \theta_2$$
$$1.643 \sin \theta_1 = 1.00 \sin 90°$$

$$\sin \theta_1 = \frac{1.00}{1.643} = 0.608$$
$$\theta_1 = 37.4°.$$

3. LENSES AND OPTICAL INSTRUMENTS

The optics of thin lenses may be understood using Snell's law. Again, one must always draw a careful ray diagram in attacking the problem. From Snell's law, a relation called the thin lens equation can be derived:

$$1/s + 1/s' = 1/f$$

where

$$1/f \equiv (n - 1)\,(1/R_1 - 1/R_2)$$

is the reciprocal of the focal length.

This thin lens equation applies to both concave (diverging) and convex (converging) lenses. A convex lens has a positive focal length f (see Figure 63 for a typical ray diagram), whereas in a concave lens, $f < 0$. The object seen by the lens is said to be real if the object distance is positive. The image is said to be real if the image distance is positive. Otherwise, the object or image is called virtual. The image is right-side up if the magnification (m_1) is positive, and the image is inverted if $m_1 < 0$.

The simple microscope consists of one lens placed near the eye, with the object just inside the focal point of the lens and the image at the near point of the eye. Using the thin lens equation gives $\frac{1}{s} = \frac{1}{f} + \frac{1}{25}$ or, for the magnification,

$$m_1 = \frac{h'}{h} = -\frac{s'}{s} = 1 + \frac{25}{f}$$

FIGURE 63

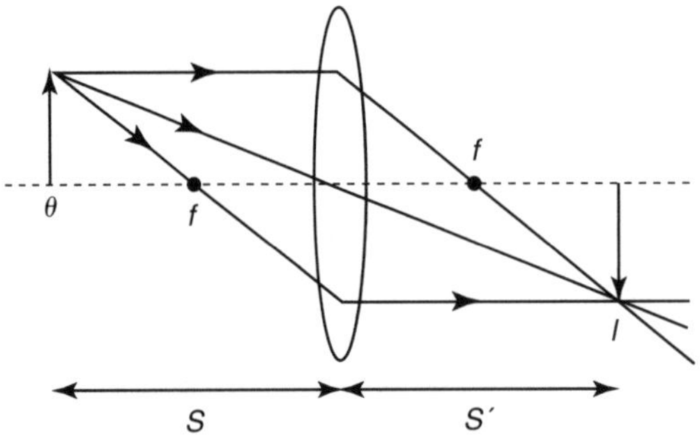

When the eye is relaxed, the object at the focal point of the lens and the image is at infinity. In that case, a smaller magnification of $m_1 = \frac{25}{f}$ is obtained.

The compound microscope consists of two lenses, an objective and an eyepiece. The two lenses are separated by a distance l very much greater than f_e or

$$f_0 : 1 >> f_0, f_e.$$

The object is placed just outside the focal length of the objective, forming an image close to the focal length of the eyepiece. The eyepiece serves as a simple magnifier for this first image. The net magnification is thus

$$m_1 = m_0 m_e = -\frac{1}{f_0} \times \frac{25}{f_e}.$$

The telescope also makes use of an objective and an eyepiece separated by a distance l. In this case,

$$l = f_0 + f_e.$$

The first image is formed at the focal point of the objective because the object is at infinity. The magnification is then

$$m_1 = -\frac{f_0}{f_e}.$$

Therefore, it is essential for the telescope that the objective focal length be greater than the eyepiece focal length.

Problem

A converging lens with a focal length of 3 m forms an image of an object placed 9 m from it. Using the diagram in Figure 64, find the position of the image and the magnification.

FIGURE 64

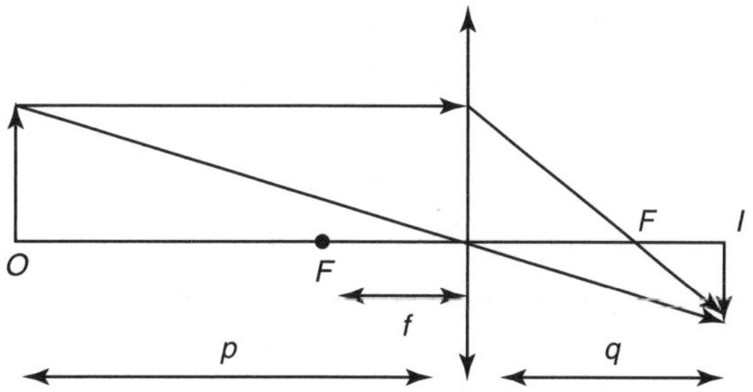

Solution

The simple lens equation for the covering lens of this problem is

$$\frac{1}{f} = \frac{1}{p} + \frac{1}{q}$$

where f, p, and q are, respectively, the focal length of the lens and the distances of the object and the image from the lens. The image is real and inverted, as shown in the figure. Substituting the given values in the above equation gives

$$\frac{1}{f} = \frac{1}{p} + \frac{1}{q} = \frac{1}{3\text{ m}} - \frac{1}{9\text{ m}} = \frac{2}{9}\text{m}^{-1}$$

and

$$q = \frac{9}{2}\text{m} = 4.5\text{ m}$$

Because the value of q is positive, the image occurs on the right side of the lens. The magnification M is

$$M = \frac{q}{p} = \frac{4.5\text{ m}}{9\text{ m}} = 0.5,$$

so the image is one-half as high as the object.

Problem

When an object is placed 10 in. from a certain lens, its virtual image is formed 10 in. from the lens. Determine the focal length and character of the lens.

Solution

Because the image is virtual, on the same side of the lens as the object, its distance from the lens, q, is negative. Substitution in the general equation for lenses yields

$$\frac{1}{p}+\frac{1}{q}=\frac{1}{f}$$

$$\frac{1}{20\text{ in}}+\frac{1}{-10\text{ in}}=\frac{1}{f}$$

$$\frac{1}{f}=\frac{-10\text{ in}+20\text{ in}}{(20\text{ in})\times(-10\text{ in})}=-\frac{10}{200\text{ in}}$$

$$f=-20\text{ in.}$$

The negative sign for the focal length indicates that the lens is diverging. Diverging lenses are concave. **See Biology Review, Vision, page 202.**

The extremes of the range over which vision is possible are called the far point and the near point of the eye. The far point of the normal eye is at infinity.

Problem

The near point of a certain eye is 100 cm in front of the eye. What lens should be used to see clearly an object 25 cm in front of the eye?

Solution

$s = +25\text{ cm} \qquad s' = -100\text{ cm}$

$$\frac{1}{f}=\frac{1}{s}+\frac{1}{s'}=\frac{1}{25}+\frac{1}{-100}$$

$$f=+33\text{ cm}$$

A converging lens of focal length of 33 cm is required.

4. POLARIZATION

Polarized light is light that has waves in only one plane. This light can be obtained by passing unpolarized light through a material that allows light to pass through in only one plane, as shown in Figure 65.

FIGURE 65

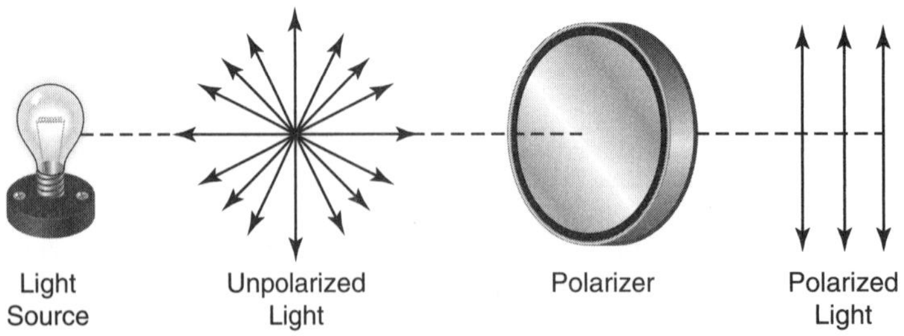

5. DISPERSION

Because for some transparent materials the index of refraction depends on frequency, the speeds of the various wavelengths of light will not be the same when passing through these transparent materials. That the speeds of wavelengths of light are different in a refracting medium is called dispersion.

6. VISUAL SPECTRUM, COLOR

Color	Wavelength (angstroms)
Ultraviolet	< 4,000
Violet	4,000–4,250
Blue	4,250–4,900
Green	4,900–5,750
Yellow	5,750–5,850
Orange	5,850–6,500
Red	6,500–7,000
Infrared	> 7,000

XI. ATOMIC AND NUCLEAR PHYSICS

1. QUANTUM THEORY

A. Work of Einstein and Planck

In the preceding section, the properties of light were discussed within the context of classical optics. Classical physics alone can explain many properties of light, but not all. Einstein postulated that a beam of light consisted of small bundles of energy. These energy bundles are light quanta, or photons. The energy E of a photon is proportional to its frequency f.

$$E = hv$$

where h = Planck's constant = 6.63×10^{-34} J·sec.

Problem

What is the energy of a photon of green light (frequency = 6×10^{14} vps)?

Solution

Planck's hypothesis states that $E = hv$, where v is the frequency of the radiation and h is Planck's constant. Therefore,

$$E = (6.63 \times 10^{-34}\text{ J·sec})\,(6 \times 10^{14}\text{ vps})$$
$$E = 3.98 \times 10^{-19}\text{ J.}$$

This observation by Einstein explained the photoelectron effect. In this phenomenon, when a photon collides with an electron in, for example, the surface of a metal, the energy of the photon may be transferred to the electron. This is an all-or-none process. The work function is the minimum energy to free the electron.

Problem

Will photoelectrons be emitted by a copper surface of work function 4.4 ev when illuminated by visible light?

Solution

$$\gamma = \frac{c}{f} = \frac{hv}{hf} = \frac{6.63 \times 10^{-34}\,\text{J·sec} \times 3 \times 10^{8}\,\text{m/sec}}{4.4(1.6 \times 10^{-19})\,\text{J}} = 2.82 \times 10^{-7}\,\text{m} = 2{,}820 \text{ angstroms}$$

Because the wavelength is too short, visible light cannot eject photoelectrons from copper.

B. Bohr's Model of the Hydrogen Atom

An explanation for the line spectrum of the hydrogen atom was required. Because of this, Niels Bohr proposed a mechanical model of the hydrogen atom. To account for the observation that negatively charged electrons revolve around the positively charged nucleus, Bohr postulated that the electrical attraction provided the necessary centripetal force. He then postulated that an electron in an atom revolves in certain stable orbits. An orbit has a defined associated energy. The Bohr theory of the hydrogen atom also states that if an electron goes from one orbit to another orbit of energy, a photon of energy is radiated. The concept of definitive electronic orbits has been subsequently discarded by wave mechanics, but the idea of different energy levels for the atom remains. **See Chemistry Review, Electronic Structure, page 274.**

FIGURE 66

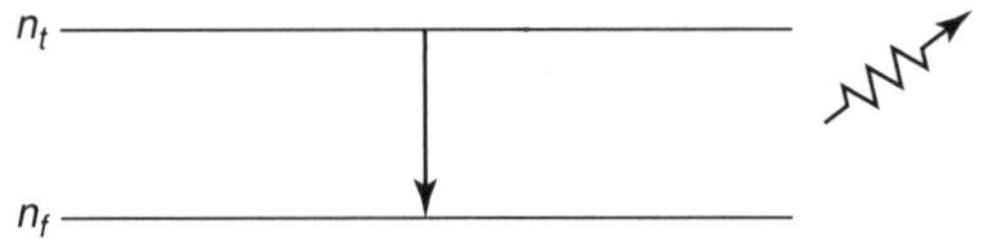

2. NUCLEAR REACTIONS

In ordinary chemical reactions, the identity of the atoms as reactants and products does not change. In these reactions, the outer electrons of atoms are transferred from one to another. In contrast, in nuclear reactions the atomic nuclei of the reactants are changed by either the emission of a particle or absorption of a particle. As a result, the atomic number and the identity of the reacting atoms are changed.

In a typical nuclear reaction $I + T \rightarrow R + E$, where an incident particle interacts with a target particle to produce an emitted particle and a residual particle, a Q value can be defined as follows:

$$Q = (m_I + m_t - m_i - m_R)\, C^2.$$

If $Q > 0$, the reaction is exoergic; if $Q < 0$, the reaction is endoergic or requires energy. This approach is useful in the radioactive decay of one particle by taking $m_I = 0$.

The nuclei of the elements consist of protons and neutrons. A proton has a + 1 charge and by definition is equal to the atomic number of an element. The atomic weight is equal to the sum of the masses of the protons and neutrons in the nucleus of an atom. From the periodic table, the number of protons in the element carbon is 6 because the atomic number is 6. The atomic weight is 12, and so the most common isotope of carbon has 6 neutrons and 6 protons. Carbon-14 has 8 neutrons.

When dealing with nuclear reactions, the key is to keep track of which particles are emitted and how much of the mass of the elements involved changes. Each particle in a reaction is assigned a symbol with a superscript giving the mass number and a subscript for the atomic number. Also, some reactions will involve the loss of energy in the form of gamma rays. In this case, the particles involved do not change mass but instead change in energy.

Problem

B^{10} is bombarded with neutrons, and particles are observed to be emitted. What is the residual nucleus?

Solution

Only alpha particles (helium nuclei) are observed to be emitted in the reaction. The reaction can be described as follows:

$$^{10}_{5}B + ^{1}_{0}n \rightarrow ^{A}_{Z}(X) + ^{4}_{2}He,$$

where the superscript gives the mass number A. It is the total number of protons and neutrons in that nucleus. In a nuclear reaction the total nucleon number and the total charge is conserved; therefore, the mass number A of the unknown nucleus must be such that

$$10 + 1 = A + 4.$$

Therefore, $A = 7$.

The subscripts refer to the atomic numbers, the total number of protons in each nucleus. Because the reaction involves protons and neutrons only, the protons carry the total charge. The conservation of total electric charge in that case reduces to the conservation of the total number of protons. Therefore,

$$5 + 0 = Z + 2 \text{ or } Z = 3.$$

The nucleus with $A = 7, Z = 3$ is $^{7}_{3}Li$. See **Chemistry Review, Nuclear Chemistry, page 328.**

3. EINSTEIN'S RELATION

$$E = mc^2$$

An object's mass can also be described as an amount of energy.

Problem

What is the energy content of 1 gm of water?

Solution

If the mass of the gram of water were completely converted to energy, the amount of energy released would be

$$\begin{aligned} E &= mc^2 \\ &= 1 \times 10^{-3}\,\text{kg} \times (3 \times 10^8\,\text{m/sec})^2 \\ &= 9 \times 10^{13}\,\text{joules} \end{aligned}$$

4. RADIOACTIVE DECAY AND HALF-LIFE

Radiation is pervasive in various forms: light (4,000- to 8,000-angstrom photons), radio waves, black-body photons, cosmic ray particles, among others. Many forms of radiation, especially particles, follow an exponential law:

$$N = N_0 e^{-\lambda t}$$

where γ is the decay constant.

This exponential decay can be related to the half-life $t_{1/2}$ because

$$N_0 / 2 = N_0 e^{-\lambda t1/2}$$

Using the natural logarithm gives

$$t_{1/2} = \ln \frac{2}{1}$$

Problem

The half-life of radon is 3.80 days. After how many days will only one-sixteenth of a radon sample remain?

Solution

A half-life of 3.80 days means that every 3.80 days, half the amount of radon present decays. Because one-sixteenth is a power of one-half, this problem can be solved by counting. After 3.80 days, one-half the original sample remains. In the next 3.80 days, one-half of that decays; thus, after 7.60 days one-fourth of the original amount remains. After 11.4 days, one-eighth of the original amount remains, and after four half-lives (15.2 days), one-sixteenth the original amount remains.

As an alternative solution, the formula for decaying matter can be used:

$$\frac{N}{N_0} = e^{-\lambda t_{\frac{1}{2}}}$$

λ is an experimental constant that can be determined from the half-life. Therefore, for

$$\frac{N}{N_0} = \frac{1}{2},$$

$$\ln \frac{N}{N_0} = \lambda t_{\frac{1}{2}}$$

$$\lambda = \frac{\ln \frac{N}{N_0}}{t_{\frac{1}{2}}} = \frac{\ln 2}{t_{\frac{1}{2}}} = \frac{0.693}{3.80 \text{ days}} = 0.182 \text{ day}.$$

For $N/N_0 = 1/16 = e^{-\lambda t} = e^{-0.182t}$,

$$\frac{N}{N_0} = \frac{1}{16},$$

$$\ln \frac{N}{N_0} = -0.182t$$

$$\frac{\ln \frac{N}{N_0}}{0.182} = t$$

$$\frac{\ln 16}{0.182} = \frac{2.77}{0.182} = 15.2 \text{ days}.$$

MCAT

MEDICAL COLLEGE ADMISSION TEST

Biology Review

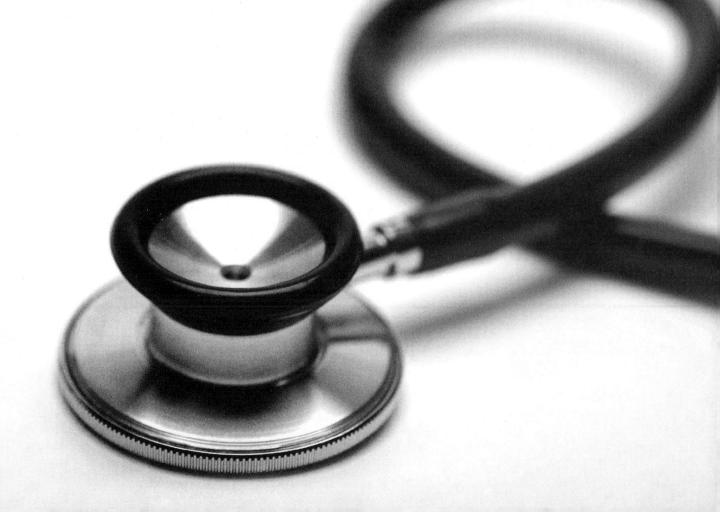

I. MOLECULAR BIOLOGY

1. PROPERTIES OF WATER

Water is essential to life, and wherever water is found, it is likely that life is present as well. Three-quarters of the earth's surface is covered by water, and water constitutes 80–90% by weight of any living thing. Water has some unique chemical and physical properties that make it an extraordinary liquid, and one that is required for life.

Chemically, water consists of hydrogen and oxygen linked by polar covalent bonds. The lone electron pairs on oxygen form a dipole, and water is characterized by areas of partially negative and partially positive charges. Hydrogen bonds are formed between the partially positive hydrogen atom and the electronegative oxygen atom. See Chemistry Review, Bonding, page 286.

In water, the shape determined by the central oxygen is called bent, and the bond angle is 109° (Figure 1).

FIGURE 1. Water Molecule

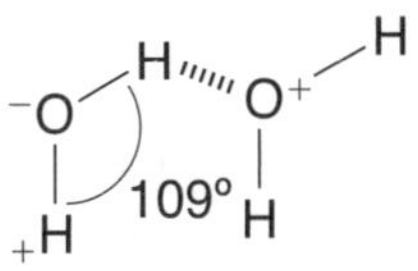

Water is a polar solvent, and because "like dissolves like," water is a good solvent for polar biological macromolecules as well as inorganic substances. A number of inorganic ions are essential to biological systems. See Chemistry Review, Solution Chemistry, page 300.

Despite its low molecular weight, water exists as a liquid at room temperature. A large amount of energy is required to convert liquid water into gaseous water or water vapor, and this phenomenon is reflective of the strength of the hydrogen bond in water. The specific heat of water is quite high, so a great deal of heat is required to raise the temperature of water. Consequently, the temperatures of living systems, which are mainly water, are relatively constant. See Chemistry Review, Thermodynamics and Thermochemistry, page 317.

Water has its greatest density at 4°C and is less dense when frozen. Consequently, ice floats and water sinks at 4°C. In aquatic systems, water usually freezes from the top of the body of water to the bottom. Organisms living near the bottoms of lakes and ponds are protected. See Physics Review, Fluids and Solids, page 107.

Problem

What property of water is most responsible for its unique characteristics?

A. Boiling point
B. Density
C. Specific heat
D. Hydrogen bonding

Solution

D. Hydrogen bonding is the phenomenon that is most responsible for the boiling point, density, and specific heat of water. Choices A, B, and C are consequences of hydrogen bonding.

2. BIOLOGICAL MOLECULES

There are four major classes of biological molecules: carbohydrates, lipids, proteins, and nucleic acids. These molecules differ systematically in their structure and function. Six elements make up 99% of all living organisms: carbon, hydrogen, nitrogen, oxygen, phosphorus, and sulfur.

A. CARBOHYDRATES

Carbohydrates have two important functions in the cell: (1) They are the principal energy source for most living things, and (2) they are the material that forms the basis for other types of material.

Carbohydrates are called sugars and, as the name *carbohydrates* implies, contain only carbon, hydrogen, and oxygen. In every carbohydrate, the proportion of carbon to hydrogen to oxygen is CH_2O. There are three kinds of carbohydrates: monosaccharides, or "simple sugars"; disaccharides, or "two sugars"; and polysaccharides, or "many sugars." Examples of monosaccharides are glucose, fructose, and ribose. Examples of disaccharides are sucrose, maltose, and lactose. The suffix *ose* means "sugar." Representatives of the polysaccharides are cellulose and starch.

By virtue of the equal number of oxygen atoms for every carbon atom, carbohydrates are polar molecules and are, for the most part, soluble in water. The oxygen atoms are mainly bonded to form alcohols, and the high numbers of hydroxyl groups make carbohydrates water soluble. The remaining oxygen atoms are either aldehydes or ketones. In solution, these carbonyl groups react with the hydroxyl groups to from cyclic etherlike structures. **See Organic Chemistry Review, Functional Groups, page 334.**

The six-membered ring that glucose forms has hydroxyl groups above and below the plane of the ring. When the hydroxyl group attached to the carbon bearing the ether linkage is on the same side as the substituent at carbon-6, the anomer is designated as beta glucose. When the hydroxyl group is on the opposite side of the substituent at carbon-6, the isomer is called alpha glucose. In solution, all three forms are present and are in equilibrium with one another. The process by which the beta form changes into the alpha form, and vice versa, is called mutorotation (Figure 2). **See Chemistry Review, Equilibrium, page 324.**

FIGURE 2. Mutorotation of Glucose

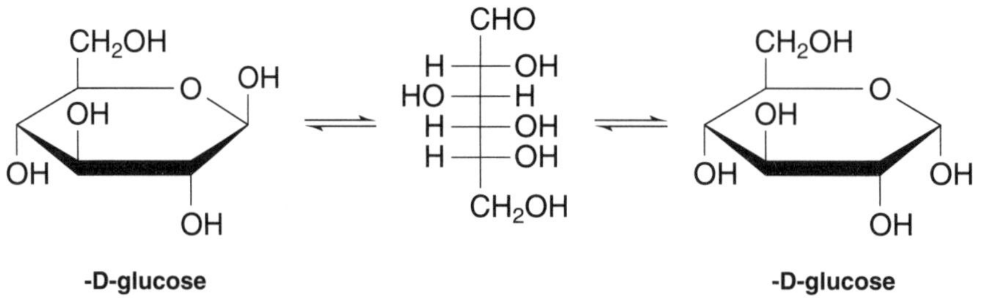

See Organic Chemistry Review, Aldehydes and Ketones, page 345.

Important disaccharides include sucrose (cane sugar), maltose (malt sugar), and lactose (milk sugar). Sucrose consists of glucose and fructose. Maltose is formed from two glucose units, and lactose consists of glucose and galactose. Disaccharides are formed by the removal of water from two monosaccharides. The addition of water splits sucrose into its glucose and fructose units. Chemically, this process is acid catalyzed, and the splitting is called hydrolysis.

When many monosaccharides are joined together, polysaccharides are formed. Three important polysaccharides that consist only of glucose units are starch, glycogen, and cellulose. Starch is used as the stored energy source in plants, whereas glycogen is the stored energy source in animals. Cellulose is the structural polysaccharide in plants, and approximately 50% of wood is cellulose. The difference between these polysaccharides rests in the way the glucose units are bonded together. Cellulose has only beta linkages, and starch and glycogen have only alpha linkages.

Problem

Sucrose is table sugar and has the molecular formula of $C_{11}H_{20}O_{10}$. Sucrose is freely soluble in water. Which of the following characteristics is the principal reason that sucrose is very soluble in water?

A. Mutorotation
B. Hydrolysis
C. Hydrogen bonding
D. Combustion

Solution

C. Although sucrose has 11 carbons, the significant number of oxygen atoms present renders the compound water soluble. These oxygen atoms are mainly in the form of hydroxyl groups. Hydrogen bonds between the water molecules and the hydroxyl groups make sucrose water soluble. In the absence of an acid catalyst, the hydrolysis of sucrose to glucose and fructose is very slow.

B. Lipids

Lipids are a family of substances found in living organisms that are insoluble in water. They are nonpolar materials and are soluble in nonpolar solvents. Lipids span a variety of structural types that include fatty acids, triglycerides, phospholipids, glycolipids, terpenes, steroids, and prostaglandins.

In the body, lipids play three major roles: (1) They store energy in fat cells, (2) they form parts of cell membranes and serve to separate cellular solutions from one other, and (3) they function as chemical messengers.

Fatty acids are long-chain carboxylic acids, and only a small proportion of lipids are free carboxylic acids. Animal fats and vegetable oils are triglycerides. Triglycerides are esters of glycerol (Figure 3) and fatty acids. Saturated fatty acids have only single bonds in the hydrocarbon chain, and unsaturated fatty acids have at least one double bond in the chain.

FIGURE 3. Glycerol

CH_2OH
|
$CHOH$
|
CH_2OH

See Organic Chemistry Review, Carboxylic Acids, page 350.

In triglycerides, all three hydroxyl groups are esterified (Figure 4).

Saturated fats typically come from animal sources and are solids at room temperature. Oils are vegetable in origin and contain unsaturated fatty acids.

Complex lipids are the phospholipids and the glycolipids. Glycolipids are complex lipids that contain carbohydrates. Phospholipids contain an alcohol, two fatty acids, and a phosphate group. In glycerophospholipids, the alcohol is glycerol.

FIGURE 4. Triglyceride

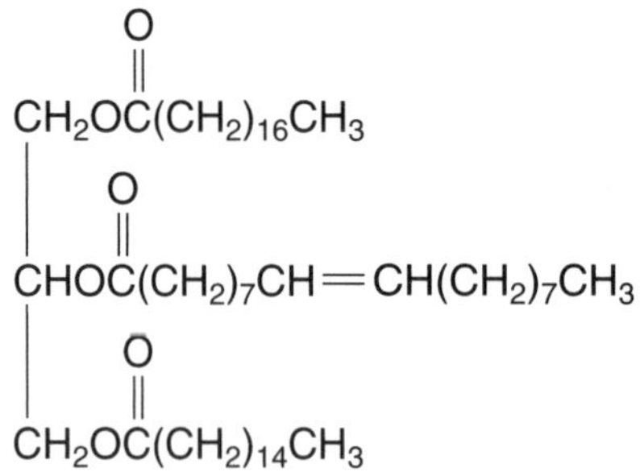

Phospholipids are important components of many cellular membranes. In a phospholipid, one end of the molecule is polar because of the presence of the water-soluble phosphate group, and the other portions are very nonpolar because of the long fatty acid chain.

Terpenes are characteristically odoriferous and are thus known as essential oils. Structurally, they contain isoprene subunits. Isoprene is 2-methyl-1, 3-butadiene. Vitamin A is a terpene and a fat-soluble vitamin important in vision.

Steroids have four carbon-containing rings, and the ring system is exemplified by the well-known substance cholesterol (Figure 5).

FIGURE 5. Cholesterol

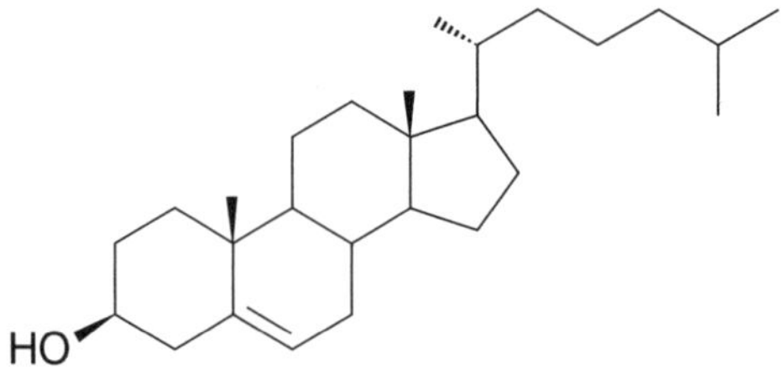

Cholesterol serves two functions in the body: (1) It is a component of plasma membranes in most animal cells; and (2) it is the precursor for the synthesis of other steroids, such as the steroidal hormones testosterone and estrogen, and bile salts.

Prostaglandins are C_2O-carboxylic acids that contain a five-membered ring, at least one double bond, and several oxygen-containing functionalities (Figure 6). Prostaglandins are very potent in small amounts, and their activity results in a broad spectrum of effects. They can lower or raise blood pressure, cause inflammation and blood clotting, and induce labor.

FIGURE 6. Prostaglandin

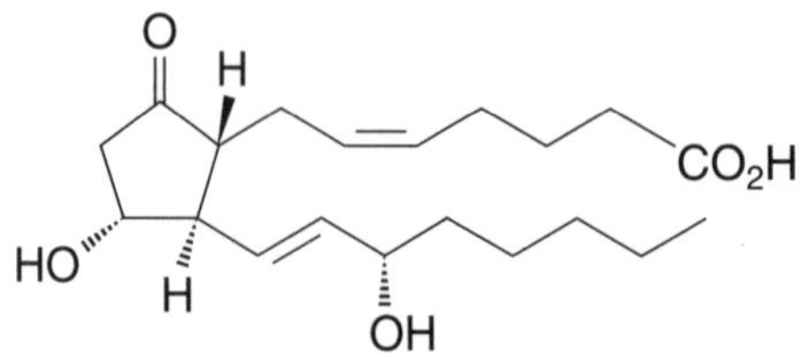

Problem

Whale blubber consists mainly of

A. fatty acids.　　　B. triglycerides.　　　C. glycerophospholipids.　　　D. steroids.

Solution

B. Whale blubber is fat tissue and therefore composed of triglycerides.

C. PROTEINS

The most important of the biological macromolecules are proteins. A protein is a large molecule that consists of amino acids. Amino acids are the fundamental component of proteins, and amino acids have some unique features.

There are 20 naturally occurring amino acids (Table 1), and combinations of these 20 amino acids make up proteins. As the name *amino acid* implies, an amino acid contains an amine functional group and a carboxylic acid. The structure of an amino acid is shown in Figure 7, and the 20 amino acids in nature fit this structure.

TABLE 1. The 20 Amino Acids

Amino Acid	Three-Letter Abbreviation	One-Letter Symbol	Formula
Aliaphatic Amino Acids			
Glycine	Gly	G	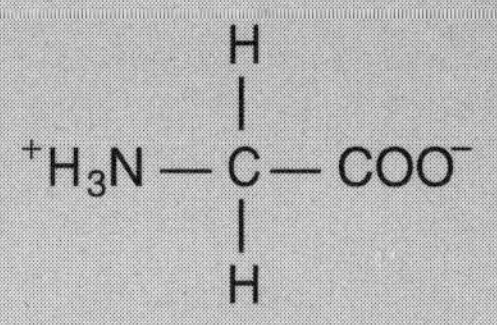 $^+H_3N-C(H)(H)-COO^-$
Alanine	Ala	A	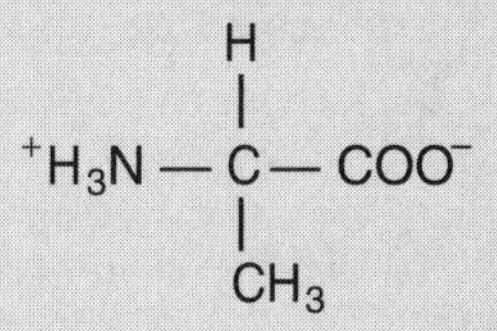 $^+H_3N-C(H)(CH_3)-COO^-$
Valine*	Val	V	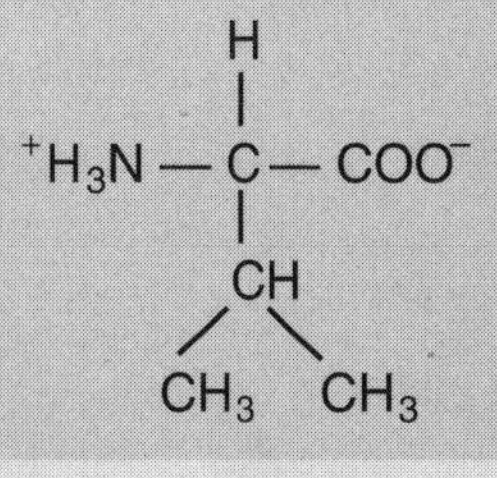 $^+H_3N-C(H)(CH(CH_3)_2)-COO^-$
Leucine*	Leu	L	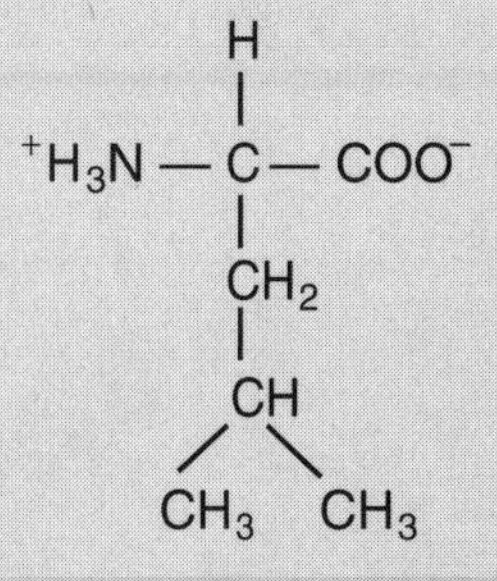 $^+H_3N-C(H)(CH_2CH(CH_3)_2)-COO^-$

(Continued)

TABLE 1. *Continued*

Amino Acid	Three-Letter Abbreviation	One-Letter Symbol	Formula
Isoleucine*	Ile	I	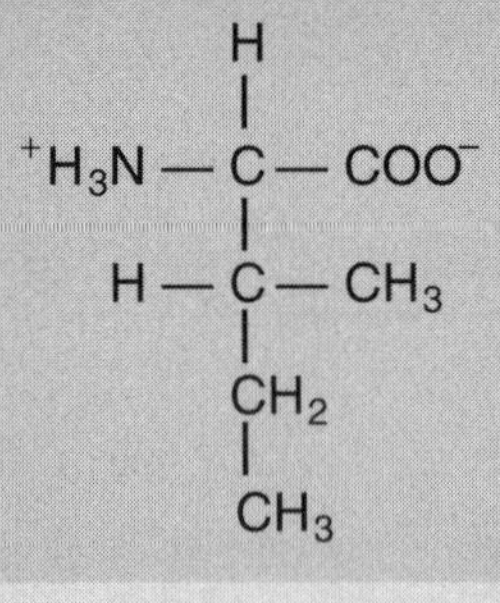
Aliphatic Hydroxyl Side Chains			
Serine	Ser	S	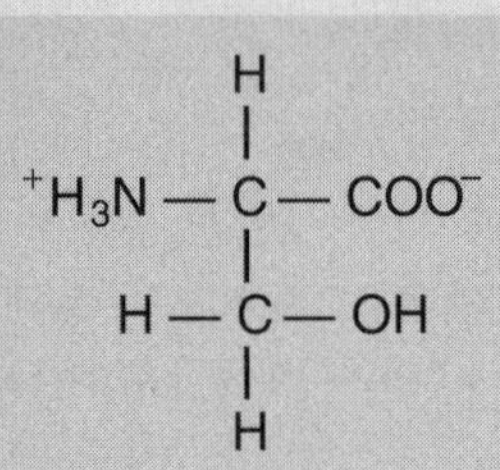
Threonine*	Thr	T	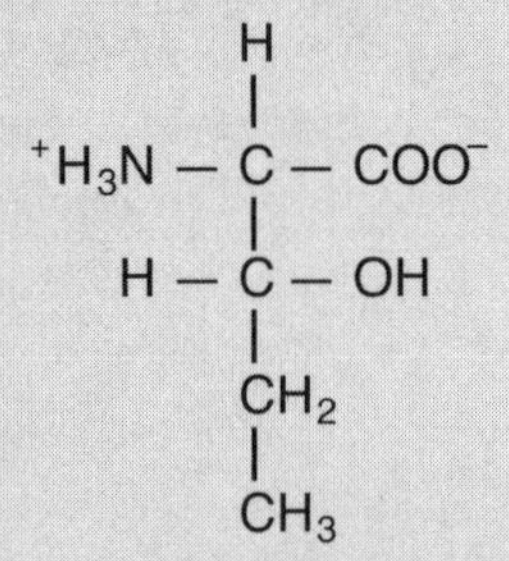
Aromatic Side Chains			
Phenylalanine*	Phe	F	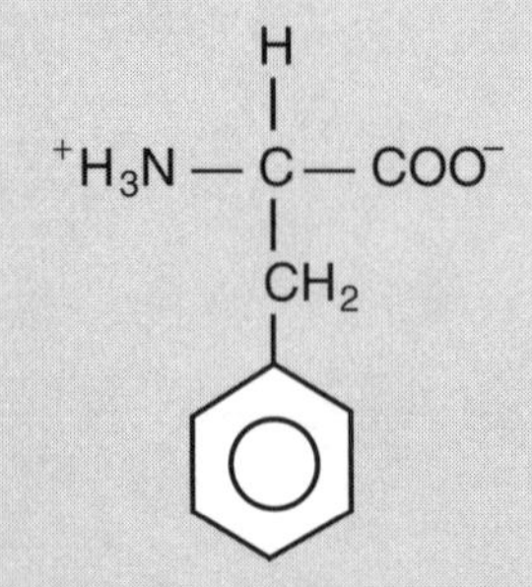
Tyrosine	Tyr	Y	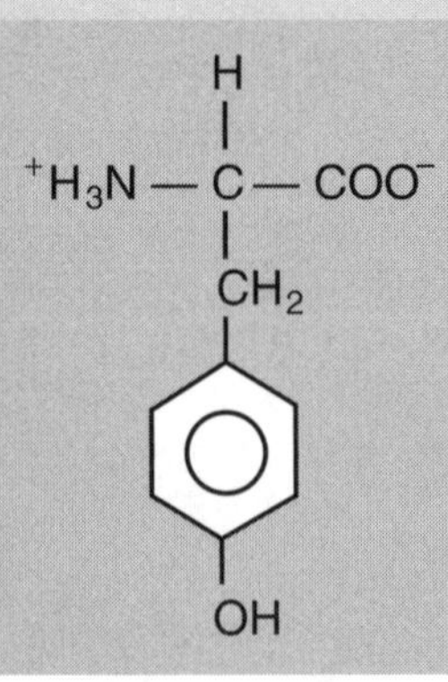

Amino Acid	Three-Letter Abbreviation	One-Letter Symbol	Formula
Tryptophan*	Trp	W	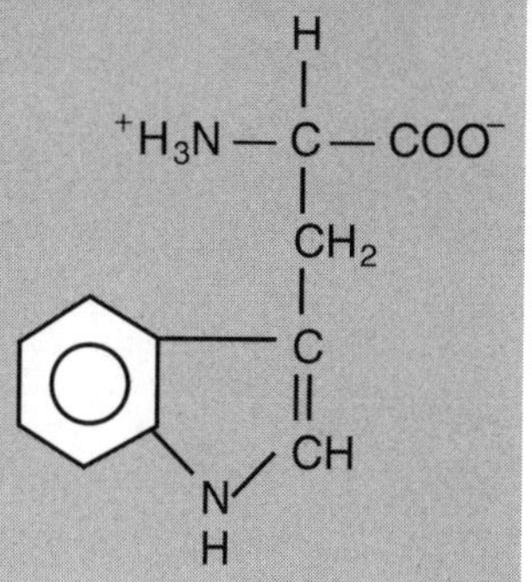
Basic Amino Acids			
Lysine*	Lys	K	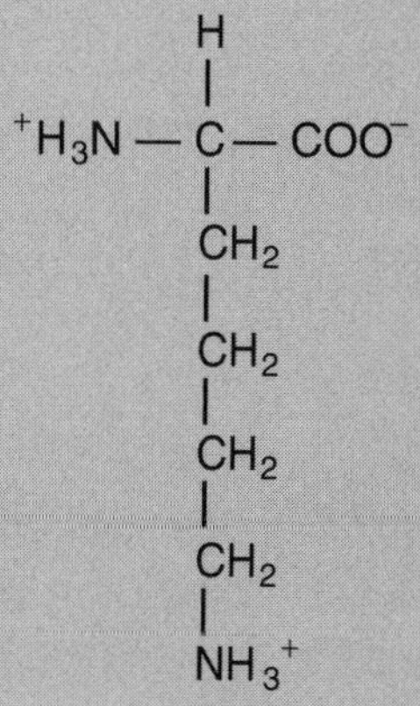
Arginine*	Arg	R	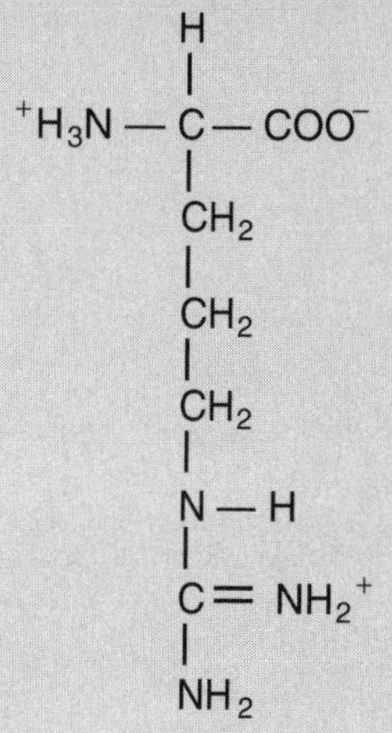

(Continued)

TABLE 1. *Continued*

Amino Acid	Three-Letter Abbreviation	One-Letter Symbol	Formula
Histidine*	His	H	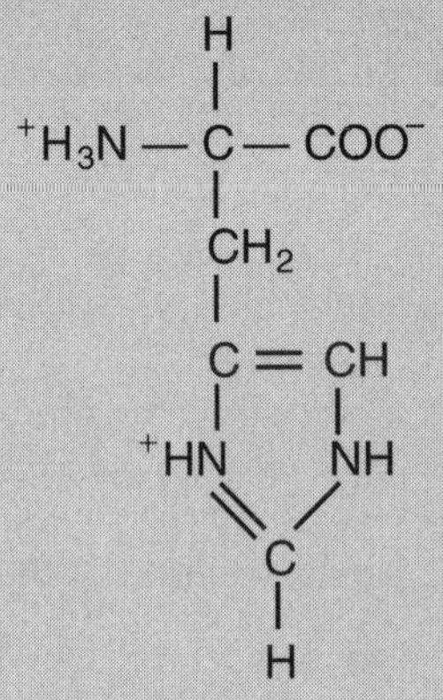
Acidic Amino Acids			
Aspartate (or Aspartic Acid)	Asp	D	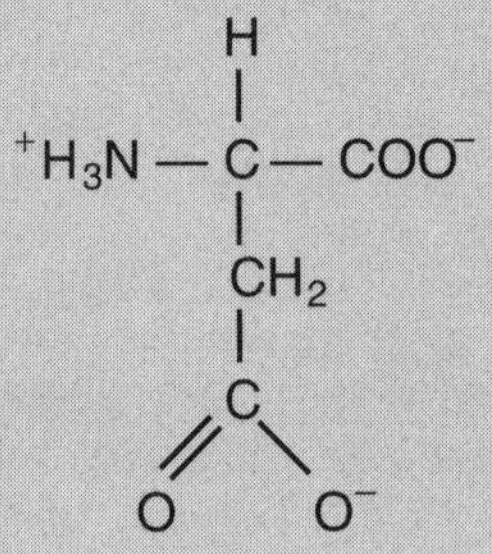
Glutamate (or Glutamic Acid)	Glu	E	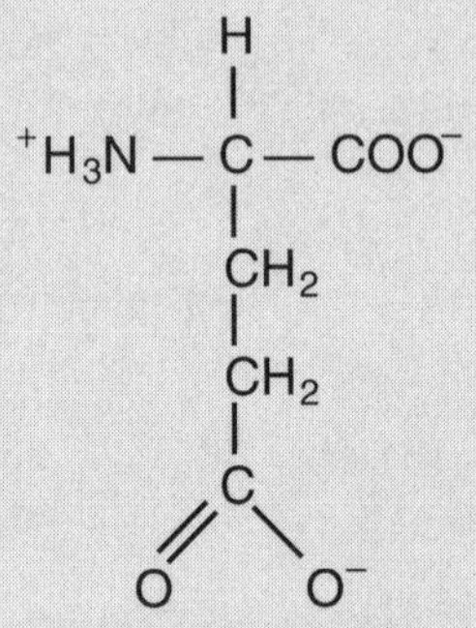
Amide-containing Amino Acids			
Asparagine	Asn	N	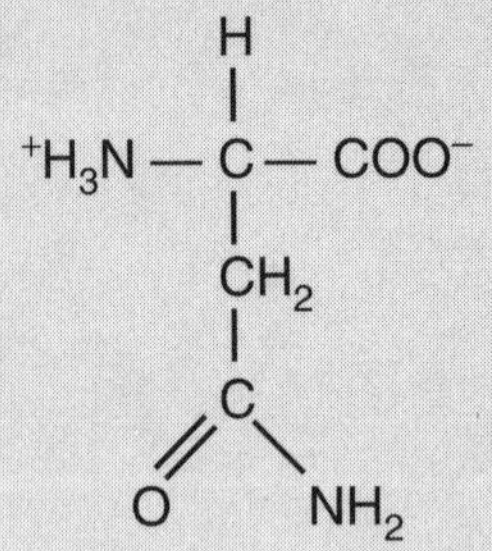

Amino Acid	Three-Letter Abbreviation	One-Letter Symbol	Formula
Glutamine	Gln	Q	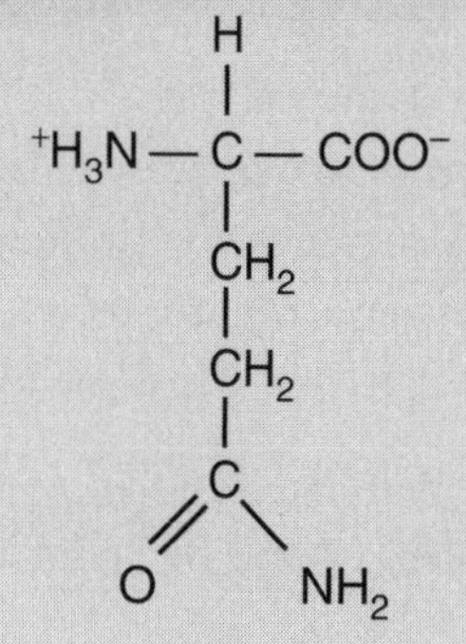
Sulfur-containing Amino Acids			
Cysteine	Cys	C	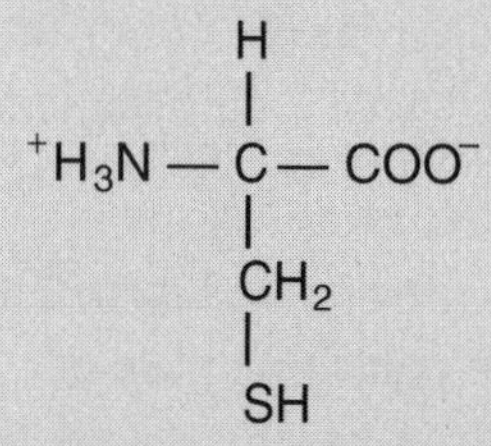
Methionine*	Met	M	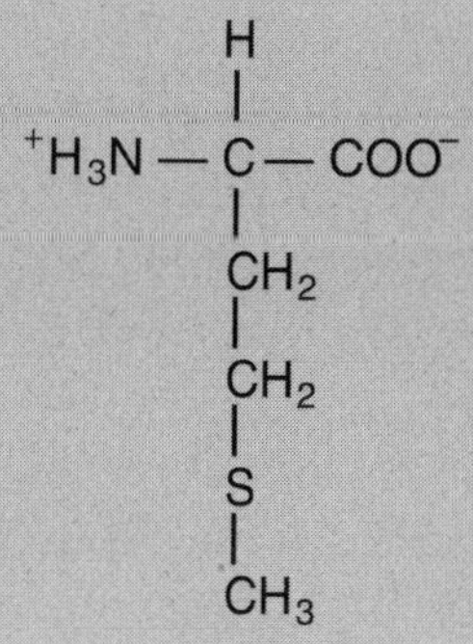
Other Amino Acids			
Proline	Pro	P	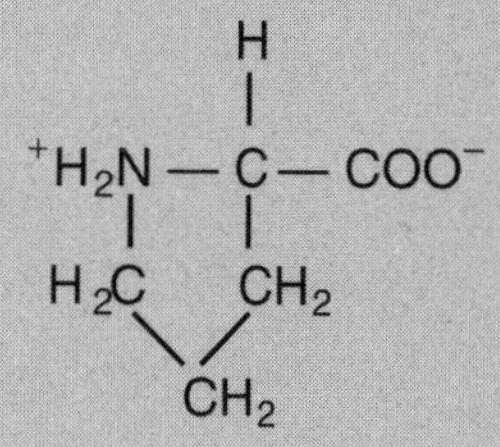
*Essential for *homo sapiens*			

FIGURE 7. Amino Acid

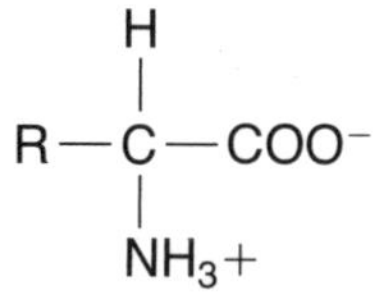

See Organic Chemistry Review, Functional Groups, page 334.

The 20 amino acids found in proteins are called alpha amino acids. The term *alpha* means that the amino group is next to (alpha) the carboxylic acid group. The amino group is bonded to the same carbon as the carboxylic acid group.

An amino group is basic and a carboxylic acid group is acidic; thus, an amino acid has the structure of an amine group protonated by the carboxylic acid. Because the carboxylic acid group is acidic, it donates its proton to the amine. Compounds that have a positive charge on one atom and a negative charge on another atom are called zwitterions. The pH at which an amino acid has an equal number of positive and negative charges is called the isoelectric point. **See Chemistry Review, Acids and Bases, page 304.**

Amino acids have physical properties that indicate their ionic character. Glycine, the simplest amino acid, has a melting point of 262°C. Amino acids are also soluble in water because of their ionic character.

In humans, not all the amino acids required for protein synthesis are made by the body. Eight amino acids are essential: valine (Val), leucine (Leu), isoleucine (Ile), lysine (Lys), phenylalanine (Phe), tryptophan (Try), threonine (Thr), and methionine (Met). Histidine (His) is required in infants but not in adults. The essential amino acids must come from dietary sources.

Because an amino acid is a zwitterion, its structure depends on the pH of the medium. In an acidic medium, the carboxylate ion will accept a proton from an acid and be protonated (Figure 8). The carboxylate ion is the conjugate base of a weak acid and is a relatively strong base.

FIGURE 8. Amino Acid in an Acidic Medium

$$R-\underset{\underset{NH_3+}{|}}{\overset{\overset{H}{|}}{C}}-COO^- + H_3O+ \longrightarrow R-\underset{\underset{NH_3+}{|}}{\overset{\overset{H}{|}}{C}}-COOH + H_2O$$

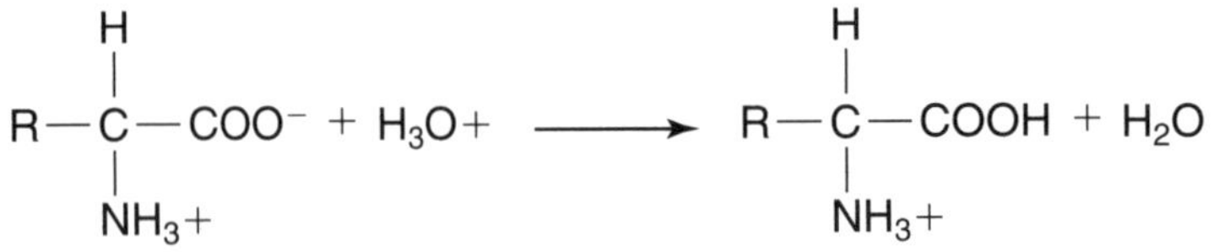

A different result is observed when a base, or a hydroxide ion, is added to a solution of an amino acid (Figure 9). In this case, the weakly acidic ammonium ion donates a proton to the hydroxide ion and water is formed.

FIGURE 9. Amino Acid in a Basic Medium

$$R-\underset{\underset{NH_3+}{|}}{\overset{\overset{H}{|}}{C}}-COO^- + OH^- \longrightarrow R-\underset{\underset{NH_2}{|}}{\overset{\overset{H}{|}}{C}}-COO^- + H_2O$$

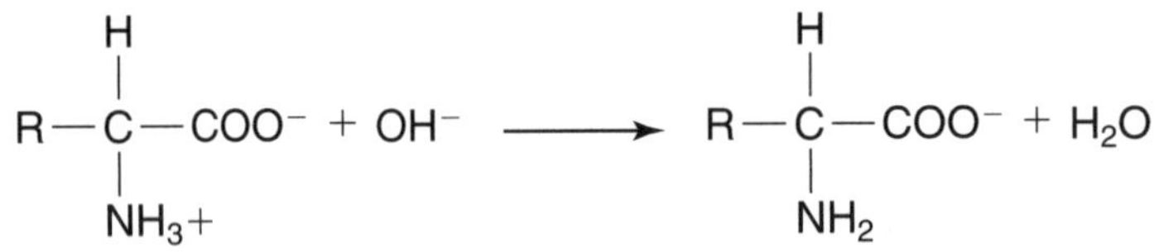

All amino acids except for glycine are chiral and have at least one stereocenter. L-glyceraldehyde (or S-glyceraldehyde) has the same configuration as L-alanine (Figure 10). The predominant configuration of the natural amino acids is an S shape.

FIGURE 10. Stereochemistry of Amino Acids

$$HO-\underset{\underset{CH_2OH}{|}}{\overset{\overset{CHO}{|}}{C}}-H \qquad +H_3N-\underset{\underset{CH_3}{|}}{\overset{\overset{COO^-}{|}}{C}}-H$$

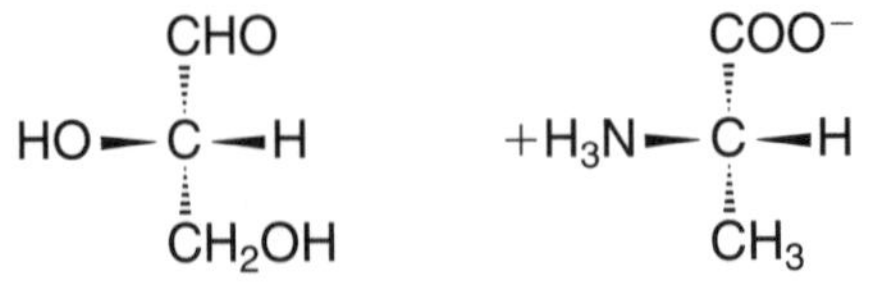

L-Glyceraldehyde　　　　　**L-Alanine**

See Organic Chemistry Review, Stereochemistry, page 333.

The amino acid cysteine has a chemical property that the other 20 amino acids do not possess. Cysteine will react with another mole of cysteine to form cystine, a dimer of cysteine. This reaction occurs through the use of mild oxidizing reagents and can be reversed by the use of reducing agents (Figure 11).

FIGURE 11. Oxidation of Cysteine

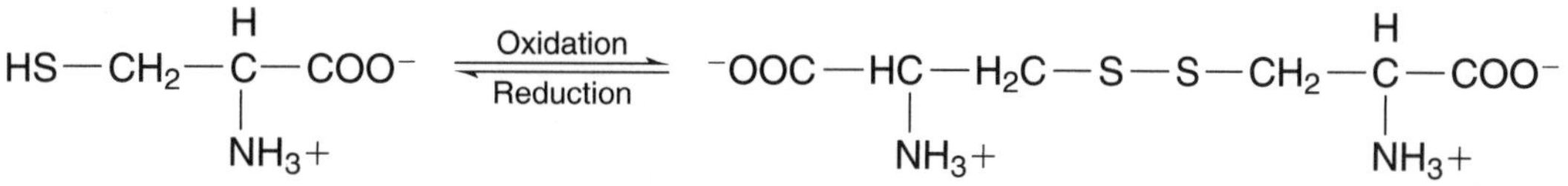

When two amino acids combine, peptides are formed (Figure 12). Peptides are formed via peptide bonds, and a peptide bond is an amide bond. Water is a by-product of the reaction, and the process is known as dehydration. When a peptide bond is broken, water is required, and the process is known as hydrolysis.

FIGURE 12. Peptide Formation

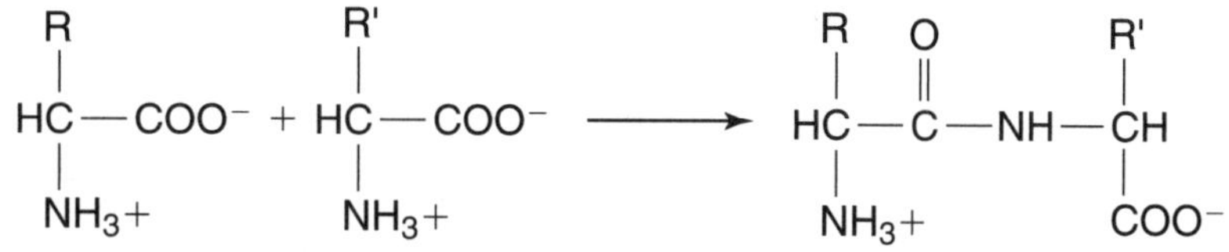

In a polypeptide chain, the amino acid units are linked by peptide bonds. The peptide bond is formed between the carboxyl group of one amino acid and the amino group of the next amino acid. As shown in Figure 13, the peptide bond has a partial double-bond character that restricts rotation about the C−N peptide bond. This restricted rotation limits the number of possible conformations obtainable by a polypeptide.

FIGURE 13. Partial Double-Bond Character of a Peptide Bond

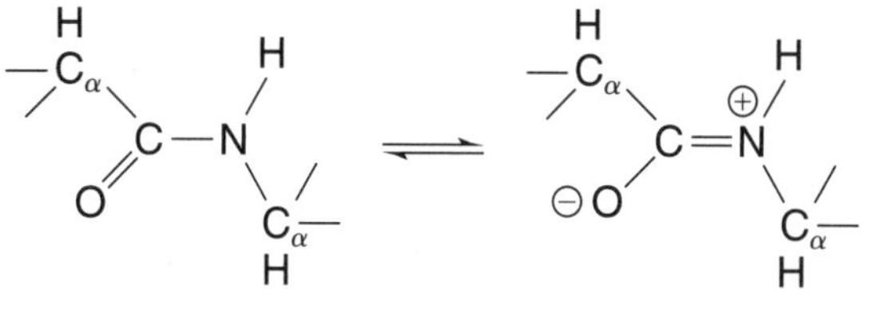

Problem

Proteins are least soluble in water at their isoelectric point. What will occur when a small amount of hydrochloric acid is added to a protein at its isoelectric point?

A. The protein will remain out of solution because the isoelectric point is a constant.

B. The protein will dissolve because the amino groups are protonated.

C. The protein will dissolve because the carboxylic acid is deprotonated.

D. The protein will remain out of solution because the pH is below the isoelectric point of the protein.

Solution

B. The protein will dissolve because a net positive charge has been obtained.

When many amino acids are linked by peptide bonds, polypeptides or proteins are formed. Proteins have many functions in the body, including structure, catalysis, movement, transport, hormones, protection, storage, and regulation. Proteins have hierarchical structural features that enable these functions. These structural features are called the primary, secondary, tertiary, and quaternary structures.

The primary structure describes the linear sequence of amino acids. Because there are 20 amino acids, the linear sequence can be very different from one protein to another. The disease sickle cell anemia results from a single substitution in the primary sequence of valine for glutamic acid in the protein hemoglobin.

The secondary structure describes the folding of the linear sequence of amino acids. Two distinct patterns have emerged: an alpha helix and the beta sheet. These patterns arise because of hydrogen bonding between the $-C{=}O$ of a peptide bond and the $H{-}N$ of another peptide linkage. A hydrogen bond exists between the electronegative oxygen atom of the peptide bond and the electropositive hydrogen atom of an amide amine group (Figure 14). This hydrogen bonding occurs in the backbone of the protein. Random coils are a third kind of secondary structure where no distinctive pattern emerges as a result of hydrogen bonding.

FIGURE 14. Hydrogen Bonds Between Polypeptides

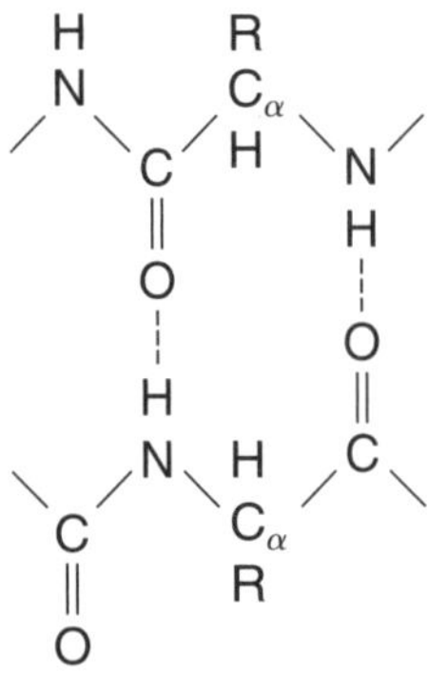

In contrast to the secondary structure, the tertiary structure arises because of interactions with the R group of the amino acids. Covalent bonds can be formed with the amino acid cysteine and the formation of a disulfide bridge.

Hydrogen bonding is also important in tertiary structures, except that the hydrogen bonding occurs between polar groups on the side chain. When the polar R groups contain an acidic amino acid ($-COO^-$) and another contains a basic amino acid ($-NH_3^+$ or $=NH_2^+$), a salt bridge or ionic bond can be formed between these groups.

The amino acids that contain nonpolar groups can form interactions. Although weak, these interactions, called hydrophobic interactions, are sufficiently strong to stabilize a loop or some other tertiary structure.

Certain proteins have more than one polypeptide chain, and the interaction between these chains determines the quaternary structure. The individual subunits are held together by hydrogen bonds, salt bridges, and hydrophobic interactions. Hemoglobin is an example of a protein with a quaternary structure because it contains two alpha subunits (a) and two beta subunits (b), as in a_2b_2.

Proteins can be either water soluble or bound to biological membranes. For water-soluble proteins, the hydrophilic amino acid side chains are generally found near the outer surface of the protein. The hydrophobic amino acid side chains are found in the interior of the protein where they are out of contact with water. Hydrophobic amino acid side chains (Cys, Val, Ile, Leu, Met, Trp, and Phe) are relatively nonpolar and do not interact with water molecules. Hydrophilic amino acid residues (Lys, Arg, His, Asp, Glu, Asn, and Gln) are polar and interact favorably with water.

Membrane proteins are associated with the lipid bilayer of biological membranes. There are two general categories of membrane proteins: intrinsic membrane proteins and extrinsic membrane proteins. Intrinsic membrane proteins are strongly associated with the biological membrane and can be removed only with a denaturing detergent such as sodium dodecyl sulfate (SDS). Intrinsic membrane proteins often have a sequence containing numerous hydrophobic amino acid side chains that are strongly associated with the hydrophobic domain of the lipid bilayer. Extrinsic membrane proteins are only loosely associated with biological membranes and can be removed by alterations in the ionic strength or by a chelator such as EDTA.

Problem

Which interactions in a protein would be most influenced by the pH of the medium?

A. Hydrogen bonding
B. Peptide bonding
C. Hydrophobic effect
D. Disulfide bonding

Solution

A. Hydrogen bonding depends on the ionization state of the groups such as COO^- and NH_3^+.

D. Nucleic Acids

The final group of biological molecules is the nucleic acids. Nucleic acids are polymers. The monomers that make up the nucleic acid polymers are nucleotides. Nucleotides consist of a five-carbon sugar, a phosphate group, and a nitrogenous base. There are two important nucleic acids: deoxyribonucleic acid (DNA) and ribonucleic acid (RNA). DNA contains the five-carbon sugar deoxyribose, a phosphate group, and a nitrogenous base (Figure 15). As shown in Figure 16, the nitrogenous base of DNA consists of adenine (A), thymine (T), cytosine (C), and guanine (G). RNA contains the five-carbon sugar ribose, a phosphate group, and three of the same nitrogenous bases as DNA (A, C, and G), but RNA has uracil instead of thymine.

FIGURE 15. Nucleotide from DNA

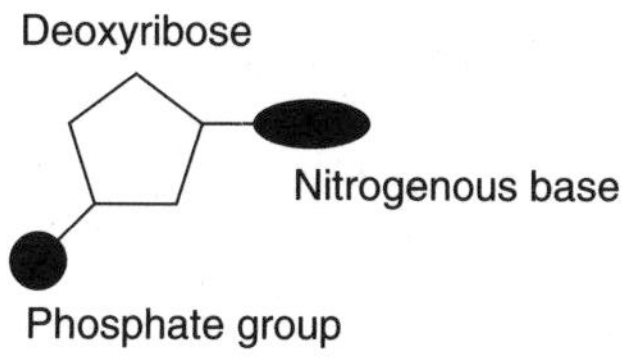

FIGURE 16. DNA Nucleotide Strand

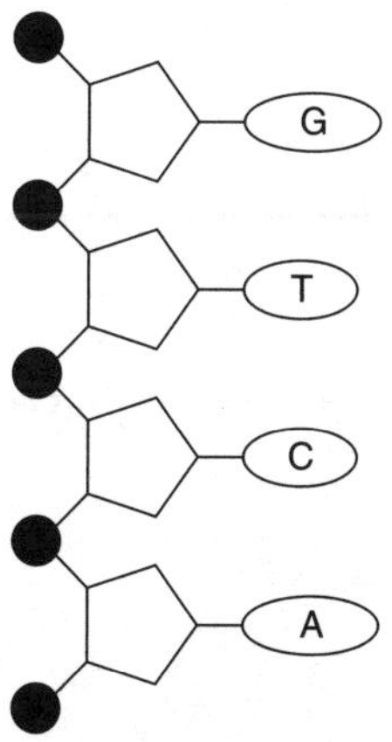

Individual nucleotides are linked together by bonds between the sugar and the phosphate group. The phosphate ester linkage is attached from the 5' end of the sugar of one nucleotide to the 3' hydroxyl group of the sugar from another nucleotide. A nucleoside contains a nitrogenous base and the sugar, either deoxyribose or ribose. The phosphate group is not present in a nucleoside.

DNA is double stranded, and one of the distinguishing features of the nitrogenous bases in DNA is that on the complementary strand, the nitrogenous base adenine is always found hydrogen-bonded to thymine, and the nitrogenous base guanine is always found hydrogen-bonded to cytosine. There are two kinds of nitrogenous bases: the pyrimidines and the purines. Adenine and guanine are purines, and thymine and cytosine are pyrimidines. The nitrogenous base uracil, which is found only in RNA, is a pyrimidine. The structure of the nitrogenous bases is characterized by a location for a covalent bond to the sugar molecule and atoms in the molecules that can either accept or donate hydrogen bonds (Figure 17).

FIGURE 17. Nitrogenous Bases

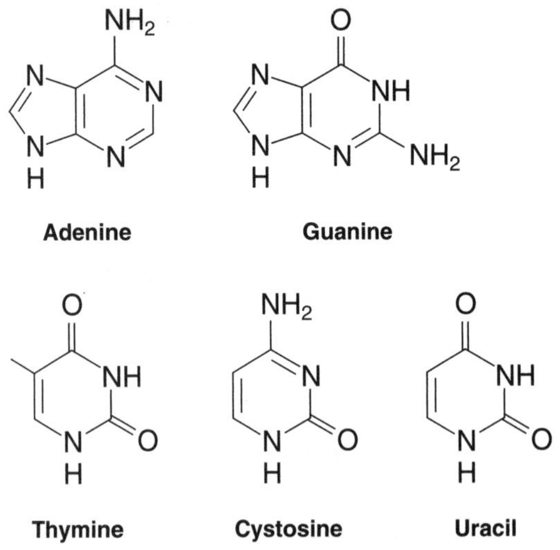

See Amines, Organic Chemistry Review, page 353.

The base pairings of adenine and thymine have two hydrogen bonds, and the base pairing of guanine and cytosine cause three hydrogen bonds to form. During RNA synthesis, the RNA base uracil hydrogen-bonds to adenine via two hydrogen bonds. The secondary amines on these structures can donate a hydrogen to either the electronegative oxygen atom of a carbonyl group of the complementary base or to a tertiary amine. Only selected tertiary amines in these bases are involved in hydrogen bonding. Selected secondary amines are used to form the covalent bond in the sugar and, in doing so, become tertiary amines that are not involved in hydrogen bonding

The structure of the sugars deoxyribose and ribose differ in that the 2' hydroxyl group is absent in deoxyribose but is present in ribose. The prefix *deoxy* means "without oxygen." Both deoxyribose and ribose form the backbone of DNA and RNA by the formation of phosphate linkages between the 5' hydroxyl group of one sugar to the 3' hydroxyl group of the next sugar (Figure 18). In a nucleoside, the anomeric 1' hydroxyl group has been replaced by the nitrogenous base, and a covalent bond is formed.

FIGURE 18. Structural Differences in DNA and RNA Nucleotides

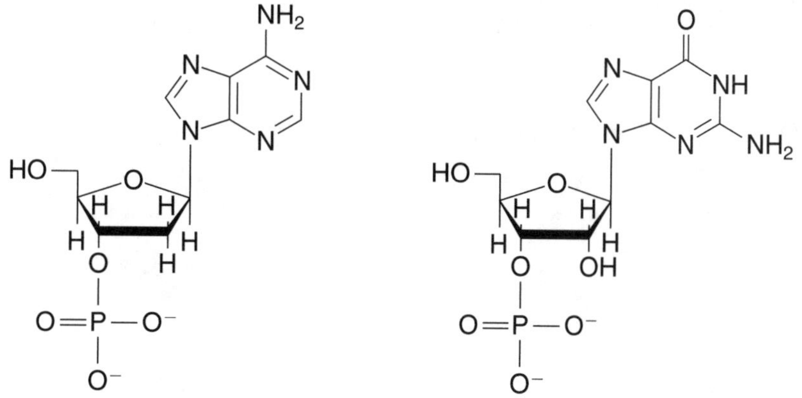

A DNA nucleotide An RNA nucleotide

3. ENZYMES AND CELLULAR METABOLISM

A. Enzyme Structure and Function

An enzyme is a protein that performs a metabolic function. Enzymes are catalysts and affect the rate but not the overall change in free energy of a chemical reaction. Most enzymes have molecular weights exceeding 10,000 daltons. The function of an enzyme is determined by its structure. The three-dimensional structure of enzymes and other proteins and nucleic acids can be found at the worldwide Protein Data Bank (http://www.pdb.org/).

All enzymes are complex proteins. For example, some proteins play only a structural role and have no metabolic functions. Proteins are polypeptides—that is, linear polymers with amino acids serving as the repeating units. Proteins are composed of one or more polypeptide chains and often contain a nonprotein moiety such as carbohydrate (as in glycoproteins), lipid (as in lipoproteins), or a metal ion (as in metalloproteins). The function of an enzyme is determined by its structure.

Problem

Enzymes are

A. proteins.
B. catalysts.
C. carbohydrates.
D. both proteins and catalysts.

Solution

D. Enzymes are proteins that act as catalysts. Carbohydrates are not proteins and therefore cannot be enzymes.

B. Control of Enzyme Activity

For the proper regulation of metabolism, it is necessary for all organisms to exert considerable control over the location, amount, and activity of enzymes. An enzyme (E) forms a complex with its substrate (S) at a well-defined region called the active site. Subsequently, the enzyme-substrate complex (ES) is converted into a product (P), and the enzyme (E) is released.

$$E + S \rightleftharpoons ES \rightarrow E + P$$

The activity of an enzyme can be regulated by changing or blocking the active site. As shown in Figure 19(a), a competitive inhibitor reversibly binds to the active site and competes with the substrate for binding at this same locus. For competitive inhibition, the activity of the enzymatically catalyzed reaction depends on the concentration of both substrate and inhibitor.

FIGURE 19. (a) Competitive Inhibition; (b) Noncompetitive Inhibition

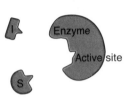

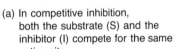

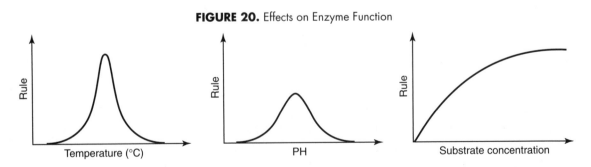

(a) In competitive inhibition, both the substrate (S) and the inhibitor (I) compete for the same active site.

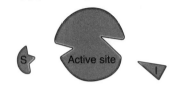

(b) In noncompetitive inhibition, the inhibitor (I) binds at a site different from the active site and does not prevent binding of the substrate (S). The inhibitor does decrease enzymatic activity.

Many enzymes have two (or more) alternative conformations, and the binding of ligands (substrates or other molecules) can influence which conformation the enzyme assumes. For allosteric proteins, one conformation is enzymatically active and the other is inactive. Allosteric enzymes are very important in the regulation of metabolic reactions (as discussed in the next section).

Because enzymes are proteins, there are optimal conditions for maximum activity for both pH and temperature, and they exhibit similar profiles as the pH and temperature are increased from low values to high values. A maximum rate of activity is observed. Enzyme reaction increases with temperature because any chemical reaction will increase with temperature. However, there is an optimal value for maximum activity because the protein can be become denatured at high temperatures.

The process of denaturation is a general phenomenon for proteins and can be experimentally observed for enzymes by changes in the reaction rate as a function of temperature and pH. At temperature values above the optimal, the protein—that is, the enzyme—undergoes irreversible conformation changes. As a result of these changes, the enzyme's activity is diminished. At temperature values below the optimal, the loss of activity is more related to changes in reaction rate kinetics as a result of the lower temperature. Enzymes have an optimal pH because conformational effects in, for example, the tertiary structure, such as salt bridges, depend on the ionization state of the functional groups of the amino acids.

An effect on enzymatic rates that does not have an optimal value but instead reaches a maximum value is substrate concentration. Enzymes are catalysts and are present in only small amounts. At high substrate concentrations, all the enzyme molecules have been complexed to substrate, and no free enzymes are available. With respect to substrate concentration, enzymes exhibit saturation kinetics.

FIGURE 20. Effects on Enzyme Function

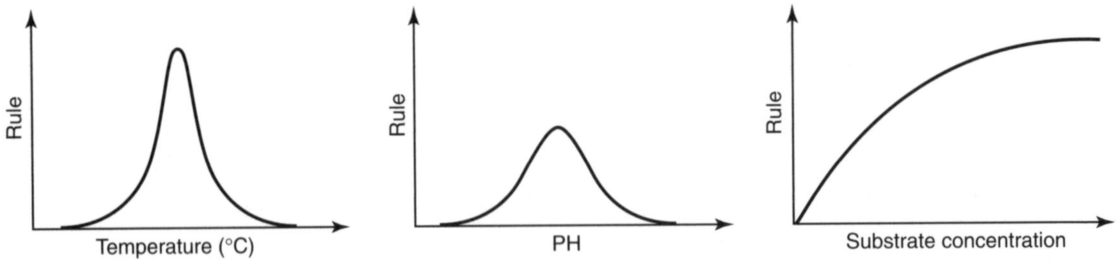

See Mathematics Review, Graphs, page 41.

Problem

Organisms can control all the following EXCEPT

A. location of enzymes.
B. type of enzymes.
C. amount of enzymes.
D. activity of enzymes.

Solution

B. Organisms control the activity of enzymes by changing or blocking active sites. Location and amount of enzymes may be controlled through feedback. Types of enzymes are determined genetically and cannot be altered.

Problem

Pickling preserves food by what mechanism?

A. Temperature
B. Food type
C. pH
D. Vitamins

Solution

C. Pickling causes the environment of the food to be acidic, thereby inactivating microbial enzymes and preserving the food.

C. Feedback Inhibition

Cells are required to synthesize an enormous number of essential compounds for their survival. Bacteria, although structurally simple compared with eukaryotic cells, can use glucose to provide their energy needs and to synthesize necessary organic components. The synthesis of these organic compounds is accomplished by specific metabolic pathways in which a precursor molecule is converted to a product by a series of enzyme-catalyzed reactions. The flow of metabolites in a metabolic pathway is often regulated by controlling the activity of key enzymes in the pathway. Usually, the first enzyme in a metabolic pathway is controlled by the end product of the pathway. This type of regulation is called feedback inhibition. In negative feedback inhibition (Figure 21), the end product of a pathway inhibits a previous enzyme in the pathway.

FIGURE 21. Feedback Inhibition of a Metabolic Pathway

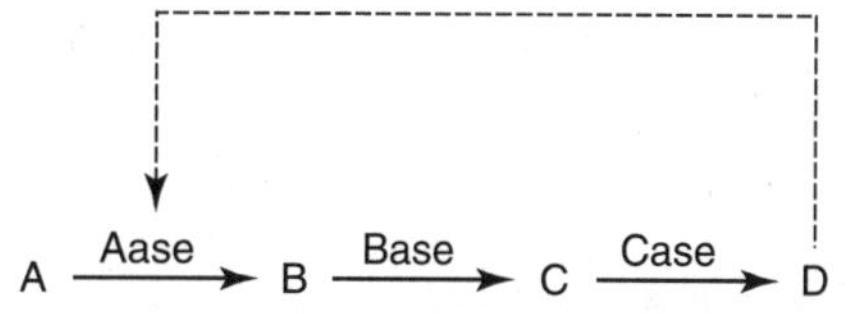

Metabolite D inhibits Aase.

The first enzyme in a metabolic pathway is usually an allosteric enzyme. The end product of the pathway binds to a regulatory site on the enzyme, causing it to assume an inactive conformation. The regulatory site is different from the active site. In the case of negative feedback inhibition, the pathway end product is usually a noncompetitive inhibitor. As shown in Figure 19(b) in the previous section, a noncompetitive inhibitor binds to the enzyme at a locus different from the active site. Further, for noncompetitive inhibition, the rate of the enzymatically catalyzed reaction depends only on the concentration of the inhibitor and not on the concentration of substrate. In summary, feedback regulation

- usually involves an allosteric enzyme,
- is very rapid, and
- can involve enzymatic inhibition or enzymatic activators (positive feedback inhibition).

Feedback regulation also provides an efficient method of conserving cellular energy and preventing the build-up of metabolic intermediates that at high levels could be toxic.

Problem

In feedback inhibition of metabolic pathways, which are controlled directly?

A. End products B. Metabolites C. Enzymes D. Precursor molecules

Solution

C. In feedback inhibition the flow of metabolites is often regulated by controlling the activity of key enzymes in a pathway. Usually, the first enzyme in a metabolic pathway is controlled by the end product of the pathway.

D. Cellular Respiration

The body converts food energy (stored in the bonds of glucose) into bonds of adenosine triphosphate (ATP), the carrier of energy used by the body in a process called cellular respiration. Although cellular respiration is a continuous process, it is conveniently divided into three stages: glycolysis, Krebs cycle, and electron transport. Some yeasts and bacteria use only glycolysis to obtain ATP. However, most organisms have higher ATP requirements and produce additional ATP via the Krebs cycle and electron transport.

Glycolysis

The sequence of energy-producing catabolic reactions called glycolysis takes place in the cytoplasmic fluid of all living cells. Glycolysis results in the production of ATP, which provides cells with a source of chemical energy. Catabolism is the chemical breakdown of food molecules to provide energy and building blocks for the synthesis of macromolecules. The first step in catabolism is the breakdown of macromolecular polymers to their monomeric units. Polysaccharides are broken down into sugars such as glucose. Glucose is further catabolized by the process of glycolysis.

Glycolysis does not require the presence of oxygen. This metabolic pathway is ancient, having evolved when the earth's atmosphere contained very little oxygen. In eukaryotes and many prokaryotes, glycolysis results in the net production of two molecules of ATP, two molecules of NADPH, and two molecules of pyruvate per molecule of glucose:

$$\text{D-glucose} + 2HPO_4^{2-} + 2ADP + 2NAD^+ \rightarrow$$
$$2CH_3C—CO_2 + 2ATP + 2\,NADPH + 2H^+.$$

The 10 steps in the glycolytic pathway are detailed in Figure 22. The first three steps of glycolysis convert glucose to fructose 1,6-diphosphate (FDP) at the cost of two ATPs. Fructose and glucose are both six-carbon sugars (hexoses). The second stage results in the splitting (by aldolase) of FDP into two three-carbon sugars (trioses)—that is, dihydroxyacetone phosphate (DHAP) and D-glyceraldehyde 3-phosphate.

FIGURE 22. Glycolysis

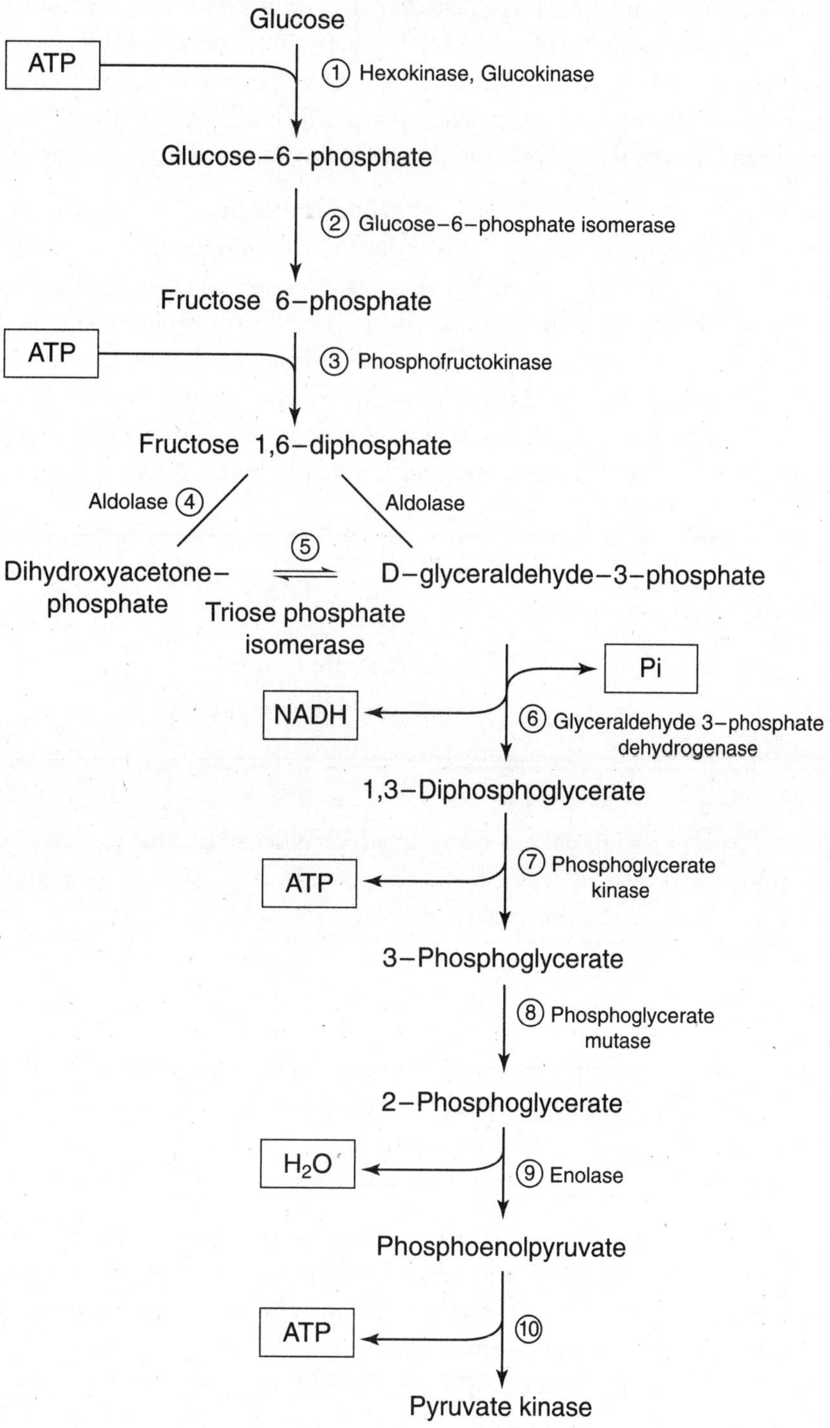

DHAP is converted to D-glyceraldehyde 3-phosphate by triose phosphate isomerase. The third phase of glycolysis produces ATP by converting D-glyceraldehyde 3-phosphate into metabolites that can transfer phosphoryl groups to adenosine diphosphate (ADP). The pyruvate produced by glycolysis is a key branch-point metabolite. Under anaerobic conditions, yeast converts pyruvate to ethanol and carbon dioxide, and animals convert pyruvate to lactic acid. Some prokaryotes utilize different pathways than the one described here. All function to generate ATP, NADH, and pyruvate, but some are less efficient than glycolysis.

The key regulatory enzyme in glycolysis is phosphofructokinase. Its activity is inhibited by ATP, citrate, and fatty acids and is activated by ADP, adenosine monophosphate (AMP), cyclic AMP, and FDP. When cells that are undergoing anaerobic glycolysis are switched to aerobic conditions, the rate of glycolysis rapidly drops. This is called the Pasteur effect. The effect is explained by the fact that under aerobic conditions, the pyruvate produced by glycolysis can undergo further oxidation via the citric acid cycle (discussed in the next section). This results in the production of 18 ATP molecules per pyruvate. Thus, the energy needs of the cell are met with a considerably reduced rate of glycolysis. The decreased rate of glycolysis with higher levels of ATP is consistent with phosphofructokinase being inhibited by ATP.

Problem

Glycolysis does NOT

A. occur in the cytoplasm.

B. require oxygen.

C. produce ATP.

D. break down glucose.

Solution

B. Glycolysis is the series of metabolic reactions by which glucose is converted to pyruvate (a three-carbon compound) with the concurrent formation of ATP. Glycolysis occurs in the cytoplasm of the cell and, for this process, the presence of oxygen is unnecessary.

Krebs (Citric Acid) Cycle

For most eukaryotic cells and aerobic bacteria, the pyruvic acid produced by glycolysis is completely oxidized to CO_2 and H_2O. This process produces reducing power in the form of NADH and $FADH_2$. NADH and $FADH_2$ are then utilized by the electron transport system to produce ATP. Electron transport occurs in the mitochondria of eukaryotic cells and in the membrane of aerobic bacteria.

In eukaryotic cells, the pyruvate produced by anaerobic glycolysis enters the mitochondrion and is decarboxylated. This leaves behind an acetate residue. NAD^+ accepts one hydrogen from pyruvic acid and one from coenzyme A (CoA). This allows the CoA and the acetate to condense, forming acetyl CoA. The primary function of the citric acid pathway is to oxidize acetyl groups to CO_2 and H_2O while producing reducing equivalents in the form of NADH and $FADH_2$. The overall reaction is

$$\text{acetyl CoA} + 2H_2O + 3NAD^+ + FAD + GDP + HPO_4^- \rightarrow$$

$$2CO_2 + 3NADH + FADH_2 + GTP + 3H^+ + CoA$$

and the enzymatically catalyzed steps are shown in Figure 23. The citric acid (or Krebs) cycle occurs in the mitochondrial matrix (see Figure 26 in the next section).

It is noteworthy that molecular oxygen (O_2) does not enter the citric acid cycle. The additional oxygen atoms required for CO_2 production come from H_2O. The one GTP produced by step 7 is easily converted to ATP (GTP + ADP = GDP + ATP). The oxidation of one NADH molecule by the electron

FIGURE 23. Krebs Cycle

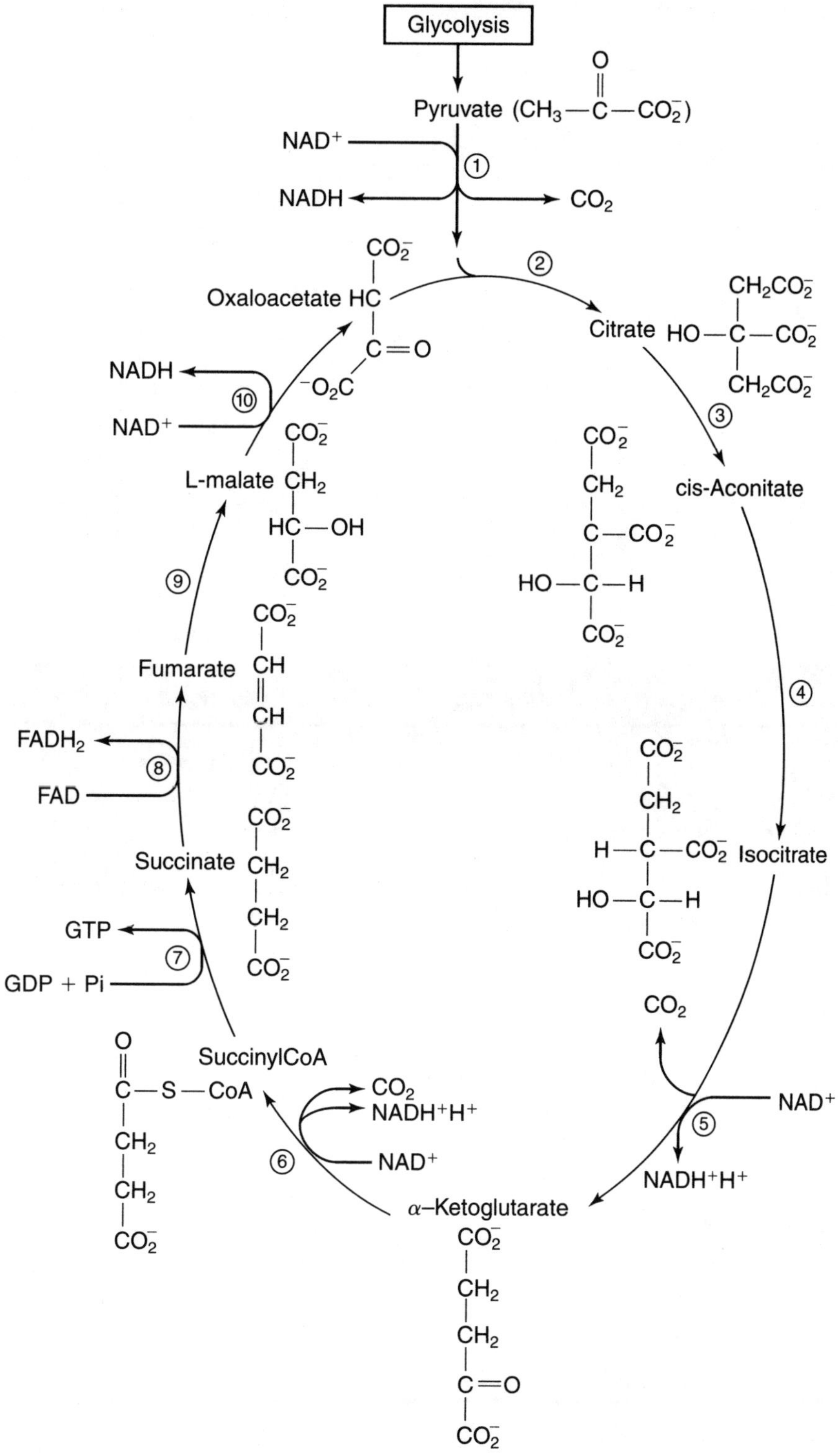

(1)	pyruvate carboxylase	(6)	alpha-ketoglutarate dehydrogenase
(2)	citrate synthetase	(7)	succinyl CoA synthetase
(3)	aconitase	(8)	succinate dehydrogenase
(4)	aconitase	(9)	fumarase
(5)	isocitrate dehydrogenase	(10)	malate dehydrogenase

transport system produces three ATPs and, similarly, the oxidation of one $FADH_2$ produces two ATPs. The complete oxidation of glucose yields 38 ATPs.

Problem

In the Krebs cycle, all the following occur EXCEPT the

A. oxidation of succinate.
B. formation of $FADH_2$.
C. formation of NADH.
D. transformation of NADH to NAD.

Solution

D. NADH is converted to NAD during oxidative phosphorylation, yielding three ATPs.

Electron Transport Chain and Oxidative Phosphorylation

The last steps in catabolism, called oxidative phosphorylation, result in the efficient production of ATP (Table 2). In these steps, electrons (e^-) are ultimately transferred to oxygen (Figure 24) with the generation of ATP. Oxidative phosphorylation is dependent on the structure of mitochondria.

TABLE 2. ATP Yield from the Complete Oxidation of Glucose

Reaction Sequence	ATP Yield per Glucose
Glycolysis: Glucose to Pyruvate (in the cytoplasm)	
Phosphorylation of glucose	−1
Phosphorylation of fructose 6-phosphate	−1
Dephosphorylation of 2 molecules of 1, 3-DPG	+2
Dephosphorylation of 2 molecules of phosphoenolpyruvate	+2
2 NADH are formed in the oxidation of 2 molecules of glyceraldehyde 3-phosphate	
Conversion of Pyruvate to Acetyl CoA (inside mitochondria)	
2 NADH are formed	
Citric Acid Cycle (inside mitochondria)	
Formation of 2 molecules of guanosine triphosphate from 2 molecules of succinyl CoA	+2
6 NADH are formed per 2 molecules of pyruvate	
Oxidation Phosphorylation (inside mitochondria)	
2 NADH formed in glycolysis; each yields 2 ATPs (not 3 ATPs each because of the cost of the shuttle)	+4
2 NADH formed in the oxidative decarboxylation of pyruvate; each yields 3 ATPs	+6
2 FADH formed in the citric acid cycle; each yields 2 ATPs	+4
6 NADH formed in the citric acid cycle; each yields 3 ATPs	+18

FIGURE 24. Electron Transport

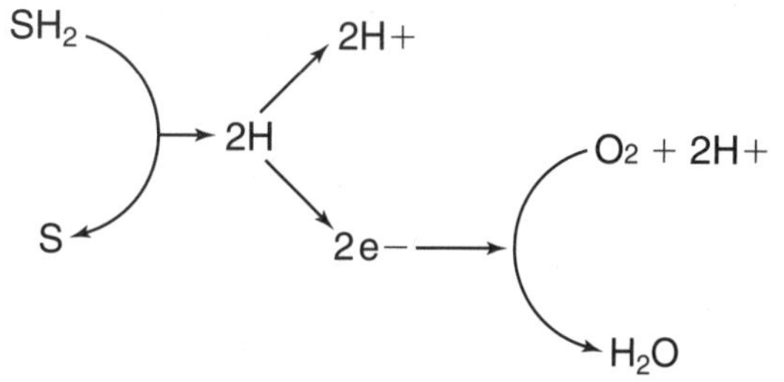

Substrates (SH_2) contain H atoms consisting of a proton (H^+) and an electron (e^-). The energy locked in H^+ and e^- is harnessed during oxidative phosphorylation to produce ATP.

Oxidative phosphorylation generates ATP by harnessing the energy of the electron transport chain to phosphorylate ADP. The enzyme catalyzing this reaction is a (H^+) proton-driven ATP synthetase (H^+–ATP synthetase). H^+–ATP synthetase is a transmembrane protein embedded in the inner mitochondrial membrane. The energy to drive ATP formation by H^+–ATP synthetase comes from a proton gradient across the inner mitochondrial membrane. This proton gradient is generated by the movement of electrons down the respiratory chain. The respiratory chain is a series of membrane-bound redox carriers, with cytochrome oxidase being the terminal electron acceptor (Figure 25).

The electrons that ultimately reach O_2 (and form H_2O) are initially carried by the hydrogen atoms of NADH and $FADH_2$ (from glycolysis and the citric acid cycle). These hydrogen atoms can be dissociated into an electron (e^-) and a proton (H^+). The electrons are transported by the respiratory chain, and the protons are released into the aqueous medium. The released H^+ ions are translocated from the matrix space to the intermembrane space, and a pH gradient is established. The energy created by this gradient is trapped by the H^+–ATP synthetase when the H^+ flow back into the matrix (Figure 26). This process is known as chemiosmosis.

The process of oxidative phosphorylation illustrates a milestone in biochemistry because it is an example of factorial metabolism—the coupling of metabolism with transport across a membrane.

Problem

The ratio of ATP produced aerobically to anaerobically by the oxidation of one molecule of glucose is

A. 2:1.   B. 1:2.   C. 1:18.   D. 18:1.

Solution

D. The aerobic production of ATP involves the Krebs (citric acid) cycle and the oxidation of glucose. The anaerobic production of ATP takes place during glycolysis. The citric acid cycle produces 34 ATPs, and the oxidation of glucose produces 2 ATPs. This makes the total number of ATPs produced during aerobic processes 36. Glycolysis yields 2 ATPs. The net ratio of aerobic ATP to anaerobic ATP is 36:2, which equals 18:1.

FIGURE 25. Respiratory Chain

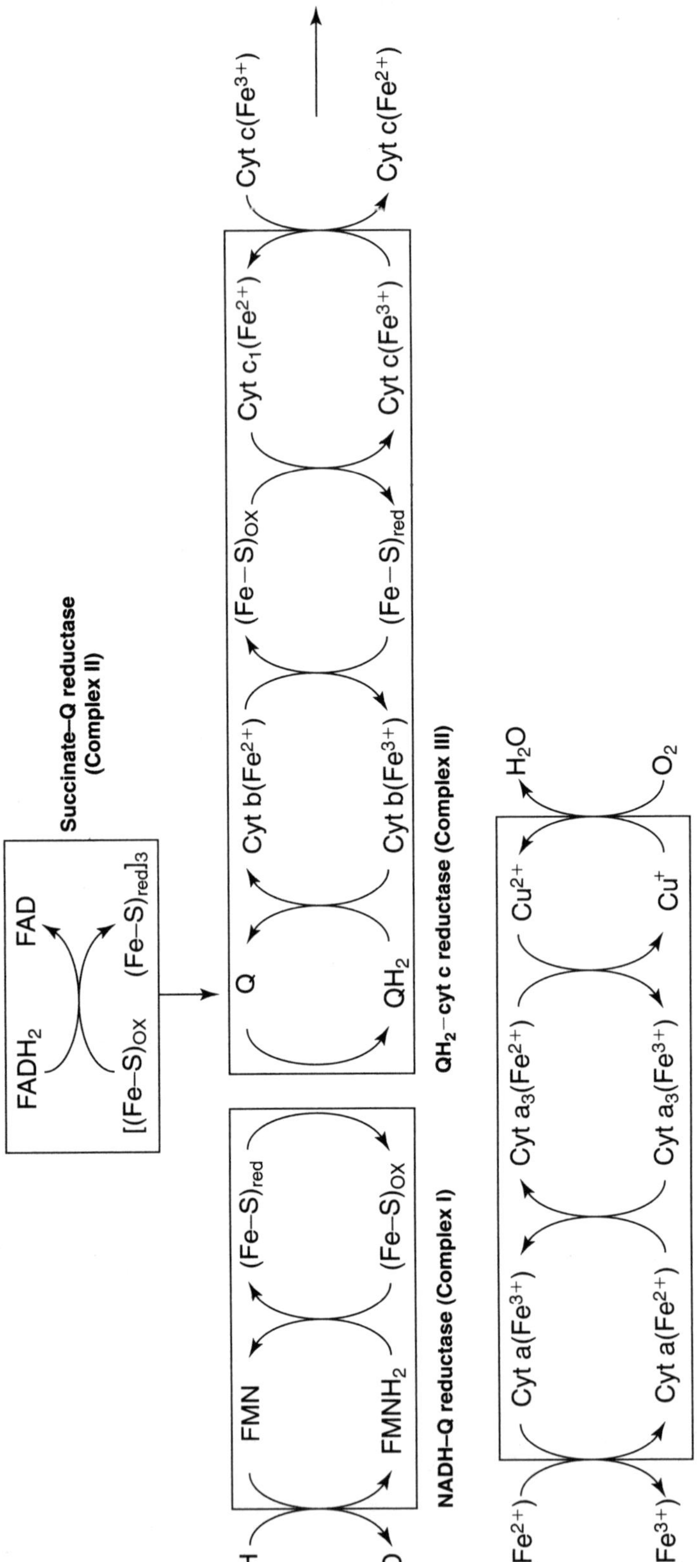

FIGURE 26. Oxidative Phosphorylation

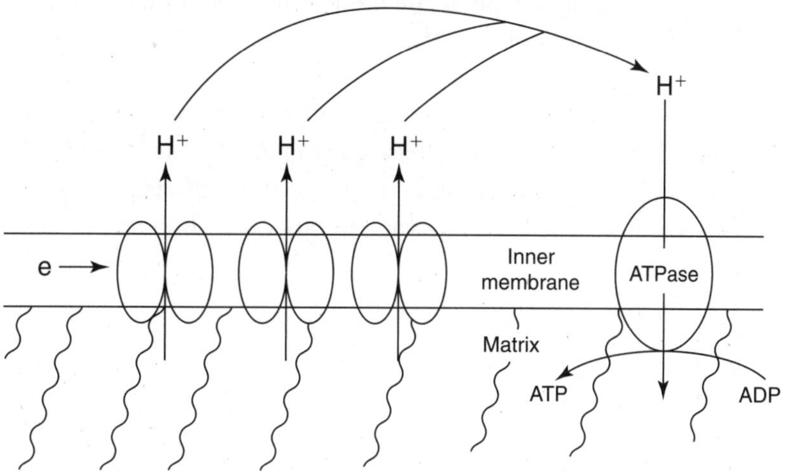

As high-energy electrons move down the respiratory chain, a proton gradient is created. H^+–ATPase uses this gradient to make ATP.

4. DNA AND PROTEIN SYNTHESIS

A. DNA Structure and Function

The information determining the sequence of amino acids in a polypeptide resides in another linear polymer called deoxyribonucleic acid (DNA). DNA, and nucleic acids in general, are polynucleotides in which the repeating units are nucleotides. DNA contains the cell's genetic information. DNA has been called an aperiodic crystal. Aperiodicity is a requirement for coding information and the "crystalline" structure of DNA provides considerable thermodynamic stability.

Nucleotides contain either a purine or a pyrimidine base attached to a five-carbon sugar-phosphate (Figure 27). In DNA, the sugar is 2-deoxyribose (dRib), and in ribonucleic acids (RNA), the sugar is ribose (Rib). Four bases are found in both DNA and RNA. Adenine and guanine are the two purine bases present in DNA. Thymidine and cytosine are the two pyrimidines. RNA also contains adenine, guanine, and cytosine, but uracil substitutes for thymine. Nucleotides are linked to each other by phosphodiester bonds between the 3' hydroxyl group of one nucleotide and the 5' end of the next (see Figure 27).

The composition of DNA provides important clues about its function and structure. Chargaff found that

- the base composition of DNA in different tissues from the same species is identical;
- the base composition of DNA from similar species is similar, and the base composition of DNA from widely divergent species is dissimilar; and
- in DNA from all species, the number of adenine bases equals the number of thymine (A = T) bases, and the number of guanine bases equals the number of cytosine bases (G = C).

The Watson–Crick model of DNA provides an immediate and simple explanation for the fact that A = T and G = C. The Watson–Crick model proposes that DNA is a double-stranded helix with the two strands running in opposite directions, or antiparallel. The purines and pyrimidine bases are stacked on top of each other, forming the inside of the double helix. The planes of the bases are essentially parallel to one another and perpendicular to the long axis of the DNA molecule. Adenine on one strand forms a specific base pair with thymine on the other antiparallel strand. The AT base pair is stabilized by two hydrogen bonds. Guanine and cytosine also form a specific base pair (GC), but it is stabilized by three hydrogen bonds. The complementary base pairing for double-stranded DNA is illustrated in Figure 28. In addition to hydrogen bonding and charge separation between phosphates along the helix, the structure of DNA is stabilized by hydrophobic interactions. The stacked bases are removed from contact with water.

FIGURE 27. Nucleic Acid Structure

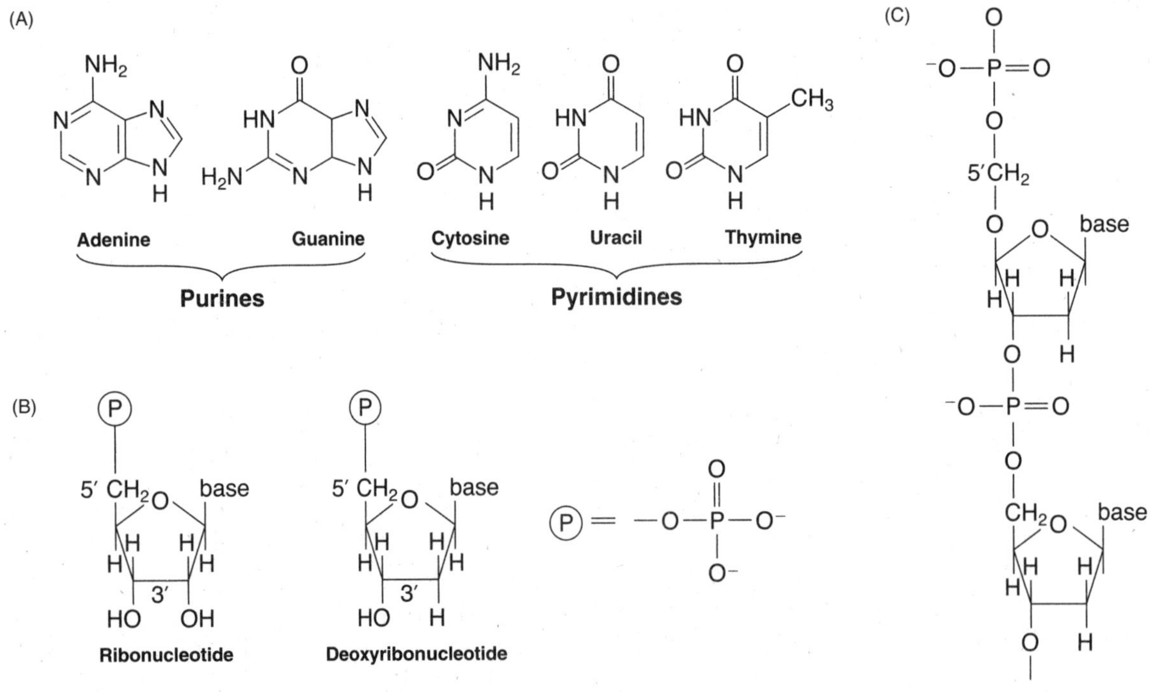

(a) Structure of bases in nucleic acids. Purines attach to ribose (or deoxyribose) at the 9′ position and pyrimidines at the 1′ position; (b) Structure of a ribonucleotide and deoxyribonucleotide; (c) Structure of single-chain DNA

FIGURE 28. Complementary Base Pairing in DNA

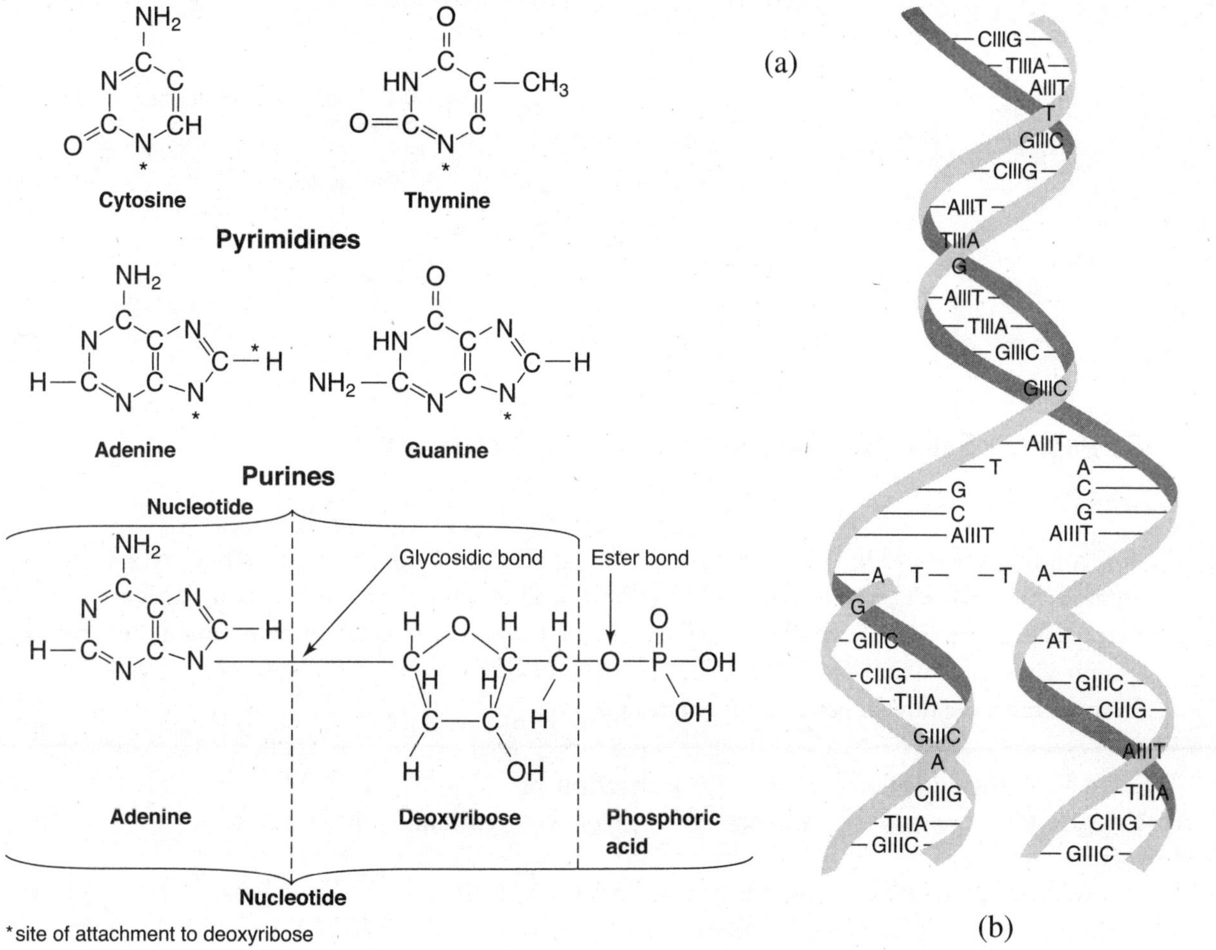

(a) Four base pairs

(b) DNA double helix, showing complementary base pairing

B. DNA as Transmitter of Genetic Information

The unique structure of DNA enables it to serve two template functions. One function is to serve as a template for its own replication. The other is to provide a template for the synthesis of RNA (transcription).

DNA replication involves

- strand separation, and
- the synthesis, via DNA polymerase, of a complementary daughter strand from each parent strand.

The biochemical details of this process are complex, involving numerous proteins. DNA replication involves a replication form in which both nascent strands are synthesized in a 5′ to 3′ direction. This results in continuous synthesis for the leading strand but discontinuous synthesis for the lagging strand (Figure 29). Discontinuous synthesis results in Okazaki fragments, which are later joined to form a continuous strand.

FIGURE 29. DNA Replication Fork with Okazaki Fragments

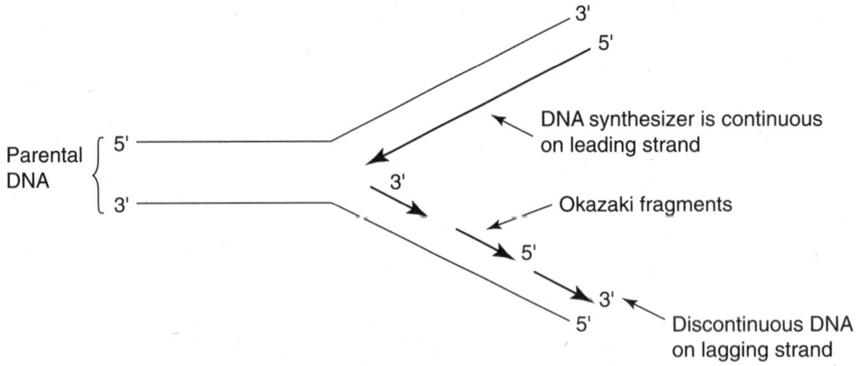

C. Protein Synthesis: Transcription and Translation

Transcription

A second function of DNA is to provide a template for the synthesis of messenger RNA (mRNA), ribosomal RNA (rRNA), and transfer RNA (tRNA), all of which are single-stranded ribonucleic acid polymers. Messenger RNA is the intermediary polymer used to transmit information about the sequence of amino acids in protein from DNA. The synthesis of RNA from a DNA template is called transcription. In most cells, the flow of genetic information is

$$\text{DNA} \xrightarrow{\text{transcription}} \text{mRNA} \xrightarrow{\text{transcription}} \text{protein}$$

In eukaryotic cells, DNA is found almost exclusively in the cell nucleus, and most of the RNA is found in the cytoplasm, where protein synthesis occurs. Both rRNA and tRNA are involved in the biosynthesis of proteins (translation) but do not carry any information coding for the sequence of amino acids in a protein. For RNA synthesis, the bases on one strand of DNA (the "sense strand") are matched with complementary ribonucleotide triphosphates and polymerized into an RNA molecule.

In prokaryotes a multi-subunit RNA polymerase is responsible for the synthesis of mRNA, tRNA, and rRNA from the DNA template. RNA polymerase cannot, however, utilize an RNA template (double stranded or single stranded) or an RNA/DNA hybrid. Transcription involves three steps:

1. Initiation
2. Elongation
3. Termination

Initiation starts at specific sites on the DNA, termed promoters. One subunit of RNA polymerase, the sigma subunit, recognizes these promoters. RNA chain elongation proceeds in a 5' → 3' direction until a termination signal is encountered on the DNA template. Some termination signals require a protein called Rho and are referred to as Rho dependent. After the polymerase encounters the signal, Rho disengages it from the template, or more specifically, promotes the dissociation of RNA polymerase from the template. Other termination signals are Rho independent.

Transcription in eukaryotic cells is mechanistically very similar to prokaryotic transcription but more complex. Eukaryotic cells contain three polymerases, denoted RNA polymerase I, II, and III. Each transcribes a unique set of genes. RNA polymerase I transcribes most of the ribosomal RNA. RNA polymerase II transcribes mRNA and most of the snRNP RNAs. RNA polymerase III transcribes small RNAs such as tRNA and the 5S ribosomal RNA. Each polymerase comprises 10 or more subunits, which is considerably more complex than *Escherichia coli* RNA polymerases. The three polymerases share common subunits, although each also has private subunits. Unlike *E. coli* RNA polymerase, eukaryotic polymerases cannot bind to promoter sequences. They require that other protein factors first bind the DNA.

The base sequence of an mRNA molecule (or of the DNA gene itself) encodes the information for the amino acid sequence of a protein. Because proteins vary greatly in molecular weight, it follows that mRNAs must also be of varying length. Each amino acid in a polypeptide is determined by a three-base codon. Three bases allow for 64 codons. However, proteins are composed of only 20 amino acids. Therefore, either some codons are not used or more than one codon can code for an amino acid (i.e., the code is degenerate). In fact, only three codons (UAA, UAG, and UGA) do not code for amino acids. They provide the termination signal for translation and are referred to as stop codons. The genetic code used in a wide variety of organisms is identical, with only minor exceptions.

In prokaryotic cells, the sequence of bases coding for a given polypeptide (the gene or cistron) are continuous. In marked contrast, the coding regions for polypeptides in eukaryotic cells can be discontinuous. The newly synthesized mRNA (the primary transcript) in eukaryotic cells contains regions, called introns, that are not expressed in the synthesized protein product. These intron regions are removed, and the regions that are expressed (exons) are spliced together to form the final functional mRNA molecule.

Translation

The process for translating an mRNA molecule into a polypeptide is very complex. Ribosomes and tRNA are of primary importance, but numerous other proteins are also required. Polypeptides are synthesized by sequentially adding amino acids to the carboxyl end of the growing polypeptide chain. The mRNA contains the codons specifying the sequence of amino acids but cannot itself associate with them. An intermediary RNA molecule called tRNA performs that task. At least one unique tRNA exists for each amino acid. The amino acid is activated and attached to its specific tRNA by an ATP-driven process utilizing the enzyme aminoacyl tRNA synthetase. A tRNA carrying its cognate amino acid is said to be "charged."

$$\text{amino acid} + \text{ATP} + \text{tRNA} + H_2O \rightarrow \text{aminoacyl–tRNA} + \text{AMP} + \text{PPi}$$

Aminoacyl–tRNA synthetase enzymes are very selective in attaching each amino acid to its cognate tRNA. Without this strict selectivity, the process of polypeptide synthesis would be compromised.

Each tRNA molecule has an anticodon consisting of three bases complementary to the bases of a codon on an mRNA molecule. The process of assembling a polypeptide from aminoacyl–tRNAs and an mRNA takes place on ribosomes. A ribosome is composed of both RNA and protein. It has two binding sites for charged tRNA: a P or peptidyl site and an A or aminoacyl site. Polypeptide synthesis involves initiation, elongation, and termination.

Prokaryote Translation

Initiation results when the mRNA and the initiator tRNA (formylmethionyl–tRNA) binds to the 30S ribosome subunit in either order. The charged initiator tRNA binds to the P site (see Figure 30). mRNA has a purine-rich sequence called the ribosome binding site (RBS), followed by the AUG codon. The RBS promotes the binding of the mRNA to RNA of the 30S ribosomal subunit. The 50S ribosomal subunit then binds to the 30S subunit, giving the 70S initiation complex. One GTP is spent to form the 70S initiation complex. Many nonribosomal proteins, termed initiation factors, are involved in establishing the 70S unit complex.

FIGURE 30. Protein Synthesis and Roles of mRNA, Ribosomes, and tRNA

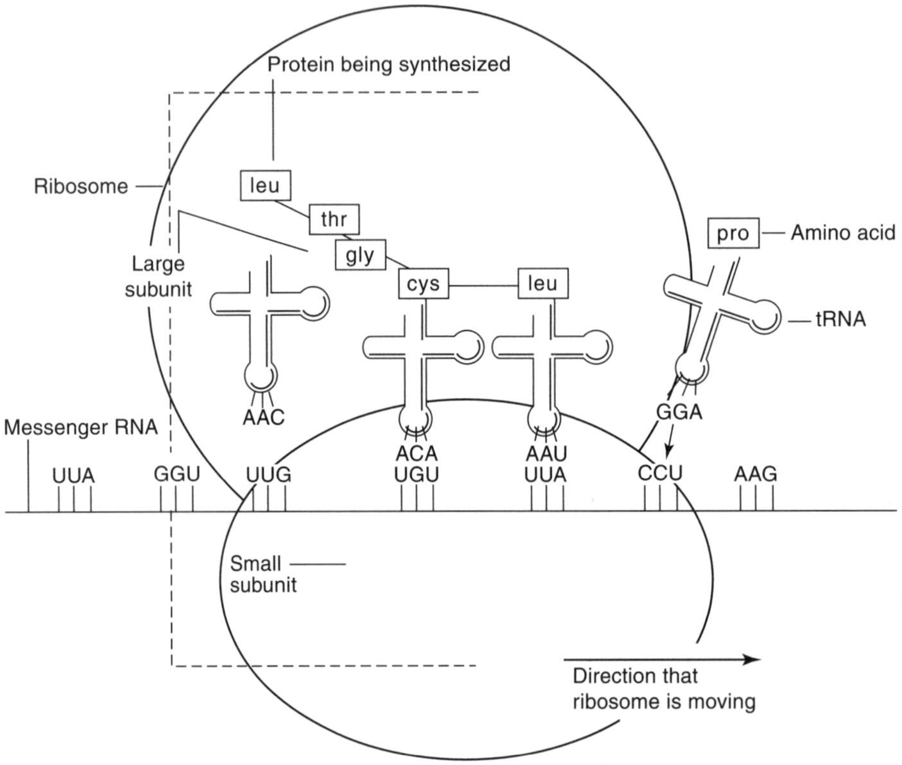

Elongation proceeds with the binding of an aminoacyl–tRNA to the A site. Formation of a peptide bond between the amino group of incoming aminoacyl–tRNA and the carboxyl group of the adjacent fmet–tRNA costs one GTP and causes the release of uncharged fmet–tRNA. The translocation of the peptidyl–tRNA from the A site to the P site moves the ribosome to the next codon and expends a second GTP. Each elongation step requires the hydrolysis of two GTPs.

Termination of polypeptide synthesis occurs when a stop codon is encountered. The stop codon is read by one of two protein release factors that cause the release of the polypeptide chain from the ribosome.

As with transcription, eukaryotic translation and prokaryotic translation are similar but have several differences. For one, eukaryotic ribosomes are relatively large. Both the small subunit (40S) and the large subunit (60S) are larger than their prokaryotic equivalents. Together they form an 80S ribosome. Also, eukaryotic initiation is notably more complex (Figure 31).

FIGURE 31. Initiation of Eukaryotic Protein Synthesis

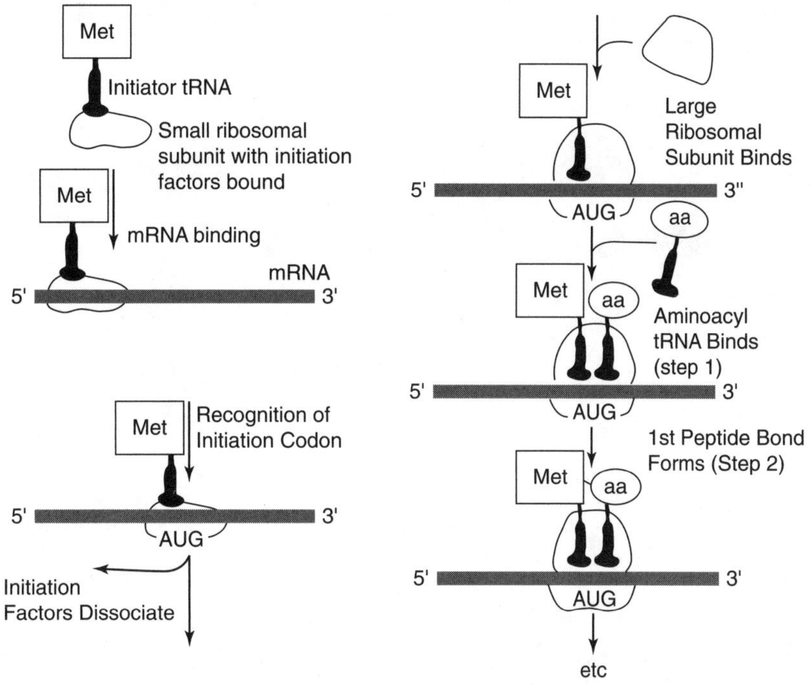

Eukaryotic initiation involves more initiation factors, many of which are themselves multi-subunited. The initiator tRNA is a special methionine tRNA (termed Met $tRNA^{Met}$), but it is not formylated. Also, the initiator tRNA always binds to the 40S subunit before the mRNA does, rather than in either order (as in prokaryotes). Furthermore, binding of the mRNA to the 40S subunit requires the hydrolysis of one ATP. With the exception of the mRNA of a few viruses, eukaryotic mRNA does not possess a ribosome-binding site but instead requires a 5' cap for efficient initiation (Figure 32). This cap is a 7-methylguanosine linked at its 5' end to the 5' end of the mRNA via a triphosphate bridge. In addition, one or two of the first nucleotide residues of the mRNA are O-methylated at the 2' position of the ribose moieties. Finally, one release factor (RF) recognizes all three stop codons.

Problem

Nitrous acid converts cytosine to uracil by deamination. This type of conversion in one DNA strand would lead to a change in the complementary base in the other strand to

A. adenine. B. cytosine. C. thymine. D. guanine.

Solution

A. Cytosine normally binds to guanine, and uracil normally binds to adenine. A conversion of cytosine to uracil would lead to a conversion of guanine to adenine in the complementary strand. Thus, a CG to AU (or AT) event has occurred.

Gene transcription is controlled by operons, and an operon is a section of DNA that regulates gene expression. The best-understood operon is called the lac operon, and in bacteria it controls gene expression for the enzyme that breaks down the sugar lactose.

FIGURE 32. Structure of Eukaryotic mRNA Cap

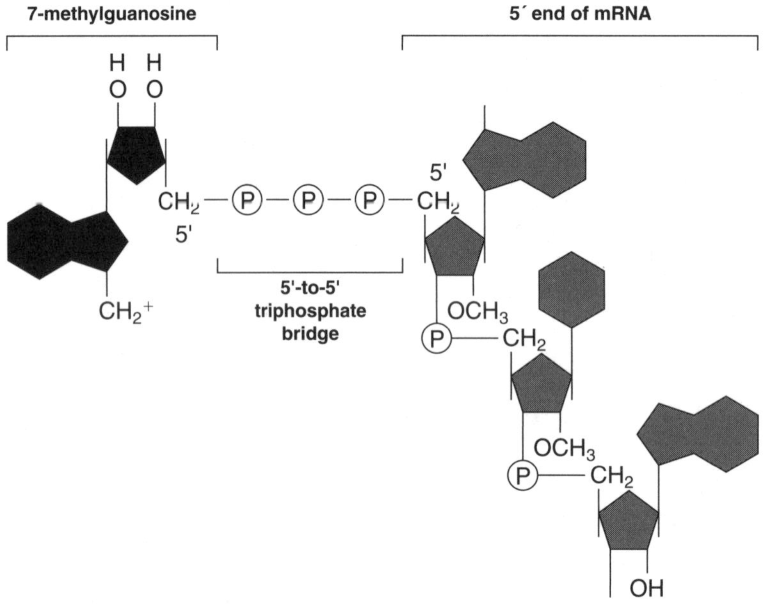

The operon consists of four major parts: structural genes, the regulatory gene, the promoter gene, and the operator. Structural genes are the sections of DNA that code for enzymes for a particular chemical reaction. For the lac operon, three enzymes are coded for and are needed to metabolize lactose. These three enzymes are beta galactosidase, galactose permease, and thiogalactoside transacetylase.

The promoter region is the region where the RNA polymerase binds to begin transcription and is upstream of the operator region. The operator is a region that controls whether transcription occurs or not. In the lac operon, the operator provides a binding site for the lac repressor protein, and the lac repressor protein is inactivated by lactose. If the lac repressor protein binds to the operator, the transcription of the genes for lactose metabolism is turned off. When lactose is present, the lac repressor protein is inactivated, and gene expression can occur. The regulatory genes code for the repressor protein.

D. DNA Technology

Recombinant DNA

Although the sequence of DNA differs from individual to individual and from one organism to another, DNA from any source consists only of the four base pairs of adenine, thymine, guanine, and cytosine. It is possible to exploit this characteristic and to engineer, for example, a particular microorganism to produce a life-saving antibiotic. The process by which this is done is called genetic engineering.

In genetic engineering, a piece of DNA from one organism is isolated by the use of restriction enzymes. Restriction enzymes are found in bacteria and are used to cleave DNA in very specific places. This cleavage produces a DNA strand that has a "sticky end" and is ready to be inserted into DNA from another source. When the same restriction enzyme is used on DNA from another source, the same cleavage occurs and a complementary sticky end is produced. When the DNA from the first source is combined with DNA from the second source in the presence of the enzyme DNA ligase, a new molecule of DNA is produced that has the DNA from the first source. If the new sequence of DNA encodes for enzymes that are used, for example, to manufacture an antibiotic, the second organism may begin producing that antibiotic.

PCR Technology

For many reasons, it might be necessary to have a sufficient amount of DNA to determine the sequence of DNA or to compare DNA from one source to another, as is done in forensic applications. The technique by which copies of DNA are made from a single strand is called PCR technology; the abbreviation PCR stands for polymerase chain reaction.

The first step in PCR is to denature the double-stranded DNA molecule and form single strands. This denaturation is caused by heat, and two strands of DNA are formed that do not recombine. Primers are added. A primer is a short sequence of known nucleotide composition. These primers are present in excess, so when the DNA is cooled, the DNA single strand does not recombine. In the presence of *taq* polymerase and in excess of nucleotides, a copy of the single strand of DNA is formed. Soon there are two molecules of double-stranded DNA.

The process of heating to denature the double-stranded DNA is repeated, and the process of cooling to activate the polymerase is repeated over and over again until sufficient copies of the original DNA plus the primer DNA have been made. The process is automated and can be repeated until a sufficient number of molecules of the DNA have been made for its specific use.

II. TAXONOMY AND MICROBIOLOGY

Knowledge of the properties and characteristics of viruses, bacteria, and fungi is essential to understanding the cause of many diseases as well as the therapeutic approaches used to alleviate diseases. Modern molecular approaches are proving to be particularly useful in this regard.

The science of taxonomy organizes animals according to their traits. In taxonomy, organisms are classified by traits and divided into hierarchical categories. These categories, from the fewest characteristics in common to the most, are as follows:

Kingdom
- Phylum
  - Class
    - Order
      - Family
        - Genus
          - Species

There are six kingdoms: Archaebacteria, Eubacteria, Protista, Fungi, Plantae, and Animalia.

Viruses are not alive because they do not live or reproduce independently. Nonetheless, their existence is very important to living things.

1. VIRAL STRUCTURE AND LIFE HISTORY

Viruses are important because they

- provide insight into evolution,
- are important tools for understanding the molecular biology of normal cells,

- are important in many diseases such as AIDS, and
- may provide powerful molecular tools for combating certain diseases.

Some viruses have been shown to cause cancer in animal models. Viruses have been obtained in a homogeneous state, and some viruses have been crystallized and their three-dimensional structure fully determined by X-ray crystallography. Recently, much emphasis has been placed on the possibility of gene therapy—using viruses to transmit selected genetic information into eukaryotic cells to correct defective genes.

A. Nucleic Acid (DNA and RNA) and Protein Components

Viruses are the simplest supramolecular complex capable of initiating replication. They contain nucleic acids (either DNA or RNA but not both) with a surrounding protein coat called the capsid that protects the encapsulated nucleic acid from damage. Some animal viruses also have an envelope of lipid and glycoprotein surrounding the capsid. An extracellular viral particle (or virion) cannot independently reproduce itself and requires a host cell for this function. It accomplishes this task by diverting the biosynthetic machinery of the host cell to synthesize its own components. In some RNA viruses, the viral mRNA preferentially binds to the host ribosomes. Thus, synthesis of viral proteins is favored over synthesis of host proteins.

Four classes of RNA eukaryotic viruses are distinguishable by the relationship of their viral RNA to their mRNA (Table 3). The designation for mRNA is (+) RNA, and its complementary RNA is designated as (−) RNA. Class I viruses contain (+) RNA, which in turn is the template (+) mRNA. The parental RNA also functions as mRNA because it is capable of polymerizing ribonucleotides from an RNA template. For class I, class II, and class III viruses, this is accomplished by a viral RNA-directed RNA polymerase (or RNA replicase).

TABLE 3. Classes of RNA Viruses

Class	Viral RNA	Flow of Genetic Information
I	(+) RNA →	(−) RNA → (+) mRNA
II	(−) RNA →	(+) mRNA
	(±) RNA → RNA	
III	(±) RNA →	(+) mRNA
IV	(+) RNA →	(−) DNA → (±) DNA → (+) mRNA

Class II viruses contain (−) RNA, which is transcribed into monocistronic mRNAs by a viral RNA transcriptase contained in the virion. One of these mRNAs codes for an RNA replicase, which generates double-stranded RNA from the parental (−) RNA. The RNA replicase also synthesizes progeny (−) RNA strands from the double-stranded RNA.

Class III viruses contain double-stranded RNA, and the (−) strand provides the template for (+) mRNA. Class IV viruses are particularly important because the flow of genetic information is from (+) RNA to DNA and then back to RNA (see Table 3). Class IV viruses are called retroviruses, and they code for an RNA-directed DNA polymerase (or reverse transcriptase). The HIV virus that causes AIDS is a retrovirus.

An important property of some RNA retroviruses (class IV RNA viruses) is their ability to induce tumors in animal models. Some DNA viruses (i.e., Simian virus 40 and polyomavirus) can also cause tumors. Cancer-causing viruses (i.e., oncogenic viruses) transform their host cells by inserting their viral-specific genes into the host chromosome. Normal cells stop multiplying when in close contact with one another; that is, contact inhibition ceases. Transformed cells no longer exhibit contact inhibition and therefore grow continuously.

In DNA or RNA viruses, the DNA provides the template for the synthesis of mRNA molecules that preferentially use the host ribosomes to synthesize viral proteins and the enzymes necessary for viral DNA synthesis.

Viruses contain very few genes (between 3 and 240) and, therefore, construct much of their molecular machinery from identical protein subunits. For example, the protein coat of the TMV (tobacco mosaic virus), which contains only 6 genes, is made up of 2,130 identical protein subunits. Coat protein subunits usually arrange themselves into either rods or spheres, or a combination of those shapes.

Problem

Viruses differ from living organisms because

A. viruses possess no bounding membrane.
B. viruses lack all metabolic machinery.
C. viruses lack all reproductive machinery.
D. All of the above

Solution

D. Viruses differ from living things in many ways. They do not have any membranes because they have no need to take in or expel material. Viruses lack all metabolic machinery and do not produce ATP because they do not perform energy-requiring processes. Viruses do possess either DNA or RNA but cannot independently reproduce. They must rely on host cells for reproductive machinery and components.

B. Bacteriophage: Structure, Function, and Life Cycle

Bacteriophages (or phages) are bacterial viruses that have either RNA or DNA genomes. Figure 33 illustrates the structure of a typical bacteriophage with a head, tail, and tail fibers. Infection of a bacterium (1–10 μm in length) begins when a phage (100–300 μm in length) attaches its tail fibers to a surface receptor on the bacterium. The DNA, which is tightly packed in the phage head, is subsequently injected through the cell wall and the cell membrane into the bacterium (Figure 34). In only a few minutes, all the metabolism of the infected bacterium is directed toward the synthesis of new phage particles. About 30 minutes after infection, the bacterium undergoes lysis, and hundreds of completed bacteriophages are released.

FIGURE 33. Structure of a Typical Bacteriophage

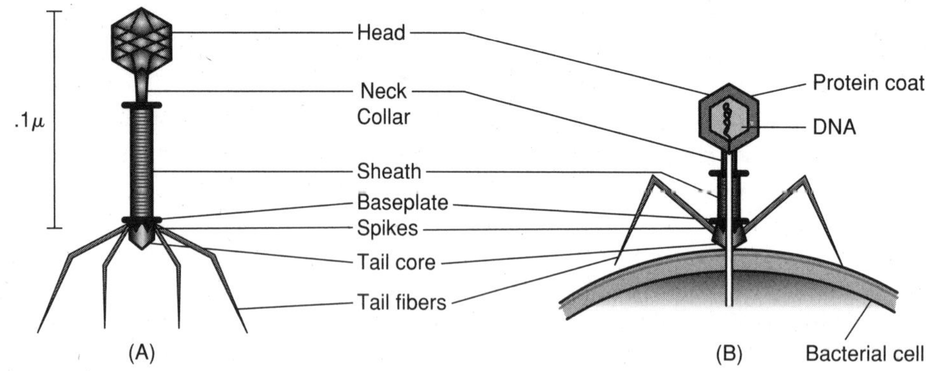

FIGURE 34. Life Cycle of a Bacteriophage

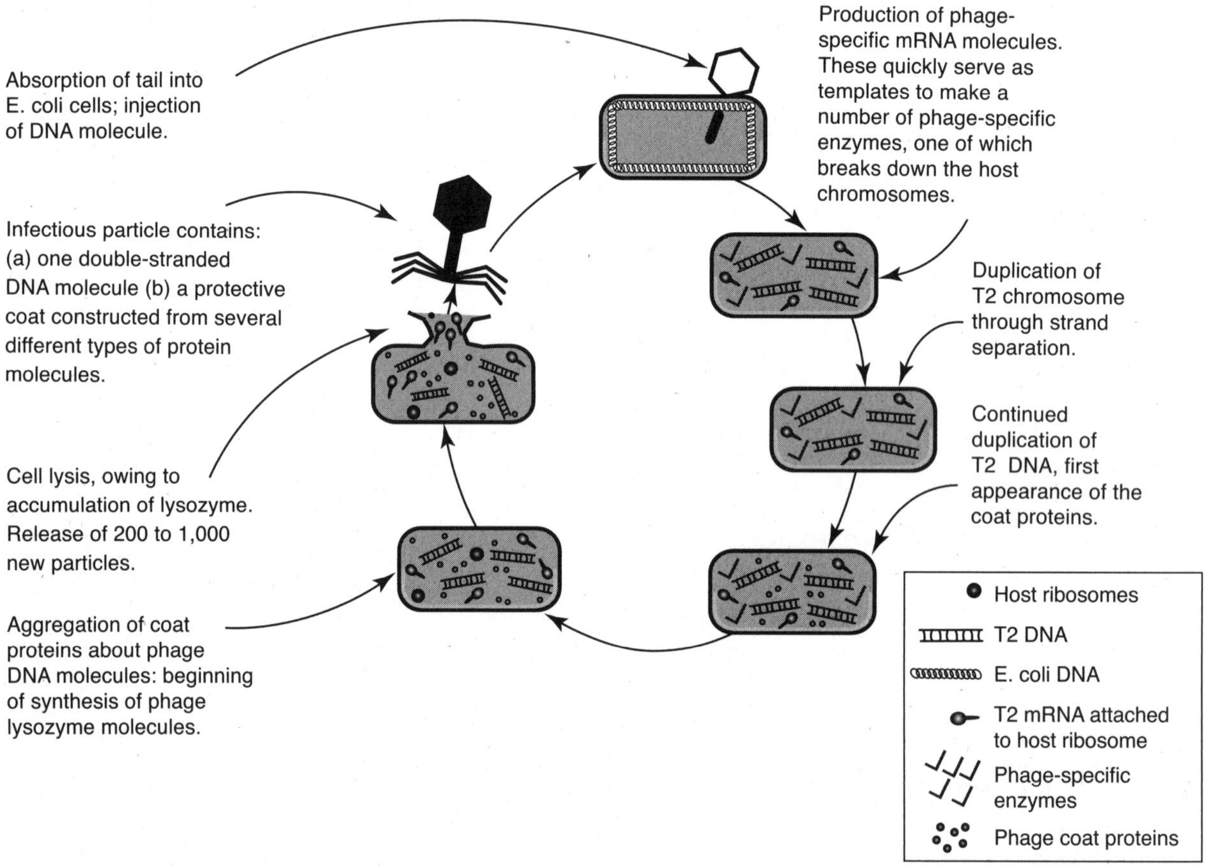

The complex coordination of the phage life cycle is a result of different phage genes being expressed at different times. The early phage genes are expressed before phage DNA synthesis begins. For many phages, some of these gene products shut down the biosynthetic capacity of the bacterium. One of the early phage gene products that helps shut down the metabolism of the host cell is a nuclease specific for bacterial DNA but not the phage DNA.

The late gene products are associated with the synthesis of viral DNA, capsid formation, packaging of the viral DNA into preformed heads, and the synthesis of lysozyme to degrade the bacterial cell wall, thus causing lysis. Not all phages cause immediate lysis of the infected bacterium. In some cases, the phage DNA incorporates itself into the bacterial chromosome and is replicated only when the host chromosome is replicated. This process is called lysogeny. Viruses that exhibit this state are called temperate or moderate viruses.

The viral DNA incorporated into the host chromosome is called a provirus or prophage. In the case of bacteriophages, this prophage can be induced to become virulent and lyse its host bacterium. The resulting infectious phages often carry small amounts of bacterial chromosome that can be transferred to newly infected bacteria. The process whereby DNA is transferred from one bacterium to another by a phage is called transduction.

Problem

Moderate viruses may

A. replace DNA only when the host replicates.
B. induce tumors.
C. cause immediate lysis of infected bacteria.
D. have both DNA and RNA.

Solution

A. In moderate viruses, the phage DNA is incorporated directly into the host chromosome and thus replicates only when the host does. RNA retroviruses may induce tumors. Most viruses, with the exception of moderate ones, cause immediate lysis of infected bacteria. Viruses may contain either DNA or RNA, not both.

2. PROKARYOTIC CELLS

A. Cell Structure and Function

All living organisms have a cell structure that can be classified as either eukaryotic or prokaryotic. The prokaryotic cell is distinguished by the absence of a membrane-bound nucleus. Prokaryotic cells (1–10 μm in length) are much smaller than eukaryotic cells (10–100 μm in length). Both types of cells can have flagella for motility, but these structures are relatively simple in prokaryotic cells. Prokaryotic cells include eubacteria, archaebacteria, blue-green algae, spirochetes, rickettsia, and mycoplasma.

In prokaryotic cells such as bacteria (Figure 35), the single chromosome is a large, single, circular, double-stranded DNA molecule that is not separated from the cytoplasm by a nuclear membrane. The prokaryotic chromosome lies in the nuclear zone. Prokaryotic cells contain less DNA than more advanced eukaryotic cells. Further, in prokaryotic cells, the processes of transcription and translation occur simultaneously.

FIGURE 35. (a) Structure of a Bacterium and (b) Bacterial Reproduction

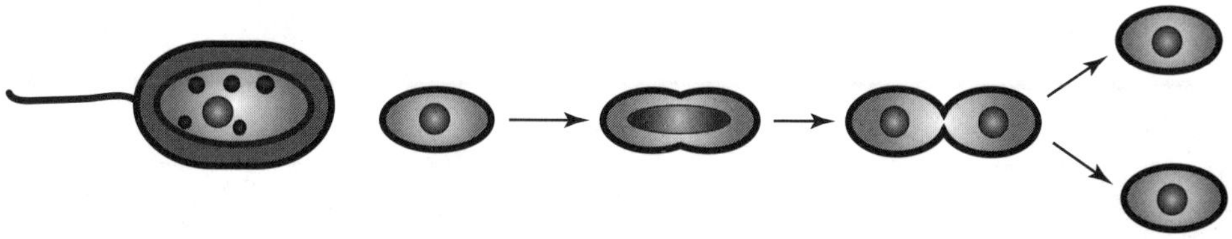

The only membranous structure present in all prokaryotic cells is the plasma membrane. Some prokaryotes have an additional membrane that is part of the cell wall. In contrast, eukaryotic cells have, in addition to the plasma membrane, membranous organelles, such as mitochondria and a membrane-bound

nucleus (Table 4 and Figure 36). The basic structure of membranes is a lipid bilayer with associated intrinsic and extrinsic membrane proteins. Ribosomes and cytosol are present in both cell types. The cytosol contains water-soluble enzymes, metabolic intermediates, and inorganic ions.

TABLE 4. Differences Between Prokaryotic and Eukaryotic Cell

Typical Bacterial Cell	
Prokaryotic	**Eukaryotic**
DNA	
No nuclear membrane	DNA contained in nucleus with surrounding nuclear membrane
No histones	DNA associated with histones
membranes	
plasma membrane	plasma membrane and other
outer membrane	membranous organelles such as mitochondria, endoplasmic reticulum, Golgi complex, peroxisomes, and lysosomes

FIGURE 36. Typical Bacterial Cell

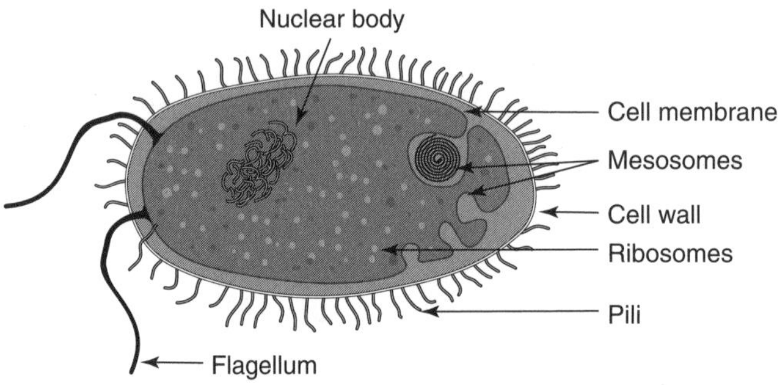

Problem

Which of the following structures is found in a bacterial cell?

A. Golgi apparatus B. Nuclear membrane C. Ribosomes D. Mitochondrion

Solution

C. Unlike eukaryotes, bacterial cells lack Golgi apparatus, endoplasmic reticulum, mitochondria, and a nuclear membrane. The lack of an endoplasmic reticulum means that the ribosomes are free (not bound to rough endoplasmic reticulum).

B. Bacterial Life History and Physiological Characteristics

Bacterial growth is the result of cellular division. For bacteria, the process of cell division is straightforward: the cell doubles in size and then divides in two. This type of growth is exponential. The time it takes for a doubling of a number of bacteria is called the mean generation time, which under ideal conditions may be less than one hour. During cellular division, the DNA of the chromosome replicates (see Figure 35), the resulting identical chromosomes separate, a cross wall forms between the chromosomes, and the cell divides and separates.

A considerable store of fundamental information about molecular biology has come from microbiological studies. Strong evidence for DNA being the genetic material comes from studies where DNA from one bacterial strain is transferred to another. The transfer of the donor DNA is accompanied by the transfer of some donor phenotype (such as virulence) to the recipient strain. DNA can be transferred from one bacterium to another by transduction, transformation, and conjugation.

Transduction is the transfer of a fragment of the bacterial genome from a donor strain to a recipient strain of bacteria using a bacteriophage as the vector. In transformation, a DNA fragment isolated from a donor strain is directly taken up by the recipient strain. In bacterial conjugation, the male and female cells adhere, chromosome or episome replication occurs in the male cell, and one copy is injected into the female cell. No transfer of DNA occurs from the female to the male bacterium.

Bacterial cells are noted for their metabolic versatility and their highly efficient regulation of metabolic and catabolic activities.

Under adverse conditions, some bacteria shift from their normal vegetative state to a dormant state; that is, they undergo sporogenesis. Sporulation is a form of cellular differentiation resulting in a metabolically dormant structure such as an endospore that is formed by the Gram-positive bacteria of the genera *Bacillus* and *Clostridium*. Under favorable conditions, the spore can undergo germination to return the cells to a vegetative state.

Problem

In transduction, a

A. male chromosome is injected into a female cell.
B. female chromosome is injected into a male cell.
C. bacteriophage transfers genetic material between bacteria.
D. DNA fragment from a donor strain is directly taken up by a recipient strain of bacteria.

Solution

C. Choice A refers to bacterial conjugation, choice B is an impossibility, and choice D refers to transformation.

3. FUNGI

A. Major Structural Types

All fungi are eukaryotic organisms, having at least one nucleus with a nuclear membrane, an endoplasmic reticulum, and mitochondria. They lack chloroplasts and chlorophyll. Fungi are spore-bearing organisms with absorptive nutrition. They reproduce sexually and asexually. The primitive plant body formed by fungi is called a thallus, but it has no true roots, leaves, stems, or vascular tissue. Although more than 100,000 species of fungi exist, only about 100 are important in human diseases. Ringworm (dermatophytoses) is a very common infectious disease caused by a fungus. Mushrooms, yeasts, and molds are examples of fungi.

B. General Life History and Physiology

Yeasts are unicellular forms of fungi with a spherical shape (3–15 μm in diameter). Yeasts reproduce by budding or binary fission. Molds grow in multicellular tubular colonies called hyphae. During growth, hyphae combine to form a mycelium.

Fungi have the ability to form "fruiting bodies," which are an effective adaptation to a land environment. The fruiting bodies serve to disperse spores or cysts. Asexual spores formed from the body (or thallus) of a fungus are called thallospores, and asexual spores formed from specialized structures are called conidia.

Fungi are also capable of sexual reproduction. Sexual reproduction causes an alteration in chromosome number. At fertilization, two haploid nuclei join to form a diploid nucleus. The diploid cells eventually give rise to haploid cells by meiosis. In lower fungi, the visible organism often exists primarily in the haploid state (haplophase) and only transiently in the diploid state (diplophase). Sexual reproduction in fungi follows this sequence:

1. Compatible haploid nuclei are brought together in the same cell of the thallus.
2. Two genetically different nuclei fuse to form a diploid nucleus.
3. Meiosis occurs to form haploid nuclei that develop into sexual spores.

Problem

All of the following are true of fungi EXCEPT they do not

A. reproduce sexually.
B. reproduce asexually.
C. produce spores.
D. produce seeds.

Solution

D. Fungi may produce spores sexually or asexually. Seeds are produced by plants, not fungi.

III. GENERALIZED EUKARYOTIC CELL

1. PLASMA MEMBRANE: STRUCTURE AND FUNCTION

A. Composition, Structure, and Movement of Proteins and Lipids

The plasma membrane surrounds the cell and separates the inside (intercellular) from the outside (extracellular) of the cell. Structurally, the plasma membrane is composed of a lipid bilayer and membrane-bound proteins (Figure 37). Lipid bilayers are also present in other organelles of eukaryotic cells, such as mitochondria and endoplasmic reticulum. Phospholipid (PL) molecules are the primary lipid constituents of most lipid bilayers (Figure 38). Cholesterol and glycolipids are also present in many biological membranes. PL molecules are amphipathic molecules; that is, they have a polar head group and two nonpolar hydrocarbon "tails." PL molecules self-aggregate to form a lipid bilayer because in that molecular arrangement, their head groups remain in contact with water, and their tails are removed from contact with water.

FIGURE 37. Lipid Bilayer

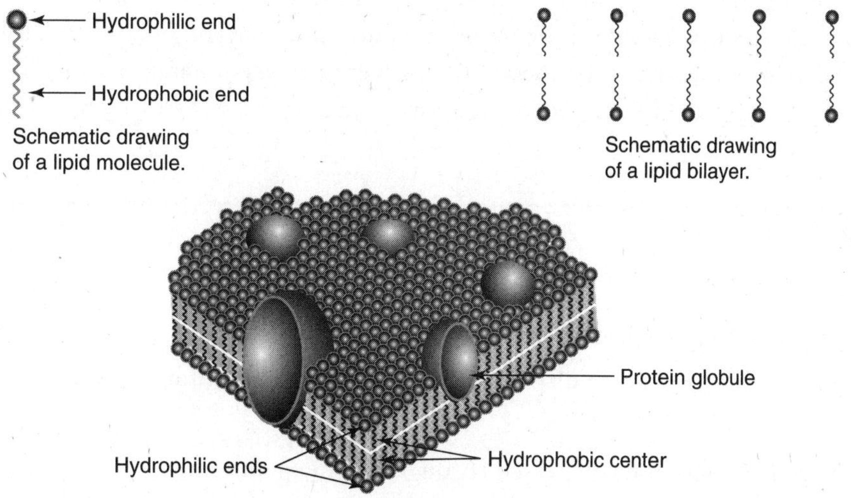

The lipid bilayer structure has two important properties:

1. It is a permeability barrier for charged molecules. Charged hydrophilic molecules cannot move through the lipid bilayer because to do so would require their giving up thermodynamically favorable interactions with polar water molecules. Water molecules, although they can permeate the bilayer, have an extremely low concentration in the hydrophobic domain of the bilayer. For charged molecules to pass through the bilayer, specific transport proteins must be present. However, hydrophobic molecules such as O_2 as well as small, uncharged polar molecules (H_2O, CO_2, and urea) are membrane permeable.

FIGURE 38. Structure of Phospholipid Molecules

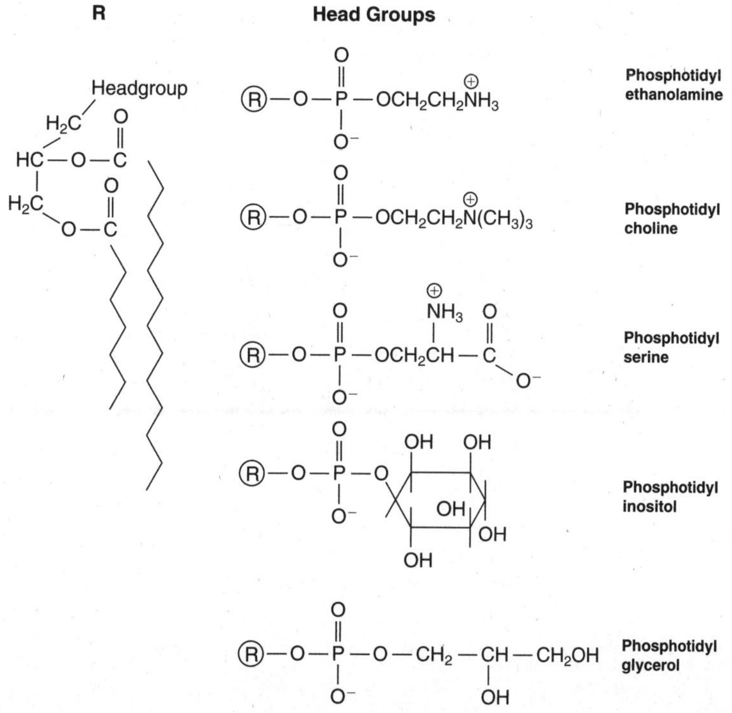

2. The individual PL molecules move rapidly in the plane of the lipid bilayer. Proteins associated with the lipid bilayer also can have rapid lateral motion. The bilayer, therefore, acts as a two-dimensional fluid, and this fluidity is necessary for diffusion of membrane-bound enzymes and receptor molecules.

The plasma membrane and the membranes of other subcellular organelles are asymmetric with respect to the head groups found on the inner and outer monolayers. In addition, the proteins associated with biological membranes are embedded in the bilayer in an asymmetric manner. For example, glycoproteins (as well as glycolipids) in the plasma membrane usually have their carbohydrate moieties facing the extracellular space.

Problem

Cell membranes are generally composed of a double layer of

A. phospholipids, with proteins dispersed throughout the membrane.

B. phosphoproteins, with glucose dispersed throughout the membrane.

C. nucleic acids.

D. proteins with phospholipids dispersed throughout the membrane.

Solution

A. The plasma membrane contains about 40 percent lipid and 60 percent protein by weight, although there is considerable variation among the various cell types. The lipid molecules of the plasma membrane are polar: one end is hydrophobic and the other end is hydrophilic. The lipid molecules are arranged in two layers so that the hydrophobic ends are near each other and the hydrophilic ends face outside. The individual lipid molecules can move laterally, so the bilayer is actually fluid and flexible. Protein molecules of the plasma membrane may be arranged at various sites and imbedded to different degrees (Figure 39). The highly selective permeability of the plasma membrane depends on the specific types and amounts of proteins and lipids present.

FIGURE 39. Protein in Plasma Membrane

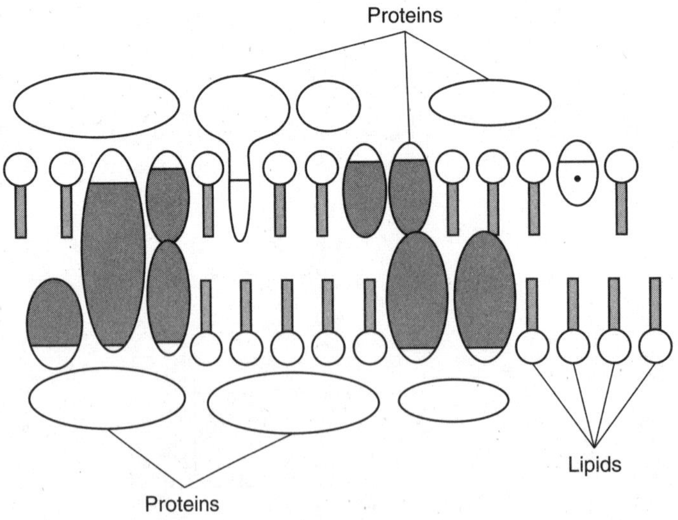

B. Membrane Transport: Passive and Active Transport

The transport of charged biomolecules across biological membranes depends on transport molecules, most of which are proteins. Transport proteins can achieve great specificity and permit only one class of molecules to be transported (e.g., only sugars or only amino acids) or one specific molecule in a class. Some transport molecules simply permit a solute to reversibly diffuse from one side of the membrane to the other. This process is called passive transport. The direction of transport for a solute will be influenced by a concentration gradient across the membrane (i.e., from high to low concentration), as well as the electric charge across the membrane (i.e., the membrane potential).

The combination of the chemical and electrical gradient is called the electrochemical gradient. Plasma membranes are more negatively charged on the cytoplasmic side than the extracellular side, and this hinders the passive transport of positively charged ions. In some cases, the passive transport of a solute is through an aqueous pore created by the transport protein. This type of transport protein is called a channel protein or porin. Transport of a solute through a channel protein is not saturable, which means that the rate of input increases in proportion to the concentration in the extracellular fluid (Figure 40). In other cases, the solute molecule binds to a transport protein that then facilitates its translocation to the other side of the membrane. This process, called facilitated diffusion, is similar to a substrate binding to the active site of an enzyme and is a saturable process.

FIGURE 40. Passive Transport

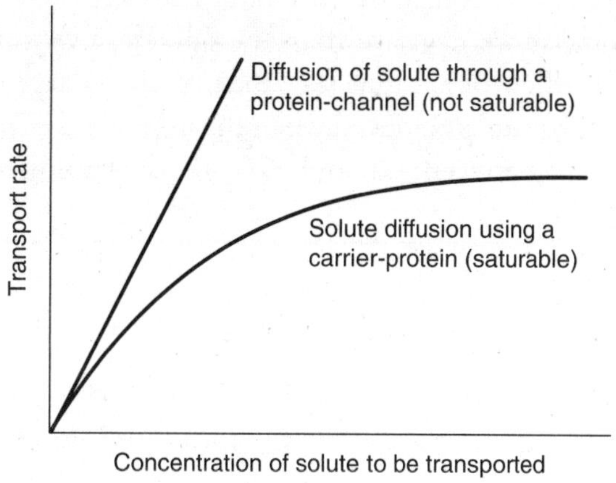

To transport a solute against an unfavorable electrochemical gradient, it is necessary to expend energy, usually ATP. This type of transport is called active transport.

Problem

Porins are important in

A. facilitated diffusion.

B. substrate binding.

C. saturable processes only.

D. passive transport.

Solution

D. Passive transport may occur when a solute passes through an aqueous pore created by a channel protein, or porin. Transport of a solute through a porin is not saturable. Facilitated diffusion occurs when a substrate binds to the active site of an enzyme.

C. The Na^+–K^+ Pump and Membrane Potential

The membrane potential of plasma membranes is generated by two important transport proteins: the Na^+,K^+–ATPase and the K^+–channel. Na^+,K^+–ATPase uses ATP to pump Na^+ ions out of the cell and K^+ ions into the cell (Figure 41). This is an example of active transport because the concentration of Na^+ outside the cell is higher than inside. The reverse is true for K^+ ions.

FIGURE 41. Membrane Potential and Active Transport

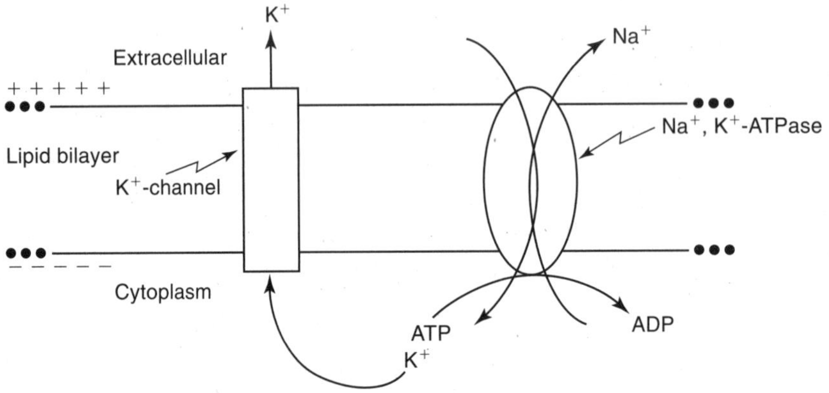

The K^+–channel permits K^+ ions to diffuse out of the cell, and this loss of positive ions causes the inside of the cell to become more negative than the outside. Eventually, the increasing negative charge inside the cell retards the outflow of K^+ ions (i.e., the negative charge inside the cell attracts the positively charged K^+ ions) and equilibrium is achieved when the inflow of K^+ ions equals the outflow. The result is a plasma membrane potential between –20 and –70 mV, depending on the cell type.

Problem

In most cells, the concentration of Na^+ is ______ in the cell than outside because of ______.

A. higher; active transport
B. higher; passive transport
C. lower; active transport
D. lower; passive transport

Solution

C. The Na^+–K^+ pump is a form of active transport in which energy is used to pump Na^+ ions out of the cell and K^+ ions into the cell.

D. Osmotic Effects and Cell Volume

The Na^+,K^+–ATPase and K^+–channel control the movement of ions and thus the level of ions inside the cell. Therefore, these elements are also the main controllers of intracellular osmotic pressure and cellular volume. The charged macromolecules (e.g., proteins) inside the cell require counterbalancing ions like Na^+, K^+, and Cl^-. This creates an osmotic pressure causing cellular swelling from the influx of water. Counterbalancing this intracellular osmotic pressure is the osmotic pressure caused by the ions in the extracellular fluid—primarily, Na^+ and Cl^-. These ions tend to move down their concentration gradient and into the cell. The cell would swell and burst if the Na^+,K^+–ATPase did not maintain a negative membrane potential and pump Na^+ out and, consequently, prevent Cl^- from leaking in.

Problem

Which ions must be transported out of the cell to prevent its rupture?

A. Na^+ B. K^+ C. Cl^- D. All of the above

Solution

D. The macromolecules inside the cell require counterbalancing ions outside the cell, such as Na^+, K^+, and Cl^-. These counterbalancing ions create an osmotic balance that prevents the influx of water into the cell, thus preventing cell rupture.

E. Membrane Receptors

The plasma membrane contains a wide variety of protein receptors to which ligands can bind. A major function of these receptors is to receive signals from the extracellular environment. Neurotransmitters and hormones are examples of ligands that bind to protein receptors on target cells and influence the behavior of the cell.

Receptor proteins (Figure 42) are usually transmembrane proteins that have an extracellular domain where signals are received, a hydrophobic domain going through the lipid bilayer, and a cytoplasmic signal-transducing domain. The initial binding of the signal molecule (i.e., the first message) alters the conformation of the protein receptor, and this activates an intracellular signal pathway. The intracellular signal is often transmitted by a second class of small and rapidly diffusible molecules called second messengers. Calcium and cyclic AMP (cAMP; Figure 43) are two important second messengers. Alternatively, the cytoplasmic domain of the receptor may have protein kinase activity, which is activated when ligand binding occurs. Thus, the receptor molecule itself can activate or inactivate certain intracellular substrates via phosphorylation.

The second messengers can then regulate a wide variety of biochemical and physiological processes. For example, the release of fatty acids from adipocytes (fat cells) is regulated by catecholamines. When catecholamines (the first messenger) bind to a surface receptor on the adipocyte plasma membrane, it causes the receptor molecule to activate an adenylate cyclase enzyme that catalyzes the production of intracellular cAMP from ATP (see Figure 42). The increased cAMP (the second messenger) activates a protein kinase that, in turn, phosphorylates the hormone-sensitive lipase enzyme. The phosphorylation activates hormone-sensitive lipase, and it then hydrolyzes triglyceride into fatty acids (Figure 44).

FIGURE 42. Cell Receptors and Signals

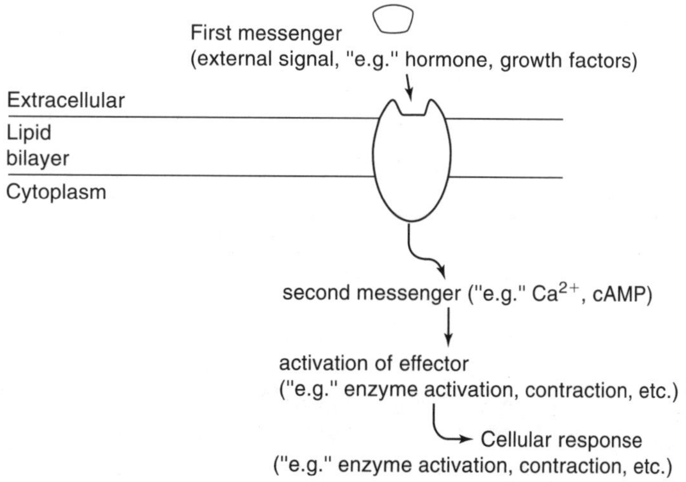

FIGURE 43. Structure of Cyclic AMP

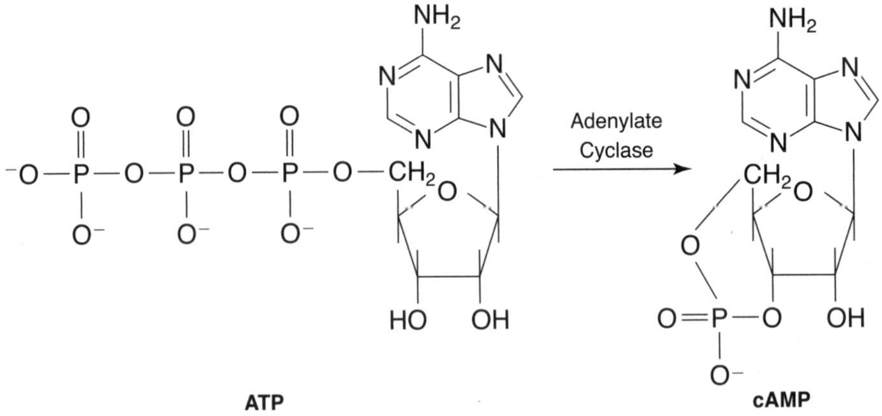

FIGURE 44. Hormone-Sensitive Lipase

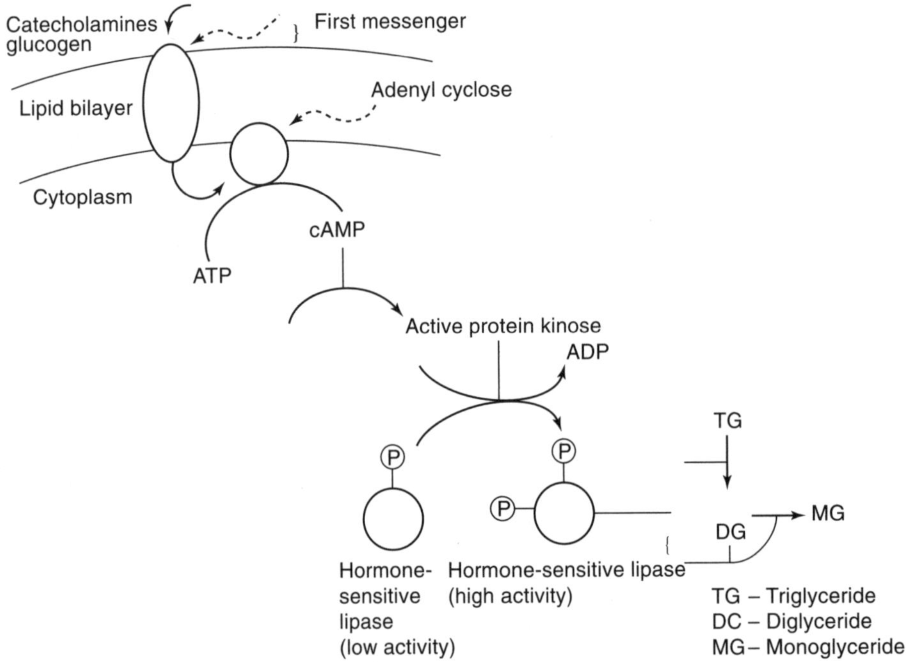

Some receptors serve to bind very large molecules brought into the cell as a source of nutrients. Most cells, for example, have receptors for low-density lipoprotein (LDL), which is a very large lipid–protein complex. The LDL receptor is called the apoB,E receptor, and it recognizes the apoB protein moiety of LDL. After binding to the apoB,E receptor, LDL is internalized by endocytosis (Figure 45) and provides the cell with an external source of cholesterol and other lipids.

FIGURE 45. LDL Uptake by Receptor-Mediated Endocytosis

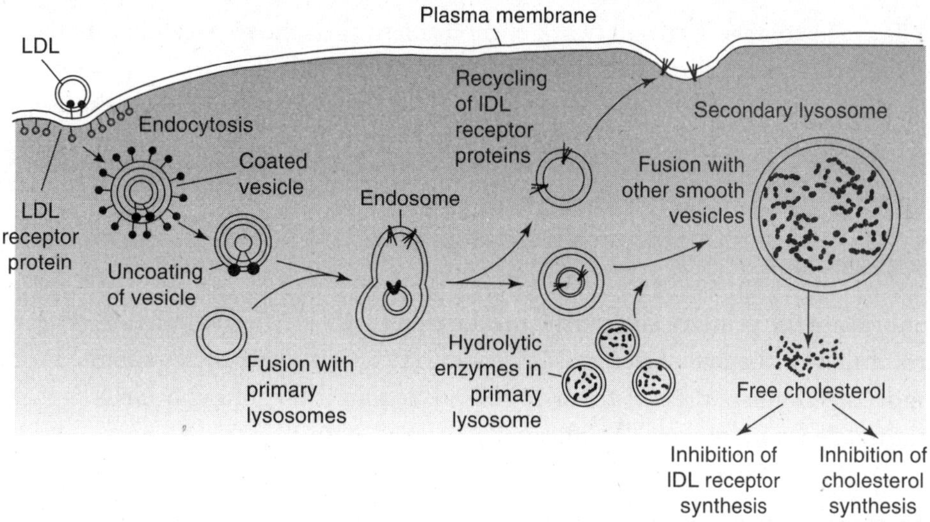

Problem

Ligands bind to

A. target cells.   B. neurotransmitters.   C. protein receptors.   D. hormones.

Solution

C. Neurotransmitters and hormones are examples of ligands that bind to protein receptors on target cells.

F. Exocytosis and Endocytosis

Macromolecules are too large to be transported through the plasma membrane by specific transport proteins. The transport of these macromolecules is accomplished by the processes of exocytosis and endocytosis. In exocytosis, an intracellular vesicle is transported to the plasma membrane where it fuses with the plasma membrane. The fusion process releases the contents of the vesicle to the extracellular space. Endocytosis is essentially the reverse of this process (see Figure 45).

Problem

Which is most likely to be transported by exocytosis?

A. Urea   B. Lipoprotein   C. Na^+ D. Hormones

Solution

B. Exocytosis is used to transport the largest molecules, macromolecules. Lipoproteins have larger molecules than any of the other materials listed.

G. Cellular Adhesion

Tissue cells are in contact with a network of molecules called the extracellular matrix. This matrix plays a major role in promoting cell-to-cell adhesion. In addition, cells that are in direct contact with each other can form cell junctions between specialized regions of their plasma membranes.

2. MEMBRANE-BOUND ORGANELLES

A. Mitochondria

Mitochondria are the primary site for the production of ATP. Mitochondria appear to be associated with the microtubules of the cytoskeleton. Mitochondria contain their own genome. Proteins from both the mitochondrial genome and the nuclear DNA are required for mitochondrial replication. In mammals, mitochondrial genes are maternally inherited.

Problem

Which of the following is responsible for the majority of cellular ATP production?

A. Endoplasmic reticulum

B. Lysosomes

C. Golgi apparatus

D. Mitochondria

Solution

D. The mitochondria are responsible for 95% of all ATP produced in the cell. For this reason the mitochondria are commonly referred to as the "powerhouse" of the cell. Mitochondria are membrane-bound organelles distributed throughout the cell. Mitochondria tend to be most concentrated in regions that require large amounts of energy, such as muscle.

B. Endoplasmic Reticulum

Eukaryotic cells contain a smooth and rough endoplasmic reticulum (ER), which represents about one-half of all the cellular membrane (Figure 46). Prokaryotic cells do not contain an ER. Structurally, the ER is one highly convoluted membrane sheet enclosing a space called the ER lumen. The cytoplasm is separated from the ER lumen by a single membrane (the ER membrane). The ER membrane is continuous with the outer nuclear membrane. The rough ER has ribosomes along the endoplasmic membrane that give it a rough appearance in an electron microscope. The two main functions of the rough ER are making membrane proteins and making secretory proteins.

Proteins that are to be secreted by the cell or sent to other intracellular organelles are delivered to the lumen of the rough ER. The polypeptides being translated on these ribosomes are transported from the cytoplasmic side of the ER membrane into the ER lumen. The ribosomes attached to the rough ER are identical to ribosomes not attached to the rough ER. Attachment of some ribosomes to the ER is directed by a small sequence of amino acids at the amino end of the polypeptide being translated (i.e., the signal sequence). The signal sequence is removed once the polypeptide has been delivered to the ER lumen. Many polypeptides undergo "core glycosylation" in the ER. Smooth ER has no attached ribosomes. Transport vesicles carrying newly synthesized lipids and proteins bud off the smooth ER for transport to the Golgi apparatus. Many important detoxification and lipid metabolism reactions take place on the smooth ER.

FIGURE 46. Generalized Eukaryotic Cell

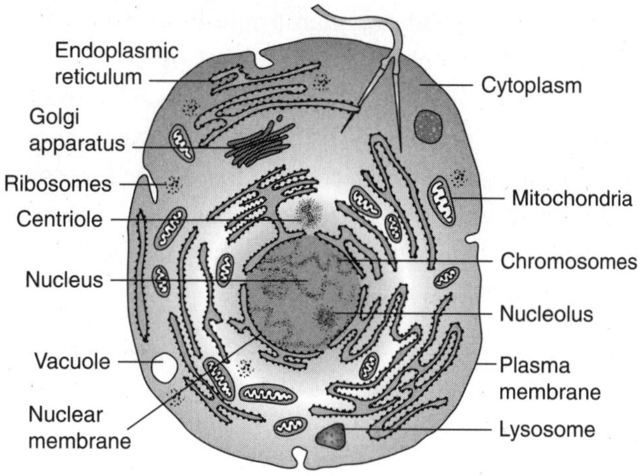

Problem

Prokaryotic cells contain

A. an endoplasmic reticulum.

B. ribosomes.

C. a nuclear membrane.

D. both an endoplasmic reticulum and ribosomes.

Solution

B. Prokaryotic cells contain ribosomes, but they do not have an endoplasmic reticulum or nuclear membrane.

C. Golgi Apparatus

The Golgi apparatus is composed of flattened membrane-bound sacs surrounded by a swarm of smaller membrane-bound vesicles called "coated vesicles." Proteins associated with the ER are transported to the Golgi apparatus by these small vesicles, which are coated with a protein called clathrin. Glycoproteins are received by the convex side of the Golgi apparatus and undergo "terminal glycosylation" in the Golgi apparatus. The sugar moieties of glycoproteins are extensively modified by enzymes in the Golgi apparatus, and the modified glycoproteins are sorted and delivered either to other organelles or to the plasma membrane where they can be secreted into the extracellular fluid. The luminal side of both the ER and the Golgi apparatus correspond to the extracellular side of the plasma membrane. Further, two membranes separate the lumen of the ER from the lumen of the Golgi apparatus.

Problem

The Golgi apparatus primarily functions in

A. packaging protein for secretion.

B. synthesizing protein for secretion.

C. packaging protein for hydrolysis.

D. synthesizing protein for hydrolysis.

Solution

A. The Golgi apparatus is an organelle that is responsible only for the packaging of protein for secretion.

D. Lysosomes

Lysosomes (250–750 nm in diameter) are membrane-bound vesicles found in the cytoplasm. These organelles are responsible for the intracellular digestion of macromolecules. A primary lysosome is a newly synthesized vesicle and contains a wide variety of hydrolytic enzymes (all are acid hydrolases), such as proteases, phospholipases, and nucleases. These hydrolytic enzymes are almost all glycoproteins and have optimal enzymatic activities at pH 5.0, the pH inside the lysosomes. The primary lysosome arises from the budding of specialized regions of the Golgi apparatus. A secondary lysosome is a lysosome that is actively digesting a substrate (see Figure 45). The substrate can be a foreign pathogen such as a bacterium or an endogenous macromolecule such as LDL.

Problem

Lysosomes contain

A. glycogen stores. B. lipids. C. acid hydrolases. D. ATP.

Solution

C. Lysosomes are cell organelles found in the cytoplasm. They are vesicles surrounded by a single membrane and contain enzymes, mostly acid hydrolases. These hydrolases are released when the membrane bursts, permitting the digestion of cellular structures and macromolecules. During the normal metabolism of the cell, enzyme release is carefully controlled by mechanisms that are still very poorly understood.

3. CYTOSKELETON

A. Microfilaments, Microtubules, and Intermediate Filaments

The cytoskeleton of eukaryotic cells plays a key role in maintaining the cellular structure and cellular motility. Microfilaments and microtubules are composed of cytoskeletal filaments. These filaments are polymers of soluble subunits and can rapidly assemble and dissemble. The assembly process is energy dependent and requires ATP or guanosine triphosphate (GTP). A third type of filament is designated as an intermediate filament because its diameter is between that of microfilaments and microtubules. Intermediate filaments are found in most animal cells. They are of a more permanent nature than either microfilaments or microtubules. The molecular mechanisms involved in the contraction actin and myosin filaments are discussed in the section on muscle tissue.

Problem

Intermediate filaments are

A. found in animal cells.
B. more permanent than microfilaments.
C. intermediate in diameter between microfilaments and microtubules.
D. all of the above.

Solution

D. Intermediate filaments, found in animal cells, are more permanent than and are intermediate in diameter between microfilaments and microtubules.

B. Cilia, Flagella, and Centrioles

Cilia are hairlike projections (0.25 μm long) that extend from the surface of many animal cells. These structures are used for cell movement (as in protozoa) or to move fluid (such as mucus) at the surface of the cell. Ciliated epithelial cells are found in the respiratory tract. Ciliary movement depends on movement of the axoneme, which is primarily composed of microtubules. It is a relatively permanent structure. The soluble subunit used to construct a microtubule is called tubulin. Ciliary motion requires ATP hydrolysis, which generates a sliding movement of microtubules.

For microtubules to perform their functions they must be attached to other parts of the cell. Cilia end in a structural unit, the basal body, located at the base of the ciliary axoneme. The cytoplasmic microtubules observed in interphase cells (period between mitoses) are attached to centrioles. Basal bodies and centrioles have very similar structures, each having a nine-fold array of triplet microtubules.

The centrosome, which is present in most animal cells, has a centriole pair at its center. Higher plants do not have centrosomes. The centrosome, also called the cell center, is adjacent to the cell nucleus. It serves to organize microtubules and plays a major role in cell division.

Flagella in eukaryotic cells have a structure very similar to cilia and generate movement using the same principle detailed for cilia. Sperm cells and protozoa are examples of flagellated eukaryotic cells. The flagella of bacteria differ markedly from those of eukaryotic cells.

4. NUCLEUS: STRUCTURE AND FUNCTION

The nucleus of the cell contains the nuclear DNA encoding the genetic information required for cellular replication, differentiation, and functions. DNA replication and RNA synthesis occur in the nucleus. The RNA in the nucleus can undergo processing (e.g., RNA splicing) before being transported to the cytoplasm.

Nuclear DNA associates with histone proteins to form nucleosomes, the unit particles of chromatin. Chromatin, in turn, is packaged to form very compact structures called chromosomes. Other proteins, called nonhistone proteins, are also associated with nuclear DNA. Most of the DNA in the nucleus does not code for protein.

A. Nuclear Envelope and Nuclear Pores

The nucleus is bound by an envelope made up of two membranes: an inner and an outer nuclear membrane. The inner and outer nuclear membranes are fused at points called nuclear pores. The nuclear pores contain a nuclear pore complex thought to permit the selective transport (in and out) of macromolecules. For example, DNA and RNA polymerases that are synthesized in the cytoplasm must be transported into the nucleus through nuclear pore complexes.

Problem

Nuclear pore complexes

A. transport micromolecules.

B. transport the nucleus.

C. fuse the nuclear and cell membranes.

D. fuse the inner and outer nuclear membranes.

Solution

D. Nuclear pore complexes fuse the inner and outer nuclear membranes to permit the transport of macromolecules to and from the nucleus.

B. Nucleolus

The nucleolus is a highly ordered structure specially designed to produce the rRNA required for ribosomes. The synthesized rRNA immediately combines with ribosomal proteins to form subunits. These subunits join to form functional ribosomes only after they have been transported from the nucleus through nuclear pores to the cytoplasm.

Problem

rRNA is made in the

A. endoplasmic reticulum.
B. nucleolus.
C. ribosomes.
D. cytoplasm.

Solution

B. rRNA is synthesized in the nucleolus and combined with ribosomal proteins.

5. MITOSIS

A. Mitotic Process, Phases of the Cell Cycle

Cells are continuously subjected to various kinds of stress that can result in cell death. For an organism to grow and survive, cells must reproduce themselves. For cellular division to occur, a cell must first double its contents, divide the nucleus, and then divide its cytoplasm. The process of nuclear division is called mitosis. A cell that is not undergoing active division is said to be in interphase. The interphase period has been further delineated based on the occurrence of DNA synthesis (Figure 47). The period of active DNA synthesis and replication (sister chromatids) is called S-phase. The gap period before S-phase is called G1-phase, and the gap period after S-phase is called G2-phase. The mitotic phase, designated M-phase, begins after the G2-phase.

FIGURE 47. Cell Cycle Phase

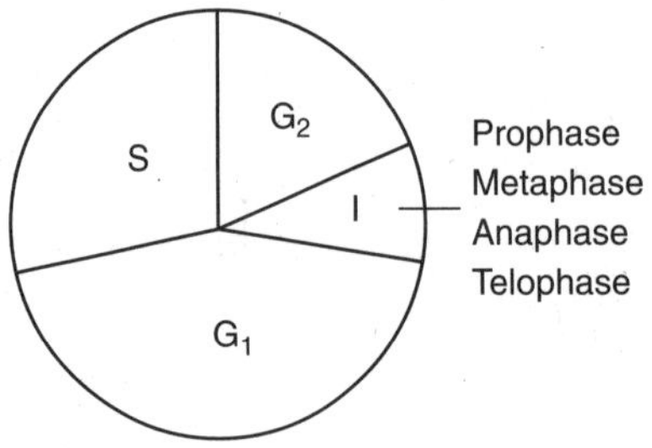

Problem

A mitotic cell produces

A. two cells with half of the chromosomes of the first cell.
B. two cells, each with the full chromosome complement of the original cell.
C. four cells with half of the chromosome complement of the original cell.
D. four cells with the full chromosome complement of the first cell.

Solution

B. Mitosis refers to the process by which a cell divides to form two daughter cells, each with exactly the same number and kind of chromosomes as the parent cell.

B. Mitotic Structures

Chromatids and Centromere

Most of the synthetic events necessary for cell division occur during interphase. In animal cells, the initiation of DNA replication (i.e., the start of S-phase) is closely associated with the replication of the cell's pair of centrioles. The centrioles are the microtubule-organizing center of the cell. Each centriole pair forms the spindle pole during mitosis. Once DNA synthesis is initiated, it continues until all the DNA is replicated. As the DNA replicates, new histones are attached and chromatin is formed. Each chromosome is duplicated in S-phase, forming two sister chromatids joined by a centromere.

Centrioles, Asters, and Spindles

G2-phase begins at the end of the S-phase. During G2-phase, cells prepare for mitosis by constructing much of the macromolecular machinery used in the mitotic spindle (as discussed in the next section). M-phase begins at the end of G2-phase. M-phase has been further divided into prophase, metaphase, anaphase, and telophase. During prophase, chromatin condenses into chromosomes. In addition, the mitotic spindle is formed. The mitotic apparatus consists of the two centrioles, a set of microtubules, and two pairs of centrioles. The microtubules form a radial array called the aster around each pair of centrioles. Some of the microtubules eventually connect each pair of centrioles. These microtubules make up the spindle. The microtubules are responsible for the movement of chromosomes during mitosis.

Kinetochore

Early metaphase starts with the dissolution of the nuclear envelope. Microtubules subsequently become attached to chromosomes at a locus called the kinetochore. During metaphase, the chromosomes become aligned at a plate halfway between the spindle poles. At anaphase, the chromosomes are broken apart by the microtubules attached to the kinetochores. During telophase, the daughter chromosomes arrive at opposite spindle poles, and the kinetochore microtubules dissociate. Further, a nuclear envelope appears around each set of new chromosomes, and nucleoli reappear. This completes the process of mitosis. The subsequent division of the cytoplasm is called cytokinesis.

Problem

Kinetochore microtubules dissociate during

A. prophase. B. metaphase. C. telophase. D. anaphase.

Solution

C. Kinetochore microtubules attach during prophase. At anaphase, they break apart the chromosomes. During telophase, the kinetochore microtubules dissociate.

6. MEIOSIS

Every organism has a certain number of chromosomes. To preserve this number, the female donates half of its chromosomes and the male delivers half of its chromosomes. In mitosis, cells of identical chromosome number are produced. By contrast, in meiosis, cells of a haploid number of chromosomes are formed. This process occurs in the specialized sex organs called gonads. The process produces four new cells with a haploid number of chromosomes. The process occurs in two rounds of cell division called meiosis I and meiosis II. In meiosis I, the number of chromosomes reduces, and in meiosis II, mitotic division occurs.

During interphase, prior to meiosis I, double-stranded chromosomes are formed. Meiosis I consists of four stages: prophase I, metaphase I, anaphase I, and telophase I. Meiosis II consists of prophase II, metaphase II, anaphase II, and telophase II and is very similar to mitosis.

In prophase I, the members of each pair of chromosomes move together and lie side by side. They do not fuse together. This pairing process is called synapsis and is different from prophase in mitosis. Exchange of pieces of chromosomes can occur between homologous chromosomes. This process is known as crossing over and allows for genetic recombination.

During metaphase I of meiosis I, the chromosome pairs line up and move to the metaphase plate. The chromosome pairs are called tetrads. The centromere does not divide.

Anaphase I is characterized by separation and movement of chromosomes. Each pair of chromosomes within a tetrad separates and moves to opposite poles.

In telophase I, two new nuclei are formed. The chromosomes are double-stranded, but the cells contain the haploid number of chromosomes. After telophase I, the two haploid cells undergo cytokinesis.

Problem

Meiosis II differs the most from mitosis in what phase?

A. Prophase II B. Metaphase II C. Interphase D. Teleophase II

Solution

C. There is no interphase between meiosis I and II because the chromosomes are already replicated.

IV. SPECIALIZED EUKARYOTIC CELLS AND TISSUES

1. NEURAL CELLS AND TISSUES

A. Structures: Cell Body, Axon, Dendrites, Myelin Sheath, Schwann Cells, and Nodes of Ranvier

The neuron is the key cell type in the nervous system. A neuron receives information from other neurons or from sensory receptors and transmits the information either to other neurons or to muscles. The structure of a typical vertebrate neuron is shown in Figure 48.

Information is transmitted by neurons either by an action potential or by synaptic transmission. The action potential is an all-or-none response, and it is a time-dependent change in the transmembrane

FIGURE 48. Structure of a Typical Vertebrate Neuron

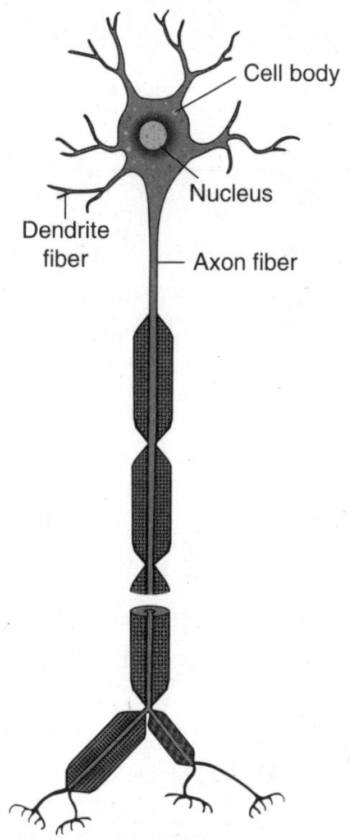

potential of the neuron. The action potential is carried away from the cell body by the axon that usually branches and has many termini, called synaptic knobs. When the action potential comes to an axon terminal, it contacts the synapse, which is a knoblike structure. The synapse is the junction between the end of the axon and the dendrites of an adjacent neuron.

In vertebrates, many axons are insulated by layers of myelin that serve to increase the speed at which an action potential is transmitted along the axon. The myelin sheath (in peripheral neurons) is formed by glial cells called Schwann or sheath cells (Figure 49). Between one Schwann cell and the next is a small region where the axon has no sheathing. This region, called the node of Ranvier, is very rich in Na^{+}–channels.

FIGURE 49. Structure of Schwann Cells and the Nodes of Ranvier

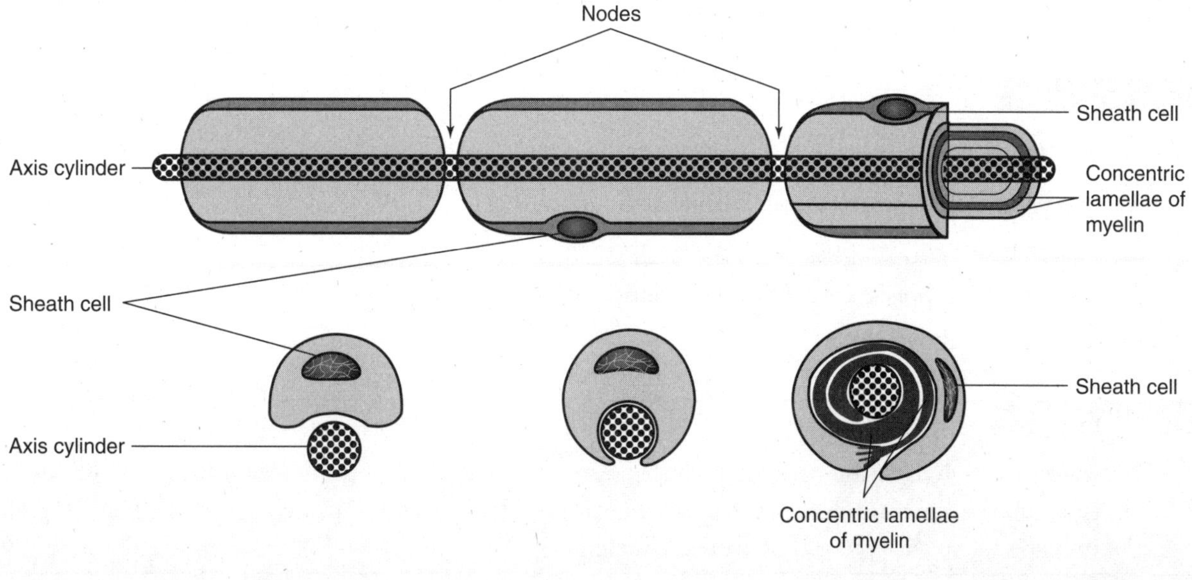

Problem

The myelin sheath of many axons is produced by the

A. node of Ranvier. B. nerve cell body. C. Schwann cell. D. astrocytes.

Solution

C. Schwann cells are the myelin-forming cells of the peripheral nervous system. Each Schwann cell forms a single myelin internodal segment around a portion of an axon. Schwann cells may also surround unmyelinated axons, without producing myelin.

B. Synapse

The structure of a synapse is shown in Figure 50. The presynaptic cell is separated from the postsynaptic cell by the synaptic cleft. The action potential in the axon triggers the release of neurotransmitter substances from storage vesicles (synaptic vesicles) in the synaptic knobs. The release of the neurotransmitter causes an electrical change in the postsynaptic cell. The postsynaptic cell sums up electrical signals induced by the release of the neurotransmitter and, when a critical total signal level is reached, an action potential is generated by the postsynaptic cell.

FIGURE 50. Structure of a Typical Synapse

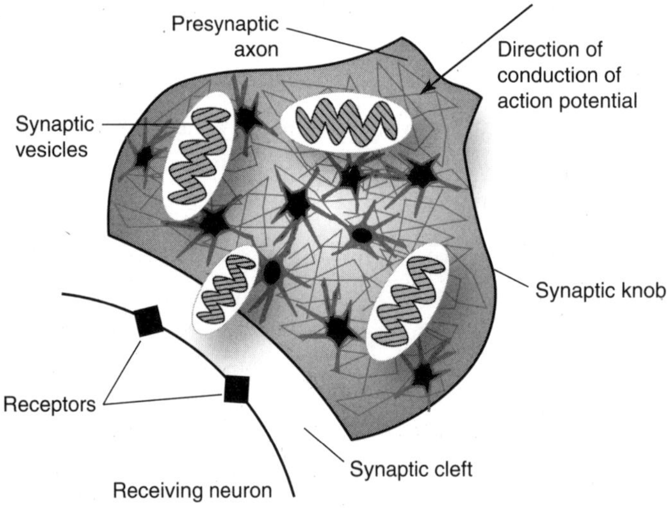

Problem

The correct sequence for signal transmission in a synapse is

A. presynaptic cell, postsynaptic cell, synaptic cleft.
B. presynaptic cell, synaptic cleft, postsynaptic cell.
C. synaptic cleft, presynaptic cell, postsynaptic cell.
D. none of the above.

Solution

B. Electrical signals in the presynaptic cell cause release of neurotransmitter substances that flow through the synaptic cleft to the postsynaptic cell. The postsynaptic cell creates an electrical signal in response to the received neurotransmitter.

C. Resting Potential and Action Potential

The resting potential of a neuron is established by the Na^+,K^+–ATPase and the K^+–channel, as described in the previous section. The action potential is generated by a voltage-gated Na^+–channel. A voltage-gated channel is one whose permeability can increase or decrease depending on the level of the membrane potential. The resting membrane potential of a neuron is about −70 mV. When the axon receives a nerve impulse, this electrical signal increases the membrane potential to about 0 mV (top panel of Figure 51). This initial increase is called membrane depolarization. Concomitant with the membrane depolarization, there is an opening of a voltage-gated N^+–channel that permits Na^+ to flow into the cell (recall that Na^+ is high outside the cell and low inside the cell). This influx of positive charge causes the membrane potential to become even more positive, and this is accompanied by a closing of the Na^+–channels. As the Na^+–channels close, the K^+–channels open and K^+ moves out of the cell (recall that K^+ is high inside the cell and low outside). Therefore, the inside of the cell becomes more negative. This part of the action potential is called repolarization. The K^+–channels close slowly so that there is a dip below −70 mV (hyperpolarization) and finally a return to the resting potential of −70 mV.

FIGURE 51. Action Potential

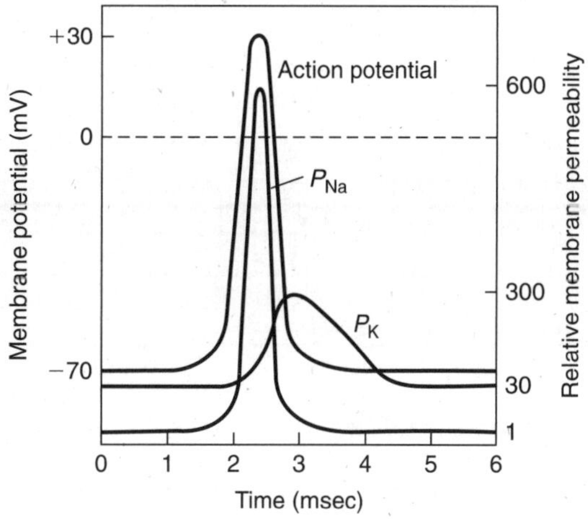

Problem

In Figure 51, membrane polarization occurs

A. before 0 msec. B. at 0 msec. C. at 1 msec. D. at 4 msec.

Solution

B. The resulting neuron potential of a neuron is about −70 mV. When the axon receives a nerve impulse, the potential reduces to about 0 mV, resulting in a membrane depolarization.

2. CONTRACTILE CELLS AND TISSUES

A. Skeletal, Smooth, and Cardiac Muscle

Vertebrates have three types of muscles: skeletal, smooth, and cardiac. The specialized muscle cells in muscle tissues all have the ability to contract using actin and myosin filaments. ATP hydrolysis provides the energy for muscle contraction. Skeletal muscles are under voluntary control and connect the bones of the skeleton. Skeletal muscles are used for complex activities such as walking. Skeletal muscles are made up of long muscle fibers (myofibers), and each fiber is considered a large, single cell that is formed by the fusion of many separate cells. Each myofiber has many nuclei and bundles of myofibrils. As shown in Figure 52, a myofiber (1–40 mm in length and 10–50 μm in width) has a striated (striped) appearance. The striated appearance results from bundles of aligned myofibrils with dark bands (A bands) alternating with light bands (I bands). A narrow line bisects each I band and is called the Z line.

FIGURE 52. (a) Structure of Two Adjacent Myofibrils; (b) Structure of a Sarcomere

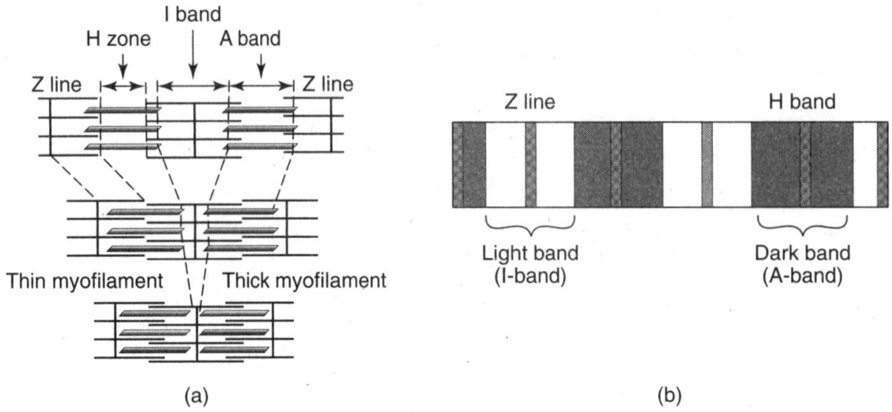

Smooth muscles are under involuntary control by the central nervous system. Smooth muscles are involved with movements of the small and large intestine and the bladder, and they control the diameter of blood vessels. Smooth muscle cells are not striated and have one nucleus per cell. Cardiac muscle is found only in the heart. The cells are striated. Cardiac muscle is under involuntary control. Cardiac muscles produce the synchronous contractions of the heart (i.e., the heartbeat).

Problem

Which of the following statements is false?

A. Cardiac muscle is uninucleate, striated, and controlled by the autonomic nervous system.

B. Skeletal muscle is multinucleate, striated, and controlled by the somatic nervous system.

C. Smooth muscle is uninucleate, nonstriated, and controlled by the autonomic nervous system.

D. None of the above is false.

Solution

D. All of the statements regarding muscle types are true. Skeletal muscle is responsible for most voluntary movements, and it is controlled by the somatic nervous system. It contains striations because of the ordered arrangement of thick and thin filaments and has many nuclei. Smooth muscle lines the stomach, intestinal tracts, and blood vessels with involuntary movements controlled by the autonomic nervous system. Smooth muscle is uninucleate and does not have striations. Cardiac muscle contains features of both types of muscle. It is striated, uninucleate, and is not under voluntary control.

B. Sarcomere

The sarcomere is the basic unit of contraction in striated muscles, and it is the region between two Z lines, as shown in Figure 52(b). Myofibrils are made up of repeating sarcomere units. The sarcomere has thick myosin filaments as well as thin actin filaments. The thin filaments are attached to the Z line. The movement of thick and thin filaments between each sarcomere leads to muscle contraction.

Problem

During muscular contraction,

A. sarcomeres move between myofibrils.
B. myofibrils move between Z lines.
C. myosin and actin filaments move between sarcomeres.
D. Z lines are made of myofibrils.

Solution

C. The sarcomere has myosin and actin filaments. The movement of these filaments between each sarcomere leads to muscular contraction. Actin filaments attach to the Z line. Myofibrils are made of sarcomeres.

C. Calcium Regulation of Contraction

The movement of skeletal muscles is under voluntary control, and muscle contraction is initiated by neurotransmitter release from a neuron. The electrical impulse from the neuron triggers an action potential in the plasma membrane of the myofiber and is rapidly spread by transverse (or T) tubules (from the plasma membrane) to the Z line of the myofibrils. The signal is then transmitted to the sarcoplasmic reticulum. The sarcoplasmic reticulum surrounds each myofibril, and when activated by the electrical impulse, it releases Ca^{+2} ions, causing all the myofibrils in the myofiber to simultaneously contract.

Problem

Which is required for muscular contraction?

A. Electrical impulse B. Ca^{+2} ions C. Na^{+} ions D. Both A and B

Solution

D. Muscular contraction is initiated by electrical impulse from a neuron. The impulse makes the sarcoplasmic reticulum release Ca^{+2} ions, which cause myofibrils to contract.

3. EPITHELIAL CELLS AND TISSUES

Epithelial cells form the inner and outer surfaces of the body. These cells have many specialized shapes and functions. Epithelial cells adhere to each other and to the basal lamina. Simple squamous epithelium cells, illustrated in Figure 53(a), form a thin layer of cells that cover the inner lining of most blood vessels. Simple cuboidal epithelium, shown in Figure 53(b), also consists of a single layer of tightly fitting cells, but they have a cubelike shape. Cuboidal epithelium cells line the ducts of many glands. A layer of elongated simple columnar epithelial cells, illustrated in Figure 53(c), form the lining of the stomach, the cervix, and the small intestine. Goblet cells are found in simple columnar epithelium, and they secrete mucus. Stratified epithelia are several cell layers thick, and they form the surface of the mouth, the esophagus, and the vagina. The outer layer of skin consists of stratified squamous epithelial cells that have undergone a process of keratinization. Intestinal epithelial cells are very specialized, and the cell surface facing the lumen of the small intestine has many microvilli that are important in the absorption of nutrients. The microvilli contain actin filaments that help maintain their rigidity.

FIGURE 53. Types of Epithelial Cells

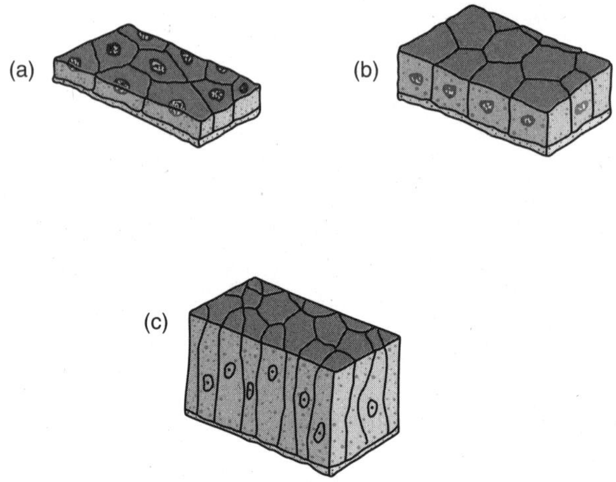

(a) Simple squamous epithelium; (b) Simple cuboidal epithelium; (c) Simple columnar epithelium

The basal lamina provides a distinct boundary between the epithelial cells and the cells that underlie the basal lamina.

Problem

Epithelial tissues perform many functions. Which of the following is a function of this tissue?

A. Absorption B. Protection C. Secretion D. All of the above

Solution

D. Epithelium exhibits a multiplicity of structural forms, all having the common role of covering the outer surface and lining the inner surfaces of the body. In some cases, as in skin, the function is mainly protective. In many other instances, however, epithelial tissue carries out functions such as surface and transepithelial transport, absorption, and secretion.

4. CONNECTIVE CELLS AND FIBER TYPES

A. Major Cell and Fiber Types

Connective tissues are characterized by the presence of relatively few cells with a large complement of extracellular matrix. The extracellular matrix typically contains collagen fibers secreted by connective tissue cells.

At least four distinct types of collagen fibers have been identified. Type IV is found exclusively in the basal lamina. Types I and III are found in skin, whereas bone contains only type I. The extracellular matrix also has polysaccharides that are primarily glycosaminoglycans. These polysaccharides are often cross-linked with protein to form proteoglycans. Bone and teeth are composed of extracellular matrix with a secondary deposition of calcium phosphate crystals.

Problem

Collagen fibers are found in

A. skin. B. blood. C. bones. D. both skin and bones.

Solution

D. Collagen is found primarily in connective tissue, such as skin and bones. Blood is not a connective tissue.

B. Loose versus Dense Connective Tissue

Connective tissue is classified as either loose or dense. Loose connective tissue forms the bed for epithelial cells and many glands. Blood vessels run through loose connective tissues. Dense connective tissue is found in bone, cartilage, and tendons.

Problem

Which of the following is not a connective tissue?

A. Bone B. Tendons C. Cartilage D. Muscle

Solution

D. Connective tissues function to support and hold together structures of the body. Bone, cartilage, tendons, ligaments, and fibrous connective tissues are all types of connective tissue. The cells of these tissues characteristically secrete a large amount of noncellular material called matrix. The nature and function of each kind of connective tissue is determined primarily by its matrix. Most of the connective tissue volume is made up of matrix.

C. Cartilage

Cartilage provides support, framework, and protection. There are three types of cartilage: hyaline, elastic, and fibrocartilage. Each contains a different kind of extracellular matrix. Hyaline cartilage is the most abundant and occurs in many joints and bone ends. During embryonic development, skeletal components are first formed from hyaline cartilage subsequently replaced by bone. Elastic cartilage is more flexible than hyaline cartilage, and it forms the external structure of the ears. Fibrocartilage is mechanically very strong, and it serves a protective role by functioning as a cushion between bones in the knees and the pelvic girdle. Cartilage cells are found in small chambers called lacunae surrounded by extracellular matrix.

Problem

Elastic cartilage is found

A. on bone ends.
B. in ears.
C. in the pelvis and knees.
D. on bone ends and in knees.

Solution

B. Elastic cartilage is found in ears. Hyaline cartilage coats bone ends. The pelvis and knees contain fibrocartilage.

D. Extracellular Matrix

The extracellular matrix, primarily composed of collagen and tropocollagen, is the basic structural unit from which collagen is constructed. Collagen fibers are extremely strong. Tropocollagen has a unique triple-helix structure, and each polypeptide strand is called an alpha chain. Intramolecular hydrogen bonds link each alpha chain to the other two alpha chains. The amino acid sequence of each alpha chain is given by a repeating series of

$$(\text{gly-pro-}X)n,$$

where every third residue is glycine (gly), *X* can be any amino acid, and *pro* is short for *proline*. In collagen fibers, the tropocollagen molecules are aligned along their long axes but are displaced by about 64 nm. The adjacent tropocollagen molecules are also cross-linked to one another. This cross-linking greatly enhances the mechanical strength of the collagen fibers.

Problem

The extracellular fibers found in all connective tissues are composed mainly of

A. collagen.
B. calcium.
C. elastin.
D. glycans.

Solution

A. The connective tissues are defined as the complex of cells and extracellular materials that provide the supporting and connecting framework for all other body tissues. The connective tissues consist of extracellular fibers, amorphous ground substance, and connective tissue cells. The fibers are composed mainly of the protein collagen. The ground substance occupies the spaces between the cells and fibers and contains proteoglycans, glycoproteins, and other molecules secreted from the cells.

V. NERVOUS AND ENDOCRINE SYSTEMS

1. NERVOUS SYSTEM STRUCTURE AND FUNCTION

Neurons are the fundamental cell type of the nervous system. Neurons can transmit information from inside and outside the body to processing centers in the brain and spinal cord. The processed signals can evoke responses, also transmitted by neurons, muscles, and glands. The coordination and integration of these events leads to behavioral adaptation to environmental changes and helps maintain a stable internal environment.

A. Organization of the Vertebrate Nervous System

The structure of the neuron, action potentials, and synaptic transmission has already been discussed. The organs of the brain and spinal cord form the central nervous system. The nerves that connect the central nervous system to other body parts are called the peripheral nervous system.

Problem

The central nervous system is composed of the

A. brain and spinal cord.
B. spinal cord and nerves.
C. neurons, synapses, and spinal cord.
D. sense organs, spinal cord, and brain.

Solution

A. The organs of the brain and spinal cord form the central nervous system. The nerves that connect the central nervous system to other body parts are called the peripheral nervous system.

B. Sensor and Effector Neurons

The sensory function of the nervous system is achieved by sensors at the ends of peripheral nerves. Neurons with a sensory function are called afferent or sensory neurons. The dendrites of these neurons either function directly as receptors for stimuli or are in close association with specialized receptor cells. Most sensor neurons have a unipolar structure, as shown in Figure 54(a).

The information from sensory neurons is transmitted in the form of a nerve impulse over peripheral nerves to the central nervous system. After integration of the sensory information, a response can be transmitted by the peripheral nerves to effectors—that is, muscles and/or glands. Interneurons are neurons that get their input from other neurons and send their output to other neurons. Interneurons are found in the brain or spinal cord and are involved with processing and integration. The interneurons are multipolar, as shown in Figure 54(b).

FIGURE 54. Neuronal Structures: (a) Unipolar Neuron; (b) Multipolar Neuron; (c) Bipolar Neuron

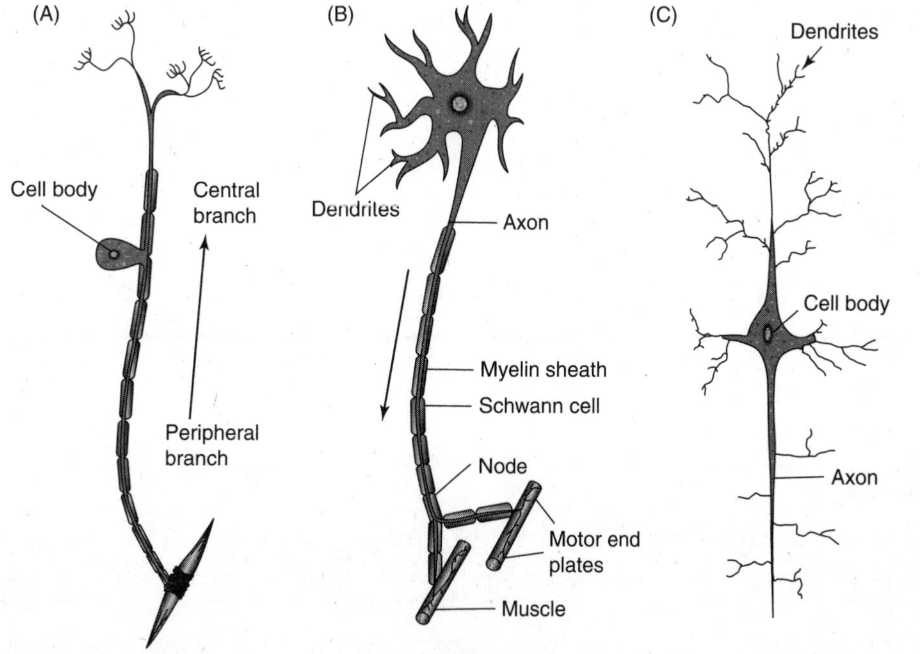

Motor neurons, also called efferent neurons, transmit nerve impulses from the brain or spinal column to effectors. Motor neurons are usually multipolar.

The axons of neurons are bundled together to form nerve fibers. Some nerve fibers contain only motor axons, some contain only sensory axons. Most nerves, however, contain both motor and sensory axons.

Problem

Bundles of axons are known as

A. interneurons. B. association areas. C. nerves. D. effectors.

Solution

C. Axons are bundled together to make nerves. Interneurons link neurons to the brain. Effectors are muscles or glands that respond to stimuli.

C. Sympathetic and Parasympathetic Nervous System

The autonomic nervous system is not under voluntary control and functions independently. The contraction of smooth muscles, blood pressure regulation, temperature regulation, and the secretory function of most glands are under the control of the autonomic nervous system. The autonomic nervous system has been further divided into the sympathetic and parasympathetic nervous systems.

In general, the sympathetic subdivision prepares an organism for energy expenditure, and the parasympathetic system restores and maintains an organism in a resting state. Organs are innervated with nerve fibers from both the sympathetic and parasympathetic divisions. The sympathetic nervous system, for example, increases heart rate and decreases intestinal secretions. These physiological adaptations are restored by the parasympathetic nervous system.

Most of the nerve fibers in the autonomic system are composed of motor neurons, and two neurons are used to connect the brain or spinal cord to the effector. The preganglionic axon comes from a neuron in the brain or spinal cord and forms a synapse with a ganglion outside the brain and spinal cord. The postganglionic axon comes from this second neuron, and it goes to the effector.

Sympathetic nerves are adrenergic and secrete the neurotransmitter called norepinephrine at the end of their postganglionic fibers. Parasympathetic nerves are cholinergic and secrete acetylcholine at the ends of their postganglionic fibers.

Problem

Which of the following is characteristic of stimulation of the sympathetic nervous system?

A. Elevated heartbeat
B. Increased saliva excretion
C. Elevated gastric secretion
D. All of the above

Solution

A. In general, the sympathetic nervous system produces the effects that prepare an animal for emergency situations, such as quickening of the heart and breathing rates and dilation of pupils.

2. SENSORY RECEPTION AND PROCESSING

A. Somatic Sensors

The specialized senses are smell, taste, hearing, equilibrium, and sight. The somatic senses are all the other senses, such as touch, heat, and pain. The somatic senses can be further divided into exteroreceptive, proprioceptive, visceral, and deep sensations. The exteroreceptive sensations arise from the surface of the body. The proprioceptive sensations arise from muscles and tendons, the visceral sensations from the internal organs, and the deep sensations from "deep" tissues (e.g., bones).

The somatic sensory receptors can be

- mechanoreceptors, which respond to mechanical movement;
- thermoreceptors, which respond to hot and cold;
- pain (or nociceptors) receptors, which signal tissue damage; or
- chemoreceptors, which respond to changes in oxygen levels, carbon dioxide levels, and pH.

A wide variety of mechanoreceptors exist. These include

- free ends of sensory nerve fibers found predominantly in epithelial cells, which respond to touch and pressure;
- Meissner's corpuscles, which respond to light touch; and
- Pacinian corpuscles, which respond to deep pressure and tissue vibrations.

Problem

Somatic sensory receptors could not detect a

A. bright light. B. hot stove. C. stomachache. D. sunburn.

Solution

A. Somatic sensory receptors transmit information from nonspecialized parts of the body. They do not transmit smell, taste, hearing, equilibrium, or sight.

B. Olfaction and Taste

The specialized sensations of smell (olfaction) and taste rely on chemoreceptors. Chemoreceptors are also present on internal tissues where they can detect changes in oxygen levels, glucose levels, and pH. In general, chemoreceptors require a threshold level of stimulation to generate a receptor potential.

The neurons in the superior part of the nasal cavity that detect odors are called olfactory receptors. These bipolar neurons, depicted in Figure 54(c), lie in a surrounding matrix of columnar epithelial cells. Bowman's glands, which secrete the mucous necessary for receptor functioning, are also embedded in the columnar epithelial cells. The mucosal ends of the olfactory neurons have many cilia that are the primary receptor sites for gaseous molecules dissolved in the mucosal fluid.

The precise mechanism whereby different gaseous molecules are distinguished is not yet clearly known. When the cilia are stimulated, a receptor potential is generated, triggering a nerve impulse in the olfactory nerve fibers. This signal is transmitted to the central nervous system. The olfactory receptors undergo a progressive adaptation; with time, the response to a stimulus diminishes. Taste cells undergo a similar adaptation.

The sense of taste is generated by taste buds located in the tongue and, to a lesser extent, on the roof of the mouth. It is thought that taste consists of different combinations of five primary tastes: sour, savory (umami), salty, sweet, and bitter. The taste receptors are microvilli that protrude from taste cells, which are specialized epithelial cells. The outer surface of the taste bud is covered with stratified squamous epithelial cells, and the microvilli from the taste cells protrude from a pore on this surface. The taste cells are replaced about every 10 days. After stimulation, the taste cells generate a receptor potential that, in turn, triggers a nerve impulse transmitted to the central nervous system.

Problem

Following exposure to a strong odor over a long period, olfactory receptors exhibit a diminished response. This is a result of

A. receptor stress.

B. progressive adaptation.

C. receptor death.

D. lack of mucosal fluid.

Solution

B. Progressive adaptation to strong stimuli reduces the response of taste and olfactory receptors.

C. Hearing

Ear Structure

The ear, which functions in both hearing and balance, has external, middle, and internal components. The external ear consists of the auricle, which is funnel shaped, and the auditory canal, which is tube shaped (Figure 55). These structures serve to funnel sound waves into the ear, where they produce pressure oscillations on the eardrum. The middle ear is in the tympanic region of the temporal bone. The eardrum, or tympanic membrane, separates the external and middle ear.

FIGURE 55. Structure of the Ear

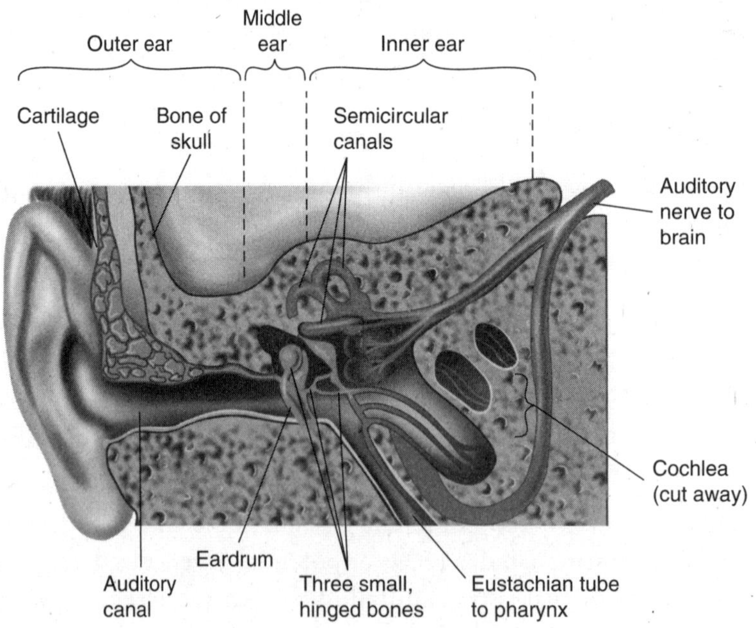

Three small bones in the tympanic cavity transmit the vibration of the eardrum to the inner ear (Figure 56). The malleus (or hammer) is attached to the eardrum. The malleus causes the incus (or anvil) to vibrate, and this movement is then transmitted to the stapes (or stirrup). It is the movement of the stapes that causes movement of fluid in the inner ear. The stapes is connected to an opening in the middle ear called the oval window.

FIGURE 56. Structures of the Middle Ear

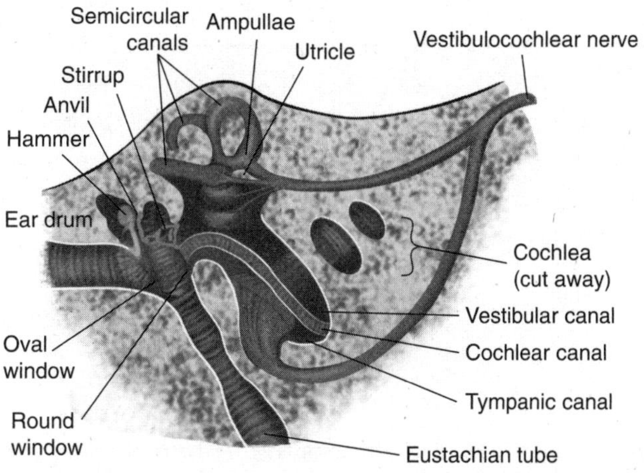

The inner ear contains the labyrinth (Figure 57), a complex set of interconnecting and coiled tubes. The labyrinth includes the cochlea and three semicircular canals. The cochlea contains a fluid moved by the impact of the stapes. The surface of the basilar membrane inside the cochlea contains the organ of Corti. The organ of Corti has the hair cells that function as the receptors for sound oscillations.

FIGURE 57. Labyrinth of the Inner Ear

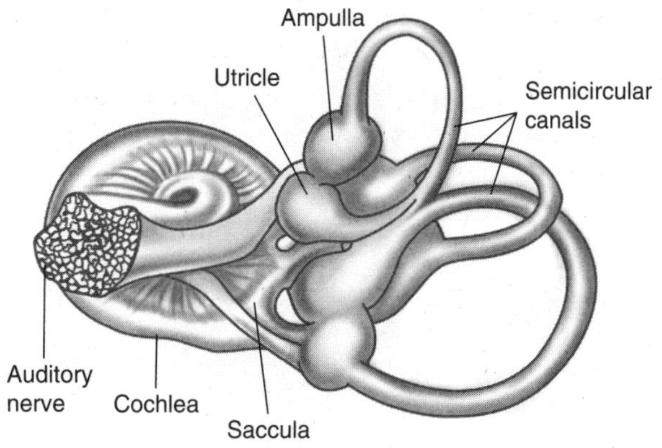

The eustachian tube connects the middle ear to the throat and permits pressure equilibration between the ear and the outside of the body.

Mechanism of Hearing

The organ of Corti generates a receptor potential when stimulated by the vibrations of the basilar membrane. The hearing receptor cells have cilia, or hairlike structures, that project into the endolymph of the cochlear canal. The sensitivity of the ear to different sound frequencies depends on the differential sensitivity of the hair cells. The movement of the hairs causes the generation of a receptor potential that is transmitted to the cochlear nerve fibers. Some of the nerve impulses from each ear reach both sides of the brain.

Problem

Which of the following items is NOT part of the human ear?

A. Malleus B. Cochlea C. Hyoid D. Oval window

Solution

C. Only the hyoid, a very small bone in the neck that supports the base of the tongue, is not a part of the human ear. The tectorial membrane is part of the cochlea, which is in the inner ear. The oval window is a membrane that separates the middle ear and the inner ear. The malleus is one of the small bones in the middle ear that conducts sound.

D. Vision

Eye Structure

The light receptors in the eye are extremely sensitive. A retinal rod cell can detect a single photon. The structure of the human eye is shown in Figure 58. The cornea is transparent, helps focus light, and provides mechanical protection to the other underlying tissues. The anterior chamber contains aqueous humor, and it lies between the cornea and the lens. The lens focuses light on the retina. The iris controls the diameter of the pupil and helps control the intensity of the light impinging on the retina. The vitreous humor (posterior chamber) in the eye cup helps control the internal pressure of the eye.

FIGURE 58. Structure of the Human Eye

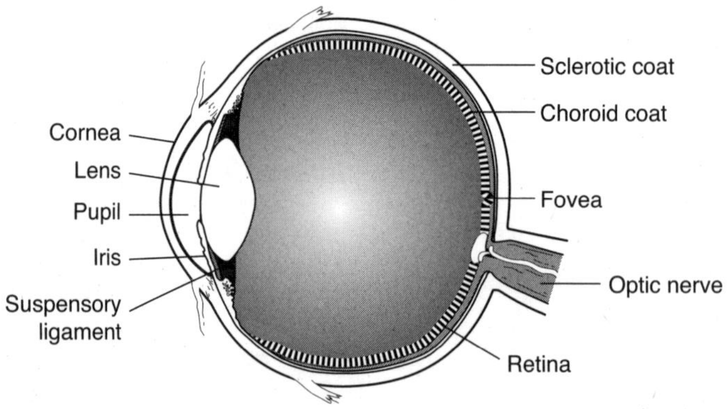

The retina contains the photoreceptor cells that are specialized either for color vision (i.e., the cones) or for night vision (i.e., the rods). In the human retina is a specialized region called the fovea that has a high density of cone cells. Before light reaches the photoreceptor cells, it must pass through a number of other retinal layers. The rod photoreceptor cells (Figure 59) are adjacent to the retinal pigment epithelium. The rod cells shed their tips each day, and these tips are phagocytized by the retinal pigment epithelium. Blood supply to the retina is by way of the choroid or by retinal blood vessels. The choroid is posterior to the retinal pigment epithelium.

FIGURE 59. Structure of the Rod Photoreceptor Cell

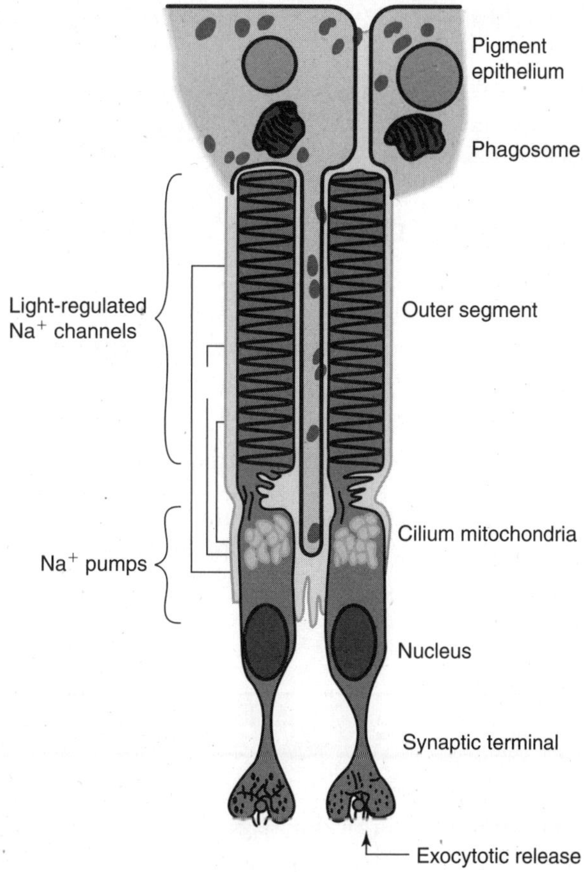

The outer segment of the rod photoreceptor cell has numerous disc membranes that are not in direct contact with the plasma membrane. A photosensitive pigment, rhodopsin, is an intrinsic membrane protein found in the disc membranes.

Light Receptors

The rhodopsin molecules in the disc membranes are covalently linked with 11-cis-retinal. Retinal is an aldehyde form of vitamin A. Light causes isomerization of the cis-retinal to the all-trans-retinal form. This isomerization triggers a change in the conformation of rhodopsin. The light-induced conformational change in rhodopsin causes Na^+–channels on the photoreceptor plasma membrane to close. In the dark, the photoreceptor cells are depolarized. This depolarization is caused by open Na^+–channels that permit a constant influx of Na^+ ions. The result of a light stimulus is to close the Na^+–channels and thereby cause the receptor cell to become hyperpolarized. This action potential causes a decreased release of inhibitory neurotransmitter.

Problem

The part of the eye that regulates the amount of incoming light is the

A. retina. B. lens. C. iris. D. cornea.

Solution

C. Light entering the eye passes through the cornea and enters the lens via a small opening called the pupil. The size of the pupil can be changed by a diaphragm-like muscular structure, the iris, so that the amount of incoming light can be regulated. The iris may contain various colored pigments. The light then falls on a light-sensitive region, the retina, which is located at the rear of the eye.

3. ENDOCRINE SYSTEM: HORMONES AND THEIR SOURCES

A. Function of Endocrine System

Bodily functions are controlled by the nervous system and the endocrine system as well as the interaction between these two systems. The nervous system, as detailed in the previous sections, relies on electrical signals. The endocrine system utilizes chemical signals, and the signal molecules are called hormones. The endocrine system refers to the set of glands, tissues, and cells that secrete hormones directly into bodily fluids.

Hormones regulate a wide variety of metabolic functions and transport functions, as well as development, growth, and reproduction. Hormones are structurally diverse and can exert physiological effects on their target tissues at very low concentrations. Hormones can be peptides, proteins, glycoproteins, biological amines, or steroids.

Problem

Hormones do NOT regulate

A. growth. B. reproduction. C. digestion. D. temperature.

Solution

D. Temperature regulation is controlled by the autonomic nervous system. Growth, reproduction, and digestion are, in part, controlled by hormones.

B. Cellular Mechanisms of Hormone Action

Many hormones exert their action by first binding to specific receptors on the cell surface. Some of the overall molecular characteristics of this type of signaling process have been discussed already (see "Plasma Membrane: Structure and Function" under Section III: Generalized Eukaryotic Cell).

Many hormones activate a cyclic AMP (cAMP) system. The first event is the binding of a hormone to a surface receptor on the plasma membrane of the target cell. The receptor–hormone complex then activates adenyl cyclase, which produces cAMP from ATP in the cytoplasm. The cAMP is the "second messenger" that relays the initial extracellular signal from the hormone (the "first messenger") to an intracellular signal (increased levels of cAMP). The increased cAMP then can activate a wide variety of physiological responses. Often a protein kinase is activated that can phosphorylate specific enzymes and thereby regulate their enzymatic activity.

Steroid hormones do not utilize a cAMP system. The steroid hormones are freely permeable to the plasma membrane and do not have surface receptors. Instead, they bind to cytoplasmic receptors, and the receptor–hormone complex then initiates a series of events leading to the activation of specific genes in the cell nucleus.

Problem

Steroid hormones are unlike other hormones because they

A. utilize the cAMP system.
B. have cytoplasmic receptors.
C. have surface receptors on the plasma membrane.
D. are secreted directly into bodily fluids.

Solution

B. Steroids have cytoplasmic receptors. Most other hormones have surface receptors on the plasma membrane and utilize the cAMP system. All hormones are secreted directly into bodily fluids.

C. Control of Hormone Secretion

The secretion of hormones into circulating blood is a very regulated process. Both negative and positive feedback loops help regulate this process (Figure 60). In a negative feedback loop, gland A secrets hormone A, which stimulates gland B to produce hormone B, which then can inhibit the secretion of hormone A by gland A. In a positive feedback loop, gland A produces hormone A, which stimulates gland B to produce hormone B, which further stimulates gland A to secrete hormone A.

FIGURE 60. (a) Positive Feedback Regulation; (b) Negative Feedback Regulation

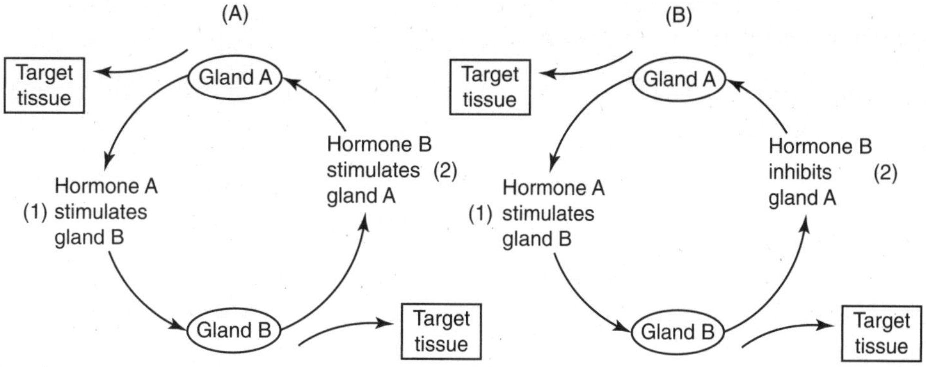

Hormonal secretions can also be controlled by the nervous system. For example, the adrenal medulla (see below) secretes catecholamines in response to nerve impulses and not by the influence of other hormones or any other stimulus.

Problem

Hormone secretion is controlled by

A. negative and positive feedback.
B. the nervous system.
C. negative feedback only.
D. both A and B.

Solution

D. Hormone secretion can be controlled by positive feedback, negative feedback, or the nervous system.

D. Major Endocrine Glands, Their Hormones, Specificity, and Target Issues

The major endocrine glands, their hormone products, their target tissues, and their functions are detailed below.

Pituitary Gland

Pituitary gland — lies at the base of the brain and is connected to and controlled by the hypothalamus. The pituitary gland is divided into the anterior and posterior pituitary gland.

Anterior Pituitary Gland

Anterior pituitary gland — produces hormones that influence other glands.

Adrenocorticotropic hormone (ACTH) — a protein hormone whose target tissue is the adrenal cortex. ACTH controls the secretion of some adrenocortical hormones and thereby influences the metabolism of glucose, fats, and proteins.

Follicle-stimulating hormone (FSH) — a protein hormone whose target tissue is the ovary. FSH stimulates the growth and reproductive activities of the gonads.

Growth hormone (GH) — a protein hormone that promotes body growth and has a major impact on formation of body protein. It increases

- the transport of amino acids through cell membranes, and
- the synthesis of proteins by ribosomes.

It also decreases the rate of protein catabolism.

Luteinizing hormone (LH) — a protein hormone that stimulates the growth and reproductive activities of the gonads.

Prolactin (PRL) — a protein hormone that stimulates growth of the mammary gland and production of milk.

Thyroid-stimulating hormone (TSH) — a protein hormone whose target tissue is the thyroid gland. TSH controls the synthesis of thyroxine in the thyroid gland. Thyroxine, in turn, controls many metabolic reactions.

Posterior Pituitary Gland

Antidiuretic hormone (ADH) — a peptide hormone, also called vasopressin, that causes a decreased secretion of water by the kidneys (i.e., antidiuresis).

Oxytocin — a peptide hormone whose target tissues include the uterus and the mammary gland. Oxytocin is thought to play a key role in the birthing process, causing contraction of the uterus. Oxytocin also stimulates the expression of milk from the mammary gland in response to suckling.

Thyroid Gland

Thyroid gland — located below the larynx and on both sides of the trachea.

Thyroxine (T4) — an iodinated amino acid derivative that increases the overall metabolic rate and, in children, promotes growth. In particular, T4 increases protein synthesis, increases the number and size of mitochondria, and stimulates both carbohydrate and fat metabolism. Secretion of T4 is controlled by TSH from the anterior pituitary gland.

Triiodothyronine (T3) — an iodinated amino acid derivative whose functions are similar to those detailed for thyroxine.

Parathyroid Glands

Parathyroid glands — located on the posterior surface of the thyroid gland. The parathyroid hormone is the only hormone secreted by the parathyroid gland.

Parathyroid hormone (PTH) — a protein hormone that causes absorption of calcium and phosphate from bone. Moreover, the PTH causes a dramatic increase in the secretion of phosphate by the kidney. The overall result of increased levels of PTH in plasma is an increase in calcium but a decrease in phosphate levels. PTH promotes the conversion of vitamin D into 1,25-dihydroxycholecalciferol, which helps promote calcium transport through cell membranes. 1,25-Dihydroxycholecalciferol is the active form of vitamin D. High levels of plasma calcium decrease the secretion of PTH.

Adrenal Glands

Adrenal glands — lie at the top of the kidney. The adrenals consist of two distinct glands that secrete different hormones. The exterior of the adrenals is the cortex, and the central region is the medulla. The cells of the medulla are modified postganglionic cells. The cells of the adrenal medulla are in contact with the sympathetic division of the autonomic nervous system.

Adrenal medulla — made up of modified postganglionic cells. The cells of the adrenal medulla are in contact with the sympathetic division of the autonomic nervous system. Nerve impulses from the sympathetic nerve fibers are the stimulus for the secretion of epinephrine and norepinephrine.

Epinephrine — a hormone, also called adrenalin, that is a biological amine. Both epinephrine and norepinephrine are catecholamines. Epinephrine prepares the body for a "fight or flight" response, in which the heart rate, metabolic rate, and systemic blood pressure increase. The liver converts glycogen into glucose, the airways dilate, and the force of cardiac muscle contraction increases.

Norepinephrine — a biological amine with a structure similar to that of epinephrine, and its biological effects are very similar.

Adrenal Cortex

Adrenal cortex — secretes a group of hormones called corticosteroids that are all synthesized from cholesterol. Corticosteroids are further divided into glucocorticoids, mineralocorticoids, and androgenic hormones. The glucocorticoids increase blood glucose, and the mineralocorticoids affect electrolytes. The androgenic hormones are precursors to testosterone.

Aldosterone — the primary mineralocorticoid that causes sodium ions to be retained and potassium ions to be excreted. This hormone also reduces urinary output, promotes water retention, and increases extracellular fluid volume. Aldosterone exerts its effects on the tubules of the kidney. The secretion of aldosterone is controlled by many factors such as the potassium concentration in extracellular fluid, the renin–angiotensin system, body sodium, and adrenocorticotropic hormone.

Cortisol — the primary glucocorticoid. This hormone has the liver as its primary target. Cortisol influences carbohydrate, protein, and fat metabolism. One effect of cortisol is to stimulate gluconeogenesis—that is, the synthesis of glucose from noncarbohydrates, particularly from amino acids. Increased gluconeogenesis, in turn, causes an increased formation of glycogen in the liver. In addition, cortisol causes an increased release of fatty acids from fat cells (adipocytes). The secretion of cortisol is first stimulated by the hypothalamus (of the brain), which secretes corticotropin-releasing hormone (CRH). CRH causes the anterior pituitary to secrete ACTH, and ACTH causes the adrenal cortex to release cortisol. Stress of almost any kind will cause the release of ACTH, which is rapidly followed by secretion of cortisol. Cortisol also exerts an anti-inflammatory effect on tissues damaged by injury.

Pancreas

The pancreas lies behind the stomach and is connected to the duodenum. The secretory cells of the pancreas play a role in the endocrine and exocrine systems. The exocrine part of the pancreas secretes digestive enzymes into the small intestine (duodenum). The role of the pancreas in digestion will be discussed later in this review. The endocrine part of the pancreas is due to the islets of Langerhans, which contain alpha, beta, and delta cells. These cells secrete their products directly into the bloodstream. The alpha cells secrete glucagon, the beta cells secrete insulin, and the delta cells secrete somatostatin. Humans with type I diabetes have beta cells incapable of secreting insulin. Insulin and glucagon work in concert to control many metabolic activities.

Insulin — a protein hormone that influences carbohydrate, fat, and amino acid metabolism. Insulin decreases the release of fatty acids and fat cells and promotes the utilization of glucose. High levels of blood glucose (e.g., after a meal) stimulate the secretion of insulin. Insulin promotes the uptake and storage of glucose by almost all tissues in the body, particularly those of the liver and muscles. In liver and muscle tissue, glucose is stored as glycogen. The glycogen in the liver is used to supply the blood with glucose when the dietary supply of glucose decreases. Insulin also causes the liver to convert glucose into fatty acids that are subsequently stored in fat cells as triglycerides. Insulin also promotes the transport of amino acids into many tissues. Low levels of insulin cause fatty acids and glycerol to be released from adipocytes into plasma. The increased plasma levels of nonesterified fatty acids stimulate the liver to synthesize triglycerides, cholesterol esters, phospholipids, and cholesterol. These lipids are secreted by the liver in the form of very low-density lipoprotein. In addition, high levels of plasma fatty acids stimulate liver mitochondrial fatty acid oxidation, producing ketone bodies (i.e., beta hydroxybutyrate and acetoacetate). Humans with the inability to secrete insulin often have high levels of very low-density lipoprotein and also develop premature atherosclerosis.

Glucagon — a protein hormone that counteracts many of the metabolic effects of insulin. In particular, glucagon promotes an increase in blood glucose levels by causing a breakdown in glycogen (glycogenolysis). The secretion of glucagon is regulated by blood glucose levels; that is, low levels of blood glucose stimulate glucagon secretion.

Ovary

See Section X, Reproductive System and Development.

Testes

See Section X, Reproductive System and Development.

Problem

The adrenal medulla is most closely associated with

A. insulin.
B. epinephrine.
C. chorionic gonadotropin.
D. vasopressin.

Solution

B. Epinephrine is a secretory product of the adrenal medulla. It causes a breakdown of glycogen to glucose in the liver and skeletal muscle, leading to a rise in blood glucose levels. Epinephrine elevates blood pressure and the heart rate. It also constricts cutaneous blood vessels and dilates skeletal muscle vessels. In addition, epinephrine causes the organs of the digestive tract to experience vasoconstriction.

VI. CIRCULATORY, LYMPHATIC, AND IMMUNE SYSTEMS

1. CIRCULATORY SYSTEM

A. Multiple Functions, Including Role in Thermoregulation

The circulatory system has a major role in maintaining the stability of the body's internal environment, or homeostasis. The fluid in the body can be divided into intracellular fluid and extracellular fluid, which have different compositions. The extracellular fluid can be further divided into interstitial fluid and the fluid of the circulatory system (i.e., plasma). The circulatory system is responsible for the movement and mixing of the extracellular fluid.

Some major roles of the circulatory system are

- the delivery of oxygen and required nutrients,
- the removal of metabolic waste products,
- the transport of regulatory molecules such as hormones,
- the transport of protective chemicals and enzymes (vitamin E is an example of a protective chemical that inhibits free-radical damage to cell membranes and macromolecules),
- the transport of molecules and cells essential to the immune system, and
- thermoregulation.

Problem

The circulatory system does all the following EXCEPT

A. deliver oxygen.
B. regulate blood pressure.
C. transport enzymes.
D. remove waste products.

Solution

B. The circulatory system transports materials to and from tissues; it does NOT regulate blood pressure. Blood pressure is, in part, controlled chemically.

B. Four-Chambered Heart, Pulmonary, and Systemic Circulation

The overall organization of the circulatory system is shown in Figure 61. In essence, the four-chambered heart, while a single organ, can be thought of as two pumps: one propels blood to the lungs, and the other drives systemic circulation.

FIGURE 61. Circulatory System

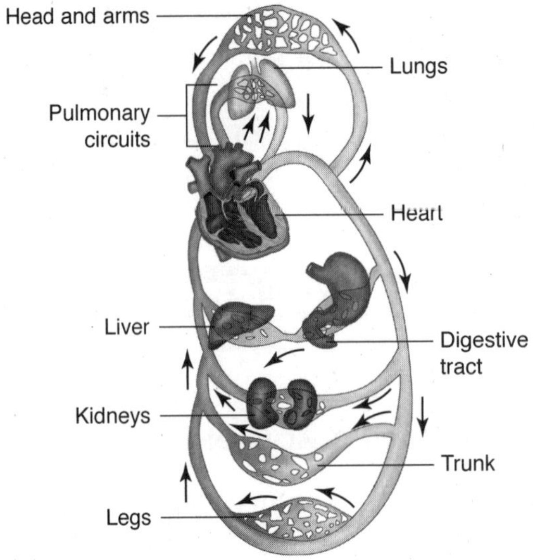

The four-chambered heart (Figure 62) is composed of two atria and two ventricles. The atria are filling chambers that pump blood to the ventricles and provide the main contractile force needed to move blood through the circulatory system. Between the atria and ventricles are the atrioventricular valves. At the exits from the heart, between the right ventricle and pulmonary artery and left ventricle and aorta, are the pulmonary and aortic semilunar valves.

FIGURE 62. Heart

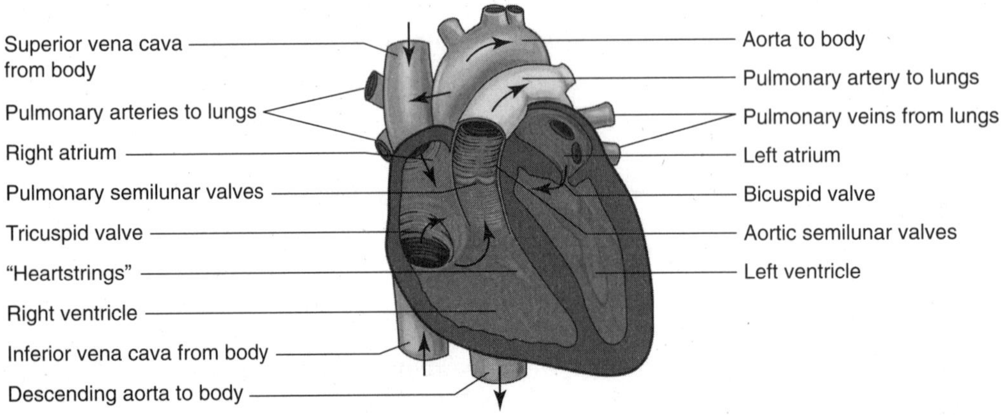

Deoxygenated venous blood from the inferior and superior venae cavae flows into the right atrium. Atrial contraction moves the blood through the atrioventricular valve (tricuspid valve) to the right ventricle. The contraction of the right ventricle pumps blood to the lungs through the pulmonary semilunar valves where the blood is oxygenated and carbon dioxide is removed. The oxygenated blood is returned to the heart via the pulmonary veins and enters the left atrium. With the contraction of the left atrium, the blood enters the left ventricle through the other atrioventricular valve (mitral or bicuspid valve). The contraction of the left ventricle pumps blood into the systemic circulatory system through the other aortic semilunar valves.

The heart is supplied with oxygenated blood by two branches of the aorta: the right and left coronary arteries. A major cause of cardiovascular disease is the accumulation of atherosclerotic plaques in the coronary arteries. This severely narrows the lumen of these arteries. A small blood clot can block these arteries, leading to cut-off of oxygenated blood to the heart muscle and thus resulting in a heart attack.

The cardiac cycle is the period from the end of contraction to the end of the next contraction. The period of relaxation is diastole, and the period of contraction is systole.

Problem

Which of the following is NOT a true statement?

A. Blood enters the heart through the superior (anterior) vena cava or through the inferior (posterior) vena cava.
B. The pulmonary artery carries oxygenated blood.
C. Oxygenated blood first enters the left atrium of the heart.
D. The systemic circulation contains oxygenated blood.

Solution

B. Blood enters the right atrium of the heart through the superior or inferior vena cava. When this chamber is filled, the blood is forced through the tricuspid valve and into the right ventricle. From there, this deoxygenated blood travels through the pulmonary artery to the lungs, where it exchanges carbon dioxide for oxygen. Once oxygenated, the blood travels to the left atrium through the pulmonary veins. It travels through the bicuspid valve to the left ventricle, goes out the aorta, and is then distributed throughout the body.

C. Arterial and Venous Systems, Capillary Beds, and Systemic and Diastolic Pressure

Arteries carry blood away from the heart under high pressure. Arteries have strong walls that pulse with heart pulsations. The maximum pressure reached during the arterial pulse is called the systolic pressure, and the lowest pressure is called the diastolic pressure. The arteries end in arterioles that control the flow of blood into the capillary beds. The capillaries have very thin walls that permit the exchange of nutrients, hormones, electrolytes, and other substances between blood and the interstitial spaces between cells. The deoxygenated blood from the capillary beds collects in the venous system and returns to the heart. The venous system is under low pressure, and veins have thinner walls than arteries.

The arterial pulse pressure is influenced primarily by the stroke volume of the heart and by the compliance of the arterial vasculature. The stroke volume of the heart is the amount of blood pumped out of the heart with each heartbeat. The greater the stroke volume output, the greater the arterial pulse pressure. The compliance of the arterial vasculature refers to the distensibility of the arteries to a pressure load. The greater the arterial compliance, the lower the arterial pulse pressure.

Problem

The only artery in the human body that carries deoxygenated blood is the

A. pulmonary artery.
B. right coronary artery.
C. left coronary artery.
D. carotid artery.

Solution

A. The pulmonary artery carries blood to the lungs to be cleaned of its carbon dioxide. All other arteries carry oxygenated blood.

D. Composition of Blood

Whole blood can be separated by low-speed centrifugation into a cell-free fluid called serum (or plasma if a blood anticoagulant is present) and a pellet containing cells and platelets. Plasma is about 92% water and contains electrolytes, lipoproteins, proteins, hormones, other nutrients, and vitamins. The lipoproteins are lipid–protein complexes. Lipoproteins are the primary transport molecules for lipids. Lipoproteins are further divided into very low-density lipoprotein, low-density lipoprotein, and high-density lipoprotein. High plasma levels of low-density lipoprotein are associated with atherosclerosis and cardiovascular disease. In contrast, high plasma levels of high-density lipoprotein are thought to protect against atherosclerosis.

The primary proteins found in plasma are albumin, globulins, and fibrinogen. Albumin is the most abundant plasma protein (about 60%) and is a carrier molecule for nonesterified fatty acids. Albumin also plays a role in maintaining the osmotic pressure of blood. The globulins are divided into alpha, beta, and gamma globulins. The gamma globulin fraction contains molecules that function as antibodies in the humoral immune system (as discussed later in this review). Fibrinogen functions in clot formation.

The red blood cell (or erythrocyte) is the primary cell found in blood. This unique cell has a plasma membrane but no other membranous organelles and does not have a nucleus. The primary function of red blood cells is oxygen transport to tissues and the removal of carbon dioxide. The oxygen-carrying molecule in the red blood cell is hemoglobin (as discussed in the next section). The red blood cell has a biconcave shape, is extremely deformable, and can move through very small capillaries. In anemia, the number of red blood cells in a given volume of blood is low, resulting in a decreased ability to deliver oxygen to tissues. Nutritional and/or genetic factors can contribute to anemia.

Blood also contains white blood cells and platelets. White blood cells (or leukocytes) include monocytes, lymphocytes, neutrophils, eosinophils, and basophils. Neutrophils, eosinophils, and basophils (all three are also called granulocytes) as well as monocytes are phagocytic cells. The role of these phagocytic cells in the immune system is discussed later in this review. Lymphocytes also play a key role in the immune system. Platelets function in clot formation.

E. Role of Hemoglobin in Oxygen Transport

Hemoglobin is the primary molecule found in red blood cells, and its primary function is transporting oxygen. The three-dimensional structure of hemoglobin is known in detail from X-ray crystallographic studies. Hemoglobin is a tetramer ($alpha_2beta_2$), with two identical alpha subunits and two identical beta subunits. Both the alpha and beta subunits have a structure similar to myoglobin. Myoglobin is the monomeric oxygen-binding protein of muscle. Each of the hemoglobin subunits has a heme group containing iron in the ferrous (Fe^{+2}) state. Each heme group can bind a single oxygen molecule. Oxygen binding does not change the oxidation state of the heme iron.

Hemoglobin is an allosteric protein. The binding of oxygen to hemoglobin is regulated by other molecules such as protons (H^+), carbon dioxide (CO_2) and 2,3-diphosphoglycerate (DPG). These molecules exert their influence on oxygen binding by binding to sites that are distinct from the oxygen-binding sites. A key feature of oxygen binding to hemoglobin is the cooperative nature of this binding (Figure 63).

Cooperative binding occurs when the binding of each oxygen molecule facilitates the binding of the next oxygen molecule. This cooperative binding results in a characteristic sigmoidal dissociation curve, as shown in Figure 63. In contrast, the binding of oxygen to myoglobin is not cooperative (and the dissociation curve is a hyperbola), but myoglobin does have a stronger affinity for oxygen than does hemoglobin.

The cooperative binding of oxygen to hemoglobin plays an important physiological role in the delivery of oxygen to tissues. Hemoglobin is almost fully saturated with oxygen at the partial pressure of oxygen found in the lung (pO_2 = 100 mm Hg). Oxygen is readily dissociated from hemoglobin and delivered to myoglobin, which has a stronger affinity for oxygen. As more oxygen is dissociated from hemoglobin, the affinity of the remaining oxygen is less. This follows because dissociation is the reverse of binding. Thus, hemoglobin is able to deliver oxygen to tissues even at the low pO_2 levels found in capillaries (pO_2 = 20–26 mm Hg).

CO_2, DPG, and H^+ shift the oxygen dissociation curve to the right—that is, the affinity of hemoglobin for oxygen is decreased. Tissues with a high metabolic activity, such as contracting muscle, generate large amounts of H^+ and CO_2. High levels of H^+ and CO_2 lower the affinity of hemoglobin for oxygen and thereby increase the delivery of oxygen to these metabolically active tissues. This is called the Bohr effect.

FIGURE 63. Oxygen Binding to Hemoglobin and Myoglobin

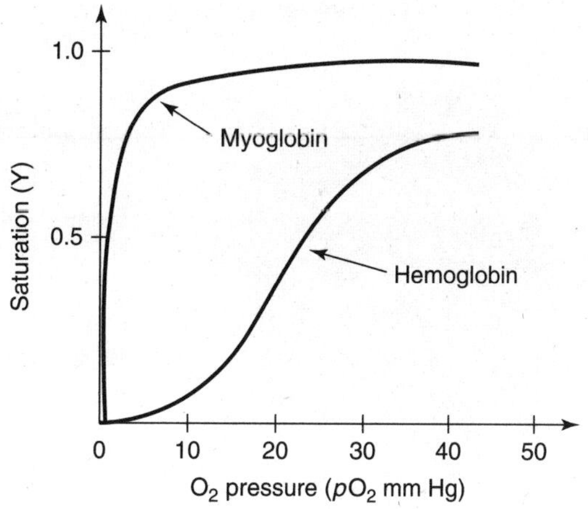

Problem

In muscles, oxygen leaves hemoglobin to bind with myoglobin because

A. the presence of H^+ and CO_2 in muscles increases the affinity of hemoglobin for oxygen.

B. the removal of oxygen from hemoglobin increases hemoglobin's affinity for the remaining oxygen.

C. myoglobin has a stronger oxygen affinity than does hemoglobin.

D. the bonding of oxygen to myoglobin is cooperative.

Solution

C. Myoglobin has a stronger oxygen affinity than does hemoglobin. Myoglobin does not have cooperative oxygen binding. The presence of H^+ and CO_2, as well as the removal of oxygen from hemoglobin, decreases the affinity of hemoglobin for oxygen.

2. LYMPHATIC SYSTEM

The lymphatic system provides an important link with the cardiovascular system and the immune system. Fluid and proteins that are lost from the cells are returned to the blood via the lymphatic system. The fluid in the lymphatic system is called lymph. The lymphatic system begins with blind-ended lymph capillaries (Figure 64) that join together and enter large veinlike lymph vessels. At certain locations, the lymph vessels are expanded into structures called lymph nodes. The lymph nodes are an important part of the body's defense system against infection. Lymph capillaries called lacteals are in the villi of the small intestine. Lacteals absorb fats and transport them from the digestive tract to the circulatory system. The lymph from the upper and lower portions of the body flows into veins in the thorax.

Lymph capillaries have many "flaps" or valves that permit the inflow of fluid and particulate matter but prevent their backflow into the interstitial spaces. Edema, which is the accumulation of fluid in tissues, can result if fluid flow through the lymphatic system is blocked.

Bacteria and viruses that have infected tissues cannot be directly absorbed via the blood capillaries. These pathogens enter lymph and are subsequently transported into lymph nodes that contain large numbers of lymphocytes and macrophages defending against these microorganisms. The role of macrophages and lymphocytes in the immune system is detailed in the next section.

FIGURE 64. Lymphatic Capillary

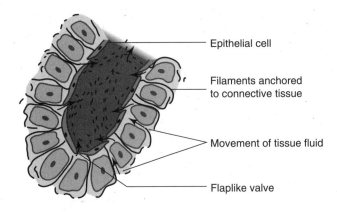

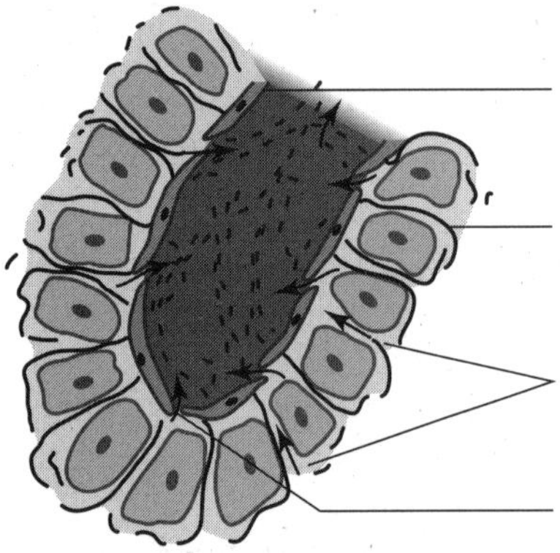

Problem

The lymphatic system transports all the following EXCEPT

A. plasma. B. interstitial fluid. C. pathogens. D. macrophages.

Solution

A. Plasma travels in the circulatory system. Interstitial fluid (lymph), pathogens, and macrophages may be transported in the lymphatic system.

3. IMMUNE SYSTEM

The primary function of the immune system is to provide resistance from attack by infectious agents such as bacteria and viruses. Most immune responses in higher organisms involve the production of antibodies (i.e., acquired immunity), but other innate mechanisms for killing infectious agents also exist. Macrophages, for example, can kill invading bacteria by phagocytosis (engulfing and digesting), and this process can occur in the absence of antibodies. The acidic digestive juice of the stomach is also effective in killing infectious agents introduced by swallowing.

A. Antigens, Antibodies, and Antigen–Antibody Reactions

Acquired immunity depends on the production of recognition molecules that can distinguish "self" from "nonself." There are two forms of acquired immunity:

1. Humoral immunity
2. Cellular immunity

Humoral immunity is the production of protein molecules that bind to the invading agent and mark it for destruction. Cellular immunity is the formation of lymphocytes that bind to the invading agent and cause its destruction.

A typical antibody consists of four polypeptide chains. There are two identical light chains and two identical heavy chains. As shown in Figure 65(a), the four chains are held together by disulfide bonds to form a Y-shaped molecule. As shown in Figure 65(b), both the heavy and light chains of an antibody are built up from a structurally similar domain, or polypeptide subunit, of about 220 amino acids. Each light chain has two such domains: a constant domain and variable domain. Similarly, each heavy chain has three (sometimes two) constant domains and one variable domain. The variable domains are at the amino-terminal ends of both heavy and light chains, as shown in Figure 65(b), and the amino acid sequence in this region is very variable. The variable regions provide the specificity that enables an antibody to bind to a very specific region of another molecule—that is, the antigen. The constant regions of antibodies provide a mechanism for binding the antibody to other cells (such as macrophages) or binding to elements of the complement system.

FIGURE 65. Structure of a Typical IgG Antibody Showing the Constant and Variable Polypeptide Segments

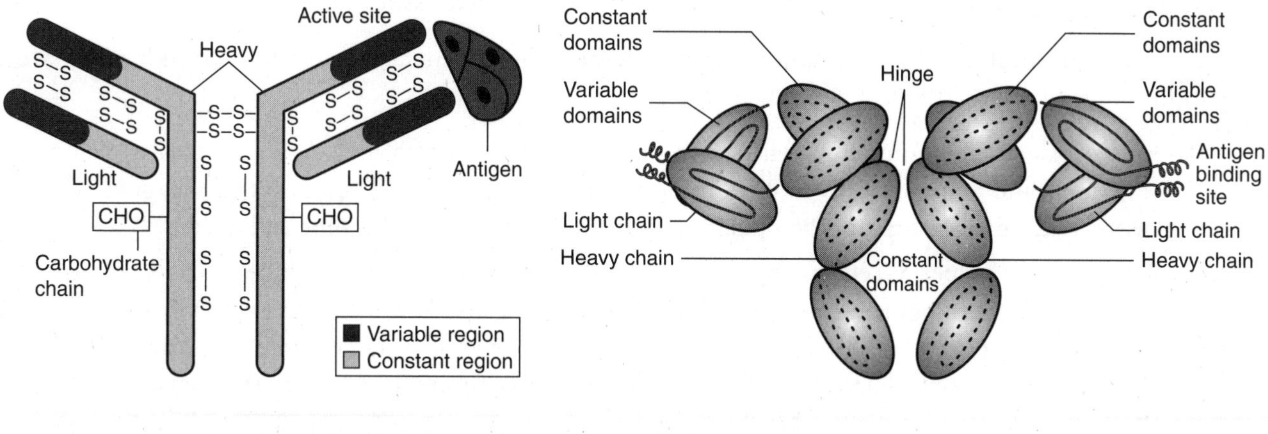

(a) Position of disulfide bonds

(b) Arrangements of domains

When antibodies bind to an antigen on an invading organism, they mark it for destruction by either the complement system or by macrophages. The proteins of the complement system destroy an invading organism by perforating its cell membrane. Antibodies can also inactivate an invading organism by agglutination (multiple antigenic sites are bound together to form a clump), precipitation (the water-soluble antigen complexes with the antibody, and the complex is insoluble), or by neutralization (the antibody binds to and covers a toxic site).

Problem

The complement system of immune response does NOT

A. agglutinate antigens.
B. precipitate antigens.
C. ingest antigens.
D. neutralize toxic sites.

Solution

C. The complement system may agglutinate, precipitate, or neutralize antigens. Macrophages ingest antigens.

B. Tissues and Cells of the Immune System

T-Lymphocytes, B-Lymphocytes, Bone Marrow, Spleen, Thymus, and Lymph Nodes

Lymphoid tissues form the "organ system" responsible for immunity. Lymphoid tissues contain a high concentration of lymphocytes. Lymphoid tissue is widely distributed throughout the body and is particularly concentrated in lymph nodes, the thymus, the bone marrow, and the spleen. Lymphocytes can move between lymphoid tissue and the blood. Acquired immunity does not develop until after contact is made with an invading agent.

T-Lymphocytes and B-Lymphocytes

Lymphoid tissues contain two types of lymphocytes: T-lymphocytes (or T-cells) and B-lymphocytes (or B-cells). T-lymphocytes form the sensitized cells of the cellular immune system, and B-lymphocytes play a key role in the production of antibodies that provide humoral immunity. T-cells have another class of recognition molecules called T-cell receptors that will only recognize cells bearing both "self" and "nonself" markers.

Both T- and B-cells arise from embryonic stem cells, but before becoming part of lymphoid tissues, they require a maturation process. For T-cells, maturation occurs in the thymus gland, and for B-cells, the exact site is not known but is thought to be in the bone marrow. After the maturation process the T- and B-cells migrate to and become imbedded in the lymphoid tissues.

The immunological events following an infection by an infectious agent such as a virus are as follows:

1. Macrophages ingest numerous viruses and display some specific viral markers or antigens on their surface. Some helper T-cells in circulation have the proper T-cell receptors to recognize the processed viral antigens on the macrophage surface, and these T-cells become activated.
2. The activated helper T-cells multiply and stimulate the multiplication of killer T-cells and activated B-cells that can recognize the same processed viral antigens. The activated B-cells multiply and differentiate into plasma cells that produce antibodies to the viral antigen. Some of the activated B-cells become memory cells that permit a rapid response to any future infection by the virus.
3. The killer T-cells will destroy host cells that have become infected with the virus and thereby will inhibit viral replication. The antibodies produced by the B-cells will also bind to the virus and prevent them from infecting additional host cells.
4. When the infection is contained, suppressor T-cells halt the immune responses, and memory T-cells and memory B-cells remain in the blood and lymphatic system.

The AIDS virus is particularly damaging to the immune system because it invades and kills helper T-cells.

Problem

The functional difference between B-cells and T-cells is that

A. B-cells differentiate from stem cells, and T-cells differentiate from lymphocytes.
B. T-cells differentiate from stem cells, and B-cells differentiate from lymphocytes.
C. T-cells secrete antibodies in response to introduced antigens, and B-cells direct the cell-mediated response.
D. B-cells secrete antibodies in response to introduced antigens, and T-cells direct the cell-mediated response.

Solution

D. T-cells and B-cells are the cells involved in the immune responses of the body. Both cell types differentiate from stem cells of the bone marrow. The stem cells that migrate to the thymus become T-cells and are responsible for cell-mediated immunity. Those stem cells that migrate to the bursa or an analogous structure become B-cells and are the cells of the humoral immune system.

VII. DIGESTIVE AND EXCRETORY SYSTEMS

1. DIGESTIVE SYSTEM

The primary role of the digestive system is to break down food into substances that can be absorbed into the body. Any substances that cannot be absorbed from the digestive tract are eliminated in the feces. The digestive system consists of the alimentary canal and the exocrine organs that secrete digestive juices into the alimentary canal. The alimentary canal starts at the mouth and includes the pharynx, esophagus, stomach, small intestine, large intestine, and anus (Figure 66). The salivary glands, pancreas, liver, and gallbladder are organs that secrete substances into the alimentary canal.

FIGURE 66. Digestive System

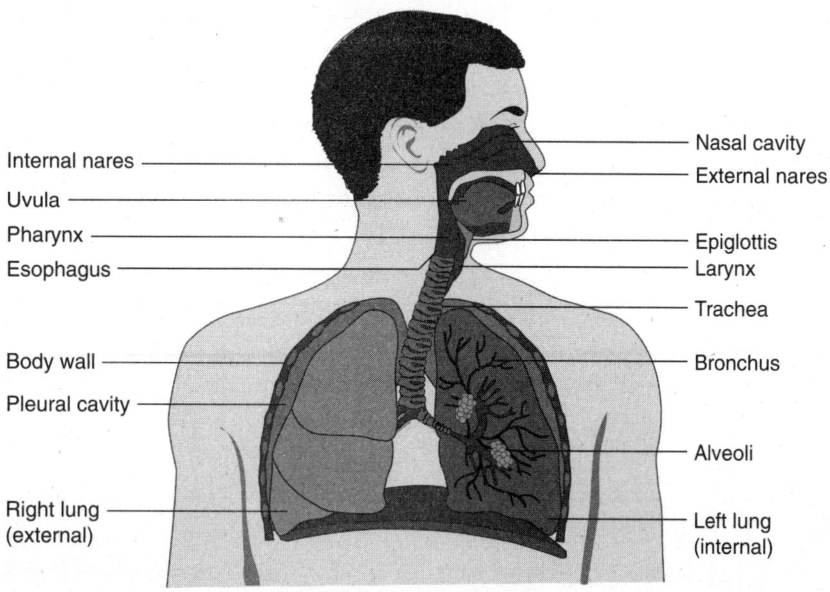

A. Ingestion: Structures and Their Functions

The first component of the alimentary canal is the mouth, which mechanically reduces the size of food materials and mixes the masticated particles with saliva from the salivary glands. The teeth are specialized structures for breaking up food particles and increasing the surface area of the food particles. The incisors cut large food sections, the canines serve to grasp and tear food, and the premolars and molars are effective in grinding food particles.

Secreted into the mouth by the salivary glands, saliva increases the moisture content of the food particles and initiates the digestion of carbohydrate. Amylase is the digestive enzyme in saliva, and it splits starch and glycogen into disaccharides. Glucose is stored as starch granules in plants and as glycogen granules in animals. The two principal components of starch are the polysaccharides amylose and amylopectin.

Problem

Which of the following organs is NOT a part of the human digestive system?

A. Esophagus B. Thymus C. Gallbladder D. Pancreas

Solution

B. All the choices are part of the digestive system except for the thymus. The thymus is part of the immune system.

B. Stomach

The food mass from the mouth passes through the pharynx and the esophagus by a peristaltic wave, and enters the stomach. In the stomach, the food mass is mixed with gastric secretions, and the digestion of protein is initiated. The gastric glands secrete pepsinogen, mucus, hydrochloric acid, and intrinsic factor. Intrinsic factor is important in promoting the absorption of vitamin B_{12}. Pepsinogen is the inactive form of pepsin.

The inactive form of an enzyme is called a zymogen. Pepsinogen is activated to pepsin by cleavage of a 44-residue peptide (from the amino terminal end). This activation occurs spontaneously at pH 2 and is catalyzed by pepsin. Pepsin is an acid protease and has maximal enzymatic activity at pH 2 to 3. The hydrochloric acid in the stomach functions to maintain an acidic pH (of 1) and denatures dietary protein to make it more susceptible to protease attack. Pepsin primarily catalyzes the hydrolysis of peptide bonds with an aromatic amino acid residue such as phenylalanine, tryptophane, or tyrosine. The polypeptides produced by pepsin digestion are transported to the small intestine for further hydrolysis. The mixture of food mass and gastric juices in the stomach constitutes chyme. Chyme enters the small intestine, which also receives the secretions of the liver and pancreas.

Problem

Which of the following is a zymogen?

A. Protease B. Tyrosine C. Chyme D. Pepsinogen

Solution

D. Pepsinogen is a zymogen, an inactive form of an enzyme. Protease is an enzyme, tyrosine is an amino acid, and chyme is the mixture found in the stomach.

C. Digestive Glands, Including Liver and Pancreas, and Bile Production

The pancreas functions in the exocrine system, as well as in the endocrine system (see Section V, Nervous and Endocrine Systems). The acinar cells, which form most of the pancreatic mass, secrete pancreatic juice that travels through the pancreatic duct to the duodenum. The bile duct from the liver and gallbladder enter the duodenum at the same site. Pancreatic juice aids the digestion of carbohydrate, fat, and protein. The pH of pancreatic juice is alkaline, and it neutralizes the acidic chyme from the stomach. Carbohydrate digestion is assisted by pancreatic amylase, which breaks down starch and glycogen into disaccharides (as discussed in the previous section). Triglycerides are hydrolyzed into glycerol and free fatty acids by the action of pancreatic lipase.

A mixture of zymogens is released into the small intestine. These zymogens include trypsinogen, chymotrypsinogen, and procarboxypeptidase, and they are converted into their active forms—trypsin, chymotrypsin, and carboxypeptidase, respectively. Trypsin hydrolyzes the carboxyl side of peptide bonds with arginine and lysine residues, whereas chymotrypsin acts on the carboxyl side of peptide bonds with aromatic residues (phenylalanine, tryptophan, and tyrosine) as well as methionine. Carboxypeptidase A releases the carboxyl-terminal amino acids, and carboxypeptidase B is restricted to peptides with an arginine or lysine carboxyl terminal. The pancreas also secretes nucleases to break down nucleic acids into nucleotides.

The liver functions in the process of digestion by secreting bile salts that act like detergents and emulsify fat. This emulsification increases the surface area of the fat droplets. Lipases can efficiently utilize triglycerides (fat droplets) that have been emulsified by bile salts. Bile salts are synthesized by hepatic cells from cholesterol and are secreted into the common bile duct. The common bile duct exits to the duodenum via a sphincter muscle (the sphincter of Oddi). Between meals, the sphincter of Oddi is closed, and bile is stored in the gallbladder.

Problem

Bile is secreted by the

A. stomach. B. liver. C. duodenum. D. gallbladder.

Solution

B. Bile is an aqueous solution that contains various organic and inorganic solutes. Among the major organic solutes are bile salts, phospholipids, cholesterol, and bile pigments. The adult human liver produces about 15 ml of bile per kilogram of body weight. The rate of synthesis and secretion depends mainly on blood flow to the liver.

D. Small Intestine and Large Intestine

The small intestine receives chyme from the stomach as well as pancreatic juice and bile. The small intestine begins at the pyloric sphincter and ends at the large intestine. The three segments of the small intestine are the duodenum, the jejunum, and the ileum. The small intestine has numerous villi that project into the intestinal lumen. These villi serve to mix chyme with intestinal juices and aid in the absorption of digested nutrients. The small intestine is the primary absorbing organ of the alimentary canal. The epithelial cells of the intestinal mucosa of the duodenum have various digestive enzymes. These include peptidases (which break down polypeptides into amino acids) and enzymes that convert disaccharides into monosaccharides. Also, the duodenum is where the pancreatic juices and bile enter the digestive tract.

The large intestine plays almost no role in the digestion of food but does reabsorb water and electrolytes. In addition, it stores feces, consisting of undigestible food components such as fiber, until defecation.

Problem

Villi are fingerlike protrusions of the

A. small intestine.
B. outer ear.
C. bronchioles.
D. capillaries.

Solution

A. Villi line the lumen of the small intestine and thereby increase the intestinal surface area. Most of the nutrient absorption during digestion occurs through the villi.

E. Muscular Control of Digestion

The smooth muscles of the alimentary canal promote both the mixing of food with gastric juices and the rhythmic wavelike movements (peristaltic contractions) that propel food through the lumen of the digestive tract. The regulation of this muscular contraction is primarily controlled by the intrinsic nervous system. This intrinsic system also regulates much of the secretory functions required for digestion. In addition, nerve fibers from the parasympathetic and sympathetic branches of the autonomic system interact with the intrinsic nervous system of the gut. In general, the parasympathetic system increases the activity of the gut, and the sympathetic system decreases that activity.

The vagus nerve, which is part of the parasympathetic system, arises from the brain and innervates the esophagus, stomach, pancreas, and proximal half of the large intestine. Parasympathetic nerve fibers also originate from the sacral segments of the spinal cord and innervate the distal segment of the large intestine. The sympathetic innervation also regulates the gastrointestinal tract. The preganglionic fibers originate in the spinal cord, and the postganglionic fibers innervate all parts of the gut. Norepinephrine secreted by the ends of the sympathetic nerves inhibits the contractions of smooth muscles in the gut and inhibits the intrinsic nervous system.

Problem

Norepinephrine inhibits all the following EXCEPT

A. smooth muscle contraction.
B. peristalsis.
C. the intrinsic nervous system.
D. the parasympathetic nervous system.

Solution

D. Norepinephrine inhibits the intrinsic nervous system and smooth muscles in the gut (which produce peristalsis). Norepinephrine does not affect the parasympathetic nervous system.

2. EXCRETORY SYSTEM

A. Role of the Excretory System in Body Homeostasis

Metabolic waste products are often toxic and must be removed from the body to prevent tissue damage. Blood and lymph are the fluids that initially receive metabolic wastes. Gaseous waste products such as CO_2 are removed from blood by the respiratory system. Salts and nitrogenous wastes are removed from the circulatory system by the urinary system. The urinary system also plays a key role in body homeostasis by helping to regulate the volume and composition of extracellular fluid, the production of red blood cells, and blood pressure. The urinary system is composed of a pair of kidneys, a pair of ureters, a urinary bladder, and a urethra (Figure 67).

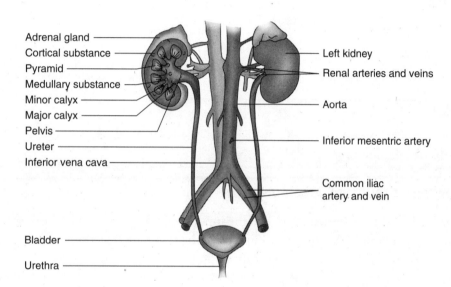

FIGURE 67. Urinary System

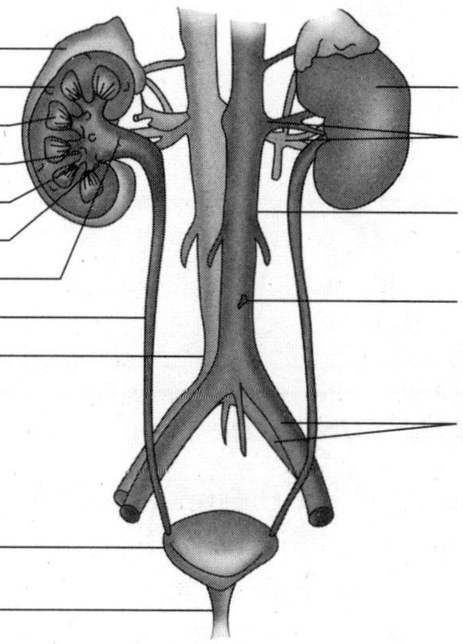

Problem

Wastes are removed from the blood by the

A. respiratory system.

B. urinary system.

C. digestive system.

D. both A and B.

Solution

D. The respiratory and urinary systems both remove wastes. The respiratory system removes gases from the blood, and the urinary system removes liquid and dissolved materials from the blood. The digestive system breaks down food but does not remove wastes.

B. Kidneys: Structure and Function

The kidneys are located on both sides of the spinal column and are behind the parietal peritoneum. The surface of the kidney facing the spinal column (the medial surface) is concave and contains a deep sinus through which the renal artery (from the aorta) and the renal vein (from the inferior vena cava) enter. The ureter, which transports urine away from the kidney, also exits from the renal sinus. The extrarenal ureter is expanded into a funnel-shaped sac (the renal pelvis) at its junction with the renal sinus. The intrarenal tubes of the ureter branch to form two major calyces, each of which further divides into minor calyces. Urine is delivered into the minor calyces by the renal papillae and then flows through the ureter into the bladder.

The interior of the kidney is divided into an inner renal medulla and an outer renal cortex. The renal medulla contains pyramidal structures whose apexes form the renal papillae. The renal cortex has a granular appearance due to the many small tubules of the nephrons (as discussed in the next section).

In addition to its role of removing metabolic wastes, the kidney secretes erythropoietin, which stimulates the production of red blood cells. Renin is also secreted by the kidney, and it helps regulate blood pressure. The inactive form of vitamin D (25-hydroxyl vitamin D) is converted to the active form of vitamin D (1,25-dihydroxy vitamin D) in the kidney. The active form of vitamin D promotes Ca^{+2} absorption.

Problem

The kidney can do all the following EXCEPT

A. remove metabolic wastes.

B. help activate vitamin C.

C. help regulate blood pressure.

D. help stimulate production of red blood cells.

Solution

B. The kidney does everything listed but help in the activation of vitamin C. The kidney helps in the activation of vitamin D.

C. Nephrons: Structure and Function

Urine is formed by the nephrons, which are the functional units of the kidney. About a million nephrons are present in each kidney. As shown in Figure 68, the two major sections of a nephron are a corpuscle (a glomerulus enclosed within Bowman's capsule) and tubules (the proximal tubule, loop of Henle, distal tubule, and collecting tubule). The glomeruli are contained in the cortex of the kidney, and some of the tubules extend into the medulla.

FIGURE 68. Nephron

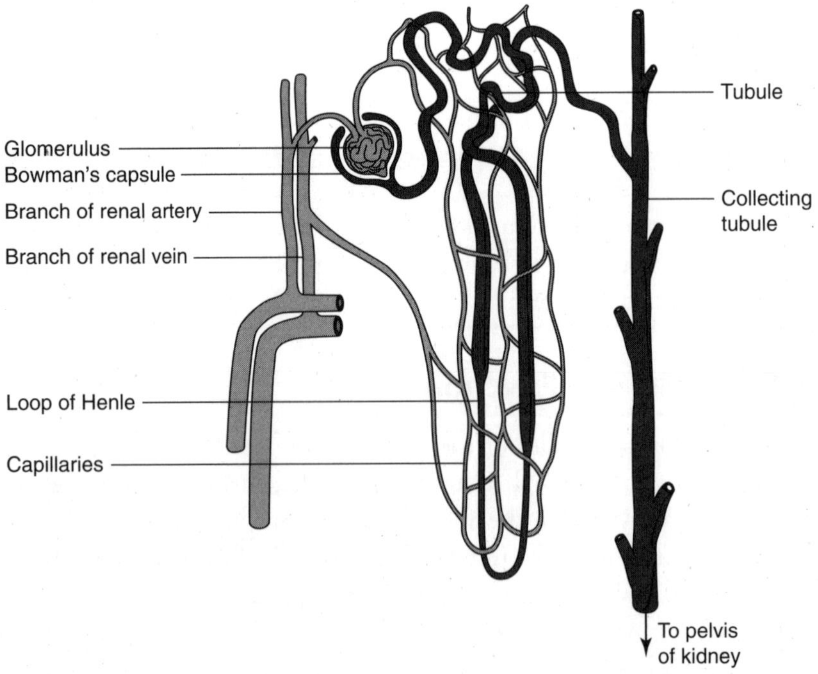

Problem

Which of the following is NOT part of the nephron in the human kidney?

A. Proximal convoluted tubule
B. Loop of Henle
C. Distal convoluted tubule
D. Major calyx

Solution

D. The nephron, which is the structural and functional unit of the kidney, consists of a corpuscle and its attached tubule. The tubule consists of the proximal convoluted portion, the loop of Henle, and the distal convoluted portion. The nephrons empty into collecting tubules. There are approximately one million nephrons in each kidney. The major calyx is not part of the nephron but rather is part of the intrarenal collecting system.

D. Formation of Urine

Blood enters the glomerulus through the afferent arteriole and exits through the efferent arteriole. The blood in the glomerulus is under pressure (60 mm Hg), and that pressure forces some fluid out of the blood and into Bowman's capsule. The fluid in Bowman's capsule flows into the following structures:

1. Proximal renal tubule (in the cortex of the kidney)
2. Loop of Henle
3. Distal tubule
4. Collecting duct, which flows into the renal pelvis

The result of this fluid movement is the creation of urine. The solute composition of urine depends on the amount of water present and the amounts of each of various solutes to be excreted from the body to maintain proper concentrations of these substances. The loop of Henle and the vasa recta provide mechanisms for regulating the osmolarity and volume of urine produced by the kidney.

The concentration of electrolytes and other substances in the fluid contained in Bowman's capsule (i.e., the glomerular filtrate) is very similar to that found in interstitial fluid. Most of the water and some of the solutes in the glomerular filtrate are reabsorbed by tubule cells; that is, a tubule cell transports a substance from the lumen of the tubule into the interstitial fluid. Substances in the interstitial fluid then easily enter the peritubular capillaries. The solutes reabsorbed into the circulation are useful, and their loss as urine would be wasteful. For example, glucose, amino acids, and many electrolytes are reabsorbed. Toxic, unwanted, or "excess" solutes are not reabsorbed and appear in urine. In addition to waste molecules that leave the blood when they are filtered into Bowman's capsule, some wastes are directly secreted by tubule cells; that is, they are transported by tubule cells from the interstitial fluid into the tubule lumen.

E. Storage and Elimination of Wastes

Urea is a by-product of amino acid metabolism, and it is a main constituent of urine. Uric acid, which is formed from the catabolism of purines, is also eliminated in urine. From the renal pelvis, urine flows through the ureter to the urinary bladder. The flow of urine through the ureter is promoted by peristaltic contraction of the muscular lining of the ureter. The process by which the urinary bladder empties is called micturition. Micturition occurs when the tension in the walls of the bladder reaches a threshold level caused by the increasing volume of urine. This triggers a reflex that results in the emptying of the bladder. The micturition reflex can also be influenced by both inhibitory and stimulatory signals from the brain. In particular, the relaxation of the urethral sphincter is necessary before urination can proceed.

Problem

Micturition is controlled by

A. reflex. B. signals from the brain. C. hormones. D. both A and B.

Solution

D. Micturition is controlled by reflex and signals from the brain, not hormones.

VIII. MUSCLE AND SKELETAL SYSTEMS

1. MUSCLE SYSTEM

A. Functions

The primary function of all muscle tissue is contraction, during which chemical energy is converted to mechanical energy. The contraction of muscle fibers causes tension on the body parts to which they are attached. Skeletal muscles function by applying tension to their attachment points on bones. Bones and muscles form lever systems that control body movements and help maintain posture. Muscles also function to control the movement of fluids in the circulatory and excretory systems and help maintain body temperature.

B. Basic Muscle Types and Locations

Almost half the body is muscle mass, with the vast majority being skeletal muscle. Smooth muscle and cardiac muscle account for about 5–10% of body mass. The structure of various contractile cells and the molecular mechanisms responsible for muscle contraction has been discussed in Section IV, Specialized Eukaryotic Cells and Tissues.

Skeletal Muscles

Skeletal muscle fibers are about 50–150 μm in diameter and extend the entire length of a muscle. The multinucleated cells of skeletal muscles are striated. Individual skeletal muscles are separated from each other by a surrounding fascia that can also extend beyond the muscle to become part of a tendon. The tendon functions to connect the muscle to bone.

Some major skeletal muscles are described in the following paragraphs:

Biceps brachii — in the upper arm, with two heads (immovable origins) that originate on the scapula. The muscle follows the humerus and is connected to the radius by a tendon. Contraction causes the arm to bend at the elbow.

Pectoralis major — a large muscle of the chest that connects the humerus (in the upper arm) to the bones of the thorax.

Deltoid — a triangular muscle located on the shoulder. Its contraction moves the upper arm at the shoulder joint.

Extensor digitorum — muscles that extend either the fingers or toes. All extensor muscles act to straighten body parts away from the main body.

Sternomastoid group — connect the sternum and mastoid and act primarily on the head, moving it to the side and flexing it.

Figures 69(a) and 69(b) show many of the major skeletal muscles.

Smooth Muscles

Smooth muscles contain fibers that are 2–5 μm in diameter and 50–200 μm in length (smaller than skeletal fibers) and have only a single nucleus. Smooth muscles contract and relax more slowly than skeletal muscles.

FIGURE 69 (a). Anterior View of Superficial Skeletal Muscles

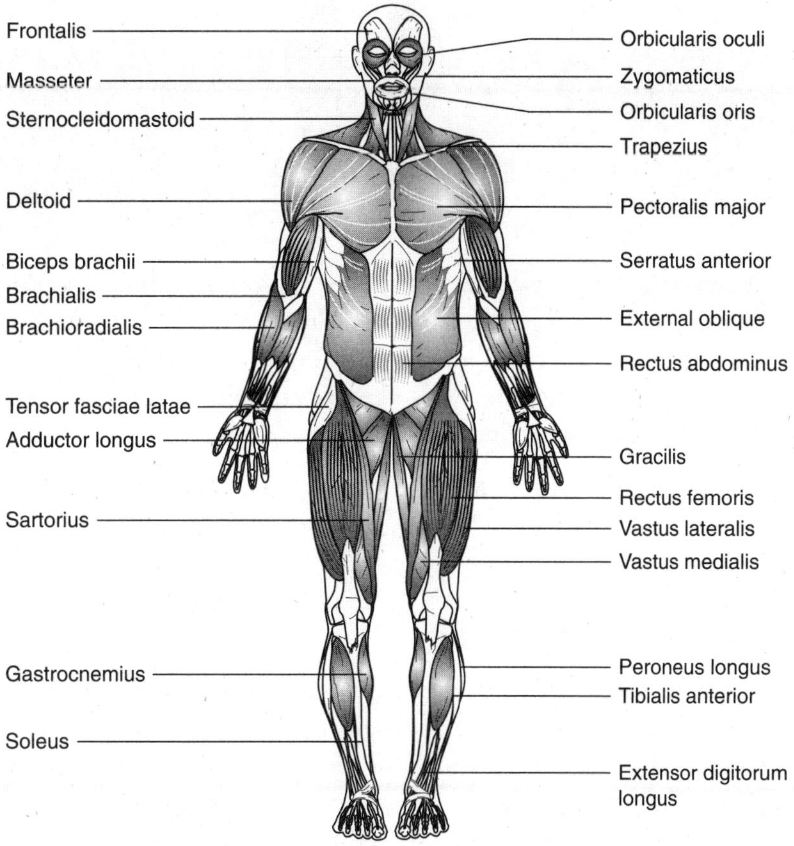

FIGURE 69 (b). Posterior View of Superficial Skeletal Muscles

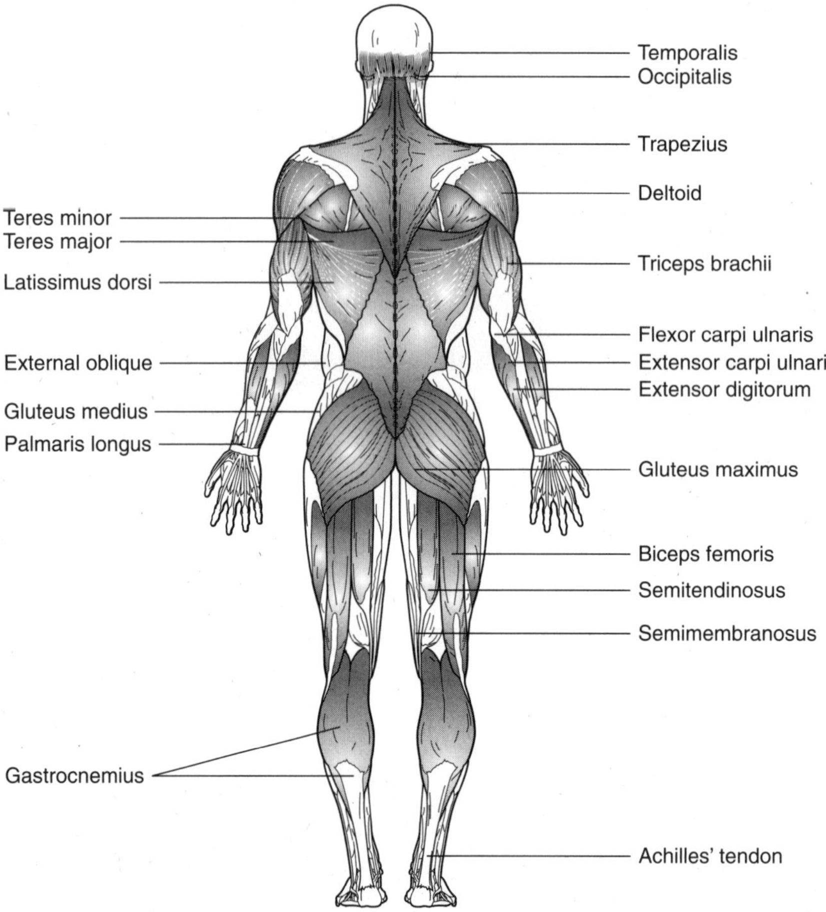

Visceral and multiunit are the two major types of smooth muscles. Visceral smooth muscle cells are in contact with each other (at points called gap junctions). When one smooth muscle cell is stimulated, the action potential can spread via gap junctions to other smooth muscle cells. Visceral smooth muscles are found in the intestines, the bile ducts, the ureters, and the uterus. Visceral smooth muscles are responsible for the peristaltic contraction of the intestinal tract.

In contrast, each multiunit smooth muscle cell acts independently and is usually innervated by a single nerve that controls its contraction. Multiunit smooth muscles are found in the walls of blood vessels and in the iris of the eye.

Cardiac Muscles

The primary function of cardiac muscles is the rhythmic pumping action of the heart. The ventricles provide the primary force for pumping blood through the blood vessels. Cardiac muscles exist only in the heart. Cardiac muscle cells are striated and have a single nucleus. Cardiac muscle fibers contain angular intercalated discs (Figure 70). These discs are specialized cell junctions that anchor cardiac cells to each other, allowing the action potential to spread from cell to cell. There are two major types of cardiac muscle: (1) contractile cells that make up the bulk of the atria and ventricles and generate the force that pumps the blood, and (2) conducting cells that are specialized for developing and conducting action potentials. The conducting cells provide a mechanism for the rapid transmission of excitatory impulses throughout the heart.

The intercalated discs of cardiac muscle fibers contain gap junctions and so allow the rapid transmission of action potentials. Action potentials rapidly propagate throughout the lattice of interconnected cells. The heart is composed of the atrial syncytium and the ventricular syncytium. These syncytia are separated by fibrous tissue, except by a band of conducting cells called the A-V bundle that allows the action potential to spread from the atria to the ventricles.

FIGURE 70. Intercalated Disc of Cardiac Muscle

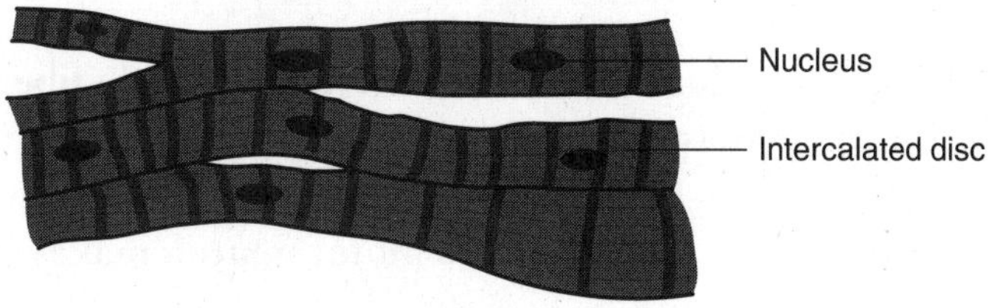

Problem

The major difference between skeletal and smooth muscles is that

A. skeletal muscles contain multinucleated cells.
B. smooth muscles have longer fibers than skeletal muscles.
C. smooth muscles contract more slowly than skeletal muscles.
D. smooth muscles relax more slowly than skeletal muscles.

Solution

A. Smooth muscles cells contain a single nucleus.

C. Nervous Control of Muscles

Motor and Sensory Control

Motor (or efferent) neurons carry nerve impulses out from the brain or spinal cord. Each skeletal muscle fiber is connected to a myelinated motor neuron at a region called the neuromuscular junction. The specialized region of the muscle fiber membrane that forms a junction with the axon of the motor neuron is called a motor end plate (Figure 71).

FIGURE 71. Motor End Plate

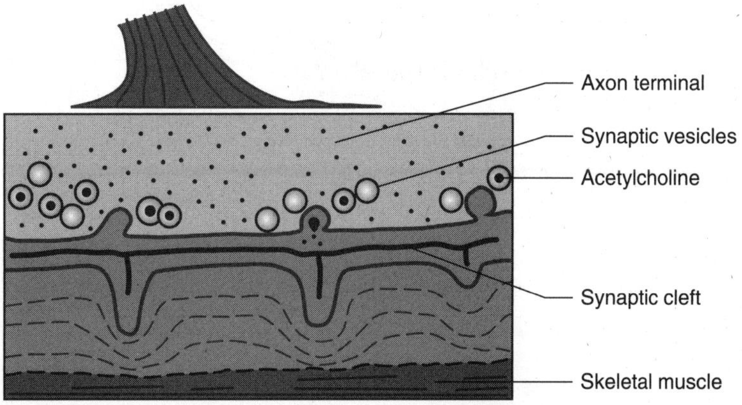

A nerve impulse (also known as an action potential) reaching the neuromuscular junction will cause the release of acetylcholine, which triggers the generation of action potential in the muscle fiber. The acetylcholine released into the synaptic cleft between an axon terminal and the plasma membrane of the muscle fiber is rapidly destroyed by acetylcholinesterase.

Motor Unit

Each motor neuron branches to form contacts with many muscle fibers. The neuron and the muscle fibers attached to it form a motor unit. When an impulse is transmitted through the motor neuron, it will cause the simultaneous contraction of all muscle fibers to which it is attached. Very fine movements require the number of connections a motor neuron makes with muscle fibers to be small (e.g., about 10).

Reflex Arc

Motor axons and sensory (or afferent) axons usually occur in the same "mixed" nerve. The simplest manner in which sensory and motor neurons are integrated to evoke behavior is in a reflex arc (Figure 72). For example, in the knee-jerk response, striking the patella stimulates a stretch receptor neuron that sends an impulse to the spinal cord. Within the gray matter of the spinal cord, the axon of the sensory neuron forms a synapse with a dendrite of a motor neuron. The impulse travels via the motor neuron axon to the quadriceps femoris muscle, which responds by contracting and causing extension of the leg.

FIGURE 72. Simple Reflex Arc That Elicits a Knee-Jerk Response

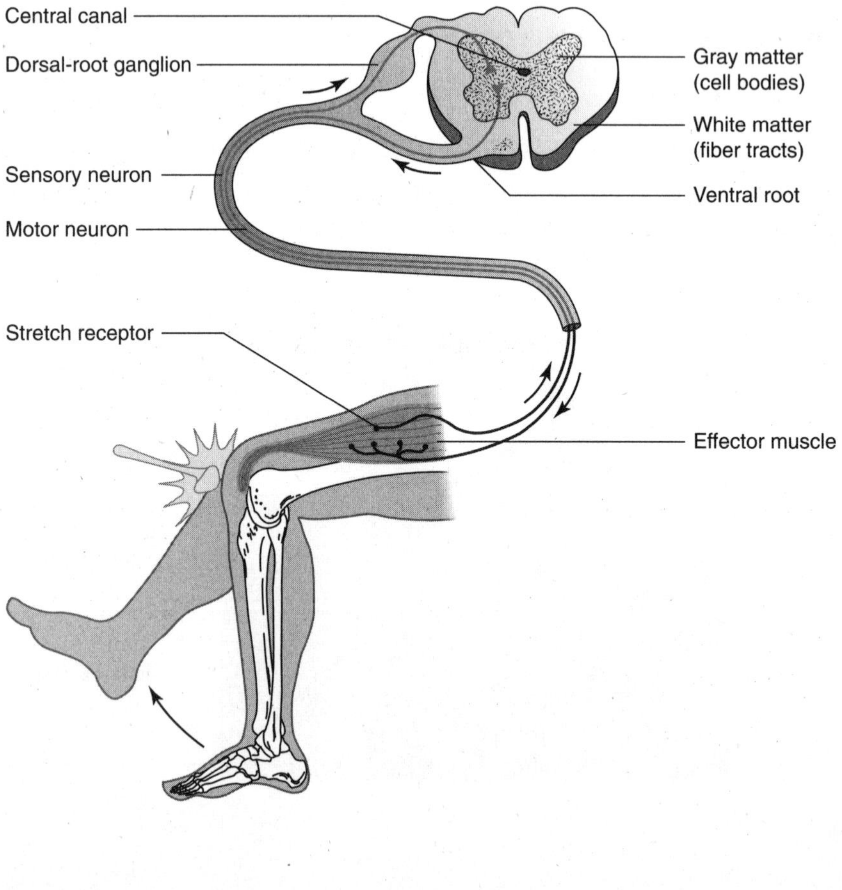

Most of the sensory neurons that enter the spinal cord do not terminate on motor neurons but rather on interneurons. Interneurons are more numerous (by a factor of about 30) than motor neurons, and they have numerous connections to each other and to motor neurons. These interconnections provide the basis for complex reflex responses such as the withdrawal reflex.

Voluntary and Involuntary Control

Reflex behavior is unconscious and automatic but plays a critical role in homeostasis. Changes in vascular tone in response to hot or cold, sweating, and some motor functions of the gut are all examples of autonomic reflexes that occur in the spinal cord.

The brain stem, which connects the cerebrum to the spinal cord, has numerous nerve pathways that help regulate the involuntary functions involved with equilibrium, respiration, cardiovascular function, eye movements, and support of the body against gravity.

"Voluntary" control of motor functions is primarily under the control of the frontal lobes of the cerebral cortex and the cerebellum of the brain. The cerebral cortex contains a pyramidal area consisting of very large pyramid-shaped cells. Motor signals from the brain originate in the pyramidal cells and travel through the brain stem and to the spinal cord via the pyramidal or corticospinal nerve tract. Most of the pyramidal fibers terminate on interneurons in the spinal cord gray matter. These interneurons form synapses with motor neurons controlling various voluntary muscles.

In addition to the corticospinal tracts, extrapyramidal tracts transmit motor signals from the brain. A specialized region of the frontal lobe that coordinates the muscular area involved with speech is called Broca's area.

2. SKELETAL SYSTEM

A. Bone Structure

Bone, like other connective tissues, consists of cells and fibers, but unlike the others, its extracellular components are calcified, making it a hard, unyielding substance ideally suited for its supportive and protective function in the skeleton.

Inspection of a long bone with the naked eye reveals two distinct forms of bone: cancellous (spongy) and compact. Spongy bone consists of a network of hardened bars having spaces between them filled with marrow. Compact bone appears as a solid, continuous mass, in which spaces can be seen only with the aid of a microscope. The two forms of bone grade into one another without a sharp boundary (Figure 73).

In typical long bones, such as the femur or humerus, the shaft (diaphysis) consists of compact bone surrounding a large central marrow cavity. In adults, the marrow in the long bones is primarily of the yellow, fatty variety, while the marrow in the flat bones of the ribs and at the ends of long bones is primarily of the red variety and is active in the production of red blood cells. Even this red marrow contains about 70% fat.

The ends (epiphyses) of long bones consist mainly of spongy bone covered by a thin layer of compact bone. In a long bone that is still growing, the epiphysis contains a cartilaginous region known as an epiphyseal plate. The epiphyseal plate and the adjacent spongy bone constitute a growth zone, in which all growth in length of the bone occurs. The surfaces at the ends of long bones, where one bone articulates with another, are covered by a layer of cartilage called the articular cartilage. This cartilage allows for easy movement of the bones over each other at a joint.

FIGURE 73. Longitudinal Section of the End of a Long Bone

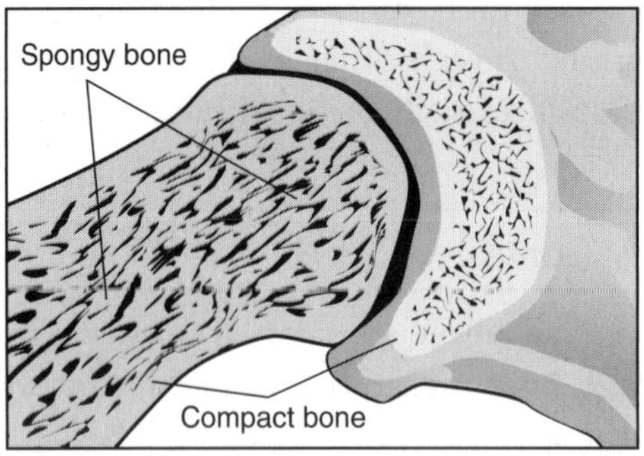

Compact bone is composed of structural units called Haversian systems. Each system is irregularly cylindrical and is composed of concentrically arranged layers of hard, inorganic matrix surrounding a microscopic central Haversian canal. Blood vessels and nerves pass through this canal, supplying and controlling the metabolism of the bone cells. The bone matrix itself is laid down by bone cells called osteoblasts. Osteoblasts produce a substance called osteoid, which is hardened by calcium, causing calcification. Some osteoblasts are trapped in the hardening osteoid and are converted into osteocytes that continue to live within the bone. These osteocytes lie in small cavities called lacunae, located along the interfaces between adjoining concentric layers of the hard matrix. Exchange of materials between the bone cells and the blood vessels in the Haversian canals is through tiny canals (canaliculi). Volkmann's canals penetrate and cross the layers of hard matrix, connecting the various Haversian canals to one another (Figure 74).

FIGURE 74. Cross-Section of a Long Bone Showing Internal Structures

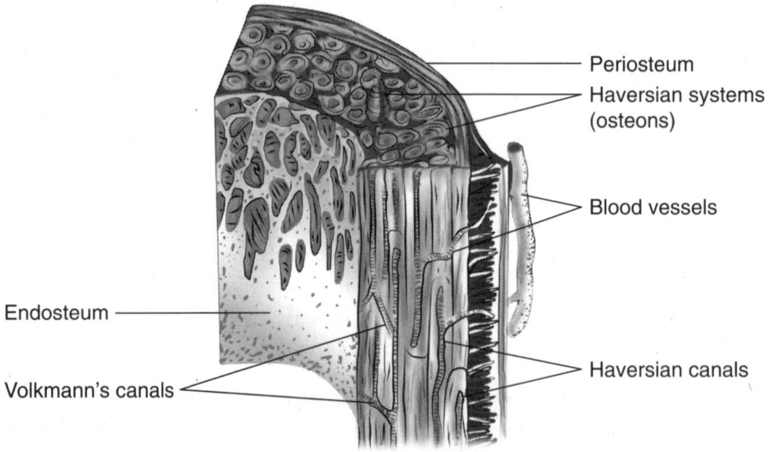

With few exceptions, bones are covered by the periosteum—a layer of specialized connective tissue. The periosteum has the ability to form bone and contributes to the healing of fractures. Periosteum is lacking on the ends of long bones surrounded by articular cartilage. The marrow cavity of the diaphysis and the cavities of spongy bone are lined by the endosteum—a thin cellular layer that also has the ability to form bone.

Haversian systems are present in most compact bone. However, certain compact flat bones of the skull, such as the frontal, parietal, occipital, and temporal bones and part of the mandible, do not have Haversian systems. These bones, termed membrane bones, have a different architecture and are formed differently from bones with Haversian systems.

Problem

A major functional difference between the long bones and the ribs is

A. color.
B. support.
C. production of red blood cells.
D. the fat content of the marrow.

Solution

C. The marrow in the ribs produces red blood cells, whereas the marrow in the long bones does not.

B. Skeletal Structure

The axial skeleton consists of the skull, vertebral column, ribs, and the sternum, as shown in Figure 75(a). The primary function of the vertebrate skull is protection of the brain. The part of the skull that serves this function is the cranium. The rest of the skull is made up of the bones of the face. In all, the human skull is composed of 28 bones, 6 of which are very small and located in the middle ear. At the time of birth, several of the bones of the cranium are not completely formed, leaving five membranous regions called fontanelles. These regions are somewhat flexible and can undergo changes in shape as necessary for safe passage of the infant through the birth canal.

The human vertebral column, or spinal column, is made up of 33 bones known as vertebrae, which differ in size and shape in various regions of the spine. The neck region comprises 7 cervical vertebrae; the thorax has 12 thoracic vertebrae; the lower back consists of 5 lumbar vertebrae; the sacral or hip region has 5 fused vertebrae forming the sacrum, to which the pelvic girdle is attached; and the coccyx or tailbone at the end of the vertebral column consists of 4, or possibly 5, small fused vertebrae. The vertebrae forming the sacrum and coccyx are separate in childhood, with fusion occurring by adulthood.

A typical vertebra consists of a basal portion, the centrum, and a dorsal ring of bone, the neural arch, which surrounds and protects the delicate spinal cord that runs through it. Each vertebra has projections for the attachment of ribs or muscles or both, and for articulating (joining) with neighboring vertebrae. The first vertebra, the atlas, has rounded depressions on its upper surface into which fit two projections from the base of the skull. This articulation allows for up and down movements of the head. The second vertebra, called the axis, has a pointed projection that fits into the atlas. This type of articulation allows for the rotation of the head.

Humans have 12 pairs of ribs, one pair articulating with each thoracic vertebra. The ribs support the chest wall and keep it from collapsing as the diaphragm contracts. Of the 12 pairs of ribs, the first 7 are attached ventrally to the breastbone, the next 3 are attached indirectly by cartilage, and the last 2, called floating ribs, have no attachments to the breastbone.

The bones of the appendages and the girdles, which attach the appendages to the rest of the body, make up the appendicular skeleton, as shown in Figure 75(b). In the shoulder region, the pectoral girdle serves for the attachment of the arms; and in the hip region, the pelvic girdle serves for the attachment of the legs. The pelvic girdle, which is wider in females so as to allow room for fetal development, consists of three fused hipbones—the ilium, ischium, and pubis—which are attached to the sacrum. The pectoral girdle consists of two collarbones, or clavicles, and two shoulder blades, or scapulas. Articulating with the scapula is the single bone of the upper arm, called the humerus. Articulating with the other end of the humerus are the two bones of the forearm, called the radius and the ulna. The radius and ulna permit the twisting movements of the forearm. The ulna has a process on its end called the olecranon but often referred to as the "funny bone." The wrist is composed of eight small bones called the carpals. The palm of the hand consists of five bones known as the metacarpals, each of which articulates with a bone of the finger, called a phalanx. Each finger has three phalanges, with the exception of the thumb, which has two.

FIGURE 75. Human Skeletal System

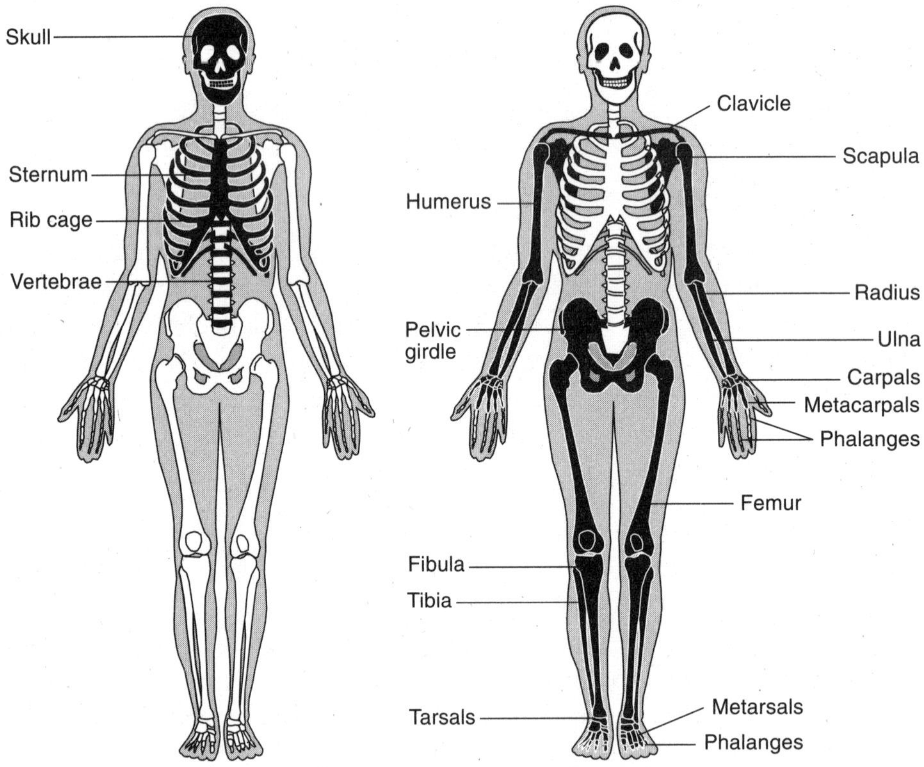

(a) Axial skeleton (b) Appendicular skeleton

The pelvic girdle consists of the two hipbones. The hipbones are attached to the sacrum. Each hipbone is formed from three fused bones: the ilium, ischium, and pubis.

The pattern of bones in the leg and foot is similar to that in the arm and hand. The upper leg bone, called the femur, articulates with the pelvic girdle. The two lower leg bones are the tibia (shinbone) and fibula. These two bones are responsible for rotation of the lower leg. Ventral to the joint between the upper and lower leg bones is another bone, the patella or kneecap, which serves as a point of muscle attachment for the upper and lower leg muscles and strengthens the joint. This bone has no counterpart in the arm. The ankle contains seven irregularly shaped bones, the tarsals, corresponding to the carpals of the wrist. The foot proper contains five metatarsals, corresponding to the metacarpals of the hand, and the bones in the toes are the phalanges, two in the big toe and three in each of the others.

The point of junction between two bones is called a joint. Some joints, such as those between the bones of the skull, are immovable and extremely strong, owing to an intricate intermeshing of the edges of the bones. Some joints are freely movable. Movable joints are of several types. Some are ball-and-socket joints, such as the joint at which the femur joins the pelvis, or where the humerus joins the pectoral girdle. These joints allow free movement in several directions. Both the pelvis and the pectoral girdle contain rounded, concave depressions to accommodate the rounded convex heads of the femur and humerus, respectively. Hinge joints, such as that of the human knee, permit movement in one plane only. The pivot joints at the wrists and ankles allow freedom of movement intermediate between that of the hinge and the ball-and-socket types (Figure 76).

FIGURE 76. Types of Joints in the Human Body

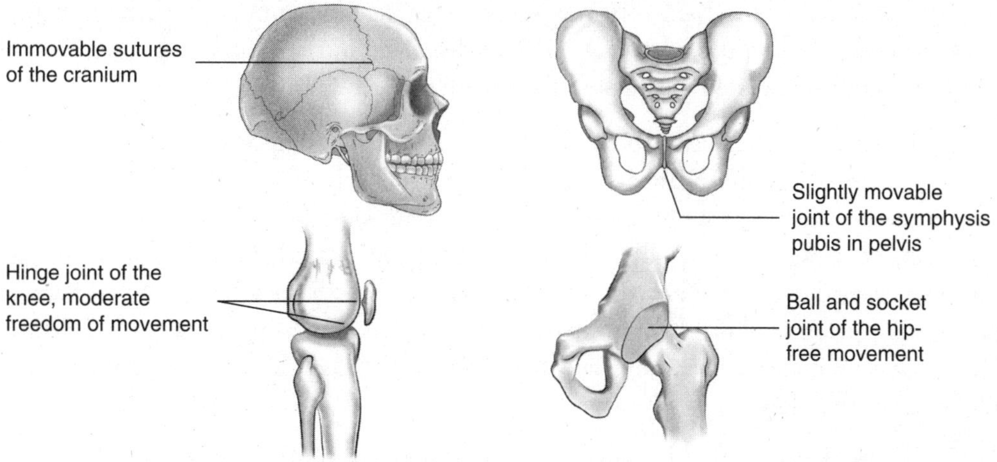

The various bones of a joint are held together by connective tissue strands called ligaments. Skeletal muscles, attached to the bones by means of another type of connective tissue strand known as a tendon, produce their effects by bending the skeleton at the movable joints. The ends of each bone at a movable joint are covered with a layer of smooth cartilage.

The joint cavity is filled with a liquid lubricant, called the synovial fluid, which is secreted by the membrane lining the cavity (Figure 77). During youth and early maturity, the lubricant is replaced as needed, but in middle and old age, the supply is often decreased, resulting in joint stiffness and restricted movement. A common disability known as bursitis is caused by the inflammation of cells lining the bursa and results in restrained movement.

FIGURE 77. Structure of a Knee Joint

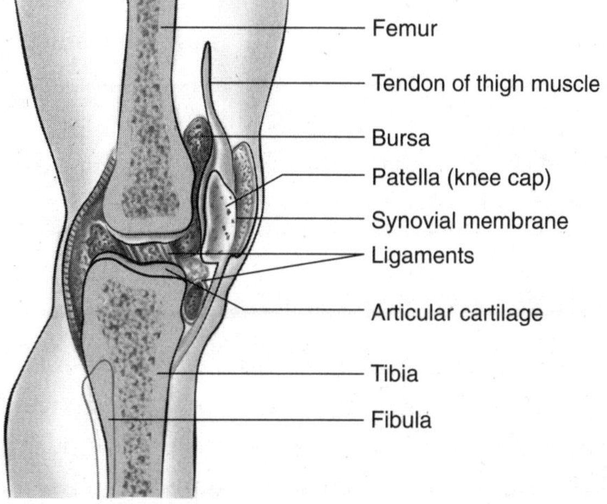

IX. RESPIRATORY AND SKIN SYSTEMS

1. RESPIRATORY SYSTEM

A. Function

Oxygen and carbon dioxide are the important respiratory gases. Although a small amount of oxygen is carried dissolved in the blood, most of the oxygen is carried by hemoglobin, an important protein found in red blood cells. Carbon dioxide (CO_2) is also dissolved in the blood and carried by hemoglobin, but most carbon dioxide is carried in the blood as bicarbonate ion (HCO_3^-).

Chemoreceptors are sensitive to changes in the chemical composition of the blood. Central chemoreceptors in the medulla oblongata are quite sensitive to levels of hydrogen ion (H^+) or CO_2. When H^+ or CO_2 increases, the receptors become excited and send signals to the breathing centers in the medulla oblongata, stimulating breathing. In addition, peripherally located chemoreceptors are located in the aortic arch and carotid arteries. They too can stimulate the medullary breathing centers when there is an increase in H^+ (decrease in pH) or an increase in CO_2, as well as when there is a decrease in oxygen in the blood. The increase in breathing will function to increase the oxygen and/or decrease the carbon dioxide levels in the blood.

The lungs are the site of gas exchange in the pulmonary circulation. The alveoli or air sacs of the lungs are thin-walled, as are the pulmonary capillaries that supply them. Hence, the respiratory gases can easily diffuse through these walls. Gases diffuse from a region of high partial pressure to one of lower partial pressure. When a person inhales, oxygen in the alveoli increases; when a person exhales, carbon dioxide in the alveoli decreases. Because the blood entering the pulmonary capillaries has a low level of oxygen and a high level of carbon dioxide, oxygen will diffuse from the alveoli into the pulmonary capillaries, and carbon dioxide will diffuse from the pulmonary capillaries into the alveoli. Thus, the blood returning to the heart from the lungs will be replenished with oxygen, and the body tissues will be rid of carbon dioxide, the major waste product of cellular metabolism.

Problem

An increase in carbon dioxide concentration will cause a decrease in the blood

A. pH.
B. oxygen concentration.
C. carbonic acid concentration.
D. lactic acid concentration.

Solution

A. An increase in carbon dioxide concentration will cause an increase in carbonic acid concentration and will lower the blood pH.

B. Breathing Structures and Mechanisms

The respiratory system in humans and other air-breathing vertebrates includes the lungs and the tubes through which air reaches them (Figure 78). Normally, air enters the human respiratory system by way of the external nares, or nostrils, but it may also enter by way of the mouth. The nostrils, which contain small hairs to filter incoming air, lead into the nasal cavities, which are separated from the mouth by the palate. The nasal cavities contain the sense organs of smell and are lined with mucus-secreting epithelium that moistens the incoming air. Air passes from the nasal cavities via the internal nares into the pharynx and then through the glottis and into the larynx. The larynx is often called the Adam's apple and is more prominent in men than women.

FIGURE 78. Human Respiratory System

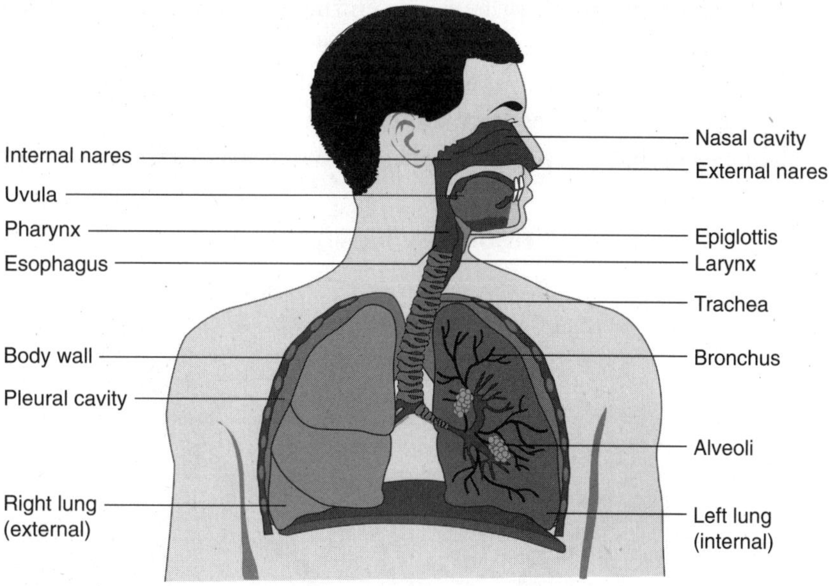

The opening to the larynx, called the glottis, is always open except during swallowing, when a flaplike structure (the epiglottis) covers it. Within the larynx are the vocal cords. The glottis is the opening between the vocal cords. Muscles of the larynx move the vocal cords together, closing the glottis, or move the vocal cords apart, allowing air to pass through the glottis. Leading from the larynx to the chest region is a long cylindrical tube called the trachea, or windpipe. In a dissection, the trachea can be distinguished from the esophagus by its cartilaginous rings, which serve to hold the tracheal tube open. In the middle of the chest, the trachea bifurcates into bronchi that lead to the lungs. In the lungs, each bronchus branches, forming smaller and smaller air tubes called bronchioles. Very small bronchioles terminate in clusters of air sacs called alveoli. Each alveolus is a cup-shaped cavity. The wall of an alveolus is covered with a rich network of capillaries. The total alveolar surface area across which gases may diffuse has been estimated to be greater than 100 square meters.

Each lung, as well as the cavity of the chest in which the lung rests, is covered by a thin sheet of smooth epithelium called the pleura. The pleurae are continuous with each other at the point at which the bronchus enters the lung. Thus, a pleura is more correctly a sac than a single sheet covering a lung. The space within this sac is filled with a thin layer of fluid; this fluid enables the lung to move without much friction during breathing.

The chest cavity is closed and has no communication with the outside. It is bounded by the chest wall, which contains the ribs on its top, sides, and back, and the sternum anteriorly. The bottom of the chest wall is covered by a strong, dome-shaped sheet of skeletal muscle called the diaphragm. The diaphragm separates the chest region (thorax) from the abdominal region and plays a crucial role in breathing by contracting and relaxing, changing the intrathoracic pressure.

2. SKIN SYSTEM

A. Composition

Human skin is composed of a comparatively thin outer layer, the epidermis, which is free of blood vessels, and an inner thick layer, the dermis, which is packed with blood vessels and nerve endings (Figure 79). The epidermis is a stratified epithelium whose thickness varies in different parts of the body. It is thickest on the soles of the feet and the palms of the hands. The epidermis of the palms and fingers has numerous ridges, forming whorls and loops in very specific patterns. These unique fingerprints and palm prints are determined genetically and result primarily from the orientation of the underlying fibers in the dermis. The outermost layers of the epidermis are composed of dead cells that are constantly being sloughed off and replaced by cells from beneath. As each cell is pushed outward by active cell division in the deeper layers of the epidermis, it synthesizes large amounts of the fibrous protein keratin and becomes a flat (squamous) scalelike epithelial cell. Keratin makes the outer layer of the skin tough and durable.

FIGURE 79. Section of Human Skin

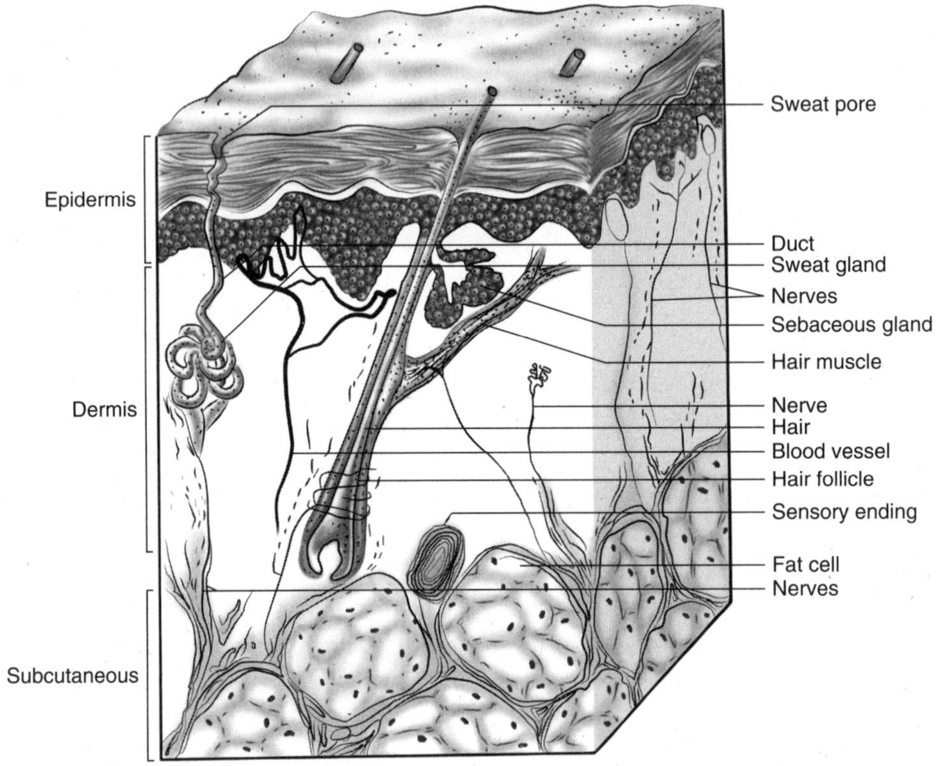

Scattered at the juncture between the deeper layers of the epidermis and the dermis are melanocytes, cells that produce the pigment melanin. Melanin serves as a protective device for the body by absorbing ultraviolet rays from the sun. Tanning results from an increase in melanin production as a result of exposure to ultraviolet radiation. All humans have about the same number of melanocytes in their skin. The difference between light and dark skin colors is genetically determined and results from the melanocytes of darker-skinned people producing more melanin.

The juncture of the dermis with the epidermis is uneven. The dermis throws projections called papillae into the epidermis. The dermis is much thicker than the epidermis and is composed largely of connective tissue. The lower level of the dermis, called the subcutaneous layer, is connected with the underlying muscle and is composed of many fat cells and a more loosely woven network of fibers. This part of the dermis is one of the principle sites of body fat deposits, which help preserve body heat. The subcutaneous layer also determines the amount of possible skin movement.

The hair and nails are keratin-based derivatives of skin and develop from the pocketing of cells from the inner layer of the epidermis (keratin is a protein). Although the hair follicles are located in the dermis, they are derived from the epidermis. Similarly, nails are derived from the epidermis. Hair follicles are found throughout the dermal layer, except on the palms, soles, and a few other regions. Individual hairs are formed in the hair follicles, which have their roots deep within the dermis. At the bottom of each follicle, a papilla of connective tissue projects into the follicle. The epithelial cells above this papilla constitute the hair root and, by cell division, form the shaft of the hair, which ultimately extends beyond the surface of the skin. The hair cells of the shaft synthesize and accumulate keratin, and then the cells die and form a compact mass that becomes the hair. Growth occurs at the bottom of the follicle only. Associated with each hair follicle is one or more sebaceous glands. The sebaceous glands secrete an oily substance that makes the surface of the skin and hair more pliable. Like the sweat glands, the sebaceous glands are derived from the embryonic epidermis but are located in the dermis. To each hair follicle is attached smooth muscle called arrector pili, which pulls the hair erect on contraction.

B. Protection and Thermoregulation

Perhaps the most vital functions of the skin are to protect the body against a variety of external agents and to help maintain a constant internal environment. The layers of the skin form a protective shield against blows, friction, and many injurious chemicals. These layers are essentially germproof and, as long as they are not broken, keep bacteria and other microorganisms from entering the body. The skin is water repellent and therefore protects the body from excessive loss of moisture. In addition, the pigment in the outer layers protects the underlying layers from the ultraviolet rays of the sun.

In addition to its role in protection, the skin is involved in thermoregulation. Heat is constantly being produced by the metabolic processes of the body cells and distributed by the bloodstream. Heat may be lost from the body in expired breath, feces, and urine, but approximately 90% of the total heat loss occurs through the skin. This is accomplished by changes in the blood supply to the blood vessels of the skin. When the air temperature is high, the blood vessels dilate, and the increased flow of blood to the skin allows for heat loss from the blood to the environment. Because of the increased blood supply, the skin appears flushed. When the temperature is low, the blood vessels of the skin are constricted, thereby decreasing the flow of blood through the skin and decreasing the rate of heat loss. Temperature-sensitive nerve endings in the skin reflexively control the blood vessels' diameters.

At high temperatures, the sweat glands are stimulated to secrete sweat. The evaporation of sweat from the surface of the skin lowers the body temperature by removing from the body the heat necessary to convert the liquid sweat into water vapor. In addition to their function in heat loss, the sweat glands serve an excretory function. The sweat glands excrete 5–10% of all metabolic wastes. Sweat contains substances similar to those in urine but is much more dilute.

Problem

The dilation of blood vessels in the skin causes

A. a minimum amount of heat loss to the environment.

B. no change in the temperature of the skin.

C. heat loss to the environment.

D. a palor to the skin.

Solution

C. The dilation of blood vessels in the skin causes a loss of heat to the environment.

X. REPRODUCTIVE SYSTEM AND DEVELOPMENT

1. MALE AND FEMALE GONADS AND GENITALIA

The successful production of offspring in higher organisms is complex and reserved for mature, fully developed organisms. The organs related to the reproductive process are called genitalia. The specific organs responsible for producing the sex cells (i.e., sperm cells in males and ova in females) are called gonads; in females, that organ is the ovary, and in males it is the testis.

A. Male Reproductive System

As shown in Figure 80, the reproductive organs in males include two testes as well as accessory internal organs (i.e., the epididymides, the ductus or vasa deferens, the seminal vesicles, ejaculatory ducts, the prostate gland, the urethra, and the bulbourethral glands) and accessory external organs (i.e., the scrotum and penis). These accessory organs primarily serve to store and deliver the sperm (or spermatozoa) to the female genitalia. Various glands secrete fluids to aid in this process.

The testes respond to hormones secreted by the anterior pituitary gland (i.e., gonadotropins). The anterior pituitary is stimulated by the hypothalamus. In addition, the testes secrete hormones such as testosterone. During puberty, testosterone stimulates testicular growth as well as the growth of the accessory male reproductive organs. Testosterone also helps to maintain secondary masculine sex characteristics (e.g., muscle mass, hair growth).

FIGURE 80. Male Reproductive System

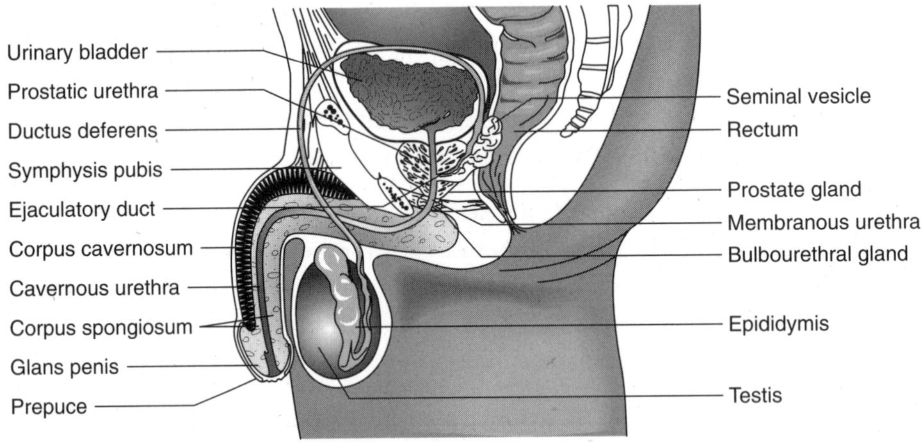

B. Female Reproductive System

The female reproductive system produces, transports, and temporarily stores ova. Ova are produced in the ovaries, which are the primary female reproductive organ. Further, the female reproductive system is specialized to accept sperm, to aid in the process of fertilization, to provide a highly controlled environment for long-term fetal development, and to deliver the newborn from an intrauterine to an extrauterine environment. Hormones are secreted by the ovaries. Figure 81 illustrates the basic structural features of the female reproductive system. The accessory internal organs of the female reproductive tract include the fallopian tubes and the vagina. The external female accessory organs include the labia majora, labia minora, clitoris, and vestibule.

FIGURE 81. Female Reproductive System

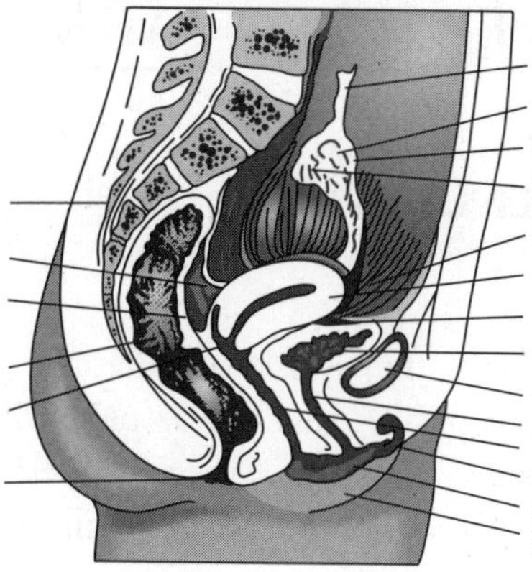

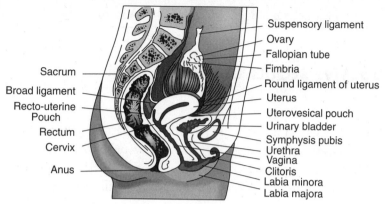

2. GAMETOGENESIS BY MEIOSIS

A. Spermatogenesis (Sperm Production)

Spermatogenesis occurs in the coiled seminiferous tubules of the testes. The seminiferous tubules have supporting columnar epithelial cells called Sertoli cells as well as spermatogenic cells. The spermatogenic cells form sperm cells. Sperm cells taken directly from the testes are neither functional nor motile. The sperm in the testes pass through ducts into the epididymis, where they become motile but still lack the ability to fertilize an ovum. To be fully functional, the sperm must incubate in the tubal fluid of the female.

After passing through the epididymis, sperm moves through the ductus deferens, a long muscular tube that ascends to the ejaculatory duct. The ejaculatory duct empties into the urethra in the penis.

B. Oogenesis (Production of Egg Cells or Oocytes)

The ovaries lie on each side of the pelvic cavity, and each ovary has an exterior monolayer of germinal epithelial cells that give rise to the ovum. At birth, these germinal epithelial cells have already differentiated into millions of primordial follicles, each of which contains an egg cell (or primary oocyte) and a surrounding single layer of follicle cells. At puberty, some of the egg cells in the follicles resume meiosis (arrested in prophase I) to form a secondary oocyte containing a haploid number of chromosomes. Further, the primordial follicles undergo a maturation process at puberty: the oocytes enlarge, and the follicular cells proliferate and form a cavity containing the oocyte and a follicular fluid. A mature follicle has an inner layer of granulosa cells and an outer layer of cells formed by ovarian stroma. The ovum is embedded in a mass of granulosa cells. During ovulation, the oocyte is discharged from the mature follicle and then travels to the opening of the uterine tube. If fertilization of the egg cell does not take place, the cell will die in a short time.

Problem

Spermatogenesis is different than oogenesis because

A. only one diploid cell is produced in spermatogenesis.
B. four viable daughter cells are produced in oogenesis.
C. polar bodies are produced in oogenesis.
D. only one haploid cell is produced in spermatogenesis.

Solution

C. Polar bodies are produced in oogenesis and only one viable egg is produced.

3. REPRODUCTIVE SEQUENCE

A. Males

The reproductive sequence in males is (1) psychic stimulation, (2) erection of the penis, (3) lubrication, and (4) emission and ejaculation (orgasm). Erection is primarily a vascular event caused by dilation of arteries and constriction of veins in response to parasympathetic impulses from the sacral portion of the spinal column. The resulting high arterial blood pressure fills the erectile tissues of the penis. There are three cylindrical masses of erectile tissues (venous sinusoids) in the penis: two corpus cavernosum and one corpus spongiosum.

The parasympathetic impulses that promote erection also stimulate the secretion of a lubricating fluid from the bulbourethral gland. This fluid lubricates the end of the penis, facilitating coitus (intercourse) and neutralizing any remaining acidity in the urethra.

Emission is the movement of sperm cells (from the testes) and secretions (from the prostate and seminal vesicles) to the urethra to form seminal fluid. Emission is a reflex that occurs in response to sympathetic impulses from the spinal cord and results in peristaltic contractions of the smooth muscles of the epididymis, the ductus deferens, and the ampulla. Sympathetic impulses also trigger the contraction of smooth muscles in the prostate glands and the seminal vesicles that force the sperm down the urethra. Ejaculation is the expulsion of seminal fluid from the urethra by a reflexive contraction of the bulbocavernosus muscle (a skeletal muscle).

B. Females

The reproductive sequence in females involves, in part, a monthly sexual cycle (normally, 28 days) that is under hormonal regulation. Follicle-stimulating hormone (FSH) and luteinizing hormone (LH) are secreted by the anterior pituitary at the beginning of the sexual cycle, and these hormones stimulate the process of ovulation. Both FSH and LH bind to cellular receptors that activate adenylate cyclase.

About two days before ovulation, a marked increase in the secretion of LH occurs, causing the mature follicle to rupture and release an oocyte that enters the uterine tube (at about day 14). Following ovulation, the follicular cells turn into the corpus luteum, which releases increased amounts of estrogen and progesterone. The increased estrogen causes a thickening of the uterine endometrium in preparation for the potential implanting of a fertilized ovum. Similarly, progesterone causes increased vascularization, swelling, and secretory activity of the endometrium, which is the innermost layer of tissue forming the uterine wall. Both estrogen and progesterone also inhibit the production of LH and FSH by the anterior pituitary gland. If fertilization does not occur, the corpus luteum stops secreting estrogen and progesterone, causing disintegration of the uterine lining (i.e., menstrual flow). If fertilization does occur, the placenta secretes chorionic gonadotropin, which extends the life of the corpus luteum to the first three to four months of pregnancy.

Coitus in the female also involves psychic stimulation, erection, lubrication, and orgasm. The clitoris (see Figure 81) contains two columns of erectile tissue, called the corpus cavernosa, that respond to parasympathetic impulses, just as the penis does, causing the clitoris to become erect. Concurrently, the Bartholin's glands located beneath the labia minor secrete lubricating mucus.

4. EMBRYOGENESIS

A. Embryonic Development

Embryonic development begins when an ovum is fertilized by a sperm and ends at parturition (birth). It is a process of change and growth that transforms a single-celled zygote into a multicellular organism.

The earliest stage of embryonic development is the one-celled, diploid zygote that results from fertilization of an ovum by a sperm. Next is a period called cleavage, in which mitotic division of the zygote results in the formation of daughter cells called blastomeres. At each succeeding division, the blastomeres become smaller and smaller. When 16 or so blastomeres have formed, the solid ball of cells is called a morula. As the morula divides further, a fluid-filled cavity is formed in the center of the sphere, converting the morula into a hollow ball of cells called a blastula. When cells of the blastula differentiate into two, and later three, embryonic germ layers, the blastula is called a gastrula. The gastrular period generally extends until the early forms of all major structures (e.g.,, the heart) are laid down. After this period, the developing organism is called a fetus. During the fetal period (the duration of which varies with species), the various systems develop further. Although developmental changes in the fetal period are not as dramatic as those occurring during the earlier embryonic periods, they are extremely important. Congenital defects may result from abnormal development during this period.

B. Germ Layers

Early forms of all major structure are laid down during the gastrula period. These forms, called primary germ layers, begin to differentiate rapidly during the fetal stage. There are three primary germ layers: ectoderm, mesoderm, and endoderm (Figure 82).

Ectoderm gives rise to the epidermis of the skin, including the skin glands, hair, nails, and the enamel of teeth. In addition, the epithelial lining of the mouth, nasal cavity, sinuses, sense organs, and the anal canal are ectodermal in origin. Nervous tissue, including the brain, spinal cord, and nerves, are all derived from embryonic ectoderm. Mesoderm gives rise to muscle tissue, cartilage, bone, and the notochord, which in humans is replaced in the embryo by vertebrae. Endoderm gives rise to the gastrointestinal and respiratory tracts and the endocrine system. Organs created from endoderm include the pharynx, liver, gallbladder and pancreas.

FIGURE 82. Early Germ Layer Development

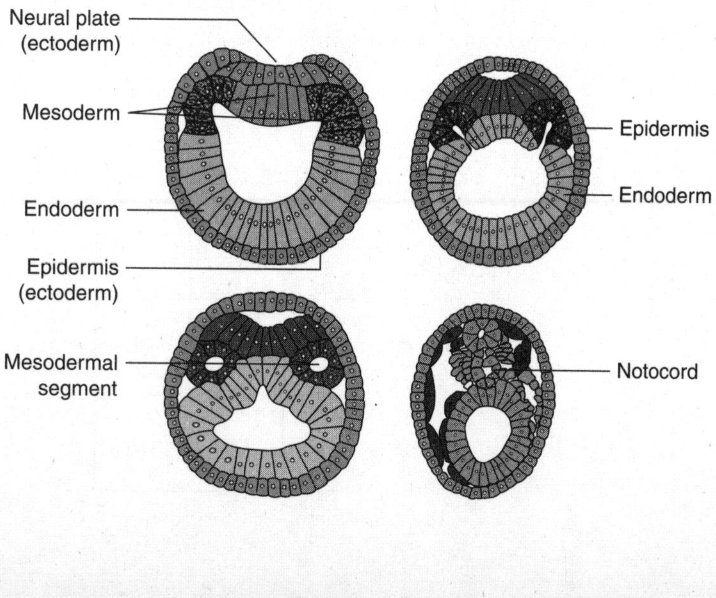

XI. GENETICS AND EVOLUTION

1. GENETICS

A. Genotype and Phenotype

Genes are the units of heredity and are located on chromosomes. Genes occur in various forms, or alleles, the combinations of which code for the specific expression of traits. Each individual inherits one allele of each gene from the mother and one from the father. If an individual inherits two identical alleles of a gene, he or she is said to be homozygous for that trait. If the alleles are different, the individual is heterozygous for that trait.

The genotype is the actual genetic constitution of the individual, but the phenotype is the expression of the genotype. For instance, there are two alleles that determine eye color. Let B represent the dominant allele, dictating brown eyes, and b represent the recessive allele dictating blue eyes. From these two alleles, there are three possible genotypes coding for eye color: BB—homozygous dominant, Bb—heterozygous, and bb—homozygous recessive. There are only two phenotypes: BB and Bb, both coding for brown eye color because B is dominant over b. Blue eyes are possible only with the genotype bb. Note that green eyes are considered blue, both genotypically and phenotypically. The phenotype includes not only physical characteristics apparent to an observer but also all characteristics that result from the genotype. For instance, an individual's blood type is part of his or her phenotype.

B. Dominant/Recessive Inheritance

There are many different types of genetic inheritance patterns. The simplest is that of dominant and recessive inheritance, as exemplified by the inheritance of eye color discussed in the previous section. Suppose two people, heterozygous for brown eyes, have children. The best way to examine the probabilities of eye color in the offspring is to use a Punnett square, in which the alleles of each parent form the axes of the square. The following Punnett square shows the mating between the two heterozygotes:

Bb × BB

	B	b
B	BB	Bb
b	Bb	bb

Phenotypically, 75% of the offspring will have brown eyes (BB and Bb), and 25% will have blue eyes (bb). The genotypes are 25% BB (homozygous dominant), 50% Bb (heterozygous), and 25% bb (homozygous recessive). The genotypic ratio is

1BB : 2Bb : 1bb.

The following Punnett square shows the cross between a blue-eyed woman and a heterozygous brown-eyed man:

bb × Bb

	b	b
B	Bb	Bb
b	bb	bb

The proportions of the offspring are 50% heterozygous (Bb) and thus brown eyed, and 50% homozygous recessive (bb) and thus blue-eyed.

C. Incomplete Dominance

Some traits show incomplete dominance, in which a dominant allele cannot fully mask the expression of the recessive allele. This is best exemplified in certain flowers, in which color is inherited as such. Let R be the dominant allele for red flower color, and let r be the recessive allele for white flower color. When a red flower (RR) is crossed with a white one (rr), the first generation will be 100% pink (Rr), as shown in the following Punnett square:

RR × rr

	R	R
r	Rr	Rr
r	Rr	Rr

If the allele for red color were fully dominant, the heterozygotes would all be red, not pink. Although the result of this one cross may appear to be a blended trait, in future generations, the dominant and recessive allele can be independently expressed again (i.e., the original traits will reemerge); thus, no blending has occurred. The subsequent cross between the pink flowers is shown in the following Punnett square:

Rr × Rr

	R	r
R	RR	Rr
r	Rr	rr

The expected probabilities of phenotypic expression are 25% red (RR), 50% pink (Rr), and 25% white (rr).

D. Codominance

In codominance, a heterozygote has two dominant alleles that are equally expressed. Codominance is best exemplified by the inheritance of blood antigens. There are multiple alleles, I^A, I^B, and i, possible at the locus that codes for ABO blood type. Of course, any one individual inherits only two alleles. I^A and I^B are dominant to i but are codominant with each other.

Type A blood is expressed by the genotypes I^AI^A and I^Ai. The person has only A antigens on red blood cells. A phenotypically type B person has the genotype I^BI^B or I^Bi. This person has only B antigens on red blood cells. The AB phenotype is expressed by the single genotype I^AI^B. These alleles are codominant, and the person has both A and B antigens on red blood cells. The homozygous recessive genotype ii is expressed phenotypically by type O blood. This person has neither A nor B antigens on red blood cells.

Punnett squares can be used to determine blood type probabilities for offspring. Suppose a heterozygous type A male mates with a heterozygous type B female. The following Punnett square shows that there will be an equal probability (25%) of each blood type in the offspring:

$I^Ai \times I^Bi$

	I^A	i
I^B	I^AI^B	I^Bi
i	I^Ai	ii

There is a 25% probability of type AB (I^AI^B), type B (I^Bi), type A (I^Ai), and type O (ii).

E. Sex-Linked Inheritance

Sex-linked inheritance is a little more complex. There are two sex chromosomes, X and Y, and 22 pairs of autosomal chromosomes. A female has two X chromosomes, one inherited from each parent. A male has an X chromosome inherited from his mother and a Y chromosome inherited from his father. The X chromosome is much larger than the Y chromosome, and the X chromosome contains genes for color blindness and hemophilia on it, both of which are recessive traits.

When a male inherits an X chromosome with the recessive allele, he will fully express the trait (hemophilia or color blindness) because his Y chromosome has no dominant homologous allele to mask it. In contrast, when a female inherits an X chromosome with the recessive allele, she might inherit the normal dominant allele on her other X chromosome. That allele will encode a functional protein, while the gene on the other X chromosome will not. Therefore, she will merely carry the trait, but will not express it. For a female to express the trait, she must inherit two recessive alleles, one on each of her X chromosomes. That means that her father must express the trait, while her mother must either be a carrier or express the trait as well. The likelihood of a mating between two individuals with this recessive sex-linked allele is low, unless the mating is between relatives.

Thus, the usual transmission of sex-linked traits is from a carrier mother to her son. The father cannot transmit the disease to his son because a male offspring has only one X chromosome, which must have come from his mother. The carrier mother has an equal chance of passing the gene on to either a son or a daughter; however, the trait is expressed more often in the son, who lacks the dominant allele to mask it. The daughter will not express the disease unless she has also acquired the recessive gene from an afflicted father.

If h represents the recessive allele for hemophilia, then a male can be represented one of two ways: an afflicted male will have the genotype X^hY, and a normal male will have the genotype X^HY. There are three possible genotypes for a female: a normal female is X^HX^H; a carrier female is X^HX^h, and an afflicted female is X^hX^h.

Suppose that C is the dominant allele for normal color vision and c is the allele for color blindness. A male is either normal (X^CY) or color blind (X^cY); a female is either normal (X^CX^C), a carrier (X^CX^c), or color blind (X^cX^c). As in hemophilia, the carrier genotype in a female means simply that she can transmit the condition, although she does not express the trait.

A cross between a carrier mother and a normal father is shown in the following Punnett square:

$X^CX^c \times X^CY$

	X^C	X^c
X^C	X^CX^C	X^CX^c
Y	X^CY	X^cY

Notice that the offspring are 25% of each of the following: normal female, carrier female, normal male, and color-blind male.

The following cross shows how a female can become afflicted when a carrier woman mates with an afflicted man:

$X^CX^c \times X^cY$

	X^C	X^c
X^c	X^CX^c	X^cX^c
Y	X^CY	X^cY

The four possible outcomes, occurring with equal probability, are carrier female, color-blind female, normal male, color-blind male.

In Figure 83, squares represent males and circles, females; shaded areas represent afflicted individuals and white areas, not afflicted. Subscripts refer to an individual within a generation. The following problems refer to the pedigree shown in the figure.

FIGURE 83. Pedigree Used in Problems

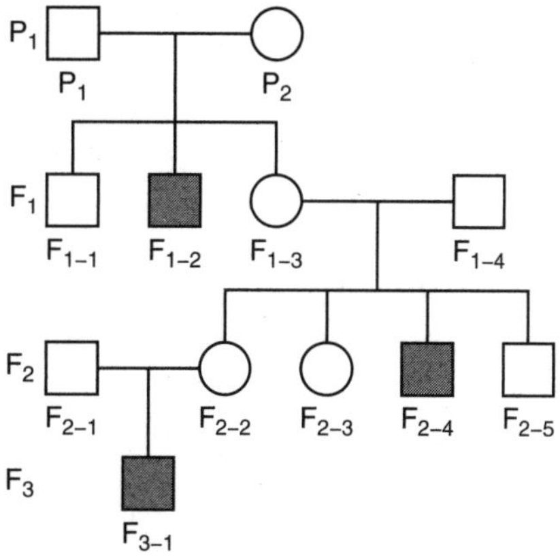

Problem

All the following statements concerning the disease in question are true EXCEPT

A. it is sex-linked.

B. it is caused by a recessive gene.

C. it may be hemophilia.

D. the afflicted boys must have received two alleles for this disease because it is recessive.

Solution

D.

Problem

If the disease is color blindness, the genotype of P1 must be

A. X^CX^c. B. X^CX^C. C. X^cX^c. D. X^CY.

Solution

D.

Problem

If F_{2-5} were to marry a woman homozygous dominant for the trait in question, the probability that they would have a child afflicted with the disease is

A. 0%. B. 25%. C. 50%. D. 100%.

Solution

A.

Problem

Different traits are characterized by different patterns of inheritance. Which of the following are incorrectly paired?

A. Eye color and dominant/recessive inheritance
B. Red, pink, and white colors in plants and incomplete dominance
C. ABO blood typing and incomplete dominance
D. Hemophilia and sex-linked inheritance

Solution

C.

2. EVOLUTION

A. Darwin's Theory: Natural Selection

In the nineteenth century, two major theories of evolution were proposed. In 1800, Jean-Baptiste Lamarck proposed a theory based on the inheritance of acquired characteristics. In other words, organs, and therefore animals, evolve through use. His classic example was his explanation for why the giraffe had such a long neck: he said that giraffes stretch their necks to reach the leaves high in trees. He assumed that an animal that stretched its neck could pass a stretched, and hence lengthened, neck on to its offspring.

Lamarck's theory was incorrect. Characteristics acquired in life (except genetic mutations in the germ cells) cannot be passed on to the next generation because the information is not in the genes. For instance, if a man develops his muscles by lifting weights, his offspring would not necessarily be muscular as well.

Charles Darwin proposed a theory of evolution largely based on his observations made during his voyage aboard *The Beagle*. While traveling about the Galapagos Islands, which lie 600 miles off the coast of Ecuador, Darwin observed that each island had similar birds—all finches. However, the finches were of different species. The most obvious anatomical distinction among the finches was the beak. Knowing that structure often dictates function, Darwin realized that the differences in beak structure were adaptations to the available food sources (i.e., insects, fruit, seeds) on the various islands. The finches all were of a common ancestor and, through many generations, differentiated into distinct species particularly suited to the environment of their islands. While the phrase was not coined at that time, this is a classic example of adaptive radiation, which refers to the emergence of several species from one species due to the segregation of habitats.

According to Darwin's theory, a giraffe would have a long neck because those giraffes that by chance had the selective advantage (long necks) could eat food in the trees and hence survive and reproduce. The offspring, like the parent, would have long necks. Giraffes with short necks would be selected against and therefore unable to survive to reproduce other short-necked giraffes.

The basic premise of Darwin's theory is that different individuals have different capacities to cope with their environment. Some individuals have characteristics that are advantageous in the environment, and those individuals will tend to survive and reproduce. The postulates of his theory were presented to the public in his book *On the Origin of Species by Means of Natural Selection* in 1859 and are reviewed below.

All organisms overproduce gametes. Not all gametes form offspring, and of the offspring formed, not all survive. Those organisms that are most competitive (in various aspects) will have a greater likelihood of survival. These survival traits vary from individual to individual but are passed on to the next generation. Therefore, over time, the best adaptations for survival are maintained in the population. The environment determines which traits will be selected for or against, but those traits may change in time. A selected trait at one time may later be disadvantageous.

Despite all of Darwin's insight, he never could explain the mechanism through which traits were passed on. This was the key drawback to his theory. At about the same time, unknown to Darwin, Gregor Mendel was experimenting with garden peas. Mendel was the first to introduce the concept of heritable factors (now called genes). However, Mendel's work was ignored by scientists at the time, only to be rediscovered early in the twentieth century.

B. Evidence for Evolution

Evidence for evolution comes from many scientific disciplines. Evidence from comparative biochemistry and molecular biology is based on the analysis of enzymes, proteins, nucleic acids, and so forth, to determine similarities in nucleotide sequences, and thus amino acid sequences. A similar molecular structure suggests a recent (by evolutionary standards) bifurcation of the original ancestral stock.

Comparative Anatomy

Comparative anatomy distinguishes between homologous structures and analogous structures. Homologous structures share an anatomical similarity resulting from a common evolutionary origin; this is exemplified by the basic bone structure in the forelimb of all vertebrates, such as the flipper of a whale and the arm of a human. Analogous structures subserve similar functions despite differences in their anatomy, and thus have no common ancestry. The wing of an insect and the wing of a bird exemplify analogous structures.

Fossil Record

The fossil record is an important clue to evolutionary origins. While fossils can actually be the preserved remnants of life (e.g., shells, skeletons), they also include imprints and molds, such as the imprint of an animal footprint. Fossil age can be estimated by the use of carbon dating. The ratio of radioactive carbon (^{14}C) to nonradioactive carbon (^{12}C) is determined. The half-life of a radioactive element is the time span during which half the atoms in a sample will have decayed. The half-life of ^{14}C (to decay to ^{12}C) is 5,730 years. The spontaneous rate of decay is constant.

C. Factors Responsible for Evolutionary Change

There are four factors that bring about evolutionary change: mutation, gene flow, genetic drift, and natural selection.

Mutation

Genetic mutations are changes in the base sequence in DNA, and thus genes, and as such are passed on to future generations. There are many different types of mutations. A point mutation is a substitution of a single nucleotide by another. This single-base substitution changes the codon to another of the 64 possible codons. Because of the degeneracy of the genetic code and because of wobble at the third position of the codon, substitution may or may not change the amino acid encoded. If the codon does call for the incorporation of a different amino acid, there still may not be a deleterious effect, especially if an amino acid is replaced by one with similar chemical characteristics, such as replacing one nonpolar amino acid with another nonpolar one. However, if the base substitution calls for an amino acid with distinct chemical characteristics, such as a difference in the charge on the amino acid, it is more likely to be deleterious. The site of the mutation is also important. For instance, if the new amino acid occurs at the functional site of a protein, such as the active site of an enzyme, it is more likely to adversely affect protein function.

Deletion or addition of a multiple of three bases results in the deletion or insertion of several amino acids, which may or may not affect protein function. Deletion or addition of one or two bases (or any other nonmultiple of three) causes a reading-frame shift. All the codons beyond the mutation will be incorrectly read, and the wrong amino acids will be incorporated. Further, an amino acid-encoding codon may be converted to a stop codon, leading to a truncated version of the protein.

Gene Flow

Gene flow is the change in allele frequency caused by migration. Migration can be immigration (entrance) or emigration (exit) of individuals (and their genes) to or from a population.

Genetic Drift

Genetic drift is a shift in allele frequency due to random fluctuation. This chance event is of special concern in small populations.

Natural Selection

Natural selection and differential reproduction are basically synonymous. This differential ability to survive and reproduce is the key factor in evolutionary change. Each individual in a population has a unique genotype (except identical twins, who have a common genotype) responsible for determining his or her phenotype. The environmental conditions at the time dictate which phenotypes are advantageous for survival. Individuals with the phenotypes that can cope best in the environment will differentially reproduce, and their genes will increase in frequency in the next generations.

D. Hardy–Weinberg Equilibrium

The Hardy–Weinberg equilibrium is an artificial state in which the proportion of alleles at a given locus remains constant. The four factors required to maintain the equilibrium are (1) no mutations, (2) isolation (and thus no migration and no gene flow), (3) large population size (and thus no genetic drift), and (4) equal viability and fertility of all genotypes (i.e., random reproduction and thus no natural selection). In real populations, these factors are not usually all met, and changes in allele frequency can occur.

In the Hardy–Weinberg equilibrium, allele frequencies and genotype frequencies are infinitely stable. For a trait with only two alleles, p and q, the frequencies are expressed by the equation

$$p + q = 1,$$

where p is the frequency of one allele at the given locus and q is the frequency of the alternative allele. The sum of the frequencies must equal 1.

Another mathematical equation holds true under a Hardy–Weinberg equilibrium:

$$(p + q)^2 = p^2 + 2pq + q^2$$

If p is the frequency of the dominant allele, p^2 is the frequency of homozygous dominants in the population. If q is the frequency of the recessive allele, q^2 is the frequency of homozygous recessives in the population. Thus, $2pq$ is the frequency of heterozygotes in the population. Note also that

$$p^2 + 2pq + q^2 = 1.$$

Suppose a teacher does a statistical analysis of eye color among students in a middle school. The analysis shows that of the 1,000 students, 910 have brown eyes and only 90 have blue eyes (or green eyes). Five years later, the analysis is repeated because the students in the first survey have graduated and other children are now in the middle school.

The results now show that of the 1,000 students, 840 have brown eyes and 160 have blue eyes. The following table summarizes the data:

Year	Brown Eyes	Blue Eyes	Total
2001	910	90	1,000
2006	840	160	1,000

In the original sample, 91% of the students had brown eyes and 9% had blue eyes. Because 9% (0.09) is equal to q^2, q must equal 0.3. Therefore, p must equal 0.7 (i.e., $p = 1 - 0.3$). The 910 brown-eyed students consisted of those that were homozygous and those that were heterozygous for the dominant allele. The homozygous-dominant population represented 49% of the total population ($p^2 = 0.7^2$), and the heterozygous population made up 42% of the total population ($2pq = 2 \times 0.7 \times 0.3$). Thus, 490 students were homozygous dominant and 420 were heterozygous, giving a total of 910 brown-eyed students.

The data for 2006 are significantly different from those gathered five years earlier. The change in allele frequencies can be accounted for by migration (immigration and emigration). In the sample, blue eyes accounted for 16% of the population (160/1,000). Thus, $q^2 = 0.16$ and $q = 0.4$. To verify this, note that

p must equal 0.6 (i.e., $p = 1 - 0.4$). Thus, the homozygous-dominant population accounted for 36% ($p^2 = 0.6 \times 0.6$) or 360 students, and the heterozygous population accounted for 48% ($2pq = 2 \times 0.6 \times 0.4$) or 480 students. Indeed, there were 840 (360 + 480) brown-eyed students in the 2006 population.

Problem

Analysis of the protein insulin shows that the only difference between porcine and human insulin is one amino acid. The scientific discipline that would make these evolutionary conclusions is

A. comparative anatomy. B. the fossil record. C. ^{14}C dating. D. molecular biology.

Solution

D.

Problem

Gene flow is a factor that brings about evolutionary change resulting from

A. natural selection. B. migration. C. chance events. D. point mutations.

Solution

B.

Problem

An equation that correctly describes a Hardy–Weinberg equilibrium is

A. $p^2 + q^2 = 1$.
B. $2p + 2pq + 2q = 1$.
C. $p^2 + 2pq^2 + q^1 = 1$.
D. $p^2 + 2pq + q^2 = 1$.

Solution

D.

Problem

If the dominant allele p has a frequency of 0.2, what is the percentage of heterozygous individuals in a population under a Hardy–Weinberg equilibrium?

A. 16% B. 4% C. 64% D. 32%

Solution

D.

3. GENETIC RESEARCH

In 1870, scientists discovered that the cell nucleus was responsible for the inherited characteristics of an individual. A later discovery revealed that threadlike materials, known as chromosomes, are contained in the nucleus. By 1900, studies showed that the number of chromosomes is constant within each species but differs from species to species. In 1920, scientists confirmed that chromosomes contain deoxyribonucleic acid (DNA). Twelve years later, an experiment involving the genetic transformation of one cell into another showed that DNA is indeed genetic material.

A. Gene Cloning

Genetics has played a critical role in the development of techniques for the creation of new organisms. The traditional methods of genetic manipulation are mutation and recombination. These processes are basically random and are required to identify the organisms with the most desirable characteristics among the other types of organisms produced.

More currently in use now is the technique known as recombinant DNA, genetic engineering, or gene cloning. Recombinant DNA procedures, however, complement earlier techniques by supplying new types of genetic variation for improvement of organisms. This technique allows for modifying the genotype of an organism in a predetermined manner. By isolating two DNA molecules and cutting them into fragments using specialized enzymes, it is possible to join these fragments in any desired combination and introduce them back into a live organism for replication and reproduction. A process for selecting the desired genotype is still necessary, but the probability of success is much higher than in earlier methods.

Gene cloning is especially important because it has many practical uses:

- Isolation of a particular gene or region of a genome
- Production of protein molecules or RNA in amounts not obtainable in the past
- Increased efficiency in the production of biochemicals such as drugs and organic chemicals with commercial use
- Creation of organisms with desirable qualities, such as animals with increased resistance to disease
- The potential correction of genetic defects in humans

An example of gene cloning is the creation in 1996 of Dolly the sheep, which was the first mammal to develop from a cell derived from adult tissue. In this particular example, a live offspring developed from a differentiated cell after nuclear transfer from an embryo-derived cell line that had been induced to become quiescent. The new population of cells was derived from an embryo, a fetus, and the mammary gland of a ewe. Nuclear transfer was carried out, and reconstructed embryos were transferred into recipient ewes. Examination of the embryos' genetic material revealed that all three cell populations were represented. The birth of Dolly, a live mammal, is consistent with the view that mammalian cell differentiation is achieved by systemic, sequential changes in the gene expression caused by interactions between the nucleus and the changing cytoplasmic environment.

B. Genetic Screening of Human Diseases

A probe, which is a radioactive DNA or RNA molecule used in DNA–RNA or DNA–DNA hybridization assays, is commonly used in prenatal detection of diseases such as cystic fibrosis, Huntington disease, or sickle cell anemia. Probes derived from the gene itself or from molecular markers genetically linked to the disease genes are utilized. If the disease gene or a region close to it in the chromosome is dissimilar from the normal chromosome in the position of one or more cleavage sites for restriction enzymes, the differences can be detected with Southern blot by using cloned DNA from the region of the probe. The genotype of the fetus can be determined directly. These techniques have a high sensitivity and can be carried out when tissue from the fetus or embryonic membrane are obtained.

MCAT

MEDICAL COLLEGE ADMISSION TEST

Chemistry Review

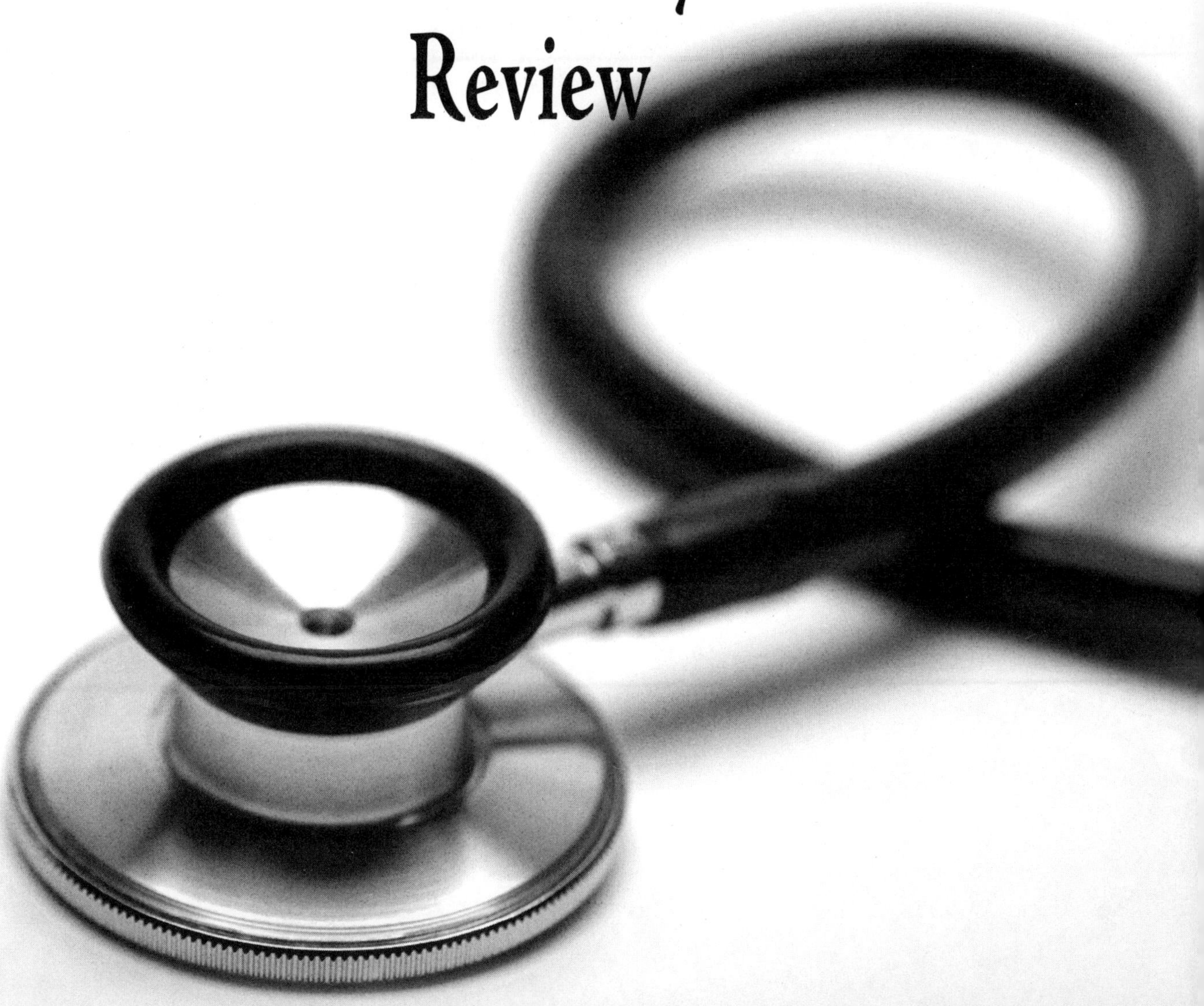

I. STOICHIOMETRY

1. MATTER

Chemistry is the study of matter. Matter can be divided into two classes: pure substances and mixtures. A mixture is a combination of two or more pure substances. Pure substances are entities that cannot be further purified. They consist of elements and compounds. Substances that contain only one kind of atom are called elements. A substance that has at least two different elements in a fixed ratio is called a compound.

2. STATES OF MATTER

There are three states of matter: solids, liquids, and gases. Gases have no definite shape or volume and they are highly compressible. Liquids also have no definite shape but possess definite volume. Solids have both definite shape and volume.

3. ATOMS

Atoms consist of subatomic particles. These particles are electrons, neutrons, and protons. Electrons have a negative and nearly negligible mass. A proton has a positive charge and a mass of 1.0073 atomic mass units (amu). A neutron has no charge and a mass of 1.0087 amu, similar to that of a proton. The nucleus of an atom consists of protons and neutrons and is surrounded by a cloud of electrons.

4. ATOMIC NUMBER

All atoms of the same element have the same number of protons. The number of protons is the distinguishing feature among the elements. In the periodic table, each element is displayed by its atomic number (Z), which equals the number of protons in the atomic nucleus. A periodic table will be available on the MCAT, and one appears in the appendix of this book. The atomic number is the integer at the top of the box for each element. For example, the atomic number for carbon is 6. Because the elements are electrically neutral, the atomic number also indicates the number of electrons in the element. These electrons will be used to form chemical bonds between the elements in compounds.

The mass number or atomic weight is equal to the number of protons and neutrons in an element. Isotopes are elements that have a different number of neutrons. For a given element, the number of protons always remains the same. For the isotope ^{14}C, the isotope has six protons and eight neutrons. The most common isotope, ^{12}C, has six protons and six neutrons.

5. ATOMIC WEIGHT

Atomic weights (or more properly, atomic masses) are given in atomic mass units, although biochemists use the dalton instead of the amu. The atomic weight is the average mass of a representative sample of atoms. For example, the atomic weight of iodine is 127, so one mole of iodine atoms will have a mass of 127 grams. The atomic weight of cobalt is 59; therefore, 59 grams of cobalt will compose one mole of cobalt atoms.

Sometimes different atoms of the same element can have different atomic weights; these are known as isotopes. For example, thallium exists in nature as two isotopes, of atomic weights 205 and 203. The atomic weight listed on the periodic table takes these differences into consideration and is an average, based on both the atomic weights of the element found in nature and on their natural abundance. For example, in nature, lead consists of the following four isotopes in the following natural abundances:

Isotope	Abundance
Pb-204	1.42%
Pb-206	24.1%
Pb-207	22.1%
Pb-208	52.4%

Using this data, we can calculate the average atomic weight of lead as

$$(0.0142)(204) + (0.241)(206) + (0.221)(207) + (0.524)(208) = 207.2.$$

That value, 207.2, is the one reported in the periodic table.

One mole of a substance contains exactly the same number of entities (atoms, molecules, or particles) as there are atoms in exactly 12 g of the isotope carbon-12. There are 6.02×10^{23} particles in one mole. This value is known as Avogadro's number.

6. MOLECULAR WEIGHT

The molecular weight of a compound is determined by simply adding up the atomic weights of all of the atoms present. Oxygen gas has the formula O_2; therefore, the molecular weight of one oxygen molecule is 32 (2×16). Molecular weights are usually given in daltons or amu, so oxygen gas has a molecular weight of 32 daltons or 32 amu. The molecular weight of water, H_2O, where H = 1 amu and O = 16 amu, is

$$(2 \times 1) + (1 \times 16) = 18 \text{ daltons.}$$

As a table showing atomic weights (sometimes called atomic masses), the periodic table is an important tool in calculating molecular weights. For instance, to find the molecular weight of copper (II) sulfate, we know that the formula is $CuSO_4$, and looking up the proper atomic weights, we get

$$(1 \times 63.5) + (1 \times 32) + (4 \times 16) = 159.5 \text{ amu}$$

Chemists weigh substances in grams rather than in amu or atoms. Therefore, it is necessary to convert the amu to grams per mole (g/mole). The molar mass is the mass in grams of 1 mole of a substance. The mass of 1 mole of calcium is 40.078 because the atomic weight of calcium is 40.078. One mole of $CuSO_4$ would weigh 159.5 grams.

Problem

A. What is the molecular weight of nitrogen gas, N_2?

B. What is the molecular weight of cobalt chloride, $CoCl_2$?

C. What is the molecular weight of benzene, C_6H_6?

Solution

A. $2 \times 14 = 28$ g/mole

B. $(58.9 \times 1) + (35.5 \times 2) = 129.9$ g/mole

C. $(12.0 \times 6) + (1 \times 6) = 78$ g/mole

For salts such as cobalt chloride and copper sulfate, the term *formula weight* is used because salts do not exist in molecular form. Do not let this term confuse you; for the purposes of the MCAT, the terms *formula weight* and *molecular weight* can be used interchangeably.

7. EMPIRICAL FORMULAS VS. MOLECULAR FORMULAS

The empirical formula is the simplest ratio of atoms present in a compound. The molecular formula shows the actual number of atoms present. From a molecular formula, a molecular weight can be determined; given an empirical formula and a molecular weight, a molecular formula can be determined. Sometimes the empirical formula and molecular formula for a compound are the same. Water has an empirical formula of H_2O (the simplest ratio) and a molecular formula of H_2O (the actual numbers present). Hydrogen peroxide has an empirical formula of HO and a molecular formula of H_2O_2.

Consider this sample calculation. If benzene has an empirical formula of CH and a molecular weight of 78, what is its molecular formula? (The atomic weight of C is 12, and the atomic weight of H is 1.)

$$12 + 1 = 13 = \text{weight of the empirical formula}$$

$$\frac{78}{13} = \frac{\text{molecular weight}}{\text{weight of the empirical formula}} = 6$$

Multiply all of the subscripts in the empirical formula by 6. The answer is C_6H_6.

Problem

A. Acetylene has an empirical formula of CH and a molecular weight of 26. What is its molecular formula?

B. Vitamin C has an empirical formula of $C_3H_4O_3$ and a molecular weight of 176 daltons. What is its molecular formula?

Solution

A. $12 + 1 = 13;\ \frac{26}{13} = 2;\ 2 \times CH = C_2H_2$ = acetylene

B. $(12 \times 3) + (1 \times 4) + (3 \times 16) = 88;\ \frac{176}{88} = 2;\ 2 \times C_3H_4O_3 = C_6H_8O_6$ = vitamin C

8. METRIC UNITS

Tables 1 and 2 list the metric units relevant to the MCAT.

TABLE 1. SI Prefixes

Fraction	Prefix	Symbol	Multiple	Prefix	Symbol
10^{-1}	deci	d	10	deka	da
10^{-2}	centi	c	10^{2}	hecto	h
10^{-3}	milli	m	10^{3}	kilo	k
10^{-6}	micro	m	10^{6}	mega	M
10^{-9}	nano	n	10^{9}	giga	G
10^{-12}	pico	p	10^{12}	tera	T
10^{-15}	femto	f			

TABLE 2. Units and Conversion Factors

Quantity	SI Unit	Symbol	Conversion Factors
Length	Meter	m	1 cm = 10^{-2} m
			1 nm = 10^{-9} m
			1 A˚ = 10^{-10} m
			1 inch = 2.54×10^{-2} m
Mass	Kilogram	kg	1 g = 10^{-3} kg
			1 mg = 10^{-6} kg
			1 lb = 0.454 kg
Time	Second	s	1 day = 8.6×10^{4} s
Temperature	Kelvin	K	0˚C = 273.15 K
Volume	Cubic meter	m^3	IL = 10^{-3} m^3
			= 1,000 cm^3
			1 mL = 1 cm^3

Problem

A. How many meters in 5.2 kilometers? How many centimeters? How many millimeters?

B. What is the mass in kilograms of 75.8 cubic centimeters of pure water at 4°C? (1 g H_2O = 1 cm^3 at 4°C.)

Solution

A. 5,200 meters, 520,000 centimeters, 5,200,000 millimeters
B. 0.0758 kilograms

9. DESCRIPTION OF COMPOSITION BY PERCENT MASS

If a substance consists of 4 grams of material A, 16 grams of material B, and 80 grams of material C, its percent composition by mass is easy to determine. It can readily be seen that the composition by mass is

4% A, 16% B, and 80% C.

Typically, we do not have the luxury of all the masses summing to 100. In such instances, we must divide the mass of each component by the sum of the masses of all components, and multiply that quotient by 100 to obtain the percent mass. For example, if analysis of a sample of baking soda showed it to consist of 35.0 grams of sodium, 1.5 grams of hydrogen, 18.3 grams of carbon, and 73.1 grams of oxygen, what is the percent composition of this baking soda? First, the mass of all of the components must be summed:

$35.0 + 1.5 + 18.3 + 73.1 = 127.9$ g of sample

To find the percentage of each component, simply divide the mass of each component by the total mass and multiply by 100:

% of sodium $= (35.0/127.9) \times 100 = 27.4\%$
% of hydrogen $= (1.5/127.9) \times 100 = 1.2\%$
% of carbon $= (18.3/127.9) \times 100 = 14.3\%$
% of oxygen $= (73.1/127.9) \times 100 = 57.1\%$

Problem

A. On analysis, a sample of calcium chloride was shown to consist of 93.0 grams of calcium and 165 grams of chlorine. What is its percent composition?
B. A sample of penicillin contained 8.62 grams of carbon, 0.808 grams of hydrogen, 2.87 grams of oxygen, 1.26 grams of nitrogen, and 1.44 grams of sulfur. What is its percent composition?

Solution

A. $93.0 + 165 = 258$ g

$$\% \text{ of Ca} = \frac{93}{258} = 36.0\%$$

$$\% \text{ of Cl} = \frac{165}{258} = 64.0\%$$

B. 57.5% carbon, 5.39% hydrogen, 19.1% oxygen, 8.40% nitrogen, 9.60% sulfur

10. MOLE CONCEPT AND AVOGADRO'S NUMBER

A mole specifies a definite quantity. Just as a dozen of anything is 12 and a gross is 144, a mole is 6.02×10^{23}. This is such a large number that usually it is used in chemistry only when large numbers of atoms and molecules are encountered. One mole of benzene would contain 6.02×10^{23} molecules of benzene. How many molecules would there be in 0.001 mole of benzene? Simple multiplication reveals the answer to be

$0.001 \times 6.02 \times 10^{23} = 6.02 \times 10^{20}$ molecules of benzene.

If there are 7.525×10^{22} atoms of neon present, how many moles are there? Knowing that there are *always* 6.02×10^{23} in a mole, the calculation is

$(7.525 \times 10^{22})/(6.02 \times 10^{23}) = 0.125$ mole, or 1/8 mole of neon.

The number 6.02×10^{23} is known as Avogadro's number. Using this definition, we can see that, if we measure out the atomic or molecular weight of a substance in grams, we will have 1 mole of atoms or molecules. For example, 1 mole of helium (atomic weight = 4) has a mass of 4 grams; half a mole, 2 grams; 10 moles, 40 grams; and so on. How many molecules (or formula units) of indium chloride are there in 1,105.0 grams of $InCl_3$ (molecular weight = 221.0 daltons)?

1,105.0/221.0 = 5.000 moles, $5.000 \times 6.02 \times 10^{23} = 3.01 \times 10^{24}$ molecules (or formula units) of $InCl_3$.

What would be the mass of 1.30×10^{22} molecules of carbon dioxide (molecular weight = 44)? First, we must find the number of moles:

$1.30 \times 10^{22}/6.02 \times 10^{23} = 0.0216$ mole of CO_2

This is multiplied by the molecular weight to find the mass:

$0.0216 \times 44 = 0.950$ g of CO_2

Problem

A. If you have 6.02×10^{23} toothpicks, how many moles of toothpicks do you have?

B. How many molecules are present in 0.002 mole of naphthalene?

C. What is the mass of 25 moles of xenon (atomic weight = 131.3)?

D. Determine the mass of 7.88×10^{25} atoms of iron (atomic weight = 55.8).

E. How much mass and how many molecules are in 3.45 moles of water (molecular weight = 18)?

Solution

A. 1 mole of toothpicks

B. $0.002 \text{ mole}\left(\frac{6.02 \times 10^{23} \text{ molecules}}{\text{mole}}\right) = 1.20 \times 10^{21}$ molecules of naphthalene

C. $25 \text{ moles}\left(\frac{131.29 \text{ grams}}{\text{mole}}\right) = 3282$ grams of xenon

D. $7.88\ \ 10^{25} \text{ atoms} \ \frac{1 \text{ mole}}{6.02\ \ 10^{23} \text{ atoms}}\left(\frac{55.85 \text{ grams}}{1 \text{ mole}}\right) = 7304$ grams of iron

E. $3.45 \text{ moles}\left(\frac{18.01 \text{ grams}}{\text{moles}}\right) = 62.1$ grams and $3.45 \text{ moles}\left(\frac{6.02 \times 10^{23} \text{ molecules}}{\text{mole}}\right) = 2.08 \times 10^{24}$ molecules of water

11. DEFINITION OF DENSITY

Density is the mass of a substance divided by its volume. For example, 34.8 mL of isobutyl iodide has a mass of 56.1 grams. What is its density? Simple division tells us the answer is

56.1/34.8 = 1.61 g/mL.

Sometimes the volume needs to be calculated. For example, if a rectangular block of pure cobalt metal measures 5.23 cm long, 10.3 cm high, and 2.01 cm wide and has a mass of 944 grams, what is the density of cobalt? First, to find the volume of a rectangular solid, we use the formula $V = l \cdot w \cdot h$:

$V = 5.23 \times 2.01 \times 10.3 = 108\ \text{cm}^3$

With a volume calculated, we proceed as before:

$944/108 = 8.72\ \text{g/cm}^3$

Sometimes, given the density, we can work backward to calculate dimensions. What is the radius of a sphere of sulfur with a mass of 26.4 grams? The density of sulfur is 2.05 g/cm^3. We find the volume as follows:

$26.4/2.05 = 12.9\ \text{cm}^3$

To determine the radius of this sphere, recall that the volume of a sphere is $4/3\pi r^3$. Solving for the radius gives a value of 1.45 cm.

Problem

A. A rectangular block of pure camphor ($C_{10}H_{15}BrO$) measures 10.0 cm in width, 50.0 cm in length, and 2.00 m in height. It contains 3.74×10^{26} molecules of camphor. What is the density of camphor?

B. How many moles of hydrogen are in 20.0 grams of $C_{17}H_{21}O_4N$? What is the weight percent of hydrogen?

C. If analysis of pyrene shows it to be composed of 95.0% carbon and 5.00% hydrogen, what is its empirical formula? If the molecular weight is found to be 202 g/mole, what is its molecular formula?

Solution

A. Calculate the volume of the box (remember, 2.00 m = 200 cm):

$200\ \text{cm} \times 50\ \text{cm} \times 10\ \text{cm} = 100{,}000\ \text{cm}^3$

Calculate the number of moles of camphor:

$3.74 \times 10^{26}/6.02 \times 10^{23} = 6.21 \times 10^2$ moles

Calculate the molecular weight of camphor:

$(10 \times 12) + (15 \times 1) + (1 \times 79.9) + (1 \times 16) = 231$ g/mole

Calculate the mass of camphor:

621 moles $\times$ 231 g/mole = 1.43×10^5 g

Calculate the density of camphor:

$1.43 \times 10^5\ \text{g}/10^5\ \text{cm}^3 = 1.43\ \text{g/cm}^3$

B. Calculate the molecular weight;

$(17 \times 12) + (21 \times 1) + (4 \times 16) + (1 \times 14) = 303$ g/mole

Calculate the number of moles in 20 grams:

$20/303 = 0.0660$ mole

Note from the formula that every mole has 21 moles of hydrogen in it:

$21 \times 0.0660 = 1.38$ moles of hydrogen

This solves the first part. The second part can be solved in two ways.

Calculate the mass of hydrogen:

$1.38 \times 1 = 1.38$ g of hydrogen

Find the weight percent hydrogen:

$(1.38/20) \times 100 = 6.93\%$ hydrogen

OR

Calculate the weight of hydrogen in 1 mole:

$1 \times 21 = 21$

Divide this into the weight of 1 mole:

$21/303 = 0.0693 = 6.93\%$

C. Assume you have 100 grams of pyrene, in which case there will be 95.0 grams of carbon and 5.00 grams of hydrogen. (Any mass will work, but obviously, when dealing with percentages, 100 is the easiest.)

Calculate the number of moles of each:

$95/12 = 7.92$ moles of carbon, $5/1 = 5$ moles of hydrogen

Divide the smallest number of moles into all the moles present, including itself:

$7.92/5 = 1.58, 5/5 = 1$

This gives a ratio of 1.58:1 (C:H).

Multiply the ratio by a common factor to eliminate decimals:

$5 \times (1.58{:}1) = 7.9{:}5$

This can be rounded off to 8:5, which means the empirical formula is C_8H_5. The weight of the empirical formula is calculated:

$(8 \times 12) + (5 \times 1) = 101$

Divide this value into the molecular weight:

$202/101 = 2$

Multiply the subscripts in the empirical formula by the value obtained in the previous step:

$2 \times (C_8H_5) = C_{16}H_{10}$,

which is the molecular formula.

12. OXIDATION NUMBER

An atom that loses electrons has undergone oxidation. The opposite process is reduction. To show the oxidation state of a particular element in a compound or reaction, chemists have invented oxidation numbers. For example, the oxidation number for aluminum in the metallic state is 0, and the salt state of aluminum, aluminum chloride, has an oxidation number of +3. There are a few simple rules for assigning oxidation numbers. (Remember, although these numbers are useful, they do not really exist in the molecules; they are artificial aids to help understand certain chemical reactions.)

Rule 1: The oxidation number of any element uncombined, or combined with itself, is always zero. For example, the oxidation numbers for He, Ne, Ar, Xe, and Rn are all 0. O_2, O_3, N_2, Gl_2, and Br_2, all have oxidation numbers of 0. Cu, Fe, Au, and Pg also have have oxidation numbers of 0. Sometimes metals are written with zero superscripts to their right to show that they are uncombined (with oxidation numbers of 0), as in Fe^0, Ag^0, and V^0.

Rule 2: The oxidation number of an ion equals the charge of an ion. For example, the oxidation number of Fe^{++} is +2 and that of Fe^{+++} is +3. The oxidation number of Cl^- is −1 and of $S^=$ is −2.

Rule 3: In all compounds, the sum of the oxidation is zero. Elements at the edges of the periodic table always have the same oxidation number in the combined state. For example, the oxidation number of lithium is always +1 and of fluorine, always −1.

Moving into the periodic table, the numbers begin to vary. Oxygen is usually −2, but it can be −1 (as it is for peroxides). Deep in the interior of the table, oxidation numbers can vary greatly and can be determined only by deduction, using the known oxidation numbers of the atoms in the compound with them. The following examples should clarify this information.

In the compound NaCl, the periodic table shows that Na will form a +1 ion and Cl a −1 ion; thus, those are the oxidation numbers for those respective atoms in the compound. It can be written as Na+1 Cl−1. Note that the sum is zero: $(+1) + (-1) = 0$. Likewise, in the compound K_2S, K forms a +1 ion and S usually forms a −2 ion. Because the compound has two K's, the total charge is +2, and again the sum of the oxidation numbers is zero: $2 \times (+1) + (-2) = 0$. This can be written $K_2S^{+1\ -2}$. For the compound PbS_2, Pb is so far into the interior of the periodic table that its oxidation number is not readily apparent. S is usually a −2, and because there are two of them, that gives us a total charge of $2 \times (-2)$, or −4. Because the sum of all of the oxidation numbers in a compound must be zero, Pb must have an oxidation number of +4 in this compound, and it would be written $PbS^{+4\ -2}$.

As a final example, consider the compound Fe_2S_3. S is usually −2, and because three of them are present, $3 \times (-2) = -6$. If the total charge on the sulfur is −6, and the sum of the oxidation numbers must equal zero for a compound, then the total charge on the iron must be +6. The total charge must be divided by the total number of iron atoms present—$(+6)/2 = (+3)$—to obtain an oxidation number of +3 for iron in this compound.

Rule 4: The sum of oxidation numbers in a polyatomic ion equals the charge of the ion. For example, in $NH^+{}_4$, hydrogen has a charge of +1, and because there are four of them, $4 \times (+1) = (+4)$. Because the total charge of the ion equals +1, the oxidation number for nitrogen in this compound is $(+1) - (+4) = (-3)$. The oxidation number of nitrogen in NO_3- will have a different value. Oxygen is usually −2, and because the compound has three of them, the total charge is $3 \times (-2) = (-6)$. Because the sum of the oxidation numbers must equal the charge of the ion, the oxidation number for nitrogen in this case is $(-1) - (-6) = (-1) + 6 = +5$.

Problem

What are the oxidation numbers of the atoms in the following compounds?

A. S_8	B. H_2O	C. MnO_2	D. Fe^{++}
E. CrO	F. Sn	G. ClO^-_4	H. $Mn_2(SO_4)_3$

Solution

A. 0	B. +1, −2	C. +4, −2	D. +2
E. +2, −2	F. 0	G. +7, −2	H. +3, +6, −2

Commonly used oxidizing agents include potassium permanganate ($KMnO_4$), potassium dichromate ($K_2Cr_2O_7$), and cerium (IV) bisulfate [$Ce(HSO_4)_4$]. Common reducing agents include tin (II) chloride ($SnCl_2$) and sodium thiosulfate ($Na_2S_2O_3$). Oxidation and reduction are collectively termed redox. A redox titration is one in which the amount of oxidizing and reducing agents are brought to an equal concentration. An example is copper (II) ions reacting with metallic iron:

$$Cu^{++} + Fe^{\circ} \rightarrow Cu^{\circ} + Fe^{++}$$

Titrations are covered in greater detail later in this review.

13. NOMENCLATURE OF INORGANIC COMPOUNDS

Ionic compounds consist of ions. An ion is an atom or group of atoms that contains a positive or negative charge. When an element loses an electron, a cation is formed, as shown in this example:

Na	→	$Na^+ + e^-$
11 protons		11 protons
11 electrons		10 electrons

If an atom gains an electron, an anion is formed, as show here:

O atom + $2e^-$	→	O^{2-} anion
8 protons		8 protons
8 electrons		10 electrons

The number of electrons that an element loses or gains depends on the row that they appear on in the periodic table. Groups 1A, 2A, and 3A form ions of +1, +2, +3, respectively. The number of electrons that remain have the same number of electrons as an atom of a noble gas. When a 7A element gains an electron, it has the same number of electrons as a noble gas. Noble gases are found in row 8A and are called noble gases because they are nonreactive substances.

Some atoms, called polyatomic ions, are always found in certain ratios and they have special names. The list of these ions and their charges is NH_4^+(ammonium ion), CN^- (cyanide), $CH_3CO_2^-$(acetate), CO_3^{2-} (carbonate) HCO_3^- (hydrogen carbonate or bicarbonate), ClO^- (hypochlorite), ClO_2^- (chlorite), ClO_3^- (chlorate), ClO_4^- (perchlorate), NO_2^- (nitrite), NO_3^- (nitrate), PO_4^{3-} (phosphate), HPO_4^{2-} (hydrogen phosphate), $H_2PO_4^-$ (dihydrogen phosphate), OH^- (hydroxide), SO_3^{2-} (sulfite), SO_4^{2-} (sulfate), HSO_4^- (hydrogen sulfate or bisulfate), CrO_4^{2-} (chromate), $Cr_2O_7^{2-}$ (dichromate), MnO_4^-(permanganate).

Inorganic compounds are named by the cation and the anion. The positively charged cation is named first, followed by the negatively charged ion. For transition metals, the oxidation state is identified by

Roman numerals. For example, Co^{2+} is the cobalt (II) ion, and Zn^{2+} is the zinc ion. A monoatomic negative ion is named by adding the suffix *-ide* to the stem of the element. For example, Cl^- becomes the chloride ion and O^{2-} becomes the oxide ion.

Problem

Provide names for the following compounds.

A. Na_2O B. $MgCl_2$ C. $CoBr_3$ D. NH_4I E. $Ca(NO_3)_2$ F. $Zn(OH)_2$

Solution

A. Sodium oxide
B. Magnesium chloride
C. Cobalt (III) bromide
D. Ammonium iodide
E. Calcium nitrate
F. Zinc hydroxide

14. DESCRIPTION OF REACTIONS BY CHEMICAL EQUATIONS

Chemical equations are written much like mathematical equations. An arrow replaces the equal sign. To the left of the arrow are the reactants, or starting materials, and to the right are the products, or final materials. The number of atoms shown on the left side of the arrow must equal the number of atoms shown on the right side. For example, to write "hydrogen and oxygen can combine to form water," the chemical equation would start with

$$H_2 + O_2 \rightarrow H_2O.$$

This shows that hydrogen and oxygen are reactants, and water is the product. However, closer inspection shows two atoms of oxygen on the left of the arrow and only one on the right. Because an atom of oxygen simply cannot disappear from the universe, something is wrong. Placing a coefficient of 2 before the H_2O would give two atoms of oxygen on the right side of the arrow, but then four hydrogen atoms would result on the right of the equation, and only two on the left. This can be remedied by placing a 2 before the hydrogen on the left side. At this point the number of atoms on both sides of the arrow are equal. Such an equation is said to be balanced. A balanced equation has an advantage over the English statement in that it shows the ratios in which the atoms (or moles of atoms) combine and form products. Thus, the balanced equation for this example is

$$2H_2 + O_2 \rightarrow 2H_2O.$$

This chemical equation shows that two moles of hydrogen combined with one mole of oxygen produce two moles of water. This will always be the ratio. Four moles of hydrogen will react with two moles of oxygen to produce four moles of water, and so on.

When working with grams of material, you must first convert to moles to use the ratios in the chemical equation. For example, $2 \times 2 = 4$ grams of hydrogen and $1 \times 32 = 32$ grams of oxygen react to form $2 \times 18 = 36$ grams of water. Notice that mass is still conserved when working in grams rather than moles. Consider the reaction of zinc carbonate with perchloric acid:

$$ZnCO_3 + HClO_4 \rightarrow Zn\,(ClO_4)_2 + H_2O + CO_2$$

It is immediately evident that only one atom of Cl is on the left side of the equation, and two are on the right. Further inspection indicates that the ClO_4 reacts as a group. Thus, putting a coefficient of 2 in front of the perchloric acid gives

$$ZnCO_3 + 2HClO_4 \rightarrow Zn(ClO_4)_2 + H_2O + CO_2,$$

which balances the equation and establishes the molar ratios for the reaction.

If we have 2.00 kilograms of $ZnCO_3$ and 100 grams of $HClO_4$, how many grams of $Zn(ClO_4)_2$ can we make? First, we must calculate the molecular weight and the number of moles present:

Molecular weight for $ZnCO_3$: $(1 \times 65.37) + (1 \times 12) + (3 \times 16) = 125.4$ g/mole

Molecular weight for $HClO_4$: $(1 \times 1) + (1 \times 35.4) + (4 \times 16) = 100.4$ g/mole

Molecular weight for $Zn(ClO_4)_2$: $(1 \times 65.37) + (2 \times 35.4) + (8 \times 16) = 264.2$ g/mole

Number of moles of $ZnCO_3$: (2.00 kg = 2,000 g); 2,000/125.4 = 15.95

Number of moles of $HClO_4$: 100/100.4 = 1.00

By looking at the molar ratios, it can be seen that for every mole of $ZnCO_3$ consumed, two moles of $HClO_4$ are needed and one mole of $Zn(ClO_4)_2$ are produced. In this instance, the $HClO_4$ is the limiting reagent because it will be used up, and the other reactant still has some material left over. Consuming the entire 1.00 mole of $HClO_4$ requires 0.500 mole of the $ZnCO_3$ (using the ratio established in the equation), leaving the remaining 15.45 moles unreacted. By the same ratio, it can be seen that 0.500 mole of $Zn(ClO_4)_2$ are produced. Converting this into grams gives $0.500 \times 264.2 = 132.1$ grams of $Zn(ClO_4)_2$ produced.

All the equations written here so far show all the atoms involved and are therefore called gross molecular equations. Some species exist in ionic form in aqueous solutions (e.g., in water). Consider this gross molecular equation:

$$Na_2CO_3 + CaCl_2 \rightarrow 2NaCl + CaCO_3$$

The only species that exists in molecular form is the $CaCO_3$ because it is insoluble. The rest are present as ions. A gross ionic equation shows this as follows:

$$2Na^+ + CO_3^= + Ca^{++} + 2Cl^- \rightarrow 2Na^+ + 2Cl^- + CaCO_3$$

Because the sodium and chloride ions do not get involved in the reaction, they are called spectator ions. They are unchanged from one side of the arrow to the other, so they can be eliminated. Such an equation is termed net ionic and would be written as follows:

$$Ca^{++} + CO_3^= \rightarrow CaCO_3$$

The following subsections describe common types of reactions and methods to balance the equations for them.

A. Direct Combination Reactions of Elements

This can be the easiest of the reaction types. Keep in mind the types of ions that the atoms in question prefer to form and deduce the formula for the product from that. For example, the reaction of zinc with sulfur can be written as

$$Zn^\circ + S \rightarrow ?.$$

The periodic table shows that Zn tends to form + 2 ions and S forms −2 ions. Thus, the resulting neutral compound is zinc sulfide, ZnS, and the reaction is written

$Zn^{\circ} + S \rightarrow ZnS$.

Notice that this equation is already balanced.

The reaction of potassium with bromine is stated as $K + Br_2 \rightarrow$? Because K and Br both form ions with a charge of 1 and are opposite in signs, the formula for potassium bromide can be deduced as KBr. The equation is written as

$K + Br_2 \rightarrow KBr$.

However, twice as many Br's are on the left side of the equation as on the right. Placing a 2 in front of the product gives the proper number of Br's but also doubles the number of K's on that side. Placing a 2 in front of the K on the left side balances the equation. The final equation is

$2K + Br_2 \rightarrow 2KBr$.

For a final example, consider the combination of aluminum and oxygen. The combination starts with

$Al^{\circ} + 0_2 \rightarrow$?.

Because Al forms +3 ions and oxygen forms −2 ions, the formula for aluminum oxide is Al_2O_3, which gives

$Al^{\circ} + O_2 \rightarrow Al_2O_3$.

In this case, the oxygen on the right-hand side can be multiplied by a fraction ($1^1/_2$) to get it to equal the value on the right side. It can be easily seen that a 2 in front of the Al on the left side puts things in balance:

$2Al^{\circ} + 1^1/_2O_2 \rightarrow Al_2O_3$

However, fractions are not generally tolerated in chemical equations. Multiplying through by 2 clears the fraction and gives

$4Al^{\circ} + 3O_2 \rightarrow 2Al_2O_3$.

Problem

Write a balanced reaction for the direct combination of the following.

A. Barium and oxygen
B. Lithium and oxygen
C. Aluminum and sulfur

Solution

A. $2Ba + O_2 \rightarrow 2BaO$, barium oxide
B. $4Li + O_2 \rightarrow 2Li_2O$, lithium oxide
C. $2Al + 3S \rightarrow Al_2S_3$, aluminum sulfide

B. Combustion Reactions

In a combustion reaction, an organic (carbon-containing) compound combines with oxygen (usually unlimited) to ultimately form carbon dioxide and water. Balancing is done as before. For example, the complete combustion of octane (C_8H_{18}, a major component in gasoline) would start with

$C_8H_{18} + O_2 \rightarrow CO_2 + H_2O$.

The 8 carbons and 18 hydrogens are easy to account for on the right side:

$$C_8H_{18} + O_2 \rightarrow 8CO_2 + 9H_2O$$

This leaves 25 oxygens to be accounted for on the left side; correcting for this gives

$$C_8H_{18} + 12^1/_2O_2 \rightarrow 8CO_2 + 9H_2O.$$

Multiplying through by 2 to remove the fraction yields the final equation:

$$2C_8H_{18} + 25O_2 \rightarrow 16CO_2 + 18H_2O$$

For the complete combustion of acetone [(CH_3COCH_3)], the beginning would be the same as before:

$$CH_3COCH_3 + O_2 \rightarrow CO_2 + H_2O$$

Again, the number of carbons and hydrogens are set equal:

$$CH_3COCH_3 + O_2 \rightarrow 3CO_2 + 3H_2O$$

All that remains to be done is to balance the oxygen atoms (remember that one oxygen is in acetone), giving a final equation of

$$CH_3COCH_3 + 4O_2 \rightarrow 3CO_2 + 3H_2O.$$

Problem

Write a balanced equation for the complete combustion of the following.

A. Xylene [$C_6H_4(CH_3)_2$]
B. Ethanol (CH_3CH_2OH)

Solution

A. $2C_6H_4(CH_3)_2 + 21O_2 \rightarrow 16CO_2 + 10H_2O$
B. $CH_3CH_2OH + 3O_2 \rightarrow 2CO_2 + 3H_2O$

C. Neutralization Reactions

According to classical acid–base theory, an acid forms H^+ ions (or more properly, H_3O^+ ions) when dissolved in water, and a base yields OH^- ions when in water. When such an acid and base are mixed in equivalent quantities, a neutralization reaction occurs, and the products are water and a salt (i.e., the combination of a metal and nonmetal). The complete neutralization of sulfuric acid and sodium hydroxide would start with

$$H_2SO_4 + NaOH \rightarrow ?.$$

A look at the ions present shows

$$H^+, SO_4^=, Na^+, \text{and } OH^-.$$

Obviously the Na^+ and H^+ do not want to combine, nor do the $SO_4^=$ and OH^-. Because of the (-2) charge on the sulfate ion, two sodium ions are needed to electrically balance the charges, resulting in sodium sulfate, Na_2SO_4. The H^+ and the OH^- combine to form H_2O. The equation can now be written as

$$H_2SO_4 + NaOH \rightarrow H_2O + Na_2SO_4.$$

To start balancing the equation, two sodiums are needed on the left side:

$$H_2SO_4 + 2NaOH \rightarrow H_2O + Na_2SO_4$$

Balancing for the hydrogen and oxygen now gives the final equation:

$$H_2SO_4 + 2NaOH \rightarrow 2H_2O + Na_2SO_4$$

Consider the neutralization of nitric acid with magnesium hydroxide. Of course, the start is

$$HNO_3 + Mg(OH)_2 \rightarrow ?.$$

From this it is evident that the salt will be magnesium nitrate, $Mg(NO_3)_2$, and of course, water will still be formed. This gives

$$HNO_3 + Mg(OH)_2 \rightarrow H_2O + Mg(NO_3)_2.$$

To balance this equation, two nitrates are placed on the left side:

$$2HNO_3 + Mg(OH)_2 \rightarrow H_2O + Mg(NO_3)_2$$

Balancing the oxygen and hydrogen gives the final equation:

$$2HNO_3 + Mg(NO_3)_2 \rightarrow 2H_2O + Mg(NO_3)_2$$

Problem

Write a balanced equation for the following neutralization reactions.

A. Orthophosphoric acid and sodium hydroxide, $H_3PO_4 + NaOH$

B. Radium hydroxide and hydrochloric acid, $Ra(OH)_2 + HC1$

C. Hydrogen sulfide and silver hydroxide, $H_2S + AgOH$

Solution

A. $H_3PO_4 + 3NaOH \rightarrow Na_3PO_4 + 3H_2O$; the salt is sodium phosphate

B. $Ra(OH)_2 + 2HCl \rightarrow RaCl_2 + 2H_2O$; the salt is radium chloride

C. $H_2S + 2AgOH \rightarrow Ag_2S + 2H_2O$; the salt is silver sulfide

D. Oxidation and Reduction Reactions

Oxidation and reduction are known collectively as redox. In any chemical system, an oxidation cannot occur unless a reduction also occurs, and vice versa. Recall from a previous section that oxidation is loss of electrons, and gaining electrons is reduction. A reducing agent causes another atom to be reduced, and in the process, the reducing agent is oxidized. In a like manner, an oxidizing agent causes another atom to be oxidized, while the agent itself is reduced. There are two main methods used to balance redox equations. The first method is to use oxidation numbers, introduced earlier in this review. Oxidation numbers have been assigned to the reactants and products of the following unbalanced equations:

$$\overset{+1}{Na}\overset{-1}{Cl} + \overset{+4}{Mn}\overset{-2}{O_2} + \overset{+1}{H_2}\overset{+6}{S}\overset{-2}{O_4} \rightarrow \overset{0}{Cl_2} + \overset{+2}{Mn}\overset{+6}{S}\overset{-2}{O_4} + \overset{+1}{Na_2}\overset{+6}{S}\overset{-2}{O_4} + \overset{+1}{H_2}\overset{-2}{O}.$$

From these numbers, it can be seen that Mn changes from a +4 to a +2; that is, it has been reduced. Cl has changed from −1 to 0; that is, it has been oxidized. Short, partial equations can be written to show these changes:

$$\overset{+4}{Mn} \rightarrow \overset{+2}{Mn}, \text{and } \overset{-1}{Cl} \rightarrow \frac{1}{2}\overset{0}{Cl_2} \; (\text{ or } 2\overset{-1}{Cl^-} \rightarrow \overset{0}{Cl_2})$$

Thus, Mn changes by −2, and Cl by +1. A multiplier must be found for each change in oxidation number so that the two products will have the same absolute value. For example, if −2 (Mn) is multiplied by 1 and +1 (Cl) is multiplied by 2, the absolute value of both products is 2. Hence, the compound containing Mn has a 1 placed in front of it, and the compound containing Cl has a 2 in front of it, as follows:

$$2NaCl + (1)MnO_2 + H_2SO_4 \rightarrow Cl_2 + MnSO_4 + Na_2SO_4 + H_2O$$

(Note that the 1 before the MnO_2 is not really necessary.) This balances the Na, Cl, and Mn. Balancing now is done as for previous problems. Placing a 2 in front of the H_2SO_4 balances the sulfur but causes problems with hydrogen and oxygen. Placing a 2 in front of the H_2O alleviates the problem, resulting in the final equation:

$$2NaCl + MnO_2 + 2H_2SO_4 \rightarrow Cl_2 + MnSO_4 + Na_2SO_4 + 2H_2O$$

An alternative method is to solve this equation using half-reactions: one to describe the oxidation reaction, and the other to describe the reduction. These two reactions are then summed to get the correct balanced equation. First, a half-reaction is written for the oxidation of chlorine:

$$2Cl^- \rightarrow Cl_2 + 2e-$$

(Note that the fate of the electrons is not important.) Another half-reaction is written for the reduction of manganese. This presents a slight problem at first. On the left side is MnO_2, a precipitate in molecular form; on the right side is $MnSO_4$, which is ionic. The first step is to eliminate the spectator ions:

$$MnO_2 \rightarrow Mn^{2+}$$

Obviously, this is not the final form. The overall reaction shows that the oxygen ends up as water. This can be accomplished only by having it bond to the hydrogen ions from the acid. This leads to

$$MnO_2 + H^+ \rightarrow Mn^{2+} + H_2O.$$

Adding the two electrons that the Mn gains and balancing the elements gives

$$MnO_2 + 4H^+ + 2e^- \rightarrow Mn^{2+} + 2H_2O.$$

Notice that one equation involves the loss of two electrons, and the other a gain of two. Had they not dealt with the same number, a multiplier would have to have been found for each equation, so the number of electrons dealt with in each would be equal. The two equations are now added:

$$2Cl^- + MnO_2 + 4H^+ + 2e^- \rightarrow 2e^- + Cl_2 + Mn^{2+} + 2H_2O$$

The two electrons can be eliminated because they are on both sides of the arrow, and the spectator ions can be added to give the form

$$2NaCl + MnO_2 + 2H_2SO_4 \rightarrow Cl_2 + MnSO_4 + Na_2SO_4 + 2H_2O,$$

which is the same result as in the first method. For some equations, one method is easier than the other. Sometimes, redox equations will deal with ions. In such instances, in the final form, not only do the elements have to balance, but so do the charges (i.e., the net charge on the left must equal the net charge on the right). These equations can still be balanced by either of the two previously described methods. For example, the net ionic form of the previous equation is

$$2Cl^- + MnO_2 + 4H^+ \rightarrow Cl_2 + 2Na^+ + 2H_2O.$$

As was stated, the net charge of the left side is

$$[(-2) + (+4)] = +2,$$

which equals the net charge of the right side (+2).

For a final example, consider this equation:

$$Cr_2O_7^{2-} + H^+ + Fe^{2+} \rightarrow Cr^{3+} + Fe^{3+} + H_2O$$

The first step in solving this by oxidation numbers is

$$\overset{+6}{Cr_2}\,\overset{-2}{O_7} + \overset{+1}{H^+} + \overset{+2}{Fe^{++}} \rightarrow \overset{+3}{Cr^{+++}} + \overset{+3}{Fe^{+++}} + \overset{+1}{H_2}\overset{-2}{O}.$$

Chromium is reduced from a +6 to a +3 state, and iron is oxidized from a +2 to a +3 state. Multiplying the chromium equation by 1 and the iron equation by 3 gives a common change in oxidation number of 3 for both species. Putting these coefficients into the equation yields

(1) $Cr_2O_7^{2-} + H^+ + 3Fe^{2+} \rightarrow Cr^{3+} + 3Fe^{3+} + H_2O.$

Here a 2 is needed in front of the Cr on the right side. The 7 oxygens on the left side can be accounted for in the water on the right side, which then requires 14 hydrogen ions on the left side. The supposed final balanced equation is

$$Cr_2O_7^{2-} + 14H^+ + 3Fe^{2+} \rightarrow 2Cr^{3+} + 3Fe^{3+} + 7H_2O.$$

Note that the net charge on the left side,

$$[(-2) + (+14) + (3 \times (+2))] = +18,$$

should equal the net charge on the right,

$$[(2 \times (+3)) + (3 \times (+3))] = +15,$$

when an equation is properly balanced. This shows that an error was made here, because 15 and 18 are not equal. First the calculations are checked and found in order. What was overlooked? Closer inspection shows that two Cr atoms have a charge of −3 in their oxidation numbers, for a total change of −6. Multiplying the iron equation by this factor yields a new equation:

$$Cr_2O_7^{2-} + 14H^+ + 6Fe^{2+} \rightarrow 2Cr^{3+} + 6Fe^{3+} + 7H_2O$$

Checking the net charges again gives

$$[(-2) + (14 \times (+1)) + (6 \times (+1))] = +24$$

for the left side and

$$[(2 \times (+3)) + (6 \times (+3))] = +24$$

for the right side. It is now balanced.

The half-reaction method is as follows. The oxidation equation is easy to write:

$$Fe^{2+} \rightarrow Fe^{3+} + e^-$$

The reducing equation is a little more difficult. Starting with

$$Cr_2O_7^{2-} \rightarrow Cr^{3+}$$

reveals that two Cr's are needed on the right side. Two Cr's will yield a total of six e^-'s (the change in oxidation number is 3, and $2 \times 3 = 6$). The 7 oxygens present can react with hydrogen to give water, which would require 14 hydrogen ions on the left. This gives

$$Cr_2O_7^{2-} + 14H^+ + 6e^- \rightarrow 2Cr^{3+} + 7H_2O.$$

Because the reduction requires six electrons and the oxidation only gives one, six times more of the oxidant is needed (sometimes both half-reactions must be multiplied by a different number to obtain a common number of electrons). Multiplying the iron equation by 6 and adding it to the chromium equation yields

$$Cr_2O_7^{2-} + 14H^+ + 6e^- + 6Fe^{2+} \rightarrow 2Cr^{3+} + 7H_2O + 6e^- + 6Fe^{3+}$$

Canceling the six electrons yields the same solution as before.

Problem

Balance the following equations.

A. $H_2O_2 + H^+ + Fe^{2+} \rightarrow H_2O + Fe^{3+}$
B. $Cl^- + Cr_2O_7^{2-} + H^+ \rightarrow Cl_2 + Cr^{3+} + H_2O$
C. $I_2 + OCl^- + OH^- \rightarrow IO_3^- + Cl^- + H_2O$

Solution

A. $H_2O_2 + 2H^+ + 2Fe^{2+} \rightarrow 2H_2O + 2Fe^{3+}$
B. $6Cl^- + Cr_2O_7^{2-} + 14H^+ \rightarrow 3Cl_2 + 2Cr^{3+} + 7H_2O$
C. $I_2 + 5OCl^- + 2OH^- \rightarrow 2IO_3^- + 5Cl^- + H_2O$

Problem

A. In the past, German airships condensed the water out of their engines' exhaust to use as ballast. Otherwise, the ship would drift higher as the fuel was consumed. A good rule of thumb was that for every gallon of gasoline burned, a gallon of water was produced. Find out how accurate this is on a mass basis. Assume gasoline to be 100% octane (C_8H_{18}), combustion to be 100%, and the recovery of the water to be 100%. The density of octane is 0.706 g/mL. How many grams of water are produced for each gram of octane consumed?

B. A sample of iron (atomic weight = 55.8) has a mass of 156 g. The iron is 95.1% pure and is reacted with hydrochloric acid by the unbalanced reaction,

$Fe° + HCl \rightarrow FeCl_3 + H_2.$

The impurities do not react with HCl, all the iron is consumed, and all the hydrogen is recovered. How many grams of hydrogen are produced? If the hydrogen is produced in one large spherical bubble, what is its diameter (H_2 has a density of 0.0898 g/L under these conditions)?

C. A lump of solid sodium hydroxide (NaOH) has a mass of 15.3 grams. To neutralize it, 19.9 grams of pure nitric acid (HNO_3) are needed. What is the weight percent purity of the NaOH sample?

Solution

A. Write a balanced equation for the combustion of octane: 8 carbons and 18 hydrogens give

$C_8H_{18} + O_2 \rightarrow 8CO_2 + 9H_2O.$

This requires a total of $12^1/_2$ O_2's. Multiplying the entire equation by 2 to eliminate the fraction yields

$2C_8H_{18} + 25O_2 \rightarrow 16CO_2 + 18H_2O.$

Find the molecular weights of octane and water:

$(12 \times 8) + (18 \times 1) = 114, (1 \times 2) + (16 \times 1) = 18$

Convert 1 g of octane into moles of octane:

$1/114 = 0.00877$ mole of octane

Use the balanced equation to go from moles of octane to moles of water:

$$0.0877 \text{ moles of octane} \left(\frac{18 \text{ moles of water}}{2 \text{ moles of octane}}\right) = 0.0789 \text{ moles of water}$$

Convert moles of water to grams of water:

$0.0789 \times 18 = 1.42$ g of water

Note that the density of octane was never used in these calculations. The final answer is 1.42 grams of water are produced for every 1.00 g of octane consumed.

B. Calculate the total mass of iron:

$156 \times 0.951 = 148$ g pure iron

Calculate the number of moles of iron:

$148/55.8 = 2.65$ moles of iron

Balance the equation by either method:

$$\overset{0}{Fe^{\circ}} + \overset{+1\ -1}{HCl} \longrightarrow \overset{+3-1}{FeCl_3} + \overset{0}{H_2} \quad Fe \longrightarrow \overset{-3}{Fe^{--+}},$$

a change of +3.

$$\overset{+1}{2H^{+}} \longrightarrow \overset{0}{H_2}$$

a change of −2 (2 atoms involved).

To obtain a common change in oxidation number (absolute value), multiply the Fe by 2 and the H by 6. This gives

$$2Fe^{\circ} + 6HCl \rightarrow 2FeCl_3 + 3H_2$$

OR

$Fe^{\circ} \rightarrow Fe^{3+} + 3e^{-}$, and $2H^{+} + 2e^{-} \rightarrow H_2$.

Notice that 3 electrons are supplied by the iron and 2 are consumed by the hydrogen. Multiplying the Fe by 2 and the H by 3 results in a total of 6 e^{-}'s swapping atoms:

$2Fe^{\circ} \rightarrow 2Fe^{3+} + 6e^{-}$, and $6H^{+} + 6e^{-} \rightarrow 3H2$

Adding these equations, including spectator ions, and canceling electrons yields

$2Fe^{\circ} + 6HCl \rightarrow 2FeCl_3 + 3H_2$.

Calculate moles of H_2 produced per mole of Fe consumed:

$$2.65 \text{ moles of Fe} \left(\frac{3\text{moles of H2}}{2\text{moles of Fe}}\right) = 3.98 \text{ moles of H2.}$$

Convert to grams of H_2: $3.98 \times 2.00 = 7.96$ grams of hydrogen. This answers the first part.

Calculate the volume of hydrogen:

$$7.96 \text{ g of H2} \left|\frac{1\text{L of H2}}{0.0898 \text{ g H2}}\right| = 88.6 \text{ L ofH2}$$

Convert to cm^3:

88.6 liters = 88,600 cm^3

The volume of a sphere is $V = 4/3\pi r^3$, and solving for *r* gives 27.6 cm.

The question asked for diameter, which is twice the radius, so

$2 \times 27.6 = 55.2$ cm.

C. Determine molecular weights for NaOH and HNO_3:

$(1 \times 23) + (1 \times 16) + (1 \times 2) = 40.0$ amu

and

$(1 \times 1) + (1 \times 14) + (3 \times 16) = 63.0$ amu, respectively

Write a balanced equation:

$HNO_3 + NaOH \rightarrow$ water + salt

The salt in this case must be sodium nitrate:

$HNO_3 + NaOH \rightarrow H_2O + NaNO_3$

Looking at the elements on both sides of the arrow shows that the equation is already balanced. Calculate the moles of HNO_3 used:

$$19.9 \text{ grams of } HNO_3 \left(\frac{1 \text{ mole } HNO_3}{63.0 \text{ grams of } HNO_3} \right) = 0.316 \text{ moles of} HNO_3$$

Calculate the number of moles of NaOH present:

$$0.316 \text{ mole } HNO_3 \left(\frac{1 \text{ mole NaOH}}{1 \text{ mole } HNO_3} \right) = 0.316 \text{ mole NaOH}$$

Calculate the grams of NaOH present:

$$0.316 \text{ mole NaOH} \left(\frac{40.0 \text{ g NaOH}}{1 \text{ mole NaOH}} \right) = 12.6 \text{ grams}$$

Calculate the weight percentage of NaOH of the sample's mass:

$(12.6/15.3) \times 100\% = 82.4\%$ purity

II. ELECTRONIC STRUCTURE AND THE PERIODIC TABLE

1. ELECTRONIC STRUCTURE

The model of the hydrogen atom that Niels Bohr introduced early in the twentieth century, showing an electron orbiting a central nucleus in a manner analogous to a planet–sun system, is quite outdated and inaccurate. The exact location of a particular electron about a nucleus at any given time cannot be accurately known. Instead, predictions can be made as to the most likely location of an electron about a nucleus. These predictions can be made because the electrons occupy definite energy levels about the nucleus.

Within these definite energy levels are regions where the probability of finding an electron is high. These areas are often thought of in terms of a cloud of negative charge, called an electron cloud. Electron clouds are denser in areas of high probability and more diffuse in areas of lower probability. Another name for electron clouds is atomic orbitals. The definite energy levels that contain atomic orbitals are often referred to as shells. Shells surround the nucleus much like the layers of an onion. Each shell is given a number, with the one closest to the nucleus being 1, and is also designated by a letter of the alphabet, with the shell closest to the nucleus given the letter K. The maximum number of electrons that each energy level can hold is determined by the formula

$$N = 2n^2,$$

where N is the maximum number of electrons for the given energy level, and n is the shell's number. Table 3 summarizes these data for the first seven shells.

TABLE 3. Electron Energy Levels

Letter Designation	Numeric Value (n)	Maximum Number of Electrons ($N = 2n^2$)
K	1	2
L	2	8
M	3	18
N	4	32
O	5	50*
P	6	72*
Q	7	98*

* The number given is hypothetical; it should be confirmed when atoms of large-enough atomic number to fill these shells are produced.

Energy shells can be divided into subshells. Electron transitions between subshells are possible. Subshells are further divided into orbitals. The maximum number of electrons that can occupy any orbital at one time is two. To help predict the most probable location of these electrons, the following four quantum numbers are used.

The principal quantum number, n, is used to designate the volume of space in which the electron moves and the energy of the electron. The n number refers to the energy shell in which the electron is residing. The n number is always an integer and can vary from 1 to infinity, in theory. In all known atoms, it is never above 7. As mentioned previously, sometimes the letters K, L, M, and so on, are used in place of the n numbers 1, 2, 3, and so on.

The angular momentum quantum number (l) designates the shape of the region that the electron is most likely to occupy. The number is equal to $n - 1$ and can vary from 0 to infinity, in theory. In all known atoms, it is never more than 3. Just as letters are sometimes used for the n number, so they are used for the angular momentum quantum number. The letters s, p, d, f, g, h, i and so on, are used in place of 0, 1, 2, 3, 4, 5, 6, and so on.

The magnetic quantum number, m, is used to designate the vector, or the general orientation of the region of high electron probability in space. The m can vary in value from -1 to $+1$ and every integral value in between (meaning m can be zero).

The spin quantum number, *s*, specifies the direction of the electron spin about a nucleus. An electron orbiting a nucleus is limited to only two possible spins:

$$+\frac{1}{2}\text{h}/2\text{p and } -\frac{1}{2}\text{h}/2\text{p},$$

where *h* is Planck's constant. Usually the spin term is simply shortened to +½ and −½.

No two electrons in a particular atom can have the same four quantum numbers. Thus, for two electrons to occupy the same orbital, they must have opposite spin. This concept is known as the Pauli exclusion principle.

A. Ground vs. Excited States

When all the electrons in an atom are in the orbitals of lowest possible energy, the atom is said to be in the ground state. If energy is somehow imparted to these electrons, they are boosted to higher energy orbitals. Such an atom is said to be in an excited state. When the electrons return to the ground state, the energy is given off in the form of electromagnetic radiation.

B. Conventional Notation for Electronic Structure

Electronic notation involves the use of the first two quantum numbers. For example, hydrogen has only one electron. It is in the first energy level ($n = 1$) and part of the s subshell. To designate this, it is written $1s^1$; the superscript 1 means that one electron is in the s orbital. Helium has a total of two electrons in the same orbital. The electronic notation for helium is $1s^2$, where 1 represents the first energy level, s denotes the subshell (s subshells are spherical), and the superscript 2 denotes two electrons occupying that subshell.

According to the Pauli exclusion principle, the two electrons in a helium atom must have opposite quantum spin numbers. To represent this, sometimes boxes with arrows are used. Each box represents a different subshell, and the arrows represent electrons. Arrows of different direction represent electrons of different spin. Thus, hydrogen is represented as

1s
↑

The electronic structure of helium is

1s
↑↓

Note that the arrows are going in opposite directions to denote the opposite spins of the electrons. The first energy level contains only the single spherical s subshell. Proceeding to the next element, lithium, a structure of

$$1s^22s^1$$

is obtained. This denotes that the 1s orbital is filled, as in helium, and the 2s subshell has one electron in it. This is shown as

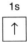

1s	2s
↑↓	↑

Note that beryllium has four total electrons:

$1s^2 2s^2$

Beryllium is represented as

1s	2s
↑↓	↑↓

Notice the paired electrons of opposite spin and a total of four electrons, although only two valence electrons.

Starting with the next element, boron, another subshell of the second energy level begins to fill. The p subshell is shaped like a dumbbell. There are actually three p's, each lying in a plane at right angles from the other two. Using the conventional terminology of Cartesian coordinates, these are known as p_x, p_y, and p_z, the subscript denoting the plane they are lying in. All three p's are of equal value; the x, y, and z terms are arbitrary. Note that these orientation factors are determined by the *m* number. (Because l = 1, and *m* equals all integers between −1 and +1, we get m values of −1, 0, and +1. That indicates three subdivisions of the p subshell, and that is what is observed.)

The notation for boron is

$1s^2 2s^2 2p^1$,

and is shown as

1s	2s	$2p_x$	$2p_y$	$2p_z$
↑↓	↑↓	↑		

Notice the unoccupied p orbitals.

As can be predicted, carbon is

$1s^2 2s^2 2p^2$,

and is shown as

1s	2s	$2p_x$	$2p_y$	$2p_z$
↑↓	↑↓	↑	↑	

The p subshell fills each orbital with a single electron before it pairs an orbital with two electrons of opposite spin. This is true of any subshell; the electrons enter each orbital of a given type singly and with identical spins before any pairings of electrons of opposite spin occur within those orbitals. This is known as Hund's rule.

Nitrogen will follow this as

$1s^2 2s^2 2p^3$.

(For review, notice that nitrogen will have a total of seven electrons, five of them valence electrons.) Nitrogen is depicted as

1s	2s	$2p_x$	$2p_y$	$2p_z$
↑↓	↑↓	↑	↑	↑

With oxygen, the p orbitals begin to pair up:

$1s^2 2s^2 2p^4$

1s	2s	$2p_x$	$2p_y$	$2p_z$
↑↓	↑↓	↑	↑	↑

Fluorine adds another electron to pair up, and with neon the second energy level is filled, giving

$1s^2 2s^2 2p^6$.

(Of the 10 total electrons, 8 are valence.) Neon is shown as

1s	2s	$2p_x$	$2p_y$	$2p_z$
↑↓	↑↓	↑↓	↑↓	↑↓

All the elements in the same vertical row in the periodic table have the same outer electron configuration. For example, sodium has the same outer configuration as lithium but is one energy level higher, with the inner electron configuration matching that of neon:

$1s^2 2s^2 2p^6 3s^1$

1s	2s	$2p_x$	$2p_y$	$2p_z$	3s
↑↓	↑↓	↑↓	↑↓	↑↓	↑

Silicone's outer electrons match those of carbon:

$1s^2 2s^2 2p^6 3s^2 3p^2$

1s	2s	$2p_x$	$2p_y$	$2p_z$	3s	$3p_x$	$3p_y$	$3p_z$
↑↓	↑↓	↑↓	↑↓	↑↓	↑↓	↑	↑	

Argon will match that of neon:

$1s^2 2s^2 2p^6 3s^2 3p^6$

1s	2s	← 2p →			3s	← 3p →		
↑↓	↑↓	↑↓	↑↓	↑↓	↑↓	↑↓	↑↓	↑↓

As the fourth energy level begins to fill, the electron notation follows the predictable rule previously mentioned for potassium ($\ldots 4s^1$) and calcium ($\ldots 4s^2$). However, at scandium, a new rule needs to be introduced. Recall that the quantum number is equal to $n - 1$. When $n = 3$, the l quantum number is 2, which is a d orbital. Although this is in the fourth row of the table, it is the third row that is filling with electrons in these transition metals. Therefore, the number of valence electrons does not change. Also, recall that the m quantum number can have any integral value from -1 to $+1$ when $l = 2$. This gives $m = -2, -1, 0, 1, 2$, which gives five sublevels (orbitals) for the d subshell. These five orbitals are all of equal value and follow Hund's rule for pairing.

The nomenclature for scandium is

$1s^22s^22p^63s^23p^63d^14s^2$,

which shows 21 total electrons but only two valence electrons, just like magnesium. This is represented as

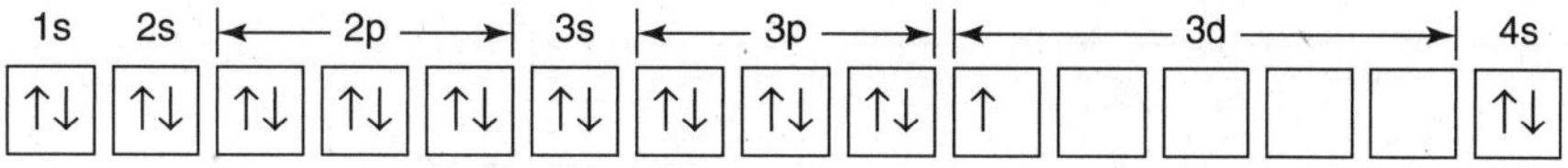

Using Hund's rule as introduced, the electron configuration of titanium is

$1s^22s^22p^63s^23p^63d^24s^2$,

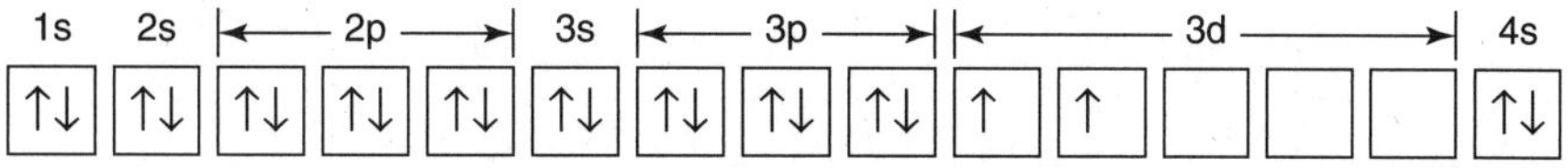

The same rule can be used for vanadium. At chromium, another aspect of electron behavior must be revealed. The predicted configuration is

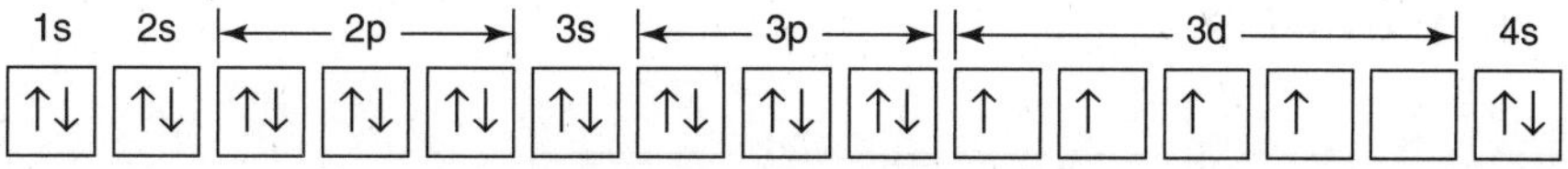

However, the attraction of four electrons in the 3d is strong enough to pull in an electron from the 4s, so the proper configuration is

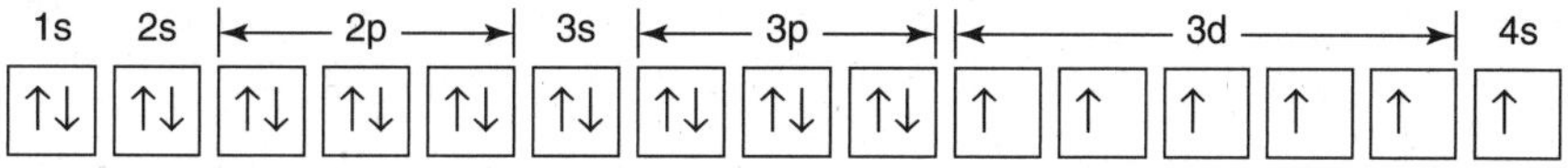

represented by

$1s^22s^22p^63s^23p^63d^54s^1$

(22 total electrons, 1 valence.) At the next element, manganese, the 4s fills up again:

$1s^22s^22p^63s^23p^63d^54s^2$

(2 valence electrons out of a total of 25).

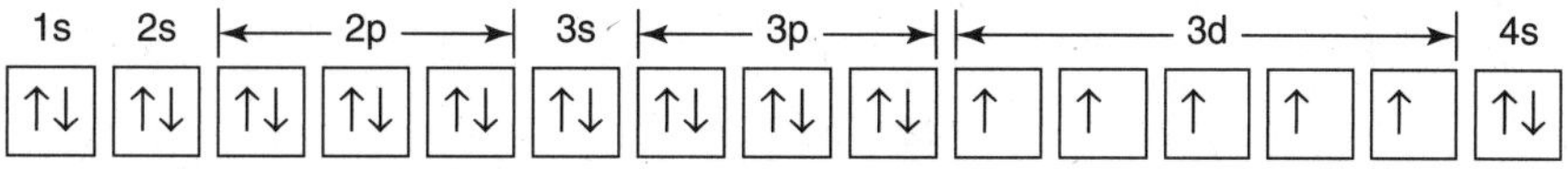

At iron, the d orbitals begin pairing:

$1s^22s^22p^63s^23p^63d^64s^2$

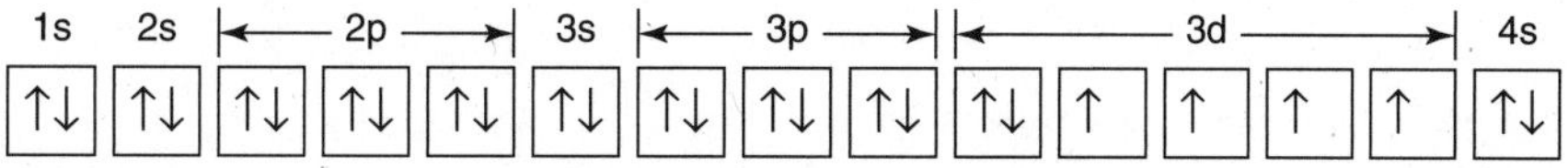

This continues up to copper. The force of nine electrons in the d level is strong enough to pull in an electron from the 4s, giving

$1s^22s^22p^63s^23s^23p^63d^{10}4s^1$

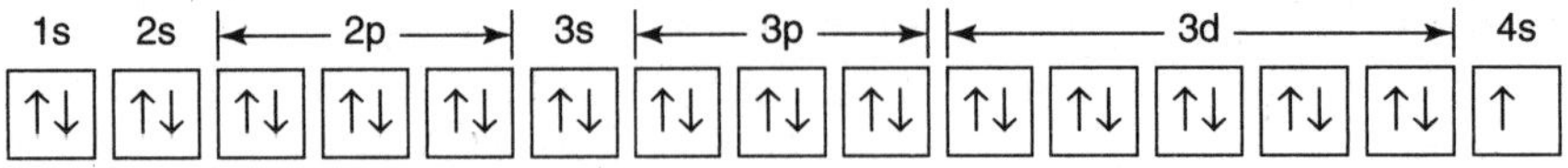

At zinc, the 4s fills up again:

$1s^22s^22p^63s^23p^63d^{10}4s^2$

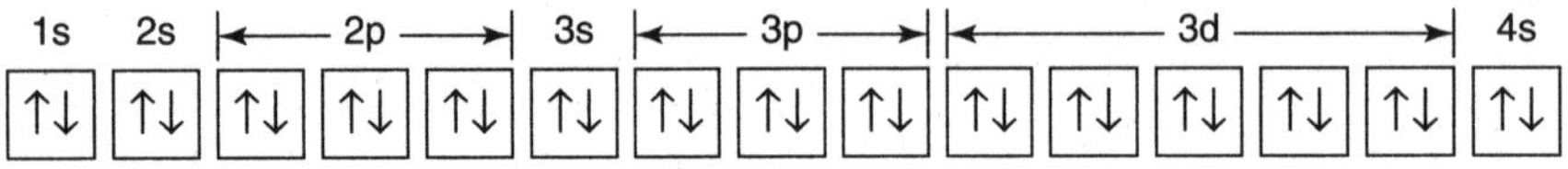

With gallium, the 4ps begins filling, following the rules given for them. For example, selenium is

$1s^22s^22p^63s^23p^63d^{10}4s^24p^4$, shown as

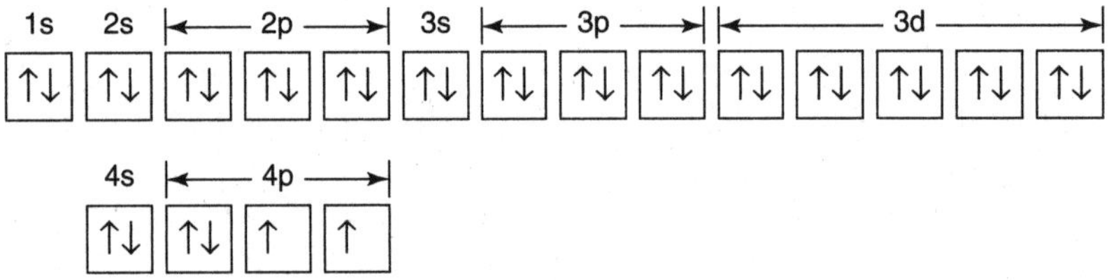

Again, these rules apply when moving down vertically in the periodic table. Remember, when dealing with d subshells, they are one energy level lower than the outer energy level of the atom. For example, niobium (atomic number 41), starting with a neon core, is

$3s^23p^63d^{10}4s^24p^64d^35s^2$,

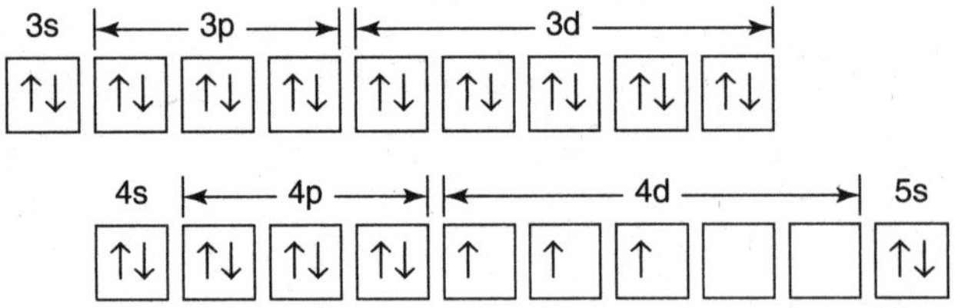

Silver, starting with a neon core, is

$3s^23p^63d^{10}4s^24p^64d^{10}5s^1$, or

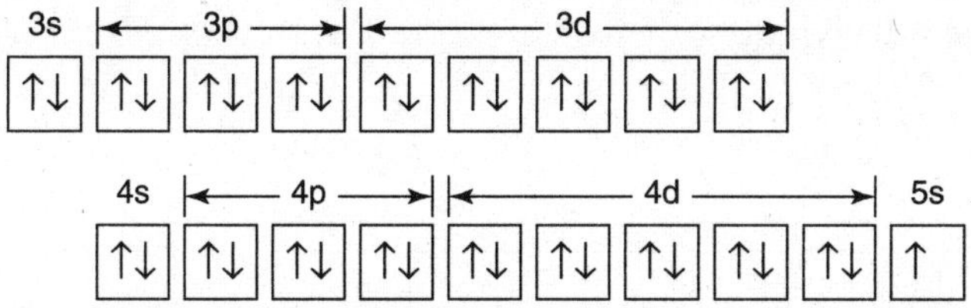

Iodine is

$3s^2 3p^6 3d^{10} 4s^2 4p^6 4d^{10} 5s^2 5p^5$, or

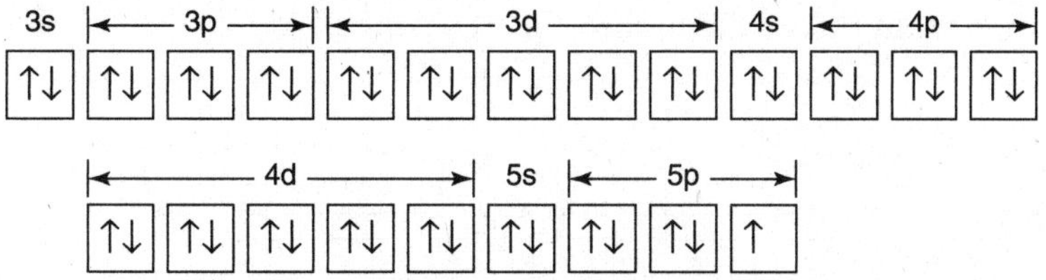

The last set of orbitals that involves another set of rules are those of the lanthanide and actinide series. Again, looking at the quantum numbers, when $n = 4$, $l = 3$, which corresponds to an f subshell. The m number of an f subshell can have a value of $-3, -2, -1, 0, 1, 2,$ or 3, which gives a total of seven orbitals in the f subshell, at two electrons each—that is, 14 electrons. Lanthanum, predictably, is (starting with a xenon core) $5d^1 6s^2$. With the next element, cerium, the f orbitals begin to fill, observing Hund's rule. This is a 4f that is filling, two energy levels below the outer level. This rule holds true for all these series. Cerium, the first of the lanthanoid series, begins to fill the 4f orbitals. However, the force of one electron in the 4f is enough to pull the electron out of the 5d. The 5d electron joins the 4f. Thus, cerium (starting with a xenon core) is

$4f^2 5d^0 6s^2$, or

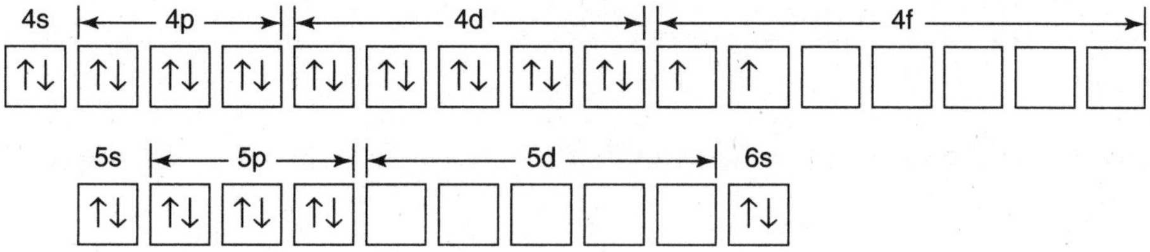

The 4f orbitals continue to fill, obeying Hund's rule, and the 5d remains empty. Neodymium is

$4f^4 5d^0 6s^2$

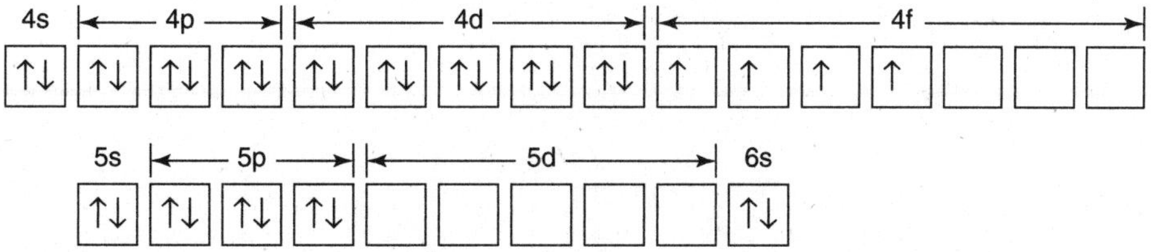

At gadolinium, an electron again goes to the 5d, giving

$4f^7 5d^1 6s^2$

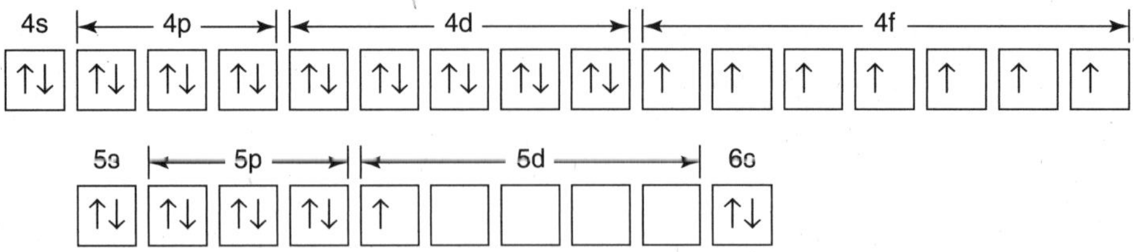

With terbium, the lone 5d electron is again pulled down into the 4f, giving

$4f^9 5d^0 6s^2$

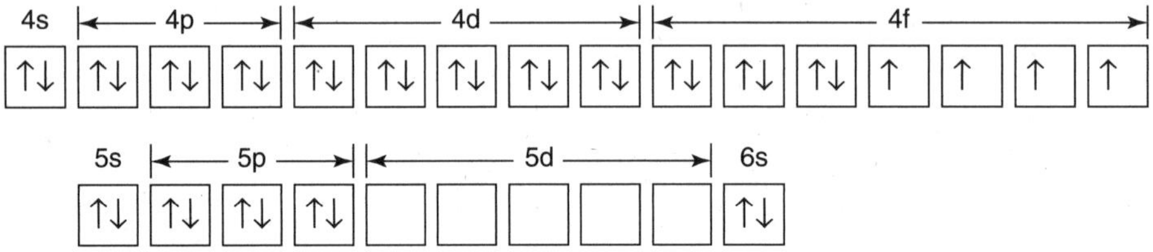

At lutetium, an electron again goes to the 5d, giving

$4f^{14} 5d^1 6s^2$,

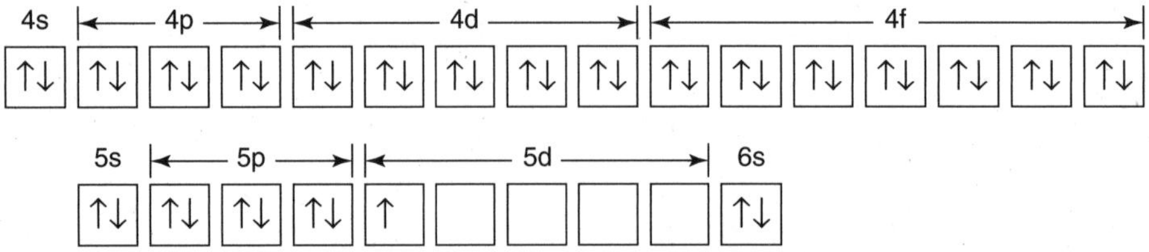

Next is hafnium, where the 5d subshell continues to fill. The notation for tungsten, starting with a xenon core, is

$4f^{14} 5d^5 6s^1$.

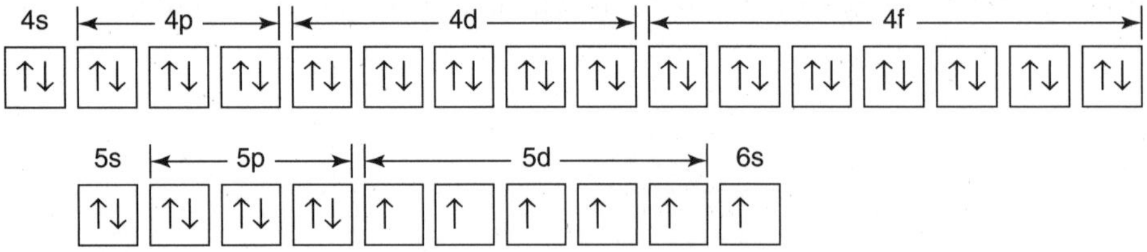

Polonium is

$4f^{14} 5d^{10} 6s^2 6p^4$.

The same rules can be applied to the actinoid series. Uranium, starting with a xenon core, is

$4f^{14} 5d^{10} 5f^4 6d^0 7s^2$,

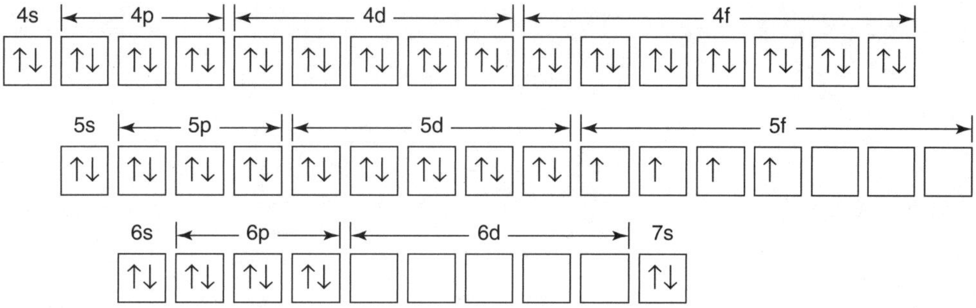

Problem

Write the complete electronic notation and representations showing Hund's rule for the following elements. Write an abbreviated form of the electronic configuration.

A. Osmium B. Cadmium C. Calcium

D. Strontium E. Curium

Solution

A. Os — $1s^2 2s^2 2p^6 3s^2 3p^6 3d^{10} 4s^2 4p^6 4d^{10} 4f^{14} 5s^2 5p^6 5d^6 6s^2$

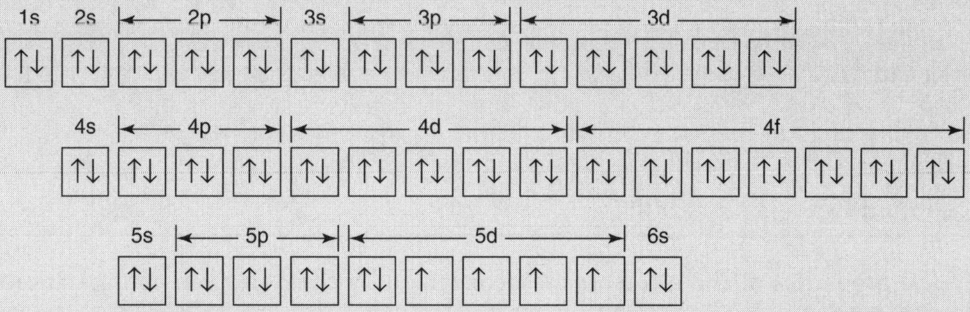

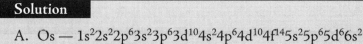

B. Cd — $1s^2 2s^2 2p^6 3s^2 3p^6 3d^{10} 4s^2 4p^6 4d^{10} 5s^2$

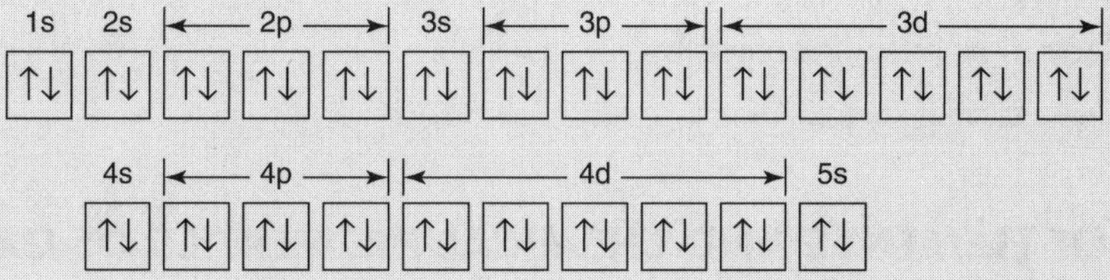

C. Ca — $1s^2 2s^2 2p^6 3s^2 3p^6 4s^2$

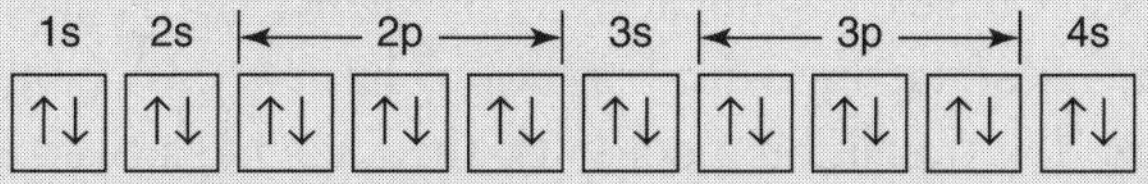

D. Sr — $1s^2 2s^2 2p^6 3s^2 3p^6 3d^{10} 4s^2 4p^6 5s^2$

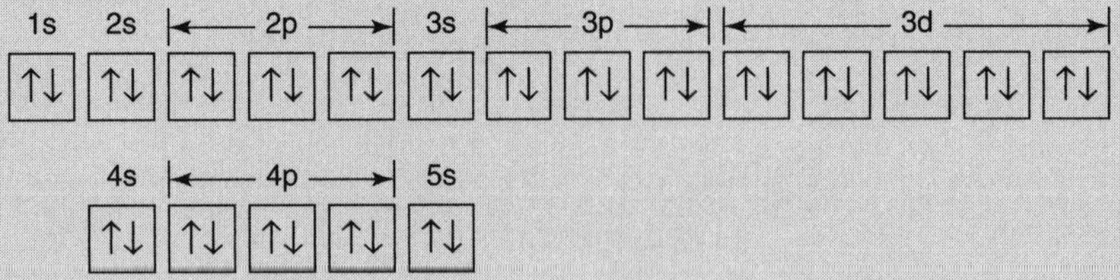

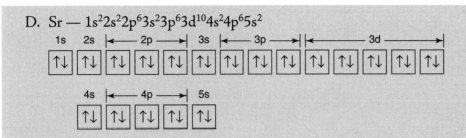

E. Cm — $1s^2 2s^2 2p^6 3s^2 3p^6 3d^{10} 4s^2 4p^6 4d^{10} 4f^{14} 5s^2 5p^6 5d^{10} 5f^7 6s^2 6p^6 6d^1 7s^2$

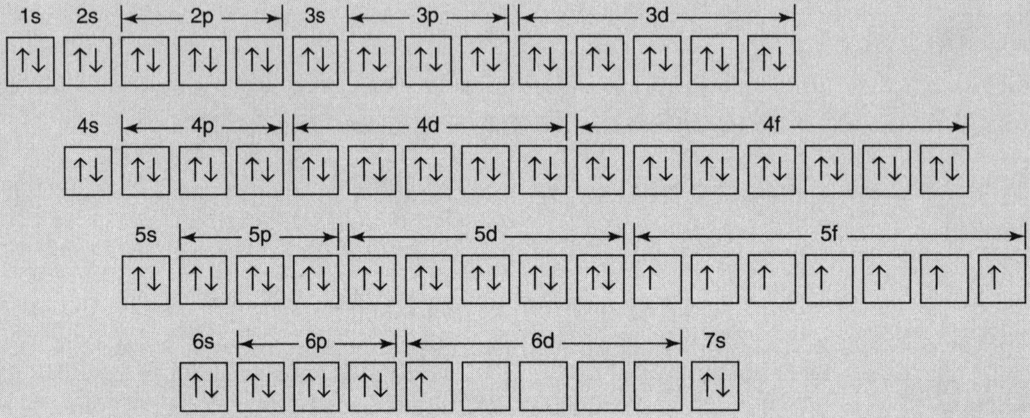

The abbreviated forms extract the configuration for the closest noble gas and show the valence electrons.

A. Osmium [Xe] $4f145d^6 6s^2$

B. Cadmium [Kr] $4d^{10} 5s^2$

C. Calcium [Ar] $4s^2$

D. Strontium [Kr] $5s^2$

E. Curium [Rn] $5f^7 6d^1 7s^2$

Many physical properties of the elements are determined by their electron configurations. On the other hand, much of the chemistry of the elements involves the formation of cations and anions. Electrons are lost or gained, and in doing so, stable electron configurations are formed in which the cations or anions have electron configurations identical to those of a noble gas. For example, the sodium ion is formed by removal of one electron from sodium metal:

$$Na: [1s^2 2s^2 2p^6 3s^1] \rightarrow Na^+: [1s^2 2s^2 2p^6] + e^-$$

2. CLASSIFICATION OF ELEMENTS AND CHEMICAL PROPERTIES OF GROUPS AND ROWS

Elements in the same vertical row of the periodic table have the same number of valence electrons. Group 1A (starting with hydrogen) has one valence electron, 2A (starting with beryllium) has two, 3A (starting with boron) has three, and so on, for all of the A groups. The transition metals (1B through 3B) as well as the lanthanide and actinide series usually have two valence electrons. The few exceptions to this can easily be predicted using the electron orbital notation discussed in the last section.

FIGURE 1. Allowed Quantum Numbers for the First Four Energy Levels

Energy level – n	1	2				3								
Subshell – l	0 (s)	0 (s)	1 (p)			0 (s)	1 (p)			2 (d)				
Orbital – m	0	0	−1	0	+1	0	−1	0	+1	−2	−1	0	+1	+2
Spin – S $(\frac{h}{2\pi})$	$+\frac{1}{2} -\frac{1}{2}$	$+\frac{1}{2} -\frac{1}{2}$	$+\frac{1}{2} -\frac{1}{2}$	$+\frac{1}{2} -\frac{1}{2}$	$+\frac{1}{2} -\frac{1}{2}$	$+\frac{1}{2} -\frac{1}{2}$	$+\frac{1}{2} -\frac{1}{2}$	$+\frac{1}{2} -\frac{1}{2}$	$+\frac{1}{2} -\frac{1}{2}$	$+\frac{1}{2} -\frac{1}{2}$	$+\frac{1}{2} -\frac{1}{2}$	$+\frac{1}{2} -\frac{1}{2}$	$+\frac{1}{2} -\frac{1}{2}$	$+\frac{1}{2} -\frac{1}{2}$

Energy level – n	4															
Subshell – l	0 (s)	1 (p)			2 (d)					3 (f)						
Orbital – m	0	−1	0	+1	−2	−1	0	+1	+2	−3	−2	−1	0	+1	+2	+3
Spin – S $(\frac{h}{2\pi})$	$+\frac{1}{2} -\frac{1}{2}$	$+\frac{1}{2} -\frac{1}{2}$	$+\frac{1}{2} -\frac{1}{2}$	$+\frac{1}{2} -\frac{1}{2}$	$+\frac{1}{2} -\frac{1}{2}$	$+\frac{1}{2} -\frac{1}{2}$	$+\frac{1}{2} -\frac{1}{2}$	$+\frac{1}{2} -\frac{1}{2}$	$+\frac{1}{2} -\frac{1}{2}$	$+\frac{1}{2} -\frac{1}{2}$	$+\frac{1}{2} -\frac{1}{2}$	$+\frac{1}{2} -\frac{1}{2}$	$+\frac{1}{2} -\frac{1}{2}$	$+\frac{1}{2} -\frac{1}{2}$	$+\frac{1}{2} -\frac{1}{2}$	$+\frac{1}{2} -\frac{1}{2}$

A. First and Second Ionization Energies

All atoms strive to have a full outer shell. For hydrogen and helium, this means two outer electrons. For all other atoms, it means eight outer electrons. The energy required to remove one electron from an atom is known as its first ionization energy. The energy required to remove a second electron is known as the second ionization energy, and so on. Because the elements in group 1A need to lose only one electron to have a full outer shell, their first ionization energy is fairly low, ranging from 3.9 electron volts (eV) for cesium to 5.4 eV for lithium. However, giving up a second electron is much more difficult for these atoms because that loss will keep their outer shells from being full. The second ionization energies for this group range from 25.1 eV for cesium to 75.6 eV for lithium—significantly higher than the first ionization energy. The group 2A elements want to lose two electrons; thus, their secondary ionization energy are lower than that of the 1A group.

The first and secondary ionization energies for beryllium are 9.3 and 18.2 eV, respectively. It takes more energy to form a +2 ion from a 2A element than it does a +1 ion from a 1A element. From this rule, it is logical and correct to deduce that it takes even more energy to form a +3 ion from a 3A element. These ionization energies increase moving across the periodic table. At the far right side of the table, the noble gases are the most difficult to ionize because they already have full outer shells. The first and second ionization energies for neon are 21.6 and 41.1 eV, respectively. Ionization energy decreases slightly moving vertically down the table. For all practical purposes, the ionization energies of the transition metals can be treated as if they belong to group 2A.

B. Electron Affinities

The opposite of losing electrons is gaining. The measure of energy released when an electron is added to an atom to form a negative ion is called electron affinity. As can be expected, the noble gases have zero electron affinity because their outer shells are full, and they want to neither gain nor lose electrons. The metals, which tend to lose electrons, have very low electron affinities. For example, lithium needs to lose only one electron to have a full outer shell, whereas it would have to gain seven. Thus, its electron affinity is only 0.54 eV. Contrast this with fluorine, which obtains a full outer shell by either gaining just one electron or losing seven. Its electron affinity is 3.45 eV (remember, this is energy given up, not required). Electron affinity increases moving to the upper-right corner of the periodic table (the noble gases are not included in this).

C. Electronegativity

Electronegativity is the attraction of an atom for the electrons in its outer shell. It is related to ionization potential and electron affinity. Electronegativity is discussed later in this review in reference to predicting the bonding and polarity of molecules. If the noble gases were removed from the periodic table, electronegativity would increase moving to the upper-right corner of the table and would decrease moving to the lower-left corner. Therefore, among the nonradioactive elements, fluorine is the most electronegative and cesium is the least.

III. BONDING

Bonds can be formed between atoms in a compound and between atoms in different molecules. The bonds that are formed between atoms in a compound are called intramolecular, and those that are formed between different molecules are called intermolecular bonds. Intramolecular bonds are much stronger than intermolecular bonds. However, as discussed in the Biology Review, intermolecular bonds such as hydrogen bonding and hydrophobic interactions are very important in determining the tertiary structure of proteins.

1. TYPES OF BONDS

A. Ionic Bonds

If the difference in electronegativities between atoms is great, an ionic bond will occur. An ionic bond involves an actual transfer of electrons from one atom to another, creating ions held together by electrostatic attraction. For example, cesium has one valence electron and fluorine has seven. Because of the difference in electronegativities, fluorine can pull the outer electron off cesium and incorporate it into its own outer shell. The result is a Cs+ cation and a F− anion. Opposite charges attract, so the two ions come together to form CsF.

Sometimes more than two ions are needed. In the case of potassium and sulfur, K^+ and S^{-2} are formed. To balance out the charges, two sulfurs are needed for every potassium; therefore, the formula is K_2S. Ionic bonds are the strongest chemical bonds known. It takes a great deal of energy to dissociate them.

B. Polar Covalent Bonds

When bonding atoms have different electronegativities, an unequal sharing of electrons occurs, and the resultant bond is neither ionic nor truly covalent. This type of bond is known as a polar covalent bond because it has a slightly positive end and a slightly negative end resulting from the unequal sharing of electrons. For example, in a molecule of iodine fluoride, the atom of fluorine is more electronegative than the atom of iodine. As a result, the electrons spend more time with the fluorine, giving it a slightly negative charge. The iodine atom consequently has a slightly positive charge. The unequal charge distribution gives the overall molecule a dipole moment.

A better-known example of a polar covalent bond is the oxygen hydrogen bond in water. The difference in electronegativities of hydrogen and oxygen and the unequal sharing of the electron pair in the bond between the atoms cause a partial negative charge to form on oxygen and a partial positive charge to form on hydrogen. These dipoles cause intermolecular bonds to form between water molecules. See Biology Review, Properties of Water, page 135.

C. Covalent Bonds

If the difference in electronegativities between atoms is slight or nonexistent, a covalent bond will form. A covalent bond involves sharing of electrons from one atom to another. Covalent bonds are weaker than ionic bonds. An example of a covalent bond is the formation of a chlorine molecule, Cl_2, from individual chlorine atoms. Covalent bonding is very important in organic chemistry. See Organic Chemistry Review, Bonding, page 335.

D. Hydrogen Bonding

When hydrogen is involved with the dipole forces described previously, interacting with atoms such as fluorine, nitrogen, or oxygen, a much stronger bond is established than in ordinary dipole interactions.

The attractive force exerted between these atoms is so great that it has been given the special name of hydrogen bonding. The hydrogen bond is greater than the ordinary dipole for two reasons:

1. The difference in electronegativity between hydrogen and the elements nitrogen, oxygen, and fluorine is quite large. As a result, the electrons are markedly displaced from the hydrogen.
2. The small size of the hydrogen atom allows it to approach the other atoms very closely.

E. Dipole Interactions

Recall that in polar bonding, a dipole moment is established. If there is not another dipole in the same molecule to cancel it, the resulting molecule is polar (having a positive and a negative end). In polar molecules, the negative end of one molecule is attracted to the positive end of another. An example of this is iodine chloride. Because of the differences in electronegativity, the chlorine atom has the shared electrons for a longer time than does the iodine atom, placing a negative charge on the chlorine atom and a positive charge on the iodine. In solid ICl, the molecules are tightly aligned in a manner similar to the sodium chloride crystal.

Iodine is attracted by electrostatic forces on all sides of the neighboring chloride atoms, and the chlorine is equally attracted on all sides by the neighboring iodine. Unlike the very strong ionic bonds in NaCl, the dipole forces holding the crystal structure of ICl together are much weaker. As a result, when ICl is heated only to 27°C, the relatively weak dipole forces are no longer able to hold the crystal together, and the solid melts.

F. Van der Waals Forces

The positively charged nucleus of an atom can attract and alter the electron cloud of a neighboring atom. The momentary shift in the electron creates a momentary dipole moment that can induce a similar momentary dipole in an adjacent molecule. These very weak forces work among not only polar molecules but also nonpolar molecules. They are termed van der Waals forces, or London forces, and increase with the mass of the molecule. Helium is a good example to show how very weak these forces are.

In helium, the only attractive force is a very weak van der Waals force. The attraction of one helium atom for another is so slight that even at absolute zero (0 K), helium remains a liquid (at normal pressure). The attraction of one helium atom for another is so slight that helium atoms never get close enough at ordinary pressure to form a solid.

2. LEWIS ELECTRON DOT STRUCTURES

The Lewis structure simply shows the valence electrons of an atom or ion. Here are a few examples showing sodium, strontium, sulfur, iodine, and xenon, respectively:

Na· Sr :S̈: :Ï: Xe

Returning to the problem of the covalent bonding of chlorine, note from the Lewis structure,

:C̈l:

that each Cl atom has one unpaired electron. Were two Cl atoms to come together and share their unpaired electron with the other, a covalent bond would be formed, and each Cl atom would have a full outer shell. Each atom is surrounded by an octet of eight electrons. An octet of electrons is a stable state, and the tendency of molecules and polyatomic ions to have structures in which there are eight valence electrons is known as the octet rule. This can be shown as

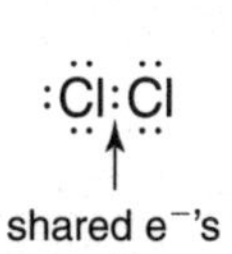

Another example is oxygen gas, O_2. The Lewis structure for O is

To form a covalent bond, two pairs of electrons must be shared, creating what is appropriately called a double bond and the resulting structure of

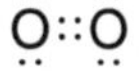

There are exceptions to the octet rule, and hydrogen almost always has two valence electrons in its outer shell.

Sometimes lines are used rather than dots; in this case, each line represents a pair of electrons. Such a structure for Cl_2 and O_2 is

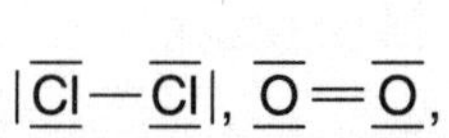

respectively. Often, unshared electron pairs are not shown, giving the representations as follows

$$Cl - Cl, O = O.$$

A. Resonance Structures

Sometimes a single structure cannot accurately represent a molecule or ion. An example is sulfur dioxide, SO_2, which can have either oxygen double-bonded to the sulfur, represented as

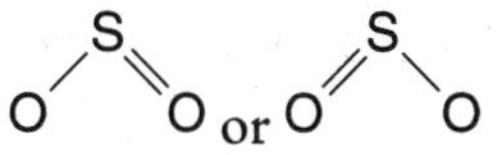

The "real" structure is neither of these but a hybrid structure between the two. The concept is called resonance, and the structure is called a resonance hybrid. It is best represented by

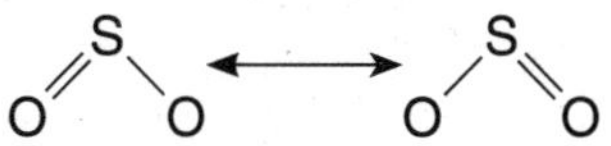

It must be stressed that SO_2 does not spend part of the time in one state and the remainder in the other; it is in a state that is a hybrid between the two.

B. Formal Charge

Often, a group of atoms can covalently bond and, as a group, needs to gain or lose electrons to fill all outer shells. As a result of these excess or deficient electrons, the group of atoms has an overall charge and is called a polyatomic ion. An example of such is sulfate, SO_4^{2-}, which needs two additional electrons to fill the outer shells, giving an overall charge of -2. It can be represented as

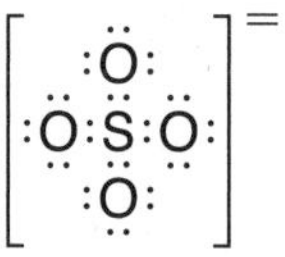

Another example is ammonia, NH_4^{+}, which has to give up an electron to have all outer shells full, resulting in a $+1$ charge. It can be represented as

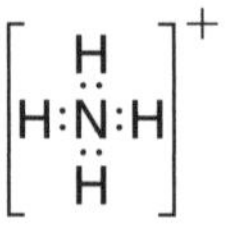

C. Lewis Acids and Bases

A Lewis acid is anything that can accept a pair of electrons, such as Cu^{2+}. A Lewis base is anything that can donate a pair of electrons, such as O^{2-}.

D. Valence Shell Electrons and the Prediction of Shapes of Molecules

Often in covalent bonding, electrons from an s orbital will join those from a p orbital. As can be expected, the shape of the resultant hybrid orbital will help determine the shape of the molecule that is formed. Recall that the s is spherical and the p is dumbbell in shape. Obviously, the more p orbitals present, the more the resultant hybrid orbital will resemble a p than an s. Such is the case in methane, CH_4, where one s electron is blended with three electrons from p orbitals. This is called sp^3 hybridization. The resultant orbital is in the shape of a tetrahedron, and so is the shape of a methane molecule. In boron trifluoride, BF_3, one s electron is blended with two electrons from p orbitals. This is known as sp^2 hybridization, and the resultant orbital has less p character than the sp^3 hybrid. The sp^2 hybrid is a flat, triangular-shaped (trigonal planar) orbital, and so is the resultant molecule, with a fluorine atom at each corner of the triangle. This model is called the valence shell electron pair repulsion (VSEPR) model. Lone electrons and bond electrons in the valence shell of an element repel one another, and they seek to be as far apart as possible.

Problem

Draw a Lewis structure for the nitronium ion NO_2^+.

Solution

A polar covalent bond is formed between nitrogen and oxygen

O—N—O

Oxygen has six valence electrons, and there are two oxygen atoms. Nitrogen has five valence electrons. A double bond is formed between the oxygen and nitrogen with the concomitant formation of a positive charge.

$[O{=}N{=}O]^+$

The total number of valence electrons is 16: 5 from nitrogen and 12 from oxygen and one less due to the positive charge.

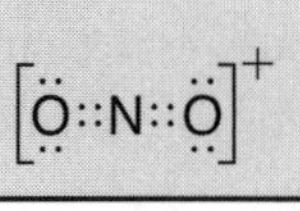

IV. PHASES AND PHASE EQUILIBRIA

1. STANDARD TEMPERATURE, PRESSURE, AND STANDARD MOLAR VOLUME

Gases will assume not only the shape but also the volume of their container. Because of this, standard conditions that can be easily replicated in any laboratory have been agreed on. Standard temperature is the temperature of melting ice, which is 0°C, or 273 K. Standard pressure is the pressure of the earth's atmosphere at sea level, which is one atmosphere, or 760 torr. Collectively, standard temperature and pressure are known as STP. One mole of ideal gas at STP will occupy a volume of 22.4 liters. Another important set of conditions is known as STAP (standard temperature ambient and pressure). This is defined as a pressure of 1 atmosphere and a temperature of 25°C (298.15 K). The ideal gas can be used to calculate pressure, temperature, volume, or number of moles of a gas, provided three of these four parameters are known.

The equation for the ideal gas law is

$$PV = nRT,$$

where P is the pressure in atmospheres (atm), V is the volume in liters, n is the number of moles, R is the universal gas law constant, and T is the temperature in kelvin (K). R, like π or e, always has the same value. In the case of this equation, it is 0.0821 L · atm/mole K. For example, the ideal gas law can verify the molar volume of an ideal gas. Putting standard conditions into the equation $PV = nRT$ gives

$$(1 \text{ atm})(V) = (1 \text{ mole})(0.0821 \text{ L} \cdot \text{atm/mole} \cdot \text{K})(273 \text{ K}).$$

Solving for V yields 22.4 liters. When using this law, it is important to keep the pressure in atmospheres, volume in liters, and temperature in kelvin. With the ideal gas law, almost all gas problems can be solved. However, there are simpler laws of more limited applicability that can be easier to use and are not so stringent with the units used. The first is Boyle's law, which states that the volume of a given gas held at constant temperature is inversely proportional to the pressure under which it is measured. Stated mathematically,

$$P_1V_1 = P_2V_2,$$

where P_1 and V_1 are the initial pressure and volume, respectively (in any units), and P_2 and V_2 are the final pressure and volume, respectively (in the same units as P_1 and V_1). For example, if a gas has a volume of 200 mL at 760 torr pressure, and the temperature remains constant, what will its volume be if the pressure were lowered to 190 torr? By simple logic, it can be deduced that the new volume should be greater than the original. Plugging the values into the formula for Boyle's law gives

$$(760 \text{ torr})(200 \text{ mL}) = (190 \text{ torr})(V_2).$$

Solving for V_2 gives a new volume of 800 mL, which is in agreement with the deduction made earlier.

Another useful law is Charles' law, which states that the volume of a given mass of gas is directly proportional to its temperature on the kelvin scale when the pressure is constant. Mathematically stated, this is

$$V_1/T_1 = V_2/T_2,$$

where V_1 and T_1 are the initial volume and temperature (volume can be in any units, but temperature must be in kelvin), and V_2 and T_2 are the final volume and temperature (in whatever units are used for V_1 and kelvin). For example, if a gas has a volume of 300 mL at 283 K, and the pressure is kept constant, what is the new volume if the temperature is raised to 303 K? As before, logic suggests that at a higher temperature and a constant pressure, the volume should increase. Thus, the new volume should be greater than 300 mL. Plugging the values into the above equation gives

$$(300 \text{ mL})/(283 \text{ K}) = (V_2)/(303 \text{ K}).$$

Solving for V_2 gives

$$V_2 = 321 \text{ mL},$$

which agrees with the logical speculation.

The kinetic molecular theory of gases can be summarized in the following three statements developed from the five postulates for kinetic theory:

1. Gases are composed of separate particles called molecules. The volume occupied by these individual molecules is quite insignificant compared with the total volume of the gas. These gas molecules are relatively far apart and have little attraction for one another.
2. Gas molecules are in constant motion. The molecules can vary in speed. They travel in straight lines in all directions and have perfectly elastic collisions with the walls of their containers and each other. The average number of collisions with the walls of their container determines the pressure of the gas.
3. The average kinetic energy of different gas molecules is the same at the same temperature. This kinetic energy increases and decreases with the temperature. Because

$$\text{Kinetic energy} = \frac{1}{2}mv^2,$$

where m is the mass of the molecule and v is the velocity of the molecule, molecules of small mass (e.g., hydrogen) must move at higher speeds compared with more massive molecules (e.g., chlorine) to have the same kinetic energy.

The laws previously mentioned apply to ideal gases that do not exist. Real gases differ from ideal gases in several ways:

1. Their molecules are not geometric points; that is, they do occupy space.
2. Real gas molecules do experience a slight attraction for one another.
3. The collisions of real gas molecules are not perfectly elastic. Real gases can behave very much like ideal gases under conditions of low pressure and high temperature.

When a mixture of gases is present, the molar fraction of each gas present exerts its own pressure. These individual gas pressures can be summed to find the total pressure of the system. For example, in a closed system, He, Ar, CO_2, and H_2 are present at pressures of 450, 230, 86, and 3 torr, respectively. The total pressure of the system is

$$(450 + 230 + 86 + 3) = 769 \text{ torr}.$$

Problem

A. A gas has a volume of 30.0 mL and a pressure of 420 torr. What is its new pressure if the temperature is held constant and the volume is changed to 500 mL?

B. A gas occupies 6.0 liters at 200 K. What is its new temperature if the pressure is kept constant and the volume changed to 10 liters?

C. Helium is present in a container at a pressure of 5 atm. Xenon is introduced until the total pressure is 25 atm. What is the pressure of the xenon?

D. How many moles of carbon monoxide are present in a volume of 20.0 liters at 300 K and 2.00 atm of pressure?

Solution

A. $P_1V_1 = P_2V_2 \quad P_2 = \dfrac{P_1V_1}{V_2} = \dfrac{420 \text{ torr} \times 30 \text{ mL}}{500 \text{ mL}} = 25.2 \text{ torr}$

B. $\dfrac{V_1}{T_1} = \dfrac{V_2}{T_2}; \; T_2 = \dfrac{V_2T_1}{V_1}; \dfrac{200 \text{ K}(10 \text{ L})}{6 \text{ L}} = 333 \text{ K}$

C. Total pressure $= P_{He} + P_{Xe}$; 25 atm = 5 atm + P_{Xe}; P_{Xe} = 20 atm

D. $PV = nRT; \; n = \dfrac{PV}{RT} = \dfrac{2 \text{ atm}(20.0 \text{ L})}{0.0821(300 \text{ K})} = 1.62$ moles CC

Problem

A. Hydrochloric acid can react with sodium carbonate to form carbon dioxide by the following unbalanced reaction:

$HCl + Na_2CO_3 \rightarrow NaCl + CO_2 + H_2O$

290.0 grams of 80.0% pure HCl are reacted with 82.0 grams of pure Na_2CO_3. The impurities will not react at all. What volume of CO_2 will be produced by this reaction at 80°C and 700 torr pressure?

B. How many grams of steam at 100°C and 1 atm pressure will fill a 55.0-gallon drum? (1 gallon = 3.88 liters.) How many grams will it hold if the temperature of the steam is raised to 200°C?

C. Oxygen gas can be produced by the decomposition of potassium chlorate by the following unbalanced reaction:

$KClO_3 \rightarrow KCl + O_2$

2.00 liters of oxygen gas are collected over water at 15°C. The vapor pressure of water at this temperature is 22.0 torr. The pressure of the wet gas is 1.00 atm. How many grams of pure potassium perchlorate must decompose to produce the 2.00 liters of O_2?

D. Calculate the density of radon gas at 25°C and 1.00 atm.

Solution

A. Calculate the molecular weights:

HCl = (1 + 35) = 36 amu

Na_2CO_3 = [(2 × 23) + 12 + (3 ×16)] = 106 amu

Calculate total grams of HCl:

290.0 × 80.0% = 232 g of HCl

Calculate moles of HCl:

$$232\,\text{g}\left(\frac{1\ \text{moleHCl}}{36\ \text{gHCl}}\right) = 6.44\ \text{moles HCl}$$

Calculate moles of Na_2CO_3:

$$82\ \text{grams}\ Na_2CO_3\left(\frac{1\ \text{mole}\ Na_2CO_3}{106\ \text{grams}\ Na_2CO_3}\right) = 0.774\ \text{moles}\ Na_2CO_3$$

Balance the equation:

$$2HCl + Na_2CO_3 \rightarrow 2NaCl + CO_2 + H_2O$$

Determine the limiting reagent; in this case, it is Na_2CO_3 because it will be used up and HCl will be left over.

Calculate the moles of CO_2 produced. The balanced equation shows that for every mole of Na_2CO_3 consumed, one mole of CO_2 is produced; thus, 0.774 mole of CO_2 is produced.

Convert Celsius to kelvin:

$$(80 + 273) = 353\ \text{K}$$

Convert torr to atmospheres:

$$(700/760) = 0.921\ \text{atm}$$

Calculate volume of CO_2:

$$PV = nRT;\ (0.921)(V) = (0.774)(0.0821)(353);\ V = 24.4\ \text{liters}$$

OR

Calculate CO_2 volume at STP:

$$0.744 \times 22.4 = 17.3\ \text{liters}$$

Change pressure to 700 torr:

$$P_1V_1 = P_2V_2;\ (760)(17.3) = (700)(V_2);\ V_2 = 18.8\ \text{liters at 273 K}$$

Change temperature to 353 K:

$$V_1/T_1 = V_2/T_2;\ (18.8/273) = (V_2/353);\ V_2 = 24.4\ \text{liters}$$

B. Calculate number of liters in 55.0 gallons:

$$(55.0 \times 3.88) = 213\ \text{liters}$$

Convert Celsius to kelvin:

$$(100 + 273) = 373\ \text{K}$$

Calculate moles of steam (assuming steam is an ideal gas):

$$PV = nRT;\ (1)(213) = n\,(0.0821)(373);\ n = 6.96\ \text{moles of steam}$$

OR

Change conditions to STP:

$V_1/T_1 = V_2/T_2$; $(213/373) = (V_2/273)$; $V_2 = 156$ liters

Calculate number of moles:

$22.4/156 = 6.96$ liters.

Calculate the molecular weight of steam:

H_2O, $(2 \times 1) + (1 \times 16) = 18$ daltons

Calculate the mass of steam:

$$6.96 \text{ moles of steam}\left(\frac{18 \text{ g steam}}{1 \text{ mole}}\right) = 125 \text{ grams of steam}$$

Repeating these calculations at 200°C (473 K), a mass of 98.7 grams is obtained.

C. Convert vapor pressure of water to atm: $22/760 = 0.029$ atm.

Subtract water pressure from total pressure to get the pressure of O_2:

$1.00 - 0.029 = 0.971$ atm of O_2

The balanced equation is

$2KClO_3 \rightarrow 2KCl + 3O_2$.

Find moles of O_2 using $PV = nRT$:

$(0.971)(2) = n(0.0821)(288)$; $n = 0.0821$ mole of O_2

molecular weight of $KClO_3 = (1 \times 39.1) + (1 \times 35.4) + (3 \times 16) = 122.5$ amu

$$\text{Moles of } KClO_3 = 0.0821 \text{ moles } O_2\left(\frac{2 \text{ moles } KClO_3}{3 \text{ moles } O_2}\right) = 0.0548 \text{ moles } KClO_3$$

$$\text{Grams of } KClO_3 = 0.0548 \text{ moles}\left(\frac{122.5 \text{ g}}{1 \text{ mole}}\right) = 6.7 \text{ grams}$$

D. Any amount of radon can be used, but 1 mole is the easiest to work with. One mole of radon will have a mass of 222 grams under any conditions (look at the atomic weight).

Convert Celsius to kelvin:

$(25 + 273) = 298$ K

Using $PV = nRT$ gives the volume:

$(1)\ V = (1)(0.0821)(298)$; $V = 24.4$ liters

Calculate density:

$(222/24.4) = 9.10$ g/liter

2. PHASE EQUILIBRIA

In a solid, the molecules are packed tightly together with no room for movement other than slight vibration. When the solid is heated, the vibrations increase until the molecules can break away from one another. At that point, the molecules are moving fairly rapidly with a fair amount of distance between them. Under such conditions, it is said that the solid has melted. If heated further, the molecules move farther apart and travel at greater speeds until they are at relatively great distances from one another and traveling at fairly high speeds. At that point, the liquid has become a gas. A change of state—such as liquid to gas or solid to liquid—is termed a phase transition.

Figure 2 shows the changes of state of water. As energy is added to the system, the temperature of the ice increases until it reaches 0°C. At that point, energy is still absorbed by the system, but there is no further increase in temperature because the energy is used to melt the ice. Ice and water can both exist at 0°C. After the ice has totally melted, addition of further energy results in an increase in the water's temperature until it reaches 100°C. Again, energy is absorbed without any increase in temperature. This time the energy is used to convert the liquid to a gas. Water and steam can both exist at 100°C. After all the water has been converted to steam, addition of further energy increases the temperature of the steam.

FIGURE 2. Changes of State of Water

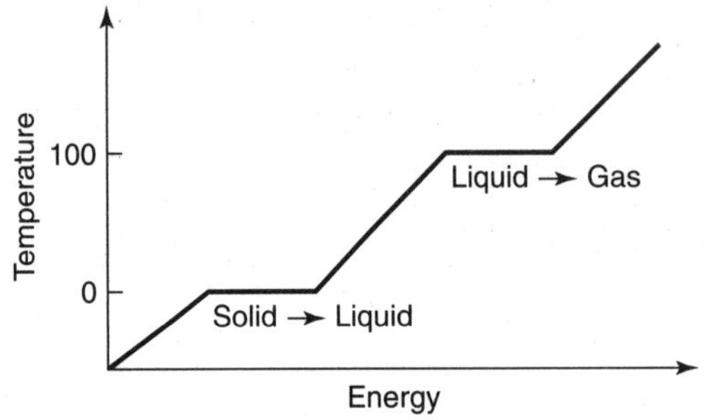

At standard pressure, water boils at 100°C and ice melts at 0°C. However, the boiling point can change drastically at other pressures, whereas the melting point remains fairly constant, decreasing only slightly with a great increase in pressure. The vapor pressure of a liquid increases with temperature. When the vapor pressure equals atmospheric pressure, boiling occurs. Obviously, if the atmospheric pressure is lowered, the liquid does not have to be heated to as high a temperature to boil. Conversely, at a higher atmospheric pressure, the liquid will boil at a higher temperature. A plot of temperature versus pressure for a substance is called a phase diagram.

A phase diagram for water is shown in Figure 3. At the pressures and temperatures in the upper-left corner, water can exist only as ice and is thus labeled "solid." Moving to the right, crossing the vertical line at 0° but not crossing the line that curves up to the right, are the temperatures and pressures where water exists only as a liquid; thus, it is labeled as such. Beyond the line that curves up, water exists as a gas. The intersection of the two lines, at 0.01°C and 4.6 torr for water, is called the triple point. At that pressure and temperature, water can exist in equilibrium in all three states of matter.

FIGURE 3. Phase Diagram for Water

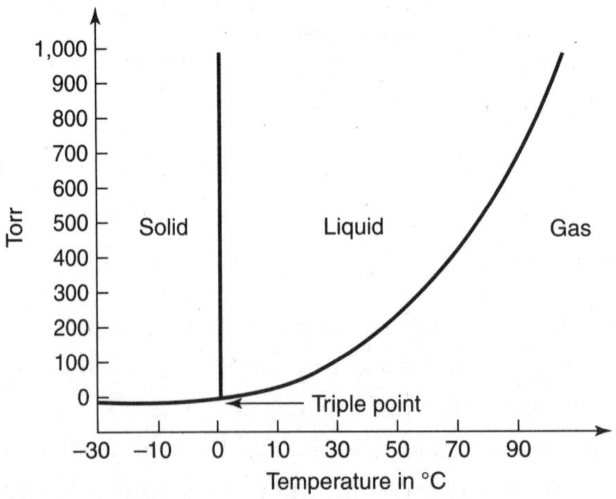

As mentioned earlier, the melting and boiling points of pure substances are constant and can be used to aid in identifying the substances. However, if other materials are present, these and other properties can be altered. The material present in the greatest quantity is called the solvent, and the material present in the least quantity is called the solute. Together they make what is called the solution. In a solution, several colligative properties of the solvent are altered. Among these are vapor pressure lowering, freezing point depression, and boiling point and osmotic pressure elevation. Vapor pressure lowering follows Raoult's law, which states that

$$P = XP^{\circ},$$

where P is the vapor pressure of the solvent over the solution, X is the mole fraction of solvent in the solution, and P° is the vapor pressure of the pure solvent at the same temperature. The osmotic pressure is the minimum pressure that must be applied to a solution bound by a semipermeable membrane to keep osmosis from occurring. This osmotic pressure is denoted by the symbol π and is calculated as

$$\pi = MRT,$$

where M is the number of moles of solute found per liter of solution, R is the universal gas law constant (0.0821 atm × liter/mole × K), and T is the temperature in kelvin.

At this point, it is useful to introduce a unit of concentration: molality (abbreviated m). Molality is defined as the number of moles of solute per kilogram of solvent. For example, if 2.00 moles of sodium chloride are dissolved in water, and the total mass of the solvent is 1 kg, the resulting concentration is 2.00 m. If 0.01 mole of camphor is dissolved in benzene with a mass of 0.150 kg, the concentration is (0.01/0.150) = 0.0667 m.

For every mole of solute dissolved per kilogram of solution, the boiling point of the solution is raised a constant amount above that of the pure solvent, and the freezing point is lowered by a constant amount below that of the pure solvent. For water, the boiling point elevation, k_b, is 0.52°C, and the freezing point depression, k_f, is 1.86°C. Thus, a 1.00 m solution of sugar in water boils at 100.52°C and freezes at −1.86°C. A 2.00 m solution of sugar in water would boil at

$$BP + \Delta T = \text{new boiling point}$$
$$\Delta T = k_b m_{\text{solute}}$$
$$[100 + (2 \times 0.52)] = 101.04^{\circ}\text{C},$$

and would freeze at

$$MP - \Delta T = \text{new melting point}$$
$$\Delta T = k_f m_{\text{solute}}$$
$$[0 - (2 \times 1.86)] = -3.72^{\circ}\text{C}.$$

If the solute dissociates to form ions in solution, the number of moles of ions formed per mole of solute is multiplied by the molality to calculate the freezing point depression and boiling point elevation. (Determining whether or not a material will dissociate into ions is discussed in more detail later in the review.) For example, if a material that dissociates into three ions when dissolved in water (three moles of ions per mole of material) is dissolved to make a 1.00 m aqueous solution, what are its boiling and freezing points? First, the number of ions formed per mole of material must be multiplied by the molality: 3 × 1 = 3. This value is now used to calculate the new boiling and freezing points:

$$\Delta T_{bp} = k_b m i$$
$$[100 + (3 \times 0.52)] = 101.56^{\circ}\text{C}$$

is the new boiling point, and

$$\Delta T_{fp} = k_f mi$$
$$[0 - (3 \times 1.86)] = -5.58°C$$

is the new freezing point.

Problem

A. Using Raoult's law, determine the vapor pressure of a solution in which the solvent is present at 95.6 molar percent. The vapor pressure of the pure solvent at the same temperature is 830 torr.

B. What is the osmotic pressure, π, of a solution at 400 K if the concentration is 0.0016 mole per liter?

C. What is the concentration in molality of 4.68 moles of $CuCl_2$ dissolved in water, so the final mass of the solution is 15.0 kg?

D. If $CuCl_2$ dissociates to form three ions when dissolved in water, what is the boiling point of the solution in question C? What is the freezing point?

Solution

A. 793 torr $= P = xP^{\circ} = 0.956 \times 830$ torr

B. 0.052 atm $= \pi = mrT = 0.0016 \times 0.0821 \times 400$

C. 0.326 m (remember, total solution mass = solvent mass + solute mass)

Molecular weight of $CuCl_2 = 63.5 + (35.5 \times 2) = 134.5$ amu

Grams of $CuCl_2 = 4.68$ moles $\times$ 134.5 g/mole = 629.4 g

$$\text{Molality} = \frac{4.68\text{ moles}}{15\text{ kg} - 0.629\text{ kg}} = 0.326\text{ m}$$

D. Boiling point = 100.51°C; freezing point = −1.82°C

$$\Delta T = k_b mi$$
$$= 0.52\ (0.326)\ 3$$
$$= 0.51°C$$
$$\Delta T = k_f mi$$
$$= 1.86\ (0.326)\ 3$$
$$= 1.82°C$$

Problem

A. What is the freezing point of 2.81 liters of water after 5.26 grams of ethanol (CH_3OH) are added to it?

B. What is the boiling point of a solution made by adding 9.32 grams of water to 2.68 kg of acetic acid (CH_3COOH)? The normal boiling point of acetic acid is 118°C, and the k_b is 2.93.

C. 10.0 grams of an unknown hydrocarbon are dissolved in 1.00 kg of cyclohexane. The freezing point of the solution is 5.09°C. What is the molecular weight of the hydrocarbon? The normal freezing point of cyclohexane is 6.50°C, and the k_f is 20.2.

Solution

A. Find the total weight of the solvent:

2.81 liters of water have a mass of 2.81 kg

Calculate the molecular weight of ethanol:

$(1 \times 12) + (4 \times 1) + (16 \times 1) = 32$ amu

Find the number of moles of ethanol:

$5.26/32 = 0.0164$ mole

Calculate molality:

$0.0164/2.810 = 0.0584$ m

Multiply by the k_f of water:

$(0.0584 \times 1.86) = 0.109°C$

Subtract this value from the normal freezing point of water:

$0 - 0.109 = -0.109°C$

B. The solvent is acetic acid:

Mass of solvent = 2.68 kg

Calculate the molecular weight of water (H_2O):

$(1 \times 2) + (16 \times 1) = 18$ amu

Calculate the number of moles of water:

$(9.32/18) = 0.518$ mole of H_2O

Calculate the molality of the solution:

$0.518/2.68 = 0.193$ m

Multiply by the k_b for acetic acid:

$(0.193 \times 2.93) = 0.565°C$

Add this to the normal boiling point:

$(0.565 + 118.000) = 118.565°C$

C. Determine the change in freezing point:

$(5.09 - 6.50) = -1.41°C$

Divide the freezing-point change by the k_f to get the molality of solution:

$(1.41/20.2) = 0.0698$ m

Determine the total moles of hydrocarbon present, using 1 kg of solvent:

$(0.0698 \times 1.00) = 0.0698$ mole of hydrocarbon

Determine the molecular weight of the hydrocarbon:

$(10.0/0.0698) = 143$ daltons

V. SOLUTION CHEMISTRY

1. IONS IN SOLUTION

Any salt that is soluble in water will dissociate into ions. Positively charged ions are called cations and negatively charged ions are called anions. Any salt that is soluble in water will dissociate into anions and cations when dissolved in water. For example, NaCl dissolved in water becomes sodium cations and chloride anions. This is represented as

$$NaCl \rightarrow Na^+ + Cl^-.$$

Notice that 2 moles of ions are produced per mole of salt dissolved. This is important to keep in mind when doing freezing-point depression and boiling-point elevation calculations, as well as molecular weight determinations using molality. Na_3PO_4 will produce four ions:

$$Na_3PO_4 \rightarrow 3Na^+ + PO_4^{\equiv}$$

Here are some rules about naming common ions:

1. Single cations are simply called by the element's name. For example Na^+ would be called a sodium ion, Al^{3+} would be called an aluminum ion.
2. The only common polyatomic cation is NH_4^+, which is called ammonium.
3. Single anions are named by dropping the ending of the element's name and adding *-ide*. For example, Cl^- is chloride, $S^=$ is sulfide, and N^- is nitride. Most of the names of polyatomic anions have to do with the number of oxygen atoms associated with them.
4. For the halogen family (F, Cl, Br, I), nitrogen, and carbon, if three oxygens are combined with the atom, the ending is changed to *-ate*. For example, ClO_3^- is chlorate, NO_3^- is nitrate, and CO_3^{2-} is carbonate. With the exception of CO_3^{2-}, all these ions have a -1 charge.
5. If four oxygens are combined with the atoms mentioned in rule 4, the prefix *per-* is placed before the name of the atom, and the suffix *-ate* is used. For example, ClO_4^- is perchlorate and BrO_4^- is perbromate.
6. If only two oxygen atoms are associated with the atoms mentioned in rule 4, the suffix *-ite* is used. For example, NO_2^- is nitrite and ClO_2^- is chlorite.
7. If the atoms mentioned in rule 4 are associated with only one oxygen atom, the prefix *hypo-* and suffix *-ite* are used. For example, ClO^- is hypochlorite and IO^- is hypoiodite.
8. $SO_4^=$ is sulfate; one less oxygen makes it $SO_3^=$, which is sulfite.
9. PO_4^- is phosphate; one less oxygen makes it PO_3^-, which is phosphite.
10. CN^- is cyanide.
11. CH_3COO^- is acetate.

2. SOLUBILITY

The concentration of solutions can be expressed in many ways. The easiest is percent composition, which can be by either volume or mass. If 5.0 mL of acetone is added to 95.0 mL of water, it is a 5.0% (V) solution. Dissolving 8.0 grams of sugar into 92.0 grams of water yields an 8.0% (W) solution. As discussed earlier, molality is the number of moles of solute per kilogram of solvent. Dissolving 78.0 moles of decane into 3.45 kg of benzene, the concentration is

$$(78.0/3.45) = 22.6 \text{ m}.$$

Molarity (abbreviated M) is the most commonly used unit of concentration in chemistry. Molarity is defined as the number of moles of solute per liter of solution. If 10.0 moles of carbon disulfide are dissolved to produce 2.00 liters of solution, the concentration is

$(10.0/2.00) = 5.00$ M.

The solubility of most common salts in water can usually be determined by the following generalizations. (Keep in mind, however, that these are generalizations!)

1. Most nitrates and acetates are soluble. Silver, chromium (II), and mercury (I) acetate are only slightly soluble.
2. All chlorates are soluble except potassium chlorate, which is slightly soluble.
3. All chlorides are soluble except those of mercury (I), silver, lead, and copper (I).
4. All sulfates are soluble except those of strontium, barium, and lead. Calcium and silver sulfate are slightly soluble.
5. Carbonates and phosphates are insoluble except for those of ammonium and the group 1A metals.
6. All sulfides other than ammonium and group I and group II salts are insoluble.
7. The hydroxides of the group 1A metals, ammonium, barium, and strontium are soluble. Calcium hydroxide is slightly soluble. All other hydroxides are insoluble. For salts considered slightly soluble, a very small amount actually does go into solution. From this can be calculated the solubility product constant, k_{sp}.

It should be noted that the k_{sp} changes with temperature, most are given at 25°C. For an insoluble salt that dissociates

$$A_xB_y \rightarrow xA^+ + yB^-$$

the k_{sp} can be calculated as follows:

$$k_{sp} = \frac{[A^+]^x[B^-]^y}{[AxBy]^1}.$$

The brackets, [ ], denote "concentration (in molarity) of the entity enclosed therein." Also note that the coefficients l, x, and y become exponents. Remember, this gives the k_{sp} only for the temperature at which the concentration measurements were made. For example, MnS has a k_{sp} of 5.6×10^{-16} at 25°C. If 25.0 grams of MnS are mixed into one liter of water and allowed to settle out, what is the concentration of Mn^{2+} ions in the water? We can begin by writing the equation for the dissociation of MnS in water, even though it occurs at a very low rate:

$$MnS \rightarrow Mn^{2+} + S^{2-}$$

Fortunately, the coefficients are all 1, which makes the exponents very easy to handle:

$$k_{sp} = \frac{[Mn^{2=}]^1[S^{2-}]^1}{[MnS]^1}$$

We can also conclude that $[Mn^{2+}] = [S^{2-}]$. As can be seen by the very low k_{sp}, most of the MnS will not be in the solution at all. When working with such highly insoluble material, its concentration is taken to be 1. Assigning the algebraic variable x to represent the $[Mn^{2+}]$, which will also equal $[S^{2-}]$, we can solve the equation:

$$5.6 \times 10^{-16} = (x \times x) / 1, \text{ or } 5.6 \times 10^{-16} = x^2, x = 2.37 \times 10^{-8}\text{M}$$

Because $x = [Mn^{++}]$, the Mn^{2+} concentration is 2.37×10^{-8} moles per liter. With such an insoluble compound, the mass added to the solvent was not even used in the calculation. It can be calculated from the information that only 2.05 micrograms of MnS went into solution that is 0.00000822% of the total salt added, a very small amount indeed. How many grams of lead are in 2.50 liters of a saturated solution of PbI_2? The k_{sp} of PbI_2 is

8.8×10^{-9} at 25°C.

A saturated solution has as much of the solute in it as possible. Any additional PbI_2 added will not go into solution. The dissociation is

$PbI_2 \rightarrow Pb^{2+} + 2I^-$.

Thus, we can write

$$K_{sp} = \frac{[Pb^{2+}]^1[I\ ]^2}{[PbI_2]^1}$$

If $x = [Pb^{2+}]$, then $2x = [I^-]$. Substituting values into the equation, we get

$8.8 \times 10^{-9} = (x) \times (2x)^2 / 1$, or $8.8 \times 10^{-9} = 4x^3$, or $x = 1.30 \times 10^{-3}M = [Pb^{2+}]$.

Multiplying by the volume of the solution gives

$(1.30 \times 10^{-3} \times 2.50) = 3.25 \times 10^{-3}$ mole of Pb^{++} present.

Converting to grams by multiplying by the atomic weight of lead, we get

$(3.25 \times 10^{-3} \times 207) = 0.670$ g of lead cations in the solution.

Return to the first example, using MnS. Suppose S^{2-} ions were added to the solution from another source. They would help to push the S^{2-} (and hence Mn^{2+}) out of the solution. This is known as the common ion effect. Repeating the example but dissolving the MnS into 0.100 M $(NH_4)_2S$, we can see how much less Mn^{2+} is in solution. From the solubility rules, we know that ammonium sulfide dissociates readily $(NH_4)_2S \rightarrow 2NH_4^+ + S^{2-}$. Thus, the $[S^{2-}]$ from the $(NH_4)_2S$ is 0.100 M. Plugging this into the equation used earlier, there are now two sources of S^{2-}: that from the MnS (x) and the $(NH_4)_2S$ (0.100).

$$k_{sp} = \frac{[Mn^{2=}]^1[S^{2-}]^1}{[MnS]^1}$$

now becomes

$5.6 \times 10^{-16} = (x)(x + 0.100)/1$.

Because we know that x for the $S^=$ from the MnS is very low, it can be neglected. (Whenever a term is very, very small, it can be neglected in an addition or subtraction operation, but NEVER in a multiplication or division operation.) This now gives us

$5.6 \times 10^{-16} = (x)(0.100) / 1$.

Solving for x gives a value of

$[Mn^{2+}] = 5.6 \times 10^{-15}$ M,

which is seven orders of magnitude smaller than the original answer because of the common ion effect.

Problem

A. What is the percent concentration of a solution made by dissolving 28.9 grams of naphthalene into 437 grams of benzene?

B. If 20.9 moles of $CuSO_4$ are dissolved into 4.89 liters of water, what is the molarity of the solution?

C. If 0.0490 mole of NaCl are dissolved in 25.5 liters of water, what is the molarity and approximate molality of the solution?

D. If 2.8 moles of $NaNO_3$ are dissolved into 4.90 liters of water, what is the $[NO_3^-]$?

E. What is the maximum concentration of $BaSO_4$ in water? The $k_{sp} = 1.08 \times 10^{-10}$.

F. What is the maximum concentration of $BaSO_4$ in a 0.200 M solution of Na_2SO_4?

G. In a saturated solution of $Tl(OH)_3$, the $[Tl^{3+}]$ was found to be 6.38×10^{-12}, and the $[OH^-]$ was 1.92×10^{-11}. Find the k_{sp} for $Tl(OH)_3$ at this temperature.

Solution

A. $6.20\%(W) = \dfrac{28.9\text{ g}}{437\text{ g} + 28.9\text{ g}} \times 100$

B. $4.27\text{ M} = \dfrac{20.9\text{ moles}}{4.89\text{ L}}$

C. $0.00192\text{ M} = \dfrac{0.049\text{ moles}}{25.5\text{ L}}$

D. $0.571\text{ M} = \dfrac{2.8\text{ moles}}{4.90\text{ L}}$

$0.00192\text{ m} = \dfrac{0.049\text{ moles}}{25.5\text{ kg}}$

E. 1.04×10^{-5} M

F. 5.40×10^{-10} M

$k_{sp} = [Ba^{2+}][SO4^{2-}] = 1.08 \times 10^{-10}$

$[Ba^{2+}] = \sqrt{1.08 \times 10^{-10}} = [BaSO4]\text{ solution}$

$k_{sp} = [Ba^{2+}][SO_4^{2-}] = 1.08 \times 10^{-10}$

$(x)(0.20) = 1.08 \times 10^{-10}$

$x = [Ba^{2+}] = [BaSO4]\text{solution}$

G. 4.52×10^{-44}

$Ti(OH)_3 \rightarrow Ti^{3+} + 3OH^-$

$K_{sp} = [Ti^{3+}][OH^-]^3$

$= [6.38 \times 10^{-12}][1.92 \times 10^{-11}]^3$

VI. ACIDS AND BASES

1. ACID–BASE EQUILIBRIA

By the Brönsted–Lowry definitions, an acid is a proton donor and a base is a proton acceptor. Consider the acid HA and the base B^-. The acid can donate its proton, and the base accepts it by the following reaction:

$$HA + B^- \rightarrow A^- + HB,$$

where HB is the conjugate acid, and A^- is the conjugate base. For example, the amino acid glycine can act as an acid or a base. In the reaction

$$H_2NCH_2COOH + H_3O^+ \rightarrow {}^+H_3NCH_2COOH + H_2O$$

it is behaving as a base, accepting a proton from a hydronium ion, and becoming a conjugate acid in the process. In the reaction

$$H_2NCH_2COOH + H_2O \rightarrow H_2NCH_2COO^- + H_3O^+$$

glycine is behaving as an acid, donating a proton to the water molecule, and becoming a conjugate base. Water can behave as both an acid and a base by the reaction

$$2H_2O \rightarrow H_3O^+ + OH^-.$$

In pure water, there is always as much H_3O^+ as OH^-. The equilibrium constant for the dissociation of water, k_w, can be calculated as

$$kw = \frac{[H_3O^+][OH^-]}{[H_2O]^2} = 10^{-14}$$

This shows that in pure water,

$$[H_3O^+] = [OH^-] = 10^{-7}$$

That is, the H_2O goes to 1.

A convenient scale for measuring the $[H_3O^+]$ in water is the pH. Any value below 7 is acidic, any value above 7 is basic, and a value of 7 is neutral:

$$pH = -\log[H_3O^+]$$

A solution with a

$$[H_3O^+] = 10^{-3}$$

will have a pH of 3, and a solution with a

$$[H_3O^+] = 10^{-11}$$

will have a pH of 11. As can be seen from the k_w, the $[H_3O^+]$ for pure water is 10^{-7}; thus, the pH of water is 7. Another important term, pOH, is defined the same way: $pOH = -\log[OH^-]$. In a solution where the

$$[OH^-] = 10^{-8},$$

the pOH is 8. The pOH of pure water is 7. The pOH and pH are related by the formula

$$14^-pOH = pH.$$

This is due to the relationship

$$k_w/[OH^-] = [H_3O^+].$$

Strong acids and bases dissociate readily in water. Strong acids include HCl, H_2SO_4, HNO_3, and $HClO_4$. Strong bases include any hydroxide of the group 1A metals. Because strong acids completely dissociate, their pH is easy to calculate. HCl dissociates by the reaction

$$HC1 + H_2O \rightarrow H_3O^+ + Cl^-.$$

If a solution of HCl is 10^{-2}M, then the $[H_3O^+] = 10^{-2}$M, and the pH is 2.0.

Sulfuric acid gives up two protons by the reaction

$$H_2SO_4 + 2H_2O \rightarrow SO_4^{2-} + 2H_3O^+.$$

If a solution is

$$2.5 \times 10^{-5}\text{M in } H_2SO_4,$$

then the $[H_3O^+]$ will be twice that, or 5.0×10^{-5}, and the pH will be 4.30. (It is necessary to have a table of common logarithms or a calculator for most pH calculations.) There are two ways to calculate the pH of a solution of a strong base. One is to calculate the pOH and convert it to pH; the other is to convert the $[OH^-]$ to $[H_3O^+]$ and calculate the pH. In a 3.8×10^{-3} M solution of NaOH, the base is entirely dissociated:

$$NaOH \rightarrow Na^+ + OH^-; [OH^-] = 3.8 \times 10^{-3}.$$

Calculating the pOH gives a value of 2.42. Substituting into the equation:

$$14 - pOH = pH,$$

we get a value of

$$(14 - 2.42) = 11.58 = pH.$$

Solving by the other method, we convert

$$[OH^-] \text{ to } [H_3O^+], (10^{-14}/3.8 \times 10^{-3}) = 2.63 \times 10^{-12} = [H_3O^+].$$

Thus, the pH is 11.58, the same as with the other method. What is the pH of a solution of HNO_3 that is 10^{-9} M? One might assume that the $[H_3O^+] = 10^{-9}$ and therefore the pH = 9. Can an acidic solution have a pH above 7.0? Obviously not. In this case, the $[H_3O^+]$ from the water (normally insignificant) must be included. The total is

$$[H_3O^+] = 10^{-9} \text{ (from the } HNO_3) + 10^{-7} \text{ (from the } H_2O) = 1.01 \times 10^{-7},$$

which gives a pH of 6.9957, or for all practical purposes, 7.0.

Weak acids do not dissociate entirely, nor do weak bases. Formic acid will dissociate somewhat,

$$HCOOH + H_2O \rightarrow HCOO^- + H_3O^+,$$

but most will stay in molecular form. The dissociation constant k_a can be calculated for a particular weak acid at a particular temperature just as one might do the solubility constant k_{sp}.

For formic acid, the equation is

$$ka = \frac{[HCOO^-][H_3O^+]}{[HCOOH]}$$

For formic acid,

$$k_a = 1.8 \times 10^{-4} \text{ at } 25°C.$$

What is the pH of a 7.28×10^{-2} M solution of formic acid at 25°C? From the dissociation equation, it can be seen that

$$[HCOO^-] = [H_3O^+].$$

As was done with the k_{sp} values, let the above ion concentrations equal x. The amount of undissociated formic acid will be

$$7.28 \times 10^{-2} - x.$$

Plugging these numbers into the equation yields

$$1.8 \times 10^{-4} = x^2/(7.28 \times 10^{-2} - x),$$

which can be solved as a quadratic:

$$x^2 + (1.80 \times 10^{-4})\,x - (1.31 \times 10^{-5}) = 0$$

Solving for x yields values of $+3.53 \times 10^{-3}$ M and -3.71×10^{-3} m for x and thus the $[H_3O^+]$.

Because an ion concentration cannot be negative, the positive value is chosen. Calculating the pH from this gives a value of 2.45. Solving quadratic equations is easier than it used to be, thanks to calculators, and often one can run into cubics and even quartics in such calculations. However, the MCAT does not allow the luxury of a calculator. Fortunately, the amount of formic acid lost to the formation of formate and hydronium ions is small, so small that it can be neglected, changing the equation to

$$1.8 \times 10^{-4} = x^2 / 7.28 \times \tilde{10}^{-2}.$$

This is easy to solve, giving

$$x = 3.62 \times 10^{-3}\text{ M} = [H_3O^+], \text{pH} = 2.44.$$

As the k_a gets even smaller, the accuracy of this method increases even more. If more H_3O^+ is added to the weak acid (e.g., in the form of a strong acid), the molecular species becomes more predominate. The pk_a is defined as $-\log(k_a)$ and is the pH at which the concentration of the molecular form is equal to the concentration of the dissociated form. For formic acid, the pk_a is

$$-\log(1.8 \times 10^{-4}) = 3.74.$$

The pH of solutions of weak bases is determined by the same method. What is the pH of a 0.200 M solution of phenylamine (aniline)? The dissociation of phenylamine in water can be written as

$$C_6H_5NH_2 + H_2O \rightleftharpoons C_6H_5NH_3^+ + OH^-.$$

From this, the equation for dissociation constant (for bases, k_b) can be written as

$$k_b = \frac{[C_6H_5NH_3^+][OH^-]}{[C_6H_5NH_2]}$$

(Note that, as with the acids, the term $[H_2O]$ does not enter into this equation because it has an effective concentration of 1.) For phenylamine, the k_b is 4.6×10^{-10}. Because $[C_6H_5NH_3^+] = [OH^-]$, the algebraic variable x can be used for the concentration of either of these. The amount lost from the original 0.200 M phenylamine, x, is so small as to be negligible. The resultant equation is

$$4.6 \times 10^{-10} = x^2 / 0.200, \text{ or } x = 9.59 \times 10^{-6} = [OH^-].$$

This gives a pOH of 5.02 and a pH of 8.98. The pH could also have been calculated by dividing the k_w by the $[OH^-]$ to obtain the $[H_3O^+]$. The pk_b of a weak base is the pH value at which half of it is dissociated and half of it is in molecular form. It is calculated as

$$pk_b = 14^- (^-\log(k_b)).$$

For phenylamine, the $pk_b = 4.66$.

Problem

What is the pH of aqueous solutions of the following?

A. 0.04 M HCl

B. 0.04 M H_2SO_4

C. 0.04 M benzoic acid

($C_6H_5COOH + H_2O \rightarrow C_6H_5COO^- + H_3O^+, k_a = 6.3 \times 10^{-5}$)

D. 4.00 M HCl

E. 0.04 M NaOH

F. 4.00 M NaOH

G. 4×10^{-14} M NaOH

H. 0.04 M ethylamine

($CH_3CH_2NH_2 + H_2O \rightarrow CH_3CH_2NH_3^+ + OH^-, k_b = 4.3 \times 10^{-4}$)

Solution

A. $1.40 = -\log[H_3O^+]$

B. $1.097 = -\log[H_3O^+] = -\log[0.04x2]$

C. 2.80; $Ka = 6.3 \times 10^{-5} = \dfrac{x^2}{0.04}$

$x = 1.59 \times 10^{-3}$

D. $-0.60 = -\log[H_3O^+]$

E. 12.60

F. 13.4

$$\begin{aligned} pH &= 14 - pOH \\ &= 14 - (-\log[0.04]) \\ &= 14 - 1.39 \end{aligned}$$

$$\begin{aligned} pH &= 14 - pOH \\ &= 14 - (-\log[4.0]) \\ &= 14 - 0.60 \end{aligned}$$

G. 7.00

H. 11.62

$10^{-7} + 4 \times 10^{-14} = [OH^-]$

$[OH^-] = 10^{-7}$

$pH = 7$

$Kb = 4.3 \times 10^{-4} = \dfrac{x^2}{0.04}$

$x = 0.004$

2. SALTS OF ACIDS AND BASES

A salt of a strong acid and strong base will yield a neutral solution when dissolved in water, no matter what its concentration is. For example, the pH of a 0.125 M NaCl solution is 7.00.

The salt of a weak acid and strong base will yield a basic solution when dissolved in water. What is the pH of a 0.125 M sodium acetate solution? The k_a for acetic acid is 1.75×10^{-5}. Sodium acetate will dissociate to form ions:

$$CH_3COONa \rightarrow CH_3COO^- + Na^+$$

The acetate ion will want to take a proton from the water:

$$CH_3COO^- + H_2O \rightarrow CH_3COOH + OH^-$$

The equilibrium constant for this can be calculated as

$$k_{eq} = \frac{[CH_3COOH]^1[OH^-]^1}{[CH_3COO^-]^1}$$

This is very similar to the expression for the k_a. By multiplying the numerator and denominator by $[H_3O^+]$, we get

$$k_{eq} = \frac{[CH_3COOH][OH^-][H_3O^+]}{[CH_3COO^-][H_3O^+]}$$

Recall that the term in the numerator $[OH^-]\,[H_3O^+] = k_w$; thus, the equation can be rewritten as

$$k_{eq} = \frac{[CH_3COOH]k_w}{[CH_3COO^-][H_3O^+]}$$

Notice the term involving concentrations is now the reciprocal of the k_a times the k_w. This can be rewritten as

$$k_{eq} = k_w\,(1/k_a) = k_w/k_a$$

The value for this can now be calculated:

$$10^{-14}/1.75 \times 10^{-5} = 5.71 \times 10^{-10} = [CH_3COOH]\,[OH^-]$$

Assigning the algebraic variable x to represent the $[OH^-]$, we can also see that

$$x = [CH_3COOH].$$

That is, for every acetate converted to acetic acid, a water molecule is converted to a hydroxide ion.

The $[CH_3COO^-]$ is equal to 0.125 M minus what was lost to form acetic acid, as in $0.125 - x$. The amount lost to this is so slight that it can be neglected. The final equation is

$$5.71 \times 10^{-10} = x^2/0.125,$$

and solving for x gives a $[OH^-] = 8.45 \times 10^{-6}$, a pOH $= 5.07$, and a pH $= 8.93$.

Calculations involving the salt of a weak base and strong acid are much the same, except the solution will be acidic. What is the pH of a 0.125 M solution of ammonium chloride? The k_b for ammonium hydroxide is 1.80×10^{-5}. Ammonium chloride will dissociate by

$$NH_4Cl \rightarrow NH_4^+ + Cl^-.$$

The ammonium ions formed will react with the water. Thus,

$$NH_4^+ + H_2O \rightarrow NH_3 + H_3O^+,$$

resulting in an acidic solution. As with the previous example, the

$$k_{eq} = \frac{[NH_3][H_3O^+]}{[NH_4^+]}$$

This time, multiplying the numerator and denominator by $[OH^-]$ yields $k_{eg} = k_w/k_b$. (See the previous paragraph for the mathematics.) We know that $[NH_3] = [H_3O^+]$ and can be assigned the value x. Thus

$[NH_4^+] = 0.125 - x$

(x being the amount lost by dissociation), and x is small enough to be neglected. The final formula is

$$\frac{10^{-14}}{1.8 \times 10^{-5}} = \frac{x^2}{0.125}$$

Solving for x gives a $[H_3O^+] = 8.33 \times 10^{-6}$, and a pH of 5.08.

For solutions of salts of weak acids and weak bases, the pH can be either acidic or basic, depending on the salt. What is the pH of a 0.125 M solution of ammonium formate? The k_b for ammonium hydroxide is

1.80×10^{-5},

and the k_a for formic acid is

1.76×10^{-4}.

To spare a lot of mathematics,

$[H_3O^+] = ((k_w k_a) / k_b)^{1/2}$.

Notice that this formula does not even concern the concentration of the salt. This is true so long as the concentration of the salt is greater than the $[OH^-]$ and $[H_3O^+]$ in pure water. If it is below these values, the pH is 7.00. Solving the previous equation yields

$$[H_3O^+] = ((10^{-14} \times 1.76 \times 10^{-4}) / 1.80 \times 10^{-5})^{1/2}$$
$$= 3.13 \times 10^{-7}, \text{ and a pH of } 6.50.$$

Problem

What is the pH of the following solutions?

A. 0.489 M potassium nitrate (KNO_3)

B. 0.0239 M sodium fluoride (NaF); the k_a for HF is 6.7×10^{-4}

C. 0.159M hydrazine chloride (H_2NNH_3Cl); the k_b for H_2NNH_2 is 1.3×10^{-10}

D. 2.65 M aniline acetate ($C_6H_5NH_4OOCH_3$); the k_a of CH_3COOH is 1.75×10^{-5}, and the k_b of $C_6H_5NH_3$ is 4.0×10^{-10}

Solution

A. 7.00

B. $F^- + H_2O \rightleftharpoons OH^- + HF$

$$K_{eq} = \frac{[OH\ \ ][HF]}{[F\ \ ]}$$

$$\frac{K_w}{K_a} = \frac{x^2}{0.0239}$$

$$x = 6.0x10\ \ ^7 = [OH\ \ ]$$

$$pOH = 6.22$$

$$pH = 7.78$$

C.
$$\frac{K_w}{K_a} = \frac{x^2}{0.159}$$
$$\frac{1\times10^{-14}}{1.3\times10^{-10}} = \frac{x^2}{0.159}$$
$$x = 3.5\times10^{-3} = [H_3O^+]$$
$$pH = 2.46$$

D.
$$[H_3O^+] = \sqrt{\frac{K_w K_a}{K_b}}$$
$$= \sqrt{\frac{(1\times10^{-14})(1.75\times10^{-5})}{4.0\times10^{-10}}}$$
$$= 2.1\times10^{-5}$$
$$pH = 4.68$$

3. BUFFERS

A buffer is solution of a weak acid with one of its salts or a weak base with one of its salts. The purpose of a buffer is to resist changes in pH. (Note that the key word is *resist*, not *prevent*.) Consider a solution of hydrofluoric acid that is 0.25 M mixed with a sodium fluoride solution of 0.5 M. What is the pH of the resultant buffer? We know that NaF will dissociate as

$$NaF \rightarrow Na^+ + F^-.$$

The dissociation of HF,

$$HF + H_2O \rightarrow H_3O^+ + F^-,$$

is not very great. The k_a for the reaction is 6.7×10^{-4}. Recall that

$$k_a = \frac{[F^-][H_3O^+]}{[HF]}$$

The [HF] will equal 0.25 M minus x, the amount that dissociates. Because x is quite small, it can be neglected. $[H_3O^+] = x$, and $[F^-]$ is the sum of the F^- from the NaF and the HF, $0.50 + X$. Again, because X is so small, it can be neglected. The final equation is

$$6.7 \times 10^{-4} = (0.50)(x) / 0.25.$$

Solving for x gives $[H_3O^+] = 3.35 \times 10^{-4}$, and pH = 3.47.

Compare the reactions of this with an unbuffered solution of the same initial pH:

3.35×10^{-4} HCl

Compare the effect on pH of the addition of 10.0 mL of 2.50 M NaOH to 200 mL of each solution. In 200 mL of the unbuffered solution, there is 6.7×10^{-5} mole of H_3O^+. This will react with the NaOH in a neutralization reaction. Of the 0.025 mole of NaOH present (0.010 liter $\times$ 2.5 M = 0.025 mole), 6.7×10^{-5} will react with the acid to form NaCl, leaving 0.0249 mole left over. The new concentration is

$$0.0249 / (0.200 + 0.010) = 0.119 \text{ M} = [OH^-].$$

The pOH is 0.925, and the pH is 13.07. Compare that to the initial value of 3.47. Now look at the same amount of the NaOH solution added to 200 mL of the buffered solution. That volume of buffer will contain 0.05 mole of HF and 0.100 mole of F^-. The 0.025 mole of NaOH will react as follows:

$$OH^- + HF \rightarrow H_2O + F^-$$

After all the OH^- has reacted, 0.025 mole of HF will be left and the total F^- will be 0.125 mole (0.100 + 0.025). With the new volume of 0.210 liter, the concentrations are 0.119 M for HF and 0.595 M for F^-. Putting this into the equation gives

$$k_a = \frac{[F^-][H_3O^+]}{[HF]}$$

which yields $[H_3O^+] = 1.34 \times 10^{-4}$ and a pH = 3.87.

Note how little this has changed from the original value. Moving in the opposite direction, compare the addition of 10.0 mL of 1.00 M HNO_3 to 200 mL first of the unbuffered HCl solution and then of the previously calculated buffer of the same pH. In 200 mL of the unbuffered solution, there are 6.7×10^{-5} moles of $[H_3O^+]$. In 10.0 mL of 1.00 M HNO_3 are 0.01 mole of $[H_3O^+]$. Adding these values together gives a new concentration of

$$(0.01 + 6.7 \times 10^{-5}) / 0.210 = 0.0479 \text{ M} = [H_3O^+], \text{ and a pH} = 1.32.$$

Adding the same amount of the HNO_3 solution to 200 mL of the buffered solution alters the pH less. The reaction is

$$H_3O^+ + F^- \rightarrow HF + H_2O.$$

The F^- and HF are initially present at 0.100 mole and 0.050 mole, respectively. After the previous reaction with 0.01 mole of H_3O^+, they are 0.090 mole and 0.060 mole, and their concentrations in the new volume of 0.210 liter are 0.428 M and 0.286 M, respectively. Plugging these values into the k_a equation yields

$$[H_3O^+] = 4.48 \times 10^{-4} \text{ and a pH} = 3.35.$$

The last example will show the effect of simple dilution on buffered and unbuffered solutions. Adding 20.0 liters of pure water to 200 mL of the unbuffered HCl solution (pH = 3.47) dilutes it. The initial 6.7×10^{-5} moles of H_3O^+ are in a new volume of 20.2 liters. The $[H_3O^+] = 3.32 \times 10^{-6}$ M and the new pH = 5.48.

Adding the same amount of pure water to 200 mL of the buffered solution changes the concentration of the F^- to 4.95×10^{-3} and the HF concentration to 2.48×10^{-3}. Plugging these values into the k_a equation gives

$$[H_3O^+] = 3.36 \times 10^{-4} \text{ M, and a pH} = 3.47.$$

Notice that the pH is unchanged from the initial value.

Problem

A. 0.298 mole of methylamine (CH_3NH_2, $k_b = 4.8 \times 10^{-4}$) is mixed with 0.602 mole of methylammonium bromide (CH_3NH_3Br) in a volume of 1.00 liter of water. What is the pH? (Clue: Find the $[OH^-]$.)

B. What is the pH of the solution when 100 mL of the buffer described in part A is mixed with 50.0 mL of 0.100 M HCl? (Clue: Remember to correct for the change in volume.)

Solution

A.

$$k_b = \frac{[CH_3NH_3^+][OH^-]}{[CH_3NH_2]}$$

$$4.8 \times 10^{-4} = \frac{(0.602)[OH^-]}{0.298}$$

$$[OH^-] = 2.4 \times 10^{-4}$$

$$pOH = 3.62$$

$$pH = 10.38$$

B. Moles of HCl = 0.05 L × 0.1 M = 0.005 mole

Moles of CH_3NH_2 = (0.1 × 0.298) − (0.005) = 0.0248 mole

Moles of $CH_3NH_3^+$ = (0.1 × 0.602) + (0.005) = 0.0652 mole

$[CH_3NH_2]$ = 0.0248/(0.1 + 0.05L) = 0.165 M

$[CH_3NH_3^+]$ = 0.0652/(0.1+ 0.05L) = 0.435 M

$$kb = \frac{[CH_3NH_3^+][OH^-]}{[CH_3NH_2]}$$

$$4.8 \times 10^{-4} = \frac{(0.435)[OH^-]}{0.165}$$

$$[OH^-] = 1.8 \times 10^{-4}$$

$$pOH = 3.74$$

$$pH = 10.26$$

4. TITRATIONS

Slowly adding small aliquots of a base of known concentration to an acid of unknown concentration, and carefully measuring the pH after each addition, yields the data needed to determine the concentration of the unknown acid. The opposite can be done with a known acid and an unknown base. Either procedure is known as a titration. When a strong acid is titrated with a strong base, and the volume of the known material added is plotted on the x-axis and the resultant pH is plotted on the y-axis, the curve is almost horizontal until it nears the equivalence point, at which point it shoots up and then levels off almost horizontal again (Figure 4).

The equivalence point will be at the middle of the almost vertical portion of the plot. At that point, the amount of base equals the amount of acid. Reading down to the x-axis shows the volume of known material used, and from that it is possible to calculate the concentration of the unknown.

Titrating a weak acid with a strong base causes the left portion of the curve to flatten out; the smaller the k_a of the acid, the flatter that portion of the curve will be (Figure 5). Titrating a weak base with a strong acid will flatten out the right portion of the curve, again, depending upon k_b of the base. Titrating a weak acid with a weak base broadens the curve on both sides, and titrating a buffered solution broadens it even more.

FIGURE 4. Titration of a Strong Acid with a Strong Base

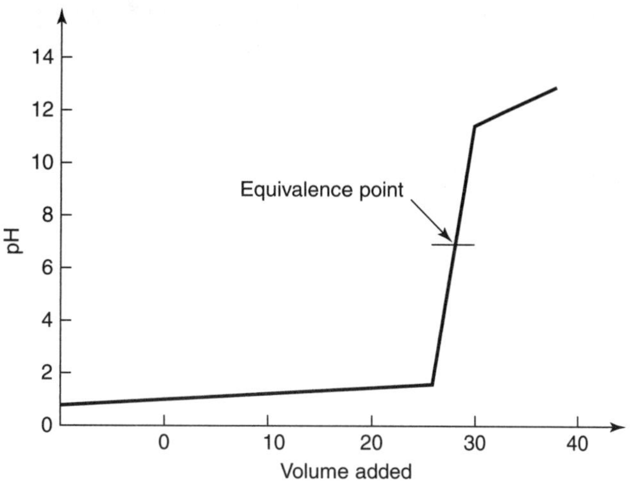

FIGURE 5. Titration of a Weak Acid with a Strong Base, with Various Values of *k*

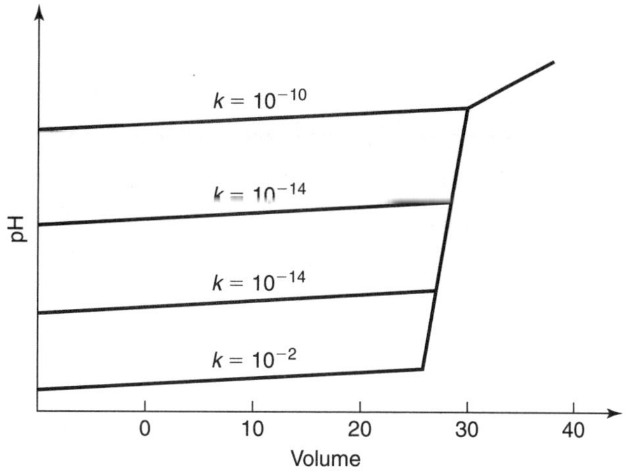

5. Indicators

Indicators are seldom used in titration anymore, having been replaced by pH meters. However, they are still included on the MCAT test. Table 4 lists various pH indicators and their color changes at various ranges.

TABLE 4. pH Indicators

Name	pH Interval	Acid Color	Base Color
Methyl violet	0.0–1.6	Yellow	Violet
Methyl yellow	2.9–4.0	Red	Yellow
Methyl orange	3.2–4.4	Red	Yellow
Methyl red	4.8–6.2	Red	Yellow

(Continued)

TABLE 4. *Continued*

Name	pH Interval	Acid Color	Base Color
Bromthymol blue	6.0–8.0	Yellow	Blue
Thymol blue	8.0–9.6	Yellow	Blue
Phenolphthalein	8.2–19.9	Colorless	Pink
Alizarine yellow	10.1–12.0	Yellow	Red

Problem

A. How many grams of BaF_2 will dissolve in 5.00 liters of water? The k_{sp} for $BaF_2 = 1.7 \times 10^{-6}$.

B. How many grams of BaF_2 will dissolve in 5.00 liters of a 0.879 M NaF solution?

C. 4.70 mL of a 4.80 M HNO_3 solution are added to 1.28 liters of water. What is the pH of the solution?

D. 4.89 grams of KOH are mixed into 28.6 liters of water. What is the pH of the solution?

E. What is the pH of a 0.249 M solution of HIO_3? The k_a for HIO_3 is 0.20.

F. What is the pH of a 0.0987 M solution of KClO? The k_a for HClO is 1.1×10^{-8}.

G. What is the pH of a 0.0987 M solution of NH_4ClO? The k_b for NH_4OH is 1.80×10^{-5}.

H. A solution of HClO has a pH of 4.65; 2.50 liters of this are mixed with 1.62 liters of the KClO solution in problem F. What is the resultant solution's pH?

I. If 1.00 gram of pure NaOH were dissolved in the solution described in H, what would the new pH be, assuming no change in volume?

Solution

A. Set up the equation for the dissociation:

$BaF_2 \rightarrow Ba^{2+} + 2F^-$

From this, the formula for the k_{sp} can be determined:

$$k_{sp} = \frac{[Ba^{2+}][F^-]^2}{[BaF^2]}$$

Using the variable x to represent $[Ba^{2+}]$, $2x = [F^-]$. The $[BaF_2]$ goes to 1. Plugging into the equation gives

$1.7 \times 10^{-6} = (x)(2x)^2 / 1.$

Simplifying yields

$1.7 \times 10^{-6} = 4x^3.$

Solving for x gives $[Ba^{2+}] = 0.00752$ M.

For every mole of BaF_2 in solution there is one mole of Ba^{2+}; thus, the $[BaF_2]$ in solution is 0.00752 M.

In 5.00 liters, there would be

$(5.00 \times 0.00752) = 0.0376$ mole of BaF_2.

Calculate the molecular weight:

$(2 \times 19) + (1 \times 137.3) = 175.3$ daltons

Calculate the mass of BaF_2 dissolved:

$(0.0376 \times 175.3) = 6.59$ g of BaF_2 in the solution

B. The same setup is used as was used in part A:

$$k_{sp} = \frac{[Ba^{2+}][F^-]^2}{[BaF^2]}$$

This time the $[F^-]$ from the BaF_2 is insignificant compared with the amount of F^- from the NaF, which is 0.879 M.

Plugging into the equation gives

$1.7 \times 10^{-6} = (x)(0.879)^2 / 1.$

Solving for x yields $[Ba^{2+}] = 2.20 \times 10^{-6}$ M.

For every mole of Ba^{2+} in solution, one mole of BaF_2 goes into solution; thus,

$[BaF_2] = 2.20 \times 10^{-6}$ M.

In 5.00 liters of solution, there are

$(5.00 \times 2.20 \times 10^{-6}) = 1.10 \times 10^{-5}$ mole of BaF_2 dissolved.

Multiplying by the molecular weight yields

$(175.3 \times 1.10 \times 10^{-5}) = 1.92 \times 10^{-3}$ g.

Therefore, 1.92 milligrams dissolve in 5.00 liters.

C. (4.70 mL = 0.0047 liter, $0.0047 \times 4.80 = 0.0226$ mole of HNO_3 present.

New volume is $1.28 + 0.0047 = 1.2847$ liters.

New concentration of HNO_3 is $0.0226 / 1.2847 = 0.0176$ M.

$[HNO_3] = [H_3O^+] = 0.0176$ M. V] pH $= -\log(0.0176) = 1.76$.

D. Molecular weight of KOH $= (39 + 16 + 1) = 56$ daltons.

Number of moles of KOH $= 4.89 / 56 = 0.0873$ mole.

$[KOH] = 0.0873 / 28.6 = 0.00305$ M.

$[KOH] = [OH^-] = 0.00305$ M. v} pOH $= -\log(0.00305) = 2.52$.

pH $= 14 - 2.52 = 11.48$.

(This could also be calculated by dividing the k_w by the $[OH^-]$ to get the $[H_3O^+]$.)

E. The dissociation is $HIO_3 + H_2O \rightarrow H_3O^+ + IO_3^-$.

The k_a is calculated as

$$\frac{[H_3O^+]^1[IO_3^-]^1}{[HIO_3]^1}$$

Plugging numbers into the equation gives

$[H_3O^+] = [IO_3^-] = x$; $[HIO_3] = 0.249 - x$.

This time the k_a is large enough that the amount lost by the HIO_3 cannot be neglected. Therefore, the next step is to solve a quadratic equation

$0.20 = (x)(x)/(0.249 - x)$.

This simplifies to $x^2 = 0.02x - 0.0498 = 0$. Solving for x yields

0.144 M or −0.344 M.

Obviously, the $[H_3O^+]$ is the positive value. Thus,

$pH = -\log(0.144) = 0.840$.

F. KClO will dissociate almost entirely:

$KClO \rightarrow K^+ + ClO^-$.

The hypochlorate ions formed will react with water:

$ClO^- + H_2O \rightarrow HClO + OH^-$

From the equations, it can be seen that

$[OH^-] = [HClO]$.

Assign values:

$[OH^-] = x$; $[HClO^-] = 0.0987 - x$

x is small enough to be ignored:

$$\frac{k_w}{k_a} = \frac{[HClO][OH^-]}{[ClO^-]}$$

Substituting values gives

$(10^{-14}/1.1 \times 10^{-8}) = x^2/0.0987$.

Solving for x yields

$[OH^-] = 3.00 \times 10^{-4}$ M.

$pOH = -\log(3.00 \times 10^{-4}) = 3.52$; $pH = 14 - 3.52 = 10.48$.

G. Concentration has nothing to do with the pH in this case.

$[H_3O^+] = ((k_w k_a)/k_b)^{1/2}$

Plugging into these numbers gives

$[H_3O^+] = (10^{-14} \times 1.1 \times 10^{-8})/(1.80 \times 10^{-5})^{1/2} = 2.47 \times 10^{-9}$ M.

$pH = -\log(2.47 \times 10^{-9}) = 8.61$.

H. The mixture described is a buffer solution. The first step in making it is finding the concentration of the weak acid solution:

$[H_3O^+] = \text{antilog}(-4.65) = 2.25 \times 10^{-5}$ M.

$$k_a = \frac{[H_3O^+][ClO^-]}{[HClO]}$$

$[H_3O^+] = [ClO^-]$

[HClO] is the unknown, which will be assigned x. This gives

$1.1 \times 10^{-8} = (2.24 \times 10^{-5})^2 / x$.

Solving for x yields

[HClO] = 0.0456 M.

In 2.50 liters, there are

(2.50 × 0.0456) = 0.114 mole of HClO.

In 1.62 liters of the KClO solution, there are

(1.62 × 0.0987) = 0.160 mole of ClO^-.

The new volume is

1.62 + 2.50 = 4.21 liters.

The new concentrations are:

for [HClO] = 0.114 / 4.21 = 0.0271 M; for [ClO^-] = 0.160 / 4.21 = 0.0380 M.

Putting these into the equation yields

$1.1 \times 10^{-8} = (x)(0.0380) / 0.0271$.

Solving for x yields

$[H_3O^+] = 7.84 \times 10^{-9}$ M

$pH = -\log(7.84 \times 10^{-9}) = 8.10$.

I. Molecular weight of NaOH = 23 + 16 + 1 = 40 amu.

In one gram of NaOH, there is 1/40 = 0.025 mole of NaOH; thus, there is 0.025 mole of OH^-. The OH^- reacts with the buffer by

$OH^- + HClO \rightarrow H_2O + ClO^-$.

The initial amounts (*not* concentrations) of HClO and ClO^- are 0.114 mole and 0.160 mole, respectively. After the OH^- is consumed, they are

0.114 − 0.025 = 0.089 and 0.160 + 0.025 = 0.185 mole.

The concentrations of HClO and ClO^- are

0.089 / 4.21 = 0.0211 M and 0.185 / 4.21 = 0.0439 M, respectively.

Plugging into the equation gives

$1.1 \times 10^{-8} = (x)(0.0439) / (0.0211)$.

Solving for x gives $[H_3O^+] = 5.29 \times 10^{-9}$.

$pH = -\log(5.29 \times 10^{-9}) = 8.28$.

VII. THERMODYNAMICS AND THERMOCHEMISTRY

1. THERMODYNAMICS

The first law of thermodynamics states that there is a constant amount of energy in the universe. If heat is added to a system and work is done, the change in energy of that particular system is equal to the heat added to the system (q) minus the work done by the system (w). Mathematically, this is

$$\Delta E = q - w.$$

The international unit of energy (and therefore of heat and work) is the joule (J), defined as the force of one newton (N) acting through the distance of one meter. Energy, potential or kinetic, can be measured in joules. This can be energy stored by position, stored in chemical bonds, or locked in the nucleus of an atom. It can also be energy due to motion, heat, or electromagnetic radiation. Other units of energy sometimes seen are listed in Table 5.

TABLE 5. Units of Energy

Unit	1 Joule = _____ of These Units
Erg	10^7
Foot · pound	0.73756
Foot · poundal	23.730
Calorie (very outdated)	0.2388
Electron volt	6.2419×10^{18}

Temperature scales have been mentioned in an earlier section. As a quick review, the two main scales in use are Celsius (formerly centigrade) and kelvin. On the Celsius scale, water freezes at 0° and boils at 100°. The kelvin scale starts at absolute zero; therefore, it has no negative temperatures. Water freezes at 273 K on this scale and boils at 373 K. When a temperature is given followed by the degree symbol but the scale is not shown, it is presumed to be Celsius (e.g., 25°). Temperature in Celsius can be converted to kelvin by adding 273.

Thermal energy (heat) can be transferred from one body to another in three ways:

1. Conduction: occurs when one body is placed in direct contact with another, and heat flows from one to the other. An example of conduction might be a block of metal at 85° placed on top of another block of metal at 0°. The heat will flow by conduction from the warmer block to the colder one.
2. Convection: occurs when a warm body heats the air surrounding it, and the air currents carry the heat to other bodies. A hot stove warms a room chiefly by convection.
3. Radiation: A warm body can emit photons of infrared wavelengths. These can travel through space and warm the bodies they strike. Heat travels from the sun through space to the earth by radiation.

When a substance is heated, its molecules move farther apart, causing the material to expand. This is quite obvious with gases, as discussed in an earlier section, and occurs to a much smaller extent in liquids and solids. The increase in volume can be calculated using the coefficient of volume expansion, ex_V, which is unique for each substance. For example, the ex_V for ethyl alcohol is $11 \times 10^{-4}/°C$. When 40.0 liters of ethyl alcohol are at 0° and then are heated to 55°, what is its new volume? First the change in temperature must be determined; $55 - 0 = 55°$. This is multiplied by the ex_V and the original volume:

$$55 \times (11 \times 10^{-4}) \times 40.0 = 2.42 \text{ liters}$$

This is added to the original volume to give the new volume of 42.4 liters. This is a change of only 6%, compared with a change of 20% had this been 40 liters of gas going from 0° to 55°. For solids, the change in volume is even less with temperature. The ex_V for ice is

$$0.5 \times 10^{-4}/°C.$$

If 4,000 cm^3 of ice is initially at $-12°$ and then cooled to $-190°$, what is its new volume? First, the temperature change is determined:

$$(-12) - (-190) = 178°$$

The change in temperature is again multiplied by the ex_V and original volume:

$$(178) \times (0.5 \times \tilde{10}^{4}) \times (4{,}000) = 35.6 \text{ cm}^3$$

This is subtracted from the original volume to give a new volume of 3,964.4 cm^3. If the solids are much larger on one axis than on any of the others (e.g., a wire), then a coefficient of linear expansion, ex_1, is used in the same manner as the ex_V to determine the change in length rather than volume. The ex_1 for silver is 2.0×10^{-5}. If a silver needle is 15.0 cm long at 25°, how long will it be at 125°? The change in temperature is 125° − 25° = 100°. Multiplying the change in temperature by the ex_1 and the original length yields

$$(100) \times (2.0 \times 10^{-5}) \times (15) = 0.03 \text{ cm.}$$

Adding this to the original length gives a new length of 15.03 cm.

A previous section showed that energy must be absorbed by a substance to convert it from a solid to a liquid and a liquid to a solid. There was an absorption of energy but no change in temperature, only a change of state. The heat of fusion is the energy required to convert a certain amount of substance from the solid to the liquid state. For example, the heat of fusion for water is 6.03 kilojoules per mole (kJ/mole). How much energy is required to melt 25.0 moles of ice at 0° to water at 0°? A simple multiplication tells us $6.03 \times 25.0 = 151$ kJ, or 151,000 J are needed to do this.

Note that the units were in kJ/mole. Sometimes they can be given in kJ/g, kJ/kg, or some other unit. Be alert to this. The energy required to convert a certain amount of a substance from the liquid to the gaseous state is the heat of vaporization. For example, the heat of vaporization of water is 40.6 kJ/mole. How much energy is required to change 29.9 grams of water at 100° to steam at 100°? First, we must convert grams to moles: 29.9 / 18 = 1.66 moles. Thus,

$$1.66 \times 40.6 = 67.4 \text{ kJ,}$$

or 67,400 joules are required.

Problem

A. If 28.7 liters of mercury are heated from −15° to 25°, what is the new volume? The ex_V for mercury is $1.8 \times 10^{-4}/°C$.

B. An iron nail is 15.0000 cm long at 35°. How long will it be at −200°? The ex_1 for iron is 1.2×10^{-5}.

C. How much energy is required to melt 29.8 grams of mercury? The heat of fusion is 2.34 kJ/mole, and the atomic weight is 200 daltons.

D. How much energy must be lost by 56.0 moles of mercury vapor to condense to liquid mercury? The heat of vaporization is 56.5 kJ/mole.

Solution

A. 28.9 liters; $\Delta V = \Delta T \times ex_V \times \text{volume} = 35°C \times 1.8 \times 10 - 4 C^{-1} \times 28.71 = 0.18$ L

B. 14.9577 cm; $\Delta V = 235 \times 1.2 \times 10 - 5 \times 15.000$ cm = 0.0423 cm

C. 349 J; moles of Hg = 0.149 mole; energy = 0.149 mole × 2.34 kJ = 0.349 kJ

D. 3,160 kJ; energy = 56.0 moles × 56.5 kJ/moles = 3,164 kJ

2. THERMOCHEMISTRY

A property of a system that is not dependent on how the system got to that state but is only dependent on the state itself is called a state function. For example, if water is heated from 0° to 15°, it makes no difference whether it is heated directly from 0° to 15° or if it is heated to 80° first, then allowed to cool to 15°; the end state (15°) is the same.

Because the universe has a finite amount of energy, energy cannot be destroyed or created—it can only change form. Endothermic reactions require energy, and they pull in heat from their surroundings. Exothermic reactions will not only run by themselves but also will give heat to their surroundings. To determine whether a reaction is endothermic or exothermic, the change in enthalpy, ΔH, is calculated. Hess's law states that for any process considered the sum of several step-wise processes, the enthalpy change for the total process must be equal to the sum of the enthalpy changes for the various steps. The ΔH for a compound can be looked up in a table. Most ΔH's are listed in kJ/mole at 298 K. For example, consider the reaction

$$CH_4 + 2O_2 \rightarrow CO_2 + 2H_2O.$$

The energy created in that reaction in forming the substances from the necessary elements is given as follows (in kJ/mole):

$$CH_4 = -74.9, O_2 = 0, CO_2 = -394, H_2O \text{ (as vapor)} = -242$$

The negative sign shows that energy is given up when these bonds are formed. Given that the result is expressed on a per-mole basis, the value for water vapor must be multiplied by 2 in this instance because 2 moles are in the equation. The energy produced by forming 1 mole of CO_2 and 2 moles of H_2O vapor is

$$[(1 \times (-394)) + (2 \times (-242))] = -878 \text{ kJ}.$$

The negative signs indicate that energy is given off. However, bonds had to be broken with the O_2 and CH_4 before the products could be made. To find the energy required to do this, the signs of the ΔH values must be reversed. This gives

$$[(1 \times (+79.4)) + (2 \times 0)] = +79.4 \text{ kJ}.$$

The positive sign shows that energy is required. Thus, for every mole of methane reacted, 79.4 kJ are required, but 878 kJ are given off, so this is a net gain of 799 kJ. Another way of showing this is by adding the sum of the ΔH's for products and reactants ($-878 + 110$ kJ—the negative sign shows that energy is being released). Repeating the previous steps for the reaction gives

$$2Ag_2S + 2H_2O \rightarrow 4Ag + 2H_2S + O_2$$

and leads to the following results. The heats of formation are

$$AgS_2 = -32.6, H_2O \text{ (liquid)} = -286; Ag = 0; H_2S = -20.1, O_2 = 0.$$

Summing up the ΔH's for the products gives

$$[(3 \times 0) + (2 \times (-20.1) + (1 \times 0)] = -40.2 \text{ kJ}.$$

Changing the signs for the reactants and summing gives

$$[(2 \times (+32.6)) + (2 \times (+286))] = +637.2 \text{ kJ}.$$

Summing the ΔH's of the products and reactants gives

$$-40.1 + 637.2 = 597 \text{ kJ}.$$

The positive signs tell us that this much energy must be applied before the reaction will run. Sometimes the ΔH value cannot be found for a particular compound. In that case, it can be approximated by the ΔH for the bond energies. For example, a single carbon–hydrogen bond has a value of −23.6 kJ/mole. Because methane has four C–H bonds, its ΔH of formation can be calculated as

$$(4 \times (-23.6)) = -94.4 \text{ kJ/mole}.$$

This agrees very closely with the observed value of −79.4. The error comes from the fact that not all C–H bonds are of equal energy because of surrounding atoms. The value given is an average. The values of a ΔH is determined experimentally using a calorimeter. The particular reaction is carried out in such a device, and the energy liberated heats a known mass of water. Measuring the increase in the temperature of the water yields data that allows the ΔH of the reaction to be calculated.

The heat capacity of a substance is the amount of energy required to raise the temperature of a body by 1°C. The specific heat is the amount of energy required to raise the temperature of 1 gram of substance 1°C. Thus, specific heat can actually be used to identify a material. For example, calculate the energy required to raise 125 grams of mercury from −10° to 120°. The specific heat of mercury is 0.138 J/gram °C. This is easily calculated, first by noting the change in temperature:

$$120 - (-10) = 130°, (130) \times (0.138) \times (125) = 2{,}242.5 \text{ J}$$

See Biology Review, Properties of Water, page 135.

Much of the energy involved in chemical reactions can be made to do useful work, but normally some of it is not available. A reaction will occur spontaneously at constant pressure and temperature only if it is capable of doing useful work. The amount of useful work that can be done by a reaction at constant temperature and pressure is referred to as the Gibbs free energy change, ΔG. If the value of ΔG for a particular reaction at a given temperature and pressure is negative, the reaction is spontaneous, and if it is positive, the reaction spontaneously runs in the opposite direction. If it is zero, the system is in equilibrium. Like enthalpy, ΔH, the Gibbs free energy change is a state function and thus can be calculated much like ΔH. Returning to a previous example of

$$2Ag_2S + 2H_2O \rightarrow 4Ag + 2H_2S + O_2,$$

we can look up the values of ΔG at 298 K and 1 atm to get

$$Ag_2S = -40.6 \text{ kJ/mole}; H_2O \text{ (liquid)} = -237 \text{ kJ/mole};$$
$$Ag = 0; H_2S = -33.5 \text{ kJ/mole}; O_2 = 0.$$

ΔG of the products is

$$(4 \times 0) + (2 \times (-33.5)) + (1 \times 0) = -67.0 \text{ kJ/mole}.$$

Reversing the signs, the ΔG for the reactants is

$$(2 \times (+40.6)) + (2 \times (+237)) = +555.2 \text{ kJ/mole}.$$

Adding together the two values gives

$$-67.0 + 555.2 = 488.2 \text{ kJ/mole}.$$

The positive sign indicates that the reaction will not run spontaneously at 298 K and 1 atm of pressure. However, the reverse reaction will, and it will liberate 488.2 kJ of energy. Compare this with the previous value of 597 kJ for the ΔH of the same reaction. ΔH gives the total energy change, and ΔG tells how much is available at the given temperature and pressure. Although ΔH is relatively constant with temperature and pressure changes, ΔG definitely is not. Neither ΔH nor ΔG is affected by the path that the reaction takes. One might correctly guess that ΔG and ΔH are related. If the free energy change is subtracted from the enthalpy change of the above reaction, a value of 423 kJ is obtained. Where has this energy gone if it did not do useful work? This energy increased the randomness or disorder of the system and is referred to as the entropy. As the entropy of a system increases, so does the disorder. The symbol for change in entropy is ΔS, and, like ΔG and ΔH, it is a state function. Values for ΔS can be looked up in tables. $\Delta G = \Delta H - T\Delta S$, where T is the temperature in kelvin. Note that a positive ΔS value denotes a spontaneous reaction, which is the opposite of ΔH and ΔG.

Problem

23.2 grams of ice are at $-15°$ and are mixed with 125 grams of water at 85° in an insulated container. Assuming that no heat is lost, what is the final temperature of the contents of the container when equilibrium has been achieved? The specific heats of ice and water are 0.116 J/mole·°C and 0.232 J/mole·°C, respectively, and the heat of fusion for water is 6.03 J/mole.

Solution

Because the values are in per-mole units, we first need to convert to moles from grams: 23.2 / 18 = 1.29 moles of ice, 125 / 18 = 6.94 moles of water.

The number of joules lost by the water will equal the number gained by the ice:

$$J_i = J_w. \quad (1)$$

The joules gained by the ice will be the number required to raise the ice from

$$-15° \ (\Delta T = 15) \quad (2)$$

to zero, plus the amount required to melt the ice at 0° to water at 0°, plus the amount required to raise the water at 0° to its final temperature:

$$T \ (\Delta T = T - 0). \quad (3)$$

The joules lost by the water will be the amount needed to lower its temperature from 85° to the final temperature:

$$T \ (\Delta T = 85 - R). \quad (4)$$

Placing these values into the equation from step (2) gives

$$(15 \times 0.116 \times 1.29) + (1.29 \times 6.03) + (1.29 \times 0.232 \times T)$$
$$= (6.94 \times 0.232 \times [85 - T]).$$

This simplifies to $10.2 + 0.299T = 136.8 - 1.61T$; $1.909T = 126.8$; $T = 66.4°$.

VIII. KINETICS AND EQUILIBRIUM

1. REACTION RATE

The rate of a chemical reaction is the amount of product produced per period of time. Most reactions do not run at a constant rate. For two reactants coming together to form a single product such as

$$mA + nB \rightarrow C,$$

where m and n are the stoichiometric coefficients, we can write the rate law as

$$R = k[A]^m[B]^n,$$

where R is the rate, k is the rate constant (which is different for each reaction), [A] is the concentration of reactant A taken to the mth power, [B] is the concentration of reactant B taken to the nth power. The reaction order depends on the exponents and with respect to which reactant the exponent is associated. For example, the reaction

$$3Mg^\circ + N_2 \rightarrow Mg_3N_2$$

will have the rate

$$R = k[Mg]^3[N_2]^1.$$

This reaction is first order with respect to N_2 and third order with respect to Mg. The overall order of the reaction is equal to $n + m$. In the case of the example, it is $(1 + 3) = 4$, or overall it is a fourth-order reaction. Most chemical reactions involve a number of individual steps between the reactants and the products. We cannot ordinarily write a correct rate equation or establish the order for an overall reaction involving several steps simply by looking at the overall balanced equation. The reaction

$$NO_2 + CO \rightarrow CO_2 + NO$$

actually occurs in two steps at temperatures below 225°. The first step is

$$NO_2 + NO_2 \rightarrow NO_3 + NO,$$

which is very slow. The second step,

$$NO_3 + CO \rightarrow NO_2 + CO_2,$$

is very fast. The first step is the slowest and thus the rate-limiting reaction.

Note that the rate of the first reaction,

$$R = k_1\,[NO_2]^2,$$

is a second-order reaction with respect to NO_2. Almost as soon as the NO_3 is formed, it reacts with the CO; thus, the [CO] has little to do with the rate of the second reaction. The rate for this would simply be $R = k_2$ (where k_2 is the rate constant for the second reaction), and this is called a zero-order reaction with respect to CO. This is not evident from simply looking at the overall equation; it has to be determined experimentally. Generally speaking, endothermic reactions increase their rate with temperature, while exothermic reactions reduce their rate as the temperature rises. Often, an activation energy barrier must be overcome to get a reaction started. If the reaction is endothermic, the activation energy is greater than that required to keep the reaction going once it is started. If the reaction is exothermic, the energy need no longer be applied once the reaction has started because it will then be giving off energy. An example of the latter is

$$2Mg + \Delta O_2 \rightarrow 2MgO.$$

Although this is very exothermic, magnesium can be in contact with oxygen for years at room temperature without any reaction occurring. However, raising the temperature to that of an ordinary match will give sufficient activation energy. Once the energy has been supplied, the match can be removed, and the magnesium will burn brightly until either it or the oxygen has all been consumed. This activation energy arranges the molecules involved in a state that is intermediate to that of the reactants and the products and of higher energy than either. This is known as the transition state. From the transition state the lower energy products are formed. The energy given off can be used to activate more reactants to the transition state, and the cycle is repeated.

The presence of a catalyst will lower this activation energy or eliminate it entirely. Enzymes are a special class of catalysts made of proteins. They also lower the activation energy of a reaction but usually operate within a narrow pH and temperature range.

2. EQUILIBRIUM

For a chemical reaction in the form

$$aA + bB \rightarrow cC + dD,$$

there will tend to be a certain amount of a back reaction:

$$cC + dD \rightarrow aA + bB$$

When the rate of the back reaction equals that of the forward reaction, the system is said to be in equilibrium. Remember, because this is a dynamic equilibrium, the forward and backward reactions are both running, and they are running at the same rate. Thus, the concentrations of the materials do not change. An equilibrium constant, k_{eq}, for any given reaction at any given temperature can be calculated. For the forward reaction given at the opening of this section, it will be

$$k_{eq} = \frac{[A]^a[B]^b}{[C]^c[D]^d}$$

This should look familiar as just another form of k_{sp}, k_a, k_b, and so on. The Le Chatelier principle states that if a stress (e.g., change in pressure, concentration, temperature, etc.) is applied to a system in equilibrium, the equilibrium is shifted in a way that tends to undo the effects of the stress. In the reaction given earlier in the section, the addition of A or B or the removal of C or D will shift the equilibrium to the right. Removal of C or D or the addition of A or B will shift it to the left. For the forward reaction, and when one of the products is removed, this is the driving force for the reaction. See **Organic Chemistry Review, Esters and Amides, page 354.**

Think of the equation as a balance. If something is added or removed from one side, material will have to be moved from one side to the other to keep it in balance. An increase in temperature will shift the equilibrium of an endothermic reaction to the right and an exothermic to the left. A decrease in temperature will do just the opposite. For a purely gaseous system, increasing the pressure will favor the side of the reaction with the fewest molecules. For example, the reaction

$$N_2 + 3H_2 \rightarrow 2NH_3$$

has four molecules on the left side and two on the right. An increase in pressure will shift the equilibrium to the right, and a decrease will shift it to the left. This rule applies only to pure gaseous systems. The presence of a catalyst will not shift the equilibrium; it will simply allow the system to attain it sooner.

As mentioned in an earlier section, when a system is at equilibrium, the $\Delta G = 0$. Knowing this, the k_{sp}, k_{eq}, and other constants can be calculated using the ΔG. The k calculated will be valid for whatever temperature the G was reported for. The relationship is

$$\Delta G = -RT \ln (k),$$

where T is the temperature in kelvin and R is the ideal gas law constant but with different units and therefore a different value: 8.314 J/mole·kelvin. For example, AgCl has a ΔG of 55.6 kJ/mole at 298 K. Solving for the k_{sp} yields

$$55.6 = -(8.314)(298) \ln (k_{sp}); -22.46 = \ln (k_{sp}); k_{sp} = 175 \times 10^{-10}.$$

Problem

What is the energy of the silver–sulfur bond in silver sulfide? The $k_{sp} = 1.0 \times 10^{-51}$ at 298 K.

Solution

The dissociation is

$$Ag_2S \rightarrow 2Ag^+ + 2S^=,$$

and from the k_{sp} value, it can be seen that it occurs to a very slight extent; thus, the bond must be fairly strong:

$$\Delta G = -RT \ln (k_{sp}); G = -(8.314)(298) \ln (1.0 \times 10^{-51})$$

Solving for ΔG gives 291 kJ/mole at 298 K.

In one formula unit, the energy would be

$291{,}000 / 6.02 \times 10^{-23} = 4.83 \times 10^{-19}$ joules per formula unit.

Each formula unit comprises two AgS bonds:

$4 \times 10^{-19} / 2 = 2.42 \times 10^{-19}$ joules per bond

IX. ELECTROCHEMISTRY

1. ELECTROLYTIC CELLS

Electrolytic cells are chemical cells that allow electrical energy to cause chemical reactions. An example is the electrolysis of water. Electrons from a source combine with hydrogen ions to form H_2 gas:

$$2H^+ + 2e^- \rightarrow H_2$$

As a result, hydrogen gas collects at the negative electrode. OH^- gives up its extra electron in the reaction:

$$4OH^- \rightarrow O_2 + 2H_2O + 4e^-$$

Thus, oxygen gas will collect at the positive electrode. In reviewing previous chemistry, it can be seen that the H^+ is reduced and the OH^- is oxidized. Rather than using the symbols + and − for electrodes, as done previously, electrochemistry uses the terms *anode* and *cathode*. The oxidation reaction always occurs at the anode, and the reduction reaction always occurs at the cathode. This is easy to remember because *cathode* and *reduction* both begin with a consonant, and *anode* and *oxidation* both begin with a vowel. An electrolyte is a material in the cell containing ions.

Figure 6 shows an electrolytic cell used to gold plate objects. The electrolyte is a solution of gold chloride ($AuCl_2$), which in solution consists of gold and chloride ions. The negative pole of a battery is connected to the anode that is the object to be electroplated. The positive pole is connected to the cathode—in this case, a gold bar. The anode and cathode are then immersed in the electrolyte. Electrons flow from the negative pole of the battery to the anode where they reduce the gold ions in the solution to gold atoms by the reaction

$$Au^{++} + 2e^- \rightarrow Au^\circ.$$

The gold metal plates out on the target. At the cathode, gold atoms on the surface of the bar lose their valence electrons by the opposite reaction and become gold ions in the solution. The electrons move to the positive pole of the battery. The flow of electrons and ions is shown in the Figure 6.

Notice that the electron flow is in the opposite direction of the positive ion flow. In the case of gold, two electrons are required to plate out one atom of gold. One mole of electrons will plate out half a mole

FIGURE 6. Electrolytic Cell

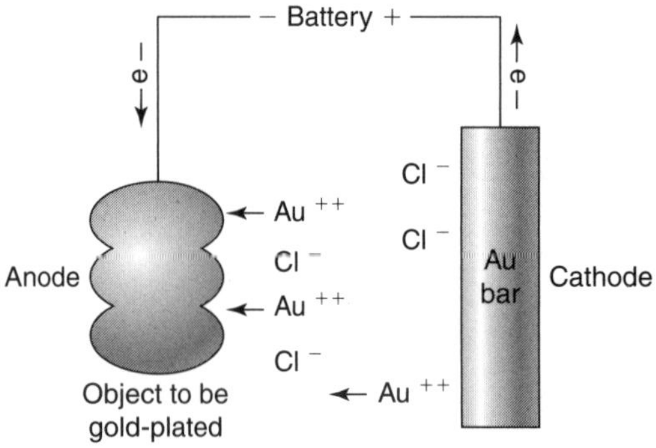

of gold, or 98.5 grams of gold. Electric charge is measured in coulombs, and one mole of electrons will have a charge of 96,487 coulombs (this value is known as Faraday's constant, or a Faraday of charge). A current of one ampere (abbreviated amp) has a charge of one coulomb passing a point every second. How much gold metal can the cell above plate out running for 8.00 hours at 0.120 amp? Assume that an unlimited amount of gold ions is available.

8.00 hours = 480 minutes = 28,800 seconds.

At 0.250 amp, this gives a total charge of

$28{,}800 \times 0.250 = 7{,}200$ coulombs of charge delivered in that amount of time.

$7{,}200 / 96{,}487 = 0.0746$ mole of electrons; $0.0746 / 2 = 0.0373$ mole of gold plated out

This corresponds with $(0.0373 \times 197) = 7.35$ grams of gold in that period. This procedure could be used to calculate the amount of any material produced by such a cell, whether it is a gas or a metal.

2. GALVANIC CELLS

A galvanic cell does just the opposite of an electrolytic cell: it uses a chemical reaction to produce an electric current. A more common name is a battery. Again, oxidation occurs at the anode and reduction at the cathode. In the cell shown in Figure 7, zinc atoms give up two electrons to become zinc ions, by the reaction

$Zn^{\circ} \rightarrow Zn^{++} + 2e^{-}$.

FIGURE 7. Galvinic Cell

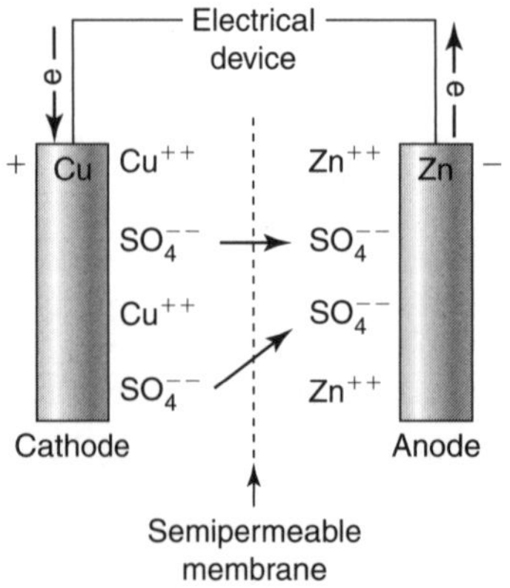

The electrons travel up the anode [the (−) pole of this battery] to the electrical device (e.g., light, meter, motor, etc.) and then to the cathode [the (+) terminal]. At the cathode, the electrons reduce the copper ions to copper atoms by the reaction

$Cu^{2+} + 2e^- \rightarrow Cu°$.

Two electrolytes are used in this cell, separated by a semipermeable membrane. The copper cathode is surrounded by a copper sulfate solution, and the zinc anode is surrounded by a zinc sulfate solution. As the reaction proceeds, the zinc anode will decrease in size, while the $ZnSO_4$ solution will increase in concentration. The copper cathode will increase in size, while the $CuSO_4$ solution becomes more dilute. As the concentration of the electrolytes change, sulfate ions are free to pass from one solution to the other via the semipermeable membrane. The direction of movement of the sulfate ions is opposite that of the electrons.

In a galvanic cell, the (+) and (−) designations for the anode and cathode are opposite those in an electrolytic cell. When the reaction has reached equilibrium, the electron flow halts and the battery is said to be dead. It can be recharged by connecting it to another source of electrons. It now becomes an electrolytic cell, the anode and cathode having exchanged positions.

The potential of a cell is measured in volts. Under standard conditions (298 K, 1 atm, 1 molar concentration) the standard potential, E°, is easily calculated. Tables of standard reduction potentials list the E°'s for standard reduction reactions. To convert the value to an oxidation potential, reverse the sign. For the cell shown in Figure 7, the following two reactions are found:

$Zn^{2+} + 2e^- \rightarrow Zn°, E° = -0.763$ volt

$Cu^{2+} + 2e^- \rightarrow Cu°, E° = +0.337$ volt

In that cell, zinc is being oxidized, so the sign is reversed, giving a potential of +0.763 volts. The total potential of the cell, E°, is determined by summing the two values:

$0.763 + 0.337 = +1.10$ volts

In other words, the cell shown in Figure 7, under standard conditions, will produce 1.10 volts of electric potential, regardless of its physical size. The positive value shows that the cell will produce electricity, but were this value zero or less, no electrical current would be produced. In fact, if the E° were negative, that would mean the cell was electrolytic, not galvanic, and a current would have to be applied to get the reaction to run.

What if concentrations are not at one molar for the electrolytes of a cell? How can the E be calculated? This is easy to do using the Nernst equation:

$$E = E^o - 0.059 / n \cdot \log \frac{\text{product}}{\text{reactant}}$$

where E is the potential under nonstandard conditions, E° is the potential under standard conditions, *n* is the number of electrons exchanged between atoms, and $\frac{[\text{product}]}{[\text{reactant}]}$ is just another equilibrium term. If in the cell shown in Figure 7,

$[CuSO_4] = 0.145$ M and $[ZnSO_4] = 1.80$ M,

what would the potential, E, be? Plugging into the equation gives

$E = 1.10 - (0.059 / 2) \times \log (1.80 / 0.145)$.

($ZnSO_4$ is produced in this reaction, it is the product; $CuSO_4$ is consumed, it is the reactant.) Continuing,

$E = 1.10 - 0.0295 \times \log (12.41); E = 1.10 - (0.0295 \times 1.09); E = 1.07$ volts.

Problem

A. How many grams of thallium metal can be plated out of a solution of Tl^{3+} ions using a current of 4.68 amp for 2.60 hours?

B. What is the standard potential of a galvanic cell that operates by the following reaction?

$Cr^{3+} + Al^{\circ} \rightarrow Cr^{\circ} + Al^{3+}$? $Cr^{3+} + 3e^{-} \rightarrow Cr^{\circ}$

$E^{\circ} = -0.74$ volt. $Al^{3+} + 3e^{-} \rightarrow Al^{\circ}$, $E^{\circ} = -1.66$ volts

C. What is the potential if the $[Cr^{3+}] = 2.50$ M and the $[Al^{3+}] = 0.178$ M?

Solution

A. 30.9 grams of thallium

4.68 amps × 2.60 hr × 60 × 60 = 4.38×10^4 coulombs

$$\frac{4.38 \quad 10^4}{9.65 \quad 10^4} = 0.454 \text{ moles of electrons}$$

$$\text{moles of } Tl^{+3} = 0.454/3$$
$$= 0.151 \text{ moles}$$

Grams of thallium = 0.151 mole × 204 = 30.9 grams

B. $E^{\circ} = 0.92$ volt $= 1.66 + (-0.74)$

C. $E = 0.94$ volt

$$E = E^{o} - 0.059/n \log \frac{[\text{products}]}{[\text{reactants}]}$$

$$E = 0.92 - 0.059/3 \log \frac{0.178}{2.50}$$

X. NUCLEAR CHEMISTRY

1. NUCLEAR REACTIONS

All the chemistry discussed to this point has involved reactions of the valence electrons of atoms, and in these reactions, the composition of the atoms in a balanced chemical equation is constant. In a series of new reactions, changes in the atoms' identities occur. These reactions are termed nuclear reactions. They cause a change in atomic number and sometimes a change in mass number as well. These reactions occur in either unstable nuclei or when stable nuclei are bombarded by particles.

Radioactive nuclei principally emit three kinds of radiation: alpha particles, beta particles, and gamma radiation. Gamma radiation is the most energetic of the three types, and alpha particles can be stopped by several layers of paper or clothing. Table 6 summarizes the various properties of these particles.

TABLE 6. Types of Radiation

Name	Symbol	Charge
Alpha	${}^{4}_{2}He$, ${}^{4}_{2}\alpha$	+2
Beta	${}^{0}_{-1}e$, ${}^{0}_{-1}\beta$	−1
Gamma	Γ	0

Uranium-238, a naturally occurring radioactive form of uranium, decays by alpha emission. Alpha emission is characterized by a change in both atomic number and mass number. Notice that the same number of protons and neutrons are present in this equation; therefore, this nuclear equation is balanced:

$${}^{238}_{92}\mathrm{U} \rightarrow {}^{234}_{90}\mathrm{Th} + {}^{4}_{2}\mathrm{He}$$

Thorium-234 decomposes by beta emission to protactinum-234. In beta emission, only the atomic number changes:

$${}^{234}_{90}\mathrm{Th} \rightarrow {}^{234}_{91}\mathrm{Pa} + {}^{0}_{-1}\beta$$

Protactinum-234 then decomposes by beta emission to uranium-234. A series of further nuclear reactions occur until the nonradioactive isotope, lead-206, is formed. A series of nuclear reactions that concludes with the formation of a nonradioactive isotope is called a radioactive decay series.

Most of the naturally occurring radioactive isotopes decompose by alpha, beta, and gamma emission. However, with the advent of the synthesis of new radioactive elements by artificial means, other modes of decomposition became known. These are positron emission and electron capture. A positron has the same mass as an electron but an opposite charge. The decay of polonium-207 to bismuth-207 is an example of positron emission. In electron capture, the mass number is unchanged, but the atomic number is reduced by 1. The conversion of beryllium-7 to lithium-7 is an example of electron capture. **See Physics Review, Atomic and Nuclear Physics, page 129.**

2. NUCLEAR FISSION

In nuclear fission, an unstable nucleus is formed as a result of neutron capture. This isotope then breaks into several fragments and releases neutrons. When uranium-235 captures a neutron, the unstable uranium-236 is formed. This step is called initiation and is similar in concept to the initiation step in free-radical chemistry. Uranium-236 then fragments into barium-141 and krypton-92 with the simultaneous release of three neutrons. These neutrons then react with more uranium-235, and a chain reaction has started. The chain eventually terminates if, for example, all the uranium-235 is consumed:

$${}^{235}_{92}\mathrm{U} + {}^{1}_{0}\mathrm{n} \rightarrow {}^{236}_{92}\mathrm{U}$$
$${}^{236}_{92}\mathrm{U} \rightarrow {}^{141}_{56}\mathrm{Ba} + {}^{92}_{36}\mathrm{Kr} + 3\,{}^{1}_{0}\mathrm{n}$$

3. NUCLEAR FUSION

In nuclear fusion, several small nuclei react to form a larger nucleus, releasing tremendous amounts of energy. Nuclear fusion is the source of energy of the sun and other stars. One example is the fusion of tritium with deuterium to form helium and a neutron:

$${}^{3}_{1}\mathrm{H} + {}^{2}_{1}\mathrm{H} \rightarrow {}^{4}_{2}\mathrm{He} + {}^{1}_{0}\mathrm{n}$$

MCAT

MEDICAL COLLEGE ADMISSION TEST

Organic Chemistry Review

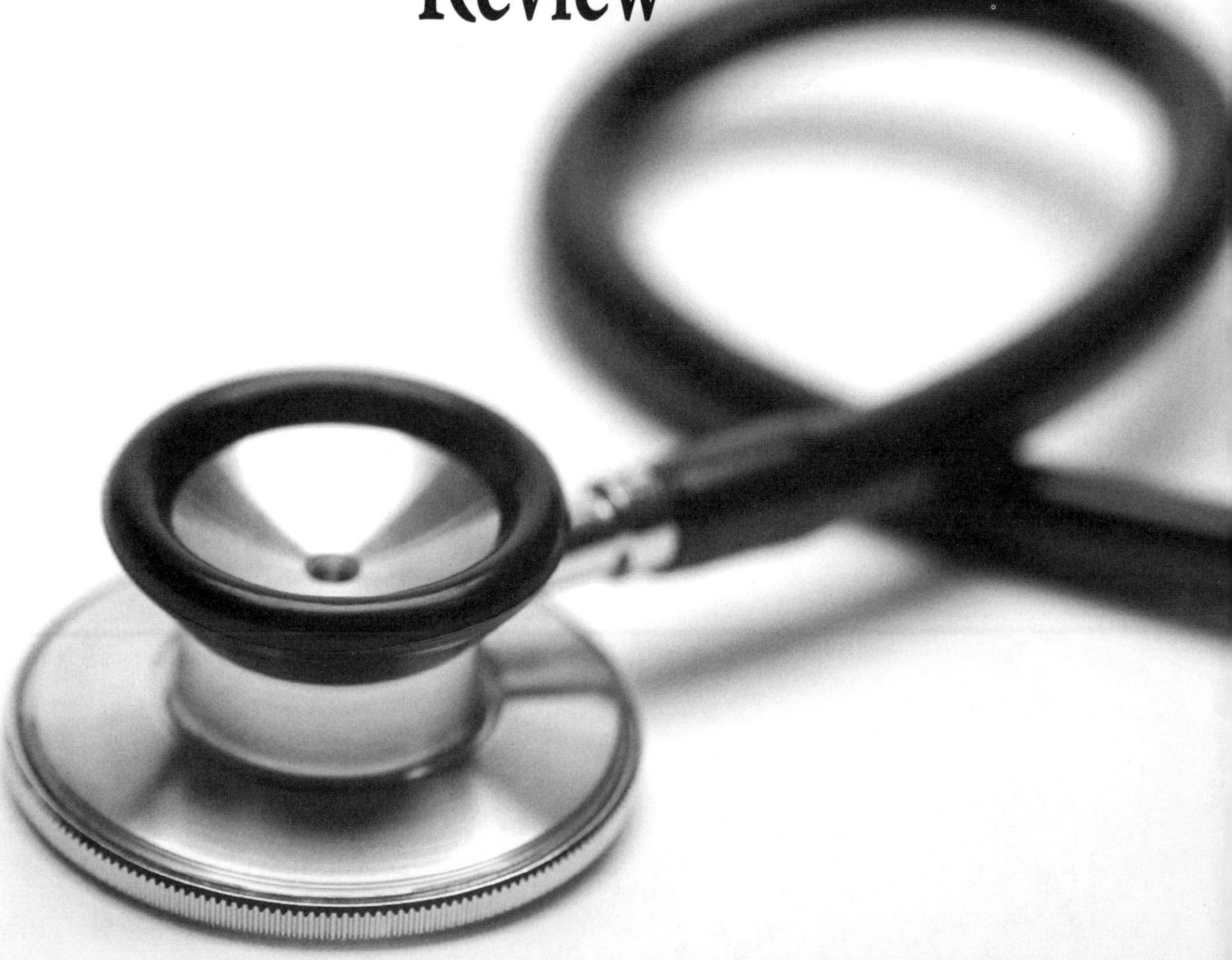

I. GENERAL PRINCIPLES

1. BONDING

Carbon is a 4A element and as such will accept four more electrons to complete its octet and to have its valence shell of electrons resemble the noble gas neon. According to the valence shell electron pair repulsion theory, any atom, including carbon, will maximize the distance between bonds. As a result, carbon has a tetrahedron shape. When carbon has single bonds attached to it, the carbon atom is sp^3 hybridized, and the bond angles are 109.5°. When the carbon atoms have double bonds, the carbon atom is sp^2 hybridized and the bond angles are 120°. A linear molecule with bond angles of 180° is observed when carbon has triple bonds. The hybridization in that case is sp. As the s character increases, the bond becomes short and more stable.

2. STEREOCHEMISTRY

Isomers are compounds, which have the same molecular formula but different physical and chemical properties. Isomers with different connectivities are constitutional isomers. Examples include 2-propanol and 1-propanol. Different isomers are possible if the isomers have the same connectivity due to stereoisomers. Even if an isomer has no stereocenter and is achiral, it can still be an isomer in the form of a cis or trans isomer. Examples of cis and trans isomers are cis-2-butene and trans-2-butene (Figure 1).

FIGURE 1

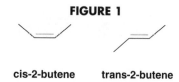

cis-2-butene trans-2-butene

Stereoisomers with stereocenters are chiral compounds, and the relationship between the isomers can be as enantiomers or diastereomers. A stereocenter is a carbon atom that has four groups bonded to it. An enantiomer has one chiral center and a mirror image that is nonsuperimposable. Such compounds are different from each other and have different optical rotations. The instrument that measures optical rotation is called a polarimeter. An equimolar mixture of two enantiomers is called a racemic mixture. A diastereomer has more than one chiral center and 2^n stereoisomers, where n equals the number of stereoisomers in the isomer. In a diastereomer, the stereoisomers are not mirror images of one another.

By convention, it is possible to identify a particular enantiomer and to differentiate it from its mirror image. This system of nomenclature is called the R, S system. The first step is to prioritize the groups on the chiral carbon, with priority assigned on the basis of atomic number. The next step is to orient the molecule so that the lowest-priority group is directed away from you. Read the groups projecting toward you from highest to lowest priority. If you read the groups in a clockwise direction, the configuration of the chiral carbon is R (Figure 2). If you read the groups in a counterclockwise direction, the configuration of the chiral carbon is S.

FIGURE 2

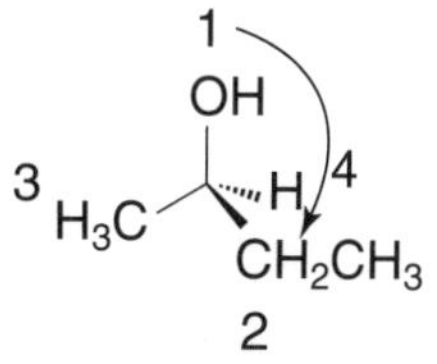

(R)-2-butanol

If a plane of symmetry exists in a diastereomer, the presence of chiral centers can be offset. The overall effect is that the compound is optically inactive despite the presence of chiral centers. Such a compound is termed a meso compound (Figure 3).

FIGURE 3

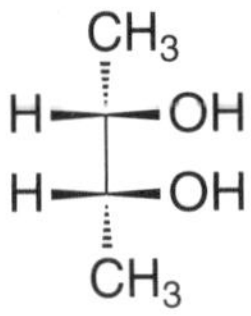

3. FUNCTIONAL GROUPS

A functional group is an atom or group of atoms within a molecule that have a characteristic set of physical and chemical properties. Functional groups form the basis for naming organic compounds. Functional groups dictate the physical properties of organic compounds, such as boiling points. Functional groups are also the sites of chemical reaction. The list of functional groups and their structures must be memorized (Table 1).

TABLE 1. Functional Groups

Name	Structure	Example
Alkane	CH_3CH_3	Ethane
Alkene	$CH_2{=}CH_2$	Ethene
Alkyne	$HC{\equiv}CH$	Ethyne
Arene	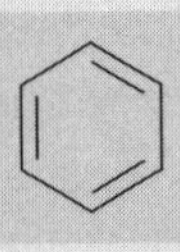	Benzene
Alcohol	CH_3CH_2OH	Ethanol
Ether	$CH_3CH_2OCH_2CH_3$	Diethyl ether
Thiol	CH_3CH_2SH	Ethanethiol
Amine	$CH_3CH_2NH_2$	Ethyl amine
Aldehyde	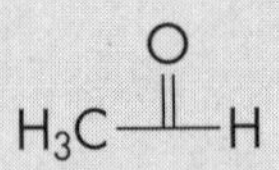	Ethanal
Ketone	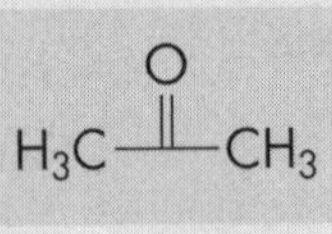	Propanone
Carboxylic acid	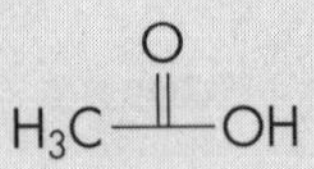	Ethanoic acid
Anhydride	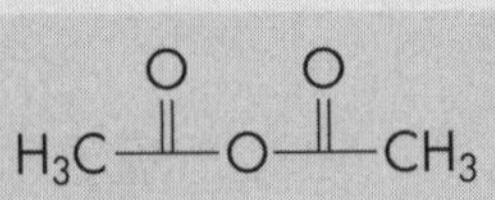	Ethanoic anhydride
Ester	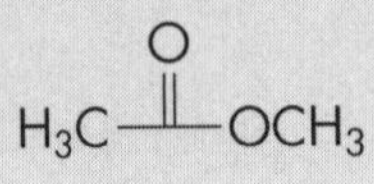	Methyl acetate

Name	Structure	Example
Amide	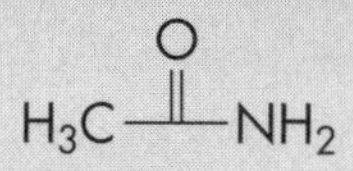	Acetamide
Nitrile	$CH_3C{\equiv}N$	Acetonitrile

II. ALKANES

Most alkanes have the general formula C_nH_{2n+2} and contain only carbon and hydrogen. They are in a general class of compounds called hydrocarbons, and because there are only single bonds in the molecule, they are known as saturated hydrocarbons. Cycloalkanes have the general formula C_nH_{2n} and have the same molecular formula as the alkenes (discussed later in this review). Only weak intermolecular forces, called London forces, are found in the alkanes, causing their boiling points to be low. In a homologous series, pentane is the first alkane to be liquid at room temperature and pressure. Branching in an alkane decreases its boiling point relative to its least branch isomer. Hexane has a boiling point of 68.7°C, whereas 2,3-dimethylbutane has a boiling point of 58.0°C. Both compounds have the same molecular formula of C_6H_{14}.

Alkanes are nonpolar and are not in soluble in polar solvents like water. This is another example of "like dissolves like." Alkanes are miscible with one another. Further, alkanes have densities less than that of water and so will float on water.

Primary hydrogens are attached to primary carbons, and primary carbons contain three or more hydrogen atoms. Secondary hydrogens are attached to secondary carbons, and they contain two or more hydrogens. Tertiary carbons have one hydrogen, and quaternary carbons have no hydrogen atoms.

Alkane nomenclature is based on the name of the longest chain of carbon in the molecule and the number of substituents in that chain. Number the longest chain nearest the first branch. Substituents should have the lowest possible number. The names of organic compounds consist of a suffix that indicates the functional group and a prefix that indicates the number of carbons (Table 2). The suffix for an alkane is *-ane*.

TABLE 2. Organic Alkane Compounds

Prefix	Number of Carbon
meth-	1
eth-	2
prop-	3
but-	4
pent-	5
hex-	6
hept-	7
oct-	8
non-	9
dec-	10

Because there is free rotation about the carbon–carbon single bond in butane, various conformations of butanes are possible. The most stable conformation is the one in which the methyl groups are furthest apart. This is termed the anticonformation (Figure 4). When rotation about the carbon–carbon single bond brings the substituents into an eclipsed conformation, the energy of the conformation is maximized. The gauche conformation arises from rotation about the carbon–carbon single bond to a conformation of intermediate energy.

FIGURE 4

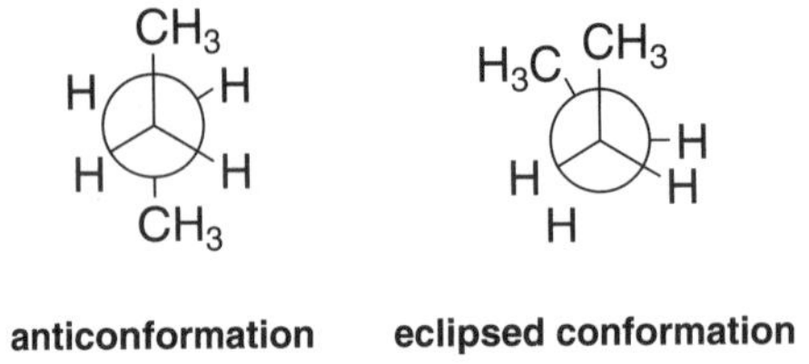

1. CYCLOALKANES

Cycloalkanes do not have the same relative stability. According to data on heat of combustion, for each CH_2 or methylene group, the heat of combustion of cyclopropane is higher than that of cyclobutane. This is a result of ring strain and the release of this energy when cyclopropane is burned.

Another important feature of the cycloalkanes is that the ring is not flat but puckered. Like the carbohydrates, such as glucose, cycloalkanes form six-membered rings. Some substituents of cyclohexane are parallel to the axis of the ring; these are called axial substituents, whereas a group found in the plane of the ring is termed equatorial (Figure 5). Because of 1,3-diaxial interactions, the most stable conformation is when the substituents are in the equatorial position.

FIGURE 5

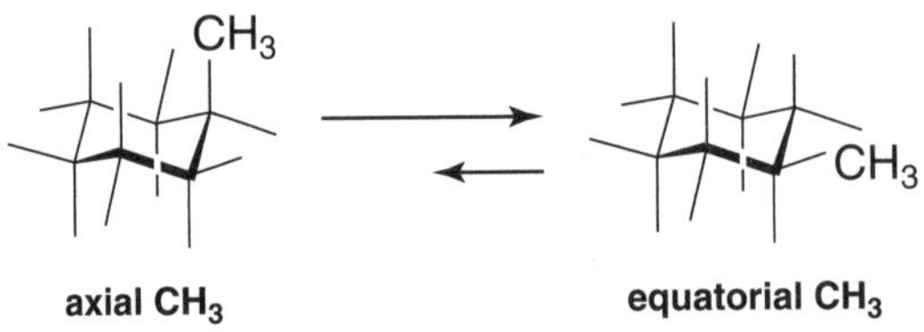

Alkanes can be synthesized from alkenes by catalytic hydrogenation (Figure 6).

FIGURE 6

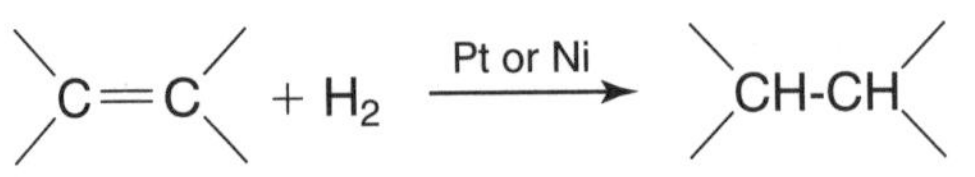

They also can be synthesized by the reaction of lithium dialkyl cuprate and an alkyl halide (Figure 7).

FIGURE 7

$$R_2CuLi + R'X \longrightarrow R\text{-}R'$$

Alkanes are generally very unreactive; however, they can be combusted to carbon dioxide and water, and they can be halogenated by a free-radical chain reaction. A free-radical chain reaction consists of the following steps:

1. Chain-initiating step
2. Chain-propagating steps
3. Chain-terminating steps

The overall reaction for the halogenation of alkanes can be shown as

$$RH + X_2 \rightarrow RX + HX.$$

The ease of halogenation decreases as the molecular weight of the halogen increases. Here the halogens are listed in decreasing order of reactivity:

$$F > Cl > Br > I$$

If ethane is mixed with chlorine gas, nothing will occur. However, if the mixture is heated or light shines on it, the halogenation reaction begins and continues even after the source of heat or light has been removed. The light or heat is involved in the chain-initiating step. In this instance, it is the dissociation of a chlorine molecule into two chlorine radicals:

$$Cl_2 + \text{light/heat} \rightarrow 2Cl^{\cdot}$$

The chlorine radicals can then react with the ethane to form hydrogen chloride and an ethane radical:

$$Cl^{\cdot} + CH_3CH_3 \rightarrow HCl + CH_3CH_2^{\cdot}$$

The ethane radical can react with a molecule of chlorine to produce chloroethane and a chlorine radical:

$$CH_3CH_2^{\cdot}\ Cl_2 \rightarrow CH_3CH_2Cl + Cl^{\cdot}$$

The last two reactions presented are chain-propagating steps. So long as they continue, so does the chain reaction. Chain-terminating steps halt the reaction. One such example is a chlorine radical reacting with an ethane radical. The result is still chloroethane, but no free radicals are generated to continue the reaction:

$$CH_3CH_2^{\cdot} + Cl^{\cdot} \rightarrow CH_3CH_2Cl$$

Other chain-terminating reactions will not only stop the chain reaction but will not create any product. For example, when two chlorine radicals come together to form a chlorine molecule, the chain is broken, but no product is formed:

$$Cl^{\cdot} + Cl^{\cdot} \rightarrow Cl_2$$

Sometimes a chain-terminating step will actually produce a contaminant. In the following example, two ethane radicals come together to produce a molecule of butane:

$$2CH_3CH_2^{\cdot} \rightarrow CH_3CH_2CH_2CH_3$$

Inhibitors can also absorb these radicals and terminate the chain reaction. For example, when oxygen enters the system, it reacts with the ethane radical:

$$CH_3CH_2^{\cdot} + O_2 \rightarrow CH_3CH_2 - O - O^{\cdot}$$

The radical formed can do very little to continue the chain reaction.

Problem

How many alkane isomers are possible from the molecular formula C_5H_{10}?

A. None B. Two C. Four D. Five

Solution

D. The five isomers are 1,1-dimethylcyclopropane, 1,2-dimethylcyclopropane, ethylcyclopropane, methylcyclobutane, and cyclopentane.

III. ALKENES

Alkenes are named in the same way as alkanes except that the suffix *-ane* is replaced with *-ene*. The carbon atoms in an alkene are numbered so that the carbon atoms bearing the double bond have the lowest possible number. Numbering of the substituents follows, and substituents are arranged in alphabetical order. Alkenes possess a carbon–carbon double bond and as a result possess two fewer hydrogens than their alkane counterparts. The more highly substituted the alkene, the more stable the alkene. The general formula for an alkene is C_nH_{2n}.

Geometric isomers can exist for alkenes because of their double bonds. If two identical functional groups are on the same side of the double bond, the molecule is referred to as a cis isomer. If they are on different sides, it is a trans isomer. If there are more than two different groups around the double bond, a different naming system is used. The atoms on each carbon are ranked according to their atomic weight. If the two higher-weight atoms are on the same side of the double bond, it is the Z isomer; if they are on the opposite sides, it is the E isomer (Figure 8).

FIGURE 8

(Z)-2-bromo-1-chloropropene (E)-2-bromo-1-chloropropene

Alkynes are named in the same way as alkanes except that the suffix *-yne* is used. Alkynes are linear molecules that do not have cis or trans isomers. The carbon hydrogen bond of terminal alkynes is acidic and can be removed by strong bases.

A notable difference between alkanes and alkenes involves the reaction of alkenes with hydrogen halides and with water. The addition of hydrogen halides destroys the double bond, and the hydrogen and halide will add to the two carbons that were once double-bonded. The hydrogen will go to the carbon atom attached to the fewest carbons. This is known as a Markovnikov addition and is illustrated in Figure 9.

FIGURE 9

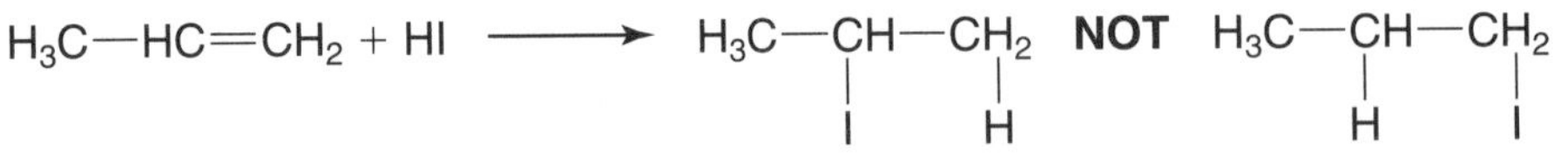

propene 2-iodopropane 1-iodopropane

Alkenes will also react with water in the presence of acids to form alcohols. A strong acid catalyst is needed to add to the double bond. Water is then added with the concomitant loss of a proton, and in doing so, the catalyst is regenerated (Figure 10). Again, if there is a difference between the two carbons, the hydrogen will add to the one attached to the fewest other carbons.

FIGURE 10

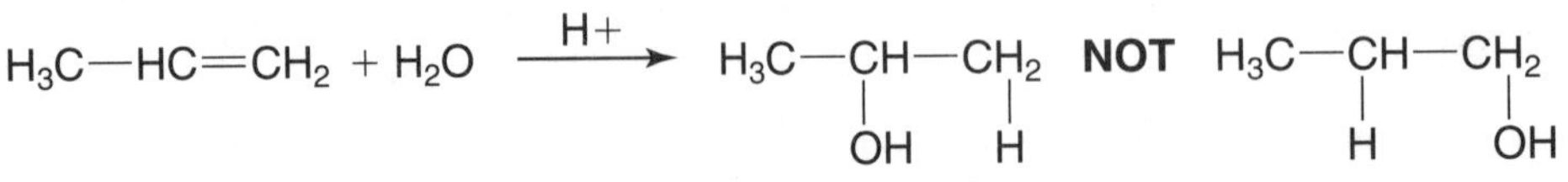

propene 2-propanol 1-propanol

Both of these reactions are reversible and can be used as a means to synthesize alkenes from either an alkyl halide or an alcohol.

Hydrogen halide addition and hydration of an alkene are examples of electrophilic addition. An electrophile carries a partial positive charge and adds to the electron-rich double bond. Other electrophiles can include +Hg (OAc) in an oxymercuration/demercuration reaction and borane in a hydroboration reaction. The alkyl borane is transformed into alcohol, so this is an example of an anti-Markovnikov addition. Alkenes also react directly with halogens to formed dihalides or with a halogen in water to form a halohydrin.

Alkenes react with ozone. When the intermediate is reacted with zinc, cleavage occurs and carbonyl compounds are produced (Figure 11).

FIGURE 11

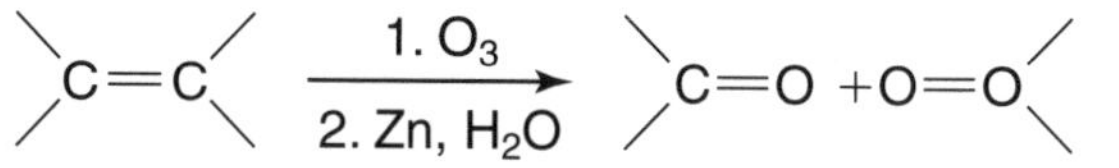

Problem

What is the correct name for the following compound?

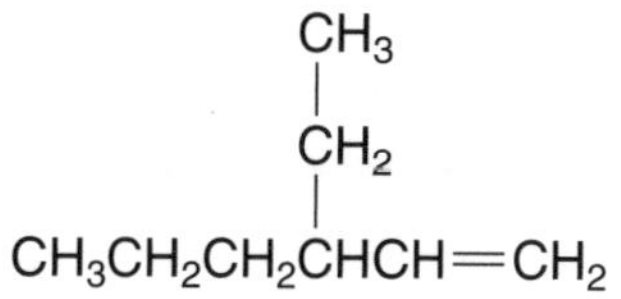

A. 4-ethyl-hex-5-ene

B. trans 4-ethyl-hex-5-ene

C. 3-ethyl-hex-1-ene

D. 3-propyl-pent-1-ene

Solution

C. This name identifies the longest chain as a six-carbon unit, and the numbering system gives the double bond the lowest possible number. There are no cis or trans isomers for this molecule.

IV. AROMATIC COMPOUNDS

Aromatic compounds are benzene and compounds that resemble benzene in behavior. Benzene is a molecule of cyclohexane with three double bonds, but it behaves so chemically different from the properties that would be predicted for "cyclohexatriene" that it has been given its own name. However, benzene and compounds resembling it do have their own category—the aromatics. Benzene is a flat molecule with all the hydrogens and carbons lying in the same plane. It is also symmetrical, with every bond angle equaling 120°. The electrons in the carbon atoms are shared in several bonds in benzene, and this delocalization of electrons makes the molecule stable. Benzene, with the three double bonds, differs greatly from its predicted properties because of the delocalization of electrons and resonance stability. Figure 12 shows the resonance hybrid representing benzene and the symbol commonly used to represent benzene, or an aromatic ring.

FIGURE 12

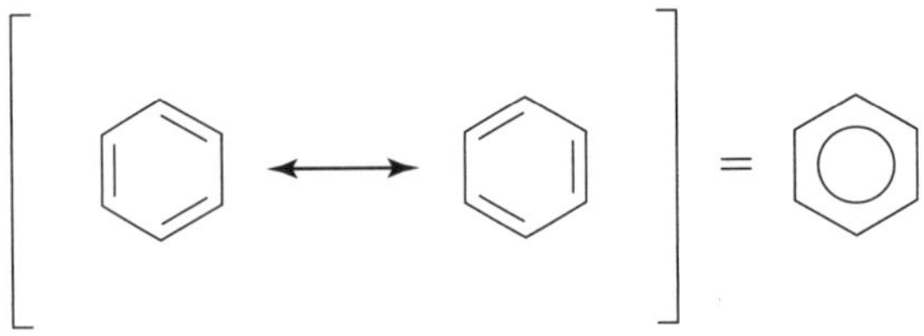

In contrast to alkenes, which undergo addition reaction with electrophiles, benzene and its derivatives react with electrophiles by substitution reactions. This process is called electrophilic aromatic substitution. Substituents on the benzene ring can influence both the rate and the location of the new substituent on the benzene ring. Electron-donating groups such as methoxy (OCH_3) will speed up the rate of electrophilic aromatic substitution because they can stabilize a positive charge. They will also direct a new substituent to be either ortho or para to the existing substituent (Figure 13).

FIGURE 13

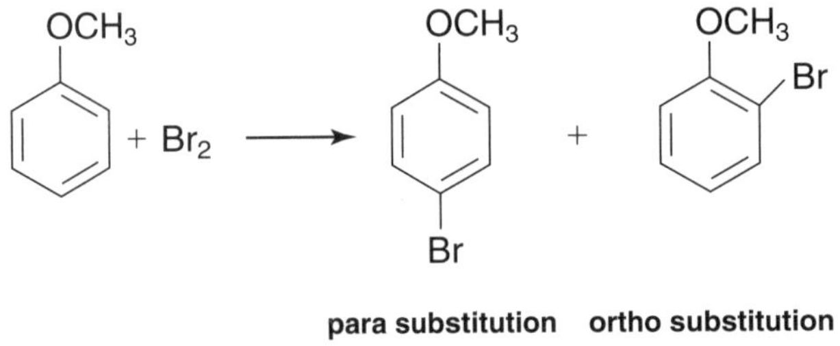

When an electron-withdrawing group such as a nitro group (NO_2) is present, the rate of electrophilic aromatic substitution is slower, and the incoming group is directed meta to the existing substituent (Figure 14).

FIGURE 14

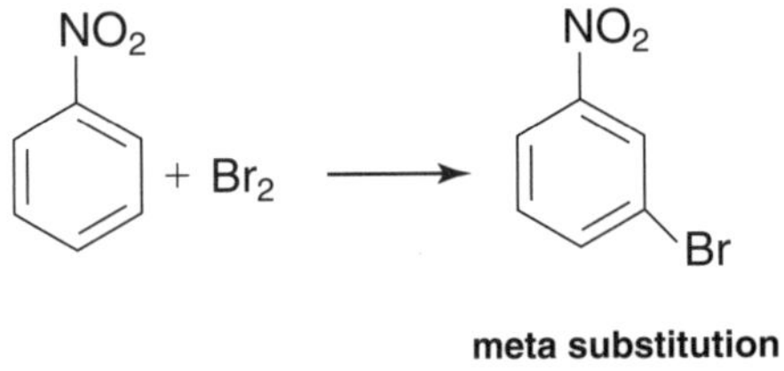

Electrophilic aromatic substitution is an important synthetic transformation. Halogen atoms, nitro groups, sulfonic acids (OSO_3H), alkyl groups, and acyl (RC=O) groups can be introduced into the benzene ring by this method.

Phenols are compounds that contain a hydroxyl group bonded to a benzene ring. They are widely distributed in nature. Vitamin E is a phenol. Intermolecular hydrogen bonding causes the boiling and melting points of phenols to be high. Phenols are weak acids, and they will react with strong bases such as sodium hydroxide and potassium hydroxide to form salts. Phenols are much stronger acids than are alcohols because of the influence of the aromatic ring. Electron-attracting groups, such as halides, or NO_2, increase the acidity of phenols, while electron-releasing groups, such as CH_3, decrease acidity (Figure 15).

FIGURE 15

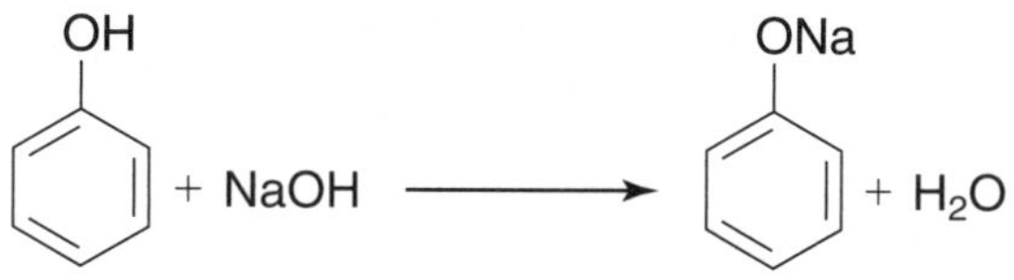

Problem

Aromatic nitro groups can be readily reduced to aromatic amines by reaction with hydrogen and a noble metal catalyst. What method can be used to prepare 4-amino-1-bromobenzene?

A. Nitration of benzene, bromination, reduction
B. Nitration of benzene, reduction, bromination
C. Bromination of benzene, reduction, nitration
D. Bromination of benzene, nitration, separation

Solution

B. Nitration of benzene will produce nitrobenzene. Reduction of nitrobenzene will afford aminobenzene or aniline. The amino group is an ortho para director and an activator and will direct the incoming halogen electrophile to the para or position four in the benzene ring.

V. ALCOHOLS AND ETHERS

Alcohols contain an –OH group, and the name of an alcohol ends in *–ol* (e.g., propanol, butanol, pentanol). An alcohol is further classified according to how many other carbon atoms are attached to the carbon atom that has the –OH group. The differences among primary (1°), secondary (2°), and tertiary (3°) alcohols are shown in Figure 16.

FIGURE 16

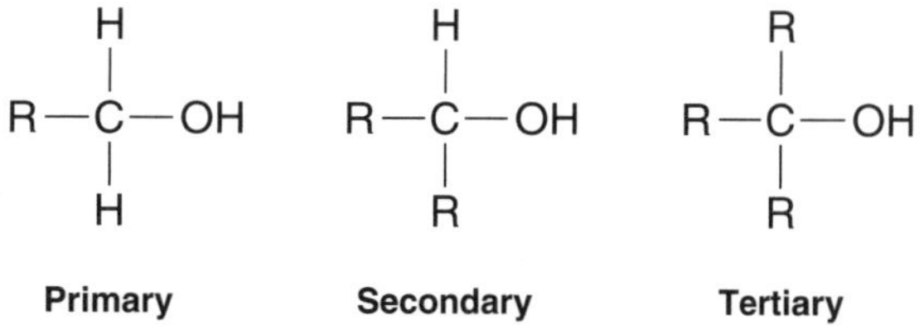

Alcohols can be dehydrated using hot acids. The ease of dehydration depends on the type of alcohol: ease is greatest for 3° alcohols and least for 1°. Following are the steps of an alcohol dehydration for ethanol.

1. The alcohol unites with a hydrogen ion (from the acid) to form a protonated alcohol.
2. The protonated alcohol dissociates into water and a carbocation (hence the name dehydration: water is removed).
3. The carbocation loses a hydrogen ion (regenerating the acid) and forms an alkene—in this case, ethene.

These steps are illustrated in Figure 17.

FIGURE 17

$$H-\underset{\underset{H}{|}}{\overset{\overset{H}{|}}{C}}-\underset{\underset{OH}{|}}{\overset{\overset{H}{|}}{C}}-H + H^+ \rightleftharpoons H-\underset{\underset{H}{|}}{\overset{\overset{H}{|}}{C}}-\underset{\underset{+OH_2}{|}}{\overset{\overset{H}{|}}{C}}-H$$

$$H-\underset{\underset{H}{|}}{\overset{\overset{H}{|}}{C}}-\underset{\underset{+OH_2}{|}}{\overset{\overset{H}{|}}{C}}-H \rightleftharpoons H-\underset{\underset{H}{|}}{\overset{\overset{H}{|}}{C}}-\underset{+}{\overset{\overset{H}{|}}{C}} + H_2O$$

$$H-\underset{\underset{H}{|}}{\overset{\overset{H}{|}}{C}}-\underset{+}{\overset{\overset{H}{|}}{C}}-H \rightleftharpoons \underset{H}{\overset{H}{\diagup}}C=C\underset{H}{\overset{H}{\diagdown}} + H^+$$

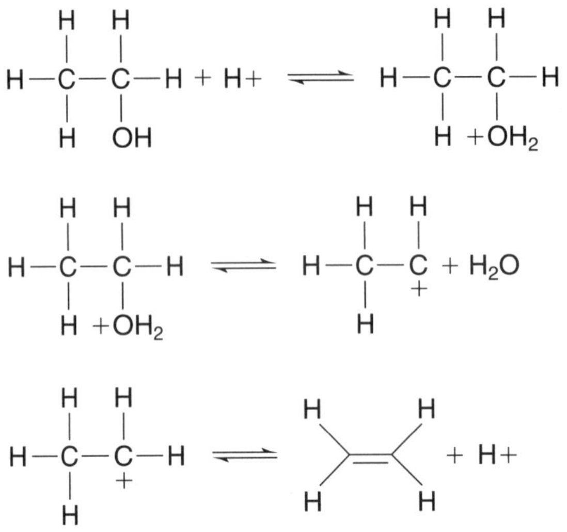

Alcohols will also react with hydrogen halides to yield alkyl halides and water. The order of reactivity of alcohols toward hydrogen halides is 3° > 2° > 1° > methanol. All alcohols except methanol and most 1° alcohols will react by what is termed an S_N1 (substitution-1) reaction, where the halide substitutes for the –OH group in its exact location, as is shown in Figure 18.

FIGURE 18

$$H_3C-\underset{\underset{OH}{|}}{\overset{\overset{CH_3}{|}}{C}}-CH_3 + HCl \longrightarrow H_3C-\underset{\underset{+OH_2}{|}}{\overset{\overset{CH_3}{|}}{C}}-CH_3 \longrightarrow$$

tert-butyl alcohol

$$H_3C-\underset{+}{\overset{\overset{CH_3}{|}}{C}}-CH_3 + Cl^- \longrightarrow H_3C-\underset{\underset{Cl}{|}}{\overset{\overset{CH_3}{|}}{C}}-CH_3$$

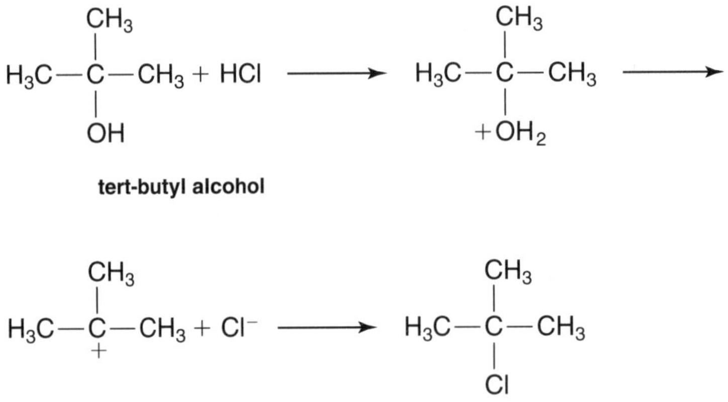

Most 1° alcohols and methanol will react by what is known as an S_N2 (substitution-2) mechanism. This yields an alkyl halide and water, but depending on the structure, there is a rearrangement of the ions formed. Thus, the halide is on a different carbon than was the –OH group. This occurs when the backside attack in a S_N2 reaction is blocked. The driving force in this reaction is the formation of the stable tertiary carbocation (Figure 19).

Primary alcohols and methyl alcohol react by an S_n2 because the kinetics of the reaction is first order with respect to the alcohol and first order with respect to the hydrogen halide concentration, while the overall kinetic order is second order. In this case, carbon halide bond formation occurs at the same time as carbon oxygen breakage (Figure 20). Arrows in organic reactions represent the flow of electrons, and so the electron pair on the halide ion is used to form the new carbon halide bond. The electron pair in the carbon oxygen bond is used to satisfy the valences of the water-leaving group.

Alcohols can be oxidized to aldehydes and ketones. Primary alcohols are oxidized (loss of hydrogen) to aldehydes. Secondary alcohols are oxidized to ketones. Tertiary alcohols are not oxidized.

FIGURE 19

$$H_3C-\underset{\underset{CH_3}{|}}{\overset{\overset{CH_3}{|}}{C}}-CH_2OH + HCl \longrightarrow H_3C-\underset{\underset{CH_3}{|}}{\overset{\overset{CH_3}{|}}{C}}-CH_2OH_2+ \longrightarrow$$

neopentyl alcohol

$$H_3C-\underset{\underset{CH_3}{|}}{\overset{\overset{CH_3}{|}}{C}}-CH_2+ \longrightarrow H_3C-\underset{+}{\overset{\overset{CH_3}{|}}{C}}-CH_2CH_3 + Cl^- \longrightarrow$$

$$H_3C-\underset{\underset{Cl}{|}}{\overset{\overset{CH_3}{|}}{C}}-CH_2CH_3$$

tert-pentyl chloride

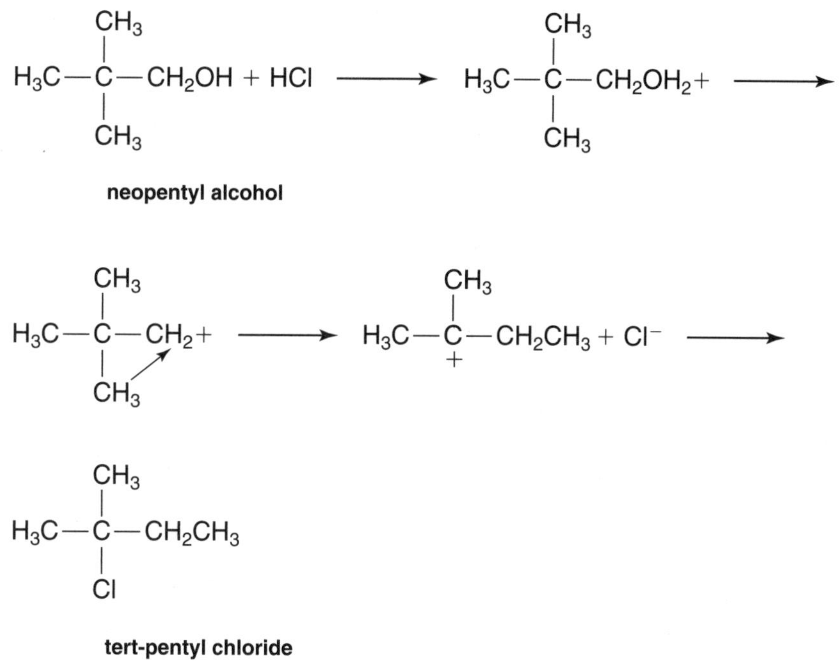

FIGURE 20

$$CH_3OH + HCl \longrightarrow CH_3OH_2+ + Cl^-$$

$$Cl^- + CH_3OH_2+ \longrightarrow CH_3Cl + H_2O$$

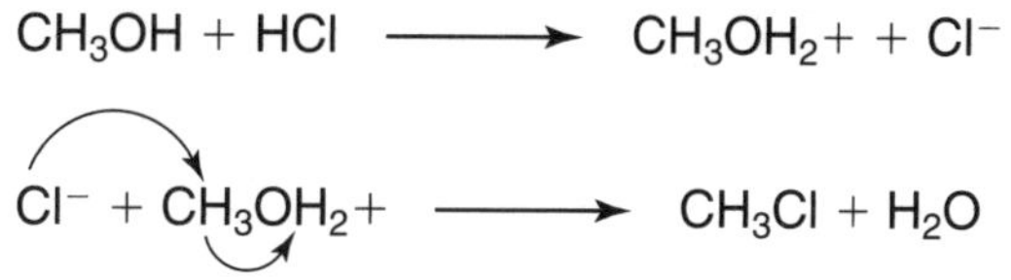

Alcohols can be prepared by a Grignard reaction. As an organometallic reagent, the Grignard reagent is reacted with a carbonyl compound to form an alcohol. In this reaction, the electron-rich nucleophilic Grignard reagent attacks the electron-deficient carbon of a carbonyl group. A new carbon–carbon bond is formed.

Hydrogen bonding affects the physical properties of alcohols, and alcohols have much higher boiling points than their alkane counterparts. Thiols have lower boiling points than related alcohols because the difference in electronegativity between hydrogen and sulfur is small and the S–H is nonpolar covalent. Generally, the more carbons in an alcohol, the lesser effect hydrogen bonding has, and the alcohol behaves more like a hydrocarbon. Branching, as in most organic compounds, decreases the melting point, boiling point, and density.

Ethers are of the general formula R–O–R′ and are named by the two groups attached to the oxygen, followed by the word *ether* (e.g., di-ethyl ether, methyl ethyl ether, butyl propyl ether). Ethers are generally very unreactive because the carbon–oxygen bond is quite stable. However, under extreme conditions (high temperatures and concentrations) ethers can be cleaved by acids to yield alkyl halides and alcohols. Hydrogen iodide (HI) is the most reactive acid used for this, followed by hydrobromic acid (HBr), followed by hydrogen chloride (HCl). Cleavage includes a nucleophilic attack by a halide ion on a protonated ether. (Because the ether accepts this proton, it is weakly basic.) The result is the displacement of the weakly basic alcohol molecule (Figure 21).

FIGURE 21

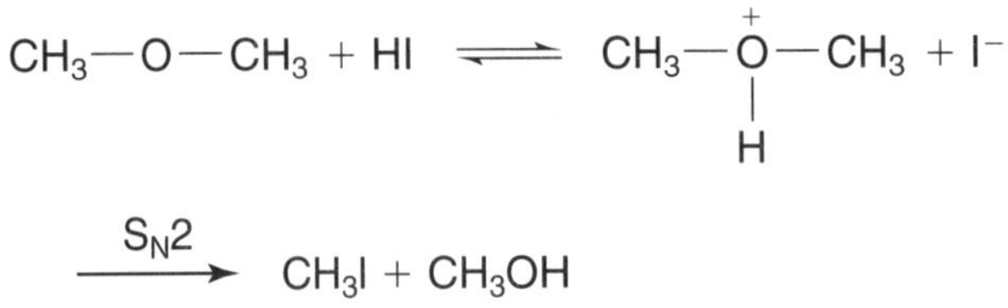

The Williamson synthesis of ethers is a general way to prepare ethers, and it involves an S_N2 reaction of a sodium alkoxide with an alkyl halide. Compounds other than an alkyl halide, which contain leaving groups such as sulfonates and sulfates, can be used. Because the mechanism is S_N2, best results are obtained when the alkyl halide is primary.

Problem

Epoxides react with water in the presence of acids to form 1,2-diols or glycols, as shown in the following figure:

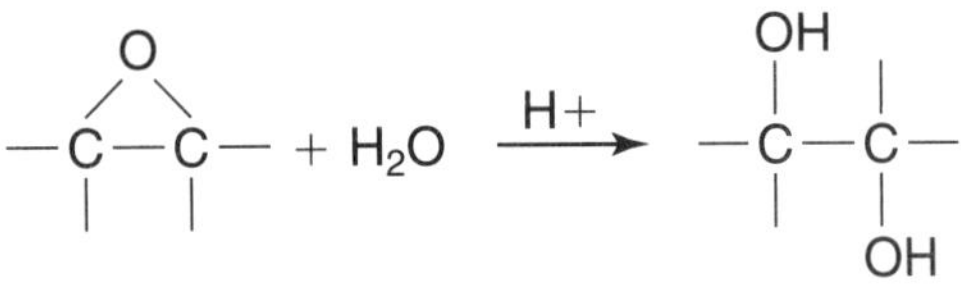

The structure of propylene oxide is as follows:

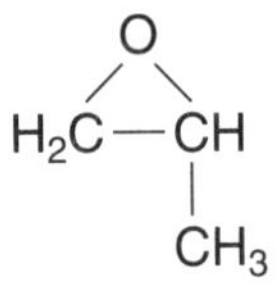

What is the product of the reaction of propylene oxide with ethanol in the presence of sulfuric acid?

A. $CH_3CH_2OCH_2CH_3$

B. 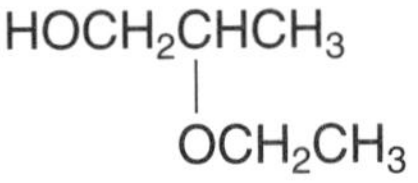

C. 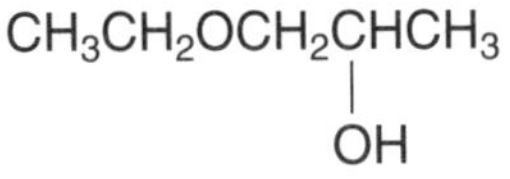

D. 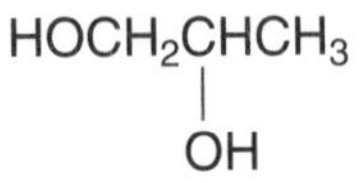

Solution

B. A tertiary carbocation is formed:

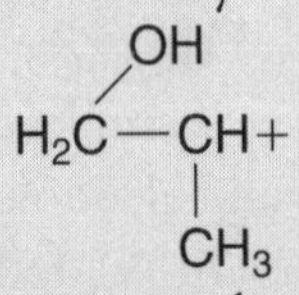

This species then reacts with ethanol as a nucleophile to form an ether. If water were the nucleophile, choice D would have been the correct answer. For choice C, the less stable primary carbocation is formed. The tertiary carbocation would always be favored.

VI. ALDEHYDES AND KETONES

Aldehydes have the general formula

$$\begin{array}{c} O \\ \parallel \\ H-C-R \end{array}$$

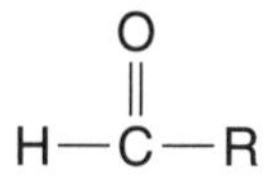

and ketones have the general formula

$$\begin{array}{c} O \\ \parallel \\ R-C-R. \end{array}$$

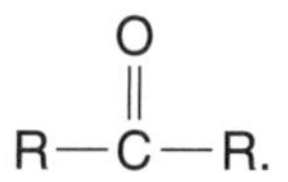

Note that they both possess the carbonyl group C=O. It is this carbonyl group that largely determines the chemistry of these compounds; thus, they are collectively known as carbonyl compounds. The names of aldehydes end in *-al* (e.g., propanal, butanal, pentanal). The names of ketones end in *-one* (e.g., 3-pentanone, 3-methyl-2-butanone, propanone). Because hydrogen bonding is not possible in aldehydes and ketones, they exhibit boiling points lower than those of the related alcohols.

Carbonyl compounds typically react by nucleophilic addition. Aldehydes undergo nucleophilic addition even more readily than ketones because of electronic and steric factors. One example of electrophilic addition is the Grignard synthesis of alcohols from carbonyl compounds.

A Grignard reagent is prepared by mixing an appropriate organic halide with metal magnesium, using dry ether as a solvent, such that

$$RX + Mg \rightarrow RMgX.$$

The C–Mg bond is highly polar, the carbon being somewhat negative and the magnesium being somewhat positive. Because of differences in electronegativity between carbon and oxygen in the carbonyl group, the carbon has a somewhat positive charge, and the oxygen is somewhat negative. The two carbons will be attracted to one another, as will the magnesium and oxygen atoms. The result is the magnesium salt of an alcohol, which, with the addition of water, becomes the alcohol itself. The Grignard synthesis with formaldehyde (methanal) yields a 1° alcohol, higher aldehydes yield 2° alcohols, and ketones yield 3° alcohols (Figure 22).

FIGURE 22

CH₃CH₂CHCH₃ + H—C=O ⟶ CH₃CH₂CHCH₂OMgBr →(H₂O) CH₃CH₂CHCH₂OH

sec-butyl magnesium bromide

A 1° alcohol
2-methyl-1-butanol

CH₃CH₂CHCH₃ + H₃C—C=O ⟶ CH₃CH₂CHCHOMgBr →(H₂O) CH₃CH₂CHCHOH

sec-butyl magnesium bromide

A 2° alcohol
3-methyl-2-pentanol

CH₃CH₂CHCH₃ + H₃C—C=O ⟶ CH₃CH₂CHCOMgBr →(H₂O) CH₃CH₂CHCOH

sec-butyl magnesium bromide

A 3° alcohol
2,3-dimethyl-2-pentanol

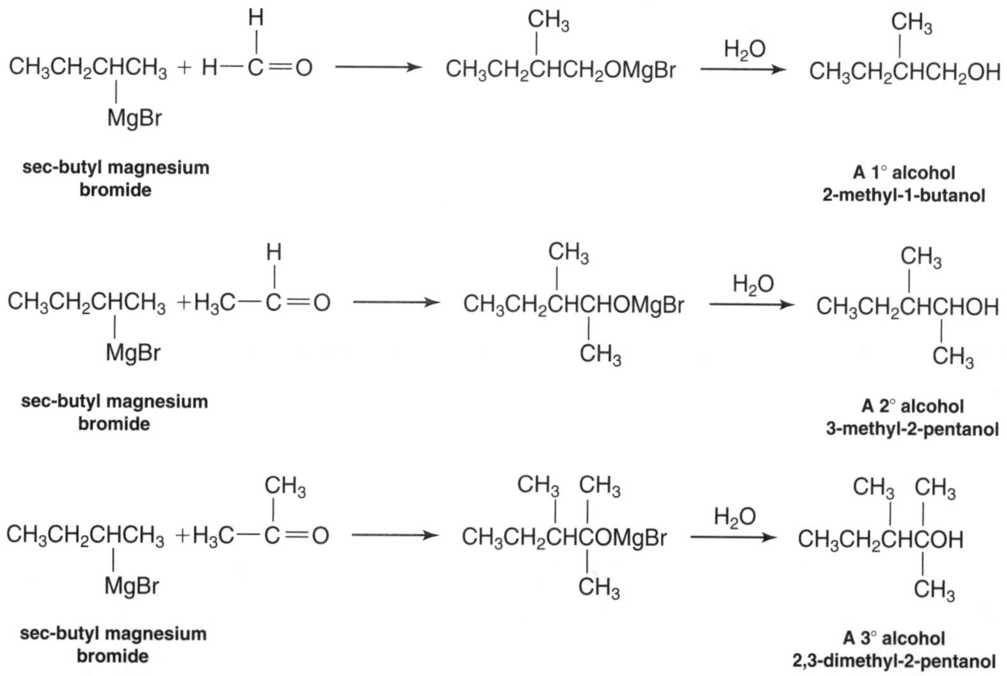

The carbonyl group of aldehydes and ketones is, in general, susceptible to nucleophilic attack and can react with various nucleophilic reagents. A good way to synthesize alcohols is the addition of a hydride to an aldehyde or ketone. An aldehyde will yield a primary alcohol, and a ketone will yield a secondary alcohol. Examples of suitable hydride reagents include sodium borohydride ($NaBH_4$) and lithium aluminum hydride ($LiAlH_4$). For these reagents, the valence on hydrogen is a negative (Figure 23).

FIGURE 23

$$ H:^- \quad + \quad {\scriptstyle\diagdown}C{=}O \quad \xrightarrow{\text{H+}} \quad HC{-}OH $$

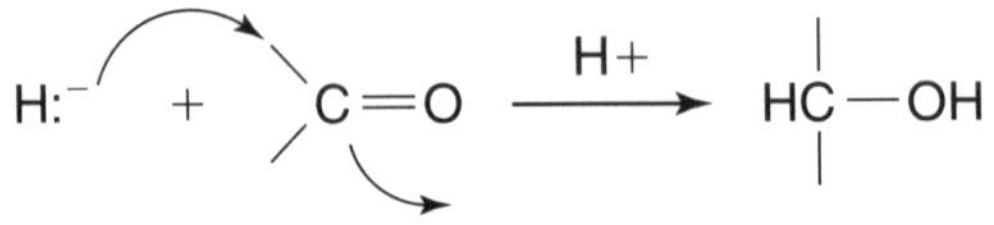

Dry alcohols, in the presence of anhydrous acids, can add to the carbonyl group of aldehydes and yield an acetal (Figure 24).

FIGURE 24

$$ CH_3CH_2CH{=}O + 2CH_2H_5OH \xrightarrow[\text{HCl}]{\text{Dry}} CH_3CH_2CH{\diagup\diagdown}^{OC_2H_5}_{OC_2H_5} + H_2O $$

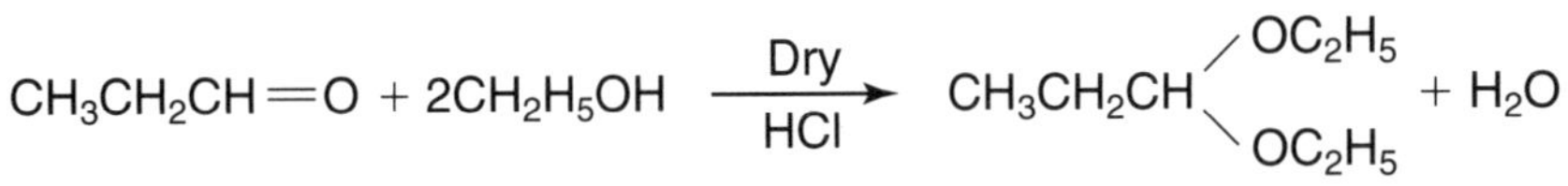

| **Propanal** | **Ethanol** | **1,1-Diethoxypropane** |

If no acid is present, the reaction will not occur.

In an alcoholic solution, there is strong evidence that an aldehyde exists in equilibrium with a compound known as a hemiacetal. A hemiacetal is formed by the addition of the nucleophilic alcohol to the carbonyl group (Figure 25). Hemiacetals are usually too unstable to be isolated.

FIGURE 25

$$ R'{-}\underset{H}{C}{=}O + ROH \xrightleftharpoons{\text{H+}} R'{-}\overset{H}{\underset{OH}{C}}{-}OR $$

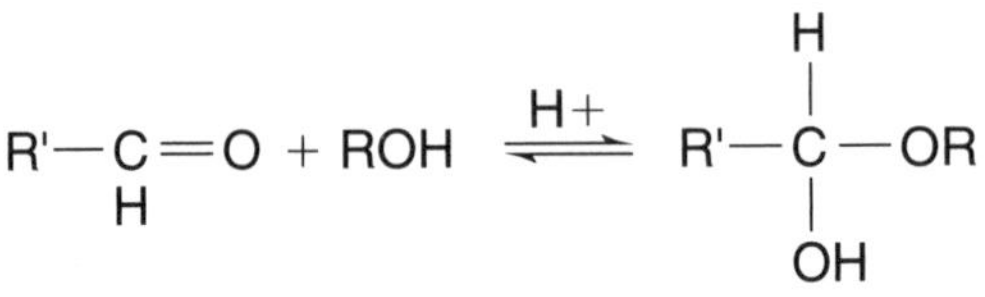

A hemiacetal

In carbohydrate chemistry, the closed form of a sugar results from the formation of a hemiacetal. Because these reactions are in equilibrium, the open-chain form is the intermediate by which the process of mutarotation occurs. The open-chain form, as either an aldehyde or an alpha hydroxy ketone, is responsible for the characteristic carbonyl reactions of carbohydrates. See **Biology Review, Biological Molecules, page 136.**

Likewise, ketals can be made using ketones. (Except for ketoses, simple ketals are more difficult to prepare through the reaction of ketones and alcohols.) The same is true of hemiketals. Ketones are more sterically hindered than aldehydes, and the additional alkyl group renders the carbonyl group less susceptible to nucleophilic attack. The basis of acetal chemistry is a carbocation, whose resonance form is shown in Figure 26.

FIGURE 26

$$ R'{-}\overset{H}{C}{+}{-}\overset{\cdot\cdot}{\underset{\cdot\cdot}{O}}R \quad \longleftrightarrow \quad R'{-}\overset{H}{C}{=}\overset{+}{O}R $$

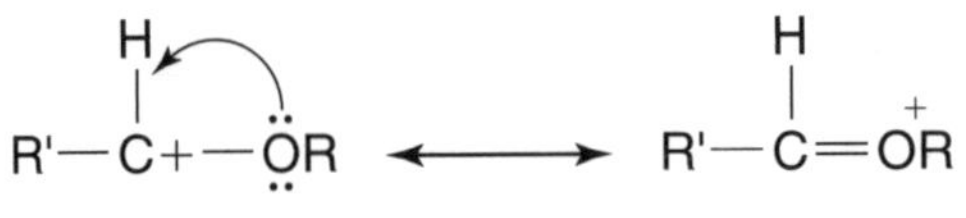

Many aldehydes and ketones are converted to amines by reductive amination, a process that involves reduction in the presence of ammonia. An intermediate compound, an imine (RCH=NH), is formed, which is then reduced to an amine. Two examples of such a procedure are shown in Figure 27. In these cases, a catalyst is not required because the amine nucleophile is very reactive.

FIGURE 27

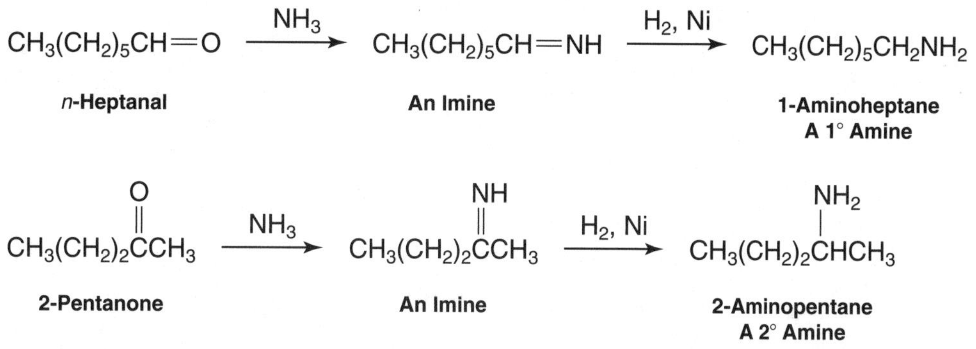

Imines can exist in tautomerization with enamines. Compounds whose structures differ markedly in arrangement of atoms, but which exist in equilibrium, are called tautomers. The term *tautomerism* describes this equilibrium. An enamine contains two double-bonded carbons, single-bonded to an amine group. An imine contains a carbon double-bonded to a nitrogen. An example of such tautomerism is shown in Figure 28.

FIGURE 28

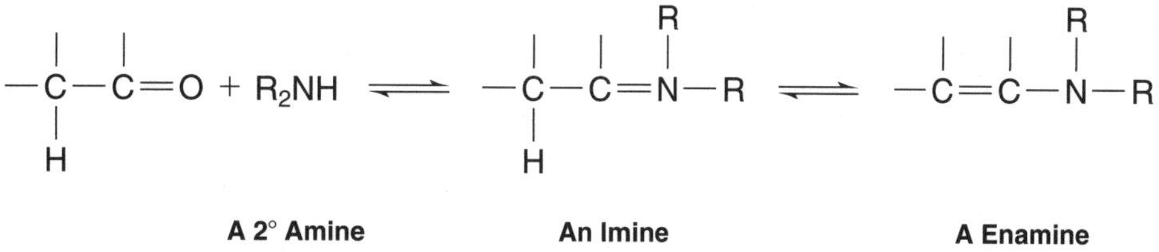

Two moles of an aldehyde or two moles of a ketone can combine with one another in the presence of a dilute base. This is known as an aldol condensation, and the product, which has the combined properties of a carbonyl (*-al*) and an alcohol (*-ol*), is called an aldol. The term *condensation* means that water is produced. An aldol condensation will not occur if an aldehyde or ketone lacks an alpha hydrogen. There is an alpha hydrogen on the carbon next to the carbonyl group, and it is the acidity of this hydrogen that causes the reaction to proceed (Figure 29). Because aldehydes contain only one alkyl group, the carbonyl group of an aldehyde is more reactive than that of the ketone in the aldol reaction and in other reactions that involve nucleophilic addition to the carbonyl group.

Another important example of a carbon–carbon bond formation reaction is the Wittig reaction. For the overall transformation, an alkyl phosphonium salt is reacted with either an aldehyde or ketone in the presence of a base to form an alkene. The first step of the Wittig reaction involves the formation of a phosphonium ylide by reaction of the phosphonium salt with a base. In the second step, the phosphonium ylide reacts with the carbonyl group resulting in elimination of triphenylphosphine oxide. The formation of a strong phosphorus oxygen bond is the driving force for this reaction (Figure 30).

FIGURE 29

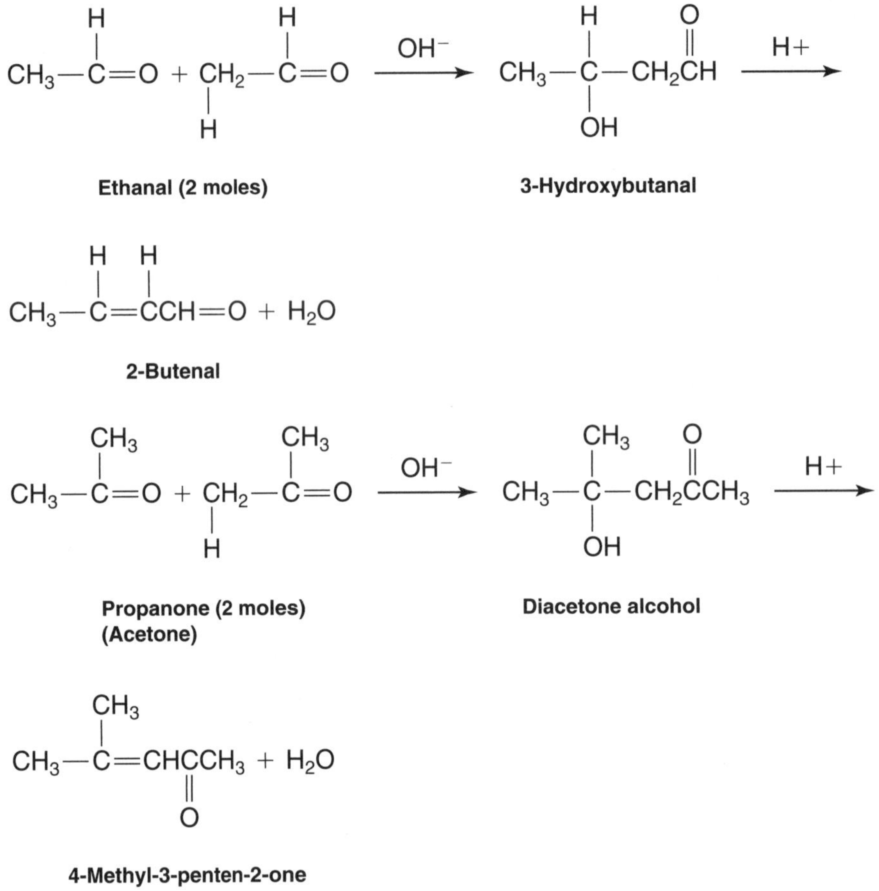

FIGURE 30

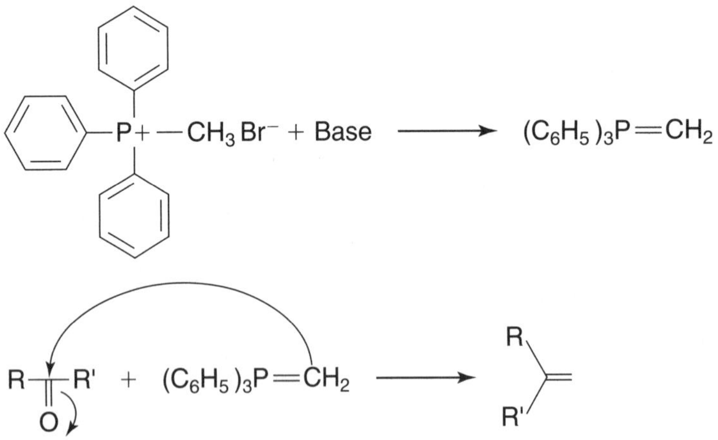

Unlike ketones, aldehydes are very susceptible to oxidation and can be oxidized to carboxylic acids by various reagents. Alkaline potassium permanganate and chromium (VI)–based reagents can accomplish this transformation. Tollens' reagent can oxidize aldehydes—but not ketones—to carboxylic acids with the formation of a silver mirror. Alpha hydroxy ketones will react with Tollens' reagents. Because monosaccharides exist as either aldehydes or alpha hydroxy ketones, aldoses or ketoses will give a positive Tollens' reagent. Aldoses and ketoses can also be oxidized by Fehling's solution. Only aldoses can be oxidized by bromine in water, nitric acid, and periodic acid.

An enol is a compound that contains two double-bonded carbons (*-ene*), and an alcohol group (*-ol*). These exist in tautomerism with ketones, with the ketone structure the most stable and thus the most preferred. The acid-catalyzed halogenation of ketones proceeds by halogenation of the enol, followed by the formation of hydrogen halide (Figure 31).

FIGURE 31

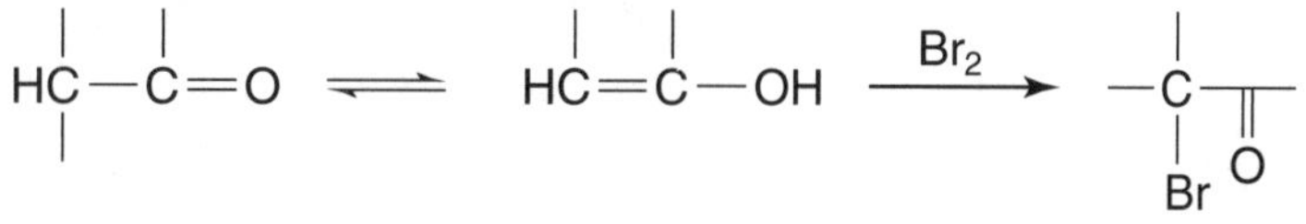

Ketone   Enol

Methyl ketones are oxidized by hypohalite to carboxylic acids. The iodoform test is the reaction of a methyl ketone with iodine and sodium hydroxide to form a yellow precipitate of iodoform CHI_3 and a carboxylic acid salt. This is a chemical test that can be used to identify the various types of carbonyl compounds present (Figure 32).

FIGURE 32

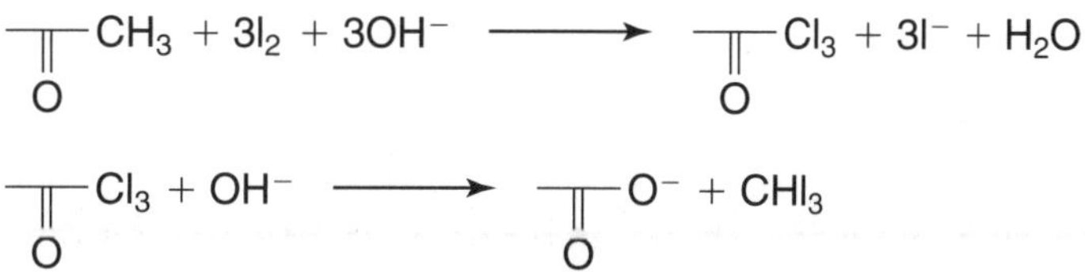

A compound that has not only a carbonyl group but also a carbon–carbon double bond has properties characteristic of both functional groups. In alpha–beta-unsaturated carbonyl compounds (containing carbon–carbon multiple bonds), the carbon–carbon double bond and the carbon–oxygen double bond are separated by just one carbon–carbon single bond (Figure 33).

FIGURE 33

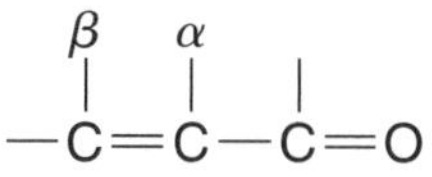

Because of this conjugation, these compounds have properties of both the carbon–carbon double bond and the carbonyl group, and some special properties as well. The presence of the carbonyl group lowers the reactivity of the carbon–carbon double bond toward electrophilic addition and controls the orientation of the addition.

Problem

Acetone is mixed with sodium hydroxide, and then the reaction mixture is treated with sulfuric acid. The result is production of product A. Product A is combined with bromine. What is the molecular formula of the final product?

A. $C_6H_{10}Br_2O$
B. $C_6H_{10}O$
C. C_6H_9BrO
D. $C_6H_{12}O$

Solution

A. The first series of reaction describe an aldol condensation and the dehydration of the alcohol to an alpha–beta-unsaturated ketone. Alpha–beta-unsaturated ketones possess a double bond and will react like an alkene with halogen to form a dibromo adduct:

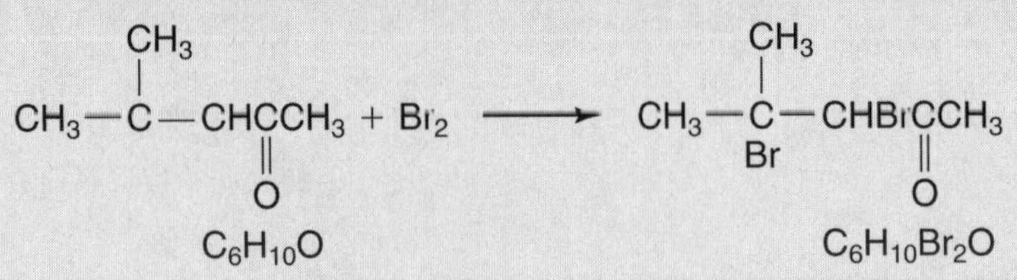

VII. CARBOXYLIC ACIDS

Carboxylic acids possess both a carbonyl and a hydroxide group (Figure 34).

FIGURE 34

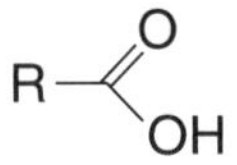

It is the –OH group that undergoes change in nearly every reaction but does so only because of the effect of the C=O. The names of these acids end with *-oic acid* (e.g., methanoic acid, ethanoic acid, propanoic acid). Common names also abound, such as formic acid and acetic acid.

Carboxylic acids can react with strong bases such as sodium hydroxide to form carboxylic acid salts. Carboxylic acids will also react with sodium bicarbonate to form sodium carboxylates. Phenols react only with sodium hydroxide to form sodium phenoxides.

Problem

A mixture of benzoic acid, benzyl alcohol, and phenol in diethyl ether is combined and the solution shaken with an aqueous solution of sodium bicarbonate. The sodium bicarbonate solution is acidified with concentrated hydrochloric acid, and a precipitate is obtained. What is the precipitate?

A. Benzoic alcohol B. Sodium chloride C. Benzoic acid D. Phenol

Solution

C. Only benzoic acid will form a salt with sodium bicarbonate and be extracted into the aqueous phase. Hydrochloric acid can protonate sodium benzoate to form benzoic acid and sodium chloride. Sodium chloride is soluble in water, and benzoic acid is insoluble in water and will precipitate from solution.

Carboxylate ions are stabilized by resonance because the negative charge can be delocalized over both electronegative oxygen atoms. Electron-withdrawing groups on the alkyl group increase the acidity of the carboxylic acid. The more electronegative the group is, the greater the acidifying effect on the carboxylic acid. Therefore, fluoroacetic acid is a stronger acid than chloroacetic acid. Hydrogen bonding, as would be expected, plays an important role in intermolecular forces in carboxylic acids. Intramolecular forces include the inductive effect of substituents on the acid chain. The inductive effect is caused by a highly electronegative or electropositive group or atom located on the chain. This effect is felt throughout the molecule, although it does decrease with the distance from the group. Electron-withdrawing groups (e.g., NO_2, halogens) increase the stability of the carboxylate ion, thereby strengthening the acid. Again, the farther this group is from the carboxylic acid functional group, the less effect it will have. An electron-releasing group, such as an amine, will destabilize the ion and weaken the acid; again, the distance rule comes into play. The carboxylate ion is further stabilized by resonance. It really has one and one-half bonds from the carbon to each oxygen (Figure 35).

FIGURE 35

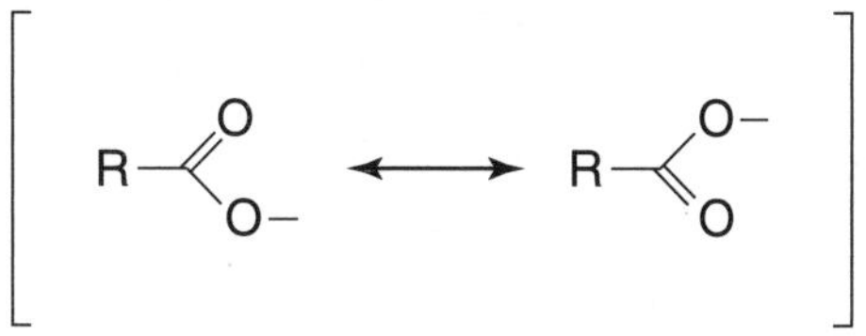

Lithium aluminum hydride can reduce an acid to an alcohol. A typical reaction might be the conversion of pentanoic acid to pentanol (Figure 36).

FIGURE 36

$$CH_3(CH_2)_3COOH \xrightarrow{LiAlH_4} CH_3(CH_2)_3CH_2OH$$

Reactions of carboxylic acid derivatives are dominated by nucleophilic substitution reactions. As a rule, carboxylic acid derivatives are more reactive toward nucleophilic substitution than are their noncarboxylic acid counterparts. In other words, for nucleophilic substitution, an acid chloride (R–COOCl) is more reactive than a comparable alkyl chloride (R–Cl), an amide ($R–COONH_2$) is more reactive than an amine ($R–NH_2$), and an ester (R–COOR′) is more reactive than an ether (R–OR′). Steric effects must also be taken into account for these reactions.

The functional group of an anhydride consists of two carbonyl groups bonded to the same oxygen atoms. The anhydride contains the same or different alkyl groups. When the alkyl groups are different, the compound is a mixed anhydride. In contrast to carboxylic acids, which do not as readily undergo substitution at the acyl carbon, anhydrides are susceptible to nucleophilic substitution at the acyl carbon. Acetic anhydride readily reacts with water to form two moles of acetic acid (Figure 37).

FIGURE 37

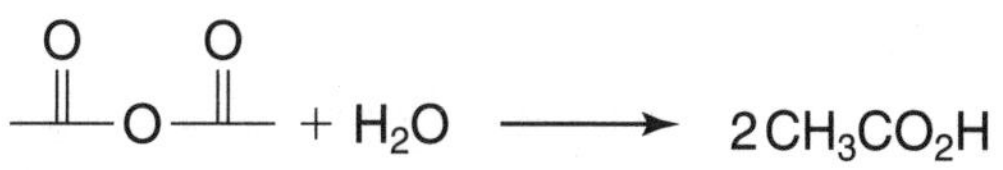

An anhydride of unique biological importance is adenosine triphosphate (ATP). ATP contains two phosphoric anhydride bonds, P–O–P, and when these bonds are hydrolyzed, they release energy (Figure 38). More energy is released in the anhydride bond than in the phosphoric-ester linkage, C–O–P.

FIGURE 38

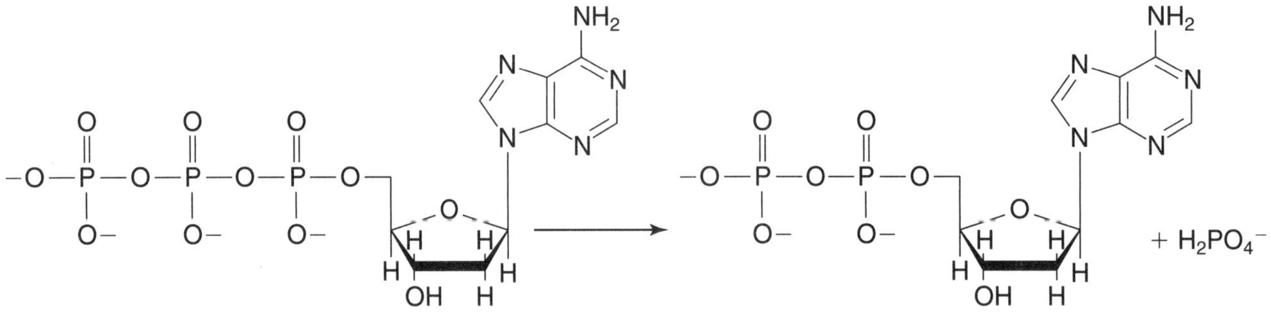

See Biology Review, Krebs (Citric Acid) Cycle, page 154.

The most reactive acid derivatives are acid chlorides. Acid chlorides are prepared from acid chlorides of inorganic acids such as thionyl chloride ($SOCl_2$) and phosphorus pentachloride (PCl_5). They react readily with water, alcohols, and amines to form carboxylic acids, esters, and amides. Because an acid chloride has a good leaving group in the chloride ion, its reaction with nucleophiles illustrates well the nucleophilic substitution reactions that are characteristic of acid derivatives (Figure 39).

FIGURE 39

$$R{-}C({=}O){-}Cl + H_2O \longrightarrow R{-}C({=}O){-}OH + HCl$$

Hydroxide is a poor leaving group compared with chloride, and the reaction is shifted to the right. The reaction is typically conducted in the presence of a base.

VIII. ESTERS AND AMIDES

Carboxylic acids react with alcohols to form esters by a process known as esterification. The reaction is acid catalyzed and is an equilibrium reaction. Typically, a large excess of the alcohol is used, and this causes the reaction to be shifted to the right. If the boiling point of the alcohol is higher than that of water, the reaction can also be driven to the right by the removal of water (Figure 40). The type of alcohol used determines the degree of the reaction, methanol being the most reactive: methanol > 1° > 2 ° >3°.

FIGURE 40

$$C_6H_5C({=}O)OH + CH_3OH \rightleftharpoons C_6H_5C({=}O)OCH_3 + H_2O$$

Benzoic acid **Methanol** **Methyl benzoate**

See Chemistry Review, Le Chatelier's Principle, page 324.

Fats, glycerides, and esters can be saponified—literally, made into soap—by using excess base of a known concentration. This is analogous to an acid–base titration. The amount of base needed to convert these materials into soap is known as the saponification equivalent and can be used to determine their equivalent weight. With the addition of an acid, the carboxylic acid is formed, and this is a general synthetic transformation in which esters can be converted into carboxylic acids (Figure 41).

FIGURE 41

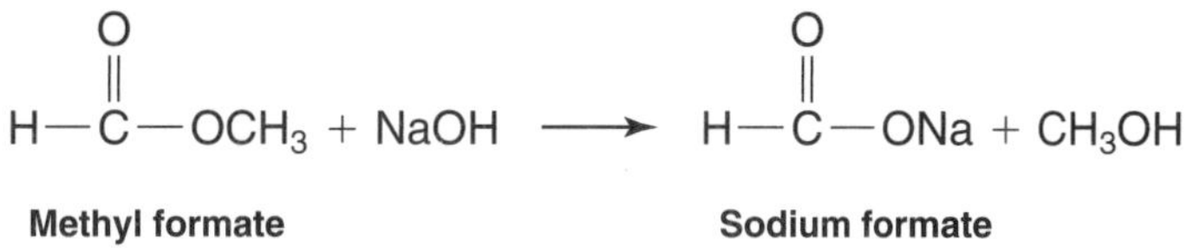

Amides are the most stable carboxylic acid derivative, and this feature is important because amide linkages form the backbone of proteins. The lone electron pair of nitrogen can be donated to the carbonyl group, and this makes the carbonyl carbon electron rich and less susceptible to attack by nucleophiles (Figure 42).

FIGURE 42

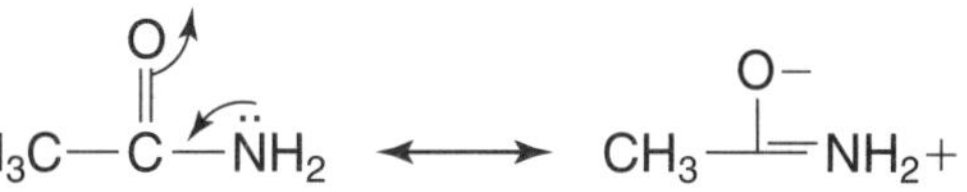

Amides can be hydrolyzed by both acids and bases, but heat is required for these transformations.

Problem

A student mixed benzoic acid, ethanol, 2-propanol, and sulfuric acid and then heated the mixture. The student analyzed the product by boiling point and determined that a mixture had been formed. The major component from the reaction would have been

A. phenyl acetate.
B. ethyl benzoate.
C. 1-methylethyl benzoate.
D. 2-methylethyl benzoate.

Solution

B. In an esterification reaction, the alcohol is a nucleophile, and the most reactive alcohols are methanol and primary alcohols. Secondary alcohols react much more slowly.

IX. AMINES

An amine has the general formula RNH_2, R_2NH, or R_3N, for a primary (1°), secondary (2°), or tertiary (3°) amine, respectively. Amines are quite basic—strong enough to turn litmus blue. They react with acids to form salts. Aliphatic amines can be extracted from an organic phase by washing the organic phase with dilute mineral acid.

An amine is named by naming the group to which it is attached and adding the suffix *-amine*. Stereoisomers of amines do exist, but the energy barrier between two possible arrangements about the nitrogen atom is so low that optical isomers are rapidly interconverted before they can be isolated. Primary and secondary amines can be converted to amides by reaction with acyl chlorides; tertiary amines will not react in this manner (Figure 43).

FIGURE 43

$$1° \ RNH_2 + R'\overset{\overset{\displaystyle O}{\|}}{-C}-Cl \longrightarrow R'\overset{\overset{\displaystyle O}{\|}}{-C}-NHR$$

$$2° \ R_2NH + R'\overset{\overset{\displaystyle O}{\|}}{-C}-Cl \longrightarrow R'\overset{\overset{\displaystyle O}{\|}}{-C}-NR_2$$

$$3° \ R_3H + R'\overset{\overset{\displaystyle O}{\|}}{-C}-Cl \longrightarrow \text{No reaction}$$

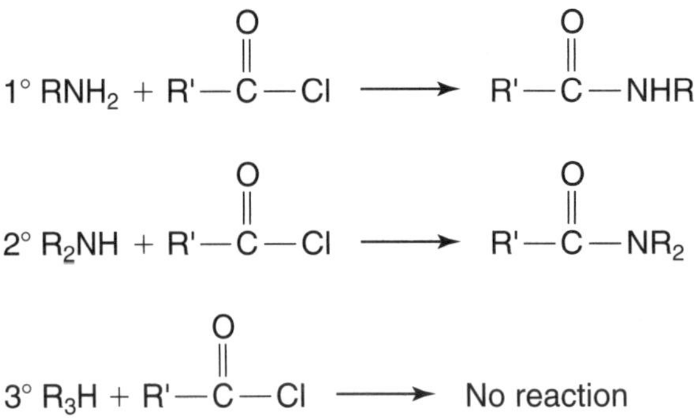

Amines can also react by alkylation. By this method, a primary amine can react with an alkyl halide to yield a secondary amine and a hydrogen halide. This process can be repeated with the secondary amine to form a tertiary amine. Finally, the tertiary amine can be converted by the same reaction to a quaternary ammonium salt (Figure 44).

FIGURE 44

$$RNH_2 \xrightarrow{RX} R_2NH \xrightarrow{RX} R_3N \xrightarrow{RX} R_4N+ \ + \ X^-$$

Quaternary ammonia salts have four organic groups covalently bonded to a nitrogen atom, and the positive charge of that ion is balanced by some negative ion. When the salt of a 1°, 2°, or 3° amine is treated with hydroxide ion, the nitrogen gives a hydrogen ion, and the free amine is liberated. The quaternary ammonium ion has no proton to give up; thus, it is not affected by hydroxide ion. The quaternary ammonium salt does react with silver oxide to form a quaternary ammonium hydroxide and a precipitate of silver halide:

$$R_4N^+ \ X^- + Ag_2O \rightarrow R_4N^+OH^- + AgX$$

Amines are more basic than water and less basic than hydroxide ions. Aliphatic amines have k_b's that are from 10^{-3} to 10^{-4}—stronger than that of ammonia. Aromatic amines have lower k_b's—10^{-9} or less—far lower than ammonia. Electron-releasing groups on the aromatic rings, such as CH_3, stabilize the cation and increase the basicity. Electron-withdrawing groups on the aromatic ring, such as COOH, halogens, destabilize the cation and decrease the basicity.

Problem

Benzamide, benzoic acid, aniline, and 1-phenylethylamine are combined with diethyl ether. Water is added and the layers are separated. What components are in the ether layer?

A. Benzamide and benzoic acid

B. Benzamide and aniline

C. Benzamide, benzoic acid, and aniline

D. Benzoic acid, aniline, and 1-phenylethylamine

Solution

B. None of the components are water soluble, so they will not be extracted. Benzoic acid and 1-phenylethylamine will react to form a salt, which will be extracted into the water layer. Aniline is too weak a base to react with benzoic acid. The nitrogen of an amide like benzamide is not basic and does not form salts with acids.

X. SEPARATIONS AND PURIFICATIONS

1. EXTRACTION

A material can be transferred from one solvent to another that is even more soluble. The only requirement is that the two solvents used must not be miscible in one another. It is standard procedure for the solvent used in the extraction to be volatile so it can be evaporated and the solute recovered. In practice, the extraction solvent is added to the solution and the container agitated. The container is then left to stand so the two phases of the immiscible solvents are completely separated. The phase containing the solute is then drained off. It is more efficient to perform several extractions using a small amount of solvent each time, rather than to perform one extraction using a large amount of solvent.

2. CHROMATOGRAPHY

Chromatography uses the differences in polarity and molecular weight to separate compounds. Any chromatography system consists of a mobile phase, such as a gas, which moves with the sample(s), and a stationary phase, which is a type of support that the samples and mobile phase move along.

In gas chromatography, the stationary phase is a liquid that is absorbed into an inert solid. The two most commonly used solid stationary phases are crushed firebrick and a similar material, kieselguhr. A variety of liquid stationary phases are used depending on the nature of the material being analyzed. Materials such as squalene, n-hexadecane, polyethylene glycol, and silicone oils and gums are commonly used. The choice depends on the polarities of the substances being separated and the maximum temperature being used for the separation.

The mobile phase is a gas that will not react with the stationary phase or the materials being separated. Helium, nitrogen, and hydrogen are commonly used, with helium by far the most common. The stationary phases are packed into a column, usually stainless steel or glass, connected to a source of gas and placed into an oven. A small amount of sample (liquid or gas) is injected into one end of the column in the direction of the gas flow. Depending on the oven temperature and differences in polarity between the stationary phase and the materials being separated, the different components of the sample will have a retention time, which is the time it takes the components to pass through the column under the given conditions.

The two most common detectors at the end of these columns—designed to distinguish the species as they leave the column—are the thermal conductivity detector (TCD, or hot-wire) and the flame ionization detector (FID). The TCD consists of a simple platinum glow-wire emitting infrared radiation (heat) that passes through the end of the column. A detector on the other side of the column records any changes in the infrared radiation passing through the column. Because the most commonly used carrier gas, helium, has a vastly different thermoconductivity than anything else (except possibly hydrogen), any material that passes through the column other than the carrier gas will absorb the infrared radiation differently, which will be registered by the detector and converted into an electronic signal.

An FID consists of a hydrogen–oxygen flame. This flame is hot enough to volatilize and ionize most substances. An ion detector above the flame registers the ions thus produced. This type of detector is about two orders of magnitude more sensitive than the TCD. It has the disadvantage of not being able to detect water because water is a product of the hydrogen–oxygen flame.

Thin-layer chromatography is a technically simpler but no less useful technique. The stationary phase is coated onto some rigid sheet in a thin layer that is usually a glass plate. Common stationary phases include starch, silica gel, cellulose, and aluminum oxide. These are applied by dissolving them in a solvent (usually water) to make a slurry and spreading a thin film on a glass plate, which is then baked in an oven to remove the solvent. The sample, in liquid form or dissolved in the mobile phase, is spotted at the bottom of the plate by a pipette and allowed to dry. The plate is then placed in a jar with a small amount of the mobile phase in the bottom. The jar is covered so the vapor pressure of the mobile phase is in equilibrium with the liquid.

The mobile phase is usually an organic solvent like benzene, chloroform, ethanol, butanol, acetone, or one of many others, or some combination of these. Differences between the polarity of the mobile phase and the substances of analysis cause the mobile phase to carry these to different heights on the plate. Once the solvent has run all the way to the top of the plate, the plate is removed from the chamber and dried. Unless the materials of interest are naturally colored, they must be stained before they can be detected. Commonly used stains include ninhydrin, pH indicators, iodine, and potassium permanganate. Sometimes ultraviolet light is used if the material fluoresces.

3. DISTILLATION

A mixture of two substances, only one of which is volatile, can be separated by distillation. A very common example is the removal of salt from water. The water will boil and vaporize at a far lower temperature than the salt. The water boils away, leaving the salt behind. The water vapor can then be condensed, and pure water can be recovered. This is known as simple distillation and is a technique that has been used for centuries.

If both components in a mixture have boiling points that are fairly close, such as benzene (b.p. = 85°C) and pentane (b.p. = 36°C), simple distillation will not do a good job of separating them. In the previous example, analysis would show that after distillation, there would be a slight enrichment of pentane (the lower-boiling material) in the distillate (the vaporized and recondensed material) and a slight enrichment of benzene (the higher boiling component) in the residue (the remains in the distillation flask), but not enough of an enrichment in either to be of any use. In such instances fractional distillation is used. A column filled with glass beads, or any other inert material offering a larger surface area, is placed between the distillation apparatus and the condenser. The less volatile vapors (in this case, benzene) will condense onto the surface of the beads and fall back into the distillation flask directly below. In such a manner, a good separation of the mixture can be realized.

4. RECRYSTALLIZATION

Recrystallization is commonly used to prepare high-purity chemicals. The original batch of impure crystals is dissolved in a "good" solvent, one in which the crystals are readily soluble. Then a "bad" solvent is added. In the bad solvent, the material of interest is insoluble but the impurities present are soluble. The substance of interest will then precipitate out of the solution.

Another method involves the use of only one solvent. The impure crystals are dissolved in a minimum amount of hot solvent. The solution is then cooled. If the solubility of the material of interest is minimal in the cold solvent but the impurities are still soluble, the material of interest will crystallize out. Doing this requires knowing the solubilities of both the material of interest and the impurities present, at various temperatures, in the solvent used.

Problem

A student measures the melting point of an unknown and finds that the melting point is 140–145°C. The student recrystallizes the unknown on a steam bath from ethyl alcohol, dries the sample, and measures the melting point again. The melting point range of the unknown will now be

A. 142–145°C. B. 140–145°C. C. the boiling point of ethanol. D. 138–145°C.

Solution

A. Recrystallization should improve the melting point and narrow the melting-point range.

XI. USE OF SPECTROSCOPY IN STRUCTURAL IDENTIFICATION

1. INFRARED SPECTROSCOPY

Infrared radiation consists of wavelengths from 0.78 to 1,000 μm. Wavelengths from 2.5 to 15 μm are most commonly used in spectroscopy, which corresponds to a frequency range of 1.2×10^{14} to 2.0×10^{13} Hz. In spectroscopy, wave number (d), which is the reciprocal of the wavelength in centimeters, is commonly used. This would correspond to a wave number of 4,000 to 670 cm^{-1}. Recall from organic chemistry that atoms attached to a carbon atom can rotate about a single bond. The bonds can also vibrate and stretch. The energy needed to excite these molecules in such a manner is present in the infrared band. For example, infrared radiation from 3,700 to 3,100 cm^{-1} (2.7 to 3.2 μm) will be absorbed by O–H and N–H bonds and cause them to vibrate. Hence, if infrared radiation is sent through an organic sample and the detector finds that the above region has been absorbed by the sample, then it is likely that the sample contains O–H and/or N–H bonds. In a like manner, triple bonds absorb between 2,700 to 1,850 cm^{-1}, and carbon–carbon double bonds absorb between 1,950 and 1,550 cm^{-1}. Tables are available that list various organic functional groups and the infrared regions that they absorb. Books are available that show the infrared spectrum of known compounds.

2. NMR SPECTROSCOPY

A strong magnetic field can cause the nuclei of certain atoms to be split into two or more quantisized energy levels. Absorption of electromagnetic energy in the range of 0.1 to 100 MHz (3,000 to 3 m) will cause transitions in the magnetically induced energy levels of the nuclei. This process is known as nuclear magnetic resonance (NMR). The sample is placed in a strong magnetic field and spun. Radio frequencies of the 0.1-to-100-MHz wavelengths are then introduced to the sample. The nucleus in question must have a quantum spin of ½ to be of any use with this procedure. Ordinary hydrogen, H^1, is the most commonly observed nuclei in this procedure; however, none of the solvents used to dissolve the sample can contain H^1. Thus, ordinary water is not suitable, nor is ordinary pentane. (However, heavy water or deuterated pentane, in which the ordinary H^1 has been replaced by H^2 [deuterium], will work fine, provided the sample is soluble in one of them.)

C^{13} is the next most commonly used atom for NMR studies. However, its natural abundance is only 1% (by comparison, H^1 is 99.99% abundant in nature), which limits its use. Other nuclei used in NMR are F^{19} and P^{31}. The frequency of the radiation absorbed (usually calibrated in parts per million) gives a clue to the surroundings of the atom of interest (e.g., for a proton, whether it is on a methyl or ethyl group, or a benzene ring). The number of splits in the absorption peak indicates how many other atoms of the same element are adjacent. The ratio of area of the peaks in the total NMR spectra shows the relative ratios of the different types of atoms present.

MCAT

MEDICAL COLLEGE ADMISSION TEST

Writing Sample Review

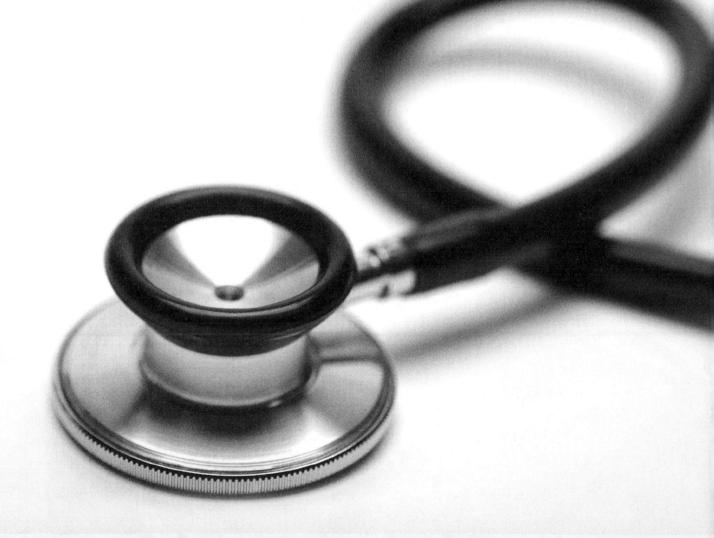

WRITING SAMPLE REVIEW

SIGNIFICANCE OF THE WRITING SAMPLE

Physicians must be able to communicate with their patients, staff, and colleagues. Not only must they be able to convey facts, findings, and their thoughts and opinions, but they must also be able to respond to important questions asked by those with whom they come into contact. Doctors must be able to receive information efficiently in oral and written form. They must be able to organize this information, give directives, and provide clear, relevant answers to questions—particularly those asked by patients. Even factual information can confuse and frighten patients—who may already be anxious, uninformed, or misinformed—if this information is carelessly presented.

Patients expect satisfactory verbal skills from their physicians. Tabulations from surveys done by the National Research Corporation show that a physician's ability to communicate effectively is of prime concern to the general public. Those surveyed deem "bedside manner" to be of greater importance than any other factor, including cost and location. *Social Science and Medicine* reports a finding that the physician's behavior (including communication) had more of an impact on patient outcome than did the patient's own behavior. The best physicians encourage the understanding and participation of their patients in their care. Clearly, effective communication is vital.

Most medical schools consider the writing ability and analytical synthesizing skills of their applicants as part of the required admission criteria. The Writing Sample section of the MCAT focuses on demonstrating those skills.

FORMAT OF THE MCAT WRITING SAMPLE

Each MCAT writing sample consists of a statement—often a direct quotation from a well-known figure or from a work of literature—and three writing tasks. The selected reading is not directly related to the biological or physical sciences, religious issues, topics that tend to generate strong emotions in readers, the application process for medical schools, or to possible rationales or motives for deciding to pursue medical school admission.

Following the quotation or statement are three specific tasks to complete in a 30-minute period. There are usually two writing samples (each with a quotation or statement and three writing tasks) on the MCAT. During a one-hour testing session, you are normally expected to complete both MCAT writing samples.

PURPOSE OF THE MCAT WRITING SAMPLES

The MCAT writing samples require you to demonstrate expository writing, a type of writing that focuses readers' attention on objects, people, events, or ideas rather than on the writer's feelings or attitudes about them. Expository writing must contain information or cover important points. This is the usual type of writing demanded on standardized exams requiring essay writing. The expository writing called for on the MCAT differs from persuasive writing, which is often called for on the Law School Admission Test (LSAT). Persuasive writing influences readers' attitudes and actions by arguing for or against a position. Consider how this differs from expository writing. Expository writing also differs from expressive writing (that emphasizes the writer's feelings and reactions to the world, people, objects, events, and ideas) and from writing done strictly for the pleasure of readers or the writer.

The writing samples included on the MCAT test many levels of knowledge. The writer is required to read at the literal level; for instance, to answer the question(s) asked, the writer must be able to demonstrate an understanding of what is asked. The writer is also required to comprehend; for example, the writer must be able to explain unusual terms. The writer must analyze (break into parts) what is expected of him or her and synthesize (put together) concepts and ideas. The writer must develop a central idea and present supporting ideas logically, using correct grammar, sentence and paragraph structure, punctuation, capitalization, and spelling.

Certain steps are necessary in preparing a good answer to the MCAT writing samples and in meeting these goals.

PREPARING TO WRITE

Writing under pressure can be frustrating. To receive a high score, you must have a realistic sense of what to expect from the writing samples. The following sections summarize essential steps in planning and writing a logical, coherent, and interesting essay.

1. Read the Statement or Question Carefully

Before beginning to write, you need to take certain preliminary steps. A few minutes spent planning will pay off: your final essay will be more focused, better developed, and clearer. You may reread the question or statement several times before and during the planning and writing of the essay. You may wish to highlight key words or phrases of the statement and/or question. If the source of the statement or question is given, you should pay attention to the author, the date or period when the statement was made, and the reference from which it was taken.

2. Consider the Audience

Essays would be pointless without an audience. An essay's success is measured by how convincing it is to its audience. Thus, successful writers determine which of the three audience types they will be addressing and address the writing specifically to that audience. An audience might be a

- general audience,
- mixed audience, or
- specialized audience.

A general audience consists of people who may not be experts on a subject but are willing to read the material. This is usually not the group that will mark the MCAT essays. A mixed audience may consist of both specialists and general readers; again, this is not likely to be the group that will score the MCAT essays. It is the third group—a specialized audience—that will likely score the essays; they have considerable knowledge of the subject and will be looking for certain things. A savvy test taker will be aware of the concerns of the specialized audience. These concerns include

- correct grammar,
- correct spelling,
- logical organization,
- generalizations supported by specific details, and
- an objective tone that is not too personal or too informal.

3. Study the Writing Tasks That Follow the Statement

Each statement or quotation is followed by three writing tasks. To receive full credit for the essay, you must address each task. It is helpful to write the essay using wording similar to that of the question so that the scorer can see immediately which task is being addressed. One of the three tasks for each essay is for you to explain what you think the statement or quotation means. The remaining two tasks ask you to describe a specific situation related to the statement or quotation and, under a given set of circumstances, whether or not the statement or quotation applies to you.

4. Prepare a Rough Outline to Fully Address Each of the Three Tasks

With a time limit of only 30 minutes, you will not be able to prepare a detailed outline as you would for an untimed essay. However, deciding how many paragraphs to have and jotting down main points (with specifics for inclusion) could help your writing go more quickly and easily. An outline helps a writer develop a logical sequence for assembling the data used in the essay. With the help of a rough outline, you are not likely to forget to include one of the writing tasks, to omit a specific supporting statement, or to remember a point you intended to make.

In a 30-minute exercise, you will probably have time for no more than four or five paragraphs. In such a format, the first paragraph will be the introduction, the next two or three paragraphs will develop the thesis with specific and relevant examples, and the final paragraph should constitute a strong conclusion.

After completing the preliminary steps of planning and outlining your essay, you are ready to begin writing the actual response to the writing task. The prewrite and organization should consume no more than five minutes.

WRITING THE INTRODUCTORY PARAGRAPH

The focus of the introduction to your essay should be the thesis statement. This statement helps readers understand the point and direction of the essay they are about to read. The thesis statement identifies the central idea of your essay and should clearly state your point of view on the subject. It also dictates the basic content and organization of your essay. The thesis is the heart of the essay; without it, readers will not be able to determine the main message or central idea of the essay. If you fail to state your thesis clearly, your entire essay will suffer.

The thesis must be something that can be argued or needs to be proven, not just an accepted fact. For example, "Animals are used every day in cosmetics and medical testing" is a fact—it needs no proof. But if you write, "Using animals for cosmetic and medical testing is cruel and should be stopped," you must support and defend this position within the confines of the three tasks given.

The thesis can be placed in any paragraph of the essay, but in a short essay, especially one written for evaluative exam purposes, the thesis is most effective when placed in the last sentence of the opening paragraph. The thesis should clearly state your opinion in a direct manner. It also serves as a blueprint for the essay. The remainder of the introduction should give two or three brief examples that support your thesis.

DEVELOPING THE PARAGRAPHS IN THE BODY OF THE ESSAY

The two or three paragraphs following the introduction will elaborate on the supporting examples you gave in your introduction. Each paragraph should discuss only one idea. Like the introduction, each paragraph should be coherently organized, with a topic sentence and supporting details.

The topic sentence is to each paragraph what the thesis statement is to the essay as a whole. It tells readers what you plan to discuss in that paragraph. It has a specific subject and is neither too broad nor too narrow. It also establishes your point of view and gives readers a sense of the direction in which you are going. An effective topic sentence also arouses readers' interest.

The topic sentence usually appears at the beginning of the paragraph, although it may occur in the middle or at the end of the paragraph. Placing it at the beginning is advantageous because it helps you stay focused on the main idea.

The remainder of each paragraph should support the topic sentence with examples and illustrations. Each sentence is supposed to progress logically from the previous one and be centrally connected to the topic sentence. Avoid including any extraneous material that does not serve to develop your thesis.

PREPARING THE CONCLUDING PARAGRAPH OF THE ESSAY

The conclusion should briefly restate the thesis and explain how it was shown to be true. The conclusion should be concise and effective for the essay to end on a strong note.

The final paragraph should not introduce any new topics that cannot be supported by further evidence. Watching a movie that suddenly shifts plot and characters at the end makes a person feel disappointed or even angry. Similarly, a conclusion must not drift away from the main focus and message of the essay. You must make sure your conclusion is clearly on the topic and represents the perspective of your essay without any confusion about its meaning. Your readers will respect you for staying true to your initial intentions.

The conclusion is your last chance to grab and impress readers. A dramatic close will remind readers of your seriousness, even passion, about the points you made in your essay. At the same time, your conclusion should not contain hyperbole or overstate the information presented.

EFFECTIVE USE OF LANGUAGE

Clear organization, while vitally important, is not the only factor the essay graders consider. Because time for the Writing Sample section is limited, minor mistakes are expected. However, you have to demonstrate clear expression of ideas and correct use of grammar, diction, usage, spelling, and punctuation. For a review of rules on grammar, usage, and mechanics, consult *The Elements of Style*, Third Edition (William Strunk Jr. and E.B. White, Boston: Allyn and Bacon, 1979.), and *REA's Handbook of English Grammar, Style and Writing* (Staff of Research & Education Association, Piscataway, NJ: Research & Education Association, 2001).

Point of View

Depending on the audience, essays may be written from one of three points of view:

1. *Subjective, Personal, or First-Person Point of View:*
   "*I* think cars are more trouble than they are worth."
   "*I* believe ..."
   "*I* feel ..."

2. *Second-Person Point of View* ("You" instead of "I" or "We"):
   "If *you* own a car, *you* will soon find out that it is more trouble than it is worth."
3. *Third-Person Point of View* (focuses on the idea, not what "I" think of it):
   "*Cars* are more trouble than *they* are worth."

It is very important to maintain a consistent point of view throughout the essay. If the writer begins writing in the first person, there should be no shift to the second or third person. Such inconsistency is confusing to readers, and the MCAT essay graders will penalize you if your essay has inconsistencies.

Tone

As a writer, the tone of your essay results from your attitude toward the subject and the audience. If your essay's topic requires a strong stand, the tone of your essay should reflect that. The tone should also be appropriate for the subject matter. A serious topic demands a serious tone. For a more light-hearted topic, you can include some humor in your essay. Whatever tone you choose, consistency is essential. Avoid sudden shifts in tone.

Transitions

Transitions are like the links of a bracelet, holding the beads or major points of an essay together. They help readers to logically follow the flow of ideas and help connect major and minor ideas. Transitions are used either at the beginning of a paragraph, or to show the connections among ideas within a single paragraph. Without transitions, readers would be distracted from the writer's ideas.

Here are some typical transitional words and phrases:

Linking Similar Ideas

again	for example	likewise
also		
for instance	moreover	

Linking Dissimilar/Contradictory Ideas

although	however	on the other hand
and		
yet		
in spite of	otherwise	

Indicating Cause, Purpose, or Result

as	for	so
as a result	for this reason	then

Indicating Time or Position

above	before	meanwhile
across	beyond	next

Indicating an Example or Summary

as a result	in any event	in other words
as I have said	in brief	in short

PROOFREADING AND REVISING THE ESSAY

Allow a few minutes at the end of the 30-minute period to proofread and (if necessary) revise your essay. The specialized audience of readers scoring the essay will read the essay as a first draft and they do not expect a perfect copy. Nevertheless, the successful examinee makes sure of the following:

- All sentences have a subject and a verb and express a clear thought.
- Run-on sentences have been avoided.
- Paragraphs have been indented, and long paragraphs have been shortened.
- The antecedent of each pronoun is clear.
- Each pronoun agrees with its antecedent in number.
- Each subject and verb agree in number.
- The same tense is used throughout the essay.
- Words are spelled correctly.
- Items in a series have been separated by commas.
- All proper nouns and the first word of each sentence have been capitalized.
- Each sentence ends with its proper mark of punctuation.
- Apostrophes have been used correctly for possession. (Contractions are avoided in formal writing.)
- Singular nouns are made to show possession by adding an apostrophe followed by an *s* ('s).
- Plural nouns ending in *s* are made to show possession by adding an apostrophe ('); plural nouns not ending in *s* are made to show possession by adding an apostrophe followed by an *s* ('s).
- *It's* is a contraction meaning "it is" and should be avoided in formal writing.
- *Its* is a possessive pronoun and requires no apostrophe.

ESSAY SCORING

The writing samples will be scored by essay graders with extensive training. Graders use a scoring guide made up of score descriptions and sample papers to score the writing samples reliably and accurately. Each grader is closely monitored throughout the scoring process to ensure fair scores for each examinee.

Essays are scored holistically, meaning that each essay is regarded as a unit and assigned a single score based on total quality. Some mistakes are expected on timed essays, so an occasional mistake will not affect the evaluation of the essay. Each paper is scored by two graders using a six-point scale. If the paper receives two scores that are more than one point apart, a third grader will determine the total score for the paper. Clarity, depth, and unity are used to determine the score. If an essay fails to address one of the writing tasks, the score cannot be higher than 3. Responses are considered not scorable if either of the two writing samples is illegible, blank, or not written in English, or if the writer totally disregards the writing task.

Score reports, percentile data, score distributions, and an explanation of the general writing characteristics of each score level are provided to the medical schools. Listed here are the typical characteristics of each of the six classifications:

6 The essay shows complexity of thought and coherent, focused organization. The ideas are thoroughly developed, and the language of the essay demonstrates superior vocabulary and sentence control.

5 The essay addresses all three writing tasks. The treatment of the topic is substantial but not thorough. Some depth of thought, control of vocabulary and sentence structure, and coherent organization are present, but major ideas are not as developed as in an essay receiving six points.

4 All three tasks are addressed; the topic is given adequate but not thorough exploration. Clarity of thought is present, but the complexity is missing. The essay is coherently organized, even though some digressions may be present. An adequate control of language is evident.

3 The essay may show some clarity of thought but may be classified as simplistic. The topic is treated coherently and major ideas are somewhat developed; however, there may be a lack of complexity and focus. The essay may neglect or distort one or more of the writing tasks. Some control of language is evident.

2 The essay seriously fails to adequately address one or more of the writing tasks. There may be problems with organization, clarity, or complexity. The essay may show several errors in mechanics, usage, or sentence structure.

1 The essay may demonstrate a lack of understanding of the writing task. Ideas are left undeveloped, and there may be serious problems with organization and clarity. Numerous errors in mechanics, usage, or sentence structure may make it difficult to follow the writer's ideas.

The number grades from the two scores are combined and assigned a letter grade from J to T. J through L scores are below average. Essays with scores of M through Q are considered average. Essays with scores of R through T are above average.

Read, plan, write, proofread, and revise! The result will be a good essay for the Writing Sample section of the MCAT.

MCAT

MEDICAL COLLEGE ADMISSION TEST

Verbal Reasoning Review

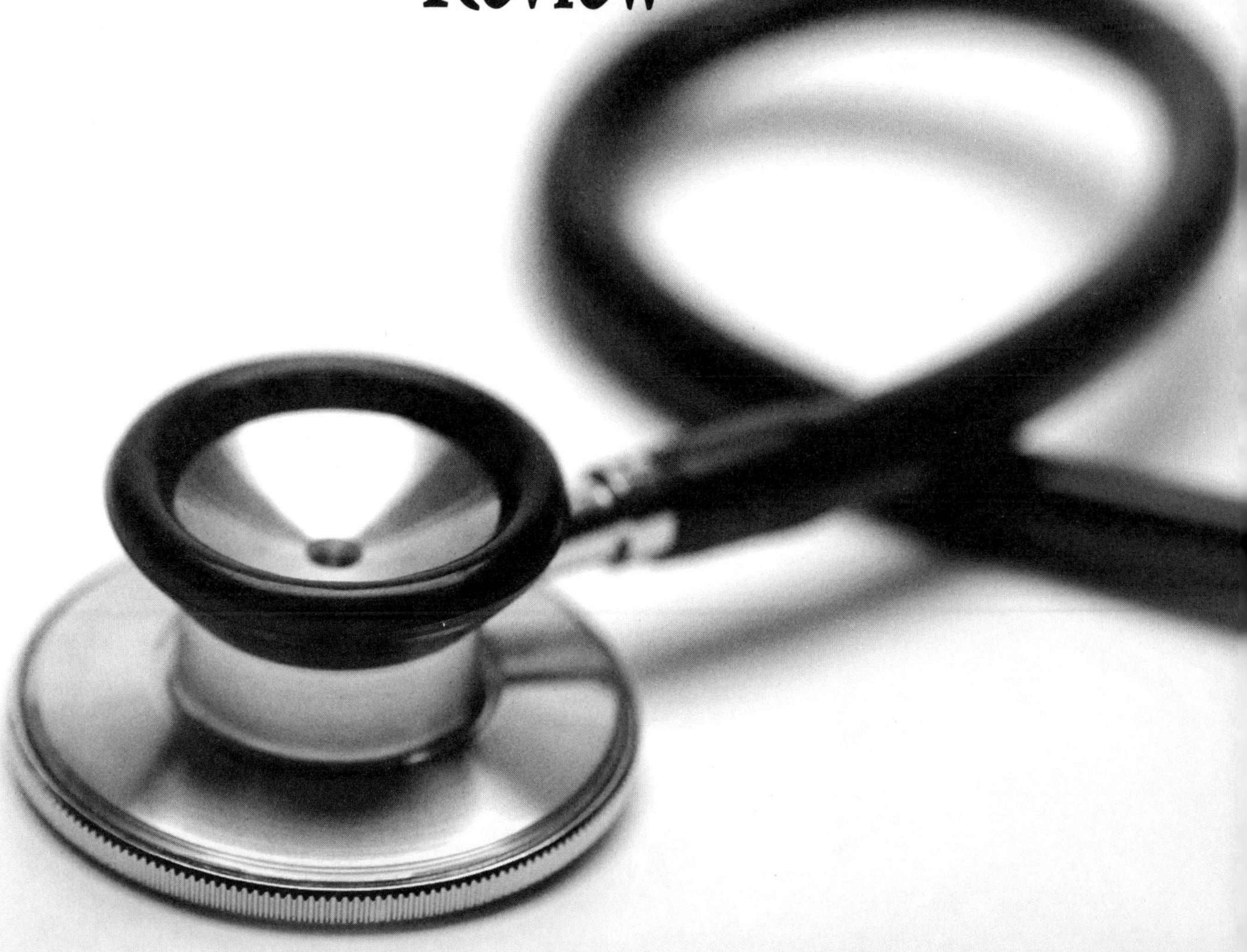

VERBAL REASONING REVIEW

PURPOSE OF THE VERBAL REASONING SECTION

In the Verbal Reasoning section of the MCAT, you are presented with several prose texts and accompanying multiple-choice questions. This part of the MCAT is designed to assess your ability to understand, evaluate, and think critically. Naturally, this is an important part of a doctor's daily routine. To obtain a thorough picture of a patient's problems, a physician must be able to comprehend medical histories and evaluate past and present symptoms and test results. In addition, a doctor has to look at a vast quantity of information and critically assess each part to establish a diagnosis and treatment for the patient.

The Verbal Reasoning section is designed to test those skills. Basically, the questions are divided into four areas:

- *Comprehension.* Comprehension questions test your ability to identify and determine the significance of, and identify the comparative relationships among, key concepts and ideas within a text passage. You have to determine the meaning of vocabulary used in the text and recognize accurate paraphrases.
- *Evaluation.* You must judge the soundness and credibility of an argument presented in the text. These questions assess your ability to distinguish between supported and unsupported claims and to judge the relevance and overall strength of an argument.
- *Application.* These test items assess your ability to predict a result or solve a specified problem and to identify general theories or models using given information. The probable cause of an event or result has to be identified, and you must evaluate the implications of any conclusions.
- *Incorporation of new information.* You are asked to recognize methods or results that challenge the presented hypotheses or theories. You have to determine if other possible solutions exist for a presented problem and how additional information affects a conclusion.

You cannot study for the Verbal Reasoning section, but you can prepare for it.

FORMAT OF THE MCAT VERBAL REASONING SECTION

The Verbal Reasoning section consists of nine passages. Each passage is followed by 5 to 10 multiple-choice questions. You have 60 minutes to answer a total of 40 questions. Each passage is 500 to 600 words long and taken from the humanities, social sciences, and areas of natural sciences not tested in the MCAT Physical Sciences and Biological Sciences sections. However, the Verbal Reasoning section is not meant to test your knowledge of specific subjects. Passages may present advanced-level topics, but the information you need to answer the questions will be in the passage or in the text of the question itself. Questions vary in difficulty, from relatively easy to difficult, and they are presented in that order.

A passage taken from the humanities might cover topics like architecture, art and art history, ethics, literary criticism, music, philosophy, and theater. A social sciences passage might come from anthropology, archaeology, economics, government, history, political science, psychology, or sociology, among other fields. A passage covering natural sciences might talk about astronomy, botany, computer science, ecology, geology, meteorology, natural history, or technology.

You will encounter passages with varying styles and content in this part of the MCAT. They are representative of the many types of written materials that college students encounter during their undergraduate coursework and thus are expected to understand. Taking undergraduate courses in the humanities and the social and natural sciences will help you become familiar with some of the types of texts and reasoning tasks presented in the Verbal Reasoning section.

THE DIRECTIONS

You should study the directions for the Verbal Reasoning section ahead of time to prevent having to take precious time to study them on the day of the test. Then you need only quickly skim the directions during the exam to refresh your memory.

Take a few minutes NOW to study the directions below:

DIRECTIONS: *The Verbal Reasoning section contains nine passages, each followed by a series of questions. Based on the information given in a passage, choose the one best answer to each question.*

Here are tips on following the directions:

Tip 1: Notice that you are instructed to choose the "best" answer based on the information given in the passage. This means that all test takers start out on equal footing in regard to knowledge of the topics because no one will have previously read the passages. Knowing this should increase your confidence.

Tip 2: Be sure to choose an answer that truly answers the question. Do not select an answer simply because it is a true statement; the answer must be the one that *best* answers the question.

Tip 3: Read all the answer choices. Often, answers that look right at first prove to be "magnet responses" meant to distract you from the correct choice.

Tip 4: Eliminate obviously incorrect answers immediately.

Tip 5: It is better to guess than not to answer at all. Even if you have absolutely no idea what the correct answer might be, you have a 25% chance of being correct by guessing. And you can increase those chances by eliminating answers you know are wrong.

READING PRACTICE

Reading many types of materials in the weeks before taking the exam can help you "shape up" for this important test. Understanding written argument—its purpose, structure, and content—is also good practice for this section. Reading newspapers, editorials, magazines, or books and answering questions afterward provides practice for the Verbal Reasoning section. Here are some questions to keep in mind while reading:

- What is the main idea of the article?
- Who is the intended audience?
- Why did the author write the article? What is the purpose?
- What is the structure of the passage?
- How does the author make the main points?
- Are there specific details? If so, what are they?
- Are there implied ideas? If so, what are they?
- Can the information be applied?
- What is the tone of the passage or the attitude of the author?

For more practice, look for questions rather than answers while reading a passage. After taking a practice test or two, you might want to begin reading passages from newspapers, magazines, scholarly journals, and books with the intent of creating MCAT-like questions based on the passages. This study technique will develop your ability to focus on key portions of a passage. In addition, your understanding of the dynamics inherent in the question-and-answer format will improve. You should develop questions with the previously listed skills in mind: comprehension, evaluation, application, and incorporation of new information.

READING SPEED

There is no *best* rate of reading. "Good" readers adjust their rate to the purpose for which they are reading. "Successful" readers, however, are aware of the strategies they use in reading. You can improve reading skills and performance on the Verbal Reasoning section by becoming aware of these successful strategies and practicing them.

The average person reads at the rate of about 250 words per minute. The reading passages on the MCAT have between 500 and 600 words. This averages out to more than two minutes to read one passage. Because nine passages appear in the Verbal Reasoning section, you should spend only about 20 of the assigned 60 minutes on actually reading the passages.

What speed should you use? Reading very slowly is not the best approach. Reading too slowly, and your mind might wander and your comprehension plummet. Reading as fast as is comfortably possible will support comprehension. You don't have to be a speed-reader to do well on the Verbal Reasoning section. In fact, reading too fast can reduce your comprehension. Most of the Verbal Reasoning passages are short enough not to require speed-reading for successful completion.

You can improve your reading speed. Articles from newspapers or magazines serve well for practice purposes. You can measure your reading speed, trying to read faster on each paragraph until you achieve an average of 250 words per minute. Because the MCAT is now computerized, you should practice reading articles from a computer screen.

A FOUR-STEP APPROACH

Following each passage on the Verbal Reasoning section of the MCAT are 5 to 10 multiple-choice questions based on the information given in the text. You have two tasks: read the passages and answer the questions.

Of those two tasks, carefully reading the passages is the most important; answering the questions is based on an understanding of the texts. Here is a four-step approach to reading:

Step 1: Previewing

Step 2: Active reading

Step 3: Reviewing

Step 4: Answering the questions

These four steps will help you successfully complete the Verbal Reasoning section.

STEP 1: PREVIEWING

A preview of the reading passage gives you the purpose and reason for reading; thus, previewing is a good strategy to use in test taking. Before reading the passage, take about 30 seconds to look over the passage and questions. An effective way to preview the passage is to read quickly the first sentence of each paragraph, the concluding sentence of the passage, and the questions—not all the answers—following the passage.

Step 2: Active Reading

After the preview, begin active reading. While reading, look for important words, topic sentences, main ideas, and words denoting the tone of the passage. If highlighting will help you save time and remember main ideas, then by all means highlight. Pay special attention to the first sentence of each paragraph because it often contains the topic of the paragraph.

Step 3: Reviewing

After finishing reading actively, take 10 to 20 seconds to look over the topic sentences and key words and phrases. Then proceed to step 4 and start answering the questions.

Step 4: Answering the Questions

Once you have completed steps 1 through 3, you are ready to answer the questions. Be careful to click the button next to the correct answer.

Don't feel bound to this technique when reading the passages. While preview, active reading, review, and answering are all necessary steps toward a respectable final score, you should experiment with strategies on practice tests.

You might feel most comfortable previewing only the questions, actively reading the passage, and then reviewing the passage while answering the questions. An alternative is to preview only the passage to become familiar with the subject matter. Then you can actively read the passage, preview the questions, review the passage, and finally answer the questions.

There is no correct answer when it comes to strategy. The four-step approach recommended here will help you gain a higher score on the MCAT. However, taking the basic four-step approach and modifying it to fit your personal needs and wants may help you even more.

Addendum to the Four-Step Approach

A modification of the four-step approach may be to actively read the passage with an initial focus on identifying the thesis statement. The thesis statement is usually expressed within the first paragraph and states the purpose of the passage. The purpose of the passage is typically to explain, prove, or demonstrate a particular point.

Subsequent paragraphs contain information that supports, tests, or refutes the thesis statement. Each paragraph contains a main topic. When reading subsequent paragraphs, you should extract the main idea and consider it in light of the thesis statement. Does the information in the paragraph support or refute the thesis statement?

When first presented with a new passage, immediately become interested in the topic. This will increase your level of comprehension and also allow you to effectively extract the thesis statement. Locating the thesis statement will help you to concentrate on the passage. Identifying the main topic of subsequent paragraphs will also serve to maintain your interest level in the passage.

The reason to actively read the passage is to answer the questions correctly. When reading the passage, try to reduce the meaning of phrases, particularly those that are very verbose, and to recognize paraphrases and synonyms.

If all subsequent paragraphs of the passage support the thesis statement, the author feels very strongly about the thesis statement. If contradictory points are presented, the author has no judgment about the thesis statement.

COMPUTERIZED MCAT FORMAT

Because the MCAT format is computerized, you read passages on a computer screen rather than a printed page. You may need to practice this skill, with its associated level of comprehension, to reach the suggested MCAT reading speed of 250 words per minute. Developing good reading skills in a computerized format will also be a benefit for other sections of the MCAT.

Highlighting selected sections of text is permitted in the computerized format. Scratch paper is also provided for you to jot down notes. All scratch paper will be collected at the end of the exam.

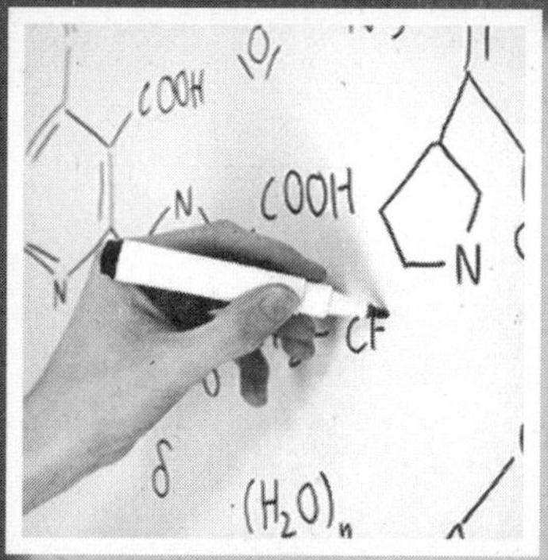

MCAT

MEDICAL COLLEGE ADMISSION TEST

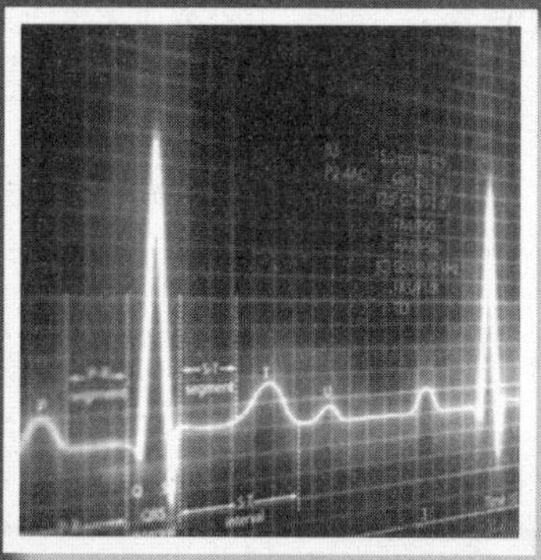

Test 1

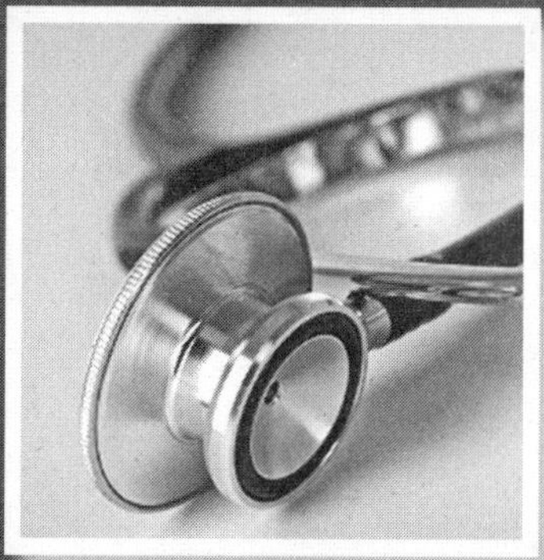

This test is also on CD-ROM in our special interactive MCAT TestWare®. It is highly recommended that you first take this exam on computer. You will then have the additional study features and benifits of enforced timed conditions, individual diagnostic analysis, and instant scoring. See page 1 for guidance on how to get the most out of our MCAT book and software.

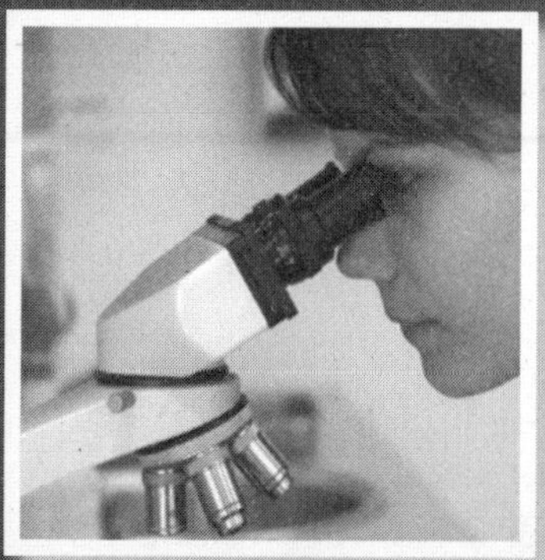

Test 1 ■ Answer Sheet

SECTION 1:
Physical Sciences

1. Ⓐ Ⓑ Ⓒ Ⓓ
2. Ⓐ Ⓑ Ⓒ Ⓓ
3. Ⓐ Ⓑ Ⓒ Ⓓ
4. Ⓐ Ⓑ Ⓒ Ⓓ
5. Ⓐ Ⓑ Ⓒ Ⓓ
6. Ⓐ Ⓑ Ⓒ Ⓓ
7. Ⓐ Ⓑ Ⓒ Ⓓ
8. Ⓐ Ⓑ Ⓒ Ⓓ
9. Ⓐ Ⓑ Ⓒ Ⓓ
10. Ⓐ Ⓑ Ⓒ Ⓓ
11. Ⓐ Ⓑ Ⓒ Ⓓ
12. Ⓐ Ⓑ Ⓒ Ⓓ
13. Ⓐ Ⓑ Ⓒ Ⓓ
14. Ⓐ Ⓑ Ⓒ Ⓓ
15. Ⓐ Ⓑ Ⓒ Ⓓ
16. Ⓐ Ⓑ Ⓒ Ⓓ
17. Ⓐ Ⓑ Ⓒ Ⓓ
18. Ⓐ Ⓑ Ⓒ Ⓓ
19. Ⓐ Ⓑ Ⓒ Ⓓ
20. Ⓐ Ⓑ Ⓒ Ⓓ
21. Ⓐ Ⓑ Ⓒ Ⓓ
22. Ⓐ Ⓑ Ⓒ Ⓓ
23. Ⓐ Ⓑ Ⓒ Ⓓ
24. Ⓐ Ⓑ Ⓒ Ⓓ
25. Ⓐ Ⓑ Ⓒ Ⓓ
26. Ⓐ Ⓑ Ⓒ Ⓓ
27. Ⓐ Ⓑ Ⓒ Ⓓ
28. Ⓐ Ⓑ Ⓒ Ⓓ
29. Ⓐ Ⓑ Ⓒ Ⓓ
30. Ⓐ Ⓑ Ⓒ Ⓓ
31. Ⓐ Ⓑ Ⓒ Ⓓ
32. Ⓐ Ⓑ Ⓒ Ⓓ
33. Ⓐ Ⓑ Ⓒ Ⓓ
34. Ⓐ Ⓑ Ⓒ Ⓓ
35. Ⓐ Ⓑ Ⓒ Ⓓ
36. Ⓐ Ⓑ Ⓒ Ⓓ
37. Ⓐ Ⓑ Ⓒ Ⓓ
38. Ⓐ Ⓑ Ⓒ Ⓓ
39. Ⓐ Ⓑ Ⓒ Ⓓ
40. Ⓐ Ⓑ Ⓒ Ⓓ
41. Ⓐ Ⓑ Ⓒ Ⓓ
42. Ⓐ Ⓑ Ⓒ Ⓓ
43. Ⓐ Ⓑ Ⓒ Ⓓ
44. Ⓐ Ⓑ Ⓒ Ⓓ
45. Ⓐ Ⓑ Ⓒ Ⓓ
46. Ⓐ Ⓑ Ⓒ Ⓓ
47. Ⓐ Ⓑ Ⓒ Ⓓ
48. Ⓐ Ⓑ Ⓒ Ⓓ
49. Ⓐ Ⓑ Ⓒ Ⓓ
50. Ⓐ Ⓑ Ⓒ Ⓓ
51. Ⓐ Ⓑ Ⓒ Ⓓ
52. Ⓐ Ⓑ Ⓒ Ⓓ

SECTION 2:
Verbal Reasoning

53. Ⓐ Ⓑ Ⓒ Ⓓ
54. Ⓐ Ⓑ Ⓒ Ⓓ
55. Ⓐ Ⓑ Ⓒ Ⓓ
56. Ⓐ Ⓑ Ⓒ Ⓓ
57. Ⓐ Ⓑ Ⓒ Ⓓ
58. Ⓐ Ⓑ Ⓒ Ⓓ
59. Ⓐ Ⓑ Ⓒ Ⓓ
60. Ⓐ Ⓑ Ⓒ Ⓓ
61. Ⓐ Ⓑ Ⓒ Ⓓ
62. Ⓐ Ⓑ Ⓒ Ⓓ
63. Ⓐ Ⓑ Ⓒ Ⓓ
64. Ⓐ Ⓑ Ⓒ Ⓓ
65. Ⓐ Ⓑ Ⓒ Ⓓ
66. Ⓐ Ⓑ Ⓒ Ⓓ
67. Ⓐ Ⓑ Ⓒ Ⓓ
68. Ⓐ Ⓑ Ⓒ Ⓓ
69. Ⓐ Ⓑ Ⓒ Ⓓ
70. Ⓐ Ⓑ Ⓒ Ⓓ
71. Ⓐ Ⓑ Ⓒ Ⓓ
72. Ⓐ Ⓑ Ⓒ Ⓓ
73. Ⓐ Ⓑ Ⓒ Ⓓ
74. Ⓐ Ⓑ Ⓒ Ⓓ
75. Ⓐ Ⓑ Ⓒ Ⓓ
76. Ⓐ Ⓑ Ⓒ Ⓓ
77. Ⓐ Ⓑ Ⓒ Ⓓ
78. Ⓐ Ⓑ Ⓒ Ⓓ
79. Ⓐ Ⓑ Ⓒ Ⓓ
80. Ⓐ Ⓑ Ⓒ Ⓓ
81. Ⓐ Ⓑ Ⓒ Ⓓ
82. Ⓐ Ⓑ Ⓒ Ⓓ
83. Ⓐ Ⓑ Ⓒ Ⓓ
84. Ⓐ Ⓑ Ⓒ Ⓓ
85. Ⓐ Ⓑ Ⓒ Ⓓ
86. Ⓐ Ⓑ Ⓒ Ⓓ
87. Ⓐ Ⓑ Ⓒ Ⓓ
88. Ⓐ Ⓑ Ⓒ Ⓓ
89. Ⓐ Ⓑ Ⓒ Ⓓ
90. Ⓐ Ⓑ Ⓒ Ⓓ
91. Ⓐ Ⓑ Ⓒ Ⓓ
92. Ⓐ Ⓑ Ⓒ Ⓓ

SECTION 4:
Biological Sciences

93. Ⓐ Ⓑ Ⓒ Ⓓ
94. Ⓐ Ⓑ Ⓒ Ⓓ
95. Ⓐ Ⓑ Ⓒ Ⓓ
96. Ⓐ Ⓑ Ⓒ Ⓓ
97. Ⓐ Ⓑ Ⓒ Ⓓ

98. Ⓐ Ⓑ Ⓒ Ⓓ
99. Ⓐ Ⓑ Ⓒ Ⓓ
100. Ⓐ Ⓑ Ⓒ Ⓓ
101. Ⓐ Ⓑ Ⓒ Ⓓ
102. Ⓐ Ⓑ Ⓒ Ⓓ
103. Ⓐ Ⓑ Ⓒ Ⓓ
104. Ⓐ Ⓑ Ⓒ Ⓓ
105. Ⓐ Ⓑ Ⓒ Ⓓ
106. Ⓐ Ⓑ Ⓒ Ⓓ
107. Ⓐ Ⓑ Ⓒ Ⓓ
108. Ⓐ Ⓑ Ⓒ Ⓓ
109. Ⓐ Ⓑ Ⓒ Ⓓ
110. Ⓐ Ⓑ Ⓒ Ⓓ
111. Ⓐ Ⓑ Ⓒ Ⓓ
112. Ⓐ Ⓑ Ⓒ Ⓓ
113. Ⓐ Ⓑ Ⓒ Ⓓ
114. Ⓐ Ⓑ Ⓒ Ⓓ
115. Ⓐ Ⓑ Ⓒ Ⓓ
116. Ⓐ Ⓑ Ⓒ Ⓓ
117. Ⓐ Ⓑ Ⓒ Ⓓ
118. Ⓐ Ⓑ Ⓒ Ⓓ
119. Ⓐ Ⓑ Ⓒ Ⓓ
120. Ⓐ Ⓑ Ⓒ Ⓓ
121. Ⓐ Ⓑ Ⓒ Ⓓ
122. Ⓐ Ⓑ Ⓒ Ⓓ
123. Ⓐ Ⓑ Ⓒ Ⓓ
124. Ⓐ Ⓑ Ⓒ Ⓓ
125. Ⓐ Ⓑ Ⓒ Ⓓ
126. Ⓐ Ⓑ Ⓒ Ⓓ
127. Ⓐ Ⓑ Ⓒ Ⓓ
128. Ⓐ Ⓑ Ⓒ Ⓓ
129. Ⓐ Ⓑ Ⓒ Ⓓ
130. Ⓐ Ⓑ Ⓒ Ⓓ
131. Ⓐ Ⓑ Ⓒ Ⓓ
132. Ⓐ Ⓑ Ⓒ Ⓓ
133. Ⓐ Ⓑ Ⓒ Ⓓ
134. Ⓐ Ⓑ Ⓒ Ⓓ
135. Ⓐ Ⓑ Ⓒ Ⓓ
136. Ⓐ Ⓑ Ⓒ Ⓓ
137. Ⓐ Ⓑ Ⓒ Ⓓ
138. Ⓐ Ⓑ Ⓒ Ⓓ
139. Ⓐ Ⓑ Ⓒ Ⓓ
140. Ⓐ Ⓑ Ⓒ Ⓓ
141. Ⓐ Ⓑ Ⓒ Ⓓ
142. Ⓐ Ⓑ Ⓒ Ⓓ
143. Ⓐ Ⓑ Ⓒ Ⓓ
144. Ⓐ Ⓑ Ⓒ Ⓓ

SECTION 1
Physical Sciences

TIME: 70 Minutes

QUESTIONS: 1–52

DIRECTIONS: Most of the questions in this section are arranged in groups, each question corresponding to a descriptive passage. Based on the information given in a passage, choose the one best answer to each question in the group. Some questions are independent of a descriptive passage and of each other. Choose the one best answer to each of these questions. If you are not sure of an answer, eliminate those choices that you know are incorrect and choose an answer from among those remaining. Fill in the corresponding circle on the answer sheet to indicate your answer. You may refer to the periodic table at any time.

PASSAGE I (QUESTIONS 1–4)

Energy production through catabolic metabolism is a fundamental process required for life. The main source of energy used in biological systems is ATP. Aerobic organisms produce ATP by the breakdown of glucose through a number of complex reactions. The production of ATP occurs through three metabolic pathways. These are glycolysis, the citric acid cycle, and oxidative phosphorylation.

In glycolysis, glucose is broken down into two pyruvate molecules according to the net reaction:

$$1\text{ Glucose} + 2PO_4^{3-} + 2ADP + 2NAD^+ \rightarrow 2\text{Pyruvate} + 2ATP + 2NADH + 2H^+ + 2H_2O$$

$$\Delta G^o = -17.5\text{kcal/mol}$$

The pyruvate produced is then oxidized to acetyl coenzyme A (acetylCoA), which is used in the citric acid cycle to produce NADH and FADH according to the net reactions:

$$1\text{Pyruvate} + CoA + NAD^+ \rightarrow \text{acetylCoA} + CO_2 + NADH$$

$$\text{acetylCoA} + 3NAD^+ + FAD + GDP + PO_4^{3-} + 2H_2O \rightarrow 2CO_2 + 3NADH + FADH_2 + GTP + 2H^+ + CoA$$

The majority of ATP production occurs during oxidative phosphorylation in the mitochondrion. Here, NADH and $FADH_2$ are oxidized, and the energy liberated is harnessed to produce ATP. The energy liberated from 1 molecule of NADH is used to produce 3 molecules of ATP. The energy liberated from 1 molecule of $FADH_2$ is used to produce 2 molecules of ATP. The process of oxidative phosphorylation requires oxygen. When oxygen levels are low, the anaerobic fermentation of pyruvate to L-lactate occurs. The removal of pyruvate competes with the production of acetylCoA, which is needed for the citric acid cycle. The equation for the fermentation of pyruvate to L-lactate is:

$$1\text{Pyruvate} + NADH + H^+ \rightarrow 1\text{ L-Lactate} + NAD^+$$

This fermentation process is not nearly as efficient in producing energy as the citric acid cycle. L-lactate is responsible for muscle aches and the burning feeling in muscles during strenuous physical activity.

1. How many moles of ATP are produced when 1 mole of glucose is converted to L-lactate?

A. 2 B. 4

C. 18 D. 36

2. How many moles of NADH are produced when 1 mole of glucose is converted to L-lactate?

   A. 4 B. 2
   C. 0 D. −2

3. Calculate the free energy change for the conversion of pyruvate to L-lactate given the following reduction potentials.

   1Pyruvate + NADH + H^+ → 1 L-Lactate + NAD^+

   Reduction potentials

   Pyruvate + $2H^+$ + $2e^-$ → lactate
   $E'_o = -0.19V$

   $NAD^+ + H^+ + 2e^- \rightarrow$ NADH
   $E'_o = -0.32V$

   1Faraday = 23.1 kcal/mol

   A. ΔG = 6 kcal/mol
   B. ΔG = 3 kcal/mol
   C. ΔG = −3 kcal/mol
   D. ΔG = −6 kcal/mol

4. Assuming the change in free energy for the conversion of pyruvate to lactate is $\Delta G = -5.0$kcal/mol, what is the change in free energy for the conversion of 1 mole of glucose to L-lactate?

   A. ΔG = −27.5 kcal/mol
   B. ΔG = −7 kcal/mol
   C. ΔG = −12.5 kcal/mol
   D. ΔG = −22.5 kcal/mol

PASSAGE II (QUESTIONS 5–8)

A chemist found an old bottle, containing a white powder, on the reagent shelf of her laboratory. The label on the bottle was partly worn away, leaving only the last three letters of the name of the contents of the bottle. These letters, "ose," suggested that the bottle might contain a sugar. In order to identify the white powder in the bottle, the chemist did several experiments.

Experiment 1. A solution was prepared by dissolving 1.500 g of the white powder in 10.00 g of water. It was noted that the temperature of the system decreased as the solution formed. The freezing point of the solution measured −1.90°C. The solution did not conduct an electric current.

Experiment 2. Qualitative elemental analysis indicated that the white powder contained only carbon, hydrogen, and oxygen. The white powder melted, with a sharp, well-defined melting point, indicating that it was a pure compound.

Experiment 3. A 30.0 mg sample of the white powder was burned with excess oxygen in a combustion analysis apparatus. The carbon dioxide and water formed were collected and weighed. The mass of carbon dioxide obtained was 44.0 mg and that of water was 18.0 mg.

5. The solubility of the white powder in water
   A. increases with increasing temperature.
   B. decreases with increasing temperature.
   C. remains the same with changing temperature.
   D. changes with changing temperature, but the nature of the change cannot be deduced on the basis of the information given in Passage II.

6. The density of the solution prepared in experiment 1 was 1.05 g/mL. What was its volume?

   A. 9.5 mL B. 10.0 mL
   C. 10.5 mL D. 11.0 mL

7. In experiment 3, what is the mass of the oxygen contained in the 30.0 mg sample of the white powder?

   A. 8 mg B. 16 mg
   C. 24 mg D. 12 mg

8. What is the simplest or empirical formula of the white powder?

   A. CHO B. CH_2O
   C. C_2H_2O D. $C_{12}H_{22}O_{11}$

PASSAGE III (QUESTIONS 9-12)

An isotope of the fictitious, transuranium element mysterium has the following properties: Atomic number: 119; Mass number: 300; First ionization energy: 300 kJ/mol; Alpha particle decay half life: 600 s.

Note that the atomic number places mysterium directly below francium, atomic number 87, in the periodic table. Mysterium was produced by bombardment of a uranium target with high-energy uranium nuclei. The target, containing unreacted uranium, mysterium, and many other reaction products, was dissolved, and the mysterium separated by a series of precipitation and ion exchange reactions. The first time mysterium was produced, the chemical separation required 30.0 minutes and the quantity of mysterium recovered was 1.0 mg.

9. If the production of mysterium involved the reaction of ${}^{238}_{92}U$ with ${}^{238}_{92}U$ and only one product in addition to the ${}^{300}_{119}My$ was produced, what is the symbol for the other product?

   A. ${}^{300}Zn$ B. ${}^{176}Tb$

   C. ${}^{191}At$ D. ${}^{258}Md$

10. Using the symbol My for mysterium, what is the formula of mysterium sulfate?

    A. My_2SO_4 B. $MySO_4$

    C. $My_2(SO_4)_3$ D. $My(SO_4)_2$

11. What is the second ionization energy of mysterium?

    A. 150 kJ/mol B. 300 kJ/mol

    C. 320 kJ/mol D. 1250 kJ/mol

12. The first time mysterium was produced, what mass of mysterium was present in the target at the end of the bombardment just before the start of the chemical separation? Assume no loss in the separation process.

    A. 0.1 mg B. 1.0 mg

    C. 3.0 mg D. 8.0 mg

QUESTIONS 13–16 are NOT based on a descriptive passage.

13. A car travels at a rate of 30 kilometers/hour for 15 kilometers. It then increases its average speed to 60 kilometers/hour for the next 30 kilometers. The overall average speed for the 45 kilometers is

    A. 30 km/hr. B. 35 km/hr.

    C. 40 km/hr. D. 45 km/hr.

14. A ball is thrown straight up into the air. When the ball is exactly at the top of its flight, the acceleration of the ball is equal to

    A. 9.8 m/s^2 up.

    B. 9.8 m/s^2 down.

    C. 0 m/s^2.

    D. It depends on the initial speed of the ball.

15. A gas placed under 1 atmosphere absolute pressure occupies a volume of 2 cubic meters at 250°K. What is the new volume if the temperature is increased to 294°K?

    A. 5.8 m^3 B. 2.35 m^3

    C. 2 m^3 D. 588 m^3

16. What is the product of the following reaction?

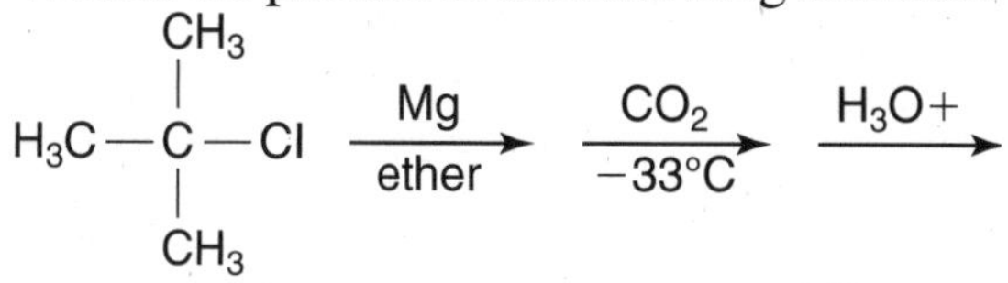

A.
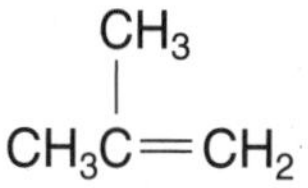

B.
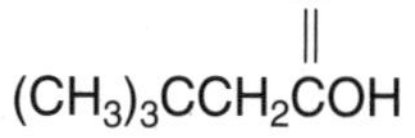

C.
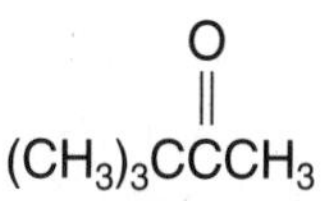

D.
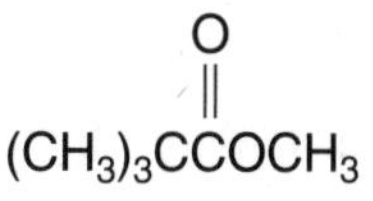

PASSAGE IV (QUESTIONS 17-21)

Magnesium has many important industrial uses. When it is combined with other metals such as aluminum or nickel, the tensile strength of the alloy is greatly increased.

Magnesium can be isolated from seawater in a multi-step process that involves precipitating the manganese from solution with base, filtering the precipitate, reacting the precipitate with HCl, and then reducing the $MgCl_2$ electrolytically to form solid magnesium metal.

$$Mg^{2+}_{\text{Seawater}} + NaOH \rightarrow Mg(OH)_{2(s)}$$

$$K_{sp} = 1.8 \times 10^{-11}$$

Filter $Mg(OH)_2$ precipitate from seawater and add to pure H_2O

$$Mg(OH)_{2(s)} + 2HCl \rightarrow Mg^{2+} + 2Cl^- + 2H_2O$$

$$Mg^{2+} + 2Cl^- \rightarrow Mg_{(s)} + Cl_{2(g)}$$

17. How many grams of NaOH are needed to precipitate $Mg(OH)_2$ from 1.0L of seawater that is 0.001M in Mg^{2+}. The K_{sp} of $MgOH_2 = 1.8 \times 10^{-11}$.
    A. 1.8×10^{-8} g NaOH
    B. 7.2×10^{-7}g NaOH
    C. 1.34×10^{-4} g NaOH
    D. 5.37×10^{-3} g NaOH

18. If the 1L of seawater above is allowed to evaporate to half its volume, how much NaOH needs to be added to induce precipitation of $Mg(OH)_2$?
    A. 1.8×10^{-7} or Δ of the original amount.
    B. 1.34×10^{-4} g NaOH, the same amount of NaOH as before.
    C. 3.79×10^{-3}g NaOH.
    D. 1.07×10^{-2}g NaOH, twice as much NaOH as before.

19. If 20.0g of $Mg(OH)_2$ is added to 1L water, what volume of 12M HCl must be added to neutralize the $Mg(OH)_2$ to form $MgCl_2$?
    A. 1.75 ml B. 5.7 ml
    C. 17.5 ml D. 57 ml

20. Calculate the cell potential for the electrolysis of Mg^{2+} to magnesium metal.

    $Mg^{2+} + 2Cl^- \quad Mg_{(s)} + Cl_{2(g)}$

    Half reaction

    $Mg^{2+} + 2e^- \quad Mg^0_{(s)}$
    $E^O = -2.38V$

    $Cl_{2(g)} + 2e^- \quad 2Cl^-_{(aq)}$
    $E^O = +1.36V$

    A. −5.1V B. −3.74V
    C. −1.02V D. 1.02V

21. Once neutralized, Mg^{2+} is in solution along with Cl^-. The magnesium ion can be electroplated to form solid magnesium metal. If 5.0 amp of current is supplied to an electrolytic cell containing Mg^{2+} and Cl^- for one hour, how many grams of magnesium are produced?
    A. 2.27g Mg B. 18.14g Mg
    C. 18.65g Mg D. 0.1865g Mg

PASSAGE V (QUESTIONS 22–25)

The rates of many biochemical reactions may be analyzed using the Michaelis-Menton mechanism for enzyme kinetics. This model uses a two-step mechanism. In the first step, the enzyme (E) reacts with the substrate (S) to form an enzyme-substrate complex (ES). In the second step, the enzyme-substrate complex decomposes to regenerate the enzyme and form the product (P).

Step 1 $E + S \underset{k'}{\overset{k}{\rightleftharpoons}} ES$

Step 2 $2ES \overset{k''}{\rightleftharpoons} E + P$

Note that the total concentration of enzyme (TE = E + ES) is constant. An expression for the rate of formation of product may be obtained using the steady state approximation. It is assumed that the rate of formation of ES is equal to its rate of disappearance.

$$k[E][S] = k'[ES] + k''[ES] \qquad \text{(Reaction 3)}$$

Substituting [TE] − [ES] for [E], rearranging, and letting Km = (k′ + k″)/k leads to:

[ES] = [TE] [S]/(Km + [S]) (Reaction 4)

The rate of product formation, from step 2, is equal to k″[ES]. Substituting for [ES] using reaction (4) gives

Rate of product formation
= k″[TE][S]/(Km + [S]) (Reaction 5)

This slightly awkward expression for the rate of product formation may be simplified for two limiting cases. If the concentration of substrate is very small, i.e., [S] << Km, then

Rate of product formation
= k″[TE] [S]/Km (Reaction 6)

On the other hand, if the substrate concentration is very large, i.e., [S] >> Km, then

Rate of product formation = k″[TE]
(Reaction 7)

22. The first step of the Michaelis-Menton mechanism is a bimolecular, second-order reaction. If the initial concentrations of both the enzyme (E) and substrate (S) are doubled, by what factor will the initial rate of formation of enzyme-substrate complex (ES) change?

 A. 2 B. 4
 C. 8 D. 16

23. Reaction (3) may be rearranged into the form of an equilibrium constant:

$$K_{eq} = [ES]/[E]\,[S].$$

 What is K_{eq} expressed in terms of rate constants?

 A. k/(k′k″) B. k′k″/k
 C. 1/Km D. Km

24. Which graph below best represents the dependence of the rate of product formation (R) on the substrate concentration ([S]) according to the Michaelis-Menton mechanism, equation (5)?

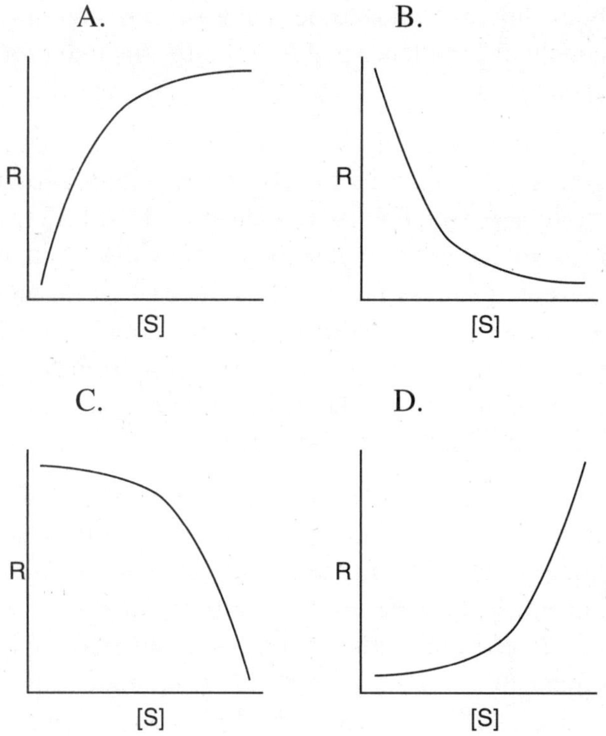

25. Reaction (6) leads to the following expression for the concentration of substrate with time:

$$\ln[S] = \ln[So] - Ct$$

 where [So] is the initial substrate concentration and C is a constant that depends on the rate constants and total enzyme concentration. What is the half life for the disappearance of substrate under these conditions?

 A. lnC/2 B. 2/lnC
 C. C/ln2 D. ln2/C

PASSAGE VI (QUESTIONS 26–29)

Almost all of the electrical energy in use today is in the form of alternating current. Alternating current can be transported over greater distances than can direct current. With the use of transformers, voltages are amplified from the power plant and transported at very high voltages, but at low currents. Some people worry about the effects of electromagnetic radiation from these power lines; however, no studies have yet provided any conclusive evidence suggesting that this radiation is dangerous.

Typical power lines use currents less than 100 A. At a distance of 20 cm away from a long straight power line with a current of 100 A, the magnetic field is equal to 1 Gauss due to that current. 1 Gauss is equal to 1×10^{-4} Tesla and is approximately equal to the magnetic field of the Earth. Therefore, magnetic fields from these power lines are not large when compared to the magnetic field of the Earth.

Another aspect of this radiation is the energy of the photon associated with the frequency (60 Hz) of the current. The 60 Hz alternating current generates photons, or particles of electromagnetic radiation, of frequency equal to 60 Hz. Using this frequency value and Planck's constant (4.14×10^{-15} electron volt-seconds), it is possible to determine the energy associated with photons of this frequency. Energy levels for photons start to become unsafe when they match the energy needed to ionize atoms.

Another issue concerning power lines is the power loss associated with the current passing through resistive wires. Part of the electrical energy is converted into thermal energy and is then unavailable for use in electric circuits at the receiving end. To minimize these losses, lower resistivity wires are used such as copper or aluminum with resistivities of 1.7×10^{-8} and 2.8×10^{-8} Ohm-meters, respectively. Other important aspects regarding the choice of wire material is the density and cost of the material. Copper has a density of 9.0 g/cm^3 and a cost of 40 ¢/kg, while aluminum has a density of 2.7 g/cm^3 and cost of 10 ¢/kg.

26. How large is the magnetic field 1 meter away from a long straight power line with a current of 100 A? Neglect the magnetic field of the Earth.
    A. 5 Gauss
    B. 1 Gauss
    C. 0.2 Gauss
    D. 0.04 Gauss

27. At what approximate frequency would a photon start to be considered unsafe?
    A. 10^{20} Hz
    B. 10^{15} Hz
    C. 10^{10} Hz
    D. 60 Hz

28. What is the mass of the section of power line from question 40?
    A. 2.8 g
    B. 450 g
    C. 28,000 g
    D. 450,000 g

29. Assume that aluminum was used for a 100-amp, 10m-long power line instead of copper and that the average power consumption was kept the same as in the copper line. (The diameter of the aluminum line would, however, be different.) What is the approximate ratio of the mass of the aluminum power line to the mass of the copper power line?
    A. 1/1
    B. 1/2
    C. 1/4
    D. 1/10

QUESTIONS 30–32 are NOT based on a descriptive passage.

30. What is the product of the following reaction?

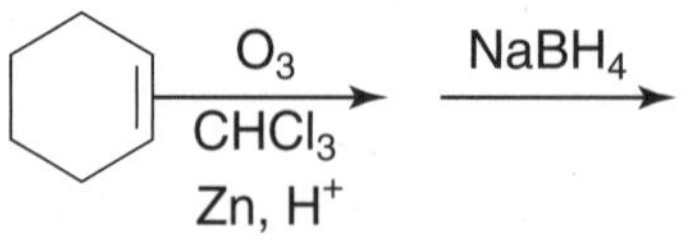

A. 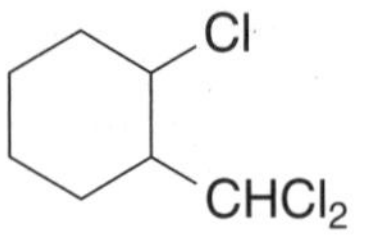

B. 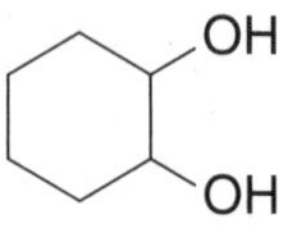

C. 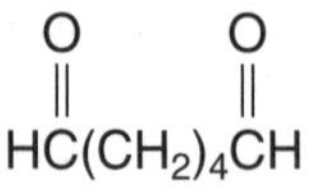

D. $HO(CH_2)_6OH$

31. All of the following share the same crystal structure EXCEPT
    A. LiCl
    B. NaCl
    C. KCl
    D. CsCl

32. Which of the following is NOT characteristic of an exothermic reaction?
    A. The potential energy of the reactants is lower than the potential energy of the products.
    B. There is a positive ΔH.
    C. There is no energy of activation.
    D. All of the above.

PASSAGE VII (QUESTIONS 33-36)

The mass spectrometer is an instrument used by scientists to determine the elemental composition of a sample. One common design is illustrated below. Initially, neutral atoms of the sample under investigation are singly ionized (that is, one electron is removed), and these ions then travel with various velocities toward the right into the velocity selector. The velocity selector consists of two parallel plates with a higher voltage on the lower plate that produces an electric field pointing upward between the plates. In addition, a magnetic field is applied perpendicular to this electric field. The purpose of the velocity selector is to provide a force on the ions in one direction, due to the electric field, and a force in the opposite direction, due to the magnetic field. For ions of a particular velocity, the forces are of exactly equal magnitude but in opposite directions so that the net force on these *selected* ions is zero. These velocity-selected ions then travel to the right undeflected and pass through the hole into the mass spectrometer chamber.

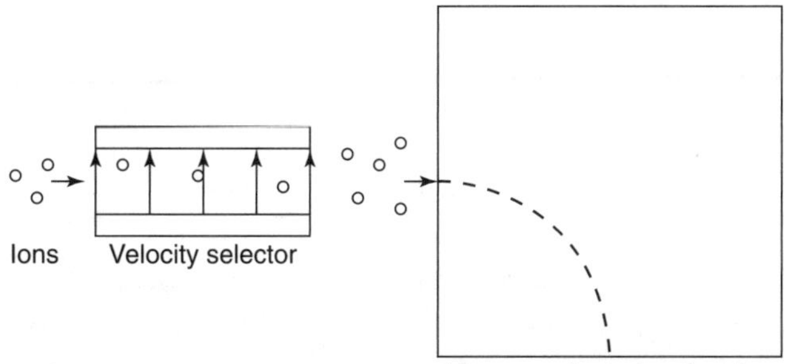

In the mass spectrometer chamber, the ions are subjected to a uniform magnetic field. The force from this magnetic field deflects the ions into a circular path, as shown by the dotted line. The radius of this circular path determines the mass of the ion, and therefore, the element.

The magnetic force on a charged ion is determined by the equation $F = qvB$. In the mass spectrometer chamber, this magnetic force is equivalent to the centripetal force that is given by $F = (mv^2)/r$. In these equations, F is the force measured in Newtons, B is the magnetic field measured in Tesla, q is the charge of the ion measured in Coulombs, v is the speed of the ion measured in meters per second, m is the mass of the ion measured in kilograms, and r is the radius of the circle measured in meters.

Other pertinent information is the charge of a proton, which is $+1.6 \times 10^{-19}$ C, and the charge of an electron, which is -1.6×10^{-19} C. The electric field in the velocity selector is equal to 4.0×10^6 N/C. The magnetic field in the velocity selector is 2.5 Tesla, and the magnetic field in the mass spectrometer chamber is 8.0 Tesla.

33. What is the magnitude of the force due to the electric field on the ions in the velocity selector?
    A. 6.4×10^{-13} N
    B. 2.5×10^{25} N
    C. 4×10^{-26} N
    D. It depends on the mass of the ion.

34. What is the direction of the magnetic field in the velocity selector?
    A. Toward the right
    B. Toward the left
    C. Into the page
    D. Out of the page

35. In relation to the electric field, E, and magnetic field, B, in the velocity selector, the velocity of the velocity-selected ions is determined by the relation
    A. $v = EB$
    B. $v = B/E$
    C. $v = E/B$
    D. $v = E + B$

36. What is the direction of the force on the ion in the mass spectrometer chamber?
    A. Pointing in toward the center of the circle
    B. Pointing outward from the center of the circle
    C. Pointing along the direction of the motion
    D. Pointing against the direction of motion

PASSAGE VIII (QUESTIONS 37–41)

In the United States, traffic accidents account for the loss of over 40,000 lives each year. Extensive research has gone into the causes of these accidents, including influences from driver behavior, vehicle safety features, and road conditions. The application of basic physics to vehicle collisions can lead to a better understanding of the pertinent elements that determine driver safety. For example, in the collision illustrated below, a 1000-kg car initially traveling to the right at a speed of 30 m/s collides head-on with a 2000-kg truck initially traveling to the left. During the collision, the bumpers lock together. Immediately after the collision, the two vehicles start skidding to the left as one mass at a speed of 6 m/s. Just before and just after the collision, conservation of momentum may be applied to the system of the two vehicles because external forces, namely, friction, have not had a chance to take effect. As always, Newton's three laws of motion also apply.

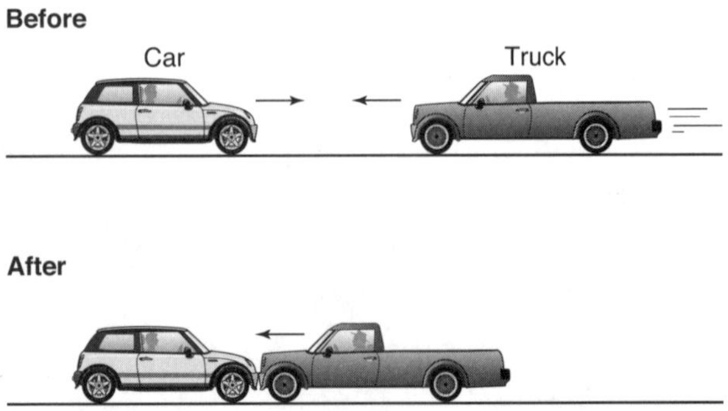

Other physics pertaining to collisions concern the concept of impulse. For an object in a collision, the impulse, I, is defined by the equation,

$$I = F\,\Delta t = \Delta p,$$

where F is the average force on the object, Δt is the interaction time or duration of the collision, and Δp is the change in momentum of the object. This concept is exploited in test collisions involving crash dummies. In one collision, a car with a padded dashboard travels at a certain speed until it crashes into a brick wall coming to a stop. The exact same experiment is repeated with the exact same car, but the padding is removed from the dashboard. In each instance, because no seat belts are used, the dummy is allowed to hit the dashboard, causing the dummy to come to a stop. Then, the damage to the dummy is measured.

Another issue influencing driver safety concerns the stopping distance of a car. Friction between the tires and the ground is the key factor in determining stopping distance. Some coefficients of kinetic (μ_k) and static (μ_s) friction between tire rubber and concrete are listed in the table below.

Surfaces	μ_k	μ_s
rubber on dry concrete	0.85	1.2
rubber on wet concrete	0.60	0.80

The speed of the car at the time the brakes are applied is another factor that strongly influences stopping distance. In fact, stopping distance is proportional to the square of the speed of the car.

37. In the illustrated collision between the two vehicles, what was the initial speed of the truck just before the collision?
    A. 6 m/s
    B. 12 m/s
    C. 24 m/s
    D. 36 m/s

38. During the collision, what is the ratio of the force of the truck on the car to the force of the car on the truck?
    A. 1/2
    B. 1/1
    C. 2/1
    D. 4/1

39. In a certain experiment, a car is driven at a speed of 10 m/s. The brakes are suddenly applied, and the car stops over a distance of

20 m. The experiment is repeated with the same car, but the speed of the car is 30 m/s when the brakes are applied. What is the new stopping distance?

A. 20 m
B. 60 m
C. 180 m
D. 900 m

40. A small town sets the speed limit so that the average car should be able to stop in a distance of 4 m. The deceleration rate of the average car is 10 m/s^2. Neglecting the reaction time needed to apply the brakes, what should be the speed limit for the average car?

A. 4 m/s
B. 9 m/s
C. 20 m/s
D. 40 m/s

41. Which graph below best illustrates the force of the padded dashboard on the dummy's head as a function of time?

A.

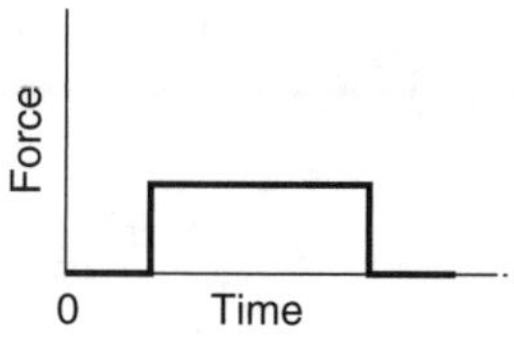

B.

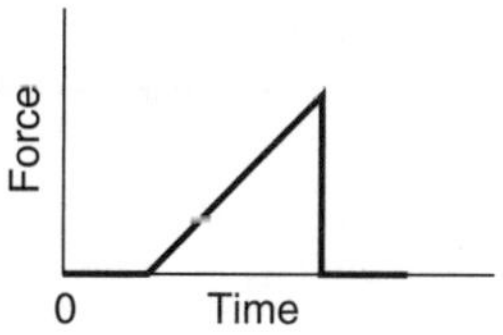

C.

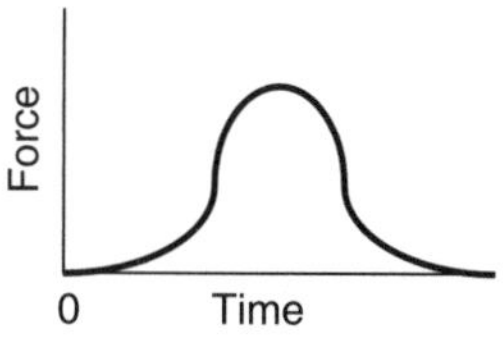

D.

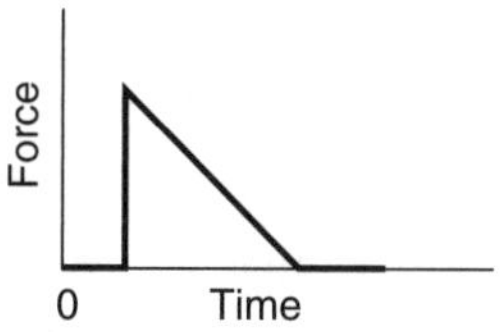

PASSAGE IX (QUESTIONS 42–45)

The electrical circuit in an X-ray room is 120 V and has a 20 A circuit breaker. The small X-ray unit plugged into this circuit draws a current of 8 A. In addition to the X-ray unit, a 1200 W coffee maker is plugged into this circuit. The X-ray unit contains both a step-up and a step-down transformer. The step-down transformer converts the 120 V to 6 V to heat the cathode of the X-ray tube to produce electrons. The step-up transformer converts the 120 V to 48000 V, which is then rectified and used to accelerate the electrons within the X-ray tube where they collide with the anode to produce the X-rays. The X-ray unit contains many electrical circuits. A small part of one of these circuits is diagrammed below. In this portion of the circuit, a 10 ohm resistor is connected in series with a 5 ohm resistor and this combination is in parallel with a 15 ohm resistor.

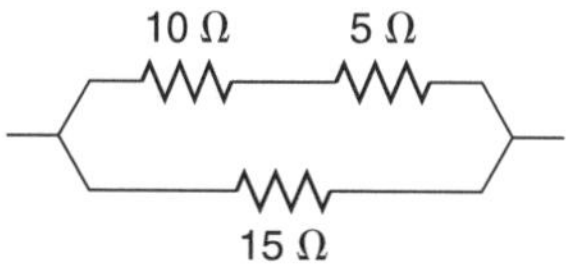

42. As stated in the passage, "the step-up transformer converts the 120 V to 48000 V, which is then rectified and used to accelerate the electrons within the X-ray tube . . . ." The meaning of the term *rectified* in this context refers to

A. the conversion of electrical energy into kinetic energy.
B. the conversion of 48000 V back to 120 V.
C. the conversion of alternating-current voltage into direct-current voltage.
D. the narrowing of the electron beam.

43. What is the resistance of the coffee maker?

A. 2 ohm
B. 6 ohm
C. 10 ohm
D. 12 ohm

44. What single resistor is equivalent to the combination of resistors described and diagrammed above?

A. 7.5 ohm
B. 15 ohm
C. 22.5 ohm
D. 30 ohm

45. Assume that a third device is plugged into the same circuit as the X-ray unit and the coffee maker. How much current would this third device need to draw to just barely trip the circuit breaker?

A. 4 A
B. 3 A
C. 2 A
D. 1 A

PASSAGE X (QUESTIONS 46–50)

Sound is a longitudinal pressure wave in the medium through which it is transmitted. The speed of sound depends on the density of the medium and temperature. For gases, the speed of sound is proportional to the square root of the absolute temperature. Approximate values of the speed of sound, near room temperature in three materials, are given in the table below.

Material	Speed of Sound (m/s)
air	340
helium	1020
tissue	1600

The human ear can detect sound over a wide range of frequencies, extending from as low as 50 Hz to as high as 20 kHz. Ultrasound, with frequencies of a few megahertz and wavelength of 0.1 mm in tissue, is used as a diagnostic tool. For example, the reflection of a focused beam of ultrasound from a tumor may be used to locate the depth and size of the tumor.

The intensity level of sound is usually measured in decibels. The intensity level in decibels (dB) is related to the intensity (I) or sound pressure (P) by dB = 10 log (I/I_0) = 20 log (P/P_0). The most commonly used reference is to take P_0 = 200 picobar = 2×10^{-5} N/m^2. The loudness of a sound, as detected by the human ear, varies with the intensity level and with the frequency or pitch of the sound. The loudness level, measured in a unit called a phon, is defined such that at a frequency of 1000 Hz, the intensity level in decibels is numerically equal to the loudness level in phons. At other frequencies, the loudness level may be greater or smaller than the intensity level. The figure below shows the variation of the intensity level with frequency for a constant loudness level of 40 phons.

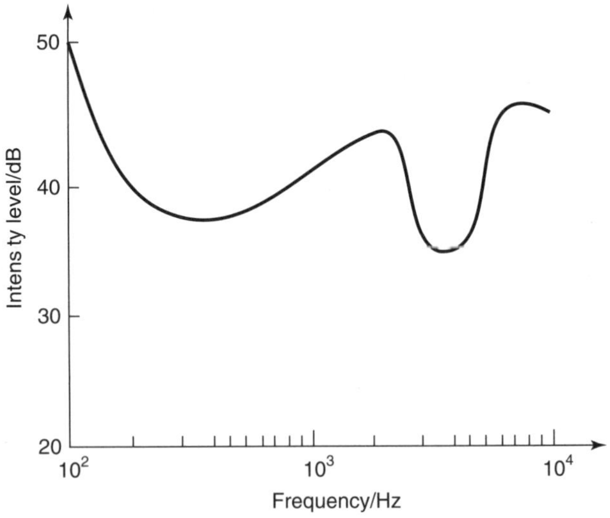

46. For a given wavelength and temperature, what is the ratio of the frequency of sound in helium to that in air?
    A. 1/3
    B. 3/1
    C. $1/\sqrt{3}$
    D. $\sqrt{3}/1$

47. The time interval between the ultrasound echoes from the front and rear surfaces of a tumor was measured to be 10 μs. What is the thickness of the tumor?
    A. 2 mm
    B. 4 mm
    C. 8 mm
    D. 16 mm

48. Tissue is denser than air, and air is denser than helium. From this information and from the preceding table for the speed of sound at room temperature in these materials, it can be said that the speed of sound
    A. is proportional to the density of the material.
    B. is proportional to the square of the density of the material.
    C. is proportional to the square root of the density of the material.
    D. may be dependent on the density of the material, but it must also depend on at least one other factor besides temperature and density.

49. A violin string of length L is plucked and vibrates as shown below:

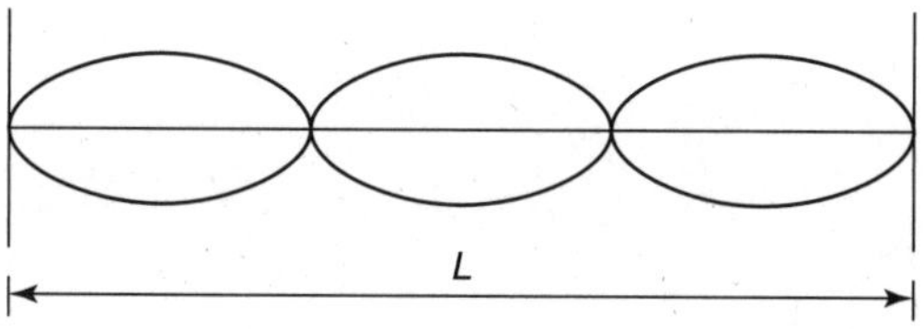

What is the wavelength of the sound wave produced by this vibration?

A. $L/3$ B. $2L/3$
C. $L/2$ D. $3L/2$

50. By what factor is the pressure of a sound wave of intensity level 40 dB greater than the pressure of a 20 dB intensity level sound wave?

A. 2 B. 5
C. 10 D. 20

QUESTIONS 51–52 are NOT based on a descriptive passage.

51. What is the kinetic energy of a 100 gram projectile traveling with a velocity of 60 m/sec?

A. 60 joules B. 80 joules
C. 100 joules D. 180 joules

52. The Newton is an expression of what relationship?

A. kg × m/s B. grams × cm/s^2
C. slugs × ft/s^2 D. kg × m/s^2

If time still remains, you may review work only in this section. When the time allotted is up, you may go on to the next section.

SECTION 2
Verbal Reasoning

TIME: 60 Minutes

QUESTIONS: 53–92

DIRECTIONS: The verbal reasoning section contains nine passages, each followed by a series of questions. Based on the information given in a passage, choose the one best answer to each question.*

PASSAGE I (QUESTIONS 53–57)

A good scientific law or theory is falsifiable simply because it makes definite claims about the world. For the falsificationist, it follows readily that the more falsifiable a theory is, the better. The more claims a theory makes, the more potential there is for showing that the world does not, in fact, behave in the way laid down by that theory. A very good theory is one that makes very wide-ranging claims about the world, and that is, consequently, highly falsifiable. This is a theory that resists falsification whenever it is put to the test.

This point can be illustrated by means of a trivial example. Consider the two laws:

(a) Mars moves in an ellipse around the sun.
(b) All planets move in ellipses around their sun.

It is clear that (b) has a higher status than (a) as a piece of scientific knowledge. Law (b) tells us what law (a) tells us and more. Law (b), the preferable law, is more falsifiable than (a). If observations of Mars should turn out to falsify (a), then they would falsify (b) also. Any falsification of (a) will be a falsification of (b), but the reverse is not the case. Observation statements referring to the orbits of Venus, Jupiter, etc., that might conceivably falsify (b) are irrelevant to (a). If we follow Popper and refer to those sets of observational statements that would serve to falsify a law or theory as potential falsifiers of that law or theory, then we can say that the potential falsifiers of (a) form a class that is a subclass of the potential falsifiers of (b). Law (b) is more falsifiable than law (a), which is tantamount to saying that, because it claims more, it is the better law.

A less-contrived example involves the relationship between Kepler's theory of the solar system and Newton's theory of the solar system. Kepler's theory consists of three laws of planetary motion. Potential falsifiers of this theory consist of sets of statements referring to planetary positions, relative to the sun, at specified times. Newton's theory, a better theory that supersedes Kepler's, is more comprehensive. It consists of Newton's law of motion, plus his law of gravitation, with the latter asserting that all pairs of bodies in the universe attract each other with a force that varies inversely as the square of their separation. Some of the potential falsifiers of Newton's theory are sets of statements of planetary positions at specified times, but there are many others. These include those referring to the behavior of falling bodies and pendulums, the correlation between the tides and the locations of the sun and moon, and so on. There are many more opportunities to falsify Newton's theory than there are to falsify Kepler's theory. As the falsificationist's theory goes, Newton's theory is able to resist falsification attempts, thereby establishing its superiority over Kepler's theory.

Highly falsifiable theories should be preferred over less falsifiable ones, provided they have not, in fact, been falsified. This qualification is important to the falsificationist. Theories that have been falsified must be ruthlessly rejected. The enterprise of science consists in the proposal of highly falsifiable hypotheses, followed by deliberate and tenacious attempts to falsify them.

"We learn from our mistakes. Science progresses by trial and error." Falsifications become important landmarks, striking achievements, and major growing-points in science because of this logical process. This renders impossible the derivation of universal laws and theories from observation, but makes possible the deduction of their falsity.

Adapted from A. F. Chalmers. *What Is This Thing Called Science*? 2nd edition. New York: University of Queensland Press, 1982, pp. 42–43.

53. According to the author, the most important advances in science occur by
    A. proposing highly falsifiable theories.
    B. falsifying existing theories.
    C. finding general theories of motion.
    D. identifying theories of planetary motion.

54. Based on the passage, which of the following is a *potential falsifier*?
    A. An observation statement that falsifies an existing theory
    B. A description of a general theory
    C. A statement describing a narrowly defined theory
    D. A statement describing the shape of Mars' orbit

55. Based on the passage, it can be reasonably inferred that a bad scientific theory does which of the following?
    A. Limits the advance of scientific knowledge
    B. Fails to make definite claims about the world
    C. Has been falsified
    D. Inaccurately describes planetary motion

56. Based on the passage, which of the following would a falsificationist consider necessary for a very good scientific theory?
    I. A theory making wide-ranging claims about the world
    II. A theory that resists falsification
    III. A theory containing false claims
    A. I only
    B. I and II
    C. I and III
    D. II and III

57. According to the passage, which of the following would not be considered a potential falsifier of Kepler's theory?
    A. An observation that Mars was not in the correct place at a given time
    B. An observation that neither Mars nor Venus were in the predicted places at a specified time
    C. An observation that there was no correlation between the tides and the positions of the sun and moon
    D. An observation that none of the planets in the solar system conformed to their predicted positions at any point in time

PASSAGE II (QUESTIONS 58–62)

It is a fundamental claim of feminism that women are oppressed. The word *oppression* is a strong word that repels and attracts. It is dangerous, dangerously fashionable, and in danger of losing its meaning. It is also misused intentionally in many instances.

The statement that women are oppressed is frequently met with the claim that men are also oppressed. We hear that the act of oppressing is oppressive to those who oppress, as well as to those who are oppressed. Some men cite as evidence of their oppression their much-advertised inability to cry. It is difficult, women are told, to be masculine. When the stress and frustration of being a man are cited as evidence that they, as oppressors, are oppressed by their oppressive actions, the word *oppression* is being stretched to meaninglessness. It is treated as though its scope includes any and all human experience of limitation or suffering, no matter the cause, degree or consequence. Once such usage has been put on us, if we ever deny that any person or group is oppressed, we seem to imply that we think they never suffer or have feelings. We are accused of insensitivity; even of bigotry. For women, such accusation is particularly intimidating, since sensitivity is one of the few virtues that have been assigned to us. If we are found insensitive, we may fear we have no redeeming traits at all, and perhaps are not real women. Thus, we are silenced before we begin: the name of our situation, drained of meaning, and our guilt mechanisms tripped.

But this is nonsense. Human beings can be miserable without being oppressed. It is perfectly consistent to deny that a person or group is oppressed without denying that they have feelings or that they suffer.

One is marked for application of oppressive pressures by one's membership in some group or category. Much of one's suffering and frustration befalls one partly, or largely, because one is a member of that category. In the case at hand, it is the category, "woman." "Being a woman is a major factor in my not having a better job than I do; being a woman selects me as a likely victim of sexual assault or harassment; it is my being a woman that reduces the power of my anger to a proof of my insanity." If a woman has little, or no, economic or political power, and/or achieves little of what she wants to achieve, a major causal factor is that she is a woman. For any women of any race or economic class, being a woman is significantly attached to whatever disadvantages and deprivations she suffers, be they great or small.

This is not the case with respect to a person being a man. Simply being a man is not what stands between him and a better job. Whatever assaults and harassments a man is subject to, being male is not what selects him for victimization. Being male is not a factor that would make his anger impotent; in fact, quite the opposite. If a man has little, or no, material or political power, and/or achieves little of what he wants to achieve, his being male is not part of the explanation. Being male is something he has working for him, even if race, class, age, or disability work against him.

Women are oppressed for being women. Members of certain racial and/or economic groups and classes, both the males and the females, are oppressed for being members of those races and/or classes. But men are not oppressed for being men.

Adapted from Marilyn Frye. *The Politics of Reality: Essays in Feminist Theory*. Trumansburg, New York: The Crossing Press, 1983, pp. 1–2, 15–16.

58. Based on the passage, which of the following is an accurate statement of the author's feeling about the word *oppression*?
    A. It should not be used to describe what has happened to women.
    B. It can never be applied to men.
    C. It loses meaning when applied to describing mere misery.
    D. It has no application to feminist theory.

59. Based on the passage, which of the following does the author argue?
    A. Men are never oppressed.
    B. Men do not oppress women.
    C. Women never oppress men.
    D. Men are not oppressed simply due to their gender.

60. Which of the following problems does the author claim is caused in large part by her being a woman?
    I. Not having a better job
    II. Being subject to sexual harassment
    III. Suffering any deprivations
    A. I only
    B. II only
    C. I and II
    D. I, II, and III

61. The author argues one is marked for oppression due to which of the following?
    A. Because one is a man
    B. Due to membership in some group
    C. Because one is a woman
    D. Due to individual characteristics

62. The author notes women may fear they have no redeeming traits if they are considered insensitive. To be true, this argument must be based on the assumption that
    A. women see themselves as being sensitive.
    B. men see women as being sensitive.
    C. women have only one redeeming trait.
    D. women are insensitive.

PASSAGE III (QUESTIONS 63–68)

In the first quarter of the twentieth century, two momentous theories were proposed: the theory of relativity and the quantum theory. From them sprang most of twentieth-century physics. But the new physics soon revealed much more than simply a better model of the physical world. Physicists began to realize that their discoveries demanded a radical reformulation of the most fundamental aspects of reality. They learned to approach their subject in totally unexpected and novel ways that seemed to turn common sense on its head and that found accord with mysticism rather than materialism.

The fruits of this revolution are only now starting to be plucked by philosophers and theologians. Many ordinary people too, searching for a deeper meaning behind their lives, find their beliefs about the world very much in tune with the new physics. The physicist's outlook is even finding sympathy with psychologists and sociologists, especially those who advocate a holistic approach to their subjects.

In giving lectures and talks on modern physics, I have discerned a growing feeling that fundamental physics is pointing the way to a new appreciation of man and his place in the universe. Deep questions of existence — "How did the universe begin and how will it end? What is matter? What is life? What is mind?" — are not new. What is new is that, at last, we may be on the verge of answering them. This astonishing prospect stems from some spectacular recent advances in physical science — not only the new physics, but its close relative, the new cosmology.

For the first time, a unified description of all creation could be within our grasp. No scientific problem is more fundamental or more daunting than the puzzle of how the universe came into being. Could this have happened without any supernatural input? Quantum physics seems to provide a loophole to the age-old assumption that "you can't get something for nothing." Physicists are now talking about "the self-creating universe": a cosmos that erupts into existence spontaneously, much as a subnuclear particle sometimes pops out of nowhere in certain high energy processes. The question of whether the details of this theory are right or wrong is not so very important. What matters is that it is now possible to conceive of a scientific explanation for all creation. Has modern physics abolished God altogether?

Yet, this is not a book about religion. Nor is this a science book. Rather, it is about the impact of the new physics on what were formerly religious issues. In particular, I make no attempt to discuss religious experiences or questions of morality. This is a book about science and its wider implications. Inevitably, it is necessary to explain some technicalities in careful detail, but I do not claim that the scientific discussions are either systematic or complete. The reader should not be deterred by the thought that he or she is in for some punishing mathematics or strings of specialist terminology. I have tried to avoid technical jargon as much as possible.

The central theme of the book concerns what I call the Big Four Questions of Existence. Toward the end of the book, tentative answers to these questions begin to emerge — answers based on the physicist's conception of nature. The answers may be totally wrong, but I believe that physics is uniquely placed to provide them. It may seem bizarre, but in my opinion, science offers a surer path to God than religion. Right or wrong, the fact that science has actually advanced to the point that, what were formerly religious questions can be seriously tackled, in itself indicates the far-reaching consequences of the new physics.

Adapted from Paul Davies. *God and the New Physics*. New York: Simon & Schuster, 1983, pp. vii–ix.

63. Which of the following does the author suggest about quantum theory and the theory of relativity?
    A. Relativity proved useless after quantum theory was discovered.
    B. They caused a re-examination of fundamental theories of reality.
    C. Their implications were confined to the physical world.
    D. They had little impact on the scientific community.

64. According to the author, which of the following groups have benefited from the new physics?
    I. Theologians
    II. Psychologists
    III. Ordinary people
    A. I and II
    B. I and III
    C. II and III
    D. I, II, and III

65. Which of the following does the author assert with respect to answers to the Big Four Questions of Existence?
    A. He has the correct answers to these questions.
    B. These questions are unanswerable.
    C. Physics is in a good position to attempt to answer them.
    D. These questions are irrelevant to the new physics.

66. By suggesting the physicist's outlook is finding sympathy with sociologists, the author means which of the following?
    A. Sociologists feel sorry for physicists.
    B. Some sociologists agree with the physicist's outlook.
    C. Physicists agree with the sociological viewpoint.
    D. Sociologists now study the new physics.

67. The author asks whether the new physics has abolished God. Based on the passage, what does the author most likely believe about the question?
    A. The author believes it is true.
    B. The author believes it is false.
    C. The author believes this will be the eventual conclusion reached by the new physics.
    D. The author believes the question bears no relevance to the new physics.

68. According to the author, new discoveries in physics forced physicists to do which of the following?
    A. Concentrate their energies on particle physics
    B. Begin to examine religion
    C. Reject psychological notions of mind and matter
    D. Examine physics in ways contrary to common sense

PASSAGE IV (QUESTIONS 69–72)

Each year millions of people die from malnutrition and related health problems. For those of us in affluent countries, this poses an acute moral problem. We spend money on ourselves, not only for the necessities of life, but for innumerable luxuries. The problem is that we could forgo our luxuries and give the money for famine relief instead. The fact that we don't suggests that we regard our luxuries as more important than feeding the hungry.

Instead of asking the question, "Why do we behave as we do?" we should ask, "What is our duty? What should we do?" We might think of this as the "common-sense" view of the matter: morality requires that we balance our own interests against the interests of others. It is understandable, of course, that we look out for our own interests, and no one can be faulted for attending to his own basic needs. But at the same time, the needs of others are also important, and when we can help others, especially at little cost to ourselves, we should do so.

But, one person's common sense is another person's naive platitude. Some thinkers have maintained that, in fact, we have no "natural" duties to other people. Ethical Egoism is the idea that each person ought to pursue his or her own self-interest exclusively. This is different from Psychological Egoism, which is a theory of human nature concerned with how people do behave — Psychological Egoism says that people do in fact always pursue their own interests. Ethical Egoism, by contrast, is a normative theory — that is, a theory about how we ought to behave. Regardless of how we do behave, Ethical Egoism says we have no moral duty except to do what is best for ourselves.

Ethical Egoism does not say that one should promote one's own interests as well as the interests of others. That would be an ordinary, unexceptional view. Ethical Egoism is the radical view that one's only duty is to promote one's own interests. According to Ethical Egoism, there is only one ultimate principle of conduct: the principle of self-interest. This principle sums up *all* of one's natural duties and obligations.

However, Ethical Egoism does not say that you should avoid actions that help others, either. It may very well be that in many instances your interests coincide with the interests of others, so that in helping yourself you will be aiding others. Or it may happen that aiding others is an effective means for creating some benefit for you. Ethical Egoism does not forbid such actions; in fact, it may demand them. The theory insists only that in such cases the benefit to others is not what makes the act right. What makes the act right is, rather, the fact that it is to one's own advantage.

Finally, Ethical Egoism does not imply that in pursuing one's interests, one always ought to do what one wants to do, or what gives one the most pleasure in the short run. Someone may want to do something that is not good for himself or that will eventually cause himself more grief than pleasure — he may want to drink a lot or smoke cigarettes or take drugs or waste his best years at the race track. Ethical Egoism would frown upon all this, regardless of the momentary pleasure it affords. It says that a person ought to do what really is in his or her own best interest over the long run. It endorses selfishness, but it doesn't endorse foolishness.

Adapted from James Rachels. *The Elements of Moral Philosophy*. New York: Random House, 1986, pp. 65–67.

69. According to the author, the common-sense view of morality holds which of the following?
    A. Act to provide the greatest good to the most people.
    B. Act to help others, especially when it costs us little.
    C. Consider only the interests of others in deciding how to act.
    D. Act according to our own common sense.

70. Based on the passage, which of the following would the author most probably say is our duty with respect to world hunger?
    A. Give up our luxuries and give the money to the world hunger relief effort.
    B. Continue to enjoy our luxuries.
    C. Ignore the problem.
    D. The passage gives no indication as to how the author thinks we should act.

71. Based on the passage, which of the following is most likely to be consistent with Ethical Egoism?
    I. Playing video games
    II. Opening a savings account
    III. Smoking cigarettes
    A. I only
    B. II only
    C. III only
    D. I, II, and III

72. Which of the following problems is most likely to occur when applying Ethical Egoism in real-world situations?
    A. Identifying long-term and short-term interests
    B. Avoiding helping others
    C. Eliminating common-sense actions
    D. Logistical interpretation of natural duty

PASSAGE V (QUESTIONS 73–77)

A nurse I know believes that more babies are born during the full moon than at any other time. She recently told me, "The moon was full last week, and we had double the normal number of births. It happens all the time." Someone else I know canceled a trip to Europe this past summer for fear of a terrorist hijacking but thinks nothing of commuting to work every day. An acquaintance who has played the stock market for two decades swears by a certain fund: "Any money manager who can consistently outperform the market eight years in a row gets my money!"

The foregoing examples illustrate various forms of "math abuse": the inability or unwillingness to apply a simple logical analysis to certain situations that arise in everyday life. Someone who cannot deal with simple numerical ideas is innumerate, just as someone who cannot read or write is illiterate. I prefer the term "math abuse" because it has a wider scope. It includes errors that are not strictly numerical, and it also has a moral dimension. We abuse mathematics by failing to apply even the little we know of it to the false or questionable ideas that we encounter. We do not want to be duped, but most of us are fooled on a regular basis by politicians, the media and even friends.

What is wrong, for example, with the notion that more babies are born during the full moon? The idea certainly has charm, and I, for one, would not be upset in the slightest if it turned out to be true. Suppose for the moment, though, that it is not true. Why might the nurse still claim that the peak baby-delivery period comes during the full moon?

Suppose that after watching the delivery of 15 babies in one day, the nurse looks out the window and sees a full moon. A month later, the maternity ward is relatively quiet, but the nurse does not bother to check the phase of the moon. If one watches only for the events that reinforce a belief, one is screening out all the events that falsify it. This phenomenon of belief is what Paulos calls a filter.

Filters can be found everywhere. Casinos that contain dozens of slot machines ring with the sound of winning. Every time the three little cherries line up, a machine disgorges a bunch of quarters that clatter into a tray. Losing makes no sound. Someone entering a casino may well be overwhelmed by the impression that everyone is winning. Yet even a few quarters won every 10 tries on average would produce a more or less continuous clatter from just 10 active machines.

The filtering phenomenon accounts for a good deal more than the "charitable casino" illusion. It can misguide us in our investment strategies. Was my friend right to place such confidence in a fund that beat the odds eight years in a row? Here is a simple way to judge the issue. First assume that the success of a fund depends on just plain luck — say, the flip of a coin. If the coin comes up heads one year, the fund will outperform the market index. If the coin comes up tails, on the other hand, the fund will drop below the index. Now if 1,024 funds were operating in 1982, consider their fate over eight years. By 1983, say, out of one-half of the funds, 512 had outperformed the index. By 1984 half of these, 256, had again beaten the index. Each year the number of funds that continued to show superior returns was halved: 128, 64, 32, 16, 8, 4. The last number represents the "hot funds," those that produced unusually good profits every year from 1982 through 1989.

It was amusing to watch a television interview of the manager of a hot fund. To what did he attribute his unusual success? The manager carried on at some length about waves, cycles, bulls and bears. But the fact is that his success might just have been luck. A simple probabilistic model accounts for the hot-fund phenomenon quite well. In the face of this model, investors are well advised to view any and all claims with a certain degree of skepticism.

Adapted from A. K. Dewdney. "Mathematical Recreations." *Scientific American*, March 1990, pp. 118–119.

73. Based on the passage, which of the following can we reasonably conclude about the author's beliefs concerning birth rates?
    A. The nurse is in a position to know the details of birth rate cycles.
    B. It is more likely that fewer, rather than more, babies are born during a full moon.
    C. It is unlikely there is any statistical basis for the nurse's belief.
    D. Birth rates have nothing to do with math abuse.

74. According to the passage, which of the following best describes the role filters play in math abuse?
    A. They cause people to avoid mathematics.
    B. They cause people to ignore events that are contrary to what they want to believe.
    C. They cause people to lose money.
    D. Filters have nothing to do with math abuse.

75. According to the author, what is the filtering process that occurs in casinos?
    A. Gamblers tend to win more often playing slot machines.
    B. There is a low probability of winning at slot machines.
    C. It is only obvious when people win playing slot machines.
    D. Casinos make the least amount of money on slot machines.

76. What is the author suggesting by drawing an analogy between the probability of coin tosses and hot funds?
    A. That investing is based on chance
    B. That the laws of probability do not apply to investing
    C. That investing in hot funds is a wise strategy
    D. That some hot funds will occur simply by chance

77. If the suggestion about hot funds is correct, which of the following is most likely to be the author's advice about investing in a fund that has beaten the market for eight years in a row?
    A. Invest in it immediately.
    B. Do not invest in it for the sole reason that it is hot.
    C. Invest only a small amount in the hot fund.
    D. Wait a year before investing.

PASSAGE VI (QUESTIONS 78–82)

Opponents of abortion often profess deep concern for the health of women. In literature and speeches, they suggest that abortion poses greater physical and psychological risks than childbirth. John C. Willke, president of the National Right to Life Committee, recently reiterated these claims to *Scientific American*. He said his belief in them rests on his experience as an obstetrician and on anecdotal reports, which are primarily written by others in the anti-abortion movement. "There are no good, hard statistics on this," he said, "but there are none on the other side either."

In fact, government statistics clearly show legal abortion to be safer than giving birth. Data compiled by the National Center for Health Statistics from 1981 to 1985 indicate that abortion was 11 times less likely than childbirth to lead to a woman's death. Researchers at the Centers for Disease Control reported in 1982 that women undergoing abortions are 100 times less likely to have complications requiring major abdominal surgery than women bearing children.

The question of psychological harm has been more difficult to assess. Indeed, C. Everett Koop, the former Surgeon General, judged past studies to be inconclusive. Now, however, a group at the Johns Hopkins School of Hygiene and Public Health has provided "hard statistics" on this issue.

The researchers studied 334 black urban teenagers who entered clinics in Baltimore to be tested for pregnancy. The homogeneity of the group reduced the chances that the study's results would be skewed by other variables, according to Laurie Schwab Zabin, who performed the study with Marilyn B. Hirsch. The teenagers were initially interviewed before they or the researchers knew the results of the pregnancy tests. They were then divided into three groups — those who bore a child, those who had an abortion and those who were not pregnant — and tracked for two years.

The investigators' report in *Family Planning Perspectives* concluded that those who chose abortion were less likely to undergo adverse psychological episodes (as measured by three separate psychological tests) than either those who bore children or those who had not been pregnant. They were also more likely to remain in school and less likely to become pregnant again.

"The right-to-lifers have been saying that it is terrible to let young women go through abortions," Zabin says. "Our study shows we should lay that ghost to rest. Not only is abortion a medically safe procedure; we now know it is psychologically safe."

Poor urban teenagers represent an important minority of all those who elect to have abortions, Zabin notes. They are the most likely to be affected by laws proposed in a number of states that would limit the use of public funds for abortion, require minors to gain consent from parents or otherwise restrict the practice of abortion.

Moreover, such laws could help give more substance to Willke's claims if they hinder women from obtaining timely abortions. Numerous studies show that the risks of medical complications rise significantly when abortions are performed after 16 weeks of pregnancy.

Adapted from John Horgan. "Right to Lie?" *Scientific American*, April 1990, pp. 14, 18.

78. Based on the passage, which of the following types of abortion statistics were gathered without difficulty?

    I. Death due to abortions versus childbirth
    II. Medical complications following abortions versus childbirth
    III. Psychological effects following abortions versus childbirth

    A. I and II
    B. I and III
    C. II and III
    D. I, II, and III

79. Based on the passage, which of the following statements best describes the findings of the National Center for Health Statistics and the Centers for Disease Control?

    A. Death and complications following an abortion are much less likely than after childbirth.
    B. Death and complications following an abortion are much more likely than after childbirth.
    C. Death and complications following an abortion are slightly less likely than after childbirth.
    D. Death is less likely following an abortion, but the probability of complications increases.

80. According to the author, which of the following is true with respect to the findings of Zabin and Hirsch?
    A. Subjects having abortions were more likely to suffer psychological episodes than those who were not pregnant, but no more likely than those who gave birth.
    B. Subjects having abortions were less likely to suffer psychological episodes than those in either of the other groups.
    C. Subjects having abortions were more likely to suffer psychological episodes than those in either of the other groups.
    D. Their findings were inconclusive.

81. The Zabin and Hirsch study focused exclusively on black urban teenagers. Which of the following was not specifically mentioned as an advantage of such a limited focus?
    I. Avoid the influence of other variables
    II. Extension of the findings to other groups
    III. This group is most likely to be affected by certain anti-abortion laws
    A. I only
    B. II only
    C. III only
    D. I and II

82. Based on the passage, why does the author suggest anti-abortion laws might actually cause the problems claimed by Willke?
    A. They will force those wanting an abortion to commit crimes.
    B. They will allow the performance of illegal abortions.
    C. They will keep women from obtaining abortions before it becomes dangerous.
    D. They will force women to lose their privacy when they request public funding to have an abortion.

PASSAGE VII (QUESTIONS 83–86)

Although democratic nations are founded on the principle of individual liberties and rights, there clearly must be a balance between the scope of individual freedom and the needs of government. Theoretically, individual rights must be curtailed where their exercise constitutes a threat to the very preservation of the nation or to the states and local communities within it. Whether a nation, a state, or a locality, the community at large does have a public interest that it can and should pursue with diligence. In the broadest sense, the decisions made by legislative majorities reflect community interests, although such interests are also represented by the executive and the judiciary. Only at the federal level is the judiciary independent of direct political control, under the system of separation of powers and checks and balances. At the state and local levels, judges are still mostly elected, making them directly accountable to the people. An elected judiciary is less likely to stand apart from the political process in making its decisions on the scope of individual liberties and rights. Such rights, therefore, are more likely to be limited if there is a public clamor for their restriction (for example, when the elected officials of localities respond to local public opinion by demanding controls over "obscene" magazines, movies, and books).

While there may be political excesses that threaten to limit civil liberties and rights, there are also legitimate governmental needs that may call for a modification of individual freedoms. This occurs when these civil freedoms are used, or misused, in order to attack the very foundations of the system itself. This problem becomes most acute during times of war or civil unrest. During such times, the Supreme Court has given the government wide powers to curb individual freedom.

Perhaps the most extraordinary abridgment of the rights of citizens occurred in 1941, when a Japanese attack was considered by large numbers of people within and outside the government, including military leaders, to be an imminent possibility on the West Coast. An even more likely probability considered was sabotage and subversion by

Japanese infiltrators. These fears eventually led to the establishment of concentration camps for Japanese-Americans. This was largely based upon an executive order by President Roosevelt, a decision that was upheld by the Supreme Court, against constitutional challenges in *Korematsu v. United States* in 1944. Writing for the majority of the Court, Justice Hugo Black said that during wartime, military necessity justified the order, which excluded Japanese-Americans from the West Coast. Did the exclusionary order constitute racial discrimination? No. The Court said that, although only the Japanese-Americans were excluded, the reason was not of race but of military necessity. *Korematsu* was an extreme case, but it illustrates the degree to which civil rights have been denied on the basis of the public interest.

In drawing the line between public interest and individual freedom, the Supreme Court has relied upon the "balancing test," which attempts to weigh the needs of government against the rights of individuals to determine the proper balance between permissible government restraints and individual freedom. One of the most important spheres of civil liberties where the balancing test has been applied regards the civil liberties and rights enumerated in the First Amendment, particularly the liberties of speech, press, and the right of assembly. In addition to the balancing test, the "clear and present danger" test is used in determining the permissible scope of political speech, press, and assembly. In this political sphere, the clear and present danger test is used to judge the extent to which Congress or the state legislatures may regulate and control the expression of political ideas.

Adapted from Pete Woll and Robert H. Binstock. *America's Political System*, 4th edition. New York: Random House, 1984, pp. 95–96.

83. Based on the passage, with which of the following statements would the authors be most likely to agree?
   A. Individual rights are superior to governmental needs.
   B. Governmental needs are superior to individual rights.
   C. A balance must be struck between individual rights and governmental needs.
   D. Political excesses can never limit civil liberties.

84. Based on the passage, we can reasonably infer which of the following?
   A. Local judges are mostly elected.
   B. Federal judges are mostly elected.
   C. State judges are not accountable to the people.
   D. Federal judges are not elected.

85. According to the authors, which of the following are in a better position to protect individual liberties?
   A. Members of Congress
   B. Federal judges
   C. State judges
   D. The president

86. Which of the following liberties is not specifically mentioned in the passage as a First Amendment liberty?
   A. Speech
   B. Press
   C. Religion
   D. Assembly

PASSAGE VIII (QUESTIONS 87–90)

That the area of obscenity and pornography is a difficult one for the Supreme Court is well-documented. The Court's numerous attempts to define obscenity have proven unworkable and left the decision to the subjective preferences of the justices. Perhaps Justice Stewart put it best when, after refusing to define obscenity, he declared, "But I know it when I see it." Does the Court literally have to see it to know it? Specifically, what role does the fact-pattern, including the materials' medium, play in the Court's decision?

Several recent studies employ fact-pattern analysis in modeling the Court's decision making. These studies examine the fact pattern or case characteristics, often with ideological and attitudinal factors, as a determinant of the decision reached by the Court. In broad terms, these studies owe their theoretical underpinnings to attitude theory. As the name suggests, attitude theory views the Court's attitudes as an explanation of its decisions.

These attitudes, however, do not operate in a vacuum. As Spaeth explains, "the activation of an attitude involves both an object and the situation in which that object is encountered." The objects to which the Court directs its attitudes are the litigants. The situation — the subject matter of the case — can be defined in broad or narrow terms. One may define the situation as an entire area of the law (e.g., civil liberties issues). On an even broader scale, the situation may be defined as the decision to grant certiorari or whether to defect from a minimum-winning coalition.

Defining the situation with such broad strokes, however, does not allow one to control for case content. In many specific issue areas, the cases present strikingly similar patterns. In examining the Court's search and seizure decisions, Segal found a relatively small number of situational and case characteristic variables explain a high proportion of the Court's decisions.

Despite Segal's success, efforts to verify the applicability of fact-pattern analysis in other issue areas and using broad-based factors have been slow in forthcoming. Renewed interest in obscenity and pornography by federal and state governments, the academic community, and numerous anti-pornography interest groups indicates the Court's decisions in this area deserve closer examination.

The Court's obscenity and pornography decisions also present an opportunity to study the Court's behavior in an area where the Court has granted significant decision-making authority to the states. In *Miller v. California* (1973), the Court announced the importance of local community standards in obscenity determinations. The Court's subsequent behavior may suggest how the Court will react in other areas.

87. According to the author, the Court's obscenity decisions have relied on
   A. personal judgments.
   B. objective legal analysis.
   C. fact-pattern analysis.
   D. established definitions.

88. The tone of the author is
   A. ironic.
   B. hostile.
   C. sarcastic.
   D. concerned.

89. From the passage, *judicial attitudes* can probably be defined as
   A. attitude objects.
   B. subjective preferences.
   C. case characteristics.
   D. fact patterns.

90. The author's attitude toward the study of the Court's decisions is that such a study
   A. is unnecessary.
   B. has been successful.
   C. should avoid attitude theory.
   D. may shed light on the Court's behavior.

PASSAGE IX (QUESTIONS 91–92)

The judicial branch is a co-equal part of the United States government, and yet it has escaped the degree of scientific scrutiny given to the executive and legislative branches. This is not to say the judicial branch has lacked all scrutiny, only that it has traditionally been viewed from a perspective different from the other two branches of government. The executive and legislative branches have traditionally been viewed as political entities. Judges and the judicial branch have fostered the idea that they are non-political arbiters of the law. In *Marbury v. Madison*, the landmark United States Supreme Court case that established judicial review under the United States Constitution, Chief Justice John Marshall rhetorically asked who should determine the meaning of the Constitution. He answered himself by pointing to the fact that members of the other two branches were politically motivated, and that only judges were qualified to be truly non-political arbiters of the law. These statements by Chief Justice Marshall were certainly not the beginning of what is generally known as the "cult of the robe," but they are a classic example in American jurisprudence.

Following Marshall's reasoning, the study of the judiciary has traditionally used the case analysis method, which concentrates on individual cases. Each case must be decided on the basis of cases that have preceded it. Although it may be acknowledged that each case differs from every other case in many ways, past cases must still be examined to find the general principles, which are then applied to the present dispute.

This reliance on precedent, known in legal terms as *stare decisis*, and its accompanying detailed examination of each case has caused legal scholars, to paraphrase Wieland, to not be able to see the forest for the trees. To get a more accurate picture of the workings of the judiciary, it is necessary to step back from the cases. One must remain cognizant of the details, but not to such a degree that they inhibit the ability to see the greater whole. This is not to say analysis of individual cases has no place in the scientific study of the judiciary. Indeed, as was pointed out by Joyce Kilmer, there is always a place to appreciate the beauty of a tree, but there are also times when we must consider the tree as a part of the greater forest.

Although judicial scholars by and large do not subscribe to the myth that judges are non-political arbiters of the law, there is substantial interest in judicial biographies and in case studies. Judicial biographies and case studies are certainly useful in interpreting particular judicial decisions, examining the opinions of a particular judge, or discussing specific points of law. However, to optimize the results of such efforts, in terms of scientific study, such research must be viewed within the framework of a more comprehensive theory of judicial decision making.

91. The primary purpose of the passage is to
    A. suggest that judges are political decision makers.
    B. complain that no one studies the judiciary.
    C. advocate another way of studying the judiciary.
    D. describe the case analysis method.

92. Chief Justice Marshall's argument assumes
    A. judges are better educated than executives or legislators.
    B. politically motivated individuals are biased.
    C. only judges understand the Constitution.
    D. it is better to study individual cases.

STOP! If time still remains, you may review work only in this section. When the time allotted is up, you may go on to the next section. STOP!

SECTION 3
Writing Sample

TIME: 60 minutes

2 essays, separately timed

30 minutes each

DIRECTIONS: This section tests your writing skills by asking you to write two essays. You will have 30 minutes to write each one.

During the first 30 minutes, work only on the first essay. If you finish it in less than 30 minutes, you may review what you have written, but do not begin the second essay. During the second 30 minutes, work only on the second essay. If you finish it in less than 30 minutes, you may review what you have written for that essay only. Do not go back to the first essay.

Read each assigned topic carefully. Make sure your essays respond to the topics as they are assigned.

Make sure your essays are written in complete sentences and paragraphs, and are as clear as you can make them. Make any corrections or additions between the lines of your essays. Do not write in the margins.

On the day of the test, you are given three pages to write each essay. You are not required to use all of the space provided, but do not skip lines so you will not waste space. Illegible essays cannot be scored.

PART 1

Consider this statement:

"That government is best which governs least."

From *On The Duty of Civil Disobedience*, by Henry David Thoreau.

Write a comprehensive essay in which you accomplish the following objectives. Explain what you think the above statement means. Describe one or two specific situations in which the powers of government should be increased. Discuss what you think should be the basis for increasing or decreasing a government's powers.

PART 2

Consider this statement:

"[Humans] cannot subsist on the scanty satisfaction which they can extort from reality."

From *Introductory Lectures on Psychoanalysis*, by Sigmund Freud.

Write a comprehensive essay in which you accomplish the following objectives. Explain what you think the above statement means. Describe one or two specific situations in which individuals have remained human while experiencing extreme frustration. Discuss what you think is the possibility of living a meaningful life while confronting the reality of suffering.

SECTION 4
Biological Sciences

TIME: 70 Minutes

QUESTIONS: 93–144

DIRECTIONS: Most of the questions in this section are arranged in groups, each corresponding to a descriptive passage. Based on the information given in a passage, choose the one best answer to each question in the group. Some questions are independent of a descriptive passage and of each other. Choose the one best answer to each of these questions also. If you are not sure of an answer, eliminate those choices that you know are incorrect and choose an answer from among those remaining. Fill in the corresponding circle on the answer sheet to indicate your answer. You may refer to the periodic table at any time.

PASSAGE I (QUESTIONS 93–96)

Fluids within the body account for approximately 60% of body weight and are contained within several different compartments. Two-thirds of the body fluids are located intracellularly, and the remaining one-third is extracellular. Extracellular fluid is divided into two components: the circulating blood plasma and the interstitial fluid. The body fluid compartments do not exist in isolation. Exchange of fluids can occur internally between compartments and between the external environment and the body fluid compartments as shown in Figure 1.

It is possible to measure the size of the various body fluid compartments by injecting a substance into the compartment of interest, allowing adequate time for mixing to occur and then obtaining a sample of fluid from the compartment. The concentration of the injected substance in the sample is then determined. Using this information, the volume of fluid in which the substance was distributed can be calculated. The substance used should ideally remain only in the compartment of interest, distribute quickly and uniformly within the compartment, be removed slowly from the body, be non-toxic and easy to measure.

FIGURE 1. The body fluid compartments. The arrows indicate possible sites of fluid exchange.

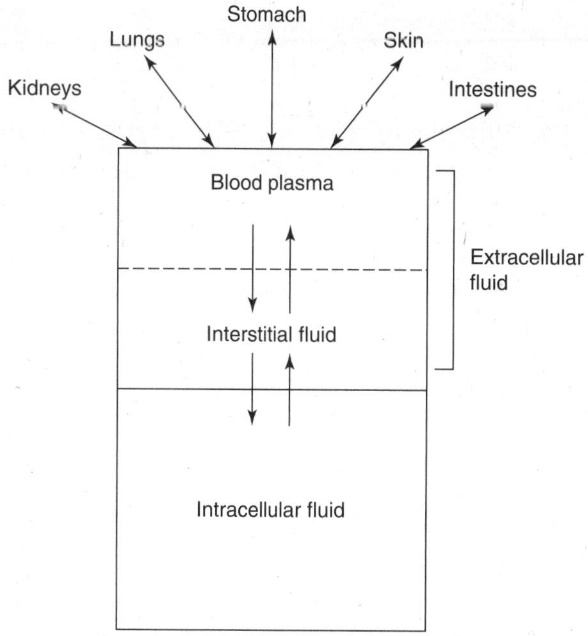

Extracellular fluid volume is difficult to measure because the boundaries of this space are difficult to define and few substances mix rapidly in all parts of the extracellular fluid (i.e., bone, cartilage). Interstitial fluid volume cannot be measured directly because substances that equilibrate in the interstitial fluid will also equilibrate in the plasma. It can, however, be calculated by subtracting plasma volume from extracellular fluid volume. In the same manner, intracellular fluid volume cannot be measured directly, but can be calculated by subtracting the extracellular fluid volume from total body water.

93. The primary force producing movement of water among the various body fluid compartments is
    A. Brownian motion.
    B. active transport.
    C. osmosis.
    D. facilitated diffusion.

94. Evans blue is an aniline dye that binds to proteins circulating in the blood. Which body fluid compartment could it be used to measure?
    A. Extracellular fluid
    B. Plasma volume
    C. Intracellular fluid
    D. Interstitial fluid

95. With the exception of blood cells, exchange of water and solutes between the intracellular compartment and the plasma
    A. can occur directly.
    B. does not take place at all.
    C. occurs only in highly perfused organs, such as the lungs and kidneys.
    D. can occur only indirectly, via movement through the interstitial fluid.

96. Normally, the various body fluid compartments are in osmotic equilibrium. Therefore, a net loss of solute from the extracellular fluid
    A. leads to hypotonicity of the extracellular fluid relative to the intracellular fluid.
    B. leads to hypotonicity of the intracellular fluid relative to the extracellular fluid.
    C. leads to hypertonicity of the extracellular fluid relative to the intracellular fluid.
    D. does not change the tonicity of the extracellular fluid or intracellular fluid.

PASSAGE II (QUESTIONS 97–100)

Protein synthesis begins in the nucleus of a cell with the transfer of the genetic code from DNA to RNA via the process of transcription. Before leaving the nucleus, messenger RNA (mRNA) often undergoes post-transcriptional modification. Once the mRNA moves out of the nucleus, it associates with ribosomes and dictates the formation of a polypeptide chain via the process of translation. After the polypeptide chain is formed, it can be post-translationally modified by a variety of reactions to produce the final protein product.

Insulin is a pancreatic hormone that undergoes the processes outlined above during its synthesis. The proinsulin gene located on chromosome 11 in humans serves as the template for mRNA synthesis in the nucleus. The mRNA is processed by removing two introns and adding a poly-A tail. In the cytoplasm, this mRNA chain serves as a template for the formation of a preproinsulin polypeptide chain. As this molecule enters the endoplasmic reticulum, its 23-amino acid leader sequence is removed. The molecule is then folded, and two disulfide bonds form between the A and B chains to make proinsulin. Cleavage of a connecting segment between the A and B chains yields the insulin molecule, which is secreted by the pancreas.

97. Actinomycin D binds to DNA, preventing the polymerization of RNA on DNA. If actinomycin D were added to a pancreatic tissue culture, which of the following molecules would be present inside the pancreatic cells one hour later?
    A. Preproinsulin
    B. Proinsulin gene
    C. Connecting peptide
    D. Insulin

98. The entire process of protein synthesis
    A. occurs only within the cell nucleus.
    B. is accomplished in a single step.

C. requires many steps, some of which modify the protein.
D. occurs only in the cell cytoplasm.

99. Post-translational modification of insulin involves
A. adding a poly-A tail to the proinsulin gene.
B. nothing; there is no post-translational modification of insulin.
C. removal of two introns.
D. removal of a leader sequence and folding.

100. In eukaryotes, the portions of the genes used for protein synthesis are usually located in several segments called exons, which are separated by segments that are not translated, called introns. The final mRNA that enters the cytoplasm
A. is an unmodified transcription of the genetic code.
B. is composed solely of introns because the exons have been removed during processing.
C. contains alternating segments of introns and exons.
D. is composed only of exons because the introns have been removed during processing.

PASSAGE III (QUESTIONS 101–104)

The long-term regulation of blood pressure is controlled by the kidneys because of an exquisite relationship that exists between blood pressure and urinary sodium output (Figure 2). If there is a rise in blood pressure above the normal resting level, sodium and water excretion (output) increases. This occurs in order to reduce blood volume, and return blood pressure to its normal level. If there is a fall in blood pressure, the kidneys retain sodium and water, and sodium excretion decreases. The retention of sodium and water causes blood volume to increase, and blood pressure rises back to its normal level. This regulatory mechanism operates around a constant level of blood pressure at which urinary sodium excretion is approximately equal to dietary sodium intake. If blood pressure deviates from this set point, the kidneys alter sodium excretion accordingly in an effort to restore blood pressure to normal. Conversely, if dietary sodium intake changes, blood pressure must adjust to restore the balance between sodium intake and output. The shape, slope and set point of the curve shown in Figure 2 vary from individual to individual.

FIGURE 2. Relationship between sodium output and blood pressure

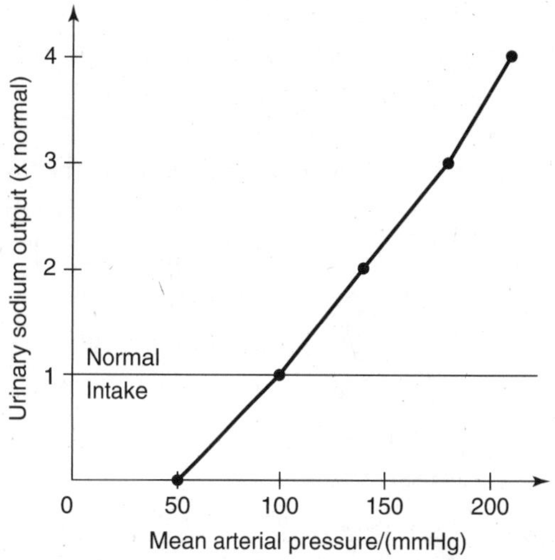

A disease, such as hypertension (high blood pressure), alters the relationship between sodium excretion and blood pressure so that a higher blood pressure is needed to excrete the same amount of sodium (i.e., sodium intake has not changed). As a result, the set point shifts upward and to the right on the curve. Diuretics, drugs that cause the kidneys to increase sodium and water excretion and, therefore, tend to lower blood pressure, are commonly used to treat hypertension.

101. If a person with high blood pressure switches to a low-sodium diet, which of the following should occur theoretically?
A. The kidneys will oppose the decrease in dietary sodium by retaining more sodium, and blood pressure will rise even further.
B. Blood pressure will remain the same.

C. To maintain sodium balance, blood pressure should decrease.

D. Blood pressure will initially increase, but then will decrease back to the original hypertensive level.

102. Angiotensin, a powerful vasoconstrictor, shifts the entire curve shown in Figure 2 to the right on the x-axis. At the same level of sodium intake, the presence of angiotensin would

A. shift blood pressure to a higher level without changing sodium output.

B. have no effect on the level of blood pressure.

C. increase urinary sodium output.

D. shift blood pressure to a lower level and decrease sodium output.

103. Patient A is more sensitive to change in dietary sodium than Patient B. When both are placed on a high-salt diet, Patient A will

A. exhibit a fall in blood pressure, while Patient B's blood pressure will rise.

B. show a rise in blood pressure similar to Patient B.

C. show no change in blood pressure, while Patient B's blood pressure will fall.

D. exhibit a greater rise in blood pressure than Patient B will.

104. If a person who is using diuretics to control blood pressure stops taking them for a period of several days, which of the following would most likely occur?

A. Blood pressure would return to a hypertensive level because the kidneys would excrete less salt and water.

B. Sodium and water excretion by the kidneys would increase, leading to a further reduction in blood pressure.

C. Renal function would remain unchanged because diuretics do not affect the kidneys.

D. Blood pressure would remain at a normotensive level because the underlying defect in kidney function would have been corrected by the prior diuretic therapy.

QUESTIONS 105–108 are NOT based on a descriptive passage.

105. The process by which gases are exchanged in the alveoli of our lungs is called

A. external respiration.

B. indirect respiration.

C. internal respiration.

D. direct respiration.

106. Vitamin A is associated with

A. blood coagulation.

B. liver function in some animals.

C. bone growth.

D. skin epithelial maintenance.

107. How do α-amino acids differ from β-amino acids?

A. They constitute an enantiomeric pair.

B. They constitute a diastereomeric pair.

C. α-amino acids exist as zwitterions.

D. The amino groups bond to different carbons.

108. Which of the following Newman projections illustrates the least thermodynamically stable conformation of iso-pentane?

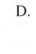

A.

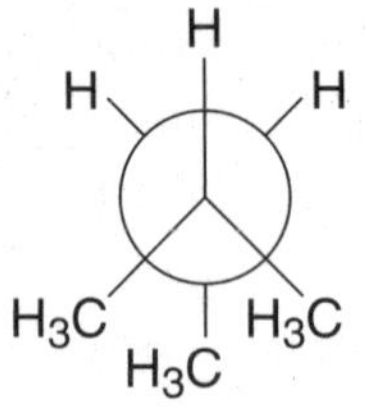

B.

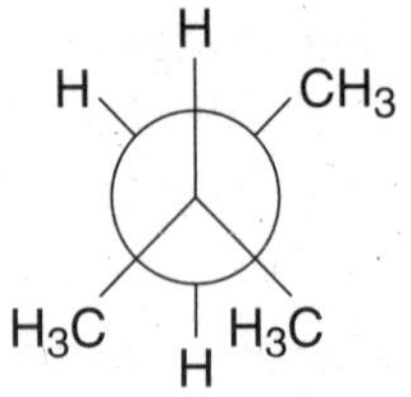

C.

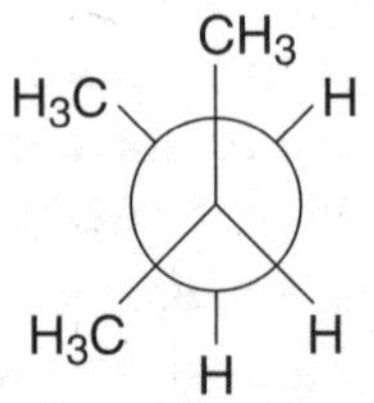

D.

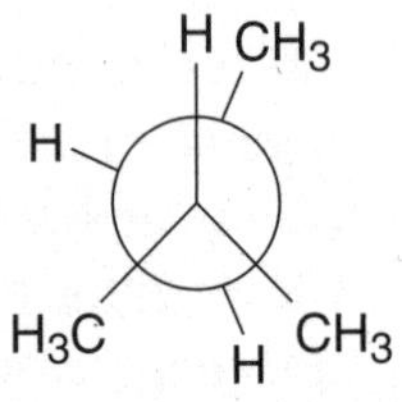

PASSAGE IV (QUESTIONS 109–111)

Skeletal muscle tissue is composed of actin and myosin filaments arranged in an orderly, overlapping fashion within each muscle fiber. When actin and myosin interact, muscle contraction occurs and tension develops. Due to the arrangement of the actin and myosin filaments, there is an optimum muscle length at which maximal tension can be developed. At muscle lengths longer or shorter than this, the tension developed is less than maximal.

To study the length-tension relationship, an isolated muscle experiment can be performed. The gastrocnemius muscle of a frog is removed from the leg and placed in an isometric transducer. The transducer measures the tension that the muscle develops when stimulated to contract. The muscle is originally placed in the transducer at approximately the same length as it would have at rest in the body. It is then shortened and lengthened in 1 millimeter increments. At each muscle length, the same stimulus is applied and the tension that develops when the muscle contracts is measured. The total tension developed can be separated into 2 components: active tension and passive tension. Active tension is generated when the muscle itself contracts. Passive tension develops as the muscle is stretched beyond its resting length. It is due to stretch of supporting structures in the muscle, such as connective tissue and elastic fibers. Total tension is equal to the sum of the active and passive tensions.

TABLE 1

Change in Muscle Length (mm)	Active Tension (kg)	Passive Tension (kg)	Total Tension (kg)
−3	0.5	0	0.5
−2	2.0	0	2.0
−1	11.0	0	11.0
0	15.0	0	15.0
+1	13.5	2.0	15.5
+2	7.0	10.0	17.0
+3	3.0	16.0	19.0

Active, passive, and total tension develops when an isolated muscle is stimulated to contract at its resting length (0) and at lengths shorter (−1, −2, −3) and longer (+1, +2, +3) than resting length.

109. If the isolated muscle used in the experiment was stretched by 5 millimeters from the resting length, which of the following would be true?
   A. Active tension = 10; passive tension = 0; total tension = 10
   B. Active tension = 0; passive tension = 20; total tension = 20
   C. Active tension = 0; passive tension = 0; total tension = 0
   D. Active tension = 10; passive tension = 20; total tension = 30

110. What is the advantage of using an isolated muscle in the experiment instead of leaving the muscle intact in the body?
   A. The properties of just the muscle itself can be studied because it is devoid of neural and hormonal influences.
   B. Muscle length can be easily changed, whereas in the body, muscles do not change length.
   C. The muscle is better able to contract and develop tension when removed from the body.
   D. There is no advantage; the results would be the same.

111. When a muscle contracts, tension develops because of
   A. interaction between the actin and myosin filaments.
   B. the overlapping arrangement of the actin and myosin filaments.
   C. a slackening within the connective tissue elements.
   D. the length-tension relationship.

PASSAGE V (QUESTIONS 112–115)

About 1.5% of body weight in an adult human is due to the mineral calcium. Calcium is necessary for important physiological processes, such as muscle contraction, nerve function and blood clotting. Approximately 99% of calcium in the body is located in the skeleton. Some of this calcium is available as a readily exchangeable reservoir, while the rest forms a large pool of stable calcium that is only slowly exchangeable. To maintain adequate plasma levels, calcium moves in and out of the readily exchangeable pool in the bone every day. Low blood calcium levels result in a condition known as hypocalcemic tetany, which is characterized by skeletal muscle spasms that can become severe enough to block the airway and lead to asphyxia.

In humans, there are usually four parathyroid glands located on the dorsal surface of the thyroid gland. Each gland has an abundant supply of blood vessels and is about 3 × 6 × 2 millimeters in size. The parathyroid glands produce and secrete parathyroid hormone (PTH). PTH is essential for life because it is involved in the regulation of calcium metabolism. Specifically, PTH acts directly on bone to mobilize calcium, leading to an increase in blood calcium levels. Secretion of PTH from the parathyroid glands is regulated by the level of plasma calcium. When plasma calcium levels fall, PTH secretion increases. When plasma calcium levels are high, PTH secretion is inhibited.

112. An excess of PTH would
    A. lead to calcium deposition in the bone.
    B. cause plasma calcium to decrease.
    C. be manifested as tetany.
    D. eventually lead to bone demineralization.

113. Calcium is extremely important because it is necessary for
    A. tetany, which is normal muscle contraction.
    B. the regulation of PTH secretion.
    C. the normal function of nerve and muscle tissue.
    D. the process of bone resorption to occur.

114. After eating a meal high in calcium, which of the following will occur?
    A. PTH secretion will increase, and calcium will be deposited in bone.
    B. PTH secretion will decrease, and calcium will be deposited in bone.
    C. PTH secretion will increase to mobilize calcium from bone.
    D. PTH secretion will remain constant, but calcium will be deposited in bone.

115. When the plasma calcium level is high, secretion of the hormone calcitonin in-creases. Calcitonin inhibits the mobilization of calcium from bone. An increase in plasma calcitonin leads to which of the following?
    A. Plasma calcium will increase due to bone resorption.
    B. Plasma PTH will decrease because these hormones have antagonistic actions.
    C. Plasma calcium will increase due to an increased secretion of PTH.
    D. Plasma calcium will decrease as a result of increased PTH activity.

PASSAGE VI (QUESTIONS 116–120)

In many species, the differences between the sexes depend primarily on a single chromosome (Y) and a single pair of endocrine structures (testes and ovaries). Of the 23 chromosomes found in germ cells, one is known as the sex chromosome. This chromosome may be one of two types, either an X or a Y. Gender is determined by the sex chromosome of the sperm that fertilizes the egg. Each ovum contains a single X chromosome. Fifty percent of normal sperm contain X chromosomes, and the other half contains Y chromosomes. The combination of two X chromosomes results in a genetic female. A genetic male is the product when an ovum combines with a Y-containing sperm.

The differentiation of the primitive gonads into testes in the case of a male, or into ovaries in the female, is determined genetically. Until the sixth week of development, the primitive gonads are identical in both sexes. They are bipotential, meaning they are capable of developing into either testes or ovaries at this point. In genetic males, the presence of a specific cell-surface protein, the H-Y antigen, stimulates the primitive gonads to develop into testes. The absence of the H-Y antigen in genetic females causes the ovaries to develop instead. The embryonic ovary does not secrete any hormones. The fetal testes, however, begin to produce and secrete the hormone testosterone in response to placental chorionic gonadotropin. The complete formation of the male internal and external genitalia depends upon the presence of testosterone. In the absence of testosterone, female internal and external genitalia develop.

After birth, both male and female gonads are quiescent until adolescence, when they are stimulated by the anterior pituitary to begin producing and secreting hormones. These hormones are responsible for the appearance of the features typical of adult males and females known as secondary sexual characteristics. The masculinizing androgens and feminizing estrogens are produced by both sexes; however, androgens predominate in males, while estrogens predominate in females.

116. A pseudohermaphrodite is an individual with the genetic constitution and glands of one sex and the genitalia of the other sex. Which of the following could result in a female pseudohermaphrodite?
   A. Exposure of a genetic female to testosterone at birth
   B. Exposure of a genetic male to estrogens during the fifth to sixth week of gestation
   C. Exposure of a genetic male to placental chorionic gonadotropin
   D. Exposure of a genetic female to androgens during the eighth to thirteenth week of gestation

117. The number of males born annually is generally slightly higher than the number of females. Which of the following statements provides a plausible explanation for this phenomenon?
   A. There are more X-containing sperm than Y-containing sperm, so an XX combination occurs more frequently than an XY combination.
   B. There are more Y-containing sperm produced than X-containing ones, so the odds of an XY combination occurring are greater than an XX combination.
   C. There are approximately equal numbers of X- and Y-containing sperm; therefore, the reason must lie elsewhere, perhaps in differences of motility between X and Y sperm.
   D. Because all eggs contain a Y chromosome, the odds of producing a male are better than the odds of producing a female.

118. The two primary functions of mature gonads are the
   A. production of germ cells and the secretion of hormones.
   B. secretion of androgens and estrogens.
   C. production of ova and the maintenance of secondary sex characteristics.
   D. secretion of testosterone and the production of sperm.

119. Up until the sixth week of gestation, the primitive gonads in both sexes are identical. What causes the internal and external genitalia to develop differently in males and females?
   A. Estrogen secreted by the immature ovaries
   B. The presence of the H-Y antigen on the surface of cells in males
   C. Testosterone and estrogen secreted by the testes
   D. Chemical signals sent from the developing brain

120. For secondary sexual characteristics to appear at the time of adolescence, the
   A. testes must secrete estrogen in males and the ovaries must secrete testosterone in females.
   B. testes must stop producing androgens.
   C. gonads must be producing and secreting hormones.
   D. ovaries must stop producing estrogens.

PASSAGE VII (QUESTIONS 121–125)

The fundamental unit of all living things is the cell. Each individual cell is capable of reproducing, metabolizing, and adapting to changes in its environment. Cells are separated from one another by their cell membranes; however, they are not isolated because materials may pass through the cell membranes to move in and out of the cells. Cells in the human body are organized into tissues and organs where they act collectively to accomplish activities basic to life such as energy production, movement, communication, and reproduction.

The two major components of a cell are the nucleus and cytoplasm. The nucleus is separated from the rest of the cell by the nuclear membrane. It is the control center of the cell because it contains the genetic material DNA. Also found within the nucleus is an RNA-producing structure called the nucleolus, which is not bound by a membrane. Filling the space between the nucleus and the cell membrane is the cytoplasm. Membrane-bound structures called organelles and a complex network of protein filaments and microtubules called the cytoskeleton are suspended in the cytoplasmic fluid. The cytoskeleton gives the cell its shape and also provides the basis for movement of the entire cell and its individual organelles.

The organelles are highly organized physical structures. They are specialized to perform a function in a more efficient manner than could be achieved simply by chemicals dispersed in the cytoplasm. The mitochondria provide energy for the cell in the form of ATP. These structures are self-replicating and can increase in number when the demand for energy increases. The endoplasmic reticulum and the Golgi apparatus are both composed of a network of flattened sacs. Rough endoplasmic reticulum (RER) has attached ribosomes and serves as a site for protein synthesis. Smooth endoplasmic reticulum (SER) does not have attached ribosomes. It is involved in lipid metabolism, steroid synthesis, and drug detoxification. Proteins and other substances formed in the endoplasmic reticulum are often transported to the Golgi, where they are modified, sorted, and packaged for delivery elsewhere in the cell or for secretion out of the cell. Lysosomes provide an intracellular digestive system. They are membrane-bound vesicles filled with hydrolytic enzymes that are capable of digesting proteins, nucleic acids, lipids and glycogen. Lysosomes remove unwanted substances from the cell, such as damaged organelles or foreign bacteria.

TABLE 2. The composition of a generalized eukaryotic cell.

Component	Percentage of cellular mass
Water	80%
Protein	15%
Lipid	3%
Carbohydrate	1%
Electrolytes and minerals	1%

121. According to Table 2, most of a cell is made up of
   A. protein, lipid, and carbohydrate.
   B. electrolytes, minerals, and water.
   C. carbohydrate.
   D. water and protein.

122. Why would cells be unable to survive for any substantial length of time without a functional lysosomal system?
   A. An accumulation of cellular debris or invasion by infectious agents would likely kill the cells.
   B. The cells would be unable to properly package and secrete proteins.

C. Reproduction could not occur because DNA is contained within the lysosomes.
D. Energy production would be too slow to sustain life.

123. Rough and smooth endoplasmic reticula are distinguished from each other by the
A. attachment of the cytoskeleton to the RER that anchors it in place.
B. fact that SER is membrane-bound, while RER is not.
C. proximity to the Golgi apparatus — RER is closer than SER.
D. presence of ribosomes on RER and their absence on SER.

124. Of all the organelles in the cell, the mitochondria are usually the most abundant. Which of the following statements best explains why?
A. Mitochondria are the control centers of the cell.
B. Digestive enzymes are contained within the mitochondria.
C. Practically all cellular processes require ATP as an energy source.
D. These structures shuttle proteins and other substances between the endoplasmic reticulum and Golgi apparatus.

125. One of the few structures in the cell that is not surrounded by a membrane is the
A. Golgi apparatus.
B. nucleus.
C. nucleolus.
D. lysosome.

QUESTIONS 126–129 are NOT based on a descriptive passage.

126. Translocation is a type of chromosomal mutation where a
A. segment of the chromosome is missing.
B. portion of the chromosome is represented twice.
C. segment of one chromosome is transferred to another non-homologous chromosome.
D. segment is removed and reinserted at another spot.

127. The thin barrier at Bowman's capsule allows for filtration of
A. whole blood.
B. ammonia.
C. plasma.
D. oxygen.

128. The phenomenon of rigor mortis is a direct result of the
A. breaking of myosin bonds by ATP.
B. breaking of actin bonds by ATP.
C. inability of the myosin cross bridges to combine with single amino acids.
D. loss of ATP in dead muscle cells.

129. Which of the following is a meta-directing, deactivating, substituted benzene?

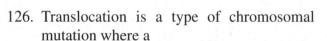

A.
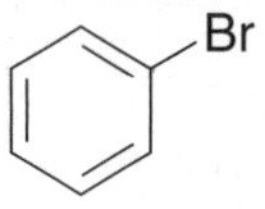

B.
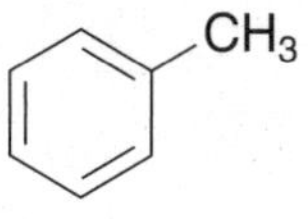

C.
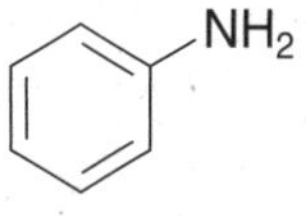

D.
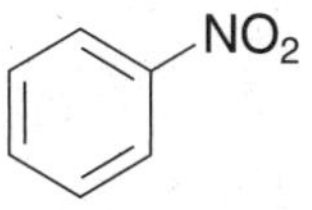

PASSAGE VIII (QUESTIONS 130–133)

Proteins are made up of various combinations of the 20 amino acids. All of the amino acids are constructed with a central carbon atom called the α carbon. Bonded to the α carbon are an amino group, carboxyl group, hydrogen atom, and one variable group called a side chain or R group. Because only the side chains vary from one amino acid to another, these groups impart individuality to each amino acid.

The amino acids can be classified conveniently using the physical properties of the side chain. At physiological pH (≈7), amino acids are grouped according to their electric charge when ionized, and according to their affinity for water. Five of the amino acids have charged side chains at pH 7. Two of these are negatively charged and are the acidic amino acids. The other three are basic amino acids that are positively charged. The non-ionic (uncharged) polar amino acids have side chains that are hydrophilic and therefore tend to be located on the surface of the protein molecule, which is exposed to the aqueous medium. Nonpolar amino acids are only slightly soluble in water and are usually confined to the interior of the protein molecule.

The α carbon is the center of asymmetry for all of the amino acids except glycine. Therefore, each amino acid can exist in two nonsuperimposable mirror image forms, or enantiomers. All of the amino acids found in proteins possess the same absolute configuration as L-alanine, which corresponds to the arrangement of analagous groups in the structure of L-glyceraldehyde. D-amino acids have an absolute configuration corresponding to D-glyceraldehyde. These are found in the cell walls of bacteria and in a number of antibiotics of bacterial origin.

130. Which of the following amino acids has a negatively charged side chain?

A. Glycine

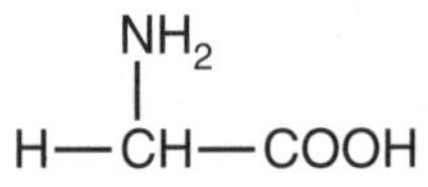

B. Alanine

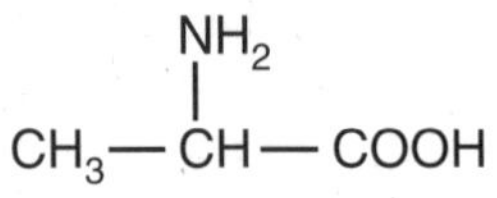

C. Aspartic acid

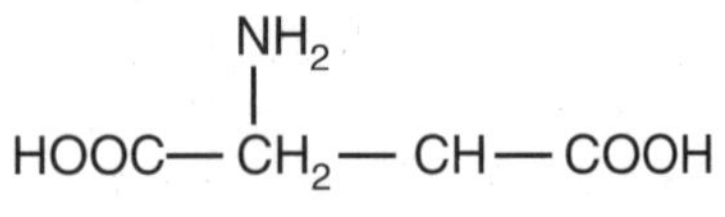

D. Phenylalanine

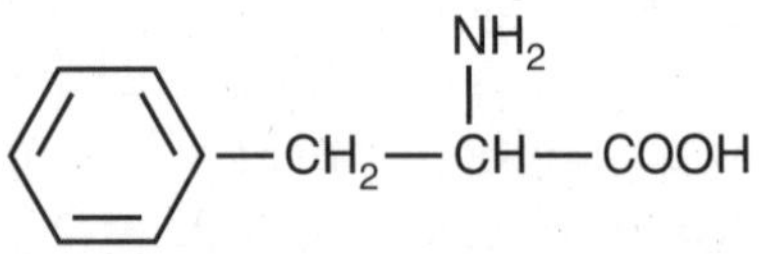

131. Amino acids with side chains that consist only of hydrocarbons are
A. hydrophobic.
B. enantiomers.
C. zwitterions.
D. hydrophilic.

132. The uncharged polar side chains of several of the amino acids are most likely involved in
A. peptide bonds.
B. hydrogen bonds.
C. covalent bonds.
D. hydrophobic interactions.

133. A particular position in a protein chain derives its physical and chemical properties from
A. the R group.
B. the α-amino group.
C. Factor XIV.
D. the carboxyl group.

PASSAGE IX (QUESTIONS 134–137)

To study a compound in isolation, it must be separated from the thousands of components with which it normally occurs. The desired substance may be quite labile and cannot be exposed to extremes of pH, temperature, or pressure. Isolation is made more difficult when only micro amounts of the substance are available and by the presence of other molecules that differ only slightly from the desired compound. This has led to the development of highly selective methods for isolating and purifying biological compounds.

Many of the separation methods involve the distribution of a mixture of solutes between two immiscible solvents. The molecules in the mixture are propelled through a channel of solvent by a force that acts equally on each molecule. Other forces retard movement of the molecules through the channel. If the retarding forces differ for different molecules in the solute mixture, separation of the molecules will occur as the mixture passes through the length of the channel.

Chromatography includes a number of separation methods based upon the technique described above that involve the percolation of a solute mixture through a porous solid support. In thin-layer chromatography (TLC), a variation of liquid-liquid chromatography, a thin film of solid support of uniform thickness, usually alumina or silica gel, is prepared on a glass or plastic surface. One of the immiscible solvents, the stationary phase, is immobilized on the inert solid support. A small amount of the solute mixture to be separated is spotted near one end of the plate. The other solvent, the mobile phase, is applied to the end of the plate closest to the spot. As the mobile phase moves along the support by capillary action, the individual components of the solute mixture will separate based upon their partition coefficients in the two phases. The order of migration of compounds can be changed by using different solvents, but in general, less polar compounds move the fastest. To increase the rate at which more polar compounds move, a more polar solvent must be used.

134. Four different samples consisting of mixtures of unknown compounds were prepared for TLC. On the right side of each plate the unknown was spotted. On the left side, a sample of a known compound A was spotted. Which of the following plates contains compound A in the unknown mixture?

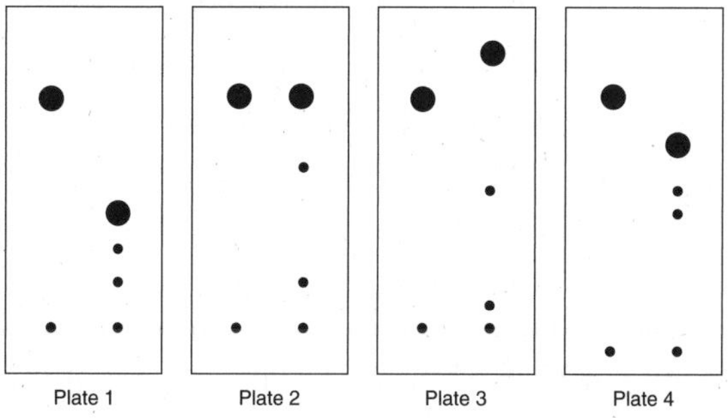

A. Plate 1
B. Plate 2
C. Plate 3
D. Plate 4

135. Which of the plates in question 134 contains the mixture with the most polar compounds?
A. Plate 1
B. Plate 2
C. Plate 3
D. Plate 4

136. To increase the rate at which more polar compounds move up the plate, which of the following solvents would be used?
A. Benzene
B. Ethanol
C. Acetic acid
D. Hexane

137. Which of the following class of compounds will move the furthest on a TLC plate?
A. Aldehydes RCH=O
B. Carboxylic acids RCOOH
C. Halogenated hydrocarbons RX
D. Alkenes $R_2C=CR_2$

PASSAGE X (QUESTIONS 138–141)

Although molecules are often drawn in only one or two dimensions, they exist in three-dimensional forms. Stereochemistry is the study of how the atoms in a molecule are arranged in space relative to one another. Isomers are two or more compounds that have the same molecular formulas. If the atoms are attached in different orders, the compounds have different structures and are called structural isomers of each other.

A second type of isomerism is geometric isomerism, which occurs in only two classes of compounds: alkenes and cyclic compounds. These compounds contain double bonds, or pi bonds, which generally cannot be broken at room temperature. The groups attached to pi-bonded carbons are therefore fixed in space relative to one another. Consider for example, the two possible structures of 1,2-dichloroethene:

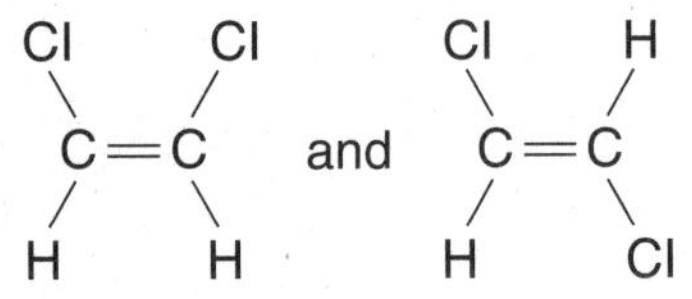

These two compounds are not structural isomers because the order of attachment of the atoms and the location of the double bond is the same in both cases. Instead, they are called stereoisomers. These isomers are different compounds that have the same structure but differ in the arrangement of the atoms in space. The structure on the left represents a *cis*-isomer in which the two Cl atoms are on the same side of the pi bond and the two H atoms are on the other side. The structure on the right is a *trans*-isomer. Here, the Cl groups are on opposite sides of the pi bond. Due to the rigidity of the double bond, the *cis*- and *trans*-isomers are not easily interconvertible.

138. Which of the following is a structural isomer of 1-propanol ($CH_3CH_2CH_2OH$)?

A. $H_2C{=}CHCH_2OH$

B. 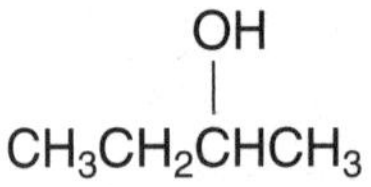

C. 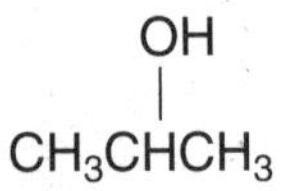

D. 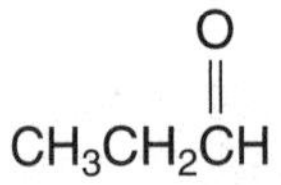

139. Which of the following pairs of formulas represent the same compound and therefore do not represent isomers?

A. 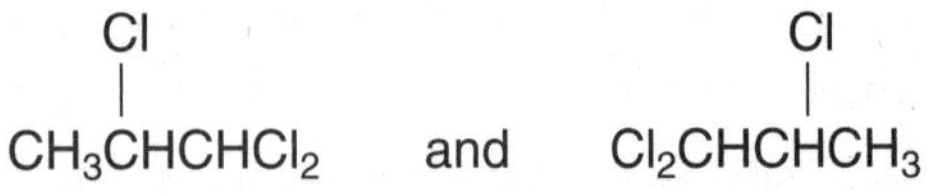

B. 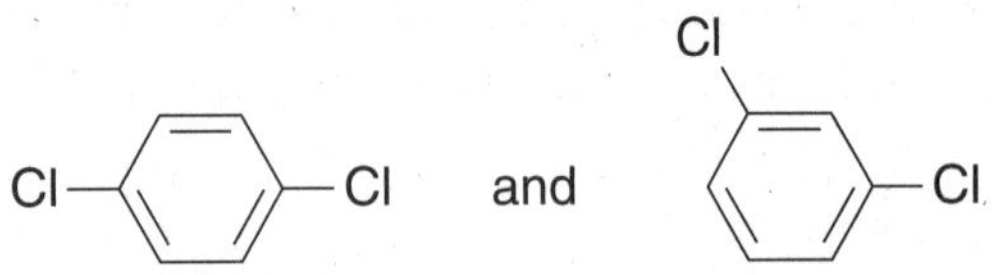

C. 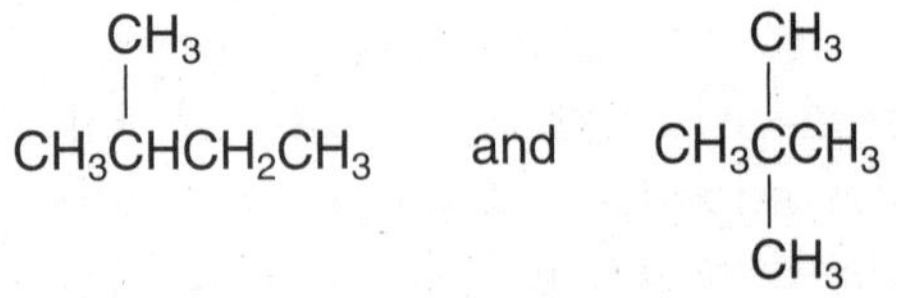

D. CH_3OCH_3 and CH_3CH_2OH

140. Which of the following pairs of structures are stereoisomers of each other?

A. 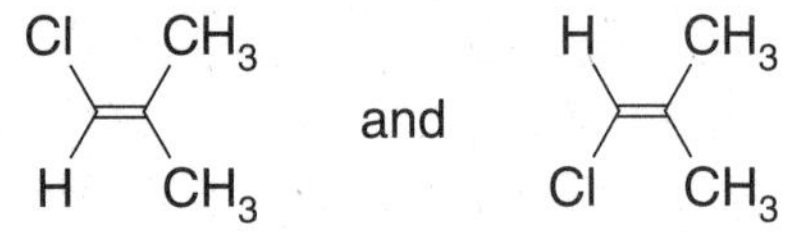

B. 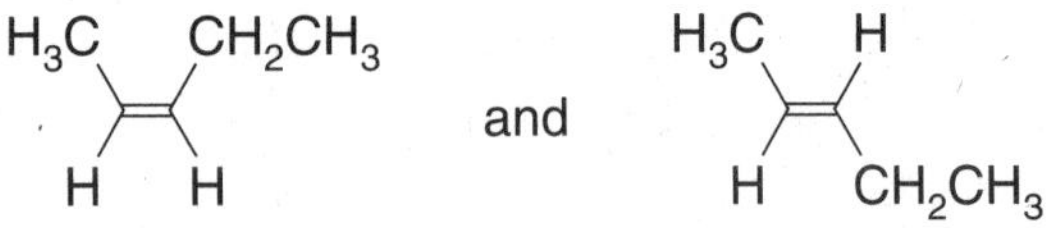

C. 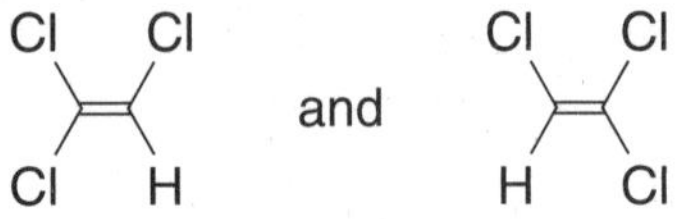

D. 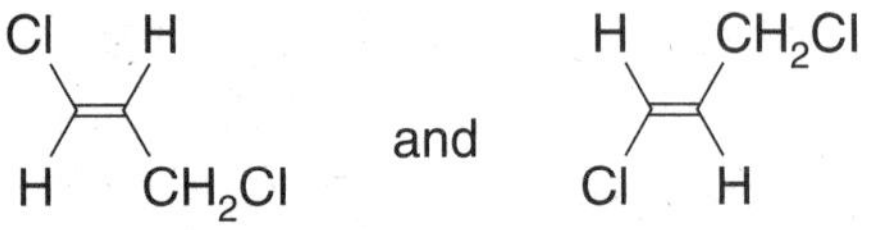

141. A requirement of stereoisomers in alkenes is that each of the carbon atoms involved in the pi bond must
A. have identical groups attached to it.
B. lie on the same side of the double bond.
C. rotate freely around the pi bond.
D. have two different groups attached to it.

QUESTIONS 142–144 are NOT based on a descriptive passage.

142. When bone formation takes place in preexisting cartilage, it is called
A. intramembranous bone formation.
B. primary ossification.
C. endochondral ossification.
D. subchondral ossification.

143. Which of the following is part of the appendicular skeleton?
A. Humerus
B. Vertebrae
C. Ribs
D. Sternum

144. Which of the following undergoes saponification?
   - A. Glucose
   - B. Starches
   - C. Glycogen
   - D. Fats

STOP!

If time still remains, you may review work only in this section. When the time allotted is up, you may go on to the next section.

STOP!

Test 1 ■ Answer Key

1.	A	37.	C	73.	C	109.	B
2.	C	38.	B	74.	B	110.	A
3.	D	39.	C	75.	C	111.	A
4.	A	40.	B	76.	D	112.	D
5.	A	41.	C	77.	B	113.	C
6.	D	42.	C	78.	A	114.	B
7.	B	43.	D	79.	A	115.	B
8.	B	44.	A	80.	B	116.	D
9.	B	45.	C	81.	B	117.	C
10.	A	46.	B	82.	C	118.	A
11.	D	47.	C	83.	C	119.	B
12.	D	48.	D	84.	D	120.	C
13.	D	49.	B	85.	B	121.	D
14.	B	50.	C	86.	C	122.	A
15.	B	51.	D	87.	A	123.	D
16.	D	52.	D	88.	D	124.	C
17.	D	53.	B	89.	B	125.	C
18.	C	54.	A	90.	D	126.	C
19.	D	55.	B	91.	C	127.	C
20.	B	56.	B	92.	B	128.	D
21.	A	57.	C	93.	C	129.	D
22.	B	58.	C	94.	B	130.	C
23.	C	59.	D	95.	D	131.	A
24.	A	60.	D	96.	A	132.	B
25.	D	61.	B	97.	B	133.	A
26.	C	62.	C	98.	C	134.	B
27.	B	63.	B	99.	D	135.	A
28.	C	64.	D	100.	D	136.	C
29.	B	65.	C	101.	C	137.	D
30.	D	66.	B	102.	A	138.	C
31.	D	67.	B	103.	D	139.	A
32.	D	68.	D	104.	A	140.	B
33.	A	69.	B	105.	B	141.	D
34.	D	70.	D	106.	D	142.	C
35.	C	71.	B	107.	D	143.	A
36.	A	72.	A	108.	B	144.	D

SECTION 1
Physical Sciences

PASSAGE I
(QUESTIONS 1–4)

1. **A.** To find out how many moles of ATP are produced, we need to find the balanced equation for the conversion of glucose to lactate. This can be found by multiplying the equation for the conversion of pyruvate to lactate by 2 and adding it to the equation for the conversion of glucose to pyruvate.

This results in:

$$\text{Glucose} + 2PO_4^{3-} + 2\text{ADP} + 2\text{NAD}^+ \rightarrow 2\text{pyruvate} + 2\text{ATP} + 2\text{NADH} + 2H^+ + 2H_2O$$

$$2 \times (\text{Pyruvate} + \text{NADH} + H^+ \rightarrow \text{L-Lactate} + \text{NAD}^+)$$

$$\text{Glucose} + 2PO_4^{3-} + 2\text{ADP} \rightarrow 2\ \text{L-Lactate} + 2\text{ATP} + 2H_2O$$

The stoichiometry of the new reaction tells us that 2 moles of ATP are produced for each mole of glucose.

2. **C.** Based on the stoichiometry of the net reaction from the previous question, zero moles of NADH are produced.

$$\text{Glucose} + 2PO_4^{3-} + 2\text{ADP} \rightarrow 2\ \text{L-Lactate} + 2\text{ATP} + 2H_2O$$

3. **D.** The free energy can be calculated using the expression $\Delta G = -nFE$, where n = mole e^-.

For pyruvate $\Delta G = -(2) \times (23.1\ \text{kcal/mol})(-0.19)$

$\Delta G = +8.76$ kcal/mol

For NADH $\Delta G = -(2) \times (23.1\ \text{kcal/mol})(-0.32)$

$\Delta G = +14.76$ kcal/mol

Combining the two reactions:

$$\text{Pyruvate} + 2H^+ + 2e^- \rightarrow \text{Lactate} \quad \Delta G = +8.76\ \text{kcal/mol}$$

$$\text{NADH} \rightarrow \text{NAD}^+ + H^+ + 2e^- \quad \Delta G = -14.76\ \text{kcal/mol}$$

$$\text{Pyruvate} + \text{NADH} + 2H^+ \rightarrow \text{Lactate} + \text{NAD}^+ \quad \Delta G = -5.99\ \text{kcal/mol} \sim -6\ \text{kcal/mol}$$

4. **A.** The balanced equations for the conversion of glucose to L-Lactate can be found by multiplying the equation for the conversion of pyruvate to lactate by 2 and adding it to the equation for the conversion of glucose to pyruvate. These same operations, when performed on the ΔGs for these reactions, should give ΔG for the whole process:

<u>ΔG</u>

$$\text{Glucose} + 2PO_4^{3-} + 2\text{ADP} + 2\text{NAD}^+ \rightarrow 2\text{pyruvate} + 2\text{ATP} + 2\text{NADH} + 2H^+ + 2H_2O \quad -17.5$$

$$2 \times (\text{Pyruvate} + \text{NADH} + H^+ \rightarrow \text{L-Lactate} + \text{NAD}^+) \quad 2(-5)$$

$$\text{Glucose} + 2PO_4^{3-} + 2\text{ADP} \rightarrow 2\ \text{L-Lactate} + 2\text{ATP} + 2H_2O \quad -27.5\ \text{kcal/mol}$$

$\Delta G = -27.5$ kcal/mol

PASSAGE II
(QUESTIONS 5–8)

5. **A.** The decrease in temperature as the white powder dissolves shows that the solution process is endothermic. Because heat is required to form the solution, adding heat to

raise the temperature will promote solution, thus increasing the solubility at the higher temperature.

6. **D.** The total mass of the solution was 1.5 g + 10.0 g = 11.5 g. The volume is this mass divided by the density. (11.5 g) (1 mL / 1.05 g) = 11.0 mL

7. **B.** In experiment 3, 30.0 mg of the sample produced 44.0 mg of CO_2 and 18.0 mg of H_2O. The molecular weight of CO_2 is 12 g/mole for C + 2(16 g/mole) for O_2 = 44 g/mole. Thus, 12 mg of the 44 mg of CO_2 is carbon. Likewise, the molecular weight of H_2O is 18 g/mole and 2 g/mole for H_2. Thus, 2 mg of the 18 mg sample of H_2O is hydrogen. The 30.0 mg sample of the white powder must contain 12 mg carbon, 2 mg hydrogen, and the remainder is 16 mg oxygen.

8. **B.** In experiment 3, it was found that 44.0 mg or 44.0 mg (1 mmol/44.0 mg) = 1.00 mmol of CO_2 and 18.0 mg or 18.0 mg (1 mmol/18.0 mg) = 1.00 mmol of H_2O were formed in the combustion of 30.0 mg of the white powder. Because one millimole of CO_2 contains one millimole of carbon, and one millimole of H_2O contains two millimoles of hydrogen atoms, the 30.0 mg of white powder contains 1.00 mmol C (12.0 mg C/mmol C) = 12.0 mg C and 2.00 mmol H (1.0 mg H/mmol H) 2.0 mgH. Experiment 2 indicated that the white powder contained only C, H, and O. The mass of oxygen can be found by difference: 30.0 mg − 12.0 mg − 2.0 = 16.0 mg O. Converting this mass to millimoles of oxygen yields 16.0 mg O (1 mmol O/16.0 mg O) = 1.00 mmol. The mole ratio of the elements in the white power is 1.00 mmol C/2.00 mmol H/1.00 mmol O, which leads to the simplest formula CH_2O.

PASSAGE III (QUESTIONS 9–12)

9. **B.** In a balanced equation for a nuclear reaction, both the sum of the mass numbers (A) and the atomic numbers (Z) for the products and reactants must be equal.

   A (reactants) = 238 + 238 = 476 = A (products) = 300 + x x = 476 − 300 = 176

   Z (reactants) = 92 + 92 = 184 + Z (products) = 119 + y y − 184 − 119 − 65

   Atomic number 65 corresponds to the element terbium, Tb.

$$2\,{}^{238}_{92}U \rightarrow {}^{300}_{119}My + {}^{176}_{65}Tb$$

10. **A.** Because mysterium is in the first column of the periodic table, it would be expected to form compounds similar to those of potassium and sodium. That is, mysterium would be expected to form ionic compounds, where it exists as a singly positive ion. Sulfate is a doubly negative ion, so two My^+ ions are required for one $SO_4^=$ ion: My_2SO_4.

11. **D.** The elements of the first group of the periodic table easily lose one electron to form singly positive ions; they have low first ionization energies. The resulting singly positive ion has a stable, noble gas–like electron configuration and a very large second ionization energy. Choices A, B, and C, because they are less than, equal to, and only very slightly greater than the first ionization energy, are all unreasonable. Choice D, more than a factor of four, greater than the first ionization energy, must be the second ionization energy of mysterium.

12. **D.** The mysterium sample goes through alpha decay with a half life equal to 600 s × 1 minute/60 s = 10 minutes. The half life is the time for half the sample to decay. After 30 minutes, the sample has undergone three half lives and therefore (1/2)(1/2)(1/2) = 1/8 of the original sample is left. Therefore, in order to have 1.0 mg of the sample remain after 30 minutes, 8.0 mg of the sample must have existed before this 30-minute period.

13. **D.** Average speed is the speed at which the car would travel the given distance in the given time:

$$t_1 = \frac{d_1}{v_1} \qquad t_2 = \frac{d_2}{v_2}$$

$$t_1 = \frac{15\ km}{30\ km/hr} = \frac{1}{2}\ hr$$

$$t_2 = \frac{30\ km}{60\ km/hr} = \frac{1}{2}\ hr$$

$t_{total} = 1/2 + 1/2 = 1$ hr to cover 45 km.

Therefore:

$$v_{avg} = \frac{d_{total}}{t_{total}} = \frac{45\ km}{1\ hr} = 45\ km/hr.$$

14. **B.** Near the surface of the earth, neglecting air resistance, all objects in free fall accelerate downward at 9.8 m/s^2. Free fall pertains to an object whose acceleration is solely influenced by the force of gravity. Even at the top of an object's flight, when the velocity is zero, the acceleration is still 9.8 m/s^2 downward. It must be remembered that acceleration is the *change* in velocity over the change in time, not velocity over the time.

15. **B.** The relationship between temperature and volume of a gas is stated in Charles' Law:

$$\frac{V_1}{T_1} = \frac{V_2}{T_2}$$

Note: All temperatures must be in ° Kelvin.

$$\frac{2m^3}{250^oK} = \frac{V}{294^oK}$$

$588\ m^3 \times {}^\circ K = 250^\circ K\ V_2$

$V_2 = 2.35\ m^3$

16. **D.** The reaction given describes the reaction of an alkyl halide with magnesium in dry ether to produce the Grignard reagent. The Grignard reagent subsequently reacts with solid CO_2, or dry ice, to produce a carboxylic acid. The reaction process is illustrated below:

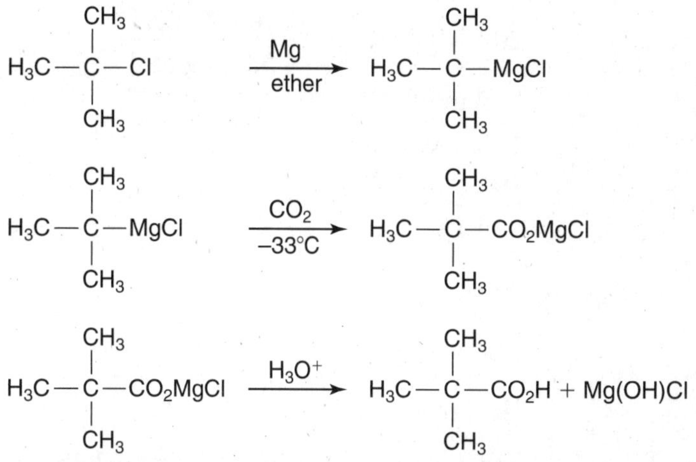

PASSAGE IV (QUESTIONS 17–21)

17. **D.** The solubility product constant (K_{sp}) is the equilibrium constant for the following reaction. Note that the solid does not appear in the equilibrium expression.

$Mg(OH)_{2(s)}\ Mg^{2+} \rightleftharpoons 2NaOH$

$Ksp = [Mg^{2+}][OH^-]^2$

$[OH^-] = (Ksp/[Mg^{2+}])^{1/2}$

$[OH^-] = (1.8 \times 10^{-11}/0.001\ M)^{1/2} = 0.000134$ mol/L

Convert to grams NaOH

1.34×10^{-4} M NaOH $\times$ (40 g NaOH/1 mol NaOH) $\times$ 1L $= 5.37 \times 10^{-3}$ g NaOH

18. **C.** Evaporating the pool reduces the volume by one half. This doubles the concentration of Mg^{2+} to 0.002 M. Plugging this value into the equation gives:

$[OH] = (1.8 \times 10^{-11}/0.002\ M)^{1/2} = 0.0000949$ mol NaOH/L

Convert to grams NaOH

9.49×10^{-5} M NaOH $\times$ (40 g NaOH/1 mol NaOH) $\times$ 1 L $= 3.79 \times 10^{-3}$ g NaOH

~4×10^{-3} g

19. **D.** Two moles of HCl are required to neutralize 1 mole of $Mg(OH)_2$. The formula weight of $Mg(OH)_2$ is = 28.28 g/mol.

$$20g\ Mg(OH)_2 \times \frac{1\,mol\ Mg(OH)_2}{58.28\ g/mol} \times \frac{2\ mol\ HCl}{1\ mol\ Mg(OH)_2} \times \frac{1L}{12\ mol\ HCl} \times \frac{1000\ mL}{1\ L} = 57mL$$

20. **B.**

$$Mg^{2+} + 2Cl^- \rightarrow Mg_{(s)} + Cl_{2(g)}$$

Half reaction

$$Mg^{2+} + 2e^- \rightarrow Mg^0_{(s)} \quad E^o = -2.38\ V$$

$$2Cl^-_{(aq)} \rightarrow Cl_{2(g)} + 2e^-$$

$$E^o = -1(+1.36\ V)$$

$$Mg^{2+} + 2Cl^- \rightarrow Mg_{(s)} + Cl_{2(g)}$$

$$E^o = -3.74\ V$$

21. **A.** From the balanced equation, 2 moles of electrons are required to form 1 mole of Mg^o.

1 Faraday = 9.65×10^4 Coulombs
= charge on 1 mole of electrons

1 Coulomb = 1 Amp × sec

So 1 hr = 3600 sec

$$60\ min \times \frac{60\ sec}{1\ min} = 3600\ sec$$

5A × 3600 sec = 18000 Coulombs

$$18000C \times \frac{1\ mol\ e^-}{9.65 \times 10^4 C} \times \frac{1\ mol\ Mg^0}{2\ mol\ e^-} \times \frac{24.3g\ Mg}{1\ mol\ Mg^0} = 2.27\ g\ Mg$$

PASSAGE V (QUESTIONS 22-25)

22. **B.** From step 1, or equation 3, the rate of formation of ES is proportional to the product [E] × [S]. If both [E] and [S] are doubled, the rate of formation of ES will increase by a factor of (2) × (2) = 4.

23. **C.** K[E] [S] = K´[ES] + k˝ [ES] = (K´ + k˝) [ES]

$$K_{eq} = \frac{[ES]}{[E][S]} = \frac{K}{K' + k''} = \frac{1}{Km}$$

24. **A.** Use equations 6 and 7 to analyze the dependence of R on [S]. Equation 6 shows that R increases in proportion to [S] for small values of [S], and equation 7 shows that R approaches a constant value for large values of [S].

25. **D.** For a first order reaction, the rate law is ln[S] = ln[So] − Ct. If t = h, the half life, then [S] = 1/2[So].

ln[1/2So] = ln [So] − Ch

ln[1/2So] = ln [So] = − Ch

ln(1/2) = ln − Ch = − ln(2)

h = ln(2) / C

PASSAGE VI (QUESTIONS 26-29)

26. **C.** The equation for the magnetic field B at a distance r from a long straight wire is $B = (\mu_0 I)/(2\pi r)$, where I is the current and μ_0 is a constant. Therefore, the magnetic field is inversely proportional to the distance. 1 meter = 100 cm = 5(20 cm), so the distance has increased by a factor of 5, and the magnetic field must decrease by a factor of 5 from 1 Gauss to 0.2 Gauss.

27. **B.** As stated in the passage, photons start to be unsafe when they ionize atoms. The photon energy necessary to ionize atoms is on the order of a few electron volts. For example, to ionize the ground state electron in the hydrogen atom requires 13.6 eV. It is not necessary to memorize this value for hydrogen, but one should have an idea of the

order of magnitude (between 1 and 100 eV). The energy of a photon is determined by the equation E = hf, where h is Planck's constant and f is the frequency. For example, a photon of frequency 10^{15} Hz has

$$E = hf = (4.14 \times 10^{-15}\ eV-s)(10^{15}\ (1/s)) \sim 4\ eV,$$

approximately the value necessary to ionize an atom.

28. **C.** Density = mass/volume, so mass = (volume)(density) = (length)(area)(density) = (length)(πr^2)(density) = (10 m)(π)(0.01 m)^2(9.0 g/cm^3)(100 cm/m)^3 ~ (10)(3)(10^{-4})(9)(10^6) g = 27 × 10^3 = 27000 g. A more precise calculation yields 28000 g. However, the approximate value is sufficient for choosing the correct answer.

29. **B.** The power and current are kept the same in each wire, so $P_c = P_a = I^2 R_c = I^2 R_a$. So $R_c = R_a = \rho_c L/A_c = \rho_a L/A_a$. Because the lengths are the same, we find that $\rho_c/\rho_a = A_c/A_a$. The mass is equal to the density times the volume so $m_c = D_c V_c = D_c A_c L$, and $m_a = D_a V_a = D_a A_a L$. To find the ratio m_a/m_c, we divide both the left and the right side of each equation and get $m_a/m_c = D_a A_a/D_c A_c = D_a \rho_a/D_c \rho_c$. Therefore, m_a/m_c = (2.7 gm/cm^3)(2.8 × 10^{-8} ohm-m)/(9.0 gm/cm^3)(1.7 × 10^{-8} ohm-m) ~ 8/15 ~ 1/2.

30. **D.** Ozonolysis is a characteristic reaction of alkenes. It degrades alkenes to aldehydes:

```
    O
    ||
R—C—H
```

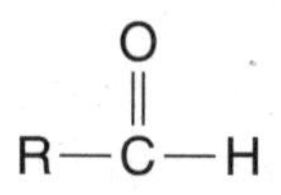

and ketones:

```
    O
    ||
R—C—R'
```

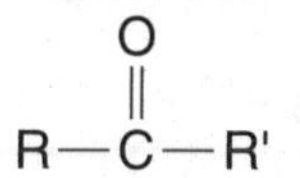

by cleaving the double bond with ozone (O_3) in the presence of zinc dust (Zn) and acid (H$^+$).

The mechanism of the reaction is as follows: ozone is passed through the alkene,

which causes the formation of an ozonide; the ozonides, which are explosive, are converted into aldehydes and ketones in the presence of zinc dust and acid:

$$R_2C{=}CR_2 + O_3 \longrightarrow R_2C\overset{O-O}{\underset{O}{\diagup\diagdown}}CR_2$$

Alkene   **Ozone**   **Ozonide**

$$R_2C\overset{O-O}{\underset{O}{\diagup\diagdown}}CR_2 \xrightarrow[H+]{Zn} R_2C{=}O + R_2C{=}O + H_2O$$

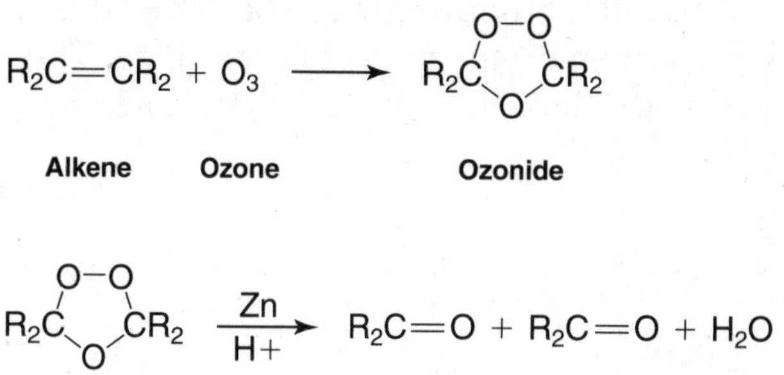

The position of the double bond in the original alkene will be indicated by the carbonyl group (C = O) formed in the products after ozonolysis. Sodium borohydride (NaBH$_4$) is a reagent used to reduce the carbonyl group of aldehydes, ketones, and carboxylic acids to the hydroxyl group of the corresponding alcohol. With the metal hydrides, the key step is the transfer of a hydride ion to the carbonyl carbon of the substance being reduced. The acidic hydrogen first reacts to liberate hydrogen gas. The carbonyl group is then attacked by the BH$_4$ q ion, and the group is reduced to the primary alkoxide. Overall, the reaction may be written as:

$$4\ RCHO + 3NaBH_4 \rightarrow 4H_2 + (RCH_2O)_4BNa \rightarrow 4\ RCH_2OH$$

In this problem, the following occurs:

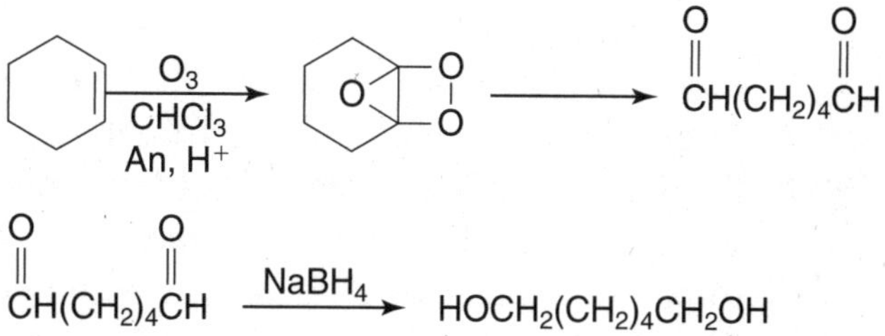

31. **D.** LiCl, NaCl, and KCl all have the 6PO(NaCl) structure. Because of the large ionic radius of Cs, CsCl takes on the 3.2PTOT(CsCl) structure.

32. **D.** All reactions, exothermic or endothermic, that involve any type of bond breaking will have an energy of activation,

though it may be very low. An exothermic reaction has a negative ΔH (change in enthalpy). Because heat is being liberated, it is only logical that the potential energy of the products should be lower than the potential energy of the reactants. This is summarized in the following diagram:

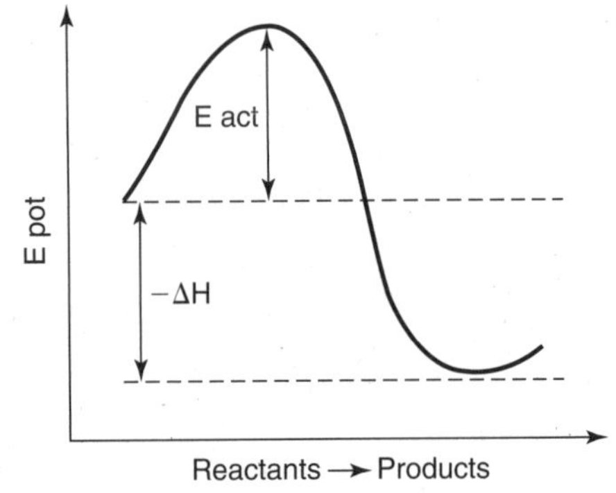

PASSAGE VII (QUESTIONS 33–36)

33. **A.** The force F on a charged particle q in an electric field E is given by the expression F = qE. Because one electron is missing from these otherwise neutral atoms, their net charge is equal to $+1.6 \times 10^{-19}$ C. So the force is $F = (+1.6 \times 10^{-19}\ C)(4.0 \times 10^6\ N/C) = 6.4 \times 10^{-13}$ N.

34. **D.** The electric force on a positively charged particle in an electric field is in the same direction as the electric field, which is up, as stated in the passage. As stated, the magnetic force is opposite to this electric force and is therefore down. To determine the direction of the magnetic field, it is necessary to use the right-hand rule. For the force on a positive charge in a magnetic field, the fingers of your right hand point in the direction of the velocity of the charge (to the right). You then sweep your fingers in the direction of the magnetic field and your thumb points in the direction of the force. For your thumb to point down (in the known direction of the magnetic force), you must sweep your fingers in the direction out of the page.

35. **C.** The velocity of selected ions is determined by the condition that the electric force qE is equal to the magnetic force qvB, or qE = qvB. Rearranging terms yields v = E/B.

36. **A.** The force on the ion in the mass spectrometer chamber is a centripetal force, which always points in toward the center of the circle. This force is always perpendicular to the direction of motion of the ion and causes it to continually change direction and thus travel in a circle.

PASSAGE VIII (QUESTIONS 37–41)

37. **C.** Using conservation of momentum, the momentum of the system before the collision must equal the momentum of the system after the collision. Referring to the initial velocity of the car, the initial velocity of the truck, and the final velocity of the car-truck combination as v_{c0}, v_{t0}, and v, respectively, we have,

$$m_c v_{c0} + m_t v_{t0} = (m_c + m_t)v$$

and

$$v_t 0 = \frac{(m_c + m_t)v - m_c v_c 0}{m_t}$$

so

$$v_t 0 = \frac{(1000\ kg + 2000\ kg)(6m/s) - 1000\ kg\,(-30m/s)}{2000\ kg}$$

$$= 24m/s$$

A very important thing to remember about momentum is that momentum is a vector, and we must assign a positive or negative value according to direction. If we define the direction to the left as positive, then we must assign a negative value to velocities to the right. This is where the −30 m/s comes from.

38. **B.** From Newton's third law, the force of the truck on the car is equal in magnitude but opposite in direction to the force of the car on the truck.

39. **C.** As stated in the passage, the stopping distance is proportional to the square of the speed of the car at the time the brakes are applied. Because the speed has increased by a factor of 3, the stopping distance must increase by a factor of $3^2 = 9$. The new stopping distance is 9(20 m) = 180 m.

40. **B.** The kinematic equation relating the final velocity v to the initial velocity v_0, the acceleration a, and distance x is $v^2 = v_0^2 + 2ax$. So

$$v^2{}_0 = \sqrt{v^2 - 2ax} = \sqrt{0 - 2(-10m/s^2)(4m)}$$
$$= \sqrt{80m^2/s^2} \sim 9m/s$$

41. **C.** In a collision, as two objects come together (in this case the dummy's head and the padded dashboard), the force gradually increases up to some maximum value and then slowly decreases. One can think of a mass approaching a spring. As the spring begins to compress, the force starts out small and then builds to the point of maximum compression. As the mass starts to move outward from the spring, the spring gradually decompresses, and the force gradually returns back to zero as the mass leaves the spring.

PASSAGE IX (QUESTIONS 42-45)

42. **C.** The voltages in the passage are all alternating current voltages. This must be the case if a transformer is used to amplify these voltages. An alternating-current voltage is one that oscillates sinusoidally between a positive and a negative value. When this voltage is finally used to accelerate the electrons, it must be made into a direct current voltage, that is, one polarity or all positive. Otherwise, it could not be used to accelerate electrons in one direction.

43. **D.** Combining Ohm's law, $V = IR$, with the power equation, $P = IV$, leads to $R = V/I = V/(P/V) = V^2/P$. Substituting $V = 120V$ and $P = 1200$W leads to $R = (120)^2/(1200) = 12$ ohms.

44. **A.** The two resistors, in series, can be replaced by a single resistor equal to their sum: $R_1 = 5$ ohm + 10 ohm = 15 ohm. The given circuit reduces to an equivalent circuit of two 15-ohm resistors, in parallel. The reciprocals of the two resistors in parallel add to give the reciprocal of the resistance of a single resistor, which is equivalent to them.

$$1/R_2 = 1/15 + 1/15 = 2/15, R_2 = 15/2 = 7.5 \text{ ohm}$$

45. **C.** The X-ray unit draws 8A and the coffee maker uses 1200W of power at 120 volts. P = VI, so the coffee maker draws I = P/V = 1200 W/120 volts = 10A of current. Therefore, to just barely trip the 20A circuit breaker, the third device would need to draw 20A − 8A − 10A = 2A of current.

PASSAGE X (QUESTIONS 46-50)

46. **B.** The product of the frequency and wavelength of sound is equal to the speed of sound. The speed of sound, in a particular medium, is therefore proportional to its frequency for a fixed wavelength.

(frequency in He)/(frequency in air)

= (speed in He)/(speed in air)
(1020 m/s)/(340 m/s) = 3

47. **C.** From the table, the speed of sound in tissue is 1600 m/s. The 10-ms travel time given is the time the sound wave needs to travel from the front to the back of the tumor and back to the front again. Therefore, the sound wave travels one length of the tumor in 5 ms. Average speed = distance/time, so distance = (average speed)(time) = (1600 m/s)(5 ms) = $(1.6 \times 10^3$ m/s$)(5 \times 10^{-6}$ s$) = 8 \times 10^{-3}$ m. A millimeter (mm) equals 1×10^{-3} meters, so the answer is 8 mm. Notice the importance

of converting to scientific notation and memorizing the powers of ten associated with prefixes such as *micro* or *milli*.

48. **D.** For any of the first three choices to be correct, the speed of sound would have to increase as the density of the material increased. If this were true, then the speed of sound should be highest in tissue and lowest in helium. From the table, we know that this is not the case. In fact, the speed of sound doesn't even *decrease* with increasing density. It does something in between. Therefore, the speed of sound must depend on something in addition to density and temperature.

49. **B.** Because the distance between nodes (points of zero wave amplitude) is one half of the wavelength, the conventional illustration shows three half-waves in the distance *L*. Thus, the wavelength must be two-thirds of *L* or $2L/3$.

50. **C.** The intensity level is $db = 20 \log(P/P_o)$. Solving for the pressure P by taking antilogarithms, gives $P = P_o\, 10^{-db/20}$. The ratio of the pressures for two intensity levels is

$$P_1/P_2 = 10^{(db1 - db2)/20} = 10^{(40 - 20)/20} = 10$$

51. **D.**

$$KE = 1/2\, mv^2$$

Using the MKS system, we obtain

$$m = 0.1 \text{ kg} \quad v = 60 \text{ m/sec}$$

then, $KE = 1/2(0.1 \text{ kg})(60 \text{ m/sec})^2$

$$KE = +1/2(0.1 \text{ kg})(3600(\text{m/sec})^2)$$

$$KE = 180 \frac{kg \cdot m^2}{\sec^2} = 180 N \cdot m$$

$$KE = 180 \text{ joules}$$

52. **D.** The Newton is that unbalanced force which acts on one kilogram mass and produces an acceleration of one meter per second squared.

SECTION 2
Verbal Reasoning

PASSAGE I (QUESTIONS 53–57)

The author of this passage describes what makes one scientific theory superior to another in terms of its falsifiability. We are given two examples to illustrate the difference. The author concludes by arguing that science proceeds by trial and error.

53. **B.** The author makes this clear in the sixth paragraph by emphasizing the words *mistakes, error*, and *falsifications*. Proposing highly falsifiable theories is preferable to proposing nonfalsifiable ones; but according to the author's claims in paragraph six, we do not learn from either type of theory until it is falsified. Thus, A is incorrect. For the same reason, D and C are incorrect and, in addition, are too narrowly phrased. Science includes more than just theories of planetary motion.

54. **A.** The author defines this term in the sixth sentence of the third paragraph by telling us, "If we follow Popper and refer to those sets of observational statements that would serve to falsify a law or theory as *potential falsifiers* of that law or theory . . . ." Answer choices B, C, and D are all incorrect because potential falsifiers are not theories themselves but statements that, if observed, would serve to falsify an existing theory.

55. **B.** The author begins the passage by telling us what a good scientific theory does: it makes definite claims about the world. By inference, a bad scientific theory does not make definite claims about the world. Answer choice A may in fact be true, but we are given no information about theories that limit the advance of scientific knowledge. One might reason that theories that do not make definite claims about the world are nonfalsifiable. Because it is the falsification of theories that leads to the striking achievements in science (sixth paragraph), we might conclude that theories that do not make definite claims about the world do limit the advance of scientific knowledge. Selecting answer choice B, however, yields the same result more directly and is thus the better answer. Although we are told in the fifth paragraph that falsified theories must be ruthlessly rejected, this does not make them *bad* scientific theories. Falsified theories have made enough definite claims about the world to be falsified and thereby advance science. Thus, answer choice C is incorrect. Answer choice D describes a theory that has not yet been falsified. However, it soon will be falsified and thus falls into the same category as C, making D incorrect.

56. **B.** The author tells us this directly in the first paragraph, and again less directly in the fifth. We are also told in the fifth paragraph why statement III is not part of a good scientific theory.

57. **C.** As described in the passage, Kepler's theory dealt exclusively with planetary motion. Because answer choice C is not an observation relating to planetary motion, it is not a potential falsifier of Kepler's theory (although it is of Newton's). A, B, and D are all statements suggesting that the locations of various planets were not as predicted. These all relate to planetary motion and are thus potential falsifiers of Kepler's theory.

PASSAGE II (QUESTIONS 58–62)

The author of this passage describes the word *oppression* and how it should be properly applied to various groups. We are given examples of how the word is misapplied and how this misapplication can lead to accusations of insensitivity and bigotry on the part of women.

58. **C.** The author first makes this point in the fifth sentence of paragraph two. She makes the point more directly in the second sentence of the third paragraph when she says, "Human beings can be miserable without being oppressed." The first sentence of the sixth paragraph shows answer choice A to be clearly incorrect. Although in the sixth paragraph, the author tells us that men are not oppressed as men, she does mention in the fourth and fifth paragraphs that men might be oppressed (just not because they are men). Thus, B is incorrect. The first sentence of the passage makes it clear that "oppression" has direct application to feminist theory, making D incorrect.

59. **D.** This point is made directly in the last sentence of the passage. In the sixth paragraph, the author allows for the possibility that men can be oppressed for reasons other than because they are men, which makes answer choice A incorrect. B and C are incorrect because the author does not specifically tell us who she thinks is oppressing women. We can reasonably infer that the author believes men oppress women; but aside from making B false, it appears that she is assuming men oppress women rather than arguing the point.

60. **D.** The author makes this point directly in the fourth and sixth sentences of the fourth paragraph.

61. **B.** The author makes this point in the first sentence of the fourth paragraph. Answer choice A is clearly incorrect due to the author's statement in the last sentence of the passage. The author does assert that she is marked for oppression, but this is because she is a member of a group that she feels has been marked for oppression, i.e., women. Therefore, although answer choice C is true, B is the better answer. D is incorrect because the author does not argue that individual characteristics, as opposed to group characteristics, are responsible for being oppressed.

62. **C.** The initial assumptions are that women see themselves as sensitive (answer choice A) and that being sensitive is a redeeming trait. If women are considered insensitive, one must also assume that they have no redeeming traits other than sensitivity in order to reach the conclusion that they have no redeeming traits at all. Although A is an assumption of the above argument, it is neither a necessary nor a sufficient condition for the conclusion to hold. Even if women did not see themselves as being sensitive, they may not think they have any redeeming traits, thus making the conclusion true (the necessary condition). Even assuming A to be correct, it does not necessarily follow that women will believe they have no redeeming traits *unless* they also believe it is their only redeeming trait. For similar reasons, B and D are also incorrect.

PASSAGE III (QUESTIONS 63–68)

The author of this passage introduces the reader to some of the broader implications and areas affected by momentous discoveries in the area of physics. In particular, he suggests that discoveries in the physical world may bring us closer to an understanding of several questions that were previously thought of as being solely religious in nature.

63. **B.** The author makes this point in the fourth sentence of the first paragraph. Answer choice A is incorrect because there is no mention in the passage of the value of the theory of relativity after quantum theory

was proposed. C is incorrect because of the author's statement in the third sentence of the first paragraph. In addition, in the second paragraph, the author tells us that the effects of these discoveries have been felt by philosophers, theologians, psychologists, and sociologists — none of whom deals exclusively with the physical world — as well. D is clearly incorrect, as demonstrated in the first paragraph.

64. **D.** In the second paragraph, the author notes that theologians have benefited from the new physics by saying that they have plucked the fruits of the scientific revolution. Later in the paragraph, he tells us that psychologists find sympathy with the new view of science. The author also indicates in the second paragraph that the beliefs of ordinary people are often in tune with the view of the world presented by the new physics. Thus, answer choice D is correct.

65. **C.** The author makes this point in the third sentence of the sixth paragraph. Answer choice A is incorrect because in the same sentence the author admits that the answers physicists find may be wrong. Despite the possibility that the answers provided by the new physics to the Big Four Questions may be wrong, there is no indication in the passage that the author believes them to be unanswerable. Thus, B is incorrect. D is clearly incorrect based on the author's statement in the third sentence of the sixth paragraph.

66. **B.** In the context of the passage, in particular the third sentence of the second paragraph, the author is using the word *sympathy* to indicate agreement. Answer choice A is incorrect because there is no indication that sociologists have any reason to feel sorry for physicists. C is incorrect because it has the relationship backward. D is incorrect because it states the physicists' view of the world, which is gaining popularity, not necessarily the study of physics. It is unlikely that sociologists will give up their discipline and turn to physics. It is more likely that they will begin to study how the implications of the new physics affect sociology.

67. **B.** This answer is reached by eliminating the other answers. Answer choices A and C are very unlikely possibilities, given the author's willingness still to consider some questions of a religious nature (fifth and sixth paragraphs), even though they may be answered by the new physics. This conclusion is supported by the author's unwillingness to discuss religious phenomena. If he believed the new physics to have abolished God, he would more likely try to explain such phenomena in scientific terms. From the sixth paragraph it should be clear the author believes the question *is* relevant to the new physics, making D incorrect.

68. **D.** The author makes this point in the fifth sentence of the first paragraph. Certainly many physicists do concentrate their energies on particle physics, but the only mention of this subarea of physics is in the form of a brief reference to subnuclear particles in the fourth paragraph. Thus, answer choice A is incorrect. In the sixth paragraph, the author argues physicists may begin to answer some questions formerly thought to be solely religious, but this does not mean physicists are examining religion. Rather, it means they are viewing physics in a new way that may have an impact on religious questions. Thus, B is incorrect. C is incorrect because we are given no information about psychological notions of mind and matter or whether they have been rejected by physicists.

PASSAGE IV (QUESTIONS 69–72)

The author of this passage is introducing the idea of Ethical Egoism. He gives an example and describes how most people would react when confronted with the problem, then suggests how an Ethical Egoist would react. He goes into some detail as to exactly what Ethical Egoism holds.

69. **B.** In the fifth sentence of the second paragraph, the author tells us that common-sense morality holds, "when we can help others — especially at little cost to ourselves — we should do so." Answer choice A is a utilitarian position and is not mentioned in the passage. C might be considered an extreme form of altruism and is also not mentioned in the passage. Although the implication of *common-sense* morality is that it is based on common sense, D is incorrect because common-sense morality assumes a specific view of what constitutes common sense (i.e., helping others when it costs us little). No individual variation is allowed.

70. **D.** In this passage, the author introduces the concept of Ethical Egoism. He does not use any language that suggests he personally believes in Ethical Egoism or that it is the correct moral view. He also gives no indication that he prefers the common-sense view of morality. Thus, because answer choice A represents the common-sense view of morality and answer choice B represents Ethical Egoism, both are incorrect. The problem of world hunger is used only as an example in the passage, and there is no indication of how the author feels about the problem, making C incorrect as well.

71. **B.** In the final sentences of the passage, the author tells us that Ethical Egoism tells us to advance our *long-term* interests. Momentary pleasure, unless, of course, it also has long-term gains, is frowned upon. The author specifically indicates in this paragraph that smoking cigarettes is not an activity condoned by Ethical Egoism (III). (I) is also an activity with only short-term pleasures. Only (II) holds any long-term advantage for the actor.

72. **A.** In the final paragraph, the author tells us that Ethical Egoism advocates only that individuals pursue their *long-term* interests. The problem is in determining their long-term interests. The smoker might argue that the years of pleasurable smoking are a long-term interest despite the likely result. For lottery winners, it was certainly in their long-term interests to have played, even though for everyone else it was not. The author speaks as if there is some objective standard that people can use to gauge whether a particular course of action *really is* in their interests. Unfortunately, people can only go by their own subjective view of what their interests are. Answer choice B is incorrect because, as pointed out in the fifth paragraph, Ethical Egoism does not suggest one should avoid helping others. Similarly, C is incorrect because there may be instances where common-sense morality and Ethical Egoism coincide. Just as Ethical Egoism does not say that we should avoid helping others, common-sense morality does not say that we cannot act in our own interests as well as help others. D is nonsense and has nothing to do with the passage.

PASSAGE V (QUESTIONS 73–77)

In this passage, the author gives us some examples of what he terms math abuse. He then tells us why these examples are abusing mathematics. Later in the passage, he begins to explain how filtering leads to math abuse. He ends the passage by giving an example of how pure luck can lead to results similar to those explained by methods that abuse math.

73. **C.** In the second sentence of the third paragraph, the author admits that it really does not matter whether more babies are born during a full moon. Nevertheless, by using births as an example of math abuse, and later explaining the filtering process using the same example, we can reasonably conclude the author is skeptical of any statistical relationship between birth rate and a

full moon. Answer choice A is incorrect because of the reasons stated above, and because there is no mention in the passage of deferring to the nurse because of her expertise. In fact, the author uses the nurse's expertise and that of the acquaintance who has invested for eight years to emphasize that these people should know better. Given the explanation for C, B is also incorrect. In addition, there is no mention in the passage of the possibility of *fewer* babies being born during a full moon. D is clearly incorrect. If it were true, the author would not have selected it to illustrate the problem.

74. **B.** This is summed up in the third sentence of the fourth paragraph, where the author says, "If one watches only for the events that reinforce a belief, one is screening out all the events that falsify it." Answer choice A is incorrect because there is no indication that filtering necessarily avoids mathematics, but only abuses it. Consider the casino example. One may very well know that probabilities are involved in slot machines, but the filtering process acts to distort our perception of the actual probability of winning. Although it may be true that filtering *can* work to lose money, it does not necessarily *cause* such losses. For example, the nurse does not lose money directly as a result of her belief (unless she makes bets or investments based on her belief). D is clearly incorrect. The point of the author's fourth, fifth, and sixth paragraphs is that filtering is a major cause of math abuse.

75. **C.** We can reach this conclusion based on the fifth paragraph. In particular, by telling us, "Losing makes no sound," the author's implication is that winning does. It is the sound of winning, quarters hitting the tray, that people hear and use as a filter to distort their expectations of winning. Answer choice A is incorrect because there is no information in the passage that gamblers win more often at slot machines than other people, nor is there any suggestion that gamblers win more often at slot machines than other games. B is incorrect because the *actual* probability of winning at a slot machine does not matter. The point is that filtering causes the *perceived* probability to be higher than the actual probability. D is incorrect because we are given no information on how much money casinos make on slot machines or any other games.

76. **D.** The discussion in the sixth paragraph makes this point. If the determination of whether a fund succeeds or fails is based on pure luck, and there is an even chance of doing either, each year about half the funds will succeed and the other half will fail. If one begins with a large enough number of funds, even after several years, some of them, simply by chance, will have succeeded every year. Answer choice A is incorrect because the author is not suggesting that investing *is* based on chance, only that chance *might* be the explanation for a hot fund rather than the expertise of the fund manager. B is simply a restatement of A and therefore is also incorrect. C is incorrect for two reasons. First, the author makes no judgment about investing in hot funds. The author's concern lies in the reasons why one chooses one fund over another. The author wants the investor to avoid math abuse in making an investment decision. Second, if hot funds can be explained by chance, the investor is better off not investing in them after they become hot.

77. **B.** If we continue the author's example in paragraph six, of the four mentioned hot funds, only two would be expected to succeed in the following year, only one in the year after that, and maybe none in the year after that. Thus, if chance determines which funds are successful, in any given year there is a 50 percent chance that any fund will gain, *and* a 50 percent chance that the same fund will lose. Our expectations cannot guarantee that exactly half of all successful funds will fail the next year, but based

on the results of many trial periods, this has become the expectation. Thus, we can reasonably expect hot funds to eventually lose money and therefore, one should not invest in hot funds for the sole reason that they are hot. (One should also not avoid them just because they are hot. This would be a form of math abuse known as the Gambler's Fallacy.) Answer choices A, C, and D are all incorrect to the extent that the suggested strategy is based on whether the fund is hot. Even though they do not solely determine whether the fund is hot, they are specific examples of B, making B the better answer.

PASSAGE VI (QUESTIONS 78–82)

The author of this passage is concerned about what he believes to be misinterpretations of abortion statistics that are being spread by John C. Willke, president of the National Right to Life Committee. Specifically, the author argues that there are hard statistics to support the claim that legal abortions are medically safer than childbirth. In addition, the author describes a study that found, in a select group of teenagers, there were fewer adverse psychological episodes among those having abortions as opposed to those giving birth.

78. **A.** In the second paragraph, the author tells us of statistics relating to deaths and medical complications due to abortions versus childbirth. In the first sentence of the third paragraph, the author tells us that psychological harm "has been more difficult to assess." Nowhere in the passage is there any indication that the other statistics were difficult to obtain. Thus, (I) and (II) are true and (III) is not.

79. **A.** In the second paragraph, we are told that data compiled by the National Center for Health Statistics indicate "abortion was 11 times *less* likely than childbirth to lead to a woman's death" (emphasis added). In the same paragraph, the author notes that the Centers for Disease Control reported "women undergoing abortions are 100 times *less* likely to have complications requiring major abdominal surgery than women bearing children" (emphasis added). The factors 11 and 100 justify the use of the word *much* rather than *slightly,* as the latter is used in answer choice C. Thus, C is incorrect. Because both institutions found abortions less likely to lead to the indicated problem, B, which uses the word *more,* is incorrect. D suggests the results were mixed, which is also incorrect.

80. **B.** In the fifth paragraph, the author tells us of Zabin and Hirsch's findings. According to the author, they report "those who chose abortion were *less* likely to undergo adverse psychological episodes . . . than *either* those who bore children or those who had not been pregnant" (emphasis added). From paragraph four, we know there were only three groups in the study: those who had abortions, those who bore a child, and those who were not pregnant. The results were not mixed for those who had abortions compared to the other two groups, which makes answer choice A incorrect. The author clearly states adverse psychological episodes were *less* likely for those who had abortions compared to the other two groups, making C incorrect. D is incorrect because the Zabin and Hirsch study was not one of the studies declared inconclusive by Koop. In addition, there is no indication in the passage that the author believes the results to be inconclusive. On the contrary, in introducing the Zabin and Hirsch study, the author indicates the study provides hard statistics on psychological harm (last sentence of the third paragraph).

81. **B.** In the fourth paragraph, we are told the homogeneity of the group studied (black urban teenagers) reduced the chances that the results were skewed by the influence

of other variables. As a result, avoiding the influence of other variables is considered an advantage (I). In the seventh paragraph, we are told this group consists of those "most likely to be affected by laws . . . that would limit . . . abortion." If the findings of Zabin and Hirsch are correct, it is important to know what the psychological effects will be on this group if access to abortions is restricted. Thus, (III) is an advantage. (II) is in fact a disadvantage. The homogeneity of the group studied will make extension of the findings to other groups difficult.

82. **C.** In the last paragraph, the author suggests that restrictions on the access of abortions will hinder women from obtaining them quickly. The author notes that despite the findings presented earlier in the passage, the risks associated with having an abortion increase significantly when the abortion is performed past the sixteenth week of pregnancy. Willke's argument is that abortions are more harmful than bearing a child. Consequently, by advocating legal restrictions that slow down the process, Willke is causing his arguments to come true. Answer choices A and B are incorrect because the passage does not draw a connection between restrictions and the surge of illegal abortions. The implication is that even legal abortions performed later in the pregnancy are riskier than those performed early. D is incorrect because there is no indication in the passage that privacy rights will be hampered by restrictions on abortion. In addition, this is not an argument credited to Willke in the passage.

PASSAGE VII (QUESTIONS 83–86)

The authors of this passage explain the balance between governmental needs and individual rights and liberties. We are told that neither can dominate, but there are times when one must give way to the other. We are given an example where several abridgements of individual rights were justified on the basis of military necessity. The authors end the passage by identifying two tests used by the Supreme Court to strike the necessary balance.

83. **C.** The authors tell us this in the first sentence of the passage: ". . . There clearly must be a balance between the scope of individual freedom and the needs of government." The authors note there may be instances when either individual rights or governmental needs dominate, but these are extreme cases (e.g., *Korematsu*) and the usual case is to strike a balance between the two. Thus, both answer choices A and B are incorrect. D is incorrect because the authors admit in the first sentence of the second paragraph that "there may be political excesses that threaten to limit civil liberties and rights . . . ." Although it is true that a threatened limitation is not necessarily a limitation, if it did not sometimes occur, the author would have been remiss in mentioning the possibility without indicating it hasn't happened. (In addition, anyone with a general understanding of the political process knows that political excesses quite often limit individual rights; yet this should be taken into account.)

84. **D.** In the fourth sentence of the first paragraph, the authors tell us that federal judges are independent of direct political control. In the next sentence, the authors contrast this by telling us most state and local judges are elected, "making them directly accountable to the people." We can thus infer that federal judges are not elected (which is true). Thus, answer choice B is incorrect. This same statement also makes C incorrect. Although A is true, we do not have to *infer* that local judges are mostly elected. We are told directly that this is the case in the fifth sentence of the first paragraph.

85. **B.** In the first sentence of the second paragraph, the authors mention the concern of political excesses. In the sixth sentence

of the first paragraph, the authors suggest elected judges might be influenced by the political process in making its decisions. In the fourth sentence of the first paragraph, we are told federal judges are not subject to direct political control. Therefore, federal judges are better able to make decisions protecting individual liberties, even though such decisions may run counter to public preferences. Answer choices A, C, and D are all incorrect because each of these groups is elected and, as a result, subject to political influences.

86. **C.** The second sentence of the fourth paragraph indicates, "One of the most important spheres of civil liberties, where the balancing test has been applied, regards the civil liberties and rights enumerated in the First Amendment, particularly the liberties of *speech, press,* and *the right of assembly*" (emphasis added). Although the free exercise of religion *is* a First Amendment liberty, it is *not* specifically mentioned in the passage. Because answer choices A, B, and D are all mentioned, they are all incorrect.

PASSAGE VIII (QUESTIONS 87–90)

87. **A.** In the passage, the author argues that the Court's obscenity decisions should be studied using fact-pattern analysis. In the second and third paragraphs, we are told that the theoretical underpinnings of fact-pattern analysis lie in attitude theory. Attitude theory, we are told in the last sentence of the second paragraph, "views the Court's attitudes as an explanation of its decisions." As used in the passage, "the Court" is clearly intended to mean the justices who collectively cast their votes to render a decision. This position is emphasized by the quote by Justice Stewart. Because the decisions rely on personal judgments, they cannot also rely on objective legal analysis, which makes answer choice B incorrect. C is incorrect because fact-pattern analysis is described in the passage as a method of *analyzing* the Court's decisions, not *making* them. D is incorrect because we are told in the first paragraph that the Court's definitions have proven unworkable, and no other definitions are mentioned in the passage.

88. **D.** If you used the tips given earlier, you know that *concerned* is a good word choice for tone. It is the correct choice. The other choices — (A) ironic, (B) hostile, and (C) sarcastic — are poor and incorrect in view of the tips and in view of the passage itself.

89. **B.** The conclusion is reached from the definition of the *attitudes* in attitude theory, and the example provided by Justice Stewart's comment on how he determines whether materials are obscene. Answer choice A is incorrect because attitude *objects* are described as part of what judicial attitudes are directed toward, the other part being the attitude situation. Consequently, A is incomplete. C and D are essentially the same things (at least within the context of this passage). As explained by the Spaeth quotation, the *activation* of an attitude requires both an object and a situation. From the definitions of these terms, and the plain meaning of "case characteristics" and "fact patterns," it should be clear these characteristics and patterns are the objects and situations that activate the judicial attitudes, but they are not the attitudes themselves. Therefore, both C and D are incorrect.

90. **D.** The author makes this suggestion in the final paragraph by indicating that the analysis of the Court's post–*Miller v. California* behavior may yield insight into how the Court will behave in other areas, "whether it has chosen to defer to the states." Answer choice A is clearly incorrect because the author's entire argument is that the Court's obscenity decisions should be studied. To

support this argument, the author notes in the fifth paragraph that there has been renewed interest in obscenity and pornography by "federal and state governments, the academic community, and numerous anti-pornography interest groups." B is incorrect because the author's argument that the Court's obscenity decisions need to be studied *assumes* that they have not been previously studied according to the author's standards or that they have not been studied successfully (but the passage contains no information on any unsuccessful studies). C is also incorrect, based on the author's primary argument. The author *wants* the Court's obscenity decisions to be studied using fact-pattern analysis, which is related to attitude theory.

PASSAGE IX (QUESTIONS 91–92)

91. **C.** The passage begins by suggesting the courts have not received sufficient scientific scrutiny because they have not been viewed as political bodies. The passage continues by noting the traditional use of case analysis. The author argues that this method has too narrow a focus and does not allow one to see the broader aspects of court procedures. The author admits that case studies have some merit but advocates broader, more scientific studies. Answer choice C is correct because the first two sentences of the passage suggest that the judiciary is not studied properly. Next, the author describes why the judiciary is studied, using the case analysis method, then continues by pointing out the problems of this method. The author concludes the passage by suggesting greater benefits would occur if the judiciary were studied differently. A is incorrect because by stating it is a "myth that judges are nonpolitical arbiters of the law" (fourth paragraph), the author shows a belief that judges are political and notes that most judicial scholars are also aware that judges are political actors. The author's assertion that judges are political actors is only one piece of evidence in support of his more general thesis. B is incorrect because the author clearly states, "This is not to say the judicial branch has lacked all scrutiny, only that it has traditionally been viewed from a perspective different from the other two branches of government" (first paragraph). D is incorrect because very little information on the case analysis method is given. It is mentioned only as supporting evidence for the broader proposition that study of the judiciary must be more scientific.

92. **B.** Marshall's conclusion is that judges should interpret the Constitution because they are nonpolitical. Based on this, one can infer that one's political affiliation will determine how one interprets the Constitution. Marshall's assumption in choosing the courts for this task rests on the idea that political actors such as executives and legislatures cannot be impartial. Answer choice A is incorrect because there is no mention in the passage of education levels. The reference to qualifications in the passage concerns the questions of whether decision-makers are politically motivated, not how well educated they are. C is incorrect because there is no mention that Marshall believes judges to have a greater understanding of the Constitution. Again, Marshall emphasizes the *political* differences between judges and other members of government. D is incorrect because Marshall's statements do not relate to the study of the judiciary. Marshall is concerned with interpretation of the Constitution. It is the author of the passage who is concerned with the study of the judiciary. The author only uses Marshall's comments as an example of the kind of thinking that led to the emphasis on studying individual cases.

SECTION 3
Writing Sample

SAMPLE ESSAY 1

This statement reflects the suspicion of government, which has been so common throughout the history of the United States. The statement suggests that government is essentially in opposition to the interests of the free individual, and that, at best, a government's use of power is a necessary evil. Ideally, each individual would take care of his or her own affairs, without interference from anyone. In reality, however, individuals need to be protected from others who attempt to violate their rights. Government, then, has the right to protect individuals from interference but no right to extend its powers and activities beyond this function. In other words, government should not interfere in the lives of individuals, except to prevent them from infringing on the rights of one another. Any other exercise of power, the statement implies, would be excessive.

Since the beginnings of this nation, citizens of the United States have been on the lookout for government interference in their lives. The Revolutionary War was fought to gain independence from excessive governmental power. With this experience behind them, the framers of the Constitution of the United States sought to limit the power of government. The Bill of Rights lists ways in which individual freedom is guaranteed against such interference. The legislative, judicial, and executive branches of government were separated so that each might prevent the others from becoming too powerful. More recently, the tenure in office of a president was limited to two consecutive terms, to prevent any individual from gaining too much personal power over the government of its citizens. Because government can overpower individual interests, it has been treated with the same caution and constraint that one might use when handling a dangerous animal.

This attitude toward government is not always healthy because there are circumstances in which the powers of government should be enhanced, rather than limited. In periods of national emergency, such as in time of war, or after a natural disaster, the federal government must assume extraordinary powers for the good of citizens who otherwise would not be able to help themselves. During a war, for the good of everyone in the nation, the government must be able to conscript troops for battle, and to impose severe penalties on individuals who, without very good reason, refuse to obey. After a community has been devastated by a flood, the federal government should provide aid to those who would not be able to recover without it. In such instances, it seems clear that government should do more than just protect individuals from one another. It must, in addition, use its power to provide aid and to compel individuals to engage in activities required for the good of everyone.

The quote above, then, expresses a view of government that is too extreme. While we can sympathize with a desire to restrain government from becoming too powerful, we can still agree that there are circumstances in which individuals can only be helped by an increase in governmental power. No simple formula can decide what the correct amount of governmental power should be. The statement could be revised in the following manner, to express a more reasonable understanding of government: "That government is best which governs for the well-being of the governed." This statement subordinates government to "the governed," without suggesting that government would ideally not exist. Whether the power of government in any specific circumstance should be great or small would depend on the circumstances in which its power is to be exercised.

EXPLANATION OF ESSAY 1

This essay directly addresses the issue of the statement and accomplishes the required tasks. Paragraphs 1 and 2 explain clearly the fundamental meaning of the statement, indicated as the first task ("Explain what you think the above statement means"). The second task ("Describe one or two specific situations in which the powers of government should be increased") is accomplished in the third paragraph. Finally, the third task ("Discuss what you think should be the basis for increasing or decreasing a government's powers") is accomplished in the fourth paragraph.

The essay develops the theme of the statement with insight, explaining not only the fundamental meaning of the statement, but exploring other important implications as well. The first three sentences indicate the attitude of rugged individualism, which is the basis for distrusting governmental power. The fourth sentence indicates a basis for properly coercing individuals, and as a result provides a basis, made explicit in the fifth sentence, for the coercive power of government. The final two sentences of the first paragraph return to the topic of distrust of governmental power, basing this, again, on the right of individuals to independence. The second paragraph provides historical examples of the attitude toward individuality and government, expressed in the first paragraph. The third paragraph looks at governmental power in a more positive light, and apparently, contradicting the almost purely negative attitude toward it, expressed in the first two paragraphs. This sets the stage for a criticism, in the fourth paragraph, of the statement and allows for a reasonable correction of the statement.

The ideas in this essay are clearly and logically developed. Each paragraph leads naturally into the next, so that the ideas developed in each seem spontaneously to call forth the ideas that follow. The idea of government interference, for example, expressed in sentence 1 of paragraph 2, is anticipated by sentence 6 of the first paragraph. The basic attitude toward government, expressed in the statement, is expressed again in the last sentence of paragraph 2, setting the stage for the criticism of the statement expressed in paragraph 3. The essay thus acquires structural unity.

The essay uses correct grammar and, while using sentences that are clearly organized, it varies their length and cadence to provide an interesting flow. For example, the final sentence of paragraph 1 is short and to the point, driving home the ideas developed through the longer and more complex sentences that precede it. The vocabulary employed is appropriate for expressing the ideas clearly and accurately, neither drawing attention to itself by being pretentious, nor giving the impression of talking down to the reader by being too stinted or simplistic (for example, in sentence 1 of paragraph 3: "the powers of government should be enhanced . . . "; and in sentence 4 of paragraph 3: "After a community has been devastated . . . ").

SAMPLE ESSAY 2

Humans require more for life than simply sustaining a heartbeat. Someone could, for example, have enough food to keep from starving to death and still be unable to live humanly. Without a variety of gratifying experiences, human life can become monotonous and even hopeless. An individual unable to do more than stay alive physically would be dead psychologically and emotionally. The brain of such a person might be physically sound, but it would be operating only at a level required to sustain a monotonous, repetitious existence. It would not be surprising if such a person were unable to sustain, for very long, even a biological existence because we need to experience more satisfaction from life than that we can receive from barely surviving.

The statement asserts that it is impossible for people generally to find what they need for a satisfying human existence through reality and the world around them. History seems to support this assertion, with its accounts of war and human suffering in all regions and throughout all periods of the world. Great literature such as the *Iliad*, or *Madame Bovary*, has portrayed human destruction through frustration in love. Our own personal experiences, if carefully and honestly reviewed, indicate that few, if any, of our dreams have been fully realized. Being "realistic" or "facing reality" means becoming resigned to the great distance between what we want and what we can realistically get. It may seem only reasonable, then, that great numbers of people must resign themselves to a life barely lived, if lived at all, in a human manner.

Such pessimism hardly seems justified, however, when we recall the masses of people who left their homelands to settle in this country, looking for a new and better life. Not all were successful, but many were able to improve their condition, and most, at least, were enlivened by new hopes and dreams. Recently, masses in Eastern Europe have fought for, and won new opportunities for a fuller life. If such people have had to confront a real world that has not easily yielded to their efforts, nevertheless, they have been able to discover, in this world, opportunities for imagining and attempting to realize efforts for improving their lives.

It must be admitted that frustration and suffering are constant features of human life, and that it is only in fantasy that they are absent for long. It is also true that, no matter how much suffering humans experience, they often, in large numbers, find the power to resist being dominated by their pain and are able to struggle with their reality in the hope of changing it. If the statement is correct in assuming that reality for most people is harsh, it nevertheless incorrectly assumes that most people are crushed by reality. Undoubtedly, the reality of some individuals' lives has been so frustrating as to destroy their humanity. However, reality is, for most people, a varied interweaving of fulfillment and frustration, providing many, if not most, individuals the ability to plan and struggle beyond periods of frustration toward periods of greater fulfillment.

EXPLANATION OF ESSAY 2

This essay directly addresses the central issue of the statement and addresses each of the three writing tasks. The first task is addressed in the first two paragraphs, the second in the third paragraph, and the final task is addressed in the fourth paragraph. The first paragraph clearly establishes the meaning of "subsist," as it is used in the statement, and indicates the relationship between "satisfaction" and human subsistence. The second paragraph explains the statement's reference to "reality" and the lack of satisfaction to be gained from it. The third paragraph provides clearly identifiable examples of situations in which reality is frustrating without causing loss of human subsistence. The fourth paragraph generalizes from the points made in the first three paragraphs to provide a unified view of reality as a negative, as well as a positive, influence on peoples' attempts to live humanly.

This essay proceeds logically through sentences and paragraphs that center consistently on the theme of the statement. Each paragraph leads to the one that follows, preparing for the ideas expressed in it, as well as referring to previously developed ideas. This unity is indicated in the transitions employed ("Such pessimism hardly seems justified . . . ," at the beginning of paragraph 3, and "It must be admitted that frustration and suffering . . . ," at the beginning of paragraph 4, refer back to the central issue of paragraphs 1, 2, and 3, and the fundamental issue of the statement).

The essay is written clearly and thoughtfully. Sentences directly state the ideas that they are intended to convey (for example, sentences 1, 6, 10, and 18). The language of the essay states precisely what is intended (for example, sentence 3: "Without a variety of gratifying experiences, human life can become monotonous and even hopeless"). The complexity of the issue is treated with clearly organized sentence and paragraph development.

SECTION 4
Biological Sciences

PASSAGE I (QUESTIONS 93–96)

93. **C.** This question requires an understanding of the forces that dictate the movement of water within the body. Osmosis is the movement of water from an area of greater concentration across a semipermeable barrier, to an area of less concentration. Most of the membranes in the body are semipermeable, i.e., permeable to water but not to most ions. Answer choice A is incorrect because it refers to the random movement of particles within a solution caused by collisions with fluid molecules. Answer choices B and D are incorrect because these types of movement require energy to move molecules against a concentration gradient. They also often require carrier proteins to transport the substance being moved.

94. **B.** An understanding of the various body fluid compartments is needed to answer this question. The only compartment in which there is a true circulating fluid that contains proteins is the blood plasma. Although the plasma volume is part of the extracellular fluid, answer choice A is incorrect because the extracellular fluid also includes answer choice D, interstitial fluid. Answer choice C is incorrect because intracellular fluid does not circulate, although it does contain proteins.

95. **D.** This question requires interpretation of Figure 1, which shows that exchange between intracellular fluid and the plasma must be indirect because it can occur only if the fluids have first passed through the interstitial space. Answer choice A is incorrect because fluids may be exchanged directly only between the intracellular compartment and the interstitial fluid, not the plasma. Answer B is incorrect because exchange of fluids between compartments is constantly occurring in an effort to maintain homeostasis. Exchange of fluids can occur throughout the body, not just in isolated organs, which is why answer C is incorrect.

96. **A.** To answer this question, the nature of equilibrium must be understood. Because the two compartments are initially in osmotic balance, removing solute from one of the compartments will upset this balance. The extracellular fluid will contain less solute, relative to the intracellular fluid, yet the absolute amount of water in both compartments is equal. As a result, the extracellu lar fluid has become hypotonic, meaning it has less osmotically active particles, compared to the intracellular fluid. Answer C is the exact opposite of the correct answer. Answer B is incorrect because the intracellular fluid would become hypertonic relative to the extracellular fluid. Answer D is incorrect because removing solute from one of the compartments will upset the osmotic equilibrium and, therefore, the tonicity of the compartments, relative to each other, must change.

PASSAGE II (QUESTIONS 97–100)

97. **B.** Because actinomycin D prevents the first stage of protein synthesis from occurring, only the proinsulin gene, which is part of the DNA molecule, would be present within the cell. Although mRNA molecules transcribed prior to the actinomycin D addition would

continue unimpeded through protein synthesis, the final product, insulin, is secreted (i.e., no longer in the cell). Answer choices A, C, and D are all produced during later stages of protein synthesis and would not be present if transcription never took place.

98. **C.** Protein synthesis occurs in many stages and, during some of these stages, the protein is modified by addition or elimination of amino acids, by folding, or by the formation of bridges between amino acid side chains. These modifications are important because they tend to stabilize the protein and to confer a specific configuration or conformation, which is necessary for the protein to function properly. Answer choices A and D are incorrect because the entire process of protein synthesis takes place in both the nucleus and cytoplasm.

99. **D.** Post-translational modification occurs after the polypeptide chain has been formed by translation of the genetic code carried by the mRNA. In the case of insulin, during this stage, the leader sequence is removed and the protein is folded. Answer choices A and C occur during post-transcriptional modification of the mRNA before it leaves the nucleus.

100. **D.** During post-transcriptional modification of the mRNA, the introns are removed. As a result, the mRNA that enters the cytoplasm consists only of exons. Answer choice A is incorrect because the mRNA is modified prior to leaving the nucleus. Answers B and C are incorrect because the introns are removed from the mRNA.

PASSAGE III (QUESTIONS 101–104)

101. **C.** Answering this question requires an understanding of the relationship between sodium excretion (output) and blood pressure, as depicted in Figure 2. If the amount of sodium in the diet (intake) is reduced, urinary sodium excretion must also be reduced to maintain sodium balance. When sodium excretion decreases, blood pressure will also decrease. If blood pressure remained high, sodium excretion would proceed at a greater rate than sodium intake, and depletion of total body sodium would occur. Answer choice B is incorrect because a change in sodium intake/excretion should, theoretically, produce a change in blood pressure. Answer A is incorrect because the kidneys will not avidly retain sodium unless there is a sodium deficiency. A low-salt diet can be maintained, as long as the diet contains adequate sodium. Answer D is incorrect because blood pressure should not increase, but rather it should decrease.

102. **A.** If the whole curve in Figure 2 were shifted to the right, blood pressure would rise at the same level of sodium intake. Answer B is incorrect because blood pressure must change when the entire curve is shifted either to the right or left of normal. Answer C is incorrect because urinary sodium output should not change if sodium intake does not change. Answer D is incorrect because the curve was shifted to the right, not the left, and sodium output should not change.

103. **D.** An increase in dietary sodium would cause blood pressure to rise in an effort to restore sodium balance. In a person more sensitive to the effect of sodium on blood pressure, blood pressure will increase to an even greater extent. Answer A is incorrect because an increase in dietary salt will lead to an increase in blood pressure, not a decrease. Answer B is incorrect because Patient A is more sensitive to changes in sodium than Patient B; thus, they should not have the same blood pressure response. Answer C is incorrect because both Patients A and B should exhibit a rise in blood pressure.

104. **A.** Diuretics act on the kidneys to increase sodium and water excretion. If diuretic therapy were discontinued, more salt and water would be retained by the kidneys, blood volume would increase, and blood pressure would rise. Answer B is incorrect because sodium and water excretion would decrease. Answer C is incorrect because diuretics specifically act on the kidneys to alter their function. Answer D is incorrect because even though diuretics can alter renal function, they do not correct any underlying defects in the kidneys.

105. **B.** In the alveoli, indirect respiration occurs. There are two phases of indirect respiration: the internal phase and the external phase. Direct respiration involves the direct exchange of gases by an organism with the external environment. This is done by lower organisms such as paramecia or hydra. (See the figure below.)

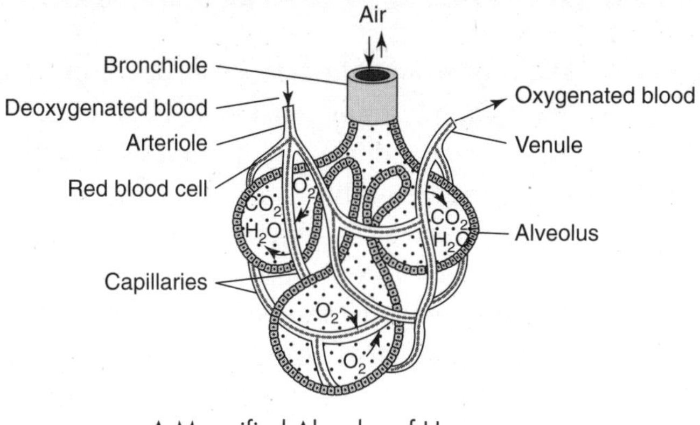

A Magnified Alveolus of Humans

106. **D.** Vitamin A is necessary for the growth and maintenance of the epithelial cells of the skin. Vitamin K assists in blood coagulation. Vitamin E is associated with liver function in some animals. Vitamin E is also responsible for male sterility in rats and possibly other animals.

107. **D.** α-amino acids have the amino group bonded to the carbon adjacent to the carboxyl group while α-amino acids have the amino group bonded to the second carbon from the carboxyl group.

108. **B.** Steric interactions between atoms in a molecule directly cause certain conformations of that molecule to be unstable. These various conformations and their steric interactions may be visualized through the use of Newman projections. Using a molecular model kit in conjunction with Newman projections is an immense help in discerning which structures will be stable and which will not.

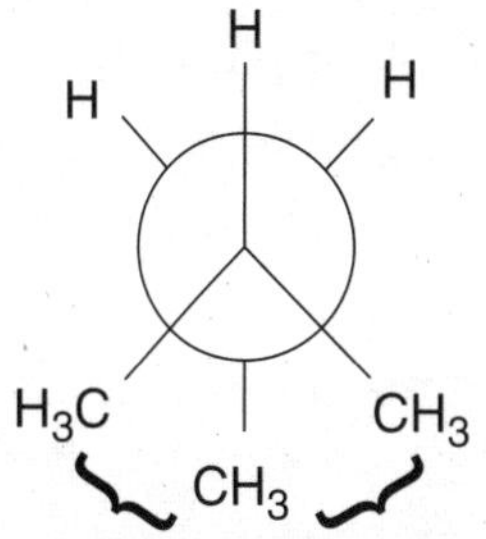

PASSAGE IV (QUESTIONS 109–111)

109. **B.** This question requires interpretation of Table 1, where the active, passive, and total tensions developed at various muscle lengths are listed. If the muscle were stretched 5 millimeters (+5) beyond its resting length, there would be no active tension. Passive tension would still develop, and total tension would equal passive tension plus 0. Answers choices A and D are incorrect because active tension would not develop. Answer C is incorrect because passive and total tensions would not be 0.

110. **A.** This question requires an understanding of the fact that relatively few processes in the body occur independently or isolated from the influences of other processes. It would be very difficult to study just the properties of skeletal muscle in the intact body because there are so many other variables that need to be controlled. There is no basis for answer choices B and C because the function of muscles is to contract and develop tension, and this can occur at a variety of different muscle lengths.

111. **A.** A basic understanding of muscle structure and function is needed to answer this question. Tension development in a muscle is a function of the interaction that occurs between actin and myosin filaments. Answer choice B is incorrect because a physical interaction must occur, not merely an overlapping of the filaments, for contraction to occur. Answer C is incorrect because slackening would not contribute to tension development at all. Answer D explains the differences in tension development at different muscle lengths, but not why tension develops.

PASSAGE V (QUESTIONS 112–115)

112. **D.** This question requires an understanding of the role played by PTH in the regulation of calcium metabolism. An overabundance of PTH would mobilize large amounts of calcium from the skeleton, hence leading to bone demineralization. Answer A is incorrect because PTH would have the opposite effect on bone. Answer B is incorrect because PTH removes calcium from bone, which then enters the plasma and thus raises plasma calcium levels. Answer C is incorrect because tetany occurs when plasma calcium levels are low, not high.

113. **C.** This question requires knowledge of the role of calcium in various physiological processes. Calcium is extremely important for proper functioning of nerve and muscle tissue. Answer A is incorrect because tetany results from a lack of calcium. Although the level of plasma calcium regulates PTH secretion, this is not the most important function of calcium; therefore, answer B is incorrect. Answer D is incorrect because calcium does not regulate bone resorption.

114. **B.** Following the ingestion of a meal that is high in calcium, PTH secretion will decrease because the level of plasma calcium regulates PTH secretion in a negative feedback fashion. Deposition of calcium in the skeleton will increase as PTH levels fall. Answers A and C are incorrect because PTH secretion will decrease. Answer D is incorrect because plasma calcium levels do regulate PTH secretion.

115. **B.** This question requires an understanding of the concept of antagonistic hormones. When plasma calcium is high, calcitonin will increase and PTH will decrease because they have opposite effects on the blood calcium level. Answer A is incorrect because plasma calcium will decrease due to calcitonin-stimulated uptake by the bones. Answers C and D are incorrect because plasma PTH will decrease.

PASSAGE VI (QUESTIONS 116–120)

116. **D.** For a genetic female to develop male genitalia, the fetus must have been exposed to androgens during the period of gestation when the genitalia form (after the seventh week). Answer A is incorrect because exposure to testosterone at birth would not affect development of the genitalia. Answer B is incorrect because estrogens are not secreted by either sex during gestation. Answer C is incorrect because exposure of a male to chorionic gonadotropin stimulates normal development of the testes.

117. **C.** Approximately half of sperm contain the X chromosome and half contain a Y. It is thought that Y-containing sperm have greater motility and therefore a better chance of fertilizing an egg. This could explain why more males are born than females. Answers A and B are incorrect because there are approximately equal numbers of X and Y sperm. Answer D is incorrect because eggs contain X, not Y, chromosomes.

118. **A.** Mature gonads produce ova and secrete estrogens in the female, and in the male they produce sperm and secrete androgens. Answer B is incorrect because the gonads also produce germ cells. Answers C and D are incorrect because they describe the functions of the gonads in one sex, but not in both.

119. **B.** Testes develop in genetic males due to the presence of the H-Y antigen. Because females lack this antigen, ovaries develop instead of testes. Answer A is incorrect because the immature ovaries do not secrete any hormones. Answer C is incorrect because the testes do not secrete estrogen. Answer D is incorrect because the brain does not control development of the genitalia in the fetus.

120. **C.** The reproductive hormones, androgens (primarily testosterone) in males and estrogen in females, stimulate the development of the secondary sex characteristics during puberty. Answer A is incorrect because the testes secrete testosterone and the ovaries secrete estrogen. Answers B and D are incorrect because the gonads must begin, not stop, producing hormones.

PASSAGE VII (QUESTIONS 121–125)

121. **D.** This question requires interpretation of Table 2. Water and protein account for 95% of the total cellular mass (80 + 15). Answer A accounts for only 19% (15 + 3 + 1), answer B accounts for 81% (1 + 80), and answer C accounts for 1%.

122. **A.** Lysosomes function as digestive organelles by removing unwanted and harmful substances from the interior of the cell. Without them, toxic materials would quickly build up and eventually kill the cell. Cells would also be unable to fight bacterial infection in the absence of lysosomes. Answers B, C, and D are incorrect because lysosomes are not involved in protein packaging, reproduction, or energy production.

123. **D.** Rough ER is characterized by the attachment of ribosomes, which gives it a rough appearance. The portion of endoplasmic reticulum that is not associated with ribosomes is smooth in appearance. Answer A is incorrect because the cytoskeleton attaches to both rough and smooth ER. Answer B is incorrect because both smooth and rough ER are bound by membranes. Answer C is incorrect because smooth ER is usually closer to the Golgi than rough ER.

124. **C.** Mitochrondia are the "powerhouses" of the cell. They provide the cell with energy in the form of ATP, so that the cell can perform basic life functions. To ensure a continual supply of ATP, there must be numerous mitochondria. Answers A, B, and D are incorrect because mitochrondia are not directly involved in these processes.

125. **C.** The nucleolus, located in the nucleus, is unique because it is not surrounded by its own membrane. Answers A, B, and D are incorrect because all of these organelles are membrane-bound.

126. **C.** When a segment of one chromosome is transferred to another non-homologous chromosome, the mutation is known as a translocation. A deletion is a mutation in which a segment of the chromosome is missing. In duplication, a portion of the chromosome is represented twice. An inversion results when a segment is removed and reinserted in the same location, but in the opposite direction. (See the figure below.)

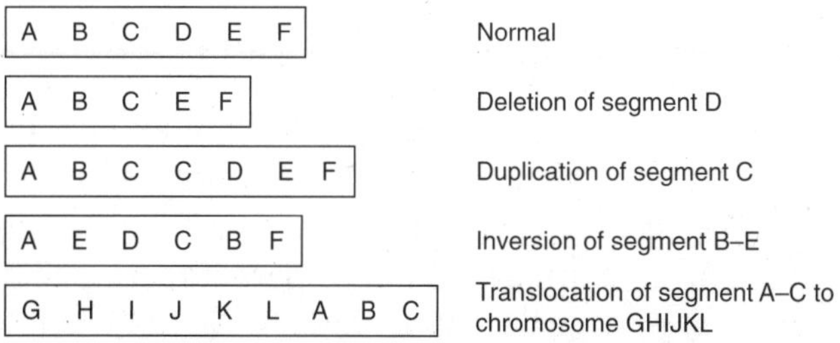

Mutations Involving Chromosome Structure

127. **C.** The thin barrier around Bowman's capsule is composed of two extremely thin layers: (1) the single-celled capillary wall and (2) the one-celled lining of Bowman's capsule. The filtration of plasma can occur through this thin barrier because plasma contains no large blood cells.

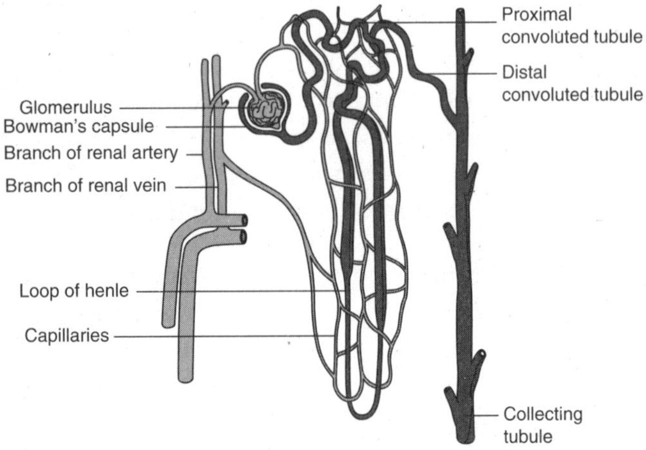

Diagram of a Single Kidney Tubule

128. **D.** Rigor mortis is a phenomenon in which the muscles become very stiff after death. It results directly from the loss of ATP in the dead muscle cells; the myosin crossbridges are unable to combine with actin and those bonds already formed cannot be broken. The rigid condition of the body results.

129. **D.** Aromatic compounds with activating groups are ortho, para directors. They are also electron-releasing groups and will direct electrophiles to add ortho and para to the substituent. Deactivating groups are meta directors, with the exception of the halogens. They are electron-withdrawing groups, and they will direct the electrophile to add meta to the substituent.

The halogens are an exception; they are deactivating groups, but they are ortho, para directors. A methyl group on a benzene ring is activating and ortho, para directing. The amino group of aniline is also activating and ortho, para directing. The nitro group of nitrobenzene is deactivating and meta directing.

PASSAGE VIII (QUESTIONS 130–133)

130. **C.** At pH 7, the amino acids exist in the following ionized forms:

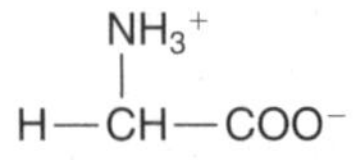

Glycine

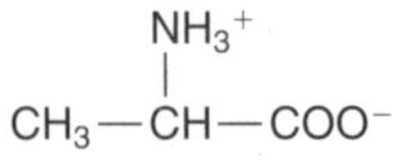

Alanine

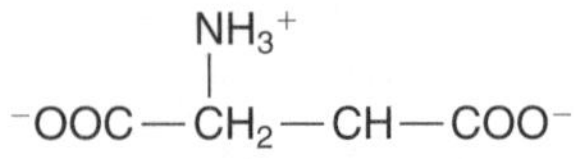

Aspartic acid

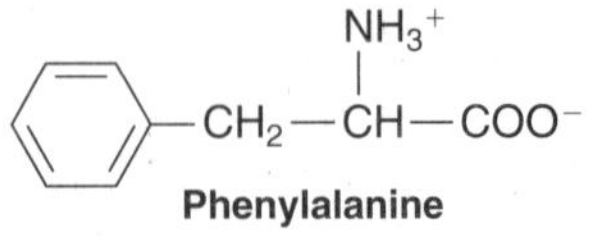

Phenylalanine

Aspartic acid is the only amino acid of the four shown that has a negatively charged side chain.

131. **A.** Hydrocarbons do not readily interact with water. Amino acids with hydrocarbon side chains will thus be hydrophobic. Answers B and C are incorrect because they are terms that may be used to describe all of the amino acids, not just those with hydrocarbon side chains. Answer D is incorrect because these amino acids will not be attracted to water.

132. **B.** Neutral or uncharged polar side chains are most likely to hydrogen bond with water. Answer A is incorrect because the side chains do not participate in peptide bond formation. Answer C is incorrect because neutral molecules will not be involved in covalent bonding. Answer D is incorrect because these amino acids will be hydrophilic, not hydrophobic.

133. **A.** Proteins are basically chains of amino acids linked end to end. Because the only part of each of the 20 amino acids that differs is the side chain or R group, this portion of the amino acid imparts the different physical and chemical properties to each position in the protein chain.

PASSAGE IX (QUESTIONS 134–137)

134. **B.** Plate 2 contains compound A in the unknown mixture because it is the only plate in which a spot from the unknown, on the right side of the plate, corresponds exactly to the known spot, on the left side, following separation.

135. **A.** More polar compounds tend to move up a TLC plate at a slower rate than less polar compounds. Therefore, the mixture that contains the most polar compounds will have spots that have moved the least from the original spot on the plate. Plate 1 contains the most polar compounds because there are more spots (3) closer to the original spot than on any of the other plates.

136. **C.** Polar compounds move at a relatively slow rate because they are more attracted to the stationary phase then to the mobile phase. To increase the rate at which a polar compound moves on a plate, a more polar mobile phase must be used. Of the compounds listed, acetic acid is the most polar. Answers A and D would be poor choices because they are nonpolar solvents.

137. **D.** Nonpolar compounds move the fastest on a TLC plate because they are more attracted to the mobile phase then to the stationary phase. Of the compounds listed, the alkenes are the only nonpolar group, and therefore will travel the fastest and furthest on a plate.

PASSAGE X (QUESTIONS 138–141)

138. **C.** This is the only possible structural isomer because it contains the same atoms found in 1 propanol (3 C, 8 H, and 1 O); however, they are arranged in different order. Answers A, B, and D all contain different atoms than 1-propanol and therefore cannot be structural isomers of it.

139. **A.** These two formulas represent the same structure because the atoms are attached in the same order; only the orientation has been changed. Answers B, C, and D are pairs of structural isomers because the order of attachment of the atoms is different for both formulas of each pair.

140. **B.** These structures differ in the arrangement of their atoms in space and are stereoisomers. The structure on the left is the *cis*-isomer, where the CH_3 and CH_2CH_3 groups are on the same side of the pi bond. The structure on the right is the *trans*-isomer, where the CH_3 and CH_2CH_3 groups are located on opposite sides of the double bond. Answers A and C are incorrect because, for stereoisomers to exist, there must be two different groups attached to each carbon of the double bond. Answer D is incorrect because both of the structures are *trans*-isomers.

141. **D.** For stereoisomers to exist, there must be two different groups attached to each of the pi-bonded carbons. Answer A is incorrect because the groups cannot be the same. Answers B and C are incorrect because the carbon atoms involved in the pi bond do not lie on either side of it or rotate around it.

142. **C.** Bone formation that takes place in preexisting cartilage is called endochondral ossification. The cartilage, which is present in infants, is replaced by bone in later years. Bones at the base of the skull in the vertebral column, the pelvis, and the limbs are all called cartilage bones because they form in this manner.

143. **A.** The appendicular skeleton is comprised of the shoulder girdle, upper extremities, pelvic girdle, and lower extremities. The humerus is the bone in the upper arm and is therefore part of the appendicular skeleton. The vertebra, ribs, sternum (breast bone), and skull are all part of the axial skeleton.

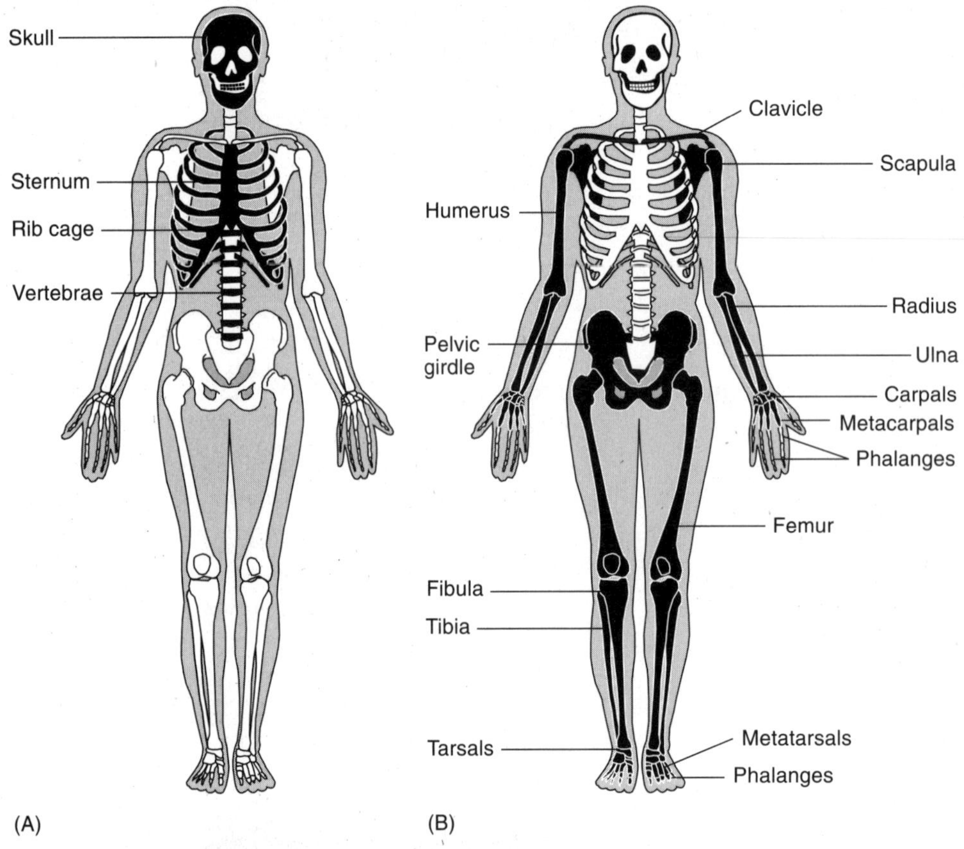

Diagrams of the Human Body Showing (A) the Bonds of the Axial Skeleton and (B) the Bones of the Appendicular Skeleton

144. **D.** Saponification is the alkaline hydrolysis of esters to produce the salt of the ester (a soap) and an alcohol. Fats are esters of glycerol, so they do undergo saponification. The general reaction for this process is:

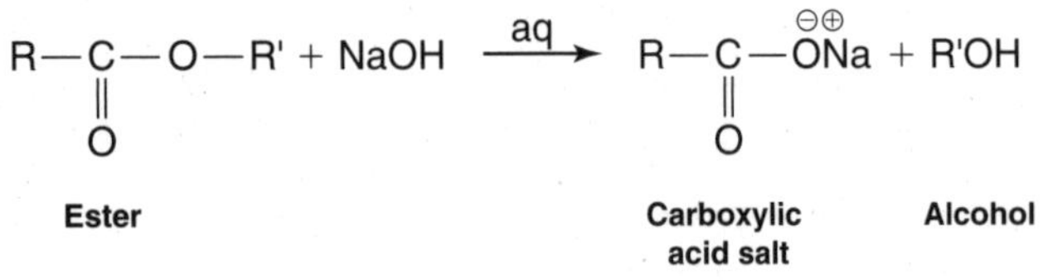

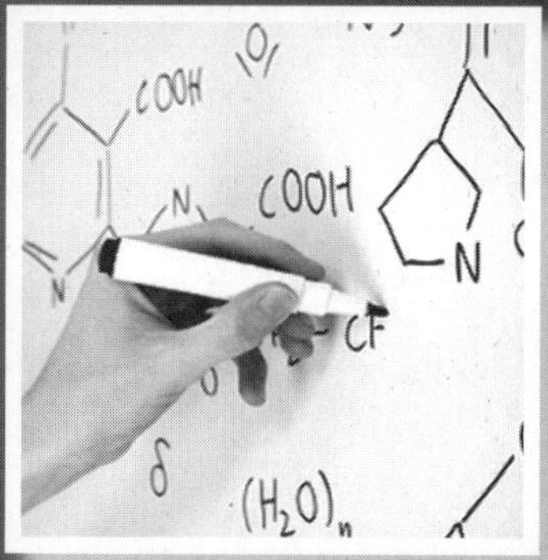

MCAT

MEDICAL COLLEGE ADMISSION TEST

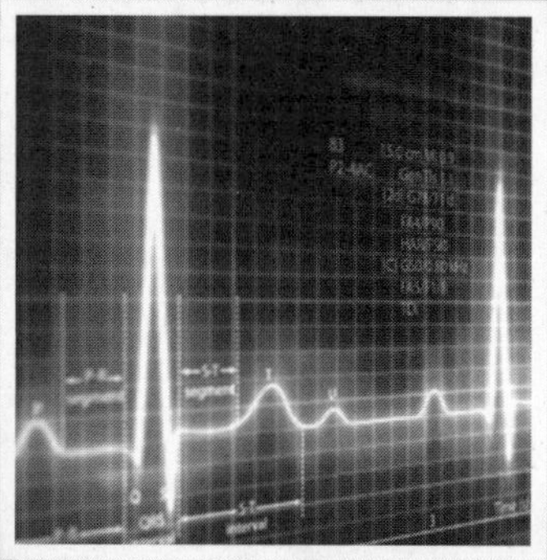

Test 2

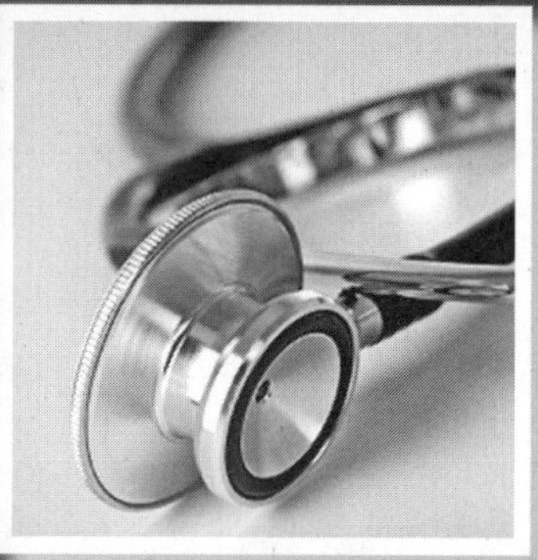

This test is also on CD-ROM in our special interactive MCAT TestWare®. It is highly recommended that you first take this exam on computer. You will then have the additional study features and benifits of enforced timed conditions, individual diagnostic analysis, and instant scoring. See page 1 for guidance on how to get the most out of our MCAT book and software.

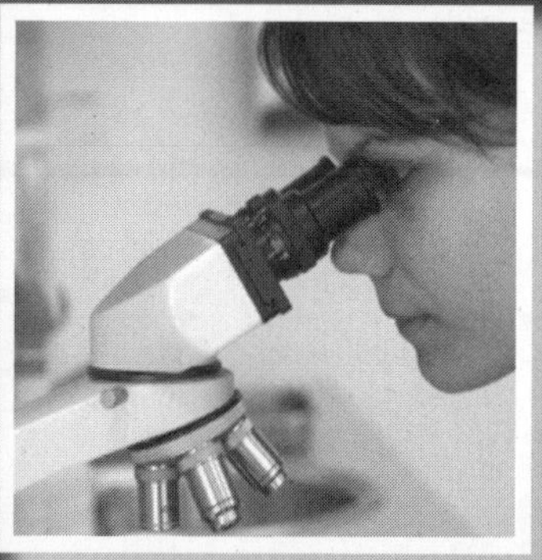

Test 2 ■ Answer Sheet

SECTION 1: Physical Sciences

1. Ⓐ Ⓑ Ⓒ Ⓓ
2. Ⓐ Ⓑ Ⓒ Ⓓ
3. Ⓐ Ⓑ Ⓒ Ⓓ
4. Ⓐ Ⓑ Ⓒ Ⓓ
5. Ⓐ Ⓑ Ⓒ Ⓓ
6. Ⓐ Ⓑ Ⓒ Ⓓ
7. Ⓐ Ⓑ Ⓒ Ⓓ
8. Ⓐ Ⓑ Ⓒ Ⓓ
9. Ⓐ Ⓑ Ⓒ Ⓓ
10. Ⓐ Ⓑ Ⓒ Ⓓ
11. Ⓐ Ⓑ Ⓒ Ⓓ
12. Ⓐ Ⓑ Ⓒ Ⓓ
13. Ⓐ Ⓑ Ⓒ Ⓓ
14. Ⓐ Ⓑ Ⓒ Ⓓ
15. Ⓐ Ⓑ Ⓒ Ⓓ
16. Ⓐ Ⓑ Ⓒ Ⓓ
17. Ⓐ Ⓑ Ⓒ Ⓓ
18. Ⓐ Ⓑ Ⓒ Ⓓ
19. Ⓐ Ⓑ Ⓒ Ⓓ
20. Ⓐ Ⓑ Ⓒ Ⓓ
21. Ⓐ Ⓑ Ⓒ Ⓓ
22. Ⓐ Ⓑ Ⓒ Ⓓ
23. Ⓐ Ⓑ Ⓒ Ⓓ
24. Ⓐ Ⓑ Ⓒ Ⓓ
25. Ⓐ Ⓑ Ⓒ Ⓓ
26. Ⓐ Ⓑ Ⓒ Ⓓ
27. Ⓐ Ⓑ Ⓒ Ⓓ
28. Ⓐ Ⓑ Ⓒ Ⓓ
29. Ⓐ Ⓑ Ⓒ Ⓓ
30. Ⓐ Ⓑ Ⓒ Ⓓ
31. Ⓐ Ⓑ Ⓒ Ⓓ
32. Ⓐ Ⓑ Ⓒ Ⓓ
33. Ⓐ Ⓑ Ⓒ Ⓓ
34. Ⓐ Ⓑ Ⓒ Ⓓ
35. Ⓐ Ⓑ Ⓒ Ⓓ
36. Ⓐ Ⓑ Ⓒ Ⓓ
37. Ⓐ Ⓑ Ⓒ Ⓓ
38. Ⓐ Ⓑ Ⓒ Ⓓ
39. Ⓐ Ⓑ Ⓒ Ⓓ
40. Ⓐ Ⓑ Ⓒ Ⓓ
41. Ⓐ Ⓑ Ⓒ Ⓓ
42. Ⓐ Ⓑ Ⓒ Ⓓ
43. Ⓐ Ⓑ Ⓒ Ⓓ
44. Ⓐ Ⓑ Ⓒ Ⓓ
45. Ⓐ Ⓑ Ⓒ Ⓓ
46. Ⓐ Ⓑ Ⓒ Ⓓ
47. Ⓐ Ⓑ Ⓒ Ⓓ
48. Ⓐ Ⓑ Ⓒ Ⓓ
49. Ⓐ Ⓑ Ⓒ Ⓓ
50. Ⓐ Ⓑ Ⓒ Ⓓ
51. Ⓐ Ⓑ Ⓒ Ⓓ
52. Ⓐ Ⓑ Ⓒ Ⓓ

SECTION 2: Verbal Reasoning

53. Ⓐ Ⓑ Ⓒ Ⓓ
54. Ⓐ Ⓑ Ⓒ Ⓓ
55. Ⓐ Ⓑ Ⓒ Ⓓ
56. Ⓐ Ⓑ Ⓒ Ⓓ
57. Ⓐ Ⓑ Ⓒ Ⓓ
58. Ⓐ Ⓑ Ⓒ Ⓓ
59. Ⓐ Ⓑ Ⓒ Ⓓ
60. Ⓐ Ⓑ Ⓒ Ⓓ
61. Ⓐ Ⓑ Ⓒ Ⓓ
62. Ⓐ Ⓑ Ⓒ Ⓓ
63. Ⓐ Ⓑ Ⓒ Ⓓ
64. Ⓐ Ⓑ Ⓒ Ⓓ
65. Ⓐ Ⓑ Ⓒ Ⓓ
66. Ⓐ Ⓑ Ⓒ Ⓓ
67. Ⓐ Ⓑ Ⓒ Ⓓ
68. Ⓐ Ⓑ Ⓒ Ⓓ
69. Ⓐ Ⓑ Ⓒ Ⓓ
70. Ⓐ Ⓑ Ⓒ Ⓓ
71. Ⓐ Ⓑ Ⓒ Ⓓ
72. Ⓐ Ⓑ Ⓒ Ⓓ
73. Ⓐ Ⓑ Ⓒ Ⓓ
74. Ⓐ Ⓑ Ⓒ Ⓓ
75. Ⓐ Ⓑ Ⓒ Ⓓ
76. Ⓐ Ⓑ Ⓒ Ⓓ
77. Ⓐ Ⓑ Ⓒ Ⓓ
78. Ⓐ Ⓑ Ⓒ Ⓓ
79. Ⓐ Ⓑ Ⓒ Ⓓ
80. Ⓐ Ⓑ Ⓒ Ⓓ
81. Ⓐ Ⓑ Ⓒ Ⓓ
82. Ⓐ Ⓑ Ⓒ Ⓓ
83. Ⓐ Ⓑ Ⓒ Ⓓ
84. Ⓐ Ⓑ Ⓒ Ⓓ
85. Ⓐ Ⓑ Ⓒ Ⓓ
86. Ⓐ Ⓑ Ⓒ Ⓓ
87. Ⓐ Ⓑ Ⓒ Ⓓ
88. Ⓐ Ⓑ Ⓒ Ⓓ
89. Ⓐ Ⓑ Ⓒ Ⓓ
90. Ⓐ Ⓑ Ⓒ Ⓓ
91. Ⓐ Ⓑ Ⓒ Ⓓ
92. Ⓐ Ⓑ Ⓒ Ⓓ

SECTION 4: Biological Sciences

93. Ⓐ Ⓑ Ⓒ Ⓓ
94. Ⓐ Ⓑ Ⓒ Ⓓ
95. Ⓐ Ⓑ Ⓒ Ⓓ
96. Ⓐ Ⓑ Ⓒ Ⓓ
97. Ⓐ Ⓑ Ⓒ Ⓓ

98. Ⓐ Ⓑ Ⓒ Ⓓ
99. Ⓐ Ⓑ Ⓒ Ⓓ
100. Ⓐ Ⓑ Ⓒ Ⓓ
101. Ⓐ Ⓑ Ⓒ Ⓓ
102. Ⓐ Ⓑ Ⓒ Ⓓ
103. Ⓐ Ⓑ Ⓒ Ⓓ
104. Ⓐ Ⓑ Ⓒ Ⓓ
105. Ⓐ Ⓑ Ⓒ Ⓓ
106. Ⓐ Ⓑ Ⓒ Ⓓ
107. Ⓐ Ⓑ Ⓒ Ⓓ
108. Ⓐ Ⓑ Ⓒ Ⓓ
109. Ⓐ Ⓑ Ⓒ Ⓓ
110. Ⓐ Ⓑ Ⓒ Ⓓ
111. Ⓐ Ⓑ Ⓒ Ⓓ
112. Ⓐ Ⓑ Ⓒ Ⓓ
113. Ⓐ Ⓑ Ⓒ Ⓓ
114. Ⓐ Ⓑ Ⓒ Ⓓ
115. Ⓐ Ⓑ Ⓒ Ⓓ
116. Ⓐ Ⓑ Ⓒ Ⓓ
117. Ⓐ Ⓑ Ⓒ Ⓓ
118. Ⓐ Ⓑ Ⓒ Ⓓ
119. Ⓐ Ⓑ Ⓒ Ⓓ
120. Ⓐ Ⓑ Ⓒ Ⓓ
121. Ⓐ Ⓑ Ⓒ Ⓓ
122. Ⓐ Ⓑ Ⓒ Ⓓ
123. Ⓐ Ⓑ Ⓒ Ⓓ
124. Ⓐ Ⓑ Ⓒ Ⓓ
125. Ⓐ Ⓑ Ⓒ Ⓓ
126. Ⓐ Ⓑ Ⓒ Ⓓ
127. Ⓐ Ⓑ Ⓒ Ⓓ
128. Ⓐ Ⓑ Ⓒ Ⓓ
129. Ⓐ Ⓑ Ⓒ Ⓓ
130. Ⓐ Ⓑ Ⓒ Ⓓ
131. Ⓐ Ⓑ Ⓒ Ⓓ
132. Ⓐ Ⓑ Ⓒ Ⓓ
133. Ⓐ Ⓑ Ⓒ Ⓓ
134. Ⓐ Ⓑ Ⓒ Ⓓ
135. Ⓐ Ⓑ Ⓒ Ⓓ
136. Ⓐ Ⓑ Ⓒ Ⓓ
137. Ⓐ Ⓑ Ⓒ Ⓓ
138. Ⓐ Ⓑ Ⓒ Ⓓ
139. Ⓐ Ⓑ Ⓒ Ⓓ
140. Ⓐ Ⓑ Ⓒ Ⓓ
141. Ⓐ Ⓑ Ⓒ Ⓓ
142. Ⓐ Ⓑ Ⓒ Ⓓ
143. Ⓐ Ⓑ Ⓒ Ⓓ
144. Ⓐ Ⓑ Ⓒ Ⓓ

SECTION 1
Physical Sciences

TIME: 70 Minutes

QUESTIONS: 1–52

DIRECTIONS: Most of the questions in this section are arranged in groups, each corresponding to a descriptive passage. Based on the information given in a passage, choose the one best answer to each question in the group. Some questions are independent of a descriptive passage and of each other. Choose the one best answer to each of these questions. If you are not sure of an answer, eliminate those choices that you know are incorrect and choose an answer from among those remaining. Fill in the corresponding circle on the answer sheet to indicate your answer. You may refer to the periodic table at any time.

PASSAGE I (QUESTIONS 1–4)

An amusement park is planning a new roller coaster. It will start at point A, travel over the first hill at point C, and then go through the loop-de-loop.

The maximum mass of a car on the ride is 2000kg.

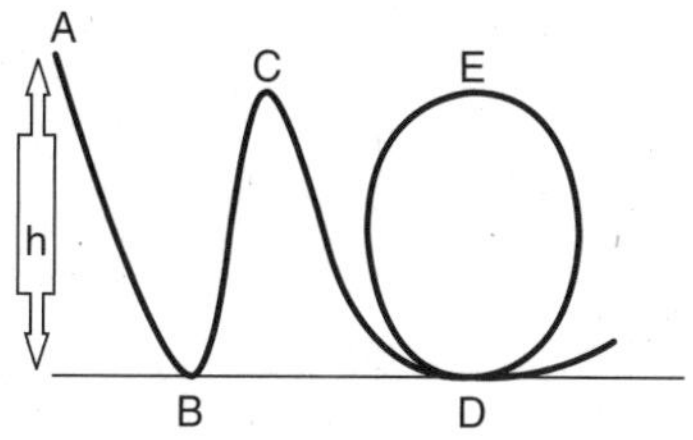

1. Calculate the potential energy at A if h = 50m
   A. 490kN B. 980kN
   C. 1960kN D. 2,500kN

2. If the height at point A were halved to save money on building supplies, the velocity at point B would be
   A. increased by a factor of 2.
   B. decreased by a factor of 2.
   C. increased by a factor of $\sqrt{2}$.
   D. decreased by a factor of $\sqrt{2}$.

3. If point C is at a height of 55m, what is the minimum height for point A?
   A. 40m B. 50m
   C. 55m D. 60m

4. Newton's Third Law says that every force has an equal and opposite reaction force. At which points does this law apply?
   A. A and C only B. B and D only
   C. A, C, and E D. At all points

PASSAGE II (QUESTIONS 5–7)

A new circuit company is investigating new multiple component circuits for use in leading-edge equipment. They are examining a multiple capacitance circuit and a multiple resistor circuit as shown on page 460 (Figures 1 and 2, respectively).

It is possible to vary a number of these components and observe interesting results. A systematic study of some of the more interesting ideas is yours to complete.

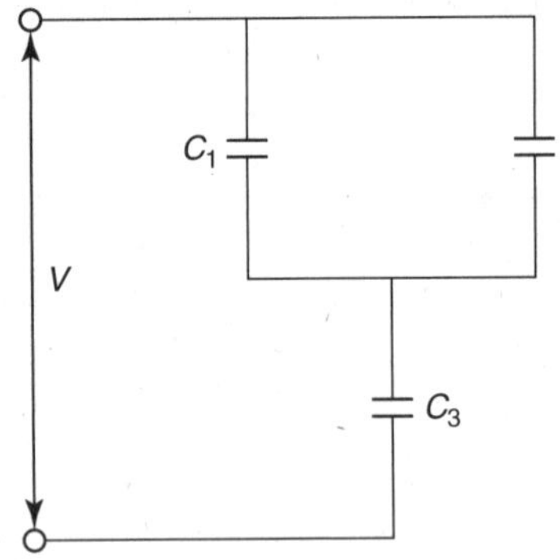

FIGURE 1

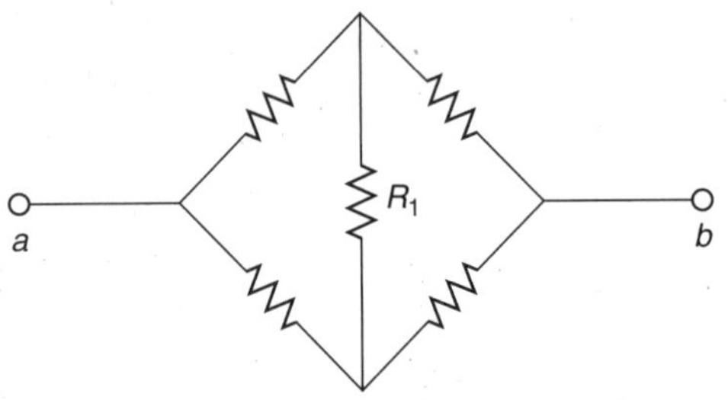

FIGURE 2

5. Find the equivalent capacitance of the combination shown in Figure 1 if you know that $C_1 = 1.10\mu F$, $C_2 = .90\mu F$, and $C_3 = 3\mu F$.
   A. 1.2μF
   B. 2μF
   C. 3μF
   D. 6μF

6. During testing, suppose that capacitor C_2 in Figure 1 is removed. What is the charge for capacitor C_3 if you assume $V = 100V$, $C_1 = 20\ \mu F$, and $C_3 = 5.0\ \mu F$?
   A. Not enough information
   B. 2.5×10^{-3}C
   C. 4.0×10^{-4}C
   D. 5.0×10^{-4}C

7. What is the equivalent resistance between points a and b of the circuit in Figure 2 if the resistor R_1 is removed? Assume each of the other resistors is 100W.
   A. 400
   B. 1.00×10^{-2}
   C. 100
   D. 50

PASSAGE III
(QUESTIONS 8–10)

As a theoretical physicist in an optics company, your responsibilities include new designs in mirrors, lenses, and filters. You know that the focal point for a thin lens is

$$\frac{1}{s} + \frac{1}{s'} = (n-1)\left(\frac{1}{r1} + \frac{1}{r2}\right)$$

where s is the object's distance from the lens, s′ is the image's distance from the lens, r1 + r2 is the curvature of radius of the surface of the lens, and n is the refractive index of the lens material. As a specialist in the area of lenses, you also know that

$$\frac{1}{s} + \frac{1}{s'} = \frac{1}{f}$$

where f is the focal length of the lens. The last thing you want to investigate is the magnification (m), which is given by $m = -(s'/s)$.

8. You have recently observed that spherical mirrors exhibit behavior similar to thin lenses. The equation

   $$\frac{1}{s} + \frac{1}{s'} = \frac{2}{r}$$

   where r = radius of curvature of the mirror holds when investigating a number of reflective surfaces. What condition must hold true to lead to the result that $r/2 = s'$?
   A. The radius of curvature is greater than the object's distance.
   B. The mirror must be flat (r approaches 0).
   C. The object's distance is greater than the radius of curvature.
   D. The object's distance is equal to the radius of curvature.

9. What does the negative sign in the magnification mean?
   A. The image is smaller than the original object.

B. The image is on the same side of the lens as the object.
C. The image is on the opposite side of the lens as the object.
D. The image is inverted compared to the original object.

10. A double convex thin lens made of glass with a refractive index of 2.0 has both radii of curvature of magnitude 25cm. Find the focal length of the lens.
A. 12.5cm
B. 25cm
C. Focal length is undefined
D. .020cm

QUESTIONS 11–13 are NOT based on a descriptive passage.

11. According to the law of inertia, an object will travel in a straight line if there is no force that pushes or pulls the object into a curved path. What is this force?
A. Centrifugal force
B. Kinetic friction
C. Moment of inertia
D. Centripetal force

12. If a 25kg object is raised 10 meters, what is the work being done?
A. 1250J B. 2400J
C. 2450J D. 250J

13. A man stands 3 meters from a small, intense source of light at the same level as his feet. If the man is 2 meters tall, how big will his shadow be on a wall 18 meters from the light source?
A. 5m B. 10m
C. 12m D. 15m

PASSAGE IV (QUESTIONS 14–16)

As the experimental physicist for the Circular Notion Pulley and Lever Company, you have been asked to investigate some lightweight, high-impact plastic, solid disk pulleys. The experiment you have set up has a nylon rope, wound around the rim of the uniform disk, pivoted to rotate around a frictionless fixed axis, through the disk's center. The mass of the disk is 515g, with a radius of 25cm. Also, a carefully measured 10N force is applied to the rope.

From previous experimentation and theory, you have established the following relationships:

Angular velocity

$$\omega = \omega_0 + \alpha_0 t$$

where α_0 is the constant angular acceleration and the applied torque

$$t = Tr$$

where T is the tension and r is the radius of the disk. Furthermore, you've shown that for a solid disk, the moment of inertia

$$I = \frac{1}{2} mr^2.$$

14. For your experiment, calculate the moment of inertia.
A. 3.2×10^{-2}kg $\times$ m^2
B. 1.6×10^{-2}kg $\times$ m^2
C. 6.4×10^{-2}kg $\times$ m^2
D. 1.6×10^{1}kg $\times$ m^2

15. From your experiment, what is the value for the applied torque?
A. 2.5N $\times$ m B. 2.5×10^2N $\times$ m
C. 4.0×10^1Nm^{-1} D. 4.0×10^{-1}Nm^{-1}

16. In a circular orbit of radius 40km around an aircraft carrier, a jet keeps a constant speed of 200km/hr. Calculate the angular acceleration of the aircraft.
A. 100km/hr^2 B. 400km/hr^2
C. 1000km/hr^2 D. 4000km/hr^2

PASSAGE V (QUESTIONS 17–20)

NASA has planned several simplified experiments for scientists who are based on Planet X to broadcast back to Earth to show students gravity at work.

Planet X has roughly 7/8 the mass of Earth and 3/4 the radius of Earth. The scientists will have a simple pendulum of length L, a spring with spring constant k, and a mass of mass M. Classrooms on Earth will need identical equipment to compare the periods of oscillations of the pendulum and the spring.

17. Calculate the gravitational acceleration on Planet X.
    A. 7/8g B. 3/4g
    C. 14/9g D. 9/14g

18. Planet X is
    A. smaller, less dense than Earth.
    B. smaller, more dense than Earth.
    C. larger, less dense than Earth.
    D. larger, more dense than Earth.

19. Calculate the force experienced by an 18kg object orbiting 1000km away, if the gravitational acceleration on Planet X is 10/9g.
    A. 19.6N B. 98N
    C. 196N D. 980N

20. If the gravitational acceleration on Planet X is $1\frac{6}{9}$g, then the period of the spring located on Planet X will be
    A. $\frac{3}{4}$ times the period of the spring on Earth.
    A. $\frac{4}{3}$ times the period of the spring on Earth.
    A. $\frac{9}{16}$ times the period of the spring on Earth.
    D. 1 time the period of the spring on Earth.

PASSAGE VI (QUESTIONS 21–25)

We are investigating the pressure versus temperature behavior of new materials for underwater applications. A phase diagram obtained through measurements of the pressure versus temperature is depicted below.

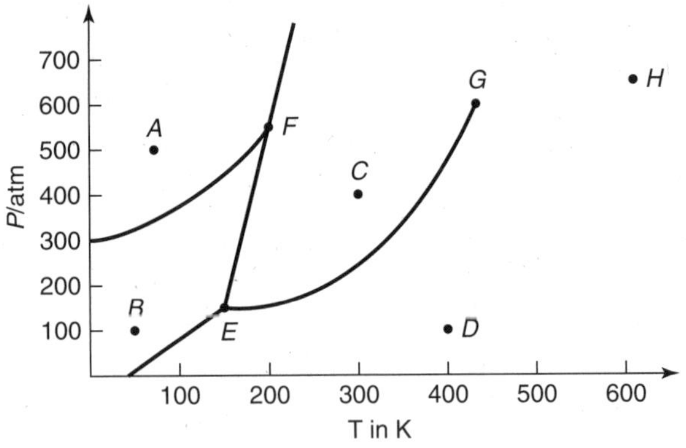

21. Which point(s) is/are defined as the triple point?
    A. Point *F* only B. Point *E* only
    C. Points *E* and *F* D. Point *G* only

22. From the plot, what is the critical temperature?
    A. 600K B. 200K
    C. 150K D. 450K

23. If you evaluate the temperature from 100K to 300K at 200atm, what occurs?
    A. The solid becomes a gas directly.
    B. The solid becomes a different solid.
    C. The solid melts and then turns into a gas.
    D. The solid melts and becomes a liquid.

24. If you hold the temperature at 300K and go from 250atm to 400atm, what do you observe?
    A. The liquid becomes a gas.
    B. The liquid becomes a solid.
    C. No physical changes are observed.
    D. The liquid freezes and then turns into a different solid.

25. What is the name of the process going directly from point *B* to point *D*?
    A. Fusion B. Sublimation
    C. Melting D. Boiling

QUESTIONS 26–28 are NOT based on a descriptive passage.

26. Which of the salts below will produce an alkaline solution when dissolved in water?

A. NH_4Cl B. $NaCl$
C. Na_2CO_3 D. $NaNO_3$

27. The work required to move 2 coulombs of charge through a potential difference of 5 volts is
   A. 10 joules. B. 2 joules.
   C. 25 joules. D. 50 joules.

28. The phenomenon that occurs when a wave spreads into the region behind an obstruction is known as
   A. refraction. B. diffraction.
   C. dispersion. D. superposition.

PASSAGE VII (QUESTIONS 29–33)

You are given the unenviable task of cleaning up a lab. You find four bottles, and you know only that they all contain 10^{-5}M solutions and that each has the following dissociative properties:

Solution I: $HNO_3 + H_2O \rightarrow H_3O^+ + NO_3^-$

Solution II: $NaOH \rightarrow Na^+ + OH^-$

Solution III: Benzenesulfonic Acid; $k_a = 2 \times 10^{-1}$

Solution IV: 5.625×10^{-3}M solution of calcium hydroxide; $k_b = 4 \times 10^{-2}$ at 30°C

($\log (5 \times 10^{-3}) = -2.3$; $\log (5 \times 10^{-4}) = -3.3$; $\log (5 \times 10^{-5}) = -4.3$; $\log (5 \times 10^{-6}) = -5.3$)

29. Calculate the pH for Solution I.
   A. 2 B. 5
   C. 9 D. 12

30. Calculate the pH for Solution II.
   A. 2 B. 5
   C. 9 D. 12

31. Each of the following graphs depicts a titration of some combination of these particular solutions. Which graph best depicts the titration of Solution II with Solution III?

A.
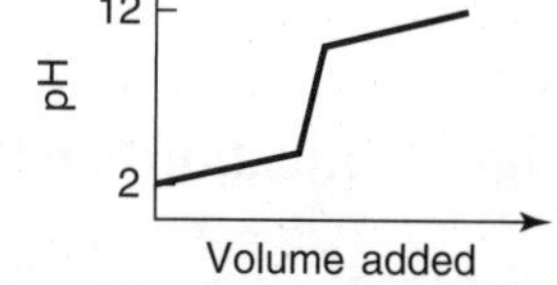

B.
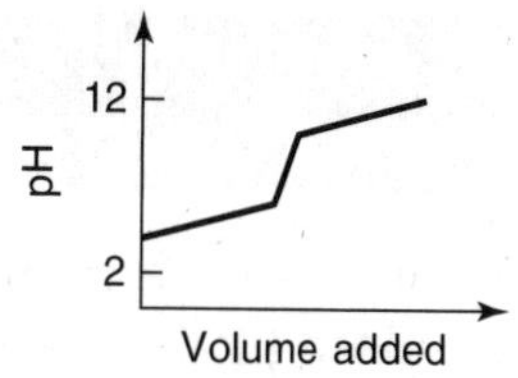

C.
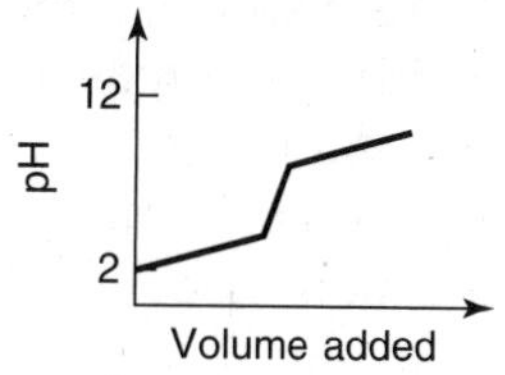

D.
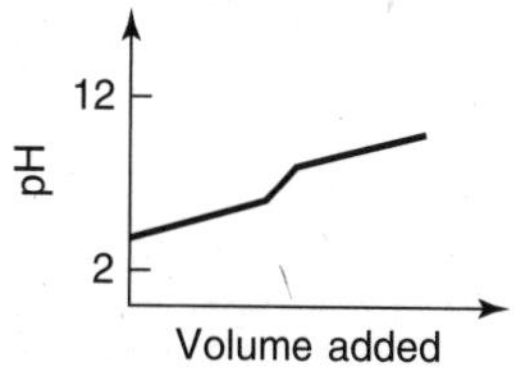

32. Calculate the pOH of Solution IV.
   A. 2.3 B. 3.3
   C. 4.3 D. 5.3

33. Each of the following graphs depicts a titration of some combination of these particular solutions. Which graph best depicts the titration of Solution IV with Solution I?

A.
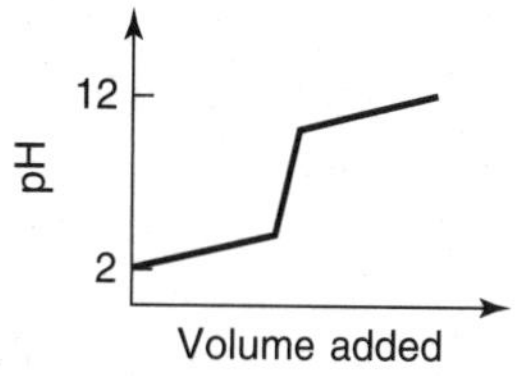

B.
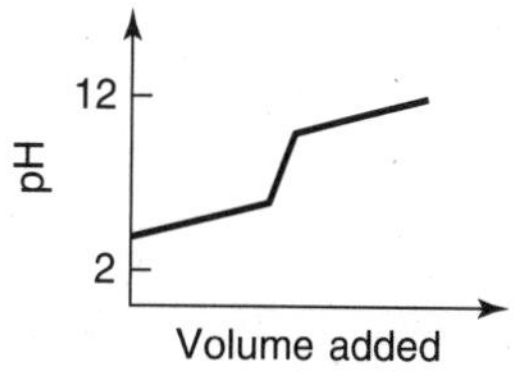

C.
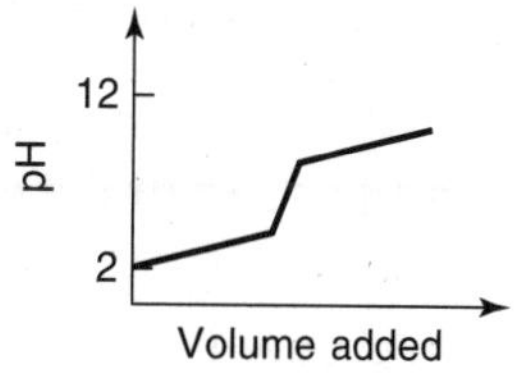

D.
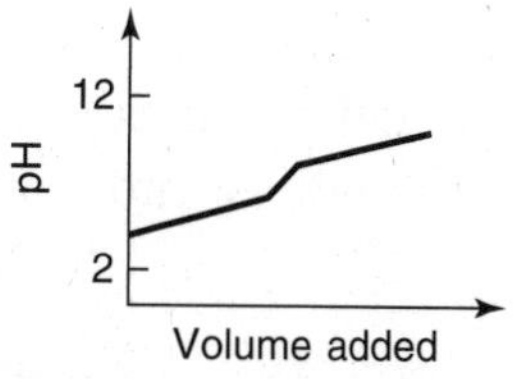

PASSAGE VIII (QUESTIONS 34–36)

Potential new molecules for refrigeration that are able to replace chlorofluorocarbons (CFCs) include a group of sulfur halide compounds. This group exhibits many different types of chemistry, including selective fluorination. A young company feels it can market chemicals like these, and it wants to learn more about their structure and possible ways to exploit the chemistry.

34. What is the correct Lewis dot structure for SF_4?

A. 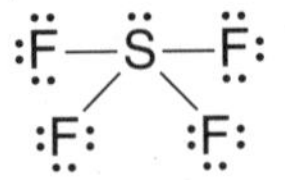

B. 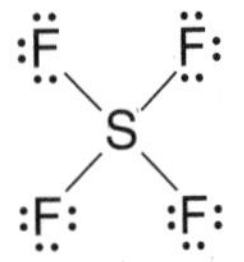

C. 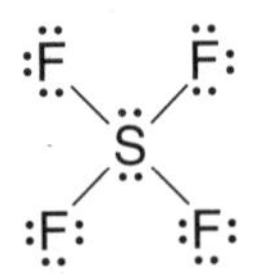

D. 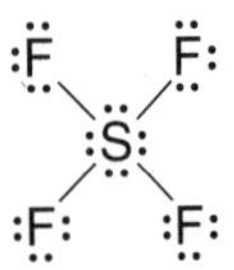

35. What structure would you predict for SCl_4, employing VSEPR theory?
    A. Square planar
    B. Tetrahedral
    C. Trigonal bipyramid
    D. See-saw

36. In SF_6, what is the hybridization of the orbitals?
    A. sp^3
    B. d^2sp^3
    C. sp^3d
    D. sp^3d^2

PASSAGE IX (QUESTIONS 37–40)

The Army Corps of Engineers is planning a dam in the town of South Plain, Idaho. Their goal is to create two lakes (one at the top of the dam and one at the bottom) and supply the local hydroelectric plant and the town with water. During the spring, the maximum water level at the top of the dam is projected to be 500m above the pipes feeding both the power and water plants.

To keep the ecosystem downriver minimally affected by the dam, the Corps not only plans to capture and relocate large numbers of wildlife annually, but will also open and close the dam to simulate actual changes in the water levels. Opponents of this plan charge that the power plant would be unable to supply the town with electricity during critical times. Proponents charge that a small town like South Plain can be supported by the excess energy made by the power plant the rest of the year. On average, the river supplies 400,000L of water a month to the plant, and the power plant can make 100kW/L. South Plain needs about 30 million kW/month.

37. Calculate the factor increase in the velocity of water if the Corps uses pipes with a radius of 4cm, and the water plant's pipes have a radius of only 2cm.
    A. 1
    B. 2
    C. 3
    D. 4

38. Calculate the maximum pressure the base of the dam is expected to withstand during the spring (r_w = $1000 kg/m^3$, pressure at the top of the dam = 1atm, g ≈ $10 m/s^2$).
    A. 499atm
    B. 501atm
    C. 4.99×10^6atm
    D. 5.01×10^6atm

39. The lake at the top of the dam will eventually become full of silt and increase in density. Calculate the ratio of final density to initial density if a square-bottom barge that previously sank 1/3 of its depth now sinks 1/6 of its depth.
    A. 2
    B. 4
    C. 6
    D. 12

40. Does the power plant make enough power in nine months to have the dam open for three months (assuming that they have the ability to store the power)?
    A. More than enough
    B. Barely enough
    C. Not enough
    D. Not enough information to tell

PASSAGE X (QUESTIONS 41–45)

The following experiments were performed to study the properties of carbon dioxide.

Experiment I:

Carbon dioxide (CO_2) and a by-product were obtained by the combustion of methane (CH_4) and oxygen (O_2). The CO_2 was then extracted from the final vapor by allowing the vapor to cool (CO_2 has a lower condensation point than the other product of this reaction).

Experiment II:

Ten liters of CO_2 at 1atm was then compressed to 4atm at constant temperature.

Experiment III:

Twenty liters of CO_2 at 45°C were then cooled to 18°C at constant pressure.

Experiment IV:

Two liters of CO_2 at 20°C and 2atm were then warmed until there were 5 liters.

41. Experiment II (constant temperature) represents which of the following laws?
    A. Ideal Gas Law B. Boyle's Law
    C. Charles' Law D. Dalton's Law

42. Calculate the final volume in Experiment II.
    A. 40 liters B. 20 liters
    C. 5 liters D. 2.5 liters

43. Experiment III (constant pressure) represents which of the following laws?
    A. Ideal Gas Law B. Boyle's Law
    C. Charles' Law D. Dalton's Law

44. Calculate the final volume in Experiment III.
    A. 40.5 liters B. 24 liters
    C. 12 liters D. 18 liters

45. What is a possible combination for final pressure and temperature in Experiment IV?
    A. 1atm; 25°C B. 1atm; 100°C
    C. 2atm; 25°C D. 3atm; 25°C

PASSAGE XI (QUESTIONS 46–50)

The following table lists the heat of fusion for several compounds.

Name	Symbol	Heat of Fusion (cal/g)
Nitrogen	N_2	6.15
Carbon monoxide	CO	7.13
Hydrogen sulfide	H_2S	16.8
Barium oxide	BaO	93.2
Sodium chloride	NaCl	123.5

46. Which bond is the weakest?
    A. The bond between barium and oxygen
    B. The bond between carbon and oxygen
    C. The bond between hydrogen and sulfur
    D. The bond between the two nitrogen atoms

47. Which bond is the strongest?
    A. The bond between the two nitrogen atoms
    B. The bond between carbon and oxygen
    C. The bond between hydrogen and sulfur
    D. The bond between barium and oxygen

48. Carbon has what electron structure?
    A. $1s^22s^12p^3$ B. $1s^22s^22p^2$
    C. $1s^22p^4$ D. $2s^22p^4$

49. Barium oxide (M.W. = 153) forms through the reaction $2Ba + O_2 \rightarrow 2BaO$. How many grams are formed if it is heated with 480 cal of energy?
    A. Less than 1 gram
    B. Less than 10 grams
    C. Less than 100 grams
    D. Less than 1000 grams

50. What is the oxidation number of each nitrogen atom in nitrogen gas?
    A. –2 B. –1
    C. 0 D. 1

QUESTIONS 51–52 are NOT based on a descriptive passage.

51. Which of the following has an effective dipole moment?

A. 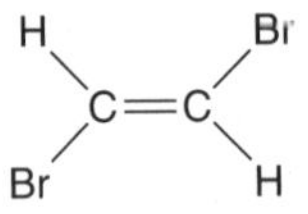

B. CCl_4

C. 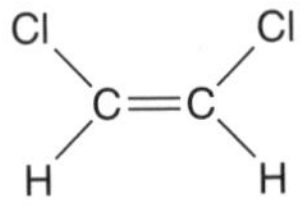

D. CO_2

52. Rainbows are caused by water droplets refracting light from the sun much the same way a prism does. Which wavelengths are diffracted the most?

A. Shorter wavelengths like blue and indigo
B. Longer wavelengths like red
C. Shorter wavelengths like red
D. Longer wavelengths like blue and indigo

STOP! If time still remains, you may review work only in this section. When the time allotted is up, you may go on to the next section. STOP!

SECTION 2
Verbal Reasoning

TIME: 60 Minutes

QUESTIONS: 53–144

DIRECTIONS: The verbal reasoning section contains nine passages, each followed by a series of questions. Based on the information given in a passage, choose the one best answer to each question.

PASSAGE I (QUESTIONS 53–57)

The philosopher Socrates is put on trial in Athens in 400 B.C. on two charges: corrupting the youth and impiety. Socrates begins his defense, as recorded in Plato's dialogue The Apology, by saying how he is going to "speak plainly and honestly," unlike the eloquent sophists the Athenian jury is accustomed to hearing. This appeal to unadorned language offends the jurors, who are expecting to be entertained.

Next, Socrates identifies two sets of accusers that he must face: past and present. The former, who filled the jurors' heads with lies about him when they were young, Socrates finds most dangerous because they cannot be cross-examined and because they influenced the jurors when they were young and their minds were impressionable. This offends the jury because it calls into question their ability to be objective and render a fair judgment.

Now Socrates addresses the charges themselves and dismisses them as being continued accusations used to mask the deeper attack on his philosophical activity. That activity, which involves questioning others until they reveal contradictions in their beliefs, will ultimately give rise to Socrates' motto, "The unexamined life is not worth living" and the Socratic method, which is still being employed in many law schools. This critical questioning of leading Athenians has made Socrates very unpopular with the people in power and, he insists, has led to his trial. Challenging the legitimacy of the legal system itself further alienates Socrates' judges.

Socrates tries to explain that his philosophical life came about quite by accident. He was content to be a humble stone mason until the day that a friend informed him that the Oracle of Delphi said that "Socrates is the wisest man in Greece." Socrates was so surprised by the statement, and so sure of its inaccuracy, that he set about disproving it by talking to the reputed wise men of Athens and showing how much more knowledge they possessed. Unfortunately, as he tells the jury, those citizens reputed to be wise (politicians, businessmen, artists) turned out to be ignorant. They possessed either no, or only very limited, knowledge in their fields of expertise, and they presumed to know everything else. Socrates had to admit, "I am wiser, because although all of us have little knowledge, I am aware of my ignorance, while they are not." But this practice of revealing prominent citizens' ignorance and arrogance did not earn Socrates their affection, especially when the bright young men of Athens became followers of Socrates and began to disgrace their elders. Hence, in his view, the formal charges of "corrupting the youth" and "impiety" were offered as a pretext to retaliate for the deeper offense of challenging the pretensions of the establishment.

Although Socrates views the whole trial as a sham, he cleverly refutes the charges by using the same method of questioning that landed him in the docket. Against the charges of corrupting the youth, Socrates asks his chief accuser, Meletus, if anyone wants to harm himself, to which Meletus answers "no." Then, Socrates asks if those with whom one associates have an effect upon one: good people for good and evil people for evil, to which Meletus answers "yes." Then, Socrates asks if corrupting one's companions makes them better or worse, to which Meletus answers "worse." Finally, Socrates springs the trap by asking Meletus if he corrupted the youth intentionally or unintentionally, to which Meletus, wanting to make the charge as bad as possible, answers "intentionally." Now Socrates shows the contradictory nature of the charge because, by intentionally corrupting, his companions he makes them worse, thereby bringing harm on himself. He refutes the second charge of impiety the same way, by showing that its two components (teaching about strange gods and atheism) are inconsistent.

Although Socrates has logically refuted the charges against him, the Athenian jury finds him guilty, and Meletus proposes the death penalty. The defendant, Socrates, is allowed to propose an alternative penalty and he proposes a state pension, so he can continue his philosophical activity to benefit Athens. He states that this is what he "deserves." The Athenian jury, furious over his presumption, votes the death penalty and one of the great philosophers of the Western heritage is executed.

53. Before beginning his defense, Socrates offends the Athenian jury
    - A. once.
    - B. twice.
    - C. three times.
    - D. four times.

54. For the Socratic method, consistency is
    - A. the hobgoblin of small minds.
    - B. the sign of a trumped-up charge.
    - C. the sign of a genuine charge.
    - D. impossible in a court of law.

55. The fact that Socrates is found guilty shows that
    - A. he did corrupt the youth.
    - B. rationality always wins.
    - C. rationality may not always win.
    - D. Athens did not have a Supreme Court.

56. Socrates' suggestion of an alternative penalty in the form of a state pension is viewed by the jury as
    - A. the ramblings of a disturbed man.
    - B. an appropriate award.
    - C. an insult to Meletus and reward to Socrates.
    - D. an insult to Socrates and reward to Meletus.

57. Socrates' trial is relevant throughout the Western heritage whenever
    - A. courts are corrupt.
    - B. defendants are intellectual.
    - C. youthful juries decide on the elderly.
    - D. established authority executes its critic(s).

PASSAGE II (QUESTIONS 58–61)

The system of American federalism will inevitably result in tension and conflict because it has established two distinct levels of government, each with its own jurisdiction. Partly because of James Madison's fear of absolute political power, the division between national and state authorities was designed to distribute sovereignty among several bodies and, thereby, prevent concentration of power and tyranny. However, this has caused historical controversies over the precise distribution of power between the central and decentralized governments. Such a controversy eventually led to the Civil War.

One interpretation of American federalism, originally held by the Anti-Federalists and later by the Confederacy, was the compact theory. According to this view, the states had entered into a compact after the Revolution and had established the national government to perform specific and limited functions (primarily foreign affairs and interstate commerce). Therefore, most of the lawmaking authority over domestic policy resided in the states. If a conflict over the division of federal and state authority arose, the compact theory held that the states could convene in order to interpret the exact meaning of the Constitution. It also implied that any state could secede from the Union.

Another view of American federalism, held by the Federalists and later the Northern advocates of the Union, argued that the Constitution was created by "The People," apart from their membership in the various states, and therefore it was not beholden to the states for its authority. This perspective, which eventually prevailed, held that the national government was separate from, and superior to, the state governments. It also believed that the United States Supreme Court should decide any disputes over the meaning of federalism in the Constitution through its power of judicial review. This view justified many incursions into state sovereignty, including most of the civil rights laws and much of police procedure, under the doctrine that the federal Bill of Rights took precedence over state law.

A third conception of American federalism, often called cooperative federalism, holds that each level of government has its own jurisdiction but that they inevitably overlap (in policies associated with health, welfare, education, etc.) and therefore the two tiers of government must work together. This view helped form many of the 1960s social welfare policies, in which the national government would design and fund programs for the poor, elderly, and so on, and the states would implement them according to local needs. The federal categorical grant programs, and later, block grants and revenue sharing programs grew out of this partnership between Washington and the states. President Reagan's New Federalism cut many of these programs, shifting authority and funding to the states alone.

The dynamism and adaptability of the American system is partly due to the ambiguous nature of American federalism, but this also necessitates continual management of tension and accommodation.

58. According to Madison, American federalism divides political power in order to
    A. give categorical grants.
    B. prevent concentration of power.
    C. allow Southern states to secede.
    D. allow the South to retain slavery.

59. According to the compact theory, the conclusion of the Civil War was
    A. unjust.
    B. just.
    C. a mistake.
    D. inevitable.

60. President Reagan's New Federalism subscribed to which notion of federalism?
    A. Compact theory
    B. Judicial federalism
    C. Dual federalism
    D. Cooperative federalism

61. The nature of American federalism makes the relationship between the United States government and the states
    A. confused but authoritarian.
    B. tense but permanent.
    C. stable but undefined.
    D. adaptable but conflictual.

PASSAGE III (QUESTIONS 62–66)

Although Plato's book *The Republic* is one of the most famous works in political theory, its vision of humanity and society are radically different from contemporary ideas. Indeed, in a twentieth-century world that values democracy, equality, and freedom, Plato's ideal state seems shocking.

Plato conceives human nature as being comprised of three elements or dispositions: (1) the philosophic, (2) the spirited, and (3) the appetitive. The philosophic part of a person is his or her desire and capacity for acquiring knowledge, the passionate search for truth fueled by curiosity. The spirited element is the love of combat and fighting — it loves the struggle of battle and the thrill of triumphing over an opponent. The appetitive side of human nature is concerned with material things: possessions, comforts, and the economy in general. For Plato, all three elements are present in everyone, but one predominates in each individual, forming his or her character. This distribution of dominant traits renders humanity essentially *unequal,* although for Plato, this inequality is not based on gender, as both men and women can be philosophic, spirited, or appetitive.

For Plato, the natural division of humanity into three dominant characteristics creates a natural class system in society. The philosophic people, whose virtue is wisdom, should govern society; the spirited people, whose virtue is courage, should form the military; and the appetitive people, whose virtue is moderation, should work in the economic sector: production, distribution, and so on. Justice, for Plato, consists of the "right ordering" of psychic and social elements and classes. The individual is subordinate to the needs of the whole society and should occupy a proper place in the social order. This explains Plato's rationale for a philosopher-king ruling over society because his or her wisdom is of the philosophic order and the virtues that accompany it.

Plato devises a "myth of the metals" that explains and justifies this class society based on internal dispositions and functional excellence. According to this myth, or "noble lie," each person born is mixed with some metal from the earth: gold with the philosophic nature, silver with the spirited nature, and bronze with the appetitive nature. This myth makes it easier for common people to understand their place in society.

However, because dominant natures are not passed on through heredity (i.e., gold parents can have a silver or bronze child, bronze parents can have a silver or gold child), Plato devises an elaborate educational system (often called communism in children) that discerns and cultivates each child's natural propensities and abilities. In this scheme, it is best for the individual to be told what his nature is by the State and to be developed in a certain way, rather than to be able to choose freely with limited knowledge of what his endeavor involves. For Plato, this social system will guarantee the most harmonious country and the happiest citizens. A democracy, by contrast, where everyone is left free to decide his own occupation, will be chaotic, leading to disorder and eventually to tyranny. Only an all-wise philosopher-king can determine each person's true capacity and order society accordingly.

Plato's inegalitarian theory, with its emphasis on individuals' fixed natures and inevitable class status, seems odd and even offensive to twentieth-century minds that value free choice, equality, democracy, and protection from authoritarian government. However, as Western democracies suffer from uncertainty, and individuals feel alienated from any secure place in society, Plato's ideas forever haunt humanity.

62. A business entrepreneur would most likely fall into the Platonic category of the
    - A. philosophic.
    - B. appetitive.
    - C. spirited.
    - D. innovative.

63. Which remark by Thomas Jefferson most contrasts with Plato's philosophy about class differences?
    - A. "The blood of patriots waters the tree of liberty . . ."
    - B. "All men are created equal."
    - C. "We are all federalists, all republicans."
    - D. "There is a natural aristocracy . . ."

64. The wisdom that characterizes the philosopher and qualifies him or her for rule is knowledge of
    - A. moderation.
    - B. combat.
    - C. the stock market.
    - D. virtue.

65. One virtue that Plato's *Republic* does not always endorse is
    - A. courage.
    - B. moderation.
    - C. honor.
    - D. truthfulness.

66. A country that recruits young people into the army by appealing to their desires for

money, benefits, and training that will help them land a job is applying which class standards to the military, in Plato's view?

A. The philosophic
B. The appetitive
C. The spirited
D. The virtuous

PASSAGE IV (QUESTIONS 67–70)

In the 1990s, America entered a social period that might be called Neo-Victorian. Like the original Victorian period of the latter nineteenth century in England and the United States, this period was characterized by an emphasis on traditional values and morality, stable families, conventional religion, and economic conservatism. The reasons for this period of Neo-Victorianism were complex, but some of the most obvious causes were: the middle-age status of the baby-boom generation, whose members now had their own children; the continuing spread of the AIDS epidemic that extended to small towns, rural areas, and those with "traditional" lifestyles; and the loss of rapid economic growth, as the decade experienced recession or slow growth. All three of these factors contributed to the emerging Neo-Victorian *zeitgeist,* or spirit of the times.

The baby-boom generation — that enormous group of Americans born during the 1950s — entered middle age during the late 1980s. Television programs like *Thirtysomething* and others characterized the mood of this graying generation, as its ages rose to late thirties and even early forties. This was the generation that experienced its adolescent rebellion *en masse* during the 1960s, causing the enormous social turmoil of the rock era, the free love movement, the drug culture, antiwar protests, radical political groups, etc. This generation then had "seen it all," had lost its innocence, and found itself experiencing a bad hangover by the 1970s. Those that survived the drug deaths, political bombings, and fractured personal relationships entered middle age as "born again"-conservatives, similar to the notorious reformed prostitute who is holier-than-thou and ready to eradicate pervasive sin and immorality. Consequently, reacting against their own past, the baby-boom generation started settling down and having babies. In 1989, there were as many births in this country as there were during the biggest year of the baby-boom era. With children came a sense of responsibility and the need for stability, reliability, and order. Graying baby boomers had experienced the destructiveness of mass rebellion, of tearing down established morality and authority. Now they repented with a vengeance. *Catcher in the Rye* may have been their Bible, but their children were raised on *Peter Rabbit.* Disney was the thing of the day. The middle-aged baby boomers became the new advocates of traditional family values, social decency, religious ethics, and especially public safety.

The AIDS epidemic threatened public safety more than any other single problem. Its association with illicit sex brought a return to traditional monogamous relationships, sex only after marriage, and a suspicion of nontraditional lifestyles. Again, the Neo-Victorian ethos of sobriety and propriety prevailed. The children growing up in the 1990s (like those of the 1890s and 1950s) were taught the sanctity of their family and the importance of fidelity.

Finally, the impending economic recession, followed by continued slow growth in the American economy, encouraged frugality and conservatism. No extravagant public spending plans or private indulgences were tolerated. The Puritan ethic of hard work and saving money descended on America.

Social trends work in cycles, however, and eventually, this Neo-Victorian period should pass. In fact, if history is a guide, the children growing up in the 1990s should have quite a wild time (à la the 1920s and 1960s) around 2008.

67. According to the author's logic, those who advocate a return to traditional values tend to be people who

A. are good Christians.
B. were raised by clergy.

C. are well educated.

D. have experienced excess and changed their lifestyles.

68. The act of raising children, as presented in this essay, leads people to become

A. neurotic. B. responsible.

C. bossy. D. irreverent.

69. If the author's views of social and psychological change are correct, the proper course to produce a *radical* adults would be to

A. give them a conservative upbringing.

B. give them a radical upbringing.

C. let them rebel as adolescents.

D. keep them from political involvement.

70. Winston Churchill's remark, "If you are not a radical at age 20, you have no heart, and if you are not a conservative at age 40, you have no head" would seem to

A. support the logic of the essay.

B. oppose the logic of the essay.

C. be irrelevant to the essay.

D. prove that the essay was written by Churchill.

PASSAGE V (QUESTIONS 71–76)

The nineteenth-century British philosopher John Stuart Mill provides arguments for intellectual liberty and against social conformity that have greatly affected American notions of free speech, free press, and academic freedom.

In his essay, *On Liberty,* John Stuart Mill argues that it is not enough to lift formal legal and ecclesiastical restrictions on freedom of thought and expression; the individual must be protected against informal *social* prohibitions on unconventional ideas. The "tyranny of society" can exert more severe penalties such as ostracism on the nonconformist than can any number of laws against unconventional or unpopular ideas. To avoid such tyranny of opinion, Mill advocates a free, tolerant atmosphere in a progressive, civilized, and humane society. The advantages of such a liberal society are manifold for Mill, especially in the advancement of knowledge.

In *On Liberty,* John Stuart Mill gives two primary reasons for allowing complete expression of all ideas, no matter how radical. First, he claims, the new ideas or viewpoints might be *correct,* and so their suppression by law or popular prejudice could rob the world of original, innovative ideas. A new and more useful conception of nature, the universe (as Galileo's), medicine, or politics could be denied humankind, and the innovator's society could fall behind the development of others. Second, Mill asserts, even if the new radical idea is wrong, the right view will be strengthened by refuting the new idea. The established truth, if it is truth, should not fear or resent challenges, but rather welcome them as another opportunity to reassert its own validity. As a result, Mill sees the ongoing debate between established beliefs and their radical challengers as clarifying and sharpening the truth. The open-minded intellectual will actually relish such contests and affirm with Mill the view that "he who knows only his own side of the case, knows little of that."

Of course, Mill does not extend this idea of complete intellectual liberty to the total freedom to *act* on all of our beliefs. It is one thing to advocate the overthrowing of the United States government through violent revolution as Marxists do, but to engage in the actual killing that such a revolution entails is rightfully prohibited, both legally and socially, for Mill. Even the verbal expression of such a belief may be suppressed if the society (such as during a depression) is in a situation where the ideas will lead people to act on them. This forms the Supreme Court's standard of a "clear and present danger" to the society that permits punishment of inflammatory speech, as enunciated by Oliver Wendell Holmes.

John Stuart Mill's conception of liberty underlies American free speech and free press where all viewpoints are permitted to be aired. The recent suppression of rock music groups on obscenity charges (based on "community standards") might concern Mill as an example of the "tyranny of the majority" squelching individual liberty of expression.

American academic freedom, where university and college professors are protected in teaching controversial ideas and theories, also rests on Mill's conception of intellectual liberty. Moves to disallow discussion of certain ideas in college classrooms because they "offend" some individual or group may seem to Mill a dangerous step away from intellectual liberty.

John Stuart Mill's ideas on liberty will always be in conflict with conformist opinions, and the struggle between conventional and radical speech will continue to occur in a free society.

71. An area of American society that might be influenced by Mill's *On Liberty* not mentioned in the essay is
    A. journalism.
    B. academia.
    C. law.
    D. religious institutions.

72. Social prohibitions on unconventional ideas and expressions may be more severe than legal restrictions for Mill because they
    A. are hidden.
    B. include the death penalty.
    C. include ostracism.
    D. are unfair.

73. Mill asserts that a free, open, and tolerant society will
    A. advance knowledge.
    B. be less humane.
    C. be less civilized.
    D. lead to civil war.

74. For Mill, the value in the expression of radical ideas that are wrong lies in their
    A. eventual acceptance.
    B. obnoxious character.
    C. sharpening of the truth.
    D. inability to persuade.

75. If a lone individual were to give a speech before an angry mob in Washington, D.C., in front of the federal courthouse, shouting, "Burn the courthouse!" American society could, according to Mill,
    A. legally prosecute him.
    B. leave him free.
    C. invoke ecclesiastical restrictions.
    D. ask if he is a communist.

76. An example of the Millian tradition might be a(n)
    A. newspaper.
    B. assembly line.
    C. news program.
    D. city council debate.

PASSAGE VI (QUESTIONS 77–81)

Organizational theory in American public administration relies on two very different approaches to understanding, structuring, and managing governmental agencies. The traditional institutional approach focuses on the organization itself: offices, positions, structures, and functions. The newer humanist approach emphasizes the people in the organization: their psychological needs, aspirations, performance, etc. Reconciling these two very distinctive approaches to public administration is not easy, but a closer examination of each theory's orientation may be helpful.

The classic structural approach to governmental organizations comes from the writings of the German sociologist Max Weber. Weber's theory of bureaucracy presents an ideal administrative structure that would produce efficient, equitable public services. Weber's bureaucracy involves a clear hierarchy of official positions, each with clearly specified duties and authority. This for Weber would make for a smooth-running organization in which everyone knows his place, his superiors, and his subordinates. These official positions would be defined and limited by specific rules and regulations so that the authority of the official would not be personal (as, for example, the authority of a prince) and less subject to abuse. All positions in the bureaucracy would be filled according to objective criteria: training, experience, etc. Salary would be tied to position; the result being that educational level, expertise, authority, and income would all correspond with each other. The organization's relations with the public, in Weber's view, would be characterized by rational, impartial, and equitable treatment of all citizens as defined by specific procedures and policies, rules and regulations. According to Weber, the internal and external workings of this kind of government agency would create a just and efficient regime.

The humanist approach to public management rejects the institutional approach to administration with its emphasis on structures and functions and offers a vision of organizations growing out of the psychology of the individuals involved. Abraham Maslow, an American psychologist, exemplifies this humanist approach with his famous "ladder of human needs." According to Maslow, human beings have a succession of needs, from lower, economic needs to higher, emotional needs that must be satisfied if one is to work effectively in any organization. Maslow identifies the first human need as basic economic sustenance: food, clothing, shelter, etc. But after this need has been fulfilled, a need for assurances of future security must be satisfied. Then, the individual needs to be loved by others. After that need is satisfied, a human need for self-esteem or a feeling of self-worth must be addressed. Finally, the person needs to be self-actualized, which entails developing and exercising all of one's talents and ability. The public administration that subscribes to this humanist theory of management cares less about organizational structures and positions, and more about the individual psychological development of the people in the organization. It sees administrative work as nurturing the people's needs and believes that this will make for a more productive and effective organization.

The traditional and humanist approaches are so radically dissimilar that it is inconceivable that they can ever be reconciled in the future.

77. A feature not common to the traditional, structural approach to organizational theory is
    A. official positions.
    B. rules and regulations.
    C. self-esteem.
    D. impartial treatment of clientele.

78. According to Max Weber, his bureaucracy would create
    A. abuses of power.
    B. excessive rules and regulations.
    C. inefficient government.
    D. smoothly operating agencies.

79. Historically, one reason that Weber may have found his ideal bureaucracy attractive was its contrast with
    A. Nazi Germany.
    B. decentralized feudal principalities.
    C. modern America.
    D. ancient Rome.

80. For a Maslowian manager, an organization full of self-actualized people would be
    A. intolerable. B. productive.
    C. chaotic. D. boring.

81. A common criticism of Maslowian theory is that it requires administrators to be
    A. efficient. B. psychologists.
    C. tyrannical. D. boring.

PASSAGE VII (QUESTIONS 82–86)

Public administration studies leadership styles and traits in order to determine which produce more effective administrative leadership and, as a result, more effective organizational relations and employee morale. This field of management leadership asks basic questions such as: Are good leaders born or made? What traits are characteristic of all good leaders? How are subordinates' abilities able to affect leadership?

A common typology of administrative leadership grew out of a study of different management styles. This involved a study conducted in the 1930s with three groups of boys, each with the assignment to complete a certain project. One group's leader was characterized as "authoritarian," which meant that he made all the decisions by himself, assigned tasks and work partners, was limited in power by neither rules nor other people, and employed a highly personal or *ad hominem* form of correction. The second group was led by a "democratic" style leader who encouraged input from the group members, established objective rules and schedules, served as a guide or facilitator rather than as a dictator, and corrected people in terms of actions rather than individualistic traits. The third group had a leader characterized as "laissez-faire," which meant that he left the group members free to do whatever they wanted individually, without orders or guidance, and basically projected a "do your own thing" attitude. The boys in this third group were free to come and go as they pleased, work with whom they pleased, and perform tasks as they pleased. At the end of the projects (which were identical), the members of each group were measured according to two variables: efficiency in completing the project and satisfaction in doing so. The first group, under the authoritarian leader, ranked high in efficiency but low in satisfaction; the second group under the democratic leader ranked high in efficiency *and* high in satisfaction; and the third group under the laissez-faire leader was low in both efficiency and satisfaction. This seemed to suggest that democratic administrators produced the best results and the highest morale, which gave rise to the participatory management school.

Another approach to leadership styles measures concern for two variables: people and production. In this model, a leader who demonstrated high concern for the people in the organization but low concern for production is termed a country club manager. An administrator who has a high concern for production but low concern for people is called an authoritarian manager. A high concern for both production and people is referred to as team leadership and a low concern for production and the organization's employees is known as impoverished leadership.

The study of leadership styles in public administration should contribute to a better understanding of what comprises effective leadership and renders America more competitive.

82. The type of leader in the first study who is most likely to correct the workers by using personal insults is
    A. impoverished. B. laissez-faire.
    C. authoritarian. D. democratic.

83. The results of the first study of leadership styles suggest that having complete freedom to do what you want in a group project is
    A. fun. B. anarchy.
    C. unfulfilling. D. unusual.

84. If the Secretary of Health and Human Services were to make the statement, "I think that most of these programs are a waste of time and money, and most of the people who work here are lazy, bureaucratic bums," this would most likely qualify that leader as
    A. country club. B. authoritarian.
    C. impoverished. D. totalitarian.

85. The team leadership model in the second typology most resembles which style in the first typology?
    A. Democratic B. Authoritarian
    C. Laissez-faire D. The New York Mets

86. The passage implies that a better understanding of effective leadership would help
    A. Eastern Europe.
    B. the American economy.
    C. Communist nations.
    D. South America.

PASSAGE VIII (QUESTIONS 87–90)

The idea that moral rules are absolute, allowing no exceptions, is implausible in light of cases such as "The Case of the Inquiring Murderer," with Kant's arguments for it being unsatisfactory. But are there any convincing arguments against the idea, apart from its being implausible?

The principal argument against absolute moral rules has to do with the possibility of conflict cases. Suppose it is held to be absolutely wrong to do A under any circumstances and also wrong to do B under any circumstances. Then what happens when a person is faced with the choice between doing A and doing B — when he must do something, and there are no other alternatives available? This case of conflict seems to show that it is *logically* untenable to hold that moral rules are absolute.

Is there any way that this objection can be met? One way would be for the absolutist to deny that such cases ever actually occur. The British philosopher P. T. Geach takes just this view. Like Kant, Geach argues that moral rules are absolute; but his reasons are very different from Kant's. Geach holds that moral rules must be understood as absolute divine commands, and so he says simply that God will not allow conflict situations to arise. We can describe fictitious cases where there is no way to avoid violating one of the absolute rules, but, he says, God will not permit such circumstances to exist in the real world.

Do such circumstances ever actually arise? "The Case of the Inquiring Murderer" is, of course, a fictitious example, but it is not difficult to find real-life examples that make the same point. During World War II, Dutch fishermen regularly smuggled Jewish refugees to England in their boats, and the following sort of thing sometimes happened. A Dutch boat, with refugees in the hold, would be stopped by a Nazi patrol boat. The Nazi captain would call out and ask the Dutch captain where he was bound, who was on board, and so forth. The fishermen would lie and be allowed to pass. Now it is clear that the fishermen had only two alternatives, to lie or to allow their passengers (and themselves) to be taken and shot.

Now suppose the two rules "It is wrong to lie" and "It is wrong to permit the murder of innocent people" are both taken to be absolute. The Dutch fishermen would have to do one of these two things; therefore, a moral view that absolutely prohibits both is incoherent. Of course, this difficulty could be avoided if one held that only one of these rules is absolute; that is, apparently Kant's way out. But this dodge cannot work in every such case; so long as there are at least two absolute rules, whatever they might be, the possibility will always exist that they might come into conflict. And that makes the view of those rules as absolute impossible to maintain.

87. The primary purpose of this passage is to
   A. discuss the role of Dutch fishermen during World War II.
   B. argue against absolute moral rules.
   C. show the difference between Kant and Geach.
   D. point out the inconsistency of moral rules.

88. The author's attitude toward Kant's position is that of
   A. agreement.
   B. disbelief.
   C. indifference.
   D. reluctant acceptance.

89. According to the author, Geach finds cases of hypothetical conflict to be
   A. irrelevant to the real world.
   B. impossible to find.
   C. unlikely to occur.
   D. proof that absolute moral rules do not exist.

90. If there are at least two absolute moral rules, the author argues that
   A. they might not come into conflict.
   B. only hypothetical cases will show potential conflict.
   C. the possibility of conflict detracts from the possibility of both being absolute.
   D. Geach's position is untenable.

PASSAGE IX (QUESTIONS 91–92)

In earlier years, during the Industrial Revolution, personnel practices of business and industry were mostly confined to hiring enough people to do the work, close supervision of employees to see that they did the work, and firing people if they did not abide by management guidelines. Labor had little influence on the system in the private sector. The management system was simple. In contrast, today's personnel practices of business and industry have become complex and subject to the influence of labor and government. Changes have occurred because society expects leaders in the private and public sectors to be sensitive to a number of social issues and to resolve difficulties that arise in the workplace.

Toward the end of the nineteenth century and early in the twentieth century, social issues were rarely considered part of the decision-making process by employers. On occasion, constituents pressed state or federal legislators to pass laws that protected the health and/or morale of employees. Immediately, the laws were challenged in court. For example, a 1923 case dealt with a law that established a board that was, among other things, authorized to determine the minimum wages of female and child workers. In that case, the Supreme Court majority stated that "adult women . . . are legally as capable of contracting for themselves as men." The law was struck down, and employer personnel practices continued to discriminate against women and children. If, in the late 1880s and early 1900s, the Supreme Court felt the legislature had overstepped constitutional boundaries, those laws were voided, and management continued its harsh policies, not only toward women and children, but also toward men.

Among the first of several court cases during the hectic years of the Industrial Revolution in America, comparison of policies showed that legislative and judicial branches were rarely unified in legal philosophy, setting national goals, and regulation policies. In a major case in 1918, the Supreme Court struck down a federal law that penalized industry when it failed to adhere to regulations that specified the ages and working hours of child employees. The children continued to work long hours. In 1923, a reporter interviewed the young man, the child plaintiff in the landmark case. At the time of the interview, the respondent was a married young man. The toll of working in a cotton mill long hours for many years had affected Reuben Dagenhart's growth and denied him the educational opportunities. His mood was somber when he told the reporter: "It would have been a good thing for all the kids in the state if that law they passed had been kept." Had Reuben read the dissenting opinion when his case was reported by the Supreme Court in 1918, he would have found that four justices also felt that the child labor law should not have been struck down. They concurred that Congress does indeed have a role in protecting the national welfare and in enforcing policy designed to "benefit . . . the nation as a whole." In contrast, the majority of the Court prevailed with a different interpretation of the Constitution and decried Congress's ulterior motive "to standardize the ages at which children may be employed . . . ."

91. Which statement best illustrates personnel management in American history?
    A. Since the beginning of the twentieth century, Congress and state legislatures have had wide latitude in correcting social ills in the private sector of business and industry.
    B. Personnel practices have been fairly stable, with little change after 1901.
    C. During the years of the Industrial Revolution, big business was highly respected by sociologists for its grave concern for the welfare of children and women employees — particularly in its standardization of working hours.
    D. Personnel management of business and industry has become increasingly complex as ideas about social welfare change.

92. What values, provided by the author, are reflected in the narrative?
    A. The author is apparently a religious person because of his emphasis on moral issues.

B. The author unfairly criticizes capitalism in the United States and is, therefore, a socialist.

C. The author unfairly criticizes justices who write dissenting opinions and, therefore, leave law unsettled.

D. The author's choice of historical facts might lead the reader to consider the motives of business and industry, such as profits, that led to hiring small children.

STOP! If time still remains, you may review work only in this section. When the time allotted is up, you may go on to the next section. STOP!

SECTION 3
Writing Sample

TIME: 60 minutes

2 essays, separately timed

30 minutes each

DIRECTIONS: This section tests your writing skills by asking you to write two essays. You will have 30 minutes to write each one.

During the first 30 minutes, work only on the first essay. If you finish it in less than 30 minutes, you may review what you have written, but do not begin the second essay. During the second 30 minutes, work only on the second essay. If you finish it in less than 30 minutes, you may review what you have written for that essay only. Do not go back to the first essay.

Read each assigned topic carefully. Make sure your essays respond to the topics as they are assigned.

Make sure your essays are written in complete sentences and paragraphs, and are as clear as you can make them. Make any corrections or additions between the lines of your essays. Do not write in the margins.

On the day of the test, you are given three pages to write each essay. You are not required to use all of the space provided, but do not skip lines so you will not waste space. Illegible essays cannot be scored.

PART 1

Consider this statement adapted from William James's "The Moral Philosopher and the Moral Life."

One could not accept a happiness shared with millions if the condition of that happiness were the suffering of one lonely soul.

Write a comprehensive essay in which you accomplish the following objectives: (1) Explain what you think the statement above means. (2) Describe a specific situation in which people *do* accept happiness based on the suffering of others. (3) Discuss the criteria under which one could find happiness without causing the suffering of others.

PART 2

Consider this statement from Jane Howard's *Families* (1978).

Good families are much to all their members, but everything to none.

Write a comprehensive essay in which you accomplish the following objectives: (1) Explain what you think the statement above means. (2) Describe a specific situation in which the good family may be everything to its members. (3) Discuss the criteria implied in the statement in order to have a "good" family, and suggest how groups other than biological or foster families may be considered families.

SECTION 4
Biological Sciences

TIME: 70 Minutes

QUESTIONS: 93–144

DIRECTIONS: Most of the questions in this section are arranged in groups, each corresponding to a descriptive passage. Based on the information given in a passage, choose the one best answer to each question in the group. Some questions are independent of a descriptive passage and of each other. Choose the one best answer to each of these questions. If you are not sure of an answer, eliminate those choices that you know are incorrect and choose an answer from among those remaining. Fill in the corresponding circle on the answer sheet to indicate your answer. You may refer to the periodic table at any time.

PASSAGE I (QUESTIONS 93–96)

It is sometimes said that the movement of molecules across cell membranes occurring in response to a concentration gradient, and termed *passive transport*, requires no metabolic energy. The term *passive transport* is misleading because no directional movement across a cell membrane can occur without the expenditure of energy by the molecules involved. If one assumes the structure of the membrane includes a lipid layer, then passage of molecules from aqueous to lipid phase, and lipid to aqueous phase, presents barriers to the molecules that can be overcome only if the molecules have appropriate energy of activation. If a molecule entering a cell has a high lipid solubility, neither its energy nor its passage through the membrane presents an obstacle. However, entry of the molecule from the membrane into the aqueous cytoplasm does present an obstacle because of the cohesive bonds it has formed with the lipid molecules of the membrane that must be broken before it can leave the membrane. If, on the other hand, a molecule entering the cell membrane is highly soluble in water, its strong hydrogen bonds with the water, in which it is dissolved outside the cell, must be broken before the molecule can enter the lipoid membrane. Its movement through the lipoid membrane also presents an obstacle. However, such a molecule readily passes from the membrane into the aqueous cytoplasm inside the cell.

Permeant	ΔH (kcal/mole)	Number of hydrogen bonds
Glycerol	24	6
Ethylene glycol	18.5	4
Diethylene glycol	18.5	4
Triethylene glycol	20.5	4
1,2,-Propandiol	19.5	4
1,3,-Propandiol	19	4
Propanol	4.5	2
Thiourea	13.5	4
Urea	6	5

93. When a molecule of high lipoidal solubility is passing through a cell membrane, what is the most energy-demanding portion of this journey?
   A. Entering the membrane from outside the cell
   B. Leaving the cell membrane, entering the cytoplasm
   C. Passing through the cell membrane
   D. Beginning movement toward the cell membrane

94. According to the table provided above, why might the transport of propanol require less energy than either of the propandiols?
   A. It lacks an -OH group.
   B. It is nonpolar.
   C. It has three carbons.
   D. It has few hydrogen bonds to break with the water.

95. Which of the following molecules would have the least problem passing through the lipoidal layer?
    A. Water
    B. Methanol
    C. Decanol
    D. Propanol

96. One can see from the table that thiourea has only one less hydrogen bond than urea to break, yet it requires 7.5kcal/mole more energy to transport. A possible explanation might be that
    A. although urea has more hydrogen bonds to break, differences in polarity between it and thiourea allow it to pass more readily through the membrane.
    B. thiourea is a larger molecule and, as a result, it requires more energy to transport a larger mass.
    C. thiourea forms a stronger hydrogen bond with water.
    D. There is no reasonable explanation for this.

PASSAGE II (QUESTIONS 97–99)

The diagram below shows a Fenn-Winterstein respirometer.

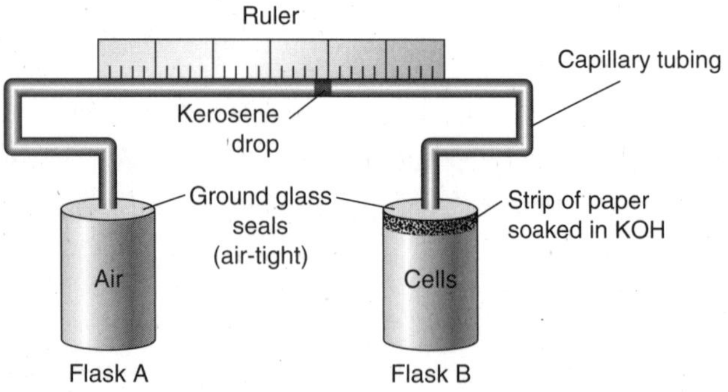

Living cells are sealed in flask B, along with a strip of paper soaked in potassium hydroxide (KOH). As the cells consume oxygen, the kerosene drop moves. If the volume of the capillary tube is known, the amount of oxygen consumed can be calculated.

97. What is the purpose of flask A, filled with air and sealed to the system?
    A. It is there in case one wishes to measure two cell cultures at once.
    B. It is there to catch the kerosene drop when it reaches the end of the tubing.
    C. It is there to cancel the effects of temperature change.
    D. Its purpose is not readily apparent.

98. Which of the following is NOT true?
    A. The above apparatus is not affected by temperature change.
    B. The above apparatus is not affected by barometric change.
    C. As oxygen is consumed, the bubble moves away from the cells.
    D. The rate the bubble moves, with regard to oxygen consumption, varies with the square of the radius of the tubing.

99. If the bubble moves 4.6mm, and the tubing has a uniform diameter of 0.20mm, how many liters of oxygen are consumed?
    A. $[(0.02/2)^{2\pi}(0.46)]/1000$
    B. $[0.2^2/2^{\pi}(4.6)]/1000$
    C. $[0.02^{2\pi} \times 4.6]/1000$
    D. $[0.2^{2\pi} \times 4.6] \times 1000$

PASSAGE III (QUESTIONS 100–102)

The spirochetes comprise a small group of non-photosynthetic and non-chemosynthetic bacteria with a very distinctive structure. Relative to their width, the helical cells are extremely long. They are capable of movement in a liquid medium by bending back and forth in broad coils and at all times retaining their fine helical structure. Reproduction is always by transverse binary fission. No resting stages are known. Some of the smaller spirochetes are so thin that they are close to the limits of resolution with the light microscope. Axial fibrils are attached to the cells' poles and wrapped around the coiled, cylindrical cell. Both the axial fibrils and the cells are surrounded by a three-layered membrane called the outer sheath. The outer sheath and axial fibrils are usually not visible by light microscopy. Depending on the type of spirochete, there are between two and more than one hundred axial fibrils present in each cell. The ultra-structure and chemical composition of the axial fibrils are similar to those of bacterial flagella. Indeed, in preserved specimens, the axial filament can become partially detached from the body of the cell and fray out into a multi-stranded structure, with the individual fibrils looking very much like eubacterial flagella. The appearance of such artifacts led early researchers to believe that some spirochetes have flagella. This is now known to be false. The free-living spirochetes are aquatic organisms, commonly found in muddy, polluted waters with low dissolved oxygen content. The largest known spirochetes live in the digestive tracts of clams and other mollusks. There is no indication that they are harmful to the mollusks. Many, but not all, of the smaller spirochetes are pathogenic and are responsible for diseases in humans and other animals.

100. What is true of all spirochetes?
   A. They are heterotrophs.
   B. They cause disease in animals.
   C. They contain axial filaments.
   D. They are heterotrophs that contain axial filaments.

101. Which statement is false about spirochetes?
   A. They have between two and more than one hundred axial fibrils.
   B. They can form spores and other vegetative stages.
   C. They do not possess flagella.
   D. Free-living spirochetes prefer brackish waters.

102. Which genus of spirochete might one be able to see without the benefit of an oil-immersion lens?
   A. *Cristispira*   B. *Spirochaeta*
   C. *Triponema*   D. *Leptospira*

QUESTIONS 103–106 are NOT based on a descriptive passage.

103. Which of the following is NOT part of a prophase chromosome?
   A. Centromere   B. Centrosome
   C. Chromatid   D. DNA

104. Albinism is a recessive trait. In a certain community of 200 people, 18 persons are albinos. How many people are normal homozygotes?
   A. 182   B. 164
   C. 100   D. 98

105. The most recent theories of the origin of life include all of the following elements in the primitive atmosphere EXCEPT
   A. free oxygen.   B. hydrogen.
   C. methane.   D. ammonia.

106. What is the product of the competing reaction of ether production through dehydration by nucleophilic substitution?
   A. Alkane   B. Alkene
   C. Alkyne   D. Alcohol

PASSAGE IV (QUESTIONS 107–111)

In the pedigree illustrated below, two autosomal, recessive traits on separate chromosomes are shown. If the top half of a figure is shaded, the individual shows trait a (possibilities: AA, Aa, aa). If the bottom half of a figure is shaded, the individual shows trait b (possibilities: BB, Bb, bb). Figures totally shaded represent individuals that show both traits, a and b. As usual, circles represent females, squares represent males, capital letters denote dominant genes, lowercase letters denote recessive genes.

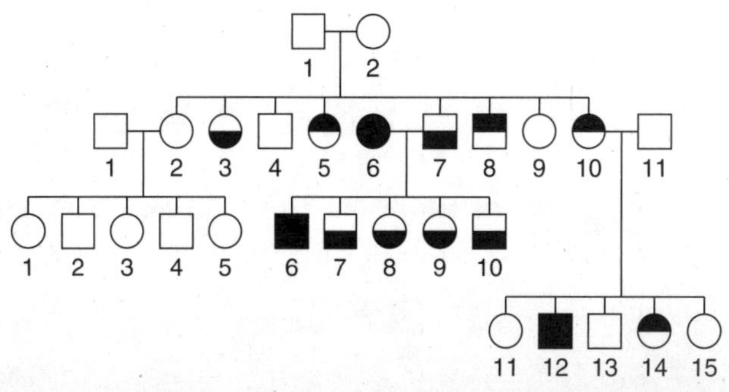

107. What is the genotype of C12?
    A. aabb
    B. AaBb
    C. AABB
    D. It cannot be determined.

108. What is the genotype of A1?
    A. aabb
    B. AaBb
    C. AABB
    D. It cannot be determined.

109. What is the genotype of B2?
    A. aabb
    B. AaBb
    C. AABB
    D. It cannot be determined.

110. What is the genotype of B11?
    A. aabb
    B. AaBb
    C. AABB
    D. It cannot be determined.

111. What are the chances of C13 being Aabb?
    A. 50%
    B. 25%
    C. 12.5%
    D. 0%

PASSAGE V (QUESTIONS 112–118)

In the pedigree shown below, trait C/c is autosomal, and trait D is on a sex-chromosome with D dominant over d, the normal condition. A figure with the upper half shaded displays trait C/c, and a figure with the lower half shaded displays trait D. A figure with both top and bottom shaded displays both traits. Assume normal mammalian sex determination. As usual, circles are females, squares are males, capital letters denote dominant genes, lowercase letters represent recessive.

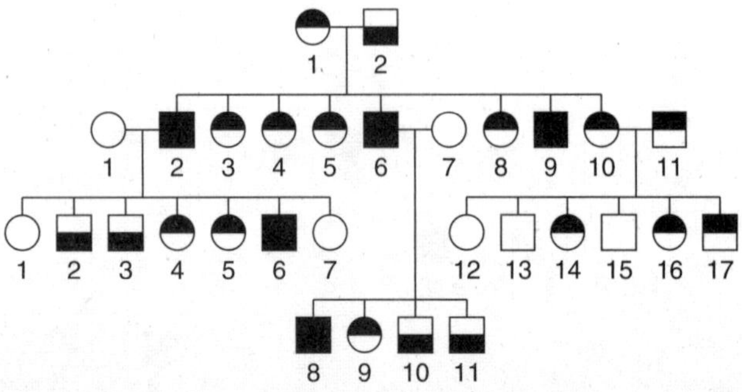

112. Trait C/c appears to be
    A. recessive.
    B. dominant.
    C. nondominant.
    D. It cannot be determined.

113. With regard to trait C/c, individual B2 must be
    A. Cc.
    B. cc.
    C. CC.
    D. It cannot be determined.

114. With respect to C/c, individual A2 must be
    A. Cc.
    B. cc.
    C. CC.
    D. It cannot be determined.

115. With respect to C/c, individual A1 must be
    A. Cc.
    B. cc.
    C. CC.
    D. It cannot be determined.

116. Trait D appears to be located on
    A. the Y chromosome.
    B. the X chromosome.
    C. both the X and Y chromosomes.
    D. It cannot be determined.

117. For trait D, individual A2 must be
    A. homozygous.
    B. heterozygous.
    C. hemizygous.
    D. It cannot be determined.

118. The genotype of C3 with respect to C/c and D must be
    A. ccDd.
    B. ccdd.
    C. ccD.
    D. It cannot be determined.

PASSAGE VI (QUESTIONS 119–122)

Cyclohexene is reacted with ozone. The product of this reaction is reacted with zinc and water to produce compound X. Cyclohexene is also reacted with $KMnO_4$ to produce compound Y.

For QUESTIONS 119 and 120, use the following choices:

A. $OHC(CH_2)_4CHO$
B. $HOOC(CH_2)_4COOH$
C. $CH_3(CH_2)_4CH_3$
D.  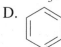

119. What is the formula for compound X?

120. What is the formula for compound Y?

121. Two ml of a 5% $AgNO_3$ solution is mixed with a drop of a 10% NaOH solution and a few drops of a 2% NH_4OH solution. If this is mixed with compound X, what will most likely happen?
A. NH_3 gas will be evolved.
B. The Ag will precipitate.
C. No reaction will occur.
D. NH_3 gas will be evolved, and the Ag will precipitate.

122. If compound X were reacted with $KMnO_4$, what product will be formed?
A. Product Y
B. There will be no further reaction.
C. $CH_3(CH_2)_4CH_3$
D. 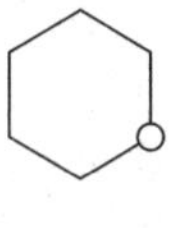

PASSAGE VII (QUESTIONS 123–125)

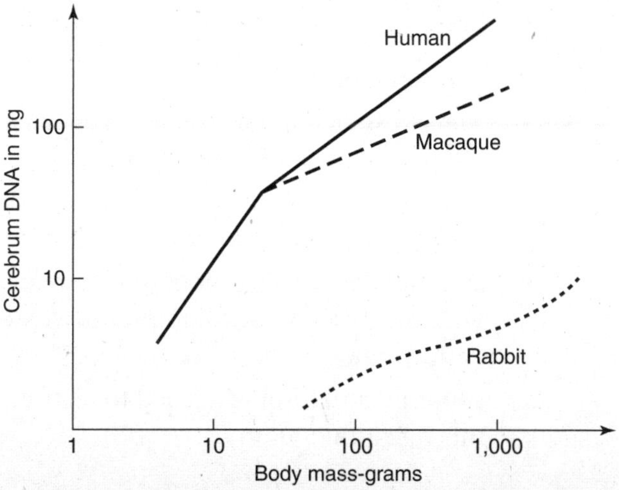

123. What is the maximum body weight where humans and macaques have the same ratio of cerebrum DNA to body weight?
A. 10 grams B. 15 grams
C. 35 grams D. 50 grams

124. In obtaining this data, what is the most important factor listed below to limit experimental error?
A. The amount of time elapsed between the killing of the animals and the extraction and measurement of their DNA
B. The diet of the animals before they were killed
C. The temperature at which the animals were kept while alive
D. The amount of RNA present in the cells

125. Where did the data in the 10-gram region on this graph come from for humans?
A. The curve is extrapolated from heavier specimens.
B. Although a person cannot weigh 10 grams, a cerebrum can.
C. The graph contains fetal data.
D. The line for humans does not go down to 10 grams.

QUESTIONS 126–129 are NOT based on a descriptive passage.

126. The nucleotide base sequence for a short section of double-stranded DNA is given below. What is the anticodon for the section of DNA that is boxed and shown in bold lettering?

5′	A	T	C	G	C	A	C	G	G	T	A	A	3′
3′	T	A	G	C	G	T	G	C	C	A	T	T	5′

A. G C A B. C G T
C. G C U D. C G U

127. In humans, which of the following is NOT contained in chromatin?
A. Histone proteins
B. DNA
C. Ribosomes
D. Nonhistone proteins

128. Which of the following items is NOT part of the human ear?
   A. Tectorial membrane
   B. Cochlea
   C. Hyoid
   D. Oval window

129. The fovea consists of
   A. equal amounts of rods and cones.
   B. more rods than cones.
   C. more cones than rods.
   D. no rods.

PASSAGE VIII (QUESTIONS 130–134)

Experiment 1:

75 grams of fresh potatoes and 500 ml of water were homogenized in a blender. Three drops of this "potato juice" were each added to: plain water, a dextrose solution, a sodium chloride solution, and a solution of pyrocathechol. After five minutes, all of the solutions remained colorless except for the pyrocathechol, which had turned yellow.

Experiment 2:

Three solutions of pyrocathechol of the same concentration were kept either on ice (0°), at room temperature (25°), or in boiling water (100°). Keeping them at these temperatures and adding three drops of the above "potato juice" to each solution gave the following results within five minutes: solution on ice — faint yellow; solution at room temperature — yellow; solution in boiling water — still colorless.

Experiment 3:

Solutions of equal concentrations of pyrocathechol were adjusted to have pH values of 4, 7, or 10. When three drops of the above "potato juice" were added at room temperature to each solution, within five minutes the solution at pH 4 was dark yellow, the solution at pH 7 was faint yellow, and the solution at pH 10 was still colorless.

Experiment 4:

Four test tubes were set up containing a pyrocathechol solution of the same concentration. Twenty drops of phenylthiourea were added to the first tube, ten drops were added to the second tube, and only one drop was added to the third tube. No phenylthiourea was added to the fourth tube. Three drops of the above "potato juice" were added to each of the above tubes. Within five minutes, the fourth tube had turned yellow, the third tube was slightly yellow, the second tube was very slightly yellow, and the first tube remained colorless.

130. The material in the potato juice that causes the pyrocathechol solutions to turn yellow is most likely a(n)
   A. enzyme.
   B. protein.
   C. catalyst.
   D. enzyme, protein, and catalyst.

131. The optimal pH for the substance in potato juice is
   A. 7.
   B. 4.
   C. 3.
   D. somewhere in the acidic range.

132. If the potato juice was boiled for ten minutes, cooled to room temperature, and then added to a pyrocathechol solution, within five minutes the solution would
   A. remain colorless.
   B. turn pale yellow.
   C. turn yellow.
   D. turn a color other than yellow.

133. When phenylthiourea was added to the pyrocathechol solution, it acted as a(n)
   A. substrate.
   B. enzyme.
   C. inhibitor.
   D. coloring agent.

134. Which statement is true?
   A. The substance in the potato juice causes the pyrocathechol to turn yellow.
   B. The substance in the potato juice aids the pyrocathechol in turning yellow.
   C. The substance in the potato juice reacts with the pyrocathechol to produce a yellow color.
   D. More information is needed to answer this question.

PASSAGE IX (QUESTIONS 135–138)

Eleven-week-old mice were given 800 rads of X-irradiation. Half of the mice were then inoculated with 2×10^6 fetal liver cells from a 12½- to 13½-day gestation mouse embryo. The fetal liver cells were given within a few hours after irradiation. The graph below shows the number of B cells found in the spleen at various times after irradiation. The remaining mice received no further treatment after irradiation. The number of B cells found in their spleen is also shown on the graph.

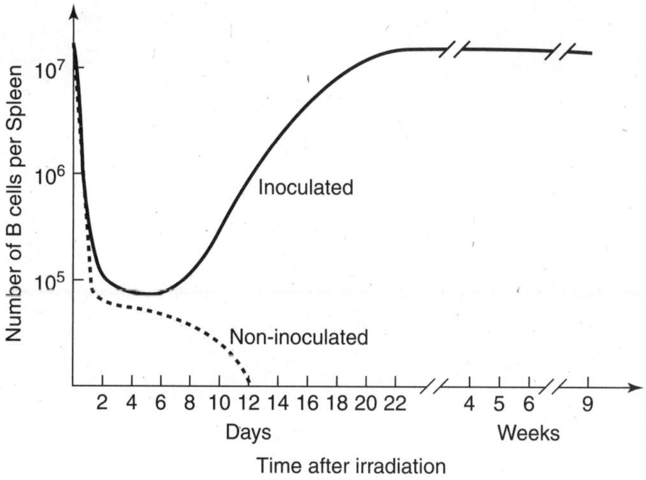

135. How long do the noninoculated mice seem to live after irradiation?
   A. No more than 12 days
   B. 12 days
   C. At least 12 days
   D. It cannot be determined from this graph.

136. In the treated group, how long does it take for the B cells in the spleen to reach half of their pre-irradiated level?
   A. 10 days
   B. 16 days
   C. 18 days
   D. 22 days

137. How long do the inoculated mice seem to live after irradiation?
   A. At least 9 weeks
   B. 9 weeks
   C. No more than 9 weeks
   D. It cannot be determined from this graph.

138. An analysis of the fetal liver cells injected into the mice shows that they contain no B cells. What is the most probable explanation for the observed regeneration of B cells?
   A. The fetal liver cells repair the radiation damage.
   B. The fetal liver cells contain a stem-cell precursor that matures into a B cell.
   C. There was an error in the analysis of the fetal liver cells; they must contain B cells.
   D. There is no explanation for this.

PASSAGE X (QUESTIONS 139–142)

Experiment 1:

A student heats 3-methyl-2-butanol in HBr. The reaction generates a single product. However, NMR spectroscopy reveals that the product was not the expected 2-bromo-3-methylbutane, but instead 2-bromo-2-methylbutane.

Experiment 2:

The student notes that if 2-methyl-3-pentanol is treated with concentrated H_2SO_4 at 107°C, the major product is 2-methyl-2-pentene. He also notes that small amounts of 2-methyl-pentene are also formed, as are trace amounts of 4-methyl-2-pentene.

Experiment 3:

The student reacts (2R, 3R) 3-methyl-3-d-2-butanol with hot HBr. The major product is a racemic mixture of 2-bromo-2-methyl-3-deuteriobutane. A small amount of (3R) 2-bromo-3-methyl-3-deuteriobutane is also produced.

139. The production of 2-bromo-2-methylbutane from 3-methyl-2-butanol in hot HBr is an example of what kind of reaction?
   A. S_n2
   B. E_2
   C. Carbocation rearrangement
   D. Carbanion rearrangement

140. In the reaction described above, why is 2-bromo-2-methylbutane the major product?
A. Tertiary carbanions are more stable than secondary carbanions.
B. Secondary carbocations are more stable than primary carbocations.
C. Secondary carbocations are less stable than tertiary carbocations.
D. Via a S_n2 reaction, Br^- attacks the 3-carbon. The hydroxyl group is simultaneously protonated, with the net effect of a loss of one molecule of H_2O per molecule of reactant.

141. What did the experiment with 3-methyl-3-D-2-butanol reveal?
A. The reaction is a S_n2 reaction.
B. There is a carbocation intermediate.
C. The hydrogen on the 3-carbon is the migration species.
D. There is a carbocation intermediate, and the hydrogen on the 3-carbon is the migration species.

142. In Experiment 2, if the student had used 2-methyl-2-pentanol instead of 2-methyl-3-pentanol, what would be the distribution of products?
A. The major product would be 2-methyl-1-pentene with a small amount of 2-methyl-2-pentene.
B. The major product would be 4-methyl-2-pentene plus a small amount of 2-methyl-2-pentene.
C. There would be no reaction. Tertiary alcohols are unreactive under these conditions.
D. The distribution of products would be very similar.

QUESTIONS 143–144 are NOT based on a descriptive passage.

143. The first stage of embryonic development, in which three distinct germ layers are seen, is the
A. morula.
B. gastrula.
C. blastula.
D. embryo.

144. The greatest similarity in structure occurs between members belonging to the same
A. class.
B. phylum.
C. family.
D. species.

STOP!

If time still remains, you may review work only in this section. When the time allotted is up, you may go on to the next section.

STOP!

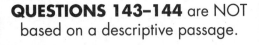

Test 2 ■ Answer Key

1. B
2. D
3. C
4. D
5. A
6. C
7. C
8. C
9. D
10. A
11. D
12. C
13. C
14. D
15. A
16. C
17. C
18. B
19. A
20. D
21. C
22. D
23. D
24. C
25. B
26. C
27. A
28. B
29. B
30. C
31. D
32. A
33. B
34. A
35. D
36. D
37. D
38. B
39. A
40. B
41. B
42. D
43. C
44. D
45. B
46. D
47. D
48. B
49. B
50. C
51. C
52. A
53. C
54. C
55. C
56. C
57. D
58. B
59. A
60. A
61. D
62. B
63. B
64. D
65. D
66. B
67. D
68. B
69. A
70. A
71. D
72. D
73. A
74. C
75. A
76. D
77. C
78 D
79. B
80. B
81. B
82. C
83. C
84. C
85. A
86. B
87. B
88. B
89. A
90. C
91. D
92. D
93. B
94. D
95. C
96. A
97. C
98. C
99. A
100. D
101. B
102. B
103. B
104. D
105. A
106. B
107. A
108. B
109. D
110. B
111. D
112. B
113. A
114. B
115. D
116. A
117. C
118. C
119. A
120. B
121. B
122. A
123. C
124. A
125. C
126. D
127. C
128. C
129. C
130. D
131. D
132. A
133. C
134. B
135. A
136. C
137. A
138. B
139. C
140. C
141. D
142. D
143. B
144. D

SECTION 1
Physical Sciences

PASSAGE I (QUESTIONS 1–4)

1. **B.** Gravitational potential energy is equal to mass times height times g.

$$PE = gmh = (9.8 \text{ m/s}^2)(2000\text{kg})(50\text{m})$$
$$= (9.8)(100{,}000) \text{ N}$$
$$= 980 \text{ kN}$$

2. **D.** By conservation of energy, PE = KE

$$PE_1 = gmh_1 = KE_1 = 1/2mv^2$$
$$v_1 = \sqrt{2gh_1}$$
$$PE_2 = mgh_2 = mg1/2h_1 = KE_2 = mv_2^2$$
$$v_2 = \sqrt{gh_1} = v_1/\sqrt{2}$$

Therefore, the velocity has been decreased by a factor of $\sqrt{2}$.

3. **C.** By conservation of energy, the potential energy at point A must be equal to or greater than the potential energy at point C.

$$mgh_A \geq mgh_C \quad \text{therefore hA} \geq h_c$$

Therefore, the minimum height at A is equal to the height at C, which is 55m.

4. **D.** Newton's Third Law applies everywhere there is a force.

PASSAGE II (QUESTIONS 5–7)

5. **A.** $\left(\frac{1}{C_1+C_2}+\frac{1}{C_3}\right)^{-1} = \left(\frac{1}{2\mu F}+\frac{1}{3\mu F}\right)^{-1}$

$$= \left(\frac{3}{6}+\frac{2}{6}\right)^{-1} = \left(\frac{5}{6}\right)^{-1} = \frac{6}{5}\mu F = 1.2\mu F$$

6. **C.** If C_2 is removed, then essentially the circuit is two capacitors in series with an equivalent capacitance given by

$$\frac{1}{C} = \frac{1}{C_1}+\frac{1}{C_3} = \frac{C_1C_3}{C_1+C_3} = \frac{(20\mu F)(5\mu F)}{(20+5)\mu F}$$
$$= 4\mu F$$

Knowing that $q = CV$ for C_3, we observe that

$$q = (4 \times 10^{-6} \text{ F})(100 \text{ V}) = 4.0 \times 10^{-4}\text{C}$$

The other three answers are incorrect.

Answer choice A is true only if you forgot how to calculate either the overall capacitance or the charge ($q = CV$).

Answer choice B is obtained if you used $C = C_1 + C_3 = 25$ mF and calculate q from this value for capacitance.

$$q = (25 \times 10^{-6} \text{ F})(100 \text{ V}) = 2.5 \times 10^{-3}C$$

Answer choice D is obtained only if you used $C = C_3$ for the capacitance.

$$q = (5 \times 10^{-6} \text{ F})(100 \text{ V}) = 5 \times 10^{-4}C$$

7. **C.** For the resistors in series, the formula for equivalence resistance is $R_{eq} = R_1 + R_2 = 100 + 100 = 200\ \Omega$. After that, solve for the two R_{eq} in parallel with the formula

$$\frac{1}{R} = \frac{1}{R_1}+\frac{1}{R_2} = \frac{R_2+R_1}{R_2R_1}$$

$$R = \frac{R_2R_1}{R_2+R_1} = \frac{(200)(200)}{200+200} = 100\,\Omega$$

The other three answers are incorrect.

Answer choice A is obtained if you simply add all four resistors together.

$$(4)(100\ \Omega) = 400\ \Omega$$

Answer choice B is obtained if you calculate $1/R$ instead of R.

$$\frac{1}{R} = \frac{200 + 200}{(200)(200)} = 1.0 \times 10^{-2}\Omega$$

Answer choice D is obtained if you calculate in parallel resistors (R) with the wrong number.

$$Re\,g = \frac{R_2R_1}{R_2 + R_1} = \frac{(100)(100)}{100 + 100} = 50\,\Omega$$

PASSAGE III (QUESTIONS 8–10)

8. **C.** When the object's distance is much greater than the radius of curvature, then the 1/s term is negligible (≈ 0).

$$\frac{1}{s} + \frac{1}{s'} \approx \frac{1}{s'} = \frac{2}{r}$$

$$\therefore \frac{r}{2} = s'$$

The other three answers are incorrect.

Answer choice A yields a non-negligible *s* term, and the equation *cannot* be further reduced.

Answer choice B yields a value of $\frac{1}{s} + \frac{1}{s'} \approx \infty$.

Answer choice D leads to a non-negligible *s* term, and the equation *cannot* be reduced further.

9. **D.** A negative sign in the magnification term tells you that an image has been inverted. The other three answers are incorrect; answer choice A would be true if the magnification term were <1.0; and B and C are a reference to the value of s', not m.

10. **A.** Using the equations in the passage with the information allows for solution by simply plugging in the numbers. (Note: r_1 and r_2 have different signs because it's a *double* convex lens.)

$$\frac{1}{f} = (n-1)\left(\frac{1}{r1} - \frac{1}{r2}\right)$$

$$= (2-1)\left(\frac{1}{25} - \left(-\frac{1}{25\text{cm}}\right)\right) = \frac{2}{25}\text{cm}$$

$$\therefore f = 12.5\,\text{cm}$$

The other three answers are incorrect.

Answer choice B is obtained if you don't subtract 1 from the index of refraction value.

$$\frac{1}{f} = (2)\left(\frac{1}{25} - \left(-\frac{1}{25\text{cm}}\right)\right) = \frac{1}{25}\text{cm}$$

Answer choice C is obtained if you don't realize that $r_1 = -r_2$, thus giving $\frac{1}{r_1} - \frac{1}{r_2} = 0$ Therefore, $1/f = 0$ or f would be undefined.

Answer choice D is obtained if you calculate $1/f$, not f, which is

$$\frac{1}{50}\text{cm or } 0.020\text{cm}$$

11. **D.** According to Newton's law of inertia, a body in motion tends to move in a straight line. To change straight-line motion into circular motion, an outside force must constantly pull the body toward the center of rotation. Such a central force is called a centripetal force.

12. **C.**

Work = Force × distance

We know the distance is 10 meters. We must, however, find F. We use the relationship:

F = mass × acceleration

$a = 9.8\text{m/sec}^2$

$m = 25\text{kg}$

$F = (25\text{kg})\,(9.8\text{m/sec}^2)$

$F = 245.0\text{kg} \times \text{m/sec}^2 = 245.0$ newtons

Now, we can substitute into the first equation:

Work = 245.0 N × 10m = 2450 N × m = 2450 joules

13. **C.** Setting up a ratio between the two similar triangles:

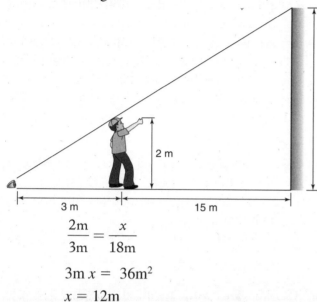

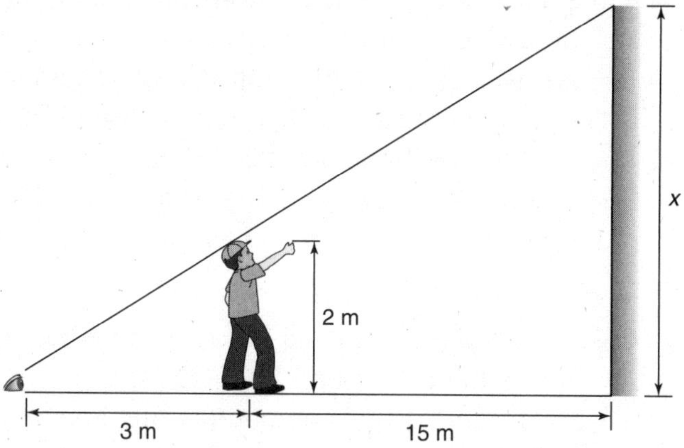

$$\frac{2\text{m}}{3\text{m}} = \frac{x}{18\text{m}}$$

$3\text{m}\,x = 36\text{m}^2$

$x = 12\text{m}$

The height of the shadow is 12 meters.

PASSAGE IV (QUESTIONS 14–16)

14. **D.** Using $\tau = Tr$ to get τ and then putting that value into the equation will yield the solution.

$\tau = (10\text{N})\,(.25\text{m}) = 2.5\text{N} \times \text{m}$

$P = \tau \times \omega = (2.5\text{N} \times \text{m})\,(3.13 \times 10^3 \text{ rad/s})$

$P = 7.8 \times 10^3 \text{ W}$

The other three answers are incorrect.

Answer choice A is obtained if you multiply the answer from D by the time (wrong units).

$P = (7.8 \times 10^3 \text{ W})(20 \text{ sec})$
$= 1.6 \times 10^5 \text{ N} \times \text{m}$

Answer choice B is obtained if you mistakenly use 10N as the applied torque (wrong units).

$P = (10\text{N})(3.13 \times 10^3 \text{ rad/s})$
$= 3.11 \times 10^4 \text{ N/s}$

Answer choice C is obtained if you miscalculate τ by not changing to *m*.

$\tau = (10\text{N})(25\text{cm}) = 250\text{N} \times \text{cm}$

$P = (250\text{N} \times \text{cm})(3.13 \times 10^3 \text{ rad/s})$
$= 7.8 \times 10^5\text{N} \times \text{cm/s}$

15. **A.** Again, simply use the equation given and the values in the passage.

$\tau = TR = (10\text{N})(.25\text{m}) = 2.5\text{N} \times \text{m}$

The other three answers are incorrect.

Answer choice B is obtained if you do not change to meters (wrong units).

$\tau = (10\text{N}) \times 25\text{cm} = 250\text{N} \times \text{cm}$

Answer choice C is obtained if you solve for *T* by dividing by *r* (units are wrong for t).

$$\tau = \frac{10\text{N}}{0.25\text{N}} = 4.0 \times 10^1 \text{Nm}^{-1}$$

Answer choice D is obtained if you make the same mistake as in C and also did not convert to meters.

$$\tau = \frac{10\text{N}}{25\text{cm}} = 4.0 \times 10^1 \text{Ncm}^{-1}$$

16. **C.** Angular acceleration is

$$\frac{v^2}{r} = \left(\frac{200\text{km}}{hr}\right)^2.$$

$$40\text{km} = \frac{40{,}000\text{km}^2}{hr^2}$$

$$40\text{km} = \frac{1.000\text{km}^2}{hr^2}$$

PASSAGE V (QUESTIONS 17–20)

17. **C.**

$$mg_E = G\frac{mM_E}{R_E^2} \Rightarrow g_E = G\frac{M_E}{R_E^2} \Rightarrow g_x = \frac{M_x}{R_X^2}$$

$$g_x = \frac{7}{8} \times \frac{19}{9} \times G\frac{M_E}{R_E^2} = \frac{14}{9}\frac{M_E}{R_E^2} = \frac{14}{9}g$$

18. **B.** Planet X has a smaller radius and is therefore smaller. It has 7/8 the mass of earth contained in only 3/4 the radius; i.e., it has more fractional mass than 3/4 of the earth. Therefore, it is denser.

19. **A.** Force equals mass times acceleration:

$$18\text{kg} \times \frac{10}{9} \times \frac{9.8\text{m}}{s^2} = (20)(9.8)\text{N} = 19.6\text{N}$$

20. **D.** The period of a spring is $T = 2\pi\sqrt{\frac{m}{k}}$, independent of gravity. Therefore, $T_x = 1(T_E)$

PASSAGE VI (QUESTIONS 21–25)

21. **C.** Three phases exist at both points *F* (solid phase I, solid phase II, and liquid) and *E* (solid phase I, liquid, and gas). The other three answers are incorrect. Answer choice A: Point *F* is a triple point, but so is point *E*. Answer choice B: Point *E* is a triple point, but so is Point *F*. Answer choice D: Point *G* is *not* a triple point.

22. **D.** At point *G*, the distinction between liquid and gas breaks down. This is known as the critical point and occurs at 450 K. The other three answers are incorrect. Answer choice A is at point *H* and is well above the critical temperature; and B and C are well below the critical temperature (several phases exist depending on the pressure).

23. **D.** You start in solid phase I, cross the equilibrium line, and finish in the liquid phase of our material. The other three answers are incorrect because answer choice A occurs only if we cross at a point below 150atm; B can occur only if we elevate the pressure at the temperature given in the problem; and in C, the solid does indeed melt but does not cross the equilibrium barrier to become a gas.

24. **C.** We've never left the liquid phase according to our phase diagram. The other three answers are incorrect because in answer choice A, we don't cross into the gas phase by increasing the pressure; and in B and D, we don't cross into either of the solid phases during these changes.

25. **B.** Going directly from a solid to a gaseous phase is by definition called sublimation. The other three answers are incorrect. Answer choice A: Fusion is the process of bringing atoms together; sublimation is the process of breaking them apart. Answer choice C: Melting is going from a solid to a liquid. Answer choice D: Boiling is going from a liquid to a gas.

26. **C.** When dissolved in water, Na_2CO_3 forms the compound $NaHCO_3$ and sodium hydroxide. Both compounds are alkaline. For example,

$$Na_2CO_3 + H_2O \rightarrow NaHCO_3 + NaOH$$

C is therefore the correct choice here.

27. **A.** The work required to move a charge through a potential difference is equal to the product of the potential difference and the charge,

$$\begin{aligned} \text{Work} &= Vq \\ &= (5 \text{ volts})(2 \text{ coulombs}) \\ &= 10 \text{ joules} \end{aligned}$$

28. **B.** Diffraction is the tendency of a wave to spread into a region behind an obstruction. This also includes a tendency of a wave to spread out when passing through a small aperture.

PASSAGE VII (QUESTIONS 29–33)

29. **B.** This is a strong acid; i.e., the dissociation is complete, so the pH = 5.

30. **C.** This is a strong base; i.e., the dissociation is complete, so the pOH = 5, and the pH = 14–pOH = 9.

31. **D.** Solution III is a weak acid with a pH = 5, so the titration starts at a pH near 5

and then has a maximum pH of 9 (i.e., the pH of solution II).

32. **A.** Solution IV is made of a weak base that does not completely dissociate.

$$k_h = \frac{x^2}{M - x} \Rightarrow x^2 + K_h x - Mk_h = 0$$

$$x = \frac{-k_h \pm \sqrt{k_h^2 + 4Mk_h}}{2}$$

$$x = \frac{-(4\times10^{-2}) \pm \sqrt{(4\times10^{-2})^2 + 4(4\times10^{-2})(5.625\times10^{-3})}}{2}$$

$$x = \frac{-(4\times10^{-2}) \pm \sqrt{(16\times10^{-4}) + 4(22.5\times10^{-5})}}{2}$$

$$x = \frac{-(4\times10^{-2}) \pm \sqrt{(16\times10^{-4}) + (9\times10^{-4})}}{2}$$

$$x = \frac{-(4\times10^{-2}) \pm \sqrt{(25\times10^{-4})}}{2}$$

$$x = \frac{-(4\times10^{-2}) \pm 5\times10^{-2}}{2} = 0.005 \text{ or } = -0.0045$$

$x = 5 \times 10^{-3}$ and $\log(5 \times 10^{-3}) = -2.3$. Therefore, the pOH = –2.3. However, we can have only positive concentrations; therefore, the pOH = 2.3.

33. **B.** Solution I is at pH of 5, so start in the middle of the graph, then follow the titration up to the maximum value of pH of solution IV (pH = 14 – pOH = 11.7).

PASSAGE VIII (QUESTIONS 34–36)

34. **A.** Sulfur has six valence e^-, and each fluorine will donate one e^- to pair with one e^- on the sulfur. Four e^- on sulfur will form the bonds, and there will be one e^- pair left over. The other three answers are incorrect because in answer choice B, the extra two electrons are not shown; in C, an extra two electrons are shown that do not belong; and in D, two extra electron pairs are shown that do not belong.

35. **D.** To put five electron pairs around sulfur (four bonding pairs and one lone pair), we start with a trigonal bipyramid structure and place the lone pair of electrons in a more stable equatorial position. This yields the see-saw structure.

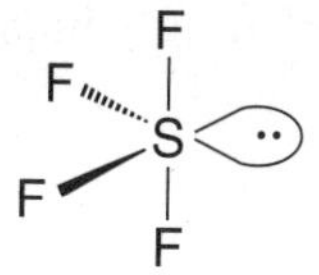

The other three answers are incorrect because, in answer choice A, the lone pair would push the other S-F bonds out of plane if square planar was exhibited; in B, tetrahedral also doesn't take into account the lone pair of e^-; and in C, you can't see the lone pair of e^-, so only the one point in the trigonal plane would be observed.

36. **D.** Boron is one of the elements in Group IIIA and has the valence electron configuration $2s^2 2p^1$. The boron atom hybridizes from its ground state as follows:

2p ↿ – – energy 2p ↿ ↿ – – → 2p –

2x ⥮ 2s ↿ sp^2 ↿ ↿ ↿

The hybrid orbitals are composed of one original s orbital and two original p orbitals. Therefore, the hybridization is sp^2.

PASSAGE IX (QUESTIONS 37–40)

37. **D.** Use the following calculation:

$$A_p v_p = A_d v_d$$

$$\frac{v_p}{v_d} = \frac{A_d}{A_p} = \frac{pr_d^3}{pr_p^2} = \frac{r_d^3}{r_p^2} = \frac{4^2}{2^2} = \frac{16}{4} = 4$$

38. **B.**

$$P_1 + r_1 g h_1 = P_2 + r_2 g h_2$$

$$P_2 = P_1 + r_1 g h_1 - r_2 g h_2 = 1atm + 0 - (1000kg/m^3)(10m/s^2)(-500m)$$

$$P_2 = 1atm + (10^3)(5 \times 10^3)(N/m) = 1atm + (5 \times 10^6)(N/m)$$

$$P_2 = 1atm + 500atm = 501atm$$

39. **A.** Density equals mass per volume.

$$\frac{r_f}{r_i} = \frac{mv_i}{mv_f} = \frac{v_i}{v_f} = \frac{Ah_i}{AH_f} = \frac{h_i}{h_f} = \frac{\frac{1}{3}}{\frac{1}{6}}$$

$$= \frac{6}{3} = 2$$

40. **B.** The power plant produces:

$$\frac{4 \times 10^5 l}{\text{month}} \times \frac{10^2 \text{kW}}{l} = \frac{4 \times 10^7 \text{kW}}{\text{month}}$$

The town uses: $\frac{3 \times 10^7 \text{kW}}{\text{month}}$

So the plant can store:

$$\frac{4 \times 10^7 \text{ kW}}{\text{month}} = \frac{3 \times 10^7 \text{kW}}{\text{month}} \frac{1 \times 10^7 \text{kW}}{\text{month}}$$

In nine months, this will add up to 9×10^7 kW.

But in three months the town uses: $3 \times 3 \times 10^7$ kW. Therefore, the power plant has barely enough power to supply the town.

PASSAGE X (QUESTIONS 41–45)

41. **B.** An ideal gas expansion/contraction at constant temperature follows Boyle's Law.

42. **D.** Boyle's Law:

$$\frac{V_1}{V_2} = \frac{P_2}{P_1} \Rightarrow V_2 = V_1 \frac{P_1}{P_2}$$

$$V_2 = 10l \frac{1atm}{4atm} = \frac{10}{4} l = 2.5l$$

43. **C.** An ideal gas expansion/contraction at constant pressure follows Charles' Law. It states that the volume of a given amount of dry ideal gas is directly proportional to the Kelvin temperature, provided the amount of gas and the pressure remain fixed.

44. **D.** Charles' Law:

$$\frac{V_1}{T_1} = \frac{V_2}{T_2} \Rightarrow V_2 = \frac{V_1}{T_1} T_2$$

$$V_2 = \frac{20l}{318K} 291K = 18l$$

45. **B.** Ideal Gas Law:

$$\frac{P_1V_1}{T_1} = \frac{P_2V_2}{T_2} \Rightarrow \frac{P_2}{T_2} = \frac{P_1V_1}{T_1V_2}$$

$$\frac{P_2}{T_2} = \frac{2atm \times 2l}{293K \times 5L} = \frac{4atm}{1500K} = \frac{1atm}{375K}$$

PASSAGE XI (QUESTIONS 46–50)

46. **D.** Nitrogen has the lowest heat of fusion and therefore the weakest bonds. Nitrogen is formed by Van der Waals bonding, which is the weakest bond.

47. **D.** Of these choices, barium oxide has the highest heat of fusion and therefore the strongest bonds. Barium oxide is formed by ionic bonding, which is the strongest bond.

48. **B.** Carbon has six electrons that must fill the lowest energy shells first. If you have trouble with this, remember that the periodic table is structured very closely according to the electron shells.

49. **B.** Use the following equation:

$$grams = \frac{energy}{heat_{fusion}} = \frac{466cal}{93.2cal/g} \approx \frac{500}{100}$$

$$= 5g < 10g$$

50. **C.** The oxidation number of any atom bonded with itself is zero.

51. **C.** When the center of negative charge does not coincide with the center of positive charge in a molecule, it is said to be polar. The molecule constitutes a dipole: two equal and opposite charges separated

in space. The molecule possesses a dipole moment that is equal to the magnitude of the charge multiplied by the distance between the centers of charge.

In (E) 1, 2-dibromoethene,

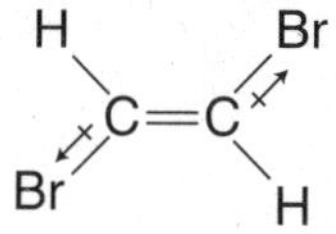

the dipole moment is zero; the individual bonds are polar but because of the symmetrical arrangement, they cancel each other out exactly. So the dipole moment of a molecule depends not only on the polarity of its individual bonds but also on the way the bonds are directed, that is, on the shape of the molecule. In carbon tetrachloride,

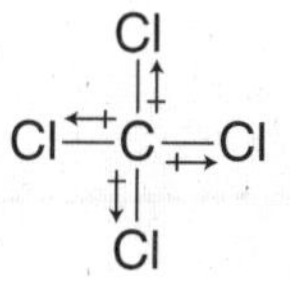

the individual bonds are also polar, but they cancel each other out because of the symmetrical arrangement of the molecule.

In (Z)-1, 2-dichloroethene,

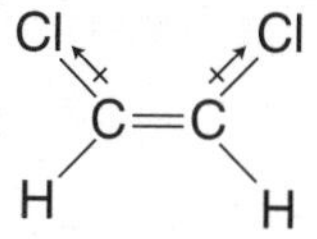

the individual bonds are polar and do not cancel each other out by the symmetrical arrangement of the dipoles. Therefore, Z-1, 2-dichloroethene has a net dipole moment.

52. **A.** Refraction bends the most energetic waves, i.e., those with the shortest wavelengths are bent the most. Red light has very long wavelengths.

SECTION 2
Verbal Reasoning

PASSAGE I (QUESTIONS 53–57)

This passage describes the trial of Socrates, as it is presented in Plato's *Apology*. It provides Socrates' explanation of his philosophical activity and his defense against the charges of heresy and corrupting the youth. The passage suggests why this philosopher and this description of his life have become classic archetypes of the conflict between wisdom and authority in the Western heritage.

53. **C.** Paragraphs 1 to 3 show how Socrates offends his jury three times even before he refutes the charges. His appeal to simple speech rejects the custom of flowery, emotional appeals in court; his reference to past accusers affecting the jurors in their youth calls into question their fair judgment; and his calling the formal charges a pretext for the real charge of embarrassing the establishment discredits the whole Athenian legal system.

54. **C.** Socrates' logical refutation of Meletus' charges by showing their internal inconsistency shows that consistency is a measure of authenticity and not a characteristic of small minds (answer choice A), false charges (answer choice B), or necessarily a court of law (answer choice D).

55. **C.** The fact that a guilty verdict follows in spite of Socrates' disapproval of the charges against him shows that reason does not always triumph (answer choice B). Because he refuted the charge of corrupting the youth, answer choice A is not correct, and a Supreme Court (answer choice D) is not mentioned.

56. **C.** The key here is that Socrates' alternative penalty of a state pension is either an insult or a proper reward, depending on who is involved. For the Athenians offended by his philosophical activity, it is an insult; to Socrates, who conducts his philosophical activity out of love for Athens in an attempt to improve it, it is a suitable compensation.

57. **D.** The essential lesson of Socrates' life, thus explaining its enduring appeal, is that all established authority resents criticism. That courts are corrupt (answer choice A), defendants are intellectual (answer choice B), or juries are youthful (answer choice C) is not relevant to that essential lesson.

PASSAGE II (QUESTIONS 58–61)

This passage describes the basic nature of the American federal system. It provides various interpretations of the relationship between national and state governments within federalism and some of the consequences of such a political system.

58. **B.** In the first paragraph, it is stated that James Madison saw the advantage of federalism as the distribution of power among several bodies, thereby preventing tyranny. Categorical grants (answer choice A) did not appear until the 1860s; the right to secede (answer choice C) and the right to retain slavery (answer choice D) were not primary components of Madison's plan.

59. **A.** Because the compact theory allows states to secede, the conclusion of the Civil War, which forced the Southern states to remain in the Union, would be considered unjust. It would not be considered just (answer choice B), inevitable (answer choice D), or merely a mistake (answer choice C).

60. **A.** By returning authority and funding to the states, Reagan's policy endorsed the compact theory. Judicial federalism (answer choice B) does not exist. Dual federalism (answer choice C) calls for shared responsibility for the social programs discontinued by Reaganism. Cooperative federalism (answer choice D) is rejected by this approach.

61. **D.** Every other pair has one incorrect characteristic: authoritarian (answer choice A), permanent (B), and undefined (C).

PASSAGE III (QUESTIONS 62–66)

This essay summarizes the political ideas in Plato's *Republic*: his division of the soul into three elements or dispositions with corresponding classes in society. It discusses some of the characteristics of Plato's thought that conflict with twentieth-century political ideas.

62. **B.** A business entrepreneur's interest in the production and distribution of goods or money and his primary motive for making a profit would place him or her in the appetitive category. The philosophic (answer choice A) loves knowledge for its own sake, while the spirited (answer choice C) loves military exploit. The innovative (answer choice D) is not one of Plato's categories.

63. **B.** Jefferson's assumption of human equality contrasts most sharply with Plato's belief in innate inequality. The revolutionary sentiments of answer choice A do not address the issue of class differences. Answer choice C about "federalists" also does not discuss class differences. The idea of a natural aristocracy (answer choice D) agrees with Plato's views on class differences.

64. **D.** The knowledge of the virtue appropriate to each class in society constitutes the philosopher's wisdom and qualifies him or her for a role in government. Answer choices A, B, and C detail the virtues of other classes (philosophic, spirited, appetitive, respectively).

65. **D.** Plato's "myth of the metals" is premised on a "noble lie" (paragraph 4) that suggests that maintaining the "just order" is more important than always telling the truth. Courage (answer choice A) and honor (answer choice C) are military virtues; moderation (answer choice B) is an appetitive virtue.

66. **B.** By appealing to material incentives for army recruiting, that country is applying appetitive or economic rather than military values of honor and courage. The virtuous (answer choice D) did not exist.

PASSAGE IV (QUESTIONS 67–70)

This passage argues that in the 1990s, America entered a Neo-Victorian social period characterized by traditional morality, stable family life, and economic conservatism. The essay details several causes of this phenomenon and its probable results in the next century.

67. **D.** Paragraph two describes the return to traditional values of the baby-boom generation as a result of a reaction to its wild youth and loss of innocence. Being Christian before this return (answer choice A) is not mentioned, nor is education level (answer choice C); being raised by clergy is irrelevant (answer choice B).

68. **B.** A primary cause of the Neo-Victorian emphasis on stability and morality is the fact that baby boomers were having children of their own, and this increased their sense of responsibility. Having children may make one neurotic (answer choice A) and bossy (answer choice C), but those are not central to the analysis. The theme of the essay suggests that parenthood does not cause people to become irreverent, so answer choice D is also incorrect.

69. **A.** If the baby boomers become conservative after a radical youth, the logic would suggest that a consistently conservative

upbringing (answer choice A) would produce a radical, unstable adulthood. A radical upbringing (answer choice B) or adolescent rebellion (answer choice C) should allow them to choose to be conservative later.

70. **A.** The passage's emphasis on life-cycle changes, with a rebellious adolescence and stable adulthood, conforms with Churchill's remark, making answer choice B incorrect. Its relevance renders answer choice C incorrect and, by itself, it does not prove Churchill's authorship.

PASSAGE V (QUESTIONS 71–76)

This passage describes John Stuart Mill's arguments for free thought and expression and shows their applicability to America.

71. **D.** All of the American institutions—journalism (answer choice A), academia (answer choice B), and law (answer choice C)—are mentioned in the essay, while religious institutions are not.

72. **D.** Mill's argument includes ostracism in the essay; it does not mention the death penalty, making answer choice B incorrect; answer choices A and D are vague, and neither is mentioned in the essay.

73. **A.** Near the end of the second paragraph, the passage shows that Mill identified tolerance and intellectual liberty with a knowledgeable, humane, and civilized society. All answer choices except A contradict his arguments.

74. **C.** In paragraph three, Mill claims that the refuting of wrong ideas will strengthen the correct ideas. He does not think that the value of wrong radical ideas lies in eventual acceptance (answer choice A) (unless they become right), or their obnoxious quality (answer choice B), or their inability to persuade (answer choice D).

75. **A.** Mill allows for prosecution, even of mere speech, if those present in a particular situation could be influenced to engage in destructive behavior. The angry crowd in front of the courthouse is one example. The state should not allow the inflammatory speaker to go free (answer choice B) and cannot invoke ecclesiastical restrictions (answer choice C); the speaker's political affiliation is irrelevant (answer choice D).

76. **D.** A city council debate encourages the expression of conflicting viewpoints in order to establish the truth, as opposed to mere reports in newspapers (answer choice A) or on television broadcast news programs (answer choice C). An assembly line (answer choice B) allows no input from individuals.

PASSAGE VI (QUESTIONS 77–81)

This passage describes two of the main approaches to organizational theory in American public administration: the traditional institutional approach exemplified in Max Weber's writings and the modern humanist school of thought displayed in Maslow's theories.

77. **C.** Paragraphs one and two show that traditional structural administrative theory includes official positions, rules and regulations, and impartial treatment of the public. It does not include self-esteem, which is characteristic of the humanist approach (paragraph three).

78. **D.** Although the current view of bureaucracy is often negative (answer choices A, B, and C), Weber saw it as rational and efficient, as stated in the second paragraph.

79. **B.** Weber wrote in the late nineteenth and early twentieth centuries, shortly after the unification of the German principalities. He drew a comparison between the bureaucracy's efficiency and rationality, which he valued, and a prince's arbitrary rule. Nazi

Germany (answer choice A) came into existence after Weber's death; modern America (answer choice C) and ancient Rome (answer choice D) were not part of his analysis.

80. **B.** At the end of paragraph three, the writer states that the Maslowian administrator wants to create a more efficient, productive organization in order to satisfy everyone's needs. Some may find this intolerable (answer choice A), chaotic (answer choice C), or boring (answer choice D), but in Maslow's theory it would be productive (answer choice B).

81. **B.** It can be assumed from the description of Maslow's theory in the passage that it expects managers to be psychologists; they should be fully aware of and promote the psychological needs and potentials of their employees. Unlike Weber, Maslow's approach does not emphasize efficiency (answer choice A) and certainly does not advocate managerial tyranny (answer choice C).

PASSAGE VII (QUESTIONS 82–86)

This passage describes management leadership studies in general and two specific administrative leadership models.

82. **C.** The authoritarian leader is mentioned as employing a "highly personal or *ad hominem* form of correction," which is most likely to involve insulting the worker. The democratic leader (answer choice D) is said to correct in terms of "actions rather than persons" and the laissez-faire leader (answer choice B) offers no correction whatsoever. Impoverished (answer choice A) does not apply because it refers to a lack of concern.

83. **C.** The laissez-faire leader who provided complete freedom for individuals to do what they wanted was ranked low in efficiency and satisfaction; therefore, complete freedom in such a setting is "unfulfilling." It may also produce anarchy (answer choice B) and it might be fun (answer choice A), but those are not measured by the study results. Unusual (answer choice D) is incorrect because the study did not focus on the frequency of the use of the leadership styles.

84. **C.** The low regard for the agency's work and its people expressed in that statement best qualifies the secretary as an impoverished leader, who, in paragraph three, is described as having low concern for production and people. Country club leaders (answer choice A) have high concern for people, and authoritarian leaders (answer choice B) have high concern for work. Totalitarian leaders (answer choice D) are not mentioned.

85. **A.** Team leadership concern for both people (implying participation) and production most resembles the high level of worker satisfaction and efficiency in the democratic leadership style presented in the first typology. The concentration of power in authoritarian leadership (answer choice B) denies a concern for people; laissez-faire's low efficiency and employee satisfaction deny team leadership's concern for production and people (answer choice C); the New York Mets are not the team mentioned in either typology.

86. **B.** When it is mentioned in the conclusion that the study of leadership styles would contribute to American competitiveness, it is implied that it would help the American economy. Better understanding of leadership might well help Eastern Europe (answer choice A), communist nations (answer choice C), and South America (answer choice D), but these are not implied in the passage.

PASSAGE VIII (QUESTIONS 87–90)

87. **B.** The author begins the passage by suggesting that absolute moral rules are implausible. He then provides evidence and examples leading to the conclusion that they are also impossible to maintain. Answer choice A is incorrect because the discussion

of Dutch fishermen is mentioned only as an example of how two absolute moral rules can come into conflict, forcing the actors (the Dutch fishermen in the example) to violate at least one of two absolute rules. The author does point out a difference between Kant and Geach, but this difference is not central to the passage (answer choice C). The author mentions the difference to show how each philosopher deals with the possibility of conflicting absolute moral rules; the author then refutes each position. The author is not arguing against moral rules in general, nor is inconsistency of paramount concern (answer choice D). The problem, according to the author, is the *absoluteness* of the rules. This is emphasized in the last sentence of the passage.

88. **B.** The author's purpose is to argue against absolute moral rules. Therefore, he cannot support Kant's position, which supports their existence. This makes both answers A and D incorrect. Given the effort the author spends refuting Kant's position, it cannot be said that he is indifferent to it (answer choice C). He merely disagrees with Kant's position and attempts to prove it wrong.

89. **A.** As stated in the third paragraph, Geach believes absolute moral rules to be of divine origin, and that God will not permit conflict to actually arise. Geach may find hypotheticals interesting, but nevertheless irrelevant to the real world. By arguing that God will not permit conflict to occur in the real world, Geach must recognize that examples of hypothetical conflict do exist, making answer choice B incorrect. Geach's position is not that examples of hypothetical conflict are unlikely to occur (answer choice C); it is that God will not allow them to occur. Answer choice D is incorrect because it is clear from the passage that, although Geach recognizes the existence of examples of hypothetical conflict between absolute moral rules, he still believes they exist.

90. **C.** The author states this directly in the last paragraph to explain why Kant's defense is untenable. In this last paragraph, the author also rejects the possibility that if two absolute moral rules exist, they will not come into conflict (answer choice A). Answer choice B is more in line with Geach's position. The author provides a real-world example of conflict by discussing the Dutch fishermen. Answer choice D is incorrect because Geach's position raises a different defense—that of divine intervention.

PASSAGE IX (QUESTIONS 91–92)

91. **D.** Answer D nicely summarizes how management practices have had to change to consider laws, agency rules, and court decisions. Answer A is incorrect. As the author explains, courts often struck down laws designed to eradicate unhealthy and unfair practices. Answer B fails to account for major changes, especially after the Supreme Court changed its interpretation of the Constitution. Answer C has missed the author's point that profit motives often led to harsh working conditions for children and women.

92. **D.** The author has apparently chosen a topic that shows how profit motives can lead to poor personnel practices. Answer A is a narrow assessment of the author's values because morality is not confined to persons of the cloth. Answer B is incorrect. One of the great freedoms in America is the ability to freely observe and express opinions about the way government has operated over the years. Critics are not necessarily socialites or socialists. Answer C offers the reader an opportunity to make a personal judgment on fairness. Actually, the author finds no problems when dissenting opinions are adopted by later courts in an effort to protect workers from poor working conditions.

SECTION 3
Writing Sample

SAMPLE ESSAY 1

At first glance, William James's observation about happiness, "One could not accept a happiness shared with millions if the condition of that happiness were the suffering of one lonely soul," sounds perfectly clear and agreeable. However, if one probes the statement at its limits, a few surprising thoughts appear. These thoughts suggest that while we may believe we act according to the statement, many of us derive happiness from the suffering of others.

Consider for a moment the statement's obvious meaning. No rational person would likely disagree with its premise. We prefer to think that any happiness we might receive from life should not be purchased at the expense of others. Most reasonable people try to live their lives without causing others to suffer. When we drive our automobiles, we try to take appropriate care so that we do not cause accidents that injure other people. In our work, we derive satisfaction, if not happiness, from a job well done and give credit, for help, to our colleagues who deserve it. When we go to a social event, we try to find happiness by enjoying the company of our friends or new acquaintances. In our personal relationships, we try to treat those we care about with concern, love, and dignity. All of these behaviors contribute to a sense of happiness in life that we gain through personal attributes, relationships with other people, and courteous and tactful treatment of others.

All well and good, but consider how each of the instances previously described could, in fact, involve "the suffering of one lonely soul" or of many other souls. Driving an automobile seems innocuous enough, but what happens if, at that social event, we imbibed too many mugs of beer? Perhaps we drive away drunk and smash another person's life to bits. Sure, we were happy at the party, even when we drove away. But we just didn't think we would cause such an "accident." Likewise, many of us feel we need to dominate other people in our personal relationships, which results in our own happiness. Doesn't it make us feel good (and happy?) when we beat our best friend at tennis? Or more darkly, we hear of, and perhaps know, people who derive their happiness from physical violence directed at a spouse or child. How about people at work? Don't we hear and, perhaps, know of people who gloat over their latest conquest? So what if one saves his six-figure-a-year income by crushing a union or by closing a plant and throwing workers into unemployment and suffering? So what if we work for a company we know is dumping toxic wastes that could cause people to suffer? That's not our problem. So what if these radioactive wastes from medical procedures end up in a dump in Mexico? We don't think we cause such things to happen, but we comply with them by not trying to stop such behavior.

So, what are we to do to live in a hostile, competitive world, one that may not allow us all that much opportunity to find happiness in the first place? We must first look to ourselves to discover our own identity so that we have a basis from which to act. We hope to find a humane self in various roles we play. We also can work toward particular outcomes. We can try to think ahead to look to the consequences of our actions. We can investigate both our own behavior and that of our work places and institutions to try to prevent inhumane acts from occurring. In short, we should discover our own ideals, form values from them that we can practice in an imperfect world, and be aware of the effects of our behavior.

From these basic and relatively simple steps we can derive happiness based on a clear conscience. We can try to avoid happiness purchased by the suffering of others. An individual embarking on such a task of self-discovery and application of values will find the journey a difficult one. But we can find true happiness only if we look for it and overcome the obstacles and temptations that cause—directly or indirectly—the sufferings of others.

EXPLANATION OF ESSAY 1

The paper as a whole focuses clearly on the topic defined by the statement and fully addresses each of the three writing tasks in the directions. The first paragraph announces the thesis or central idea of the whole piece quite clearly. Paragraph two responds to the first task ("Explain what you think the statement means"); paragraph three responds to the second task ("Describe a specific situation in which people do accept happiness based on the suffering of others"); and paragraphs four and five respond to the third task ("Discuss the criteria under which one could find happiness without causing the suffering of others").

The paper skates on relatively thin ice as it develops the topic and the implications of it in a reasonably thoughtful manner. Particularly toward the end, it almost edges into triteness or ignorant optimism. Nonetheless, the paper addresses the issues squarely and at a deep enough level (for a thirty-minute essay) to succeed. Notice how it develops a contrast between expected responses, and how the expected sometimes is actually the unexpected. The development stays at a specific level, even though it drops to the very concrete level of example and illustration only once (the "dump in Mexico"). Even so, its development clearly addresses the topic on a level that explains the meanings needed. The last two paragraphs synthesize the apparent conflict with a discussion of the basis on which one should try to achieve happiness without causing others to suffer.

One of the strengths of the essay is its unity and coherence. The essay never strays from the topic (and the tasks required) and connects the parts logically so that there is a smooth flow of thought. Each paragraph holds together around its topic, and each one also relates directly to the central idea. Transitions of various kinds (e.g., repetition of "consider" in paragraphs one and two; transitional words like "so") aid sentence-to-sentence and paragraph-to-paragraph coherence.

While the paper does not demonstrate flashes of brilliance in style and usage, it does use language appropriately and effectively. Sentence structures clarify and communicate, rather than obfuscate. Sentence variety makes the paper easy to read. A series of questions changes the pace of the essay (although this tactic can backfire, so be careful here). Occasional concrete word choices ("smash another person's life to bits") enliven the prose, as does the overall conversational tone. No significant grammar or mechanics (spelling, punctuation) errors appear.

SAMPLE ESSAY 2

Good families seem to occur few and far between, if we believe what we read and hear in the media and in sociological studies. Rapid changes occur in modern cultures, and the family, as an institution, has not escaped the ravages of change. Jane Howard's pithy observation in *Families* (1978), "Good families are much to all their members, but everything to none," sounds like an accurate description of family as we look ahead to the new century.

Ms. Howard's comment, we should note, does limit itself to "good" families; but even so, it speaks volumes to us. Good families provide a host of things to each one of their members. People derive their basic values, their customs, their rituals, their hopes for the future from their parents, which they, in turn, derived from their parents, and so on, back to the earliest ancestors. The largest part of an individual's being—from the genetic and molecular level, to the social and cultural environment—devolves from the family. A family provides a beginning—a start in life, both biologically and socially. The parent derives satisfaction from passing on both genes and values to the next generation. So, in that sense, families, good or bad, "are much to all their members."

The corollary phrase, "but everything to none," sounds contradictory, but appropriate, and even necessary. All families should prepare their young to mature and strike out on their own. Good families take that process further by actively encouraging young people to discover their identities, make decisions, act appropriately in social settings, find a vocation, and find their own future relationships. At some point in the maturing process, all children need to declare independence from their parents. Eventually they begin their own families—in whatever shape or form.

We know, of course, that many people do not have good biological or foster families. At different times in life, all people turn outward from their family for certain things even good families cannot provide. At the extreme, we find youths joining gangs that become surrogate families. These surrogate families provide *everything* the member needs—at least to that individual. Security of a sort, love of a sort, stability of a sort, even income and sustenance of a sort (often illegally obtained), all come from the gang. To gang members, no doubt, it feels as though their surrogate families provide everything. One can argue that such members deceive themselves and that these surrogate families are anything but good; however, the members feel differently. Legitimate organizations often provide virtually the same surrogate feelings for children and adults. I can remember that the Boy Scouts and, later, the Explorers, provided such a surrogate family for me. My college dormitory floor also provided a sense of family and community that seemed everything I needed at the time.

To return to Ms. Howard's original point, however, we notice that these surrogate families really do not always meet all the needs of their members. Some surrogates even contribute to the destruction of the individual; this is especially true of gangs. These surrogates—like some biological families—may encourage role playing, immaturity, and allegiance to the group over all, rather than their opposites. So a "family"—surrogate or biological—does not necessarily constitute a "good" one. A good family recognizes and instills its values within its members, but it also recognizes the need for the individual to become independent. Hitler's Nazis and the Mafia both provided strong values for their members. But they also required absolute allegiance to the group (family). No inconveniences, such as conscience, could intervene with group allegiance. Good families, on the other hand, nurture their members without demanding absolute allegiance. They pass on humane values of love and respect for all, especially the family, and also for others. In that respect, the biblical Abraham may have failed his earthly family while attempting to obey his God. Likewise, when we read of families beating their children because of allegiance to another group's—often religious—values, we certainly have to question their notions of "family."

It remains, finally, not quite as easy a task, as originally thought, to decide what good families do. Many families ignore or neglect their duties, even though they have the best of values at heart and the best of intentions in mind. Other activities—work, club, group—or duties interfere, perhaps. Unfortunately, this often results in a family providing little to all its members or nothing to some.

EXPLANATION OF ESSAY 2

The paper as a whole focuses clearly on the topic defined by the statement and fully addresses each of the three writing tasks in the directions. The first paragraph announces the thesis or central idea of the whole piece quite clearly. Paragraphs two and three respond to the first task ("Explain what you think the statement means"); paragraph four responds to the second task ("Describe a specific situation in which the good family *may be* everything to its members"); and paragraphs four, five, and six respond to the third task ("Discuss the criteria implied in the statement in order to have a ëgood' family, and suggest how groups other than biological or foster families may be considered families").

The paper develops the topic, and the implications of it, in a reasonably thoughtful manner. Toward the end, however, it almost seems to lose direction because it mixes biological family and other groups in the same breath. Nonetheless, the paper addresses the issues squarely and at a deep enough level (for a thirty-minute essay) to succeed. Notice how it develops a contrast between biological families and surrogate families, such as gangs. The development stays at a specific level, even though it drops to the very concrete level of example and illustration twice: one, the personal experience of the writer (Scouts, dormitory); and two, near the end (Hitler, the Mafia, Abraham). Even so, its development clearly addresses the topic on a level that explains the meanings needed. The last two paragraphs synthesize the apparent differences as well as can reasonably be expected, within the time limit.

One of the strengths of the essay is its unity and coherence. The essay never strays from the topic (and the tasks required) and connects the parts logically so there is a smooth flow of thought. Each paragraph holds together around its topic, and each one also relates directly to the central idea. Transitions of various kinds (e.g., repetition of "surrogate" and other phrases in paragraphs two through five; transitional words like "finally") aid sentence-to-sentence and paragraph-to-paragraph coherence.

SECTION 4
Biological Sciences

PASSAGE I (QUESTIONS 93–96)

93. **B.** Because this molecule is lipid soluble, it will be difficult to leave the lipoidal membrane and enter the aqueous cytoplasm. For the very reason that answer B is correct, answer A is incorrect because it will be easy for the molecule to leave an aqueous phase and enter a lipoidal one. Answer C is incorrect because the molecule will have no trouble passing through the lipoidal layer.

94. **D.** Propanol has half of the hydrogen bonds of the propandiols. These bonds must be broken before propanol can pass into the lipoidal membrane. Answer A is incorrect because all of these have OH groups. Answer B is incorrect because these are all polar molecules; otherwise, hydrogen bonding could not occur. Answer C is incorrect because all of the compounds in question have three carbons.

95. **C.** Answer choice A is incorrect because water is very polar and thus could not pass through the membrane easily. The remaining three choices are alcohols. Recall that the more carbons an alcohol has, the less it will behave as an alcohol, and the more it will resemble its analogous alkane. Therefore, decanol, with ten carbons, will behave much like decane, which is nonpolar and can easily pass through the lipoidal membrane.

96. **A.** Thiourea is much more water-soluble; hence it is more difficult for it to travel through the membrane. Although answer B is true, the difference in masses is so slight that it cannot explain this great of an energy difference. Answer C might be true, but again the energy difference cannot be due solely to this. Answer D is not correct because there is a possible explanation.

PASSAGE II (QUESTIONS 97–99)

97 **C.** Changes in temperature will cause changes in the volume of the gases in the capillary tubing. Flask A will experience the same temperature changes. Therefore, because they are on the other side of the bubble, they will cancel any temperature changes on the side of the cells. For this reason, the other choices are incorrect.

98. **C.** As oxygen is consumed, carbon dioxide is produced, which is absorbed by the KOH, resulting in a decrease in volume. This will cause the bubble to move toward the cells. All other choices are true. Changes in temperature will cause changes in the volume of the gases, making answer A correct. The fact that this apparatus has airtight seals shows answer B to be true. Answer choice D is simply taken from the volume of a cylinder.

99. **A.** The volume of a cylinder = $1 \times \pi \times r^2$. The given diameter must be converted to radius ($\frac{1}{2}d = r$). Converting the values in mm to cm, we get a volume in cm^3, which is converted to liters by dividing by 1,000. If one forgets to convert to cm, one ends up with answer choice B. Forgetting to change diameter to radius yields answer choice C. Answer choice D is incorrect for a number of reasons.

PASSAGE III (QUESTIONS 100–102)

100. D. The axial filaments are mentioned in the passage, which also mentions at the beginning that they are non-photosynthetic and non-chemosynthetic; therefore, they must be heterotrophic. Answer C is incorrect because many are free-living.

101. B. All the other answer choices are true, as is mentioned in the text.

102. B. Look at the dimensions given in the chart. This genus is so large that it can easily be seen under the high power lens of a microscope.

103. B. There is no centrosome present in a prophase chromosome.

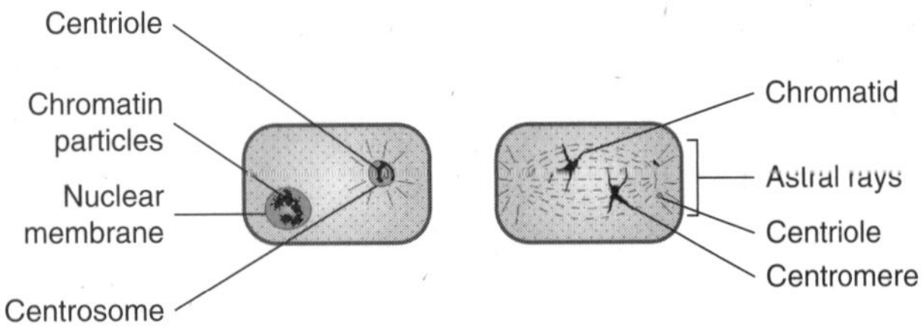

Interphase in Animal Mitosis

Prophase in Animal Mitosis without Centrosome

104. D. First, we must find the percentage of albinos in the population:

$$\frac{18}{200} \times 100 = 9\%$$

We know that albinism is a homozygous recessive trait (aa), so to find the frequency of the recessive allele, a, we take the square root of 9% (0.09) = $\sqrt{0.09}$ = 0.30. We also know that the frequency of the recessive allele (a) added to the frequency of the dominant allele (A) must equal 1. Therefore, the frequency of the nonalbino allele is 1 – 0.30 = 0.70. Squaring the frequency of the nonalbino allele will give us the frequency of homozygous nonalbinos (AA).

$$(0.70)^2 = 0.49 \text{ or } 49\%.$$

Then we multiply 0.49 × 200 and see that there are 98 homozygous dominant nonalbinos (AA).

105. A. The primitive atmosphere had essentially no free oxygen. All oxygen present was in the form of water and oxides.

106. B. Ethers have the general formula R-O-R′, where R can be aryl and/or alkyl. Ethers can be formed by two alcohol molecules in the presence of a strong acid to release a water molecule. This is called acid-catalyzed dehydration of alcohols in the formation of ethers.

The mechanism of this reaction resembles that of substitution. It involves the protonation of one alcohol and release of a water molecule to form a carbonium ion. A carbonium ion is a strong electrophile. It attacks the electron-rich oxygen of another alcohol, which releases a proton to form an ether:

$$R\text{--}O\text{--}H \xrightarrow[\text{heat}]{H_2SO_4} R^{\oplus} + H_2O$$

$$R^{\oplus} + \underset{\underset{H}{\overset{\curvearrowleft}{|}}}{:\ddot{O}\text{--}R} \longrightarrow R\text{--}O\text{--}R + H^{\oplus}$$

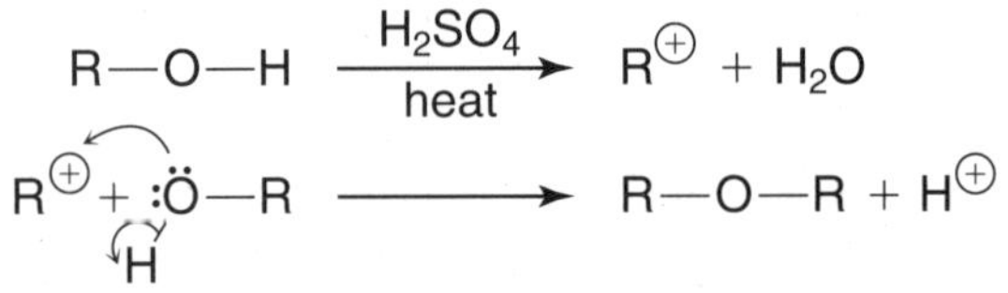

Under closer scrutiny, one can see that, in the process of strong acid protonation of an alcohol, another reaction can occur instead of the substitution attack on another alcohol. A carbonium ion is a highly reactive species and can participate in a substitution reaction, as in ether formation, or undergo an elimination reaction to form an alkene. The latter reaction is most prominent for tertiary alcohols:

$$R\text{--}\underset{R}{\overset{R}{\underset{|}{\overset{|}{C}}}}\text{--}OH \xrightarrow{H^+} R\text{--}\underset{R}{\overset{R}{\underset{|}{\overset{|}{C}}}}\text{--}O^{\oplus}H_2$$

$$R\text{--}\underset{R}{\overset{R}{\underset{|}{\overset{|}{C}}}}\text{--}O^{\oplus}H_2 \xrightarrow{-H_2O} R\text{--}\underset{R}{\overset{R}{\underset{|}{\overset{|}{C}}}}{}^{\oplus}$$

$$R\text{--}\underset{R}{\overset{R}{\underset{|}{\overset{|}{C}}}}{}^{\oplus} \longrightarrow R\text{--}\underset{R}{\overset{R}{\underset{|}{\overset{||}{C}}}}$$

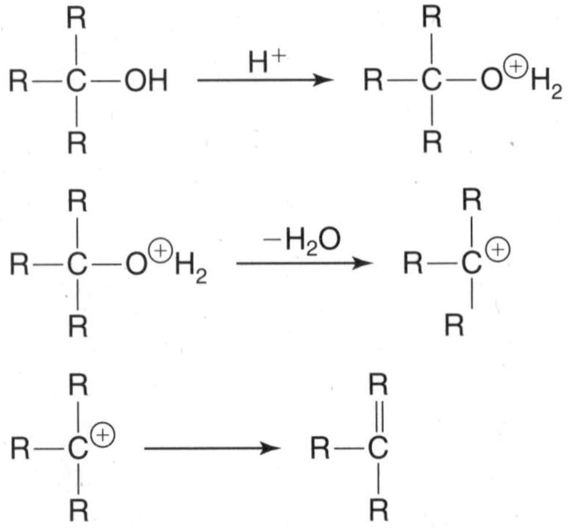

PASSAGE IV (QUESTIONS 107–111)

107. **A.** Because both traits are recessive, the individual must be homozygous to display both. Answer choices B and C would appear as a totally unshaded figure.

108. **B.** Because the figure is unshaded, it means this male individual has at least one dominant gene A and B. The fact that he has produced offspring showing traits a and b means that he must be heterozygous. The same holds true for A2.

109. **D.** B2 could be AABB, AaBB, AABb, or AaBb. The fact that she has produced five offspring without either trait a or b supports the probability that she is homozygous normal for both traits, but this fact does not prove it. Had her husband displayed one or both of the traits, it would have helped, but his genotypc is unknown.

110. **B.** This person displays no traits, yet has produced a son with traits a and b, and a daughter with trait a; therefore, he must be heterozygous for both traits.

111. **D.** One can perform a variety of probability calculations; however, if one is logical and were C13 Aabb, he would display trait b. Because he does not, he cannot possibly be this genotype. There is a 67 percent chance of him being AaBb, and a 33 percent chance of his being AaBB.

PASSAGE V (QUESTIONS 112–118)

112. **B.** Only one of the parents has trait C/c, yet all of their children display it. With the cross between B1 and B2, half of the offspring show the trait, which would be expected of a homozygous mated with a heterozygous. The cross between B6 and B7 further supports this. The mating between B10 and B11, who both show the trait, produces children that do not have it, further supporting the idea that the normal condition is recessive. Therefore, CC or Cc will show trait C/c; cc will be normal.

113. **A.** To show the trait, he can be either CC or Cc. Because he has produced normal children, he must be heterozygous, or Cc.

114. **B.** Because this is a dominant trait, the fact that A2 is normal with respect to C/c indicates that he must be homozygous normal, or cc.

115. **D.** A1 can be either CC or Cc. The fact that all of her children display trait C/c, even though her husband does not, indicates that she might be CC, but this does not prove it. However, were she to have only one child without the trait, it would prove her to be Cc.

116. **A.** It appears to be passed on from one male to all of his sons. Were it on the X chromosome, it would not show up this way because a son receives his only X chromosome from his mother.

117. **C.** Because a male has only one Y chromosome, he can be neither homo- nor heterozygous for a gene found for it; consequently, he is called hemizygous. In this case, a person with one gene, D, would display trait D; a person with one gene, d, would be normal. A female, obviously, would have neither gene D nor d because she lacks a Y chromosome.

118. **C.** Because the person does not show the dominant trait C/c, he must be homozygous normal, i.e., cc. Because trait D is shown and is on the Y chromosome, he is hemizygous for it, or D. This results in ccD.

PASSAGE VI (QUESTIONS 119–122)

119. **A.** Ozoneolysis will oxidize alkenes to aldehydes. In the case of a cyclic alkene, the ring structure is broken, and two carbonyl

groups are formed, one on each of the carbons that previously held the double-bond.

120. **B.** $KMnO_4$ will oxidize an alkene to a carboxylic acid. In the case of a cyclic alkene, the ring structure is broken and two carboxylic acid groups are formed, one on each of the carbons that previously held the double-bond. In this case, adipic acid (or by IUPAC, hexanedioic acid) is formed.

121. **B.** The solution that is prepared in the question is known as *Tollens Reagent* and is a test for aldehydes. The presence of aldehydes causes the silver to precipitate out of the solution and to form a silver mirror, by the reaction: $RCHO + 2Ag(NH_3)_2OH \rightarrow 2Ag\varnothing + RCOONH_4 + H_2O + 3NH_3$.

122. **A.** $KMnO_4$ will further oxidize an aldehyde to a carboxylic acid.

PASSAGE VII (QUESTIONS 123–125)

123. **C.** This is the point where the two lines diverge. If the logarithmic nature of the graph is neglected, answer choice D is obtained.

124. **A.** Intracellular materials begin to change as soon as a cell dies. The shorter the time between cellular death and whatever experimental parameters are measured, the better. To a lesser extent, diet (answer choice B) and temperature (answer choice C) might be able to influence DNA content, but these are slight enough that they can be neglected. Answer choice D is incorrect because RNA can readily be differentiated from DNA.

125. **C.** The graph contains data from fetal life through adulthood; therefore, the ratio of cells in the cerebrum (via DNA) can be measured against total body mass at any stage in development. For this reason, all other choices are incorrect.

126. **D.** The mRNA (codon) is synthesized from 5′ to 3′ along the DNA template strand, and the DNA template strand shown is 3′ to 5′. Therefore, the mRNA for the nucleotide sequence in bold is G C A. The anticodon is on the transfer RNA (tRNA) and is the complement of the mRNA. Therefore, the anticodon is C G U.

127. **C.** Humans are eukaryotes; in eukaryotes, chromatin is the complex of DNA and histone and nonhistone proteins. Therefore, ribosomes (answer choice C) are not found in chromatin.

128. **C.** Only the hyoid, which is a very small bone near the base of the tongue, is not a part of the human ear. The tectorial membrane is part of the cochlea, which is in the inner ear. The oval window is a membrane that separates the middle ear and the inner ear. The malleus is one of the small bones in the middle ear that conducts sound.

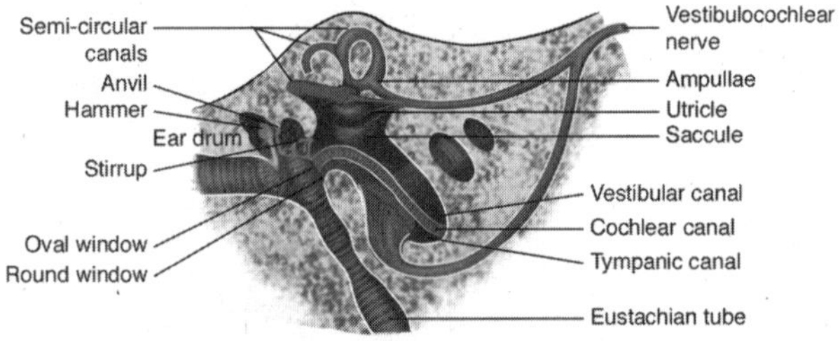

Cochlea (cutaway)

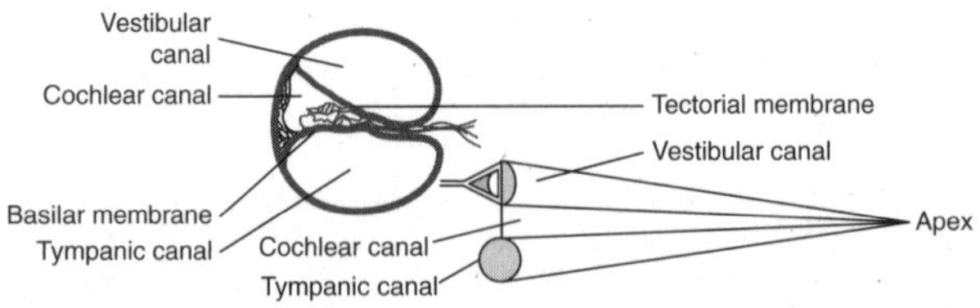

129. **C.** The fovea consists of both rods, which are used to detect objects in poor illumination and for night vision, and cones, which are the photoreceptors for day vision and are used to perceive colors. There are more cones than rods because more vision in humans takes place in the daytime or in well-lit environments.

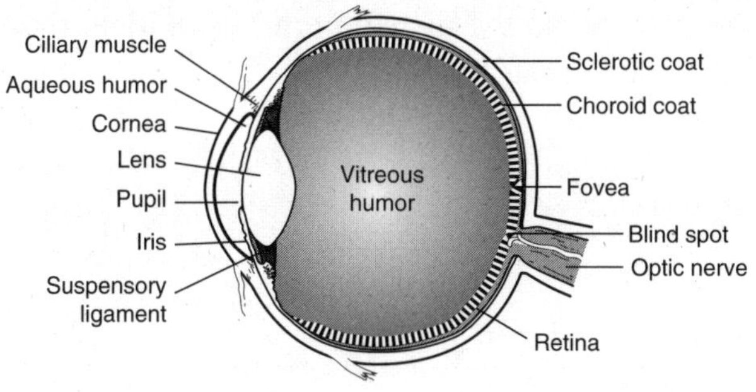

Diagrammatic section of the human eye.

PASSAGE VIII (QUESTIONS 130–134)

130. **D.** The response of the material to extreme temperatures and pH, as well as its specificity, indicate that it is an enzyme. An enzyme is a special type of catalyst made of protein; therefore, all three choices are correct. In this case, the enzyme is tyrosinase.

131. **D.** Of the pH levels tested, it worked best at pH 4. However, not enough data points were gathered to tell if this was optimum. It could work even better at a pH of 3 or 5, for example. However, it did work best within the acidic range.

132. **A.** Boiling denatures proteins and is not reversible (one cannot unboil an egg!). An inorganic catalyst can be boiled without harm.

133. **C.** The phenylthiourea was binding with the tyrosinase (enzyme), so it could not interact with the pyrocathechol (substrate).

134. **B.** Remember that an enzyme will not cause a reaction that would not naturally occur. It simply helps it attain equilibrium faster. Therefore, answer choice A is not correct. An enzyme does not chemically react with the substrate and can be used again and again. This rules out answer choice C.

PASSAGE IX (QUESTIONS 135–138)

135. **A.** No more B cells for this group are shown after day 12. Mice could have been dying before this time (and probably were), but day 12 was the last day there were any survivors. This graph does not show mortality, but from the data, it can be concluded that at least one mouse survived 12 days, and none survived any longer. Therefore, the upper limit for survival is 12 days, and the lower limit is unknown.

136. **C.** Remember that the graph is semilogarithmic, and half of the pre-irradiated level was asked for. If one treats the plot as linear, one would get answer B. If one looks for the pre-irradiation level, answer D is obtained. Answer D results from making more than one error.

137. **A.** Although this graph does not show mortality, it can be seen that there were mice still alive at the conclusion of the experiment at 9 weeks. How long they lived after that is unknown. Some of the treated mice could have died before the conclusion of the experiment, and that would not be shown on this graph.

138. **B.** B cells, as well as other lymphocytes and erythroid and myeloid cells, arise from a common stem cell ancestor. A mouse fetus of the age described in the passage does not yet have B cells.

PASSAGE X (QUESTIONS 139–142)

139. **C.** This reaction is a typical S_n1 reaction but also involves migration of a hydrogen atom.

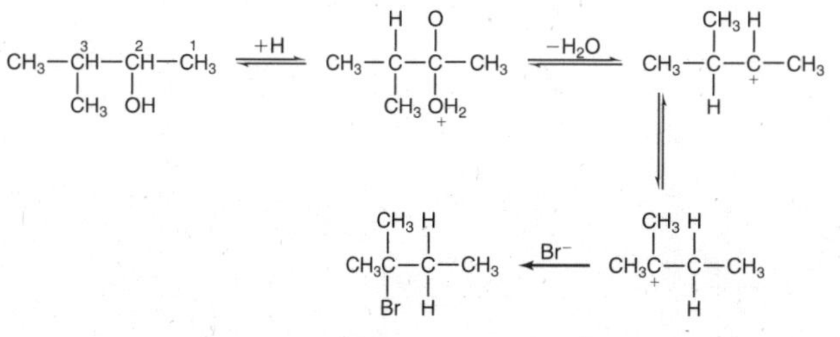

Because there is a carbocation intermediate that shifts to another carbon, this type of reaction is called a carbocation rearrangement.

140. **C.** As shown in the illustration in 139, the intermediate carbocation shifts from a secondary carbocation to the considerably more stable tertiary carbocation. Br^- reacts with this carbon, leading to 2-bromo-2-methylbutane instead of 2-bromo-3-methylbutane as essentially the sole product. Answer choice A is false because, with carbanions, the order of stability is $1^o > 2^o > 3^o$, and there is no carbanion intermediate. Answer choice B is a correct statement, but here it is the incorrect answer because the reaction does not involve a 1° carbocation. Answer choice D is incorrect because this is not an S_n2 reaction.

141. **D.** Because deuterium can be distinguished from H′ hydrogen, and its position on the carbon skeleton can be determined, it can be shown that the tertiary hydrogen moves to the secondary carbon after loss of H_2O. This has the effect of moving the carbocation from a secondary carbon to a tertiary one. Therefore, answer choice C is correct. Answer choice B is also correct because the rearrangements require an unstable intermediate. Because this is not an S_n2 reaction (due to the involvement of the carbocation intermediate), answer choice A is incorrect. Therefore, answer choice D is correct because it allows one to choose both C and B.

142. **D.** Both reactions share the same intermediate, so the distribution of products should be similar.

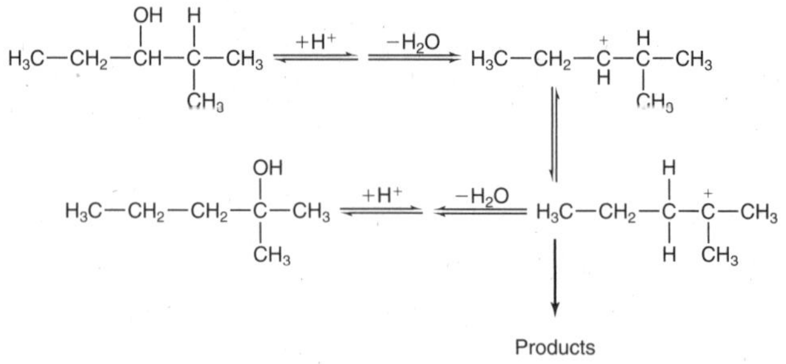

143. **B.** Though all five choices represent the development of an individual, the three primary germ layers first appear in the gastrula stage. The three germ layers are the endoderm, mesoderm, and ectoderm. These layers will eventually differentiate to form the different organs and structures of the body.

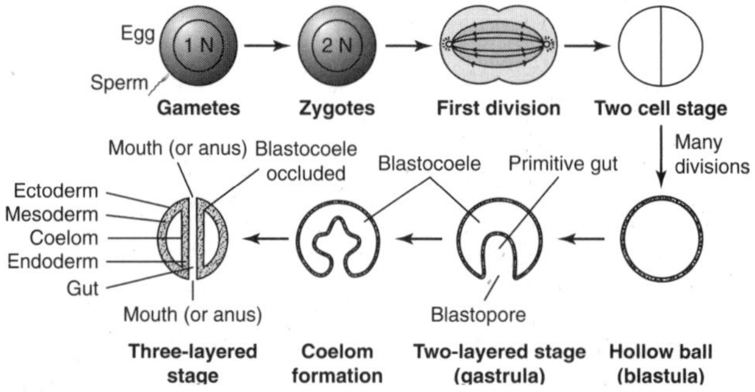

Early embryonic development in animals.

144. **D.** The greatest similarity in structure occurs between members of the same species. In order of increasing specificity, the choices are: phylum, class, family, genus, and species.

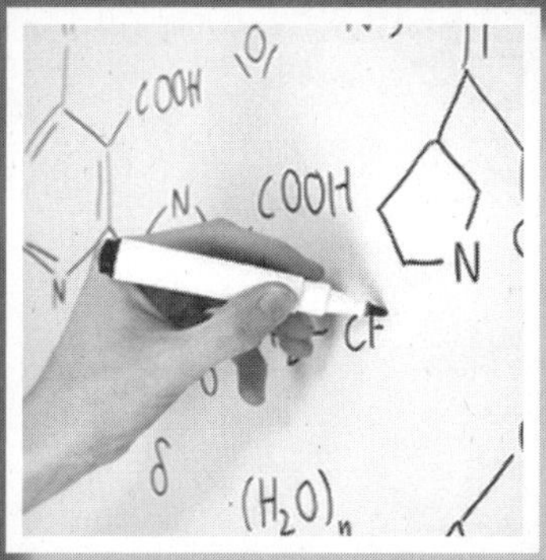

MCAT

MEDICAL COLLEGE

ADMISSION TEST

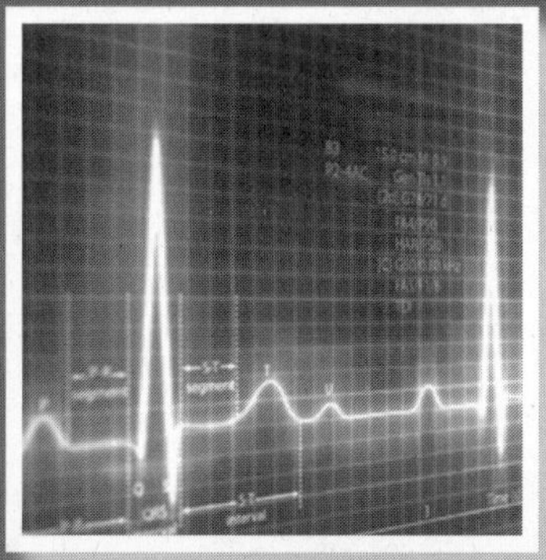

Test 3

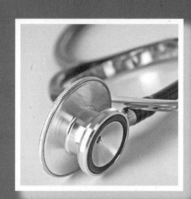

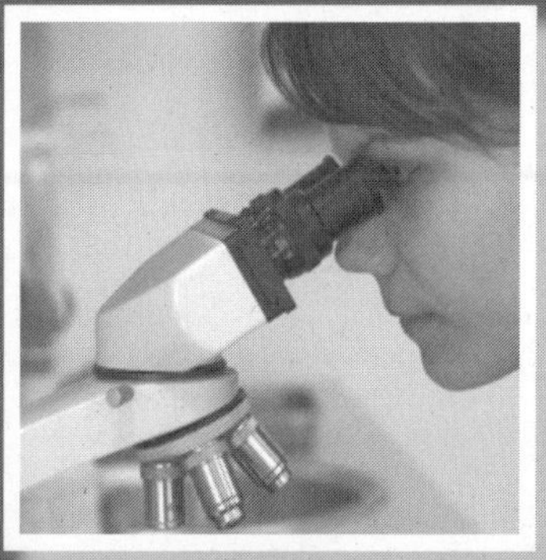

Test 3 ■ Answer Sheet

SECTION 1: Physical Sciences

1. Ⓐ Ⓑ Ⓒ Ⓓ
2. Ⓐ Ⓑ Ⓒ Ⓓ
3. Ⓐ Ⓑ Ⓒ Ⓓ
4. Ⓐ Ⓑ Ⓒ Ⓓ
5. Ⓐ Ⓑ Ⓒ Ⓓ
6. Ⓐ Ⓑ Ⓒ Ⓓ
7. Ⓐ Ⓑ Ⓒ Ⓓ
8. Ⓐ Ⓑ Ⓒ Ⓓ
9. Ⓐ Ⓑ Ⓒ Ⓓ
10. Ⓐ Ⓑ Ⓒ Ⓓ
11. Ⓐ Ⓑ Ⓒ Ⓓ
12. Ⓐ Ⓑ Ⓒ Ⓓ
13. Ⓐ Ⓑ Ⓒ Ⓓ
14. Ⓐ Ⓑ Ⓒ Ⓓ
15. Ⓐ Ⓑ Ⓒ Ⓓ
16. Ⓐ Ⓑ Ⓒ Ⓓ
17. Ⓐ Ⓑ Ⓒ Ⓓ
18. Ⓐ Ⓑ Ⓒ Ⓓ
19. Ⓐ Ⓑ Ⓒ Ⓓ
20. Ⓐ Ⓑ Ⓒ Ⓓ
21. Ⓐ Ⓑ Ⓒ Ⓓ
22. Ⓐ Ⓑ Ⓒ Ⓓ
23. Ⓐ Ⓑ Ⓒ Ⓓ
24. Ⓐ Ⓑ Ⓒ Ⓓ
25. Ⓐ Ⓑ Ⓒ Ⓓ
26. Ⓐ Ⓑ Ⓒ Ⓓ
27. Ⓐ Ⓑ Ⓒ Ⓓ
28. Ⓐ Ⓑ Ⓒ Ⓓ
29. Ⓐ Ⓑ Ⓒ Ⓓ
30. Ⓐ Ⓑ Ⓒ Ⓓ
31. Ⓐ Ⓑ Ⓒ Ⓓ
32. Ⓐ Ⓑ Ⓒ Ⓓ
33. Ⓐ Ⓑ Ⓒ Ⓓ
34. Ⓐ Ⓑ Ⓒ Ⓓ
35. Ⓐ Ⓑ Ⓒ Ⓓ
36. Ⓐ Ⓑ Ⓒ Ⓓ
37. Ⓐ Ⓑ Ⓒ Ⓓ
38. Ⓐ Ⓑ Ⓒ Ⓓ
39. Ⓐ Ⓑ Ⓒ Ⓓ
40. Ⓐ Ⓑ Ⓒ Ⓓ
41. Ⓐ Ⓑ Ⓒ Ⓓ
42. Ⓐ Ⓑ Ⓒ Ⓓ
43. Ⓐ Ⓑ Ⓒ Ⓓ
44. Ⓐ Ⓑ Ⓒ Ⓓ
45. Ⓐ Ⓑ Ⓒ Ⓓ
46. Ⓐ Ⓑ Ⓒ Ⓓ
47. Ⓐ Ⓑ Ⓒ Ⓓ
48. Ⓐ Ⓑ Ⓒ Ⓓ
49. Ⓐ Ⓑ Ⓒ Ⓓ
50. Ⓐ Ⓑ Ⓒ Ⓓ
51. Ⓐ Ⓑ Ⓒ Ⓓ
52. Ⓐ Ⓑ Ⓒ Ⓓ

SECTION 2: Verbal Reasoning

53. Ⓐ Ⓑ Ⓒ Ⓓ
54. Ⓐ Ⓑ Ⓒ Ⓓ
55. Ⓐ Ⓑ Ⓒ Ⓓ
56. Ⓐ Ⓑ Ⓒ Ⓓ
57. Ⓐ Ⓑ Ⓒ Ⓓ
58. Ⓐ Ⓑ Ⓒ Ⓓ
59. Ⓐ Ⓑ Ⓒ Ⓓ
60. Ⓐ Ⓑ Ⓒ Ⓓ
61. Ⓐ Ⓑ Ⓒ Ⓓ
62. Ⓐ Ⓑ Ⓒ Ⓓ
63. Ⓐ Ⓑ Ⓒ Ⓓ
64. Ⓐ Ⓑ Ⓒ Ⓓ
65. Ⓐ Ⓑ Ⓒ Ⓓ
66. Ⓐ Ⓑ Ⓒ Ⓓ
67. Ⓐ Ⓑ Ⓒ Ⓓ
68. Ⓐ Ⓑ Ⓒ Ⓓ
69. Ⓐ Ⓑ Ⓒ Ⓓ
70. Ⓐ Ⓑ Ⓒ Ⓓ
71. Ⓐ Ⓑ Ⓒ Ⓓ
72. Ⓐ Ⓑ Ⓒ Ⓓ
73. Ⓐ Ⓑ Ⓒ Ⓓ
74. Ⓐ Ⓑ Ⓒ Ⓓ
75. Ⓐ Ⓑ Ⓒ Ⓓ
76. Ⓐ Ⓑ Ⓒ Ⓓ
77. Ⓐ Ⓑ Ⓒ Ⓓ
78. Ⓐ Ⓑ Ⓒ Ⓓ
79. Ⓐ Ⓑ Ⓒ Ⓓ
80. Ⓐ Ⓑ Ⓒ Ⓓ
81. Ⓐ Ⓑ Ⓒ Ⓓ
82. Ⓐ Ⓑ Ⓒ Ⓓ
83. Ⓐ Ⓑ Ⓒ Ⓓ
84. Ⓐ Ⓑ Ⓒ Ⓓ
85. Ⓐ Ⓑ Ⓒ Ⓓ
86. Ⓐ Ⓑ Ⓒ Ⓓ
87. Ⓐ Ⓑ Ⓒ Ⓓ
88. Ⓐ Ⓑ Ⓒ Ⓓ
89. Ⓐ Ⓑ Ⓒ Ⓓ
90. Ⓐ Ⓑ Ⓒ Ⓓ
91. Ⓐ Ⓑ Ⓒ Ⓓ
92. Ⓐ Ⓑ Ⓒ Ⓓ

SECTION 4: Biological Sciences

93. Ⓐ Ⓑ Ⓒ Ⓓ
94. Ⓐ Ⓑ Ⓒ Ⓓ
95. Ⓐ Ⓑ Ⓒ Ⓓ
96. Ⓐ Ⓑ Ⓒ Ⓓ
97. Ⓐ Ⓑ Ⓒ Ⓓ

98. Ⓐ Ⓑ Ⓒ Ⓓ
99. Ⓐ Ⓑ Ⓒ Ⓓ
100. Ⓐ Ⓑ Ⓒ Ⓓ
101. Ⓐ Ⓑ Ⓒ Ⓓ
102. Ⓐ Ⓑ Ⓒ Ⓓ
103. Ⓐ Ⓑ Ⓒ Ⓓ
104. Ⓐ Ⓑ Ⓒ Ⓓ
105. Ⓐ Ⓑ Ⓒ Ⓓ
106. Ⓐ Ⓑ Ⓒ Ⓓ
107. Ⓐ Ⓑ Ⓒ Ⓓ
108. Ⓐ Ⓑ Ⓒ Ⓓ
109. Ⓐ Ⓑ Ⓒ Ⓓ
110. Ⓐ Ⓑ Ⓒ Ⓓ
111. Ⓐ Ⓑ Ⓒ Ⓓ
112. Ⓐ Ⓑ Ⓒ Ⓓ
113. Ⓐ Ⓑ Ⓒ Ⓓ
114. Ⓐ Ⓑ Ⓒ Ⓓ
115. Ⓐ Ⓑ Ⓒ Ⓓ
116. Ⓐ Ⓑ Ⓒ Ⓓ
117. Ⓐ Ⓑ Ⓒ Ⓓ
118. Ⓐ Ⓑ Ⓒ Ⓓ
119. Ⓐ Ⓑ Ⓒ Ⓓ
120. Ⓐ Ⓑ Ⓒ Ⓓ
121. Ⓐ Ⓑ Ⓒ Ⓓ
122. Ⓐ Ⓑ Ⓒ Ⓓ
123. Ⓐ Ⓑ Ⓒ Ⓓ
124. Ⓐ Ⓑ Ⓒ Ⓓ
125. Ⓐ Ⓑ Ⓒ Ⓓ
126. Ⓐ Ⓑ Ⓒ Ⓓ
127. Ⓐ Ⓑ Ⓒ Ⓓ
128. Ⓐ Ⓑ Ⓒ Ⓓ
129. Ⓐ Ⓑ Ⓒ Ⓓ
130. Ⓐ Ⓑ Ⓒ Ⓓ
131. Ⓐ Ⓑ Ⓒ Ⓓ
132. Ⓐ Ⓑ Ⓒ Ⓓ
133. Ⓐ Ⓑ Ⓒ Ⓓ
134. Ⓐ Ⓑ Ⓒ Ⓓ
135. Ⓐ Ⓑ Ⓒ Ⓓ
136. Ⓐ Ⓑ Ⓒ Ⓓ
137. Ⓐ Ⓑ Ⓒ Ⓓ
138. Ⓐ Ⓑ Ⓒ Ⓓ
139. Ⓐ Ⓑ Ⓒ Ⓓ
140. Ⓐ Ⓑ Ⓒ Ⓓ
141. Ⓐ Ⓑ Ⓒ Ⓓ
142. Ⓐ Ⓑ Ⓒ Ⓓ
143. Ⓐ Ⓑ Ⓒ Ⓓ
144. Ⓐ Ⓑ Ⓒ Ⓓ

SECTION 1
Physical Sciences

TIME: 70 Minutes

QUESTIONS: 1–52

DIRECTIONS: Most of the questions in this section are arranged in groups, each corresponding to a descriptive passage. Based on the information given in a passage, choose the one best answer to each question in the group. Some questions are independent of a descriptive passage and of each other. Choose the one best answer to each of these questions. If you are not sure of an answer, eliminate those choices that you know are incorrect and choose an answer from among those remaining. Fill in the corresponding circle on the answer sheet to indicate your answer. You may refer to the periodic table at any time.

PASSAGE I (QUESTIONS 1-6)

Melissyl palmitate is the major component of beeswax. Waxes are typically esters made from fatty acids and an alcohol. Hydrolysis of beeswax yields palmitic acid and melissyl alcohol. Candles made from 100 percent pure beeswax have a melting point (mp) of 61–63°C. Candlemakers have a number of additives on hand to mix with the wax to provide color and fragrance. These additives affect the melting point and hardness of the produced candle. Some common additives are camphor, citronella, and eucalyptus.

1. A 100g-beeswax candle is lit, and the CO_2 and H_2O that is produced is collected and weighed. The mass of CO_2 and H_2O produced is found to be 8.98g and 3.67g, respectively. Assuming the candle is made from pure melissyl palmitate, CO_2 and H_2O are the only products, and the mass after blowing out the candle is 97g, what is the percentage composition of C, H, and O in the wax?
   A. 81.66%C, 4.73%H, 13.61%O
   B. 81.66%C, 13.61%H, 4.73%O
   C. 89.8%C, 3.67%H, 6.50%O
   D. 89.8%C, 6.50%H, 3.67%O

2. Based on your answer to the previous question, what is the empirical formula of beeswax?
   A. $C_{23}H_{46}O$
   B. $C_{22}H_{42}O$
   C. $C_{11}H_{21}O$
   D. $C_{11}H_{23}O$

3. Melissyl palmitate has a molar mass that is 2.7 times larger than palmitic acid. The melting points of melissyl palmitate and palmitic acid are 65°C and 63°C, respectively. One would expect, based on the large difference in their molecular weights, that beeswax would have a much higher melting point than palmitic acid. How can the similar magnitude of their melting points be explained?
   A. The palmitic acid has more London force interactions in the solid.
   B. The ester functional group is polar and raises the mp of the wax so it is comparable in magnitude with palmitic acid.
   C. The hydrogen-bonding interaction present in the acid raises the melting point.
   D. The carboxylic acid is destabilizing and lowers the mp of palmitic acid, so it is comparable in magnitude with the mp of the wax.

4. The formula weight of a substance can be determined by measuring the freezing point depression of a material it is mixed with. A candlemaker mixes 1.69g of beeswax with 25.0g of camphor. The melting point of pure camphor is 179.5°C. The candlemaker measures the melting point of the camphor/beeswax mixture to be 175.5°C. What is the formula weight of melissyl palmitate if the freezing-point-depression constant for camphor is 40°C/m.?
   A. 338g/mol B. 676g/mol
   C. 15.47g/mol D. 154.7g/mol

5. Based on the formula weight and the empirical formula you found in the previous questions, what is the formula for melissyl palmitate?
   A. $C_{44}H_{84}O_2$ B. $C_{46}H_{92}O_2$
   C. $C_{23}H_{46}O$ D. $C_{22}H_{42}O_2$

6. In the pursuit of his art, a candlemaker pours 30.0g of liquid beeswax into a jar filled with 300.0ml of water. The wax solidifies and the temperature of the water increases to 5°C. Assuming no heat was lost to the surroundings, what is the temperature change of the wax when it changes from a liquid to a solid?
   $C_{water} = 4.18$ J/g°C, $C_{wax} = 5.0$ J/g°C
   A. 10 degrees B. 5 degrees
   C. 0 degrees D. 2.5 degrees

PASSAGE II
(QUESTIONS 7–10)

NASA uses a number of propellants to power its rockets. These typically consist of a fuel source and an oxidizer. The fuel and oxidizer are stored separately. When mixed, the fuel is burned (oxidized) to produce large volumes of gas. The expanding gas is released under great pressure to produce thrust. One fuel-and-oxidizer combination used is hydrogen and oxygen. Their combustion produces H_2O gas and heat.

$$2\,H_2(g) + O_2(g) \rightarrow 2\,H_2O(g)$$

$$\Delta H = -484 \text{ kJ}$$

Hydrogen/oxygen propellant mixtures produce more thrust than any other propellant mixtures used for rocket fuel. The drawback for this propellant combination is that hydrogen and oxygen are gases under normal conditions and have large volumes. To be useful, they must be liquefied to reduce their volumes for space missions. As a result, they are difficult to handle. A fuel-and-oxidizer combination that does not suffer from this limitation is dinitrogen tetroxide (N_2O_4) and hydrazine (N_2H_4). Both are liquids at normal temperatures and pressures. The balanced chemical equation for their combustion is:

$$2\,H_2NNH_{2(l)} + O_2NNO_{2(l)} \rightarrow 3\,N_{2(g)} + 4\,H_2O_{(g)}$$

7. For the reaction above, which compound is the oxidizing agent and which is the reducing agent?
   A. Oxidizing agent: H_2NNH_2 / reducing agent: N_2
   B. Oxidizing agent: O_2NNO_2 / reducing agent: N_2O_4
   C. Oxidizing agent: H_2NNH_2 / reducing agent: N_2O_4
   D. Oxidizing agent: N_2O_4 / reducing agent: H_2NNH_2

8. If 0.5kg of N_2O_4 were reacted with excess hydrazine in a 10-liter container, what is the pressure inside the container if the temperature at the end of the reaction was 700°C?
   A. 304atm B. 85atm
   C. 130atm D. 174atm

9. How much heat is released during the reaction of 2mol of hydrazine (N_2H_4) with 1mol of N_2O_4?

Substance	FW	ΔH_f kJ/mol	ΔG_f kJ/mol
$N_2H_{4(l)}$	32.05	50.6	149.43
$N_2O_{4(l)}$	92.02	−19.4	97.89
N_2	28.01	0	0
$H_2O_{(l)}$	18.01	−285.83	−237.13
$H_2O_{(g)}$	18.01	−241.82	−228.57
H_2	2.01	0	0
O_2	32.0	0	0

A. −433.5kJ B. −885.4kJ

C. −1049kJ D. −1227kJ

10. The reaction of hydrazine with dinitrogen tetroxide is exothermic. What effect will cooling the gaseous products have on the reaction if the cooling process results in the condensation of $H_2O_{(g)}$ to $H_2O_{(l)}$?
    A. The reaction will be forced to equilibrium.
    B. The forward reaction will be favored and more products will be produced.
    C. The reverse reaction will be favored and products will be consumed to produce reactants.
    D. The reaction is at equilibrium, so it is unaffected.

PASSAGE III (QUESTIONS 11–13)

Table 1 contains thermochemical data for two series of related compounds: the hydrogen halides (HF through HI) and four simple hydrocarbons. With the exception of hydrogen fluoride, there is a regular trend within each series of increasing enthalpy of vaporization, increasing normal boiling point, and increasing critical temperature with increasing molecular weight. The diatomic molecules all have nearly the same Cp, whereas the Cp of the polyatomic molecules tends to increase with the increasing number of atoms per molecule.

TABLE 1. Thermodynamic Properties of Selected Substances

Substance	Enthalpy of Vaporization, kJ/mole	Normal Boiling Point, K	Critical Temperature, K	Heat Capacity Cp, J/mol K
HF	25.2	292.8	462.1	29.1
HCl	17.5	188.3	324.6	29.1
HBr	19.3	206.6	363.2	29.1
HI	21.2	238.1	423	29.2
CH_4, methane	8.9	111.6	191.0	35.3
C_2H_6, ethane	15.7	184.6	305.4	52.6
C_3H_8, propane	19.0	231.1	369.9	73.5
C_4H_{10}, n-butane	24.3	272.6	425.1	97.4

Table 2 below gives the standard enthalpies of combustion at 273.15 K and 1 bar pressure for three substances.

TABLE 2. Standard Enthalpies of Combustion at 273.15 K

Substance	kJ/mol
C (graphite)	−393.5
H_2 (g)	−285.8
CH_4 (g)	−890.3

The combustion products consist of carbon dioxide gas and/or liquid water. The enthalpy of combustion of graphite is equivalent to the enthalpy of formation of carbon dioxide gas, and the enthalpy of combustion of hydrogen gas is equivalent to the enthalpy of formation of liquid water. The standard enthalpy of formation of water in the gaseous state is −241.8 kJ/mol at 25°C and 1 bar. The standard enthalpy of formation of water in the liquid state is −285.8 kJ/mol at 25°C and 1 bar.

11. With respect to the data in Table 1, hydrogen bonding can be used to explain which of the following?
    A. The nearly constant molar heat capacities of the diatomic molecules
    B. The unusually large molar enthalpy of vaporization of HF
    C. The trend of increasing molar enthalpy of vaporization with increasing molar mass for the hydrocarbons
    D. The trend of increasing molar heat capacity with increasing molar mass for the hydrocarbons

12. On the basis of the given enthalpies of formation of liquid water and gaseous water, calculate the enthalpy of water vaporization at 25°C.
   A. 44.0 kJ/mol B. 127.2 kJ/mol
   C. 263.8 kJ/mol D. 527.6 kJ/mol

13. On the basis of the data in Table 2, calculate the standard enthalpy for formation of methane at 25°C.
   A. +211.0 kJ/mol B. −1855.4 kJ/mol
   C. −74.8 kJ/mol D. −211.0 kJ/mol

QUESTIONS 14–17 are NOT based on a descriptive passage.

14. The law stating that the relationship between volume and temperature of an ideal gas at constant pressure is such that the volume is proportional to the absolute temperature was propounded by
   A. Charles. B. Avogadro.
   C. Boyle. D. Newton.

15. A ball is at the top of a hill. After a small amount of displacement, the ball moves to a new position. The ball was initially in
   A. equilibrium.
   B. neutral equilibrium.
   C. unstable equilibrium.
   D. natural equilibrium.

16. The change in enthalpy (ΔH) of a system is equal to the heat flow between the system and its surroundings (q) under which conditions?
   A. Constant volume
   B. Adiabatic conditions
   C. Constant pressure
   D. Constant temperature

17. A point charge +q is held at the origin (x = 0). A second point charge −3q is held at the location x = 1.00m. Determine the location on the x-axis of a third point charge, +2q, so that the net force on it will be zero.
   A. Somewhere to the right of the −3q charge, that is, somewhere at x > 1.00m.
   B. Somewhere to the left of the +q charge, that is, somewhere at x < 0 m.
   C. Somewhere between the two charges, but closer to the −3q charge.
   D. Somewhere between the two charges, but closer to the +q charge.

PASSAGE IV (QUESTIONS 18–21)

A common filling for tooth cavities is dental amalgam, a solid solution made by dissolving tin and silver in mercury. Although amalgam fillings are inert and generally do not cause health problems, they can lead to quite a surprise if one bites on a piece of aluminum foil. The electrochemical reactions between the aluminum and the components of an amalgam, with saliva and gum tissue acting as the electrolyte, can "shock" the tooth's nerve by sending a small flow of electrons to it. Some half-reactions involved, with standard reduction potentials at 25°C, include

		E°/V
Equation 1	$Al^{3+}(aq) + 3e \rightarrow Al(s)$	−1.66
Equation 2	$Sn^{2+}(aq) + 3Ag(s) + 2e \rightarrow Ag_3Sn(s)$	−0.05
Equation 3	$3Hg_2^{2+}(aq) + 4Ag(s) + 6e \rightarrow 2Ag_2Hg_3(s)$	+0.85

Aluminum is produced from its ore via an electrolytic method, the Hall-Heroult process. Aluminum oxide, Al_2O_3, is extracted from the ore, dissolved in molten cryolite, Na_3AlF_6, maintained at 980°C, and electrolized at low voltage but very high current, for example, 5.0 V and 10,000 A. In actual practice, about 7 kilowatt-hours of electric energy (excluding the energy needed to heat the furnace) is required to produce one pound of aluminum by electrolysis. This is equivalent to about 55.5 kJ/g Al.

18. What is the standard cell potential for the spontaneous reaction obtained by combining the half-reactions of equation 1 and equation 2?
   A. +1.61 V B. −1.61 V
   C. +1.71 V D. −1.71 V

19. If a galvanic or voltaic cell were constructed in which the overall, spontaneous reaction obtained by combining the half-reactions of equation 2 and equation 3 takes place,
    A. Ag_3Sn (s) is the anode, and electrons flow from Ag (s) to Ag_3Sn (s).
    B. Ag_3Sn (s) is the cathode, and electrons flow from Ag_3Sn (s) to Ag (s).
    C. Ag_3Sn (s) is the anode, and electrons flow from Ag_3Sn (s) to Ag (s).
    D. Ag_3Sn (s) is the cathode, and electrons flow from Ag (s) to Ag_3Sn (s).

20. If the half-reactions for equations 2 and 3 are combined to obtain an overall, net ionic equation for a spontaneous cell reaction, the minimum coefficient of Ag (s) in the balanced equation is
    A. 1. B. 4.
    C. 5. D. 9.

21. If the electrolytic production of aluminum were carried out with 100% efficiency at 5.0V, what energy would be required per gram of Al produced? The Faraday constant is 96,500C.
    A. 32.0kJ/g B. 58.7kJ/g
    C. 53.6kJ/g D. 55.5kJ/g

PASSAGE V (QUESTIONS 22–25)

The kinetics of the hydrolysis of methyl acetate, in the presence of hydrogen ion, was studied in a series of experiments. The overall reaction is:

$$CH_3OOCCH_3 + H_2O + H^+ \rightarrow CH_3OH + HOOCCH_3 + H^+$$

In the first set of experiments, the temperature was held constant at 25°C and the initial concentrations of methyl acetate and hydrogen ion were varied. The initial reaction rate was measured. The results are summarized in Table 1.

TABLE 1. Initial Reaction Rate at 25°C

[Methyl acetate]	[HCl]	Initial Rate (relative units)
0.1 M	0.1 M	1
0.2 M	0.1 M	2
0.3 M	0.1 M	3
0.2 M	0.5 M	10
0.2 M	1.0 M	20

In the second experiment, the concentration of methyl acetate as a function of time was measured at 25°C:

Time/min.	0.00	1.75	4.76
[methyl acetate]/M	0.30	0.20	0.10

In a third set of experiments, the half-life for the hydrolysis was measured for the same initial concentrations of methyl acetate and HCl at different temperatures.

Temperature/°C	0	10	20	30
Half-life/min	18.8	8.68	4.23	2.16

22. The hydrolysis of methyl acetate is first order with respect to methyl acetate and what order with respect to hydrogen ion?
    A. Zeroth B. First
    C. Second D. Third

23. If a reaction were half-order with respect to a reactant, by what factor would the initial rate of reaction increase if the concentration of the reactant were doubled?
    A. 0.5 B. $\sqrt{0.5}$
    C. $\sqrt{2}$ D. 2

24. The hydrolysis of methyl acetate can be followed by titrating the acetic acid produced. Which graph below best represents the change in acetic acid concentration with time?

A.

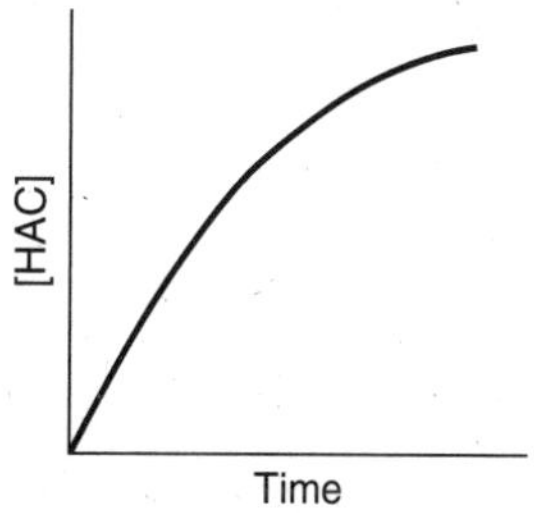

B.

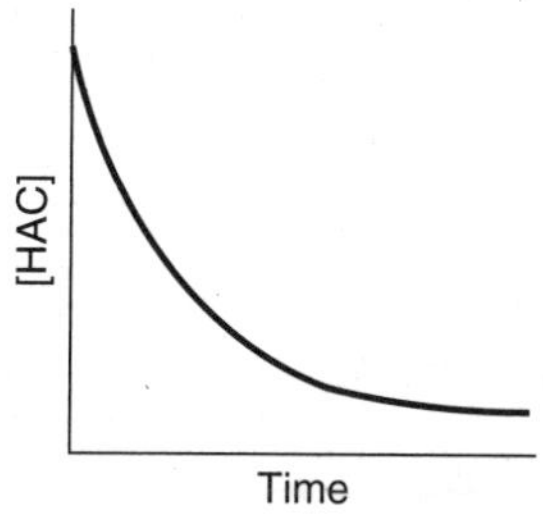

C.

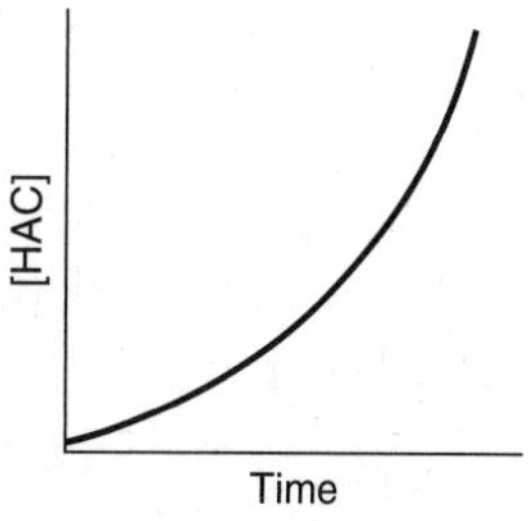

D.

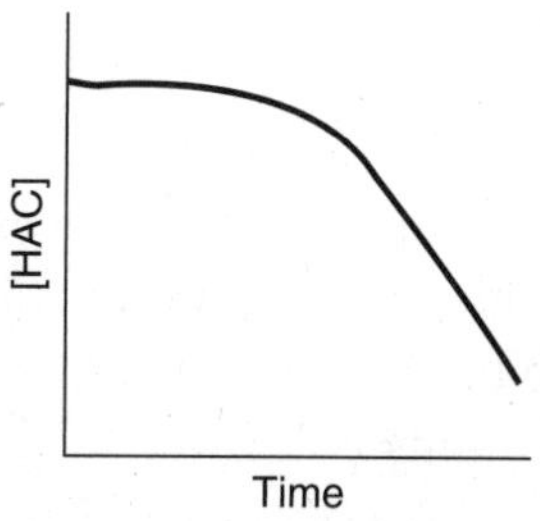

25. What is the half-life for the hydrolysis of methyl acetate at 25°C?
    A. 2.8 min B. 3.0 min
    C. 3.2 min D. 3.4 min

PASSAGE VI (QUESTIONS 26–28)

A compound microscope consists of an objective lens mounted at the bottom of the barrel and an eye lens mounted at the top of the barrel, as illustrated below. In many microscopes, the tube length, the distance from the objective lens to the real image that it forms, is 16cm.

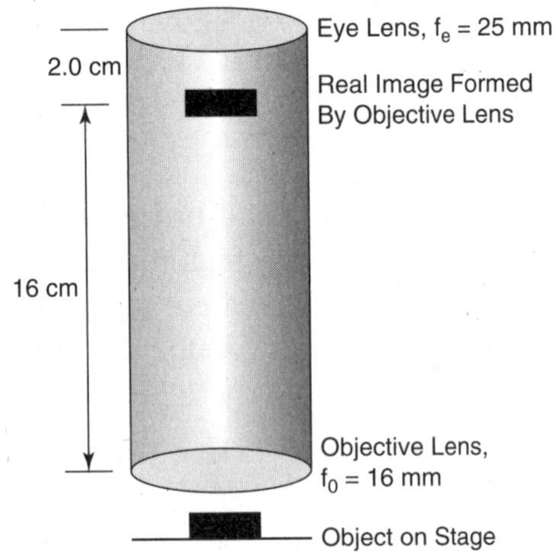

The magnification of a lens is defined as the ratio of the image size to the object size. It can be shown that the magnification M for an image distance of 16cm from a lens of focal length f (in cm) is:

$$M = (16\text{cm}/f) - 1.$$

Magnifying power is defined as the ratio of the image size as viewed with the lens to the object size as viewed at 25cm without the lens. It can be shown that the magnifying power (MP) of a lens of focal length f (in cm) is:

$$MP = (25\text{cm}/f) + 1.$$

The magnifying power of a compound microscope is the product of the magnification of the objective lens times the magnifying power of the eye lens:

$$MP_c = [(16\text{cm}/f_o) - 1][(25\text{cm}/f_e) + 1] \quad \text{Equation (1)}$$

It is useful to express the magnifying power without the "ones";

$$MP_c = (16\text{cm}/f_o)(25\text{cm}/f_e) \quad \text{Equation (2)}$$

26. The real image formed by the objective lens, as shown in the diagram, serves as the object for the eye lens. Determine the distance from the eye lens to the image formed by this object.
    A. −60mm B. −80mm
    C. −100mm D. −120mm

27. In the illustration, the focal length of the eye lens is 25mm. The object for the eye lens is the image formed by the objective lens. What type of image (with respect to the image of the objective lens, not with respect to the object below the objective lens) is formed by the eye lens for the dimensions shown in the illustration?
    A. Virtual, erect B. Virtual, inverted
    C. Real, erect D. Real, inverted

28. The object to be viewed through a microscope is usually covered with a thin glass cover slip. If the cover slip is not completely uniform in thickness, the variation in the divergence of the light when it leaves the cover slip and travels through the air to the objective lens will lead to a reduction in quality of the final image. To reduce this problem, the space between the cover slip and the objective lens is sometimes filled with oil. The oil should be chosen with an index of refraction that is
    A. nearly equal to the index of refraction of air.
    B. nearly equal to the index of refraction of the glass.
    C. much smaller than the index of refraction of air.
    D. much smaller than the index of refraction of the glass.

QUESTIONS 29–32 are NOT based on a descriptive passage.

29. In human digestion, fats are hydrolyzed to
   A. glucagon and glucose.
   B. glycerol and glucagon.
   C. xylenol and fatty acids.
   D. glycerol and fatty acids.

30. A triose may be defined as all of the following EXCEPT as a
   A. sugar.
   B. three-carbon organic compound.
   C. hydroxyaldehyde.
   D. trisaccharide.

31. Which of the following is NOT true for all waves?
   A. Their speed depends on the temperature of the transmitting medium.
   B. $v = f\lambda$
   C. They can produce interference.
   D. They can be diffracted.

32. An inclined plane is 15m long and 3m high. The force required to prevent a box weighing 120N from sliding down this frictionless plane is
   A. 8N. B. 24N.
   C. 40N. D. 45N.

PASSAGE VII (QUESTIONS 33–37)

An automobile of mass 2,000 kg is parked on a steep hill. The coefficient of static friction between the tires and the road surface is 1.00, and the coefficient of sliding friction is independent of speed. A second car, while attempting to park behind the first car, gives the first car a slight bump, which starts it sliding down the hill. At the bottom of the hill, the road curves sharply, with radius of curvature 50m. The first car slides straight down the hill and collides with a solid stone wall at the edge of the road near the foot of the hill. The car slides 200m along the road surface while descending a vertical distance of 100m. The car attains a speed of 20m/s (~45mph) just before reaching the stone wall and comes to rest 0.50s after striking the wall.

The driver of the second car sees that there is a public telephone just beyond the curve at the bottom of the hill. The second car moves down the hill, past the wreckage of the first car, rounding the curve at a speed of 13.4m/s (~30mph). The driver of the second car applies the brakes and comes to a stop by the telephone booth over a distance of 100m.

When it started, the second car accelerated from rest to 13.4m/s in the first 100m, continued at constant speed for another 200m down the hill and around the curve before starting to decelerate. The incident occurred at a place where acceleration due to gravity is 9.80m/s^2.

33. What is the approximate angle of the hill with respect to the horizontal?
   A. 10° B. 30°
   C. 45° D. 60°

34. After the first car was bumped, it started from an initial speed of zero and slid down the hill, reaching a final speed of 20m/s just before it hit the wall. Therefore, the car accelerated. What statement best describes the reason for this acceleration?
   A. After the first car was bumped by the second car, the bumping force from the second car traveled with the first car down the hill, causing it to continue to accelerate.
   B. The component of the weight down the slope of the road was greater than the sliding frictional force up the slope of the road.
   C. The sliding frictional force, unlike the static frictional force, was in the same direction as the motion of the car.
   D. After being bumped by the second car, the first car came under the

influence of no other forces besides gravity and continued down the hill with the same acceleration as an object in free fall.

35. What is the first car's potential energy, with respect to the bottom of the hill, when it is at the top of the hill?

A. 1.9MJ B. 3.1MJ
C. 3.5MJ D. 4.0MJ

36. What is the first car's kinetic energy just before it strikes the wall?

A. 0.2MJ B. 0.3MJ
C. 0.4MJ D. 0.5MJ

37. What is the magnitude of the first car's momentum just before it strikes the wall?

A. 10 Mg m/s B. 20 Mg m/s
C. 30 Mg m/s D. 40 Mg m/s

PASSAGE VIII (QUESTIONS 38–41)

An experiment was conducted to study the properties of nuclear radiation. As time progresses, radioactive nuclei decay (or change) into daughter nuclei. The general formula that determines the amount of radioactive sample still remaining (or number of parent nuclei, N, that have not yet decayed) at time t is $N = N_o e^{-lt}$, where N_o is the original number of nuclei that existed at time t = 0, and l is a decay constant. In the experiments described below, three radioactive samples were used. One was an alpha emitter, one a beta emitter, and the third sample was a gamma emitter. To detect the radiation, a Geiger-Müller (GM) tube was used and connected to a counter. The GM tube is cylindrical with a 2-cm diameter window at the end of the tube that allows radioactive decay particles to enter. Each radioactive decay particle that enters the tube ionizes the gas inside the tube and initiates an electric pulse that is recorded by the counter. These counts are recorded as a function of time, and the activity, or decay rate, is measured.

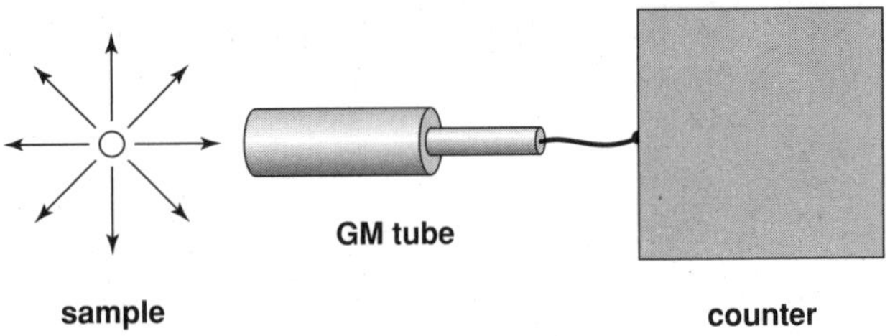

The first experiment was conducted to determine the dependence of the decay rate for gamma radiation on the distance of the source from the GM tube. These data were collected and graphed as the log of the count rate versus the log of the distance, as shown below.

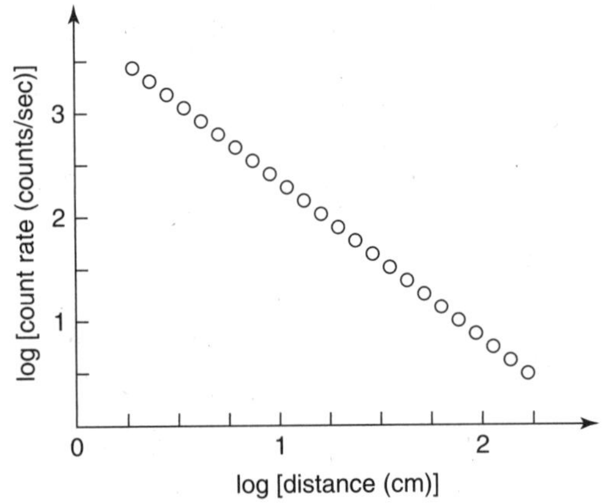

In the second experiment, the relative penetrating abilities of gamma, beta, and alpha radiation were investigated. The alpha, beta, or gamma source was placed 2cm away from the GM tube, and the count rate was measured. The experiment was repeated, first with a cardboard sheet between the tube and sample, then an aluminum sheet, and then a lead sheet. Each material had exactly the same thickness. The count rates with and without each of these three materials are listed in the table below. When comparing count rates for nuclear decay processes, it is useful to know that the standard deviation for any count rate is just the square root of that count rate.

Count rates (counts/second) for radioactive sources through various materials

Material	No barrier	Cardboard barrier	Aluminum barrier	Lead barrier
Alpha source	2250	171	165	175
Beta source	6780	2346	454	356
Gamma source	5467	5235	5003	2389

Another experiment was performed with a sample that has the extremely short half-life of just 2 days. Unfortunately, the experimenter did not realize this and left the sample on the shelf for 2 weeks before any experiments were conducted on the sample.

38. From the graph of log of count rate versus log of distance, an equation describing the dependence of count rate, DN/Dt, on distance, r, is
    A. $\Delta N/\Delta t \propto 1/r$
    B. $\Delta N/\Delta t \propto 1/r^2$
    C. $\Delta N/\Delta t \propto 1/r^3$
    D. $\Delta N/\Delta t \propto 1/r^{1.5}$

39. What can be said about the ability of alpha radiation to penetrate aluminum versus lead?
    A. Alpha radiation penetrates aluminum more easily than lead.
    B. Alpha radiation penetrates lead more easily than aluminum.
    C. There is no statistical difference between the penetrating ability of alpha radiation through aluminum versus lead.
    D. Alpha radiation would penetrate a combined barrier of lead and aluminum more easily than a barrier of just one of the materials.

40. Considering the sample with the extremely short half-life, approximately what percentage of the original sample was left after it lay on the shelf for 2 weeks?
    A. 1%
    B. 5%
    C. 10%
    D. 20%

41. Consider the exponential formula describing the decay of radioactive nuclei with time. Consider a sample that decays over many years until eventually all of the original N_0 nuclei have decayed into daughter nuclei. It can be said that
    A. for a given time period during this decay process, for example, for any given month, the same number of nuclei will decay.
    B. for a given time period during this decay process, for example, for any given month, the same fraction of nuclei will decay.
    C. as time progresses, the decay rate increases dramatically.
    D. as time progresses, the decay rate remains constant.

PASSAGE IX (QUESTIONS 42–45)

Seismic exploration is a technique used by geophysicists to obtain a picture of the Earth's subsurface. A source of disturbance, produced by a hammer blow or small explosion, is produced on the ground. Mechanical waves propagate outward from this source in all directions and are monitored by a geophone placed also on the surface at a certain distance away from the source. The diagram below illustrates the technique and shows two subsurface layers. Of the many waves

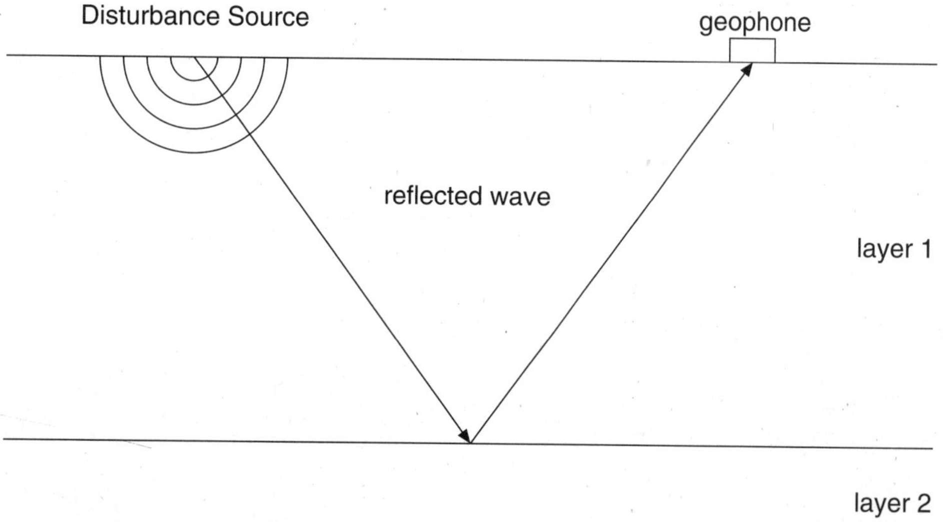

that propagate in the ground, only one is shown and consists of the sound wave that propagates through the first layer to the interface between the first and second ground layers and back up to the geophone (the reflected wave). By measuring the time between disturbance and geophone detection, it is possible to determine information such as layer thickness and wave speed in the ground. This information is useful for determining the composition of the rock or soil in the ground. In addition, submerged objects beneath the surface of the Earth can be detected by seismic waves as long as the diameter of the object is at least one fourth the wavelength of the seismic waves used to detect it.

For analyzing the physics of mechanical waves in the ground, many of the same concepts from geometrical optics that apply to electromagnetic waves are pertinent. For example, Snell's law is the same; that is, the sine of the angle of incidence of a wave in one medium divided by the speed of the wave in that medium is equal to the sine of the refracted wave in the second medium divided by the speed of that wave in the second medium. Also, total internal reflection and critical angles apply, as well as the law of reflection; that is, the angle of incidence equals the angle of reflection.

On a more global perspective, seismic waves are generated by earthquakes and detected by seismographs stationed all over the Earth. At these stations, two main mechanical waves, P and S waves, are detected. The speed of a P or S wave in a material is given by one of the following two formulas. In these formulas, Y is Young's modulus and is related to the stiffness or incompressibility of the material, r is the density of the material, and s is Poisson's ratio and is related to the anisotropy of the material. Note that 0 < s < 0.5.

$$v_P = \sqrt{\frac{Y(1-\sigma)}{\rho(1-2\sigma)(1+\sigma)}}$$

$$v_S = \sqrt{\frac{Y}{\rho 2(1+\sigma)}}$$

42. If the geophone is placed 10m away from the explosion and the reflected wave is first detected by the geophone 10ms after the explosion, what is the approximate thickness of layer 1? Assume that the wave travels at a constant speed of 2000m/s in layer 1.

A. 15m B. 12m
C. 9m D. 6m

43. In addition to the reflected wave shown, in general, there will be a transmitted wave into layer 2. Which figure below best illustrates the propagation of the transmitted wave from layer 1 into layer 2? Assume that the wave speed for layers 1 and 2 is 2000m/s and 3000m/s, respectively.

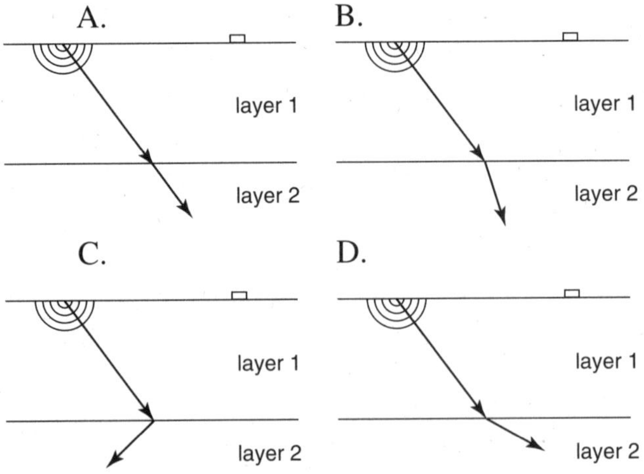

44. A seismograph detects P and S waves emanating from an earthquake. The P waves travel at a constant speed of 6000m/s and are detected 5 minutes before the S waves, which travel at a constant speed of 2000m/s. How far away did the earthquake occur?

A. 400km B. 900km
C. 1500km D. 3200km

45. For seismic waves traveling at a constant speed of 2000m/s and of frequency 30Hz, what is the minimum size object that can be detected?

A. 2m B. 15m
C. 12m D. 17m

PASSAGE X (QUESTIONS 46–50)

A centrifuge is used to separate the components of a suspension, for example, white and red blood cells from plasma, and works by spinning the suspension at high speeds. In the diagram below, a top view of the device is shown. In this example, four test tubes are suspended almost horizontally as the centrifuge spins. Typical spinning rates are 100,000 revolutions per minute. As indicated in the diagram, while spinning, the distance between the bottoms of opposite test tubes is 40cm.

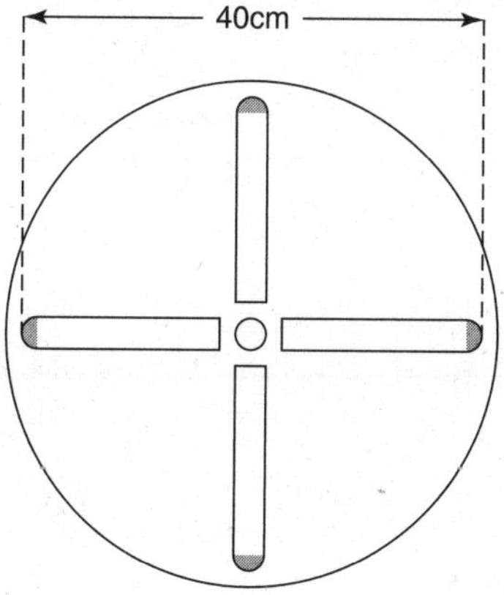

46. For a typical spinning rate, what is the speed of a particle at the bottom of the test tube?

A. 333m/s B. 925m/s
C. 2094m/s D. 4189m/s

47. For a typical spinning rate, what is the acceleration of a particle at the bottom of the test tube?

A. Zero B. $9.8 m/s^2$
C. $660{,}000 m/s^2$ D. $2.19 \times 10^7 m/s^2$

48. How does the angular speed of a particle at the bottom of the test tube, a distance of 20cm from the center of the circle, compare to the angular speed of a particle in the middle of the test tube, a distance of 10 cm from the center of the circle?

A. It is twice as much.
B. It is four times as much.
C. It is exactly the same.
D. It is half as much.

49. As the centrifuge is spinning, a small hole suddenly opens up at the base of one of the test tubes and particles begin to leak out of this hole. Which diagram best represents the subsequent travel path of these particles after they leave the hole? In each case, assume that the centrifuge is spinning counterclockwise and the hole opens up at the base of the right test tube when it is at the position shown.

A.
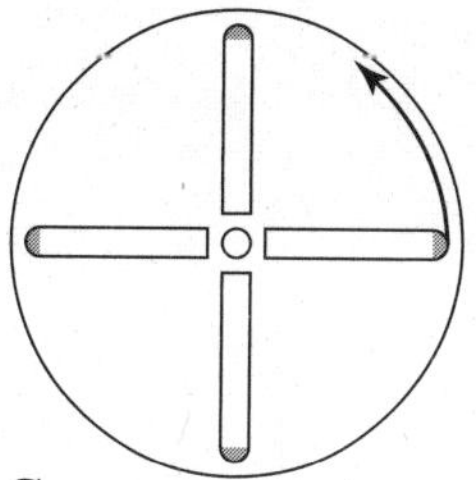

B.
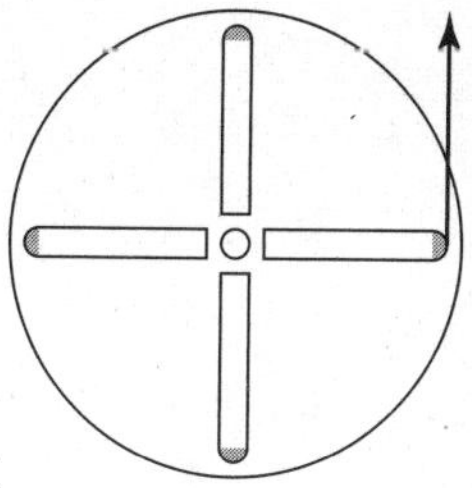

C.
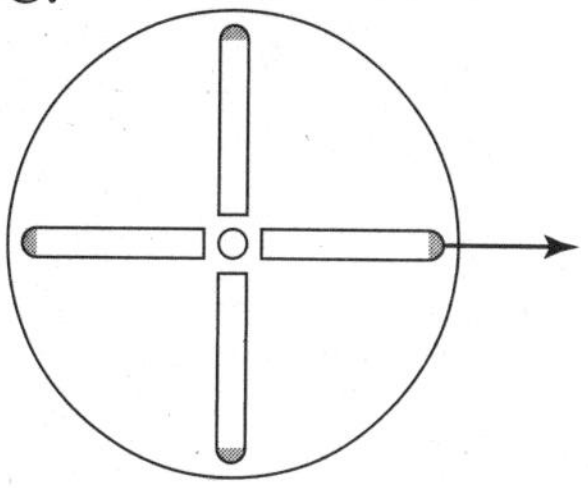

D.
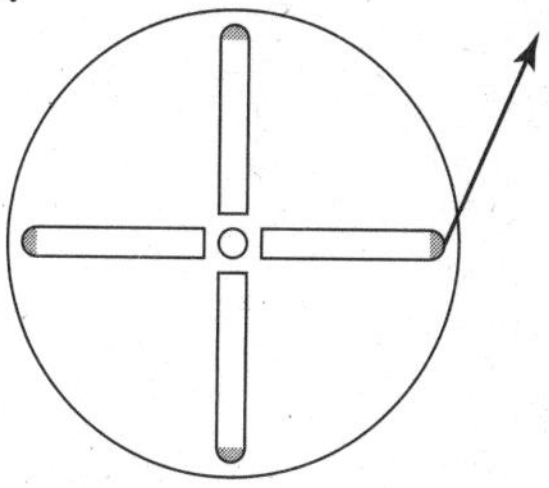

50. The relationship between the centripetal force, F, on a particle in the test tube, the mass of the particle, m, and the distance from the center of the circle, r, is given by

A. $F \propto m/r$ B. $F \propto r/m$
C. $F \propto mr$ D. $F \propto mr^2$

QUESTIONS 51–52 are NOT based on a descriptive passage.

51. A car traveling on level ground at a speed of 15 meters per second stops 10 seconds after a braking force of 3000 newtons is applied. What is the mass of the car?

A. 1,500kg B. 2,000kg
C. 2,500kg D. 3,000kg

52. Two satellites, M_1 and M_2, are in a circular orbit at a distance (s) of 6.7×10^6 meters from the center of the Earth, as indicated in the diagram below. The mass of satellite M_2 is 100 kg, and the mass of the Earth is 6.0×10^{24} kg. The speed of satellite M_1 is 7.7×10^3 m/s. $G = 6.67 \times 10^{-11}$ N-m^2. If M_2 has a mass twice as great as M_1, the orbit speed of M_2, as compared to M_1, is

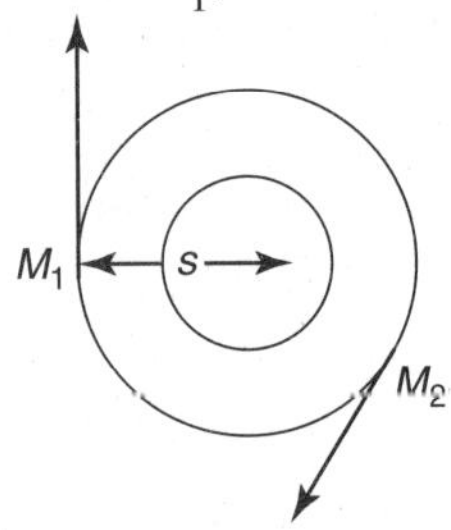

A. half as great. B. the same.
C. twice as great. D. four times as great.

STOP! If time still remains, you may review work only in this section. When the time allotted is up, you may go on to the next section. STOP!

SECTION 2
Verbal Reasoning

TIME: 60 Minutes

QUESTIONS: 53–92

DIRECTIONS: The verbal reasoning section contains nine passages, each followed by a series of questions. Based on the information given in a passage, choose the one best answer to each question.

PASSAGE I (QUESTIONS 53–58)

In May 1774, in retaliation to the "Boston Tea Party," Parliament closed the port of Boston and virtually abolished provincial self-government in Massachusetts. These actions stimulated resistance across the land. That summer, through the committees of correspondence, the Massachusetts lower house secretly invited all 13 Colonies to attend a convention. In response, on the fifth of September, 55 Delegates representing 12 Colonies, with the exception of Georgia, assembled in Philadelphia. They convened at Carpenters' Hall and organized the First Continental Congress.

Although the Delegates propounded a wide variety of political opinions, they all shared complaints against the Crown. Most of them agreed that Parliament had no right to control the internal affairs of the Colonies. Moderates, who stressed the importance of trade benefits with the mother country, believed Parliament should continue to regulate commerce. Others questioned the extent of its authority. A handful of Delegates felt the answer to the problem lay in parliamentary representation. Most suggested legislative autonomy for the Colonies. Reluctant to sever ties of blood, language, trade, and cultural heritage, at this time none openly entertained the idea of complete independence from Great Britain.

After weeks of debate and compromise, Congress adopted two significant measures. The first declared that the American colonists were entitled to the same rights as Englishmen everywhere and denounced any infringement upon those rights. The second measure passed was for the creation of the Continental Association that provided for an embargo on all trade with Britain. In order to enforce the embargo and punish violators, at the behest of Congress, counties, cities, and towns formed councils, or committees of safety—many of which later became wartime governing or administrative bodies. When Congress adjourned in late October, the Delegates resolved to reconvene in May of 1775 if the Crown had not responded by then.

In a sense, the Continental Congress acted with restraint, for while it was in session, the situation in Massachusetts verged on war. In September, just before Congress met, British troops from Boston had seized ordnance supplies at Charlestown and Cambridge, and almost clashed with the local militia. The next month, Massachusetts patriots, openly defying royal authority, organized a Revolutionary provincial assembly as well as a military defense committee. Whigs in three other colonies—Maryland, Virginia, and New Hampshire—had formed governments earlier that year. By the end of the year, all the Colonies except Georgia and New York had either set up new governments or taken control of those already in existence. During the winter of 1774/75, while Parliament mulled over conciliatory measures, colonial militia units prepared for war.

The crisis came in the spring of 1775, predictably in Massachusetts. Late on the night of April 18, the Royal Governor, Gen. Thomas Gage, alarmed at the militancy of the rebels, dispatched 600 troops from Boston to seize a major supply depot at Concord. Almost simultaneously, the Boston council of safety, aware of Gage's intentions, directed Paul Revere and William Dawes to ride ahead to warn militia units and citizens along the way of the British approach. The council of safety also alerted John Hancock and Samuel Adams, who were staying at nearby Lexington. Forewarned, the two men went into hiding.

About 77 militiamen confronted the redcoats when they plodded into Lexington at dawn. After some tense moments, the sorely outnumbered colonists dispersed; however, blood was still shed. More blood flowed at Concord and along the route the British took as they retreated to Boston; they were harassed most of the way by an aroused citizenry. What had once been merely protest had evolved into open warfare; the War for Independence had begun.

53. Which of the following statements best summarizes the main theme of the passage?
   A. The Continental Congress was an assembly of reactionary Englishmen who ignited the War of Independence.
   B. The Revolutionary War was precipitated by the British elimination of colonial self-government in Massachusetts.
   C. The first Continental Congress was made up of men with similar values and beliefs.
   D. The American Revolution was precipitated by a series of events that involved the first Continental Congress.

54. The idea of complete independence from Britain was
   A. never entertained by the colonists prior to 1775.
   B. favored by the moderates.
   C. favored by all the Delegates to the Continental Congress.
   D. never debated on the floor of the Continental Congress.

55. One of the colonies that did NOT set up a revolutionary provisional assembly was
   A. Virginia.
   B. Pennsylvania.
   C. New Hampshire.
   D. Maryland.

56. The expression *Whigs* refers to
   A. military defense committees.
   B. British troops.
   C. British sympathizers.
   D. patriots against kingly authority.

57. According to the passage, which of the following men was not involved in the Battle of Concord?
   A. William Dawes B. Thomas Gage
   C. Paul Revere D. Samuel Adams

58. In the context of the passage, the term *embargo* may be said to mean
   A. opposition. B. protection.
   C. prevention. D. proposition.

PASSAGE II (QUESTIONS 59–63)

The most serious threat organized crime poses to society is the vast sums of money criminal syndicates acquire from illicit enterprises that undermine legitimate business enterprises and political institutions. Organized crime has infiltrated labor unions, the entertainment business, manufacturing, real estate, and even the stock market. To measure its impact in terms of dollars would be a formidable, if not prohibitive, task.

In 1972, the stock brokerage industry alone estimated that stolen or missing securities of $1.2 billion were being utilized in illegal operations around the world. The loss of income tax revenue from organized crime operations is incalculable. It has been estimated that illegal betting on horse racing, lotteries, and sporting events alone totals at least $20 billion a year, with the syndicate taking about $6 to $7 billion as its share (this is about three times the amount of the annual budget for U.S. foreign aid). Loan sharks have been known to charge interest rates as high as 500 percent. Millions of dollars of cargo are pilfered from airports and piers by trucking companies and union locals working for a criminal group. Labor union pension funds have been used for loans to finance illegal or questionable enterprises, and construction companies have used shoddy materials and workmanship through kickback arrangements.

When speaking in the vernacular, the results of all this include higher prices through the monopolistic practices of organized crime, shoddy merchandise, poorly constructed and unsafe buildings, and higher taxes. More important is the threat to the free enterprise system. Organized crime operates on the local level as well, controlling businesses such as laundries, taxicab companies, paving-contract firms, travel agencies, insurance underwriting firms, vending machine companies, and restaurants.

The social costs of political corruption by organized crime are even more difficult to assess. Organized crime needs the involvement of the political system to profit from economic opportunities. The President's Commission concluded that "all available data indicate that organized crime flourishes only where it has corrupted local officials." Many times, investigations of criminal activities have discovered that respectable persons in business and public officials at all levels of government have connections to organized crime. Corruption is achieved through bribes and contributions to political campaigns; a police officer is bribed or overlooks gambling, and a state or Federal legislator's vote on a bill is bought by the criminal organization that contributed heavily to the person's campaign through a front organization. Therefore, organized crime is, in part, a subversion of the democratic process that ultimately produces a political system where the strong and powerful exist at the expense of the weak.

59. Which of the following is the main theme of this passage?
    A. Organized crime is a tale of corruption.
    B. Free enterprise is threatened by organized crime.
    C. Organized crime is controlled by public officials and big business.
    D. The people will always pay the price of the loss of free enterprise.

60. The passage states that organized crime has permeated so much of society that
    I. lotteries contribute to organized crime.
    II. bribes furnished by the syndicate are an inevitable part of the free enterprise system.
    III. it can flourish only with the support of public officials.

    A. I only
    B. I and II
    C. I and III
    D. II and III

61. Which of the following expressions fits the passage?
    A. The meek shall inherit the earth.
    B. Adaptation is the key to success.
    C. Might is right.
    D. "Survival of the fittest" is the prevailing rule.

62. Based on the passage, corruption
    A. means higher prices for every person.
    B. involves every working person.
    C. is the single cause of the loss of tax revenue.
    D. undermines the work of the President's Commission.

63. On the basis of the information given in the passage, organized crime
    A. is an economic deterrent to foreign trade.
    B. fosters growth while diminishing profits.
    C. does not distinguish between big business and the person in the neighborhood.
    D. is allowed to thrive because gambling is a national pastime.

PASSAGE III (QUESTIONS 64–67)

In his celebrated essay *On Liberty,* John Stuart Mill argued that liberty of thought and expression were central and necessary elements of well-being for both individuals and socictics. Mill argucd that the only justification for censoring self-expression is if the means of self-expression posed a threat to the freedom of others. Conformity to the prevailing opinion or lifestyle cannot be forced for any reason other than that of preventing harm to the interests of others; in which case, these interests are those that others have a right to enjoy. Mere displeasure or disapproval is not sufficient to warrant the stifling of thought and expression.

Mill argued for this liberty of expression in a two-pronged fashion, first considering the case where the stifled opinion is true, and then the case where the stifled opinion is false.

In the first case, where the opinion that is suppressed is true, we are in effect making an assumption of infallibility when we refuse to allow contrary opinions to be voiced. This assumption of infallibility does not exist in our assumption that our own beliefs are true. Rather, it exists in the undertaking to decide for others what is true and refuse to allow open debate about the truth of our own beliefs and other doctrines. Certainly, we should all have learned, both from our own experience and that of the entire human race, that we are all liable to error, even in those beliefs we hold most confidently to be true. For us to decide what will and will not be heard is to assume unwarranted infallibility.

It has been claimed that there are some beliefs that are so dangerous that we are entitled to silence them for the health and safety of the society. However, the very claim that a belief is dangerous in itself is an opinion about which we may be in error, and so it too should be subject to open debate.

In refusing to allow an opinion to be heard when it is true, though in our own belief false, we are not only assuming unwarranted infallibility but are also eliminating the opportunity to rid ourselves of our false belief.

Conversely, suppose we are correct about the beliefs we hold, and the belief that we are silencing is the one that is false. In this case, we are eliminating the opportunity for our belief system to face the challenge of honest debate, establish its truth, and expose the error of the alternatives. The challenge of debate is what adds vitality to our beliefs; in the absence of such debate, our beliefs deteriorate into dead dogmas and lose energy. Constant challenge is not a harm to truth, but a force that makes truth a living faith rather than dogma; we see and feel its merit and force.

Normally, our beliefs are a mixture of these two cases. Some of our beliefs are true and some are false; some of the beliefs that we would stifle are a mixture of the true and the false. It is for a combination of the above reasons that it is to our advantage not to stifle the free, forceful, and open expression of opinion.

64. Mill argued that the silencing of opinion can be justified when
    A. the interests of others are threatened.
    B. harm to others is threatened.
    C. harm to the entitlements of others is threatened.
    D. these opinions are disagreeable to the majority.

65. Mill accepted the idea that
    A. some restrictions on liberty of expression are warranted by the security needs of a society.
    B. no restrictions on liberty of expression are warranted by the security needs of a society.
    C. the security needs of a society are in themselves matters of opinion.
    D. the security needs of a society are not matters relating to the questions of freedom of expression.

66. According to Mill, when our beliefs are true and we know them for certain to be true, we
    A. should ensure that our beliefs are not threatened by false and seductive doctrines.

B. should ensure that our beliefs are exposed by lively and free debate.
C. will see the error of opposing beliefs.
D. will have no need for contact with opposing doctrines.

67. Based on the passage, we could expect that Mill's argument would apply to
A. governmental strictures but not the censorship imposed by private individuals or organizations.
B. any kind of stricture from either government or private agents on the holding of beliefs but not on their expression.
C. strictures on both the expression of opinion and on one's choice of lifestyle.
D. opinions that are true and only those.

PASSAGE IV (QUESTIONS 68–71)

The physical phenomenon responsible for converting light to electricity—the photovoltaic (PV) effect—was first observed in 1839 by a French physicist, Edmund Becquerel. Becquerel noted a voltage appeared when one of two identical electrodes in a weak conducting solution was illuminated. The PV effect was first studied in solids, such as selenium, in the 1870s. In the 1880s, selenium photovoltaic cells were built that exhibited 1%–2% efficiency in converting light to electricity. Selenium converts light in the visible part of the sun's spectrum; for this reason, it was quickly adopted by the then-emerging field of photography for photometric (light-measuring) devices. Even today, the light-sensitive cells on cameras that are used for adjusting shutter speed to match illumination are made of selenium. However, selenium cells have never become practical as energy converters because their cost is too high, considering the tiny amount of power they produce (at 1% efficiency).

Meanwhile, work on the physics of PV phenomena has expanded. In the 1920s and 1930s, quantum mechanics laid the theoretical foundation for our present understanding of PV. A major step forward in solar-cell technology came in the 1940s and early 1950s when a method (called the Czochralski method) was developed for producing highly pure crystalline silicon. In 1954, work at Bell Telephone Laboratories resulted in a silicon photovoltaic cell with a 4% efficiency. Bell Labs soon improved this to a 6% and then an 11% efficiency, heralding an entirely new era of power-producing cells.

A few schemes were tried in the 1950s to use silicon PV cells commercially. Most were for cells in regions geographically isolated from electric utility lines. But an unexpected boom in PV technology came from a different quarter. In 1958, the U.S. Vanguard space satellite used a small (less than one-watt) array of cells to power its radio. The cells worked so well that space scientists soon realized the PV could be an effective power source for many space missions. Technological development of the solar cell has been part of the space program ever since.

Today, photovoltaic systems are capable of transforming one kilowatt of solar energy falling on one square meter into about a hundred watts of electricity. One hundred watts can power most household appliances: a television, a stereo, or a lamp. In fact, standard solar cells covering the sun-facing roof space of a typical home can provide about 8500-kilowatt-hours of electricity annually, which is about the average household's yearly electric consumption. By comparison, a modern, 200-ton electric-arc steel furnace, demanding 50,000 kilowatts of electricity, would require about a square kilometer of land for a PV power supply.

Certain factors make capturing solar energy difficult. Besides the sun's low illuminating power per square meter, sunlight is intermittent, affected by time of day, climate, pollution, and season. Power sources based on photovoltaics require either backup from other sources or storage for times when the sun is obscured.

In addition, the cost of a photovoltaic system is far from negligible (electricity from PV systems in 1980 cost about 20 times that from conventional fossil-fuel-powered systems).

While solar energy for photovoltaic conversion into electricity is abundant, inexhaustible, and clean, it also requires special techniques to effectively gather enough of it.

68. The photovoltaic effect is the result of
    A. two identical negative electrodes.
    B. one weak solution and two negative electrodes.
    C. two positive electrodes of different qualities.
    D. positive electrodes interacting in a weak environment.

69. The most appropriate title for this passage is
    A. "Information on the Science of Edmund Becquerel."
    B. "The History of the PV Effect."
    C. "A Comparison of Selenium, Silicon, and Solar PV Cells."
    D. "The Adaptation of the PV Effect."

70. Selenium was used for photometric devices because it
    A. was the first solid to be observed to have the PV effect.
    B. is inexpensive.
    C. converts the visible part of the sun's spectrum.
    D. can adjust shutter speeds on cameras.

71. Sunlight is difficult to procure for transformation into solar energy. Which of the following statements most accurately supports this belief derived from the passage?
    A. Sunlight is erratic and subject to variables.
    B. Sunlight is steady but never available.
    C. Sunlight is not visible because of pollution.
    D. Sunlight would have to be artificially produced.

PASSAGE V
(QUESTIONS 72–76)

Old age—a difficult time for many people—can be especially so for members of racial and ethnic minority groups. Compared to the majority of Americans, these individuals are likely to have less education and money, less adequate housing, poorer health, and fewer years of life.

Many minority groups—especially black, Hispanic, Asian, and Native American—bear the added burdens of racial prejudice, language barriers, suspicion of bureaucratic processes, and difficulty obtaining needed health and other services.

In addition, minority group members who have suffered from racial discrimination all their lives are in double jeopardy in their later years because they may also be discriminated against for being old.

The number of individuals with ethnic affiliations is greater than the word *minority* might imply. According to a study supported by the National Institute on Aging (NIA), almost 40 percent of the entire U.S. population over age 65 in the 1980s will be black, or of first- and second-generation Americans belonging to various racial/ethnic subgroups.

Ethnic and racial affiliations are important in determining not only individual attitudes, problems, and needs, but the considerable strengths many minority members exhibit in adapting to old age. Yet society at large, and the research community in particular, seldom take these differences into account.

Among older blacks, for example, hypertension is twice as prevalent as it is among whites, and accidents are the leading cause of death for older Alaskan Natives and American Indians. The leading causes of death for Hispanics are not even known because those statistics are just beginning to be collected.

Such diverse populations as Samoans, Chinese, Filipinos, Koreans, Hawaiians, Japanese, and Vietnamese are lumped together as Asian and Pacific Americans. Yet lifestyles, attitudes, and other differences exist among these populations. For example, food preferences and tastes vary among these groups and, in turn, have a great impact on the effectiveness of nutrition programs.

To add to our knowledge of aging minority group members, the NIA has funded a study of about 5,000 black Americans living in 100 communities across the nation. This study, which is among the most extensive examinations ever conducted of these individuals, will focus on aging among blacks, and on the transmission of attitudes and values among generations. The study will explore regional differences among blacks in a number of important social and health-related areas, including work and retirement. Such efforts help law- and policymakers design programs that are genuinely helpful to minority groups.

For the future, the NIA is concerned with how different racial and ethnic minorities age in our society. Specifically, the research community, including investigators from minority groups, has been invited to study how family structure, social networks, occupations, lifestyles, environmental conditions, personality traits, attitudes, methods of coping, and health care practices of minority groups influence the way these individuals age.

It is clear that many concerns of the aging minority groups need further attention, not only in their own right, but because of their interrelationship with the problems of the elderly in general.

72. The central idea of this passage is
    A. the American population is aging rapidly.
    B. the NIA should continue to be funded.
    C. we have inadequate knowledge of aging minorities in our country.
    D. studies are being done to assess the needs of our aging minorities.

73. The author uses the information on Asian and Pacific Americans to
    A. discredit the value of these Americans for the study.
    B. demonstrate the value of nutritional differences in some aging minorities.
    C. compare blacks to other minorities.
    D. increase the minority studies based on nutrition for the NIA.

74. It can be inferred from the passage that the NIA
    A. needs financial support from the private sector.
    B. utilizes minority studies as an essential way of determining the needs of all age groups.
    C. has satisfactorily completed its studies.
    D. has singled out aging minorities as their sole subject of research.

75. Among the leading causes of death among certain minorities, hypertension is
    A. not present in older Alaskans.
    B. half as prevalent among older whites than it is among blacks.
    C. not present in an older Hispanic population.
    D. more of a serious concern for all blacks than it is for Alaskan Natives.

76. The passage reveals that
    A. many minorities have attitudes and values that exhibit graceful aging.
    B. adaptation to old age is exclusively a minority problem.
    C. many minorities exhibit explicit strengths in adapting to old age.
    D. ethnic and racial affiliations are important.

PASSAGE VI (QUESTIONS 77–82)

It appears that Charles Darwin first formulated the modern approach to the origins of life with a view of the circumstances, not of his present day, but of the distant past when the first life was somehow formed. He wrote in a private letter in 1871: "If we could conceive in some warm little pond, with all sorts of ammonia and phosphoric salts, light, heat, electricity, etc., present, that a protein compound was chemically formed ready to undergo still more complex changes, at the present day such matter would be instantly devoured or absorbed, which would not have been the case before living creatures were formed." In short, the logical needs for the *origin* of life include the *absence* of life: a sterile environment was exactly what was present then and what is utterly unknown in the biosphere today. But for 50 years, such large ideas lay dormant. They were ahead of the state of biology and geology. The question was too grand. Pasteur's wonderful declaration is true for our geological epoch; the ancient epoch when life originated, which is not at all the present natural life–filled environment, was not brought under study.

In 1924, a young Russian biochemist published a preliminary account of his ideas on the chemical origins of life. In a booklet entitled *Proiskhozhdenie Zhizny,* he pointed out that the complex combination of manifestations and properties so characteristic of life must have arisen in the process of the evolution of matter. A. Oparin had learned Mendeleev's ideas on the possible origin of hydrocarbons from the carbides in the crust of the Earth, and injected into his own thinking a new notion concerning the reducing nature of the early atmosphere. To Oparin's great credit, this observation was made before the astrophysicists had discovered that stars were 90% hydrogen.

In 1928, independently of Oparin, J. B. S. Haldane, the British biologist, wrote a classic paper, "The Origin of Life." Haldane speculated on the early conditions suitable for the emergence of life. According to him, when ultraviolet (UV) light acted upon a mixture of water, carbon dioxide, and ammonia, a variety of organic substances were made, including sugars and apparently some of the materials from which proteins are built up. Before the origin of life, they must have accumulated until the primitive oceans reached the constituency of a hot, dilute soup. Haldane gave us the concept of the "primordial soup."

Almost 20 years after Haldane's publication, J. D. Bernal of the University of London conjectured before the British Physical Society, in a famous lecture entitled *The Physical Basis of Life*, that clay surfaces were involved in the origin of life. He was looking for ways and means by which the primordial molecules in the hot, dilute soup could be brought together to give rise to polymers capable of replication. A physicist and crystallographer by training, Bernal was particularly attracted to the role of surface phenomena in the origin of life. He argued that favorable conditions for concentration, which may have taken place on a very large scale, were provided by the adsorption of organic molecules on the fine clay deposits. The role of clay in primordial organic synthesis is currently a lively area of investigation.

77. Based on the information in the passage, Charles Darwin
    A. believed there was a time when life was dormant.
    B. wanted to create a simulation of the origin of life.
    C. believed the origin of life required an active environment.
    D. believed that without living creatures, complex compounds would continue to exist.

78. From the passage, we can assume that A. Oparin, a Russian biochemist,
    A. utilized Mendeleev's idea that stars were 90% hydrogen.
    B. discovered the principle that natural life contracts.

C. conceived of the idea of the evolution of matter.
D. believed that Charles Darwin's theory of the origin of life was wrong.

79. From the passage, it can be concluded that
A. only Darwin, Oparin, and Haldane contributed to evolutionary theory.
B. Oparin, Haldane, and Bernal disagreed with Darwin.
C. Darwin, Oparin, Haldane, and Bernal were the only four significant contributors to evolutionary theory.
D. Darwin paved the way for the evolutionary theories of Oparin, Haldane, and Bernal.

80. It can be inferred from this passage that life
A. began from pre-existent matter.
B. had no beginning.
C. is too complex to speculate on its beginnings.
D. and its absence are but two sides of the same coin.

81. An appropriate title for this passage would be "The Evolutionary Synthesis" because
A. *synthesis* is a synonym for *origin*.
B. *synthesis* implies a contraction of matter.
C. all evolutionary theories are syntheses.
D. *synthesis* has similar meaning to *analysis*.

82. From the essay, we may infer that the relationship between the origin of life and the present study of matter
A. involves a direct cause-effect relationship to each other.
B. involves no cause-effect relationship to each other.
C. are equal.
D. are not equal.

PASSAGE VII (QUESTIONS 83–87)

Utilitarian moralists maintain that the moral value of an action depends upon the value of the consequences of that action. A person's motives in doing an action are not relevant when assessing the moral value of the action, although they may be considered in determining the moral character of the person who does the action. As a result, *consequences* determine the value of the action and *motives* are relevant only for determining the moral character of the person who does the action.

There are differences in how the consequences of an action are understood. There are those who take "consequences" in the sense of the results that come about from an action, regardless of whether or not these results were, or even could have been, foreseen. There are others who take consequences in the sense of the results that would normally come about or that should reasonably have been foreseen. Utilitarian moralists differ on their views of what kinds of consequences are relevant when assessing the moral character of an action: the actual consequences or the reasonably expected consequences.

There is yet a second way in which utilitarian moral theories differ, specifically in how they interpret the notion of an action. In one type of theory, an action is thought of as a certain way of doing something, as an action of a particular type or kind. In the other type of theory, an action is thought of as a particular performance done by a person at some place and at some time. The key difference between these two ways of construing an action has to do with the concept of *repeatability.* Is the action thought of as something that is repeatable in principle? Can one person do this very same act a number of different times, or can many different people do this very same act either at the same time or at different times? If the answer is "yes," then the act may be said to be repeatable and is then thought of as a type or kind of action. On the other hand, if the answer to these questions is "no," then the action is thought of as a particular or concrete instance of an action.

These two different ways of thinking about an action determine the type of utilitarian moral theory one holds. One stance maintains that the theory applies to types or kinds of action, while the other stance maintains that the theory applies to particular instances of types of actions. The first opinion, the one that considers actions as types, then looks to consequences as what normally results from doing a certain type of action. The actual consequences that do in fact result are not considered relevant. The other type of theory offers a choice of how the concept of consequences is conjoined with the concept of the action. We may look to either the reasonably expected consequences or to the actual consequences of a particular action in determining its moral worth.

83. Utilitarian theories evaluate the moral value of actions on the basis of
    A. the motives a person has in doing the action.
    B. a person's responsibility for the action.
    C. the actual consequences of the type of action performed.
    D. the value of an action's consequences.

84. Whether or not an action is repeatable determines whether or not it
    A. is considered by utilitarian theories.
    B. is a type of action or a particular action.
    C. has consequences.
    D. is moral.

85. A utilitarian theory that understands "consequences" as actual occurrences
    A. would be required to construe actions as types of actions.
    B. would be required to construe actions as particular actions.
    C. could construe actions as either types of or as particular actions.
    D. could, but would not be required to, construe actions as types of actions.

86. Based on the passage, utilitarian moralists agree
    A. that consequences determine the moral value of an action.
    B. on the moral values of actions.
    C. on matters of responsibility.
    D. on exactly what an action is.

87. The actual results of an action would be considered morally relevant
    A. by some but not all utilitarians.
    B. by all utilitarians.
    C. only to those who construe actions as a form of responsibility.
    D. by no utilitarians.

PASSAGE VIII (QUESTIONS 88–90)

Today, the role business and government play in solving social problems remains a controversial topic. Children no longer work in factories. Working hours for both men and women are regulated by government. Some observers feel that the New Deal legislation sponsored by President Franklin D. Roosevelt provided the major thrust for governmental regulation of private-sector personnel practices that had been the exclusive jurisdiction of industry and business management for too long. At first, the Supreme Court struck down Roosevelt-initiated statutes. But the sentiment of the country and appointment of men politically sensitive to the political goals of the president led to judicial support of laws designed to deal with social ills in the country. In the 1930s and early 1940s, Congress followed the leadership of the top executive who proposed such legislation as Social Security, workers' compensation, and mandatory minimum wages. At that time, a desire for change was ripe due to economic chaos caused by the Great Depression. Business and industry managers were suddenly cast into a different role when Congress and the Supreme Court became allies in authorizing governmental intrusion into the private sector's arena. Swift changes led to new professional expertise required for interpretation of law, additional paperwork, and implementation of personnel policies.

By the 1950s, long-standing racial discrimination was challenged. Congress had remained too long aloof and generally ignored problems associated with inequality. The NAACP bypassed the legislative branch and took its case to the judicial branch. By the 1960s, President Lyndon Johnson influenced Congress to take bold steps that eventually called for changes in the workplace. Title VII was passed, and a reduction of inequities was expected. However, the NAACP director of labor, Joann Aiggs, said in 1987, that racial discrimination remains, but federal legislation "does provide an avenue people can use to seek redress."

America has often been called a "melting pot" because of the varied ethnic, cultural, and racial heritages of its citizens. With the exception of a great flow of people from Africa before the early 1800s and the Chinese in the late 1880s, the majority of immigrants came from western Europe. The government set a national quota system. By the 1960s, laws changed, and so did the national origin of immigrants, with the majority entering the country from Asia and Latin America. The number of immigrants has grown to around nine million people coming into the country during a 10-year span. When employers hire immigrants while jobs are scarce, citizens who have been in this country for more than one generation feel threatened. Competition for jobs is a major issue. Congressional response placed a large paperwork burden on the personnel departments of business and industry. The Immigration Reform and Control Act of 1986 penalizes employers who hire illegal aliens. Today, personnel offices must report the legal status of their employees to the government. Documents must show that noncitizens have acquired authorization to work in this country. Some observers feel that governmental rules may drive illegal aliens from the workplace, and that no one else will want to perform the low-level tasks required in some of the jobs.

88. Which answer choice best summarizes the author's statements about the legislative change in the 1930s?
   A. It is evident that the author felt that President Roosevelt as chief executive should have stayed out of the legislative process and relied more on the judicial process.
   B. The author explained how President Roosevelt changed the direction of government by showing a stronger social orientation than national leaders of judicial and executive branches in earlier years.
   C. Although new legislation was passed, the laws more or less left business and industry personnel policies intact by the 1940s.
   D. At first, President Roosevelt had to rely more on the courts than on stubborn legislators in order to pass laws designed to deal with social problems.

89. Although observers may argue about what really happened during Roosevelt's term of office, interpret the factual information presented by the author by selecting the best description below.
   A. New Deal legislation received its name from the deals the president made with business and industry for the purpose of pulling the rug out from under Congress, so to speak.
   B. Evolution and transformation of labor policies increased at a rapid pace during the Roosevelt administration.
   C. The author has inferred that historically the name "Great Depression" was a phrase that caught on after the press disclosed Roosevelt's mood when the Supreme Court struck down the first three social welfare bills passed by Congress.
   D. Strange alliances are often formed in the political arena. Unorganized labor and its representatives in the legislature were seldom impressed with promises of reforms that would lead to a welfare state.

90. Below are several statements that deal with discrimination in the workplace. Choose the sentence that conforms to the author's analysis.
    A. The recent immigration act is possibly the best example of affirmative action in recent years.
    B. Illegal aliens are part of the establishment.
    C. When business and industry employers ignored social problems associated with hiring illegal aliens, government eventually stepped into the vacuum created by private-sector negligence and mandated constructive activities.
    D. Private-sector and public-sector policy-makers by and large have the same goals when trying to solve the social problems of employees.

PASSAGE IX (QUESTIONS 91–92)

Universal health coverage for all citizens is a political question staunchly supported by proponents and vigorously opposed by detractors. Both groups are emotionally committed to their idea of what is best for the nation. Today, health care coverage varies from business to business. Employees may or may not be covered by health insurance and/or retirement pension plans provided by employers. Congress has made small steps toward a national health plan through several laws. For instance, the Health Maintenance Organization Act was passed in 1973. Lobbyists have pressed for leaves of absence without fear of job loss when babies are born, children or parents are ill, or a parent experiences serious illness. The central issues for business and industry are personnel management and labor costs. Who will perform work duties for up to 26 weeks while the employee is on leave without pay?

Not surprisingly, many female employees support a leave of absence for child-rearing purposes. The National Organization for Women has worked actively to support passage of the federal law. Senator Christopher Dodd feels that the bill addresses the problems of working mothers. He cited statistics to prove his point: "half of all mothers with infants less than a year old work outside home" and "85% of all women working outside the home are likely to become pregnant at some point during their career." Dodd maintained that "we must no longer force parents to choose between their job and caring for a new or sick child." The bill has its critics. The president of the California Merchants and Manufacturers Association projects discrimination against women in hiring practices if the bill is passed. Roberta Cook of the California Chamber of Commerce said, "We're compassionate. We just don't think the issue should be the employer's responsibility. *That's* the issue."

Another social issue yet to be resolved is drug use and management/labor relations. Employers must consider the problem from several vantage points. Accidents, absenteeism, and reduction of productive labor are expensive and wasteful. The constitutional right of privacy is often argued when personnel policies for testing and/or searches are proposed. Courts have given qualified approval to some methods that employers may implement. Employers in the private sector may require drug testing as a precondition for employment. Government personnel directors must be cautious in devising new policies. Based on nothing more than the goal of a drug-free workplace in the public sector, large-scale drug testing of employees violates their right of privacy.

When comparing social issues in the late nineteenth and the early twentieth centuries with current social issues that affect personnel policies, the increasing number of complexities of labor/management relations is apparent. Yet the question can be asked: Were the emotional, physical, and economic damages experienced by workers in the early years less important than the emotional, physical, and economic damages experienced today? In his twenties, Reuben Dagenhart, plaintiff in the child labor case, was an uneducated man who weighed only about 105 pounds. Today, the "Reubens" do not quit school at a tender age and work long hours at factories, but modern-day mothers are distraught when, in some workplaces, they face job loss if they take leave to attend to a sick child or parent. In the late twentieth century, the legislative branch continues its struggles with competing pressures from labor and management while the judicial branch intercedes from time to time and makes hard decisions based on what the Constitution requires. Again, national leaders must structure social policies when legal and social philosophies collide and when economic theories clash in the marketplace of ideas.

91. Given the difficulty of legislating a universal health care plan, what appears to be the relationship between the business community and Congress?
    A. Since Congress is under pressure to expand health coverage without losing the support of business, it has passed a few laws allocating enough programs and funds to meet the immediate need of pleasing constituents who want to increase public health care.
    B. The business world has already developed a universal health plan that states that if a man or woman works, he or she has nothing to worry about.
    C. Participative management in factories where workers help choose insurance plans has been sufficient to argue against Congress moving forward on health care issues.
    D. Business has taken advantage of proponents of universal health care who follow the philosophy of Boren's testimony: "When in charge ponder;...When in doubt mumble."

92. What is the current status of leaves of absence without pay?
    A. Most employees are appalled at the idea because they do not want to be away from their jobs and because it would mean loss of income and lowering of the standard of living.
    B. Business's cry that it cannot afford to let people have a month or more off from work because it would drive up the price of products is ridiculous and is nothing more than the little boy crying wolf.
    C. Business opposes unpaid leaves of absence on the grounds that it will be burdened with training and paying replacement workers.
    D. The policy on leaves of absences seems to place an emotional hardship on families.

STOP! If time still remains, you may review work only in this section. When the time allotted is up, you may go on to the next section. STOP!

SECTION 3
Writing Sample

TIME: 60 minutes

2 essays, separately timed

30 minutes each

DIRECTIONS: This section tests your writing skills by asking you to write two essays. You will have 30 minutes to write each one. During the first 30 minutes, work only on the first essay. If you finish it in less than 30 minutes, you may review what you have written, but do not begin the second essay. During the second 30 minutes, work only on the second essay. If you finish it in less than 30 minutes, you may review what you have written for that essay only. Do not go back to the first essay.

Read each assigned topic carefully. Make sure your essays respond to the topics as they are assigned.

Make sure your essays are written in complete sentences and paragraphs, and are as clear as you can make them. Make any corrections or additions between the lines of your essays. Do not write in the margins.

On the day of the test, you are given three pages to write each essay. You are not required to use all of the space provided, but do not skip lines so you will not waste space. Illegible essays cannot be scored.

PART 1

Consider this statement:

In a world of potentially conflicting self-interests, no one can really say that one value system is better than another.

Robert N. Bellah, from *Habits of the Heart*

Write a comprehensive essay where you accomplish the following objectives: (1) Explain what you think the statement means. (2) Describe a current situation that might exemplify potentially conflicting self-interests. (3) Discuss a resolution to this dilemma.

PART 2

Consider this statement:

I am pessimistic about the human race because it is too ingenious for its own good. Our approach to nature is to beat it into submission. We would stand a better chance of survival if we accommodated ourselves to this planet and viewed it appreciatively instead of skeptically and dictatorially.

E. B. White

Write a comprehensive essay where you accomplish the following objectives: (1) Describe the conflict alluded to in this statement. (2) Take the opposite perspective and defend it. (3) Respond to whether or not you believe the two positions are reconcilable.

SECTION 4
Biological Sciences

TIME: 70 Minutes

QUESTIONS: 93–144

DIRECTIONS: Most of the questions in this section are arranged in groups, each corresponding to a descriptive passage. Based on the information given in a passage, choose the one best answer to each question in the group. Some questions are independent of a descriptive passage and of each other. Choose the one best answer to each of these questions. If you are not sure of an answer, eliminate those choices that you know are incorrect and choose an answer from among those remaining. Fill in the corresponding circle on the answer sheet to indicate your answer. You may refer to the periodic table at any time.

PASSAGE I (QUESTIONS 93–95)

FIGURE 1

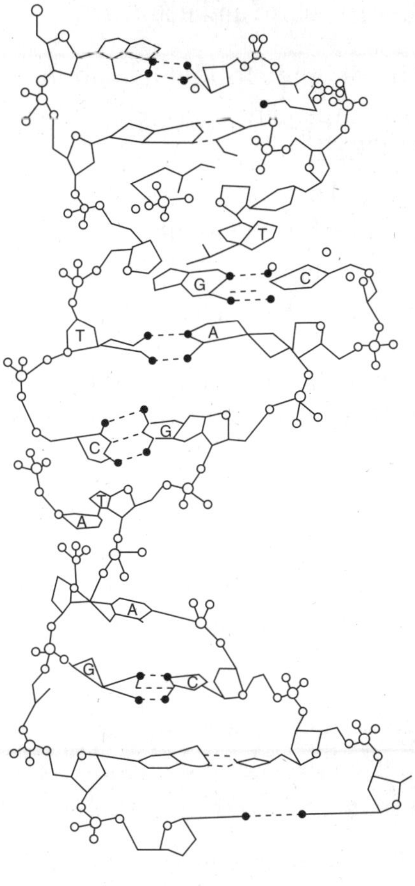

A version of the modern molecular model of DNA structure, which is a modification of the one first proposed by Francis Crick and James Watson in 1953, is depicted in Figure 1. In this view, the only atoms identified are those of oxygen and phosphorous. Using this limited information, supplemented by your knowledge of the Watson-Crick model of DNA structure, answer the following questions.

93. The polarity of a single chain of nucleic acid is such that the end known as 5′ is the end with a free

A. adenine base.
B. guanine base.
C. phosphate.
D. pentose sugar.

94. Which of the following nucleic acid bases are known as purines?

A. Adenine and guanine
B. Adenine and thymine
C. Cytosine and guanine
D. Thymine and uracil

95. According to a rule of base-pairing known as Chargaff's Principle, regardless of the source of DNA, the amounts of _____ and _____ nucleotides are always equal.

A. adenine; guanine
B. guanine; cytosine
C. cytosine; thymine
D. thymine; uracil

PASSAGE II (QUESTIONS 96–100)

Embryological development of vertebrates is initiated by fusion of sperm and egg. This fusion of gametic cells, known as plasmogamy, establishes the polarity of the future embryo (with the exception of certain groups of animals, including mammals) and is followed by karyogamy in normal development of vertebrates. The resultant zygote undergoes cleavages that begin a well-described and predictable series of major developmental events of embryology. The triggering mechanism of embryonic development is usually the fusion of egg and sperm membranes, although this can be experimentally replaced by a variety of other stimuli. Initiation of cleavage, therefore, does not depend on fertilization, and certain animals regularly utilize such parthenogenetic development in their life cycles.

The amount of yolk present in vertebrate eggs determines, in large part, the mechanics of cleavage and subsequent events. In the extreme case of telolecithal eggs of birds and reptiles, for example, the huge amount of yolk results in meroblastic cleavages and development of the embryo proceeds as a blastodisc lying on the surface of the yolk. Amphibian eggs, which contain yolk in much smaller amounts, show cleavages through the yolk material of the vegetal hemisphere. Much modern embryology is based on classic experiments that described amphibian development and the controlling influence of its immediate cellular and chemical environment on developmental patterns.

All adult structures of vertebrates, as well as the extraembryonic membranes of amniotes, develop from one or more of three germinal layers in the embryo — ectoderm, mesoderm, and endoderm. The fates of these germ layers are known from early studies and are consistent throughout the vertebrate subphylum.

96. Fertilization of a frog egg sets up the polarity of the adult organism. Accordingly, the point of penetration of the sperm will be the future _____ of the frog.
   A. dorsal surface
   B. left side
   C. ventral surface
   D. anterior end

97. The following is a correct, but not necessarily complete, sequence of stages in the development of a frog embryo:
   A. zygote, gastrula, blastula, and neural plate.
   B. blastula, gastrula, neural tube, and neural groove.
   C. gastrula, morula, blastula, and neural tube.
   D. morula, blastula, neural plate, and neural tube.

98. The spinal cord of vertebrates is derived from
   A. ectoderm only.
   B. mesoderm only.
   C. endoderm only.
   D. mesoderm and ectoderm.

99. All of the following adult vertebrate structures are derived from ectoderm EXCEPT
   A. epidermis.
   B. lining of the mouth.
   C. vertebrae.
   D. scales, hair, and feathers.

100. The influence of one group of cells on the development of another group is known as
   A. induction.
   B. determination.
   C. transformation.
   D. differentiation.

PASSAGE III (QUESTIONS 101–104)

Carbohydrates may undergo several reactions to lengthen their chains, to shorten their chains, or to modify the functional groups present.

The Kiliani-Fischer synthesis extends the chain by one carbon and creates a new chiral center.

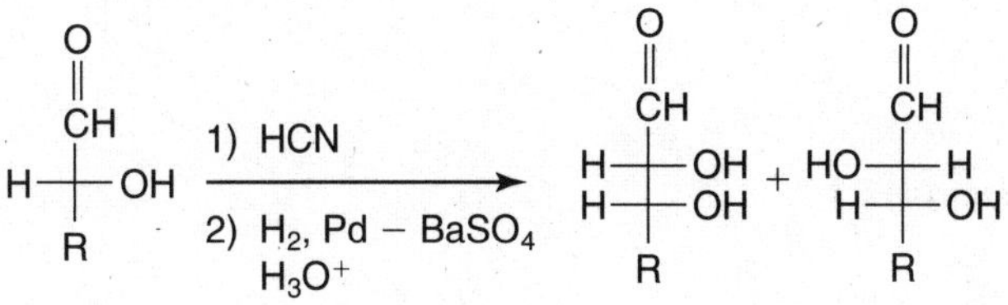

The Ruff degradation shortens the chain by one carbon at the CHO end.

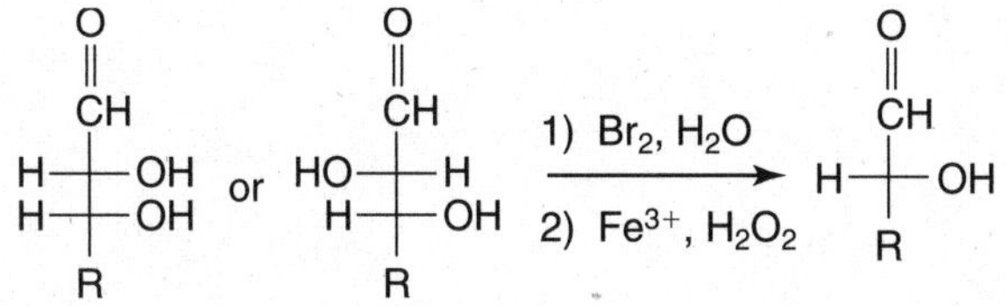

Oxidation reactions can convert carbohydrates into carboxylic acids or dicarboxylic acids.

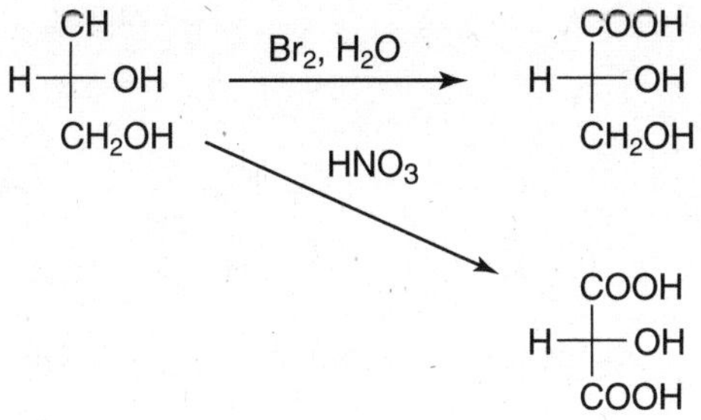

Note that chiral centers are represented as Fischer projections, where

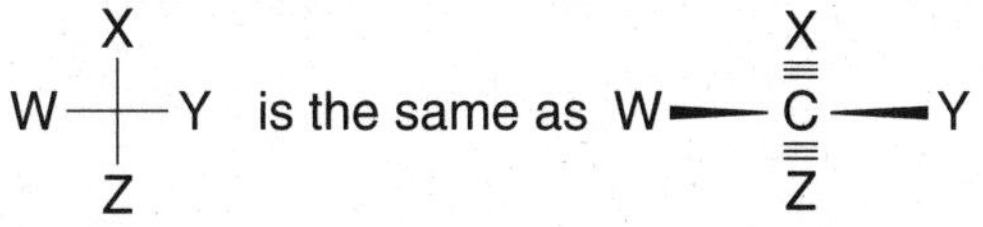

Consider the carbohydrates shown (the D - aldoses) and answer Questions 101–104.

101. Which of the aldopentoses will give a meso compound when reacted with HNO_3?
   A. Ribose only
   B. Lyxose only
   C. Lyxose and arabinose
   D. Ribose and xylose

102. Arabinose subjected to the Ruff degradation will form
   A. erythrose.
   B. erythrose and threose.
   C. glyceraldehyde.
   D. threose.

103. Xylose extended by the Kiliani-Fischer synthesis will form
   A. gulose and idose.
   B. galactose and talose.
   C. allose and altrose.
   D. glucose and mannose.

104. The aldose shown below is drawn with Fischer projection, but unconventionally.

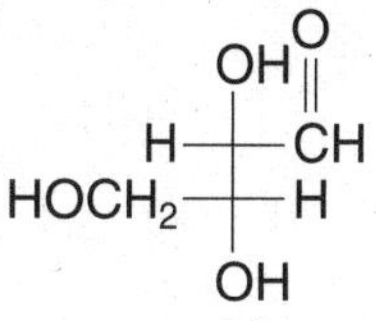

M

Which conventional figure below is identical to *M*?

A.

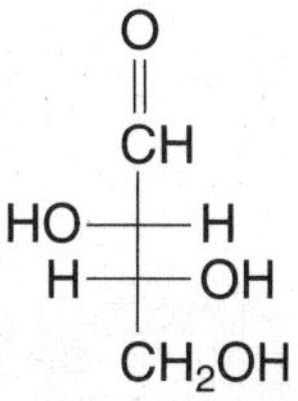

B.

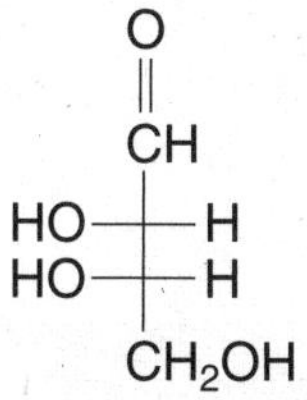

C.

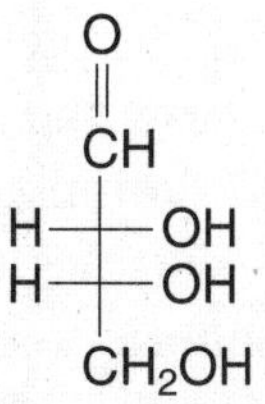

D.

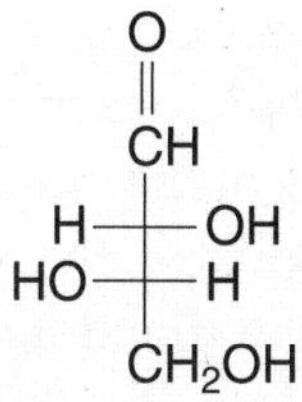

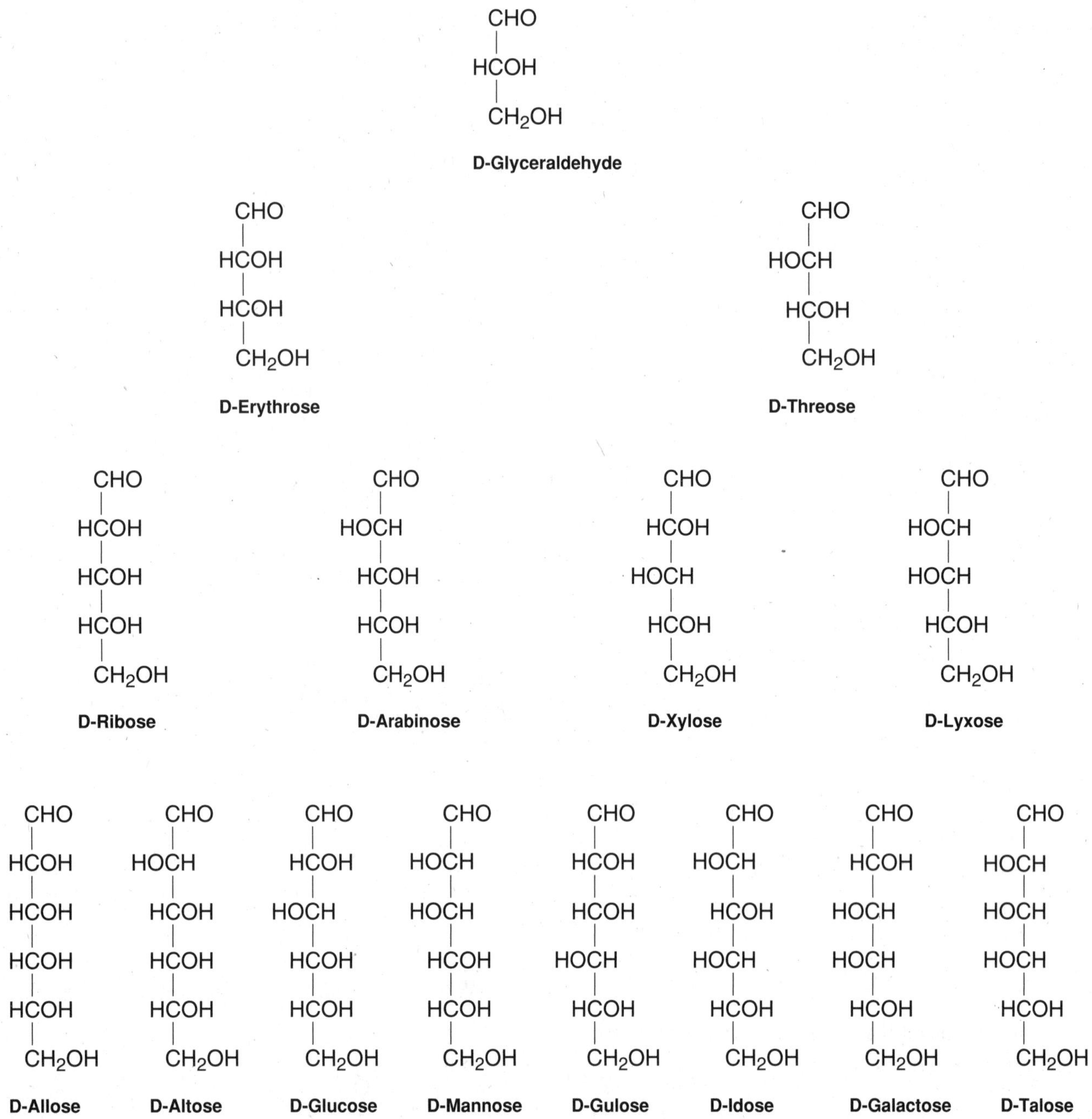

PASSAGE IV (QUESTIONS 105–108)

Ventilation of the lungs of humans and other mammals depends on changing pressure differentials between the atmosphere and the thoracic cavity of the animal. This is accomplished by contractions of the intercostal muscles of the chest and the diaphragm. Atmospheric air then moves into or out of the lungs in response to subsequent changes in intrapulmonary pressures. Figure 1 is a spirogram showing respiratory air volumes during quiet, resting breathing. Pulmonary disease may reduce vital capacity of the lungs or significantly increase the time required for expiration.

Actual gas exchange occurs across the moist membranes of air sacs known as alveoli.

No active transport of gases occurs: rather, oxygen (and other gases) first dissolves in the moist film covering the alveolar epithelium and then diffuses across the epithelium. Similarly, gases carried in the blood of the capillaries serving the alveoli diffuse across the epithelium into the lobed alveoli. Because diffusion

FIGURE 1

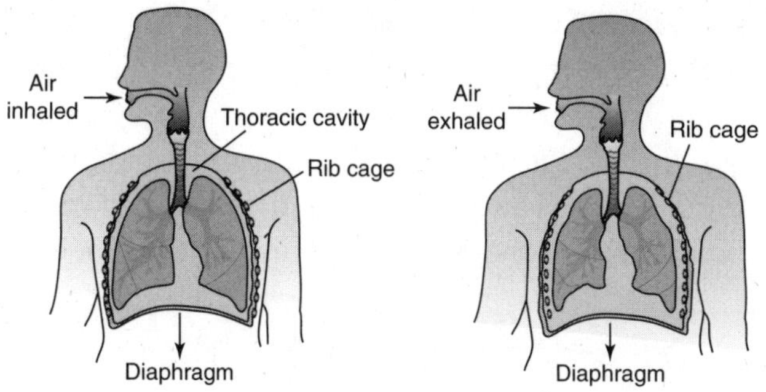

rates are a function of the differences in partial pressures of the gases involved, carbon dioxide moves from the blood into the alveoli and oxygen moves from the alveoli into the blood. Changes in partial pressures of atmospheric gases (due to changes in altitude, for example) or changes in the partial pressures of gases in the blood will thus affect gas exchange rates and amounts.

105. The partial pressure of O_2 at one atmosphere is approximately
A. 21 mmHg. B. 78 mmHg.
C. 159 mmHg. D. 760 mmHg.

106. As seen in the spirogram in Figure 2, the maximum amount of air that can be expired after a maximal inspiration is known as

FIGURE 2

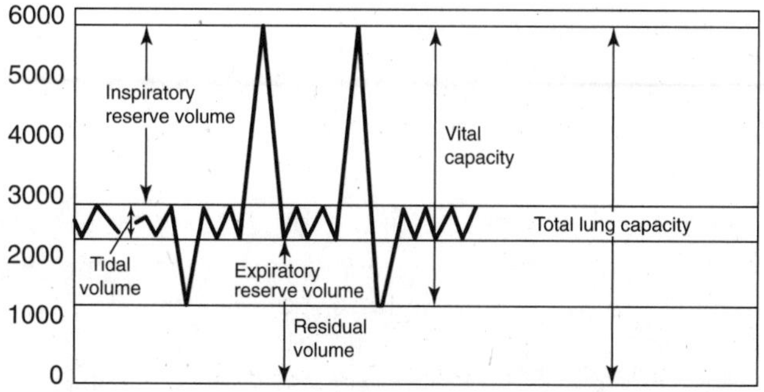

A. inspiratory reserve volume.
B. tidal volume.
C. total lung capacity.
D. vital capacity.

107. The majority of the carbon dioxide in the blood of mammals is carried as
A. carboxyhemoglobin.
B. bicarbonate.
C. dissolved carbon dioxide gas.
D. carbonic anhydrase.

108. The volume of air the patient in Figure 2 expires in each breath during quiet breathing is about
A. 6000 cc.
B. 4800 cc.
C. 500 cc.
D. 3500 cc.

QUESTIONS 109–112 are NOT based on a descriptive passage.

109. The expected product of the reaction shown below would be

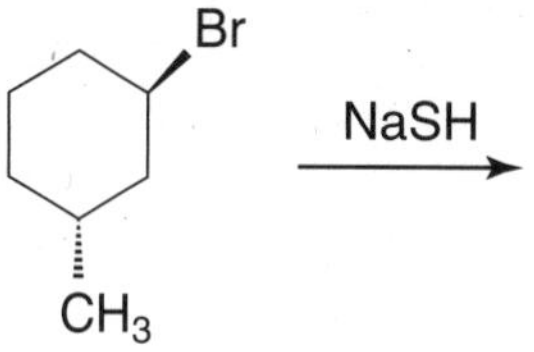

A.

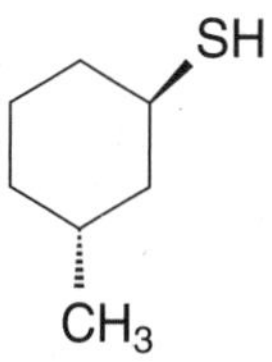

B.

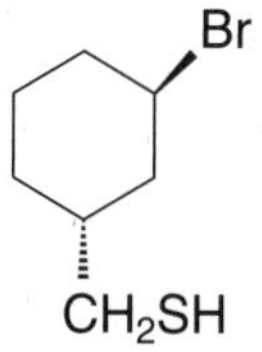

C.

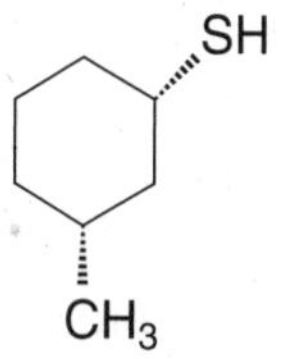

D.

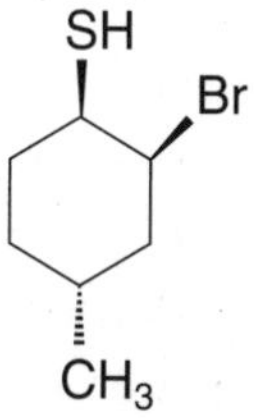

110. The main factor that determines the uptake and dissociation of oxygen and carbon dioxide in the blood is the
   A. partial pressure of oxygen.
   B. partial pressure of carbon dioxide.
   C. level of carbonic anhydrase.
   D. partial pressure of both oxygen and carbon dioxide.

111. The event necessary for the implantation of a fertilized human egg in the uterus is
   A. the disintegration of the zona pellucida.
   B. the formation of the placenta.
   C. the involution of the corpus luteum.
   D. a fall in the progesterone level.

112. The initiation of the heartbeat normally originates from the
   A. atrio-ventricular (A-V) node of the heart.
   B. sino-atrial (S-A) node of the heart.
   C. central nervous system.
   D. thyroid gland.

PASSAGE V (QUESTIONS 113–117)

The regulation of gene expression in bacteria occurs largely via operons and acts at the level of transcription. An operon is a segment of DNA that includes a regulatory gene, a promoter, an operator, and three structural genes that code for specific enzymes.

Jacob and Monad first described the lac operon. This operon regulates the production of enzymes used in the metabolism of lactose. The components of the operon act together. The regulatory gene continually produces a repressor protein. When lactose is absent, the repressor protein binds to the operator. This association of the repressor protein and the operator prevents RNA polymerase from attaching to the promoter, which in turn prevents the production of mRNA. Therefore, no enzymes for lactose metabolism are produced, as shown in the diagram below.

Lactose Absent

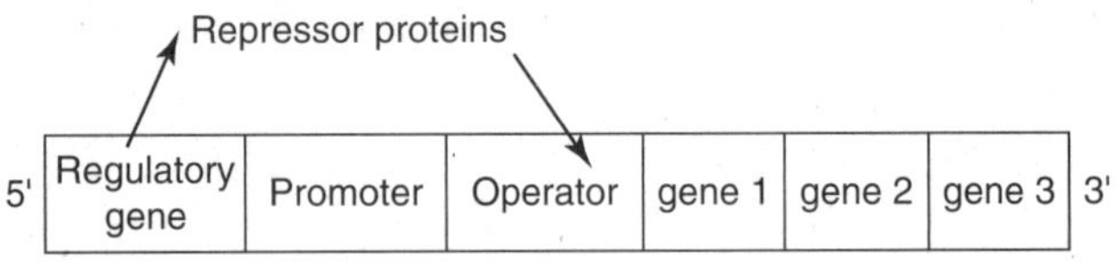

When lactose is present as the sole energy source, a derivative of lactose binds to the repressor protein and changes its shape. This prevents the repressor protein from binding to the operator. Then RNA polymerase can bind to the promoter and initiate the synthesis of mRNA from the structural genes. The mRNA provides the codons for production of the enzymes. This is shown below.

Lactose as the Energy Source

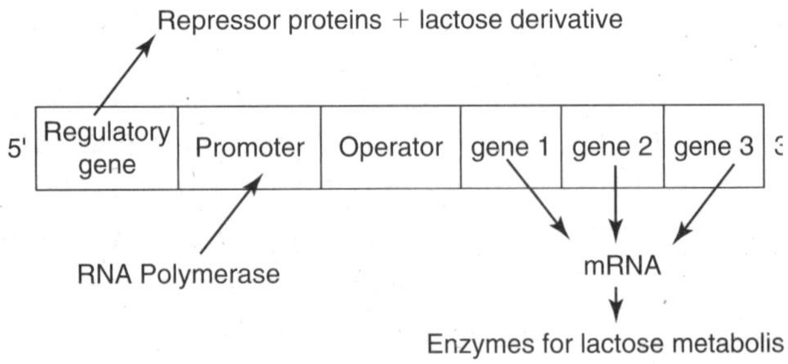

Three structural genes and three enzymes are produced. The dominant form of the structural genes must be on the same DNA strand, and the three genes must be copied together and act together. The resulting three enzymes are always produced in sequence, so that the first is required for the second and the second for the third.

113. When lactose is present as the sole energy source,
   A. the repressor protein binds to the operator.
   B. the regulatory gene is inactivated.
   C. production of repressor proteins is increased.
   D. the enzymes for lactose metabolism are produced.

114. The process initiated by RNA polymerase when lactose is present and where gene regulation occurs is called
   A. translation.
   B. dehydrogenase synthetase.

C. transcription.
D. replication.

115. Genes that are copied and that act independently are single genes. Those that are copied together and act together are called polygenic. Genes that have the dominant form on the same DNA strand are referred to as *cis*, and those on opposite strands are referred to as *trans*. The mRNA from the three structural genes is best described as
A. polytranstonic mRNA.
B. single cis mRNA.
C. polycistonic mRNA.
D. single trans mRNA.

116. Regulation of gene expression can be positive or negative. In the lac operon, the repressor protein exerts a negative effect on the expression of the structural genes if the inducer is absent. In the function of the lac operon, what is the inducer?
A. The promoter
B. The operator
C. The RNA polymerase
D. The lactose

117. Jacob and Monad were able to selectively inactivate the genes for the three enzymes. The following table shows which enzymes were produced when each of the genes was inactivated.

Enzyme	Gene Inactivated and Enzyme Produced Gene 1	Gene 2	Gene 3
permease	no	no	yes
transacetylase	no	no	no
β-galactosidase	no	yes	yes

What is the sequence of enzymes produced from gene 1, gene 2, and gene 3?

A. β-galactosidase, permease, transacetylase
B. transacetylase, permease, β-galactosidase
C. transacetylase, β-galactosidase, permease
D. permease, β-galactosidase, transacetylase

PASSAGE VI (QUESTIONS 118–122)

FIGURE 1

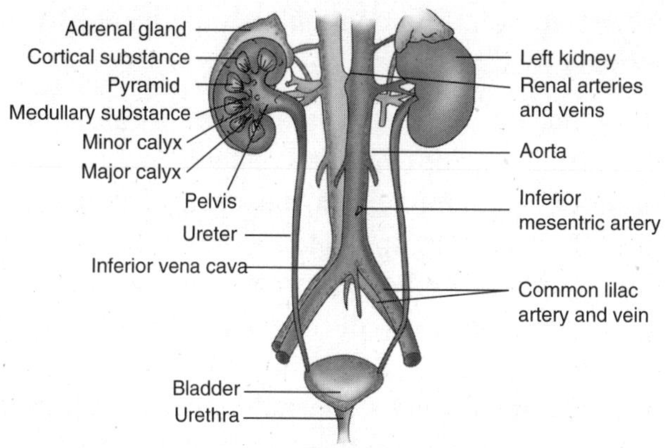

FIGURE 2

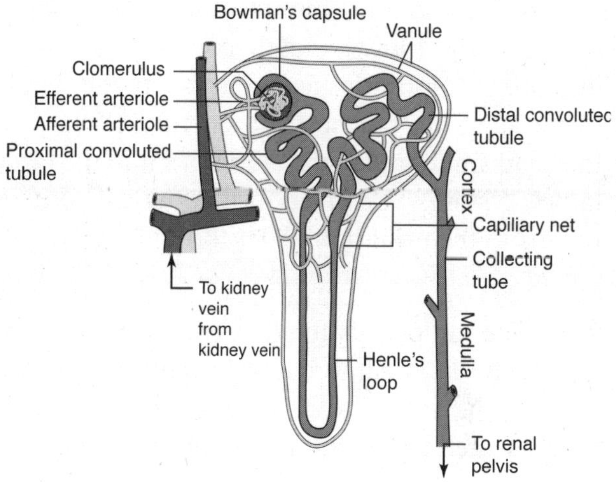

The excretory system of a vertebrate is comprised of a pair of kidneys, each connected by a ureter to the urinary bladder that is connected to a urethra through which the stored urine is eliminated. The excretory system functions to maintain homeostasis of the body through regulation of the composition and volume of blood. Consequently, the kidneys are highly vascularized. Solutes are selectively removed from blood by filtration and secretion, and carried from the body in varying amounts of water as urine.

The functional unit of a kidney is the nephron. Collectively, the nephrons of an adult human produce about 175 liters of filtrate daily. This is accomplished by forcing fluid out of glomerular capillaries and into glomerular (Bowman's) capsules using the hydrostatic pressure of the arterial system. The vast majority (99%) of this filtrate is returned to the circulatory system, and the remaining small volume of fluid containing concentrated solute is continuously delivered to the urinary bladder.

Concentration of glomerular filtrate into a hypertonic urine involves establishment of an osmotic gradient within the tissues of the kidney. This is accomplished by active pumping of ions (sodium and/or chloride) through the wall of certain portions of the nephron. As filtrate flows through the collecting tubules on its way into the renal pelvis, it encounters increasingly hypertonic tissue fluids in the medulla of the kidney. Water osmotically moves through the walls of collecting tubules into this surrounding tissue fluid and the filtrate thus becomes concentrated into urine. Capillaries associated with the tubules of the nephron reabsorb water, as well as some ions and small molecules, to return it to the circulatory system. The urine formed by this process travels to the urinary bladder through the ureter.

118. The ion pumps for Na^+ (or Cl^-) that establish the countercurrent multiplier system in the medulla of a vertebrate kidney are located in the cell membranes of the
   A. proximal convoluted tubules.
   B. distal convoluted tubules.
   C. collecting tubules.
   D. ascending loops of Henle.

119. Which of the following is a correct, but not necessarily complete, sequence of structures through which glomerular filtrate passes in a human kidney?
   A. Collecting tubule, proximal convoluted tubule, and ascending loop of Henle
   B. Proximal convoluted tubule, collecting tubule, and distal convoluted tubule
   C. Ascending loop of Henle, distal convoluted tubule, and collecting tubule
   D. Bowman's capsule, descending loop of Henle, and proximal convoluted tubule

120. Which of the following would be LEAST likely to be present in glomerular filtrate entering the proximal convoluted tubule?
   A. Glucose
   B. Platelets
   C. Amino acids
   D. Urea

121. Which one of the following processes that occurs in the kidney does NOT require active transport?
   A. Reabsorption of salts in the tubules
   B. Reabsorption of amino acids in the tubules
   C. Tubular secretion of chemicals from the blood into the urine
   D. Movement of water out of the collecting tubules

122. Which of the following correctly traces the removal of nitrogenous wastes from the human body?
   A. Conversion to urea in the liver and filtration in the kidney
   B. Conversion to ammonia in the liver and tubular secretion by the kidney
   C. Conversion to urea in the kidney and tubular secretion by the kidney
   D. Conversion to ammonia in the kidney and filtration in the kidney

PASSAGE VII (QUESTIONS 123-126)

The Hardy-Weinberg Law of population genetics predicts that if certain conditions of stability are met, the frequencies of genotypes will remain constant from generation to generation in populations of sexually reproducing organisms. The Hardy-Weinberg formula is used to determine allelic frequencies.

The conventional algebraic expression of Hardy-Weinberg equilibria assumes Mendelian inheritance (i.e., segregation of alleles and independent assortment of genes for different characters — Mendel's so-called "Laws") and assigns the symbols "p" and "q" to the dominant and recessive alleles, respectively. Because these are, by definition, the only two alleles for a given gene in a population under study, the sum of the frequencies of "p" and "q" is always 1. Expansion of the binomial $(p + q)^2$ therefore yields the formula for Hardy-Weinberg equilibria.

123. If 70% of the alleles of a given human gene are dominant and the only other known allele is recessive, what percentage of the population is heterozygous for this characteristic?

A. 30% B. 42%
C. 49% D. 70%

124. According to the Hardy-Weinberg equilibrium, $p^2 =$

A. $1 - 2pq - q^2$. B. $2pq + q^2$.
C. q^2. D. $2pq$.

125. In a population that is in Hardy-Weinberg equilibrium, the frequency of homozygous recessive individuals is 36%. What is the frequency of homozygous dominant individuals in the population?

A. 6% B. 48%
C. 13% D. 16%

126. According to Mendel's "Laws," a dihybrid cross between two heterozygotic pea plants, each producing tall plants with red flowers, would result in the classic 9:3:3:1 phenotypic ratio. In this ratio, the total number of plants showing the red flower phenotype would be

A. 1. B. 3.
C. 4. D. 12.

QUESTIONS 127–130 are NOT based on a descriptive passage.

127. DNA does not contain

A. thymine. B. adenine.
C. uracil. D. cytosine.

128. All of the following enzymes are involved in the digestion of food EXCEPT

A. pepsin. B. trypsin.
C. ribonuclease. D. ligase.

129. The peptide bond proteins are best represented as a resonance hybrid.

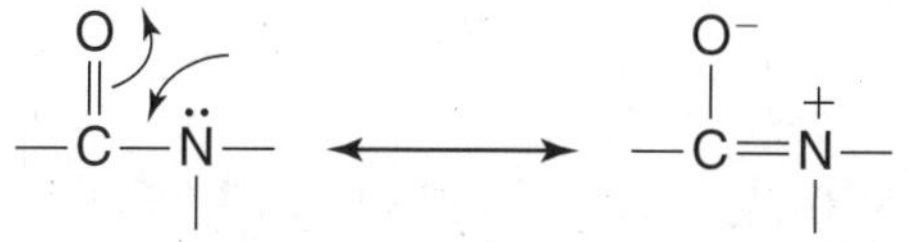

Which of the following properties is NOT attributable to the electron delocalization in the hybrid?

A. C–N bond planarity in the peptide bond
B. The optical activity of the peptide
C. Decreased basicity of the nitrogen atom in the peptide bond
D. C–N bond length in the peptide bond

130. The axon of a neuron

A. is involved in contraction.
B. contains the nucleus.
C. conducts impulses away from the cell body.
D. synthesizes neural transmitters.

PASSAGE VIII (QUESTIONS 131–133)

Amines react with p-toluenesulfonyl chloride (tosyl chloride) to give solid sulfonamide derivatives.

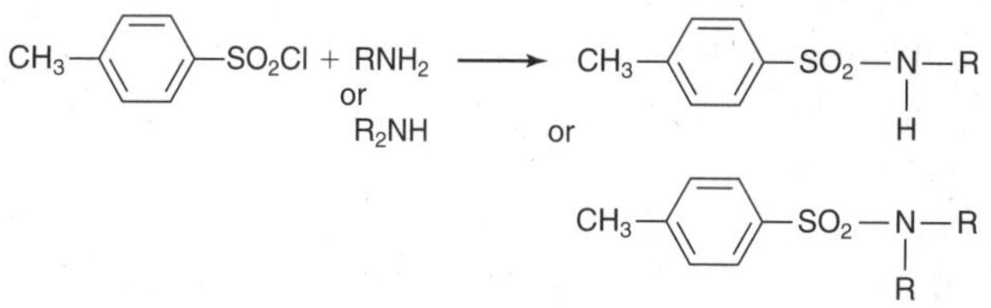

131. An amine reacts with tosyl chloride to give a solid with the NMR spectrum shown.

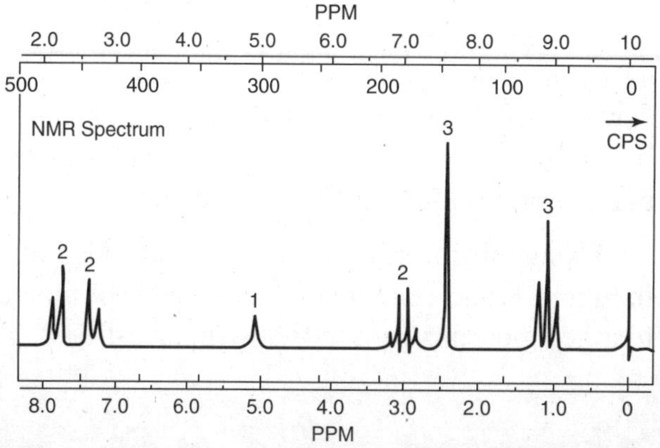

The structure of the amine is

A. $CH_3CH_2NH_2$ B. $CH_3NHCH_2CH_3$
C. $(CH_3)_2NH$ D. CH_3NH_2

132. Which class of amines will NOT react with sulfonyl chlorides?
A. Primary B. Secondary
C. Tertiary D. All will react.

133. Sulfonamides with the structure shown below will undergo an acid-base reaction with aqueous NaOH. Which hydrogen is the OH^- removing from the sulfonamide?

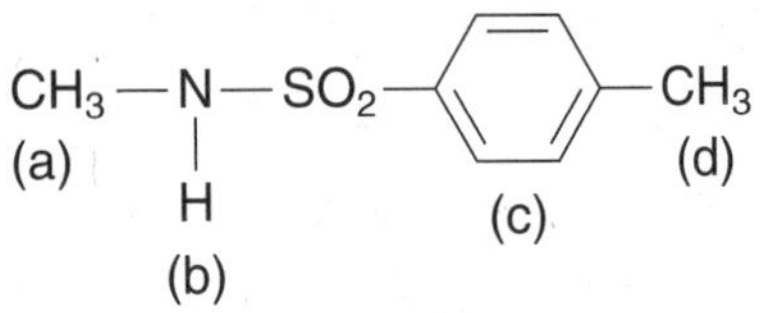

A. a B. b
C. c D. d

PASSAGE IX (QUESTIONS 134–137)

The universal genetic code consists of nonoverlapping triplets of nucleotides that are precisely coded and translated in the processes of nucleic acid replication and protein synthesis. This passage deals with protein synthesis — specifically the roles of DNA, mRNA, and tRNA in transcription and translation of the genetic code.

DNA differs from the three types of RNA in molecular size as well as in the specific nucleic acid bases and pentose sugars found in each molecule. The sequence of bases in DNA indirectly determines the sequence of amino acids that are peptide-bonded during protein synthesis by specifying the sequence of ribonucleic acid bases that make up individual mRNA molecules.

Using this information, the genetic code found in Figure 1, and your general knowledge of molecular genetics, answer the following questions.

FIGURE 1

First letter (5′ end)	Second letter: U	C	A	G	Third letter (3′ end)
U	UUU phe UUC phe UUA leu UUG leu	UCU ser UCC ser UCA ser UCG ser	UAU tyr UAC tyr UAA stop UAG stop	UGU cys UGC cys UGA stop UGG trp	U C A G
C	CUU leu CUC leu CUA leu CUG leu	CCU pro CCC pro CCA pro CCG pro	CAU pro CAC pro CAA g ln CAG g ln	CGU arg CGC arg CGA arg CGG arg	U C A G
A	AUU ile AUC ile AUA ile AUG met	ACU thr ACC thr ACA thr ACG thr	AAU asn AAC asn AAA lyx AAG lyx	AGU ser AGC ser AGA arg AGG arg	U C A G
G	GUU val GUC val GUA val GUG val	GCU ala GCC ala GCA ala GCG ala	GAU pro GAC pro GAA g ln GAG g ln	GGU gly GGC gly GGA gly GGG gly	U C A G

134. The three-base sequence of nucleotides known as an anticodon is found on molecules of
A. DNA. B. tRNA.
C. rRNA. D. mRNA.

135. Which of the following statements regarding the genetic code is correct?
A. Each of the 64 possible codons has a function in protein synthesis.
B. Some, but not all, codons code for more than one amino acid.
C. Every possible codon codes for an amino acid.
D. There is a single codon for each of the 20 naturally occurring amino acids.

136. The following is a hypothetical short mRNA sequence:
(5′) CAGGUAAAAGCGUAA (3′)
The sequence of bases in DNA that codes for this mRNA sequence is
A. (5′) CAGGUAAAAGCGUAA (3′).
B. (5′) GTCCATTTTCGCATT (3′).
C. (5′) TTACGCTTTTACCTG (3′).
D. (5′) UAAGCGAAAAUGGAC (3′).

137. The "one gene, one enzyme" principle was discovered by Beadle and Tatum. A modern

and more accurate interpretation of this would be

A. one codon codes for one enzyme.
B. one nucleic acid base codes for one protein.
C. one nucleotide codes for one enzyme.
D. one gene codes for one polypeptide.

PASSAGE X (QUESTIONS 138–140)

Animal fats and vegetable oils are triacylglycerols, triesters of glycerols with three long-chain carboxylic acids. Generally, at room temperature, fats are solid and oils are liquid. Both may be converted to glycerol and the carboxylic acids by basic hydrolosis, a reaction called saponification.

The fatty acids obtained by hydrolysis of natural triacyglycerols are unbranched, contain an even number of carbon atoms, and may be either saturated or unsaturated. The table below contains data regarding some common fatty acids.

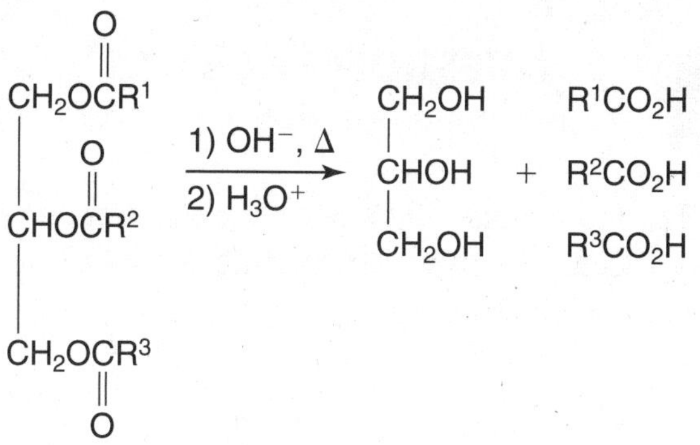

Structures of Some Common Fatty Acids

Name	Carbons	Structure	Melting point (°C)
Saturated			
Lauric	12	$CH_3(CH_2)_{10}COOH$	44
Myrustuc	14	$CH_3(CH_2)_{12}COOH$	58
Palmitic	16	$CH_3(CH_2)_{14}COOH$	63
Stearic	18	$CH_3(CH_2)_{16}COOH$	70
Arachidic	20	$CH_3(CH_2)_{18}COOH$	78
Unsaturated			
Palmitoleic	16	$CH_3(CH_2)_5CH{=\!=}CH(CH_2)_7COOH$ (cis)	32
Oleic	18	$CH_3(CH_2)_7CH{=\!=}CH(CH_2)_7COOH$ (cis)	4
Ricinoleic	18	$CH_3(CH_2)_5CH(OH)CH_2CH{=\!=}CH(CH_2)_7COOH$ (cis)	5
Linoleic	18	$CH_3(CH_2)_4CH{=\!=}CHCH_2CH{=\!=}CH(CH_2)_7COOH$ (cis, cis)	−5
Arachidonic	20	$CH_3(CH_2)_4(CH{=\!=}CHCH_2)_4CH_2CH_2COOH$ (all cis)	−50

Fatty acids are susceptible to oxidation by dioxygen. Because dioxygen has unpaired electrons, it can abstract a hydrogen atom, forming a free radical. This radical can react further with dioxygen and degrade the fats by forming odoriferous low-molecular-weight acids and aldehydes. The more unsaturated the fatty acid, the more susceptible it is to attack by dioxygen.

$$O_2 + R-CH_2-CH_2-CO_2H \longrightarrow HOO + R-CH-CH_2-CO_2H$$

$$\downarrow$$

further reaction and degradation

138. Assuming that melting tendencies of fatty acids are conferred on their triacylglycerols, which of the following will have the LOWEST melting point?

A. Glyceryl trioleate
B. Glyceryl tripalmitate
C. Glyceryl – 1 – palmitate – 2, 3 – distearate
D. Glyceryl – 1 – oleate – 2, 3 – dilinoleate

139. A fat containing a high proportion of which of the following acids would be MOST susceptible to attack by dioxygen?

A. Linoleic
B. Palmitoleic
C. Oleic
D. Stearic

140. A triacylglycerol containing which of these acids would exhibit a peak at about 3330 cm^{-1} in the infrared spectrum?

A. Palmitic
B. Lineoleic
C. Ricinoleic
D. Oleic

PASSAGE XI (QUESTIONS 141–143)

Epithelial tissue makes up the covering of internal and external body surfaces and is usually divided into simple and stratified types. The stratified types consist of two or more cell layers. Epithelial tissue is usually separated from tissues beneath it by a basement membrane. Simple types occasionally appear stratified because of irregular cell shape but, because each cell of the single layer contacts the basement membrane, this pseudostratified type is technically simple epithelium. The cells of epithelial tissues are packed very tightly and provide a boundary through which materials must pass as they leave or enter the body. Epithelial cells may be specialized in structure, having cilia, cellular processes, or glandular structures. They may also be specialized for functions such as protection from injury and invasive agents, secretion of a variety of extracellular products, absorption of nutrients, or filtration of certain substances. The permeabilities of epithelial cell membranes play an important role in regulating the movement of materials within the body and between the body and its external environment.

Connective tissues are characterized by an extensive extracellular matrix where the cells are embedded. This matrix ranges from liquid to solid and constitutes a large amount of the total tissue volume. The only connective tissues with a liquid matrix are blood and lymph. The major supportive tissues of the vertebrate body are classified as connective tissue. These supportive tissues are further divided into the categories of connective tissue proper, cartilage, and bone. The matrix of connective tissue proper always contains fibers. Cartilage has a matrix with a rubberlike consistency and contains relatively few cells that are located in cavities of the matrix. The matrix of bone is hard and the most rigid of all connective tissue. The bone matrix may have collagen fibers and contains large amounts of inorganic salts, especially calcium carbonate and calcium phosphate.

141. The epithelial tissue typically found in the walls of the urinary bladder is

A. squamous. B. transitional.
C. columnar. D. cuboidal.

142. Which of the following fibers is NOT found in connective tissue proper?

A. Elastic B. Reticular
C. Projection D. Collagenous

143. Mast cells are specialized for the production of histamine and heparin and are found in _____ tissue.

A. areolar connective
B. epithelial
C. dense connective
D. elastic cartilage

QUESTION 144 is NOT based on a descriptive passage.

144. How many ATPs are derived from one molecule of pyruvate via the Krebs cycle and the electron transport system?

A. 12 B. 14
C. 15 D. 18

STOP! If time still remains, you may review work only in this section. STOP!

Test 3 ■ Answer Key

1. B	37. D	73. B	109. C
2. A	38. D	74. B	110. D
3. C	39. C	75. B	111. A
4. B	40. A	76. C	112. B
5. B	41. B	77. D	113. D
6. C	42. C	78. B	114. C
7. D	43. D	79. D	115. C
8. A	44. B	80. A	116. D
9. C	45. D	81. B	117. A
10. B	46. C	82. B	118. D
11. B	47. D	83. D	119. C
12. A	48. C	84. B	120. B
13. C	49. B	85. B	121. D
14. A	50. C	86. A	122. A
15. C	51. B	87. A	123. B
16. C	52. B	88. B	124. A
17. B	53. D	89. B	125. D
18. A	54. A	90. C	126. D
19. C	55. B	91. A	127. C
20. C	56. D	92. C	128. D
21. C	57. B	93. C	129. B
22. B	58. C	94. A	130. C
23. C	59. B	95. B	131. A
24. A	60. B	96. D	132. C
25. B	61. C	97. D	133. B
26. C	62. A	98. A	134. B
27. A	63. C	99. C	135. A
28. B	64. C	100. A	136. C
29. D	65. C	101. D	137. D
30. D	66. B	102. B	138. D
31. A	67. C	103. A	139. A
32. B	68. D	104. A	140. C
33. B	69. D	105. C	141. B
34. B	70. C	106. D	142. C
35. A	71. A	107. B	143. A
36. C	72. D	108. C	144. C

SECTION 1
Physical Sciences

PASSAGE I (QUESTIONS 1–6)

1. **B.** The percentages of C and H are calculated from the amount of CO_2 and H_2O produced. The percentage of O is calculated by subtracting the percentage of C and H from 100%. 100g − 97g = 3g of melissyl palmitate was burned.

$$8.98\,gCO_2 \times \frac{1molCO_2}{44\,gCO_2} \times \frac{1molC}{1molCO_2} \times \frac{12.01\,gC}{1molC} = 2.45\,gC$$

$$\frac{2.45\,gC}{3.0\,gwax} \times 100 = 81.66\%C$$

$$3.67\,gH_2O \times \frac{1molH_2O}{18H_2O} \times \frac{2molH}{1molH_2O} \times \frac{1.01\,gH}{1molH} = 0.408\,gH$$

$$\frac{0.408\,gH}{3.0\,gwax} \times 100 = 13.61\%H$$

$$\%O = 100 \quad 81.66 \quad 13.61 = 4.73\%O$$

2. **A.** The empirical formula can be calculated from the percentage composition by assuming there are 100g of product. First, calculate the number of moles of each component for 100g of substance, then divide each amount by the smallest component.

$$81.66\%C \sim 81.66\,gC \times \frac{1molC}{12\,gC} = 6.81molC$$

$$\frac{6.81molC}{0.296} = 23C$$

$$13.61\%H \sim 13.61\,gH \times \frac{1molH}{1gH} = 13.61molH$$

$$\frac{13.61molH}{0.296} = 46H$$

$$4.73\%O \sim 4.73\,gO \times \frac{1molO}{16\,gO} \quad 0.296molO$$

$$\frac{0.296molO}{0.296} = 1O$$

$C_{23}H_{46}O$

3. **C.** The melting point of a compound depends on the strength and number of intermolecular interactions between molecules. The magnitude of the melting point (mp) increases with molecular weight because the number of London forces increases proportionally with the size of a molecule. Carboxylic acids form dimers that are held together by strong H-bonds. This, in effect, doubles the carboxylic acid's effective formula weight and increases its melting point.

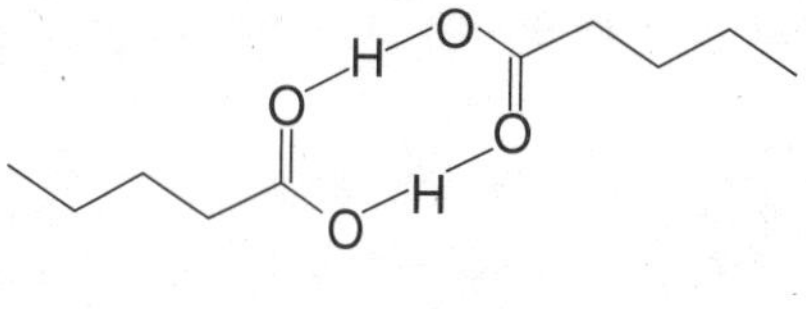

H-bonded dimer

4. **B.** The molecular weight of a compound is related to the melting point depression (same as freezing point depression) by the following formula:

$$T_{pure} - T_{mix} = K_b c$$

where c = concentration in molarity

$$c = \frac{\text{mol solute}}{\text{Kg solvent}}$$

$$FW = \frac{\text{mass substance}}{\text{mole substance}}$$

$$\frac{(Kgsolvent)\times(T_{pure} - T_{mix})}{K_b} = \text{mol substance}$$

$$\frac{(0.025\text{Kg})\times(179.5^{\circ}\text{C} - 175.5^{\circ}\text{C})}{40^{\circ}\text{C/m}}$$

$= 0.0025 mol$ beeswax

$$FW = \frac{1.69\text{g beeswax}}{0.025\text{ mol beeswax}}$$

$= 676 g$ / mol melissyl palmitate

5. **B.** The formula weight can be calculated by multiplying the empirical formula by the appropriate integer. This integer can be found by dividing the formula of a compound by the formula weight of the empirical formula.

Mass empirical formula:

$C_{23}H_{46}O = (12gC/mol \times 23) + (1gH/mol \times 46) + (16gO/mol \times 1) = 338$ g

FW = 676g beeswax/mol

676/338 = 2

$$\left.\begin{array}{l} C_{23} \times 2 = C_{24} \\ H_{46} \times 2 = H_{92} \\ O \times 2 = O_2 \end{array}\right\} = C_{46}H_{92}O_2$$

6. **C.** The wax undergoes a phase change from a liquid to a solid. The temperature change that occurs in any phase change is zero.

PASSAGE II (QUESTIONS 7–10)

7. **D.** In a redox reaction, the oxidant is oxidized by transfer of electrons from the reductant. The reductant is called the oxidizing agent. Similarly, the species that is oxidized is called the reducing agent. To determine if a species is oxidized or reduced, we must assign oxidation numbers to the reactant and product. A decrease in oxidation state is a reduction, while an increase is an oxidation.

Hydrazine (N_2H_4):

Oxidation state = 4H (+1) +2(ox #N) = 0 charge; oxidation state of N = −2

Dinitrogen teroxide (N_2O_4):

Oxidation state = 4O (−2) + 2(ox#N) = 0 charge; oxidation state N = +4

Both N_2H_4 and N_2O_4 are converted to N_2, which has an oxidation state equaling 0:

N_2H_4 (−2) going to N_2 (0) is an oxidation, so N_2H_4 is the reducing agent

N_2O_4 (+4) going to N_2 (0) is a reduction, so N_2O_4 is the oxidizing agent.

8. **A.** The pressure inside the container depends on the number of moles of gaseous product. Both N_2 and H_2O mimic gases, so we need to calculate the number of moles of each and then use this value in the equation P = nRT/V.

Calculate moles N_2 and H_2O:

$$500 gN_2O_4 \quad \frac{1molN_2O_4}{92.02 gN_2O_4} \quad \frac{3molN_2}{1molN_2O_4}$$

$$= 16.3molN_2$$

$$500 gN_2O_4 \quad \frac{1molN_2O_4}{92.02 gN_2O_2} \quad \frac{4molH_2O}{1molN_2O_4}$$

$$= 21.7 molH_2O$$

Total moles of gas = 38.0

P = nRT/V; V = 10L; T = 273 + 700 = 973K; n = 38; R = 0.082058 L atm/mol K

$$P = \frac{(38mol)(973K)(0.082058Latmmol^1K^1)}{10L}$$

$$= 30.7 atm \sim 304 atm$$

9. **C.** The answer can be calculated by applying Hess's law:

$$\Delta H = \Sigma(\Delta H_p) - \Sigma(\Delta H_r).$$

$$2\,H_2NNH_{2\,(l)} + O_2NNO_{2\,(l)} \rightarrow 3N_{2\,(g)} + 4\,H_2O_{(g)}$$

50.6kJ/mol − 19.4 kJ/mol 0 kJ/mol − 241.82kJ/mol

$$\Delta H = [(3 \times 0) + (4 \times -241.82)]_p - [(2 \times 50.6) + (1 \times -19.4)]$$

$$\Delta H = -1049 kJ$$

10. **B.** Condensing the water vapor to a liquid effectively removes the H_2O (g) product. According to Le Chatelier's principle, the forward reaction will be favored until equilibrium is restored and the ratio [products]/ [reactants] is equal to the equilibrium constant.

PASSAGE III (QUESTIONS 11–13)

11. **B.** Hydrogen bonding is a result of very polar bonds involving hydrogen and a very electronegative atom such as oxygen, nitrogen, or fluorine. Because fluorine is the most electronegative element, HF would have the strongest hydrogen bonding of the compounds listed in Table 1. Due to hydrogen bonding, the attraction among the HF molecules results in an increase in the energy needed to separate molecules from the liquid to form a gas, and therefore an unusually large molar enthalpy of vaporization. The nearly constant Cps for the HX molecules may be explained by the fact that only translational and nearly the same rotational energy must be changed to change their temperature. The increase in molar enthalpy of vaporization and increase in Cp for the hydrocarbons are associated with their increase in molar mass and increase in vibrational energy, respectively.

12. **A.** Apply Hess's Law by reversing the reaction for the formation of liquid water and adding it to the reaction for the formation of gaseous water.

$$H_2O\ (l) \rightarrow H_2\ (g) + \frac{1}{2} O_2\ (g) \quad -(-285.8\ kJ/mol)$$

$$H_2\ (g) + \frac{1}{2} O_2\ (g) \rightarrow H_2O\ (g) \quad -241.8\ kJ/mol$$

$$H_2O\ (l) \rightarrow H_2O_2\ (g) \quad +44.0\ kJ/mol$$

13. **C.** The enthalpy of combustion can be calculated from the enthalpies of formation. The expression can be solved for the enthalpy of formation of methane.

$$CH_4\ (g) + 2O_2\ (g) \rightarrow CO_2\ (g) + 2H_2O\ (l)$$

$$\Delta H\text{comb} = \Delta H_f(CO_2) + 2\Delta H_f(H_2O) - \Delta H_f(CH_4)$$

$$\Delta H_f(CH_4) = \Delta H_f(CO_2) + 2\Delta H_f(H_2O) - \Delta H\text{comb}$$

$$\Delta H_f(CH_4) = -393.5 + (2)(-285.8) - (-890.3)$$

$$\Delta H_f(CH_4) = -74.8\ kJ/mol$$

14. **A.** The relationship between the volume of a gas and its temperature was first announced by the French scientist Jacques Charles in 1787. The law states that, at constant pressure, the volume of a gas varies directly with the Kelvin temperature.

$$\frac{V_1}{T_1} = \frac{V_2}{T_2}$$

15. **C.** A body is said to be in unstable equilibrium when it does not return to its original equilibrium position after moving a small distance; rather it moves to another position.

16. **C.** Enthalpy is defined as the constant-pressure heat of reaction. The constant-volume heat of reaction is the internal energy (E or U). The two are related as shown below:

$$H = E + PV$$

$$\Delta H = \Delta E + P\Delta V + V\Delta P \ (1)$$

Taking the constant pressure case ($\Delta P = 0$) and substituting $\Delta E = q - P_{(opposing)} \Delta V$ into (1), we get:

$$\Delta H = q - P_{opp} \Delta V + P_{sys} \Delta V + 0$$

At constant pressure, the pressure of the system is equal to the pressure opposing the system throughout the reaction, that is, $P_{opp} = P_{sys}$. Therefore:

$\Delta H = q$ at constant pressure

17. **B.** The equation for the force between two point charges is $F = kq_1q_2/r^2$, where k is a constant and r is the distance between the charges. Therefore, the larger the charges, the larger the force; however, the greater the distance, the smaller the force. Like charges repel, and unlike charges attract. If the charge is placed between the two charges, each force from the other two charges will be to the right. If the charge is placed to the right of the −3q charge, it is closer to this larger charge and will receive a large force to the left from the −3q charge, but a much smaller force to the right from the +q charge. The charge must be placed to the left of the +q charge so that it can receive a moderate force to the left from the +q charge and an equally moderate force to the right from the −3q charge.

PASSAGE IV (QUESTIONS 18–21)

18. **A.** For a spontaneous reaction, the overall cell potential must be positive. Equation 1 must be reversed and added to equation 2. The overall cell potential is then the potential for equation 1 minus that for equation 2.

$E°$ cell = −.050 − (−1.66) = + 1.61 V

19. **C.** To obtain a positive cell potential, reverse equation 2 and add the result to equation 3:

$Ag_3Sn\ (s) \rightarrow Sn^{2+}\ (aq) + 3Ag\ (s) + 2e$ (oxidation)

$3Hg_2^{2+}\ (aq) + 4Ag\ (s) + 6e \rightarrow 2Ag_2\ Hg_3(s)$ (reduction)

In any cell, oxidation takes place at the anode. Tin changes the oxidation state from 0 to +2 when Ag_3Sn reacts in this cell. Therefore, Ag_3Sn is the anode. As the half-reaction shows, electrons are produced at the Ag_3Sn anode and flow to the Ag cathode.

20. **C.** Multiply the reverse of equation 2 by 3 (so that the electrons will cancel) and add the result to equation 3.

$3Ag_3Sn\ (s) \rightarrow 3Sn^{2+}\ (aq) + 9Ag\ (s) + 6e$
$3Hg_2^{2+}\ (aq) + 4Ag\ (s) + 6e \rightarrow 2Ag_2\ Hg_3(s)$

$3Ag_3Sn\ (s) + 3Hg_2^{2+}\ (aq) + 4Ag\ (s) \rightarrow 3Sn^{2+}\ (aq) + 9Ag\ (s) + 2Ag_2Sn_3\ (s)$

Cancel excess Ag (s) to obtain the net ionic equation.

$3Ag_3Sn\ (s) + 3Hg_2^{2+}\ (aq) \rightarrow 3Sn^2+\ (aq) + 5Ag\ (s) + 2Ag_2Sn_3\ (s)$

21. **C.** Note that three moles of electrons are required per mole of Al (equation 1). Find the total charge to produce one gram of Al and then multiply by the voltage to obtain the energy.

$$(1\text{g Al})\left(\frac{1\text{ mol Al}}{27\text{ g Al}}\right)\left(\frac{3\text{ mol e}^-}{1\text{ mol Al}}\right)\left(\frac{96500\text{ C}}{1\text{ mol e}^-}\right)$$

$$\left(5.0\frac{J}{C}\right) \sim \left(\frac{15}{30}\right)(100000\text{ J}) = 50\text{ kJ}$$

From this approximate solution, we know that the correct answer will not be too far from 50 kJ; therefore, we know that answer choice A cannot be correct. Also, the statement in the passage that the actual process requires 55.5 kJ/g yields another clue. The 100% efficiency process must require less energy than the actual process because, from the second law of thermodynamics; all real processes must be less than 100% efficient. The only choice that is close to 50 kJ and less than 55.5 kJ is answer choice C.

PASSAGE V (QUESTIONS 22–25)

22. **B.** Inspection of the data in Table 1 shows that the initial rate is proportional to [HCl] (to the first power) for constant methyl acetate concentration of 0.2 M (lines 2, 4, and 5). That is, rate = k [HCl], which is the rate law for a first-order reaction.

23. **C.** "Half-order" means that

$$Rate = k[A]^{\frac{1}{2}} = k\sqrt{[A]}.$$

If [A] changes by a factor of 2, then the rate must change by a factor of $\sqrt{2} = 1.4$.

24. **A.** At the start (time zero), there is no acetic acid present, so eliminate answer choices B and D. The concentration of acetic acid must increase with time, but as the methyl acetate is used up, the rate of acetic acid production must decrease, so eliminate answer choice C.

25. **B.** Use the data for the concentration of methyl acetate as a function of time at 25°C. The half-life is the time the concentration needs to change from any value to one half that value, for example, from 0.20M to 0.10M; 4.76 – 1.75 = 3.01min.

PASSAGE VI (QUESTIONS 26–28)

26. **C.** Using the lens equation 1/f = 1/p + 1/q, you can determine the image distance q from 1/q = 1/f – 1/p = 1/(25mm) – 1/(20mm) = 4/(100 mm) – 5/(100 mm) = –1/(100 mm). Therefore, the image distance is –100 mm. The minus sign indicates that the image is on the same side of the lens as the object and that it is virtual.

27. **A.** A ray diagram shows that the image is virtual and erect.

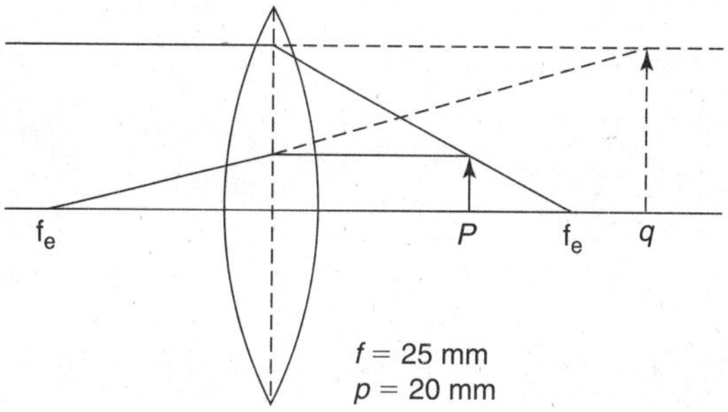

28. **B.** The purpose of the oil is to reduce the divergence when the light leaves the glass. The angles of the rays when light travels from one medium to another are related to the indices of refraction of the media by Snell's Law:

$$n_1 / n_2 = \sin (A_2) / \sin (A_1).$$

To have the angles A_1 and A_2 be the same, the indices of refraction, n_1 and n_2, must be equal. If the index of refraction of the oil equals that of the glass, there will be no divergence.

29. **D.** In human digestion, fats are hydrolyzed to glycerol and fatty acids. Fats are triacylglycerols; they are carboxylic esters derived from glycerol, $HOCH_2CHOHCH_2OH$. Fats have the general structure shown below:

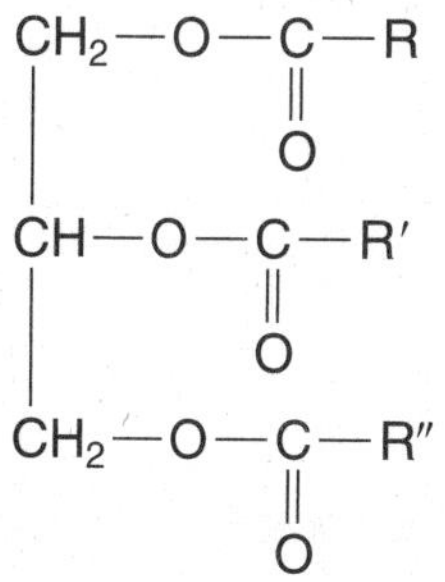

R, R′ and R′′ may represent either one, two, or three different radical groups. Hydrolysis of a fat will yield the three corresponding fatty acids and a molecule of glycerol:

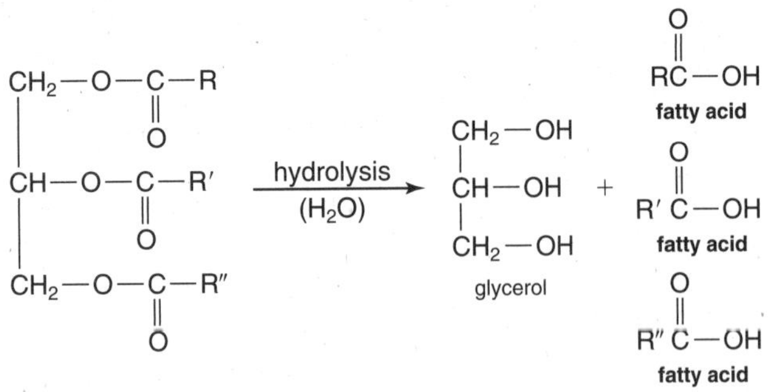

30. **D.** A triose is a three-carbon sugar. It may be referred to as a hydroxyaldehyde because it contains both a hydroxyl (OH) group and an aldehyde (HC=O) group. It is not a trisaccharide, which consists of three bonded monosaccharide units. An example of a triose is given by:

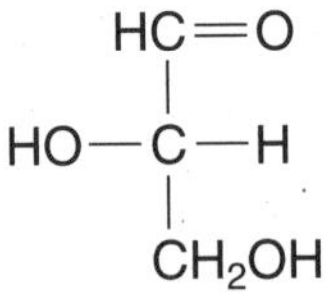

31. **A.** Unlike the speed of sound, the speed of light does not depend on temperature.

32. **B.** The effort required depends on the ratio of the length of the plane (15m) to the height (3m).

$$\frac{\text{resistance}}{\text{effort}} = \frac{\text{length}}{\text{height}}$$

$$\frac{120N}{x} = \frac{15m}{3m}$$

where x = effort required

$360 \text{ N} \times \text{m} = 15 \text{ m}x$

$x = 24 \text{ N}$

PASSAGE VII (QUESTIONS 33–37)

33. **B.** In the passage, the first car slid 200m along the road surface while descending a vertical distance of 100m. This is an example of a triangle with a hypotenuse of 200m and height of 100m, as shown below. The sine of the angle is equal to the opposite over the hypotenuse, which is 100/200 = 1/2. Therefore, the angle is 30°. It is a good idea to memorize that, for right triangles with the hypotenuse equal to twice the height, the angle opposite the height is always 30°.

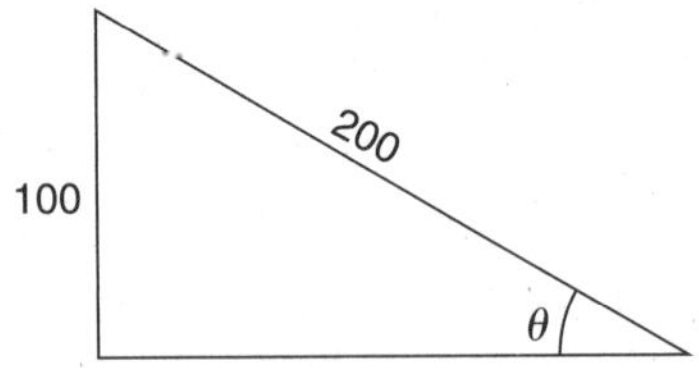

34. **B.** For an object to accelerate, there must be a net force on that object in the direction of the acceleration. The force diagram for the car is shown below. There is a downward weight of the car, an upward perpendicular (or normal) force to the ground, and a force up the slope due to sliding friction. The acceleration is along the ground, and the component of the weight down the slope must be greater than the sliding friction force up the slope for the car to accelerate down the slope.

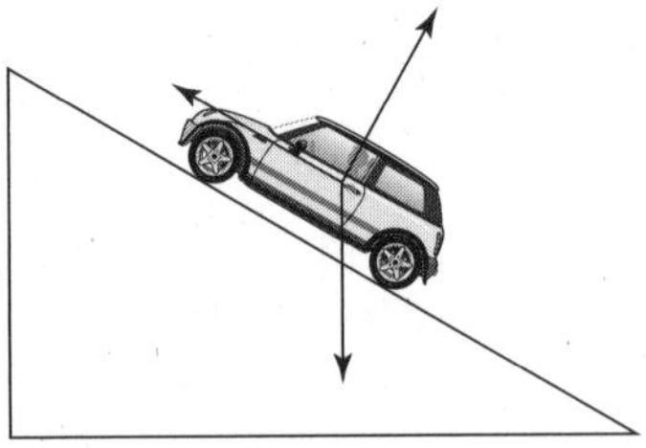

35. **A.** The potential energy is given by

$PE = mgh.$

$PE = (2000\text{kg})(9.80\text{m/s}^2)(100\text{m}) = 1.96 \times 10^6 \text{ J} = 1.9\text{MJ}.$

36. **C.** The kinetic energy is given by

$KE = \frac{1}{2} mv^2$

$KE = \frac{1}{2}(2000\text{kg})(20\text{m/s})^2 = 4.0 \times 10^5 = 0.4\text{MJ}$

37. **D.** The momentum is given by

$p = mv$

$p = (2000\text{kg})(20\text{m/s}) = 4.0 \times 10^4 \text{ kg m/s} = 40\text{Mg m/s}$

PASSAGE VIII (QUESTIONS 38–41)

38. **D.** The purpose of graphing data on a log-log plot is to determine the power law dependence between the y and x variables. For example, if $y = Cx^n$, then $\log(y) = \log(Cx^n) = \log(C) + \log(x^n) = \log(C) + n\log(x)$. This equation has the form $\log(y) = m\log(x) + b$, where the slope m is equivalent to the power exponent n. Note that you would obtain the same result even if you took the natural log (ln) rather than log base ten. In this case, the slope of the graph is $-3/2 = -1.5$, so the y variable, $\Delta N/\Delta t$, is proportional to the x variable, r, to the -1.5 power. You would obtain the same result regardless of the units used for distance or count rate.

39. **C.** As mentioned in the passage, the standard deviation for any count rate is just the square root of that count rate. The square root of the count rate for alpha radiation through aluminum, 165, or lead, 175, is about 13. The standard way to compare two values is to see whether they differ by more than one standard deviation from each other. The value 165 plus one standard deviation, 13, is 178 and the value 175 minus one standard deviation is 162. These two count rates do not differ by plus or minus one standard deviation of each other and are therefore not statistically different.

40. **A.** The half-life, 2 days, is the time for half the sample to decay, so in two weeks, the sample has undergone 7 half-lives. Therefore, $(1/2)(1/2)(1/2)(1/2)(1/2)(1/2)(1/2) = (1/2)^7 = 1/128 \sim 1\%$ of the original sample is left after 2 weeks.

41. **B.** Because the exponential function describes many natural processes, for example, population growth, compound interest, radioactive decay, it is important to know the details of this function. The negative exponential dependence of radioactive decay is shown in the graph below. At any point, the slope of this graph denotes the decay rate (DN/Dt). It is clear that the slope decreases as time increases, indicating that the decay rate is neither constant nor does it increase with increasing time. For a certain period of time, for example, $t_2 - t_1$, we can compute the relationship between decaying nuclei and time period. We have after time t_2, $N_2 = N_o\exp(-lt_2)$, and after a time t_1, $N_1 = N_o\exp(-lt_1)$. Dividing the left side of each equation and also the right side of each equation, we find $N_1/N_2 = \exp(-l[t_2-t_1])$. This implies that for any time period, t_2-t_1, the same fraction, N_1/N_2, will decay. This is similar to compound interest where, for any given time period, the percentage or *fractional* increase of money is the same rather than the additive increase.

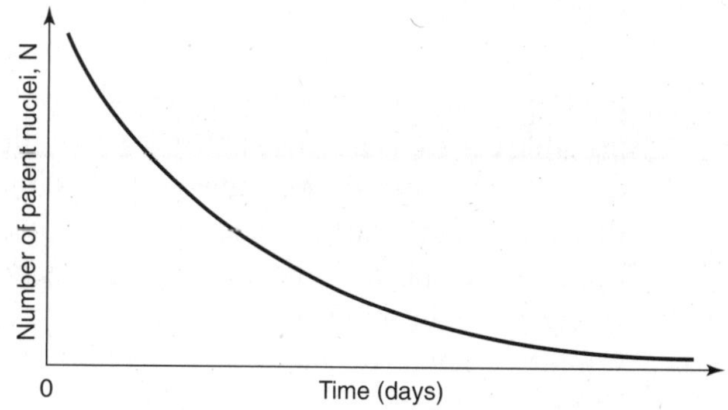

PASSAGE IX (QUESTIONS 42–45)

42. **C.** Because the angle of reflection is equal to the angle of incidence, the wave hits the interface between layers 1 and 2 at a point that is half the distance to the geophone, as shown below.

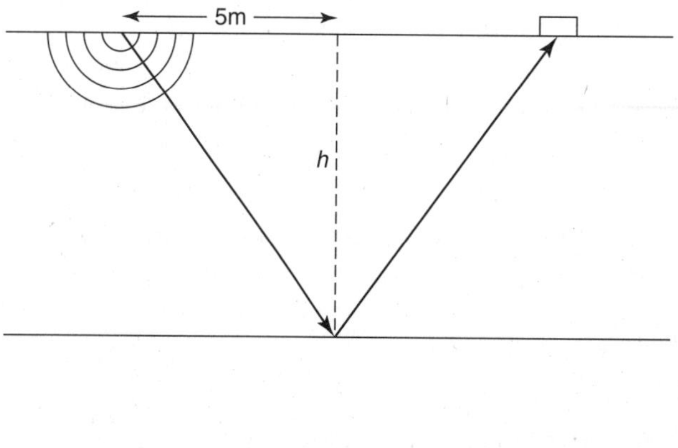

From the Pythagorean theorem, the total distance traveled for the wave is $2(5^2 + h^2)^{1/2}$, where h is the thickness of the layer. For a wave traveling at a constant speed, the total distance traveled is equal to the speed multiplied by the time elapsed. So $d = vt = (2 \times 10^3 m/s)(10 \times 10^{-3} s) = 20m$. Therefore, $2(5^2 + h^2)^{1/2} = 20m$, so $(5^2 + h^2) = 100m^2$, and therefore, $h^2 = 75m^2$ or $h \sim 9m$.

43. **D.** As stated in the passage, Snell's Law for the propagation of the wave from layer 1 into layer 2 is $\sin\theta_1/v_1 = \sin\theta_2/v_2$. Rearranging this equation, we obtain $\sin\theta_1/ \sin\theta_2 = v_1/v_2 = 2000/3000 = 2/3$. Therefore, the angle of incidence must be less than the angle of refraction. The important thing to remember is that the angles are always measured with respect to the normal (perpendicular) of the interface, as shown below. Thus, the only possible choice is D. Answer choice A would occur if the speed of the wave was the same in layers 1 and 2, and answer choice B would occur if the speed of the wave were greater in layer 1 than in layer 2. Answer choice C implies a negative angle of refraction and could never occur.

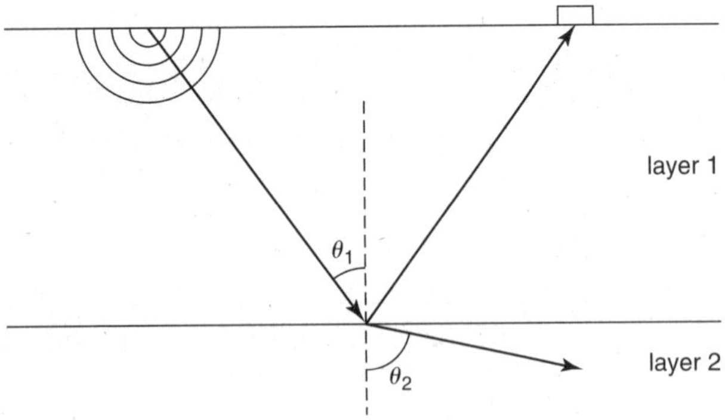

44. **B.** For waves traveling at a constant speed, the distance traveled is related to the velocity and elapsed time by $d = vt$, so that $t = d/v$. We also know that the difference in travel times is $t_S - t_P = 5$ minutes = 300 seconds. Substituting the first equation into the second, we get $d/v_S - d/v_P = 300 s = d(1/v_S - 1/v_P) = d(1/2000 - 1/6000) = d(3/6000 - 1/6000) = d(1/3000)$. Therefore, $d = (3000m/s)(300s) = (3 \times 10^3 m/s)(3 \times 10^2 s) = 9 \times 10^5 m = 900 \times 10^3 m = 900km$.

45. **D.** As stated in the passage, an object must be at least 1/4 the wavelength of a seismic wave to be detected. The relationship between wavelength l, speed v, and frequency f is given by $v = \lambda f$. Therefore, minimum size $= \lambda/4 = v/4f = (2000 m/s)/(4 \times 30\ 1/s) = 50/3m \sim 17m$.

PASSAGE X (QUESTIONS 46–50)

46. **C.** For an object traveling at a constant speed in a circle, the speed is equal to the distance traveled per revolution (the circumference) multiplied by the revolutions traveled per time (the rotational frequency). Therefore $v = 2prf = 2p$ (20cm)(100,000 revolutions/minute)(1 minute/60s) $\sim (40 \times 3 \times 10^5)/60 = 2 \times 10^5 cm/s = 2 \times 10^3 m/s = 2000m/s$. Clearly, rounding off p to 3 is sufficient for determining the correct choice.

47. **D.** Although the particles travel at a constant speed, they accelerate because their direction, and therefore their velocity, are constantly changing. This centripetal acceleration is determined by the formula $a = v^2/r$. Using the speed from the previous question, we have $a \sim (2000m/s)^2/(20cm) = (4 \times 10^6 m^2/s^2)/(0.2m) = 2 \times 10^7 m/s^2$. This approximate solution is sufficient for determining the correct answer choice.

48. **C.** The angular speed is defined as the angle swept out per unit time. As shown below, this is the same for all particles independent of the radius. The linear speed, however, is proportional to the radius because it is defined as the distance traveled per unit time.

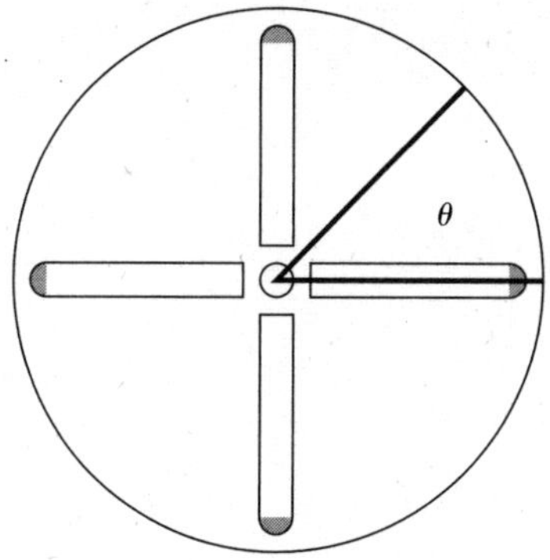

49. **B.** Once the particles leave the test tube, the net force supplied by the test tube on those particles is no longer present and the particles continue at a constant speed in a straight line. The straight line is tangent to the circle at the point when the particles first leave the test tube.

50. **C.** The centripetal force is given by the formula $F = mv^2/r$. As explained earlier, the speed v is given by the formula $v = 2\pi rf$. Substituting the second equation into the first, we obtain $F = m(2\pi rf)^2/r = 4\pi^2 f^2 mr$. The rotational frequency f is the same for all particles in the test tube, and therefore, $4\pi^2 f^2$ is a constant. Therefore, the force is proportional to the mass times the radius.

51. **B.** Using Newton's Second Law, in terms of momentum, we obtain

momentum = mv

Because mass is a scalar quantity and velocity is a vector quantity (momentum), the product of the two is a scalar quantity.

Because acceleration is defined as

$$a = \frac{vf - vi}{t}$$

Expressing a in the equation $F = ma$ as above, we obtain

$$F = m\frac{vf - vi}{t}$$

This equation states that the rate of change of momentum of a body is equal to the unbalanced force acting upon the body and is in the direction of the force.

Breaking force = − 3000 N

$$-3000N = m\frac{0 - 15m/\sec}{10\sec}$$
$$-3000N = m\frac{15m/\sec}{10\sec}$$
$$-3000kg \cdot m/\sec^2 = m(-1.5m/\sec^2)$$
$$2000kg = m$$

52. **B.** If a satellite is to remain in a circular orbit, the centripetal force required to keep it in its orbit is provided by the gravitational attraction between the satellite and the Earth. As a result, we arrive at the following equation:

$$\frac{m_s v_s^2}{r} = G\frac{m_s m_e}{r^2}$$

where m_s = mass of satellite
v_s = velocity of the satellite
m_e = mass of the Earth
r = distance between the satellite and the center of the Earth

Solving, we obtain

$v_s^2 r = Gm_e$

Because G and m_e are constants,

$v_s^2 r$ = constant

Because the mass of the satellite cancels out, this shows that a light satellite and a heavy satellite, both having the same orbital speed, will occupy the same orbit. Because M_1 and M_2 are in the same orbit, they have the same speed.

SECTION 2
Verbal Reasoning

PASSAGE I (QUESTIONS 53–58)

53. **D.** Answer choice D is correct because it represents a complete overview of the passage. Answer choice A focuses on the Continental Congress only. Answer choice B focuses only on the cause of the Revolutionary War. The passage explicitly states that the delegates held a wide variety of political opinions, so answer choice C is incorrect.

54. **A.** Answer choice B is false because moderates wanted Parliament's intervention, not exclusion, in U.S. trade. Answer choice C is inclusive and thereby false. Answer choice D contradicts the purpose of the Continental Congress.

55. **B.** This is a purely factual question testing reading ability. The passage does not mention Pennsylvania's involvement in setting up an assembly, but it does note the other states' involvement.

56. **D.** Answer choices A, B, and C are incorrect because those groups are never referred to as Whigs, although they are mentioned.

57. **B.** General T. Gage orders men to go to Concord to secure a depot. Answer choices A, C, and D all describe men who fled the scene or who warned the citizenry that the British were coming; therefore, these answer choices are incorrect.

58. **C.** An embargo prevents trade goods from leaving or entering a country. An embargo is not opposing viewpoints or extra security or a proposal, such as answer choices A, B, and D suggest, respectively.

PASSAGE II (QUESTIONS 59–63)

59. **B.** The question asks for the main theme of the passage. Answer choices A, C, and D may each be claimed to be contained in the passage, but only answer B contains the ideas collectively. The theme must be broader than any one point emphasized in the essay.

60. **B.** Because the syndicate takes a substantial share of the profit made from lotteries, option I is correct. Option II is also correct because the passage notes organized crime's infiltration into both business and politics, which includes the offering of bribes. Both options are right, so answer choice B is correct. Answer choice A is incorrect because it presents only option I. Answer choices C and D are incorrect because, here, option III is presented. This is an incorrect statement because of the word *only*, which makes the statement exclusive and universal in how it defines organized crime.

61. **C.** "Might is right" is a stoic, ethical principle that attributes mortal strength to influential power and persuasion. Organized crime reflects power and persuasion and gives the appearance of "right." Answer choice A implies the opposite of what the essay states. Answer choices B and D have little to do with power and crime and are instead biological theories.

62. **A.** Answer choice A is clearly the correct answer because it is stated in the passage. Answer B assumes every working person is involved in crime, which is incorrect. In answer C, the word *single* is

misleading. Answer D assumes organized crime has also infiltrated that specific federal commission. This is a misreading of the work of the presidential commission in the passage.

63. **C.** Answer choice A is incorrect because foreign trade is not alluded to in the passage. Answer B deceives the reader by asking about the growth rate of an unknown source. While gambling is a national pastime, one cannot conclude that gambling is an exclusive cause of organized crime. The passage gives many causes and consequences of organized crime; therefore, answer choice D is incorrect.

PASSAGE III (QUESTIONS 64–67)

64. **C.** It is not harm to others, but harm to the "rightful interests" or entitlements of others that warrants the silencing of opinion, and so both answer choices A and B are false. There is no basis at all for answer D.

65. **C.** The passage does not state that answer A is true, so it is left an open question, as is answer B. However, the question is raised, so answer D is false. Going by the information provided in the passage, C is the best answer.

66. **B.** Mill urges that lively debate helps us in the way in which we hold our beliefs and should be welcomed, so we should reject answers A and D. There is no guarantee that answer C alone, in the absence of lively debate, will be true.

67. **C.** Nothing in the passage restricts these principles to government, so there is no reason to choose answer A. Line 2 shows that Mill is concerned with both thought and expression, so answer B is false. Furthermore, the argument in line 2 applies to dealing with false opinions as well as true ones, and so we should reject answer choice D.

PASSAGE IV (QUESTIONS 68–71)

68. **D.** Answer choices A, B, and C incorrectly identify the electrodes or do not stipulate the correct kind of environment.

69. **D.** Answer choice A is limited to the initial work of Becquerel. Answer B assumes all that could be said historically has been said, and that may or may not be true. Answer C does capture much of the sense of the passage, but it does not include, by inference, the details of solar energy and its limitations.

70. **C.** Although answer choice A is a true statement, it does not reflect why selenium is used for photometric devices. Answer B is false. Answer D is a misreading of the sentence, "Even today, the light-sensitive cells on cameras that are used for adjusting shutter speed to match illumination are made of selenium."

71. **A.** Answer choice A captures the sense of both the difficulty and the availability of sunlight as a source of solar energy. Answer B negates any availability of the sun. Answer C reflects only one of the variables that affect the invisibility of the sun. Answer D does not address the question.

PASSAGE V (QUESTIONS 72–76)

72. **D.** Answer choice A is partially true, but it neglects to state anything about minorities. Funding is never addressed in the article, so answer B is incorrect. Answer C simply repeats a partially true statement, but the article is more about general knowledge than about aging minorities.

73. **B.** Answer choice B is most clearly the correct answer to a question meant to distract the reader. Answers A and C are incorrect because there is no information to confirm those statements. Answer D gives an unsubstantiated motive for including the information.

74. **B.** Many concerns of the aged belonging to a minority group need further attention and study because of their interrelationship with the problems of the elderly in general, so answer choice B is correct. Answer choice A is incorrect because the NIA gives financial support; it does not receive it. Answer choice C is incorrect because the passage states that the studies are ongoing. Because the passage does not state that the only issue studied by the NIA is aging minorities, answer D is incorrect.

75. **B.** It is another way of saying, "Among older blacks . . . hypertension is twice as prevalent as among whites . . . ." Answer choices A, C, and D cannot be known from the content of this passage.

76. **C.** The fact that many minorities have the strength to adapt to old age is clearly articulated in the passage, more so than in answer choice D, which is not the most explicit belief of those listed. Answer B has no basis in the essay. The essay does not talk about "graceful" aging; therefore, answer A is incorrect.

PASSAGE VI (QUESTIONS 77–82)

77. **D.** A careful reading of this passage unveils Darwin's belief that "a protein compound . . . would be instantly devoured or absorbed which would not have been the case before living creatures were formed." Therefore, answer choice D is the correct answer. Answer choice A is misleading because the word *dormant* does not mean "absent," which is part of a belief of Darwin. Answer choice B assumes the concept was an attempted simulation and the passage doesn't articulate that. Answer choice C is incorrect because a sterile environment is the opposite of an active environment.

78. **B.** The passage doesn't tell us who hypothesized that the stars were 90% hydrogen in answer choice A. The passage does state that Oparin had the new "notion concerning the reducing nature of the early atmosphere." Therefore, answer choice B is correct. Answer choice C is incorrect because, while Oparin contributed to the idea of the evolution of matter, the passage does not attribute the concept to him. The information in answer choice D is not given in the passage, and there is information in the passage to suggest the opposite.

79. **D.** The passage discusses only Oparin, Darwin, Bernal, and Haldane. Others may have contributed to evolutionary theory and science, but because they are not discussed here, answer choices A and C are incorrect. In addition, the passage does not indicate any disagreement among the scientists, so answer choice B is incorrect.

80. **A.** Answer choice A is incorrect because "primordial soup" is pre-existent matter. Answer choice B is blatantly refuted in the passage. Answer choice C would render the passage unnecessary or moot. D is an answer that may seem correct, but evolution implies linear progress, not a cyclical process.

81. **B.** *Synthesis* means bringing elements together, weaving a single thread. It is not a synonym for *origin* (answer choice A). Answer choice D is incorrect because the opposite of *synthesis* is *analysis*, pulling apart ideas to make conclusions. The passage speaks only of four theories, not about all theories (answer choice C).

82. **B.** B is clearly the answer and is found twice in the first paragraph: (1) "A sterile environment was exactly what was present then and what is utterly unknown in the biosphere today;" (2) "The ancient epoch when life originated, which is not at all the present life-filled environment, was not brought under study." In addition, this answer calls for an understanding of the cause-effect relationship when used in a sentence. Answers C and D refer to "equality." Nothing is inferred from or directly mentioned about the issue.

PASSAGE VII (QUESTIONS 83–87)

83. **D.** Answer choice A is incorrect because a person's motives are not important in assessing the moral value of the action. Answer choice B is incorrect because responsibility is not mentioned as a reason for evaluating actions. Answer choice C is incorrect because not all utilitarians take the actual consequences to be decisive.

84. **B.** For answer choice A, whether or not an action is repeatable does not determine whether or not it is considered, but how it is considered, as is explained in answer choice B. Answer C is incorrect because the repeatability of an action does not determine if it has consequences, but rather the type of consequences considered. Answer choice D is not a factor in the passage.

85. **B.** The passage explains that consequences in the sense of actual results can be associated only with actions thought of as particular or concrete. Types of actions will not have actual consequences but only consequences that normally occur.

86. **A.** The passage does not talk about responsibility, so answer C is incorrect. Because of the different methods of assessing morality, both answer choices B and D are false.

87. **A.** Because not all utilitarians agree on how to determine moral relevance, answer choice B is false. Actual results are not considered by those who take actions as types or kinds. Answer choice C is false because responsibility is not mentioned. Utilitarians do consider consequences relevant, so answer choice D is false.

PASSAGE VIII (QUESTIONS 88–90)

88. **B.** Certain reforms such as child labor laws and regulated work hours were instituted before President Roosevelt took office. However, the major thrust of regulation occurred under his stewardship. Although he was powerless when the Supreme Court voided several new laws, he persisted and appointed justices sympathetic to the goals of the president and the public. Eventually, judicial and congressional support followed the leadership of the chief executive. It is the proper conclusion that Roosevelt's record shows that he was more social welfare-oriented than earlier presidents while in the Oval Office. Answer A tries to figure out the author's preferences. His analysis of the judicial process does not indicate that he favored the judicial over the executive. Answer C is incorrect. The pre-1950

laws initiated tremendous change in governmental regulation of management practices previously left to the private sector. Answer D deals with chronology. After reviewing the passage, the reader will find that the judicial branch resisted change wanted by both Congress and the President.

89. **B.** Answer B correctly concludes that, although Congress had tried in earlier years to make great differences in labor policies, it was not until the Supreme Court's interpretation changed during Roosevelt's term of office that new labor laws were passed rapidly and enforced. Answer A is incorrect. The author does not imply that the term *New Deal* originated from such bizarre circumstances. Answer C is incorrect. The Great Depression dealt with the economic situation; the author does not suggest any other definition. Rather he writes of economic problems. Answer D has misinterpreted the author's analysis. Because the welfare state seeks to ensure minimum standards for all people, both workers and their representatives agreed that labor conditions and wages should be improved.

90. **C.** Answer C correctly illustrates how governmental intrusion expands when leaders in the private sector fail to make fair policies. Answer A does not consider how the act works to the detriment of illegal aliens trying to find jobs rather than protecting them against discrimination. Answer B improperly assesses the status of illegal aliens, whose political weakness lies in the fact that they have very few links with those who are in power. Answer D is erroneous, as proven by the author when he traces tensions between the two sectors.

PASSAGE IX (QUESTIONS 91–92)

91. **A.** Congress has not mustered enough votes to pass a universal health care plan; if it did, it would alienate business. Yet Congress has, on a piecemeal fashion, passed laws such as the Health Maintenance Organization Act to satisfy supporters of increased government action. Answer B is incorrect. Unfortunately, many employees in the private sector lack any kind of health coverage. Answer C overstates the situation. As the author portrays, rarely do workers, especially in non-union factories, have any bargaining power with regard to the kind of insurance coverage. Answer D is not correct. As the author shows, pro–health care people certainly are not mumbling about what they want.

92. **C.** Business's stance is to reject the leave-of-absence law because, from their point of view, such leaves will have costs of hiring and training temporaries who, as beginners, will be less productive. Answer A is incorrect. Job protection during times of stress or emergencies when employees must be away from work would be supported by most workers. Answer B is incorrect. Actually, the policy on leaves of absence would add to labor costs when production slows down due to absent employees or temporary employees. Training expenditures and expensive mistakes on the part of temporaries are examples of other costs. Answer D misunderstands the policy. The leaves are optional on the part of the employees.

SECTION 3
Writing Sample

SAMPLE ESSAY 1

The world is getting smaller and smaller, yet the understanding that one might assume would result from a smaller world seems farther and farther away. As each nation wrestles with survival and development, as in the third world countries, or with progress and growth, as in the economically powerful nations of the world, the preoccupation of each is with its own people. Each nation, with its history, culture, and pride, always prizes its values above those of other nations. Self-interest is the law of survival. It is the will to live that perpetuates values, whether those values complement other cultures or not.

Of course, it would be erroneous to assume that this very same law of survival will not create national, and often international, conflict over individual groups' rights. The heated conflict in the Middle East, though it ostensibly represents an economic conflict, is fundamentally a difference of values. This difference is so basic that it is difficult to realize an easy solution, other than one that asks the value systems to compromise. Although compromise may appear as the American way of negotiation, compromise often suggests weakness and a "soft will" to those who pride themselves on their ability to maintain control and dominance.

Conflicting value systems have coexisted peacefully at various times in history. In the Arab world, during the time of Mohammed, Jews, Christians, and Arabs coexisted because they shared a common basis for belief: they each had a holy book. Though each read it differently and interpreted it through different holy persons, each was elected to share in the truth. The vastness of the world demands the same spirit of cooperation now. When the needs of a people are satisfied, harmony is possible; when those needs are unmet, conflicting values will emerge to test the mettle of a people. Such is the dilemma the world faces in the clash of wills in the Middle East.

EXPLANATION OF ESSAY 1

The essay focuses clearly on the topic defined by the statement and fully addresses each of the three writing tasks. The first paragraph shows that the student understands the problem. It responds to the request to discuss the meaning of the statement. The next paragraph illustrates the student's interpretation of the meaning of the statement by referring to a current international example. The last paragraph shows both the difficulty in resolving the dilemma and the potential for doing so.

This is a particularly good essay because it is a thoughtful and simple approach to the idea posed in the given quote. The essay does not force the point, neither does it avoid dealing with the issue.

The writing in this essay is clear and controlled. The essay responds to the tasks at hand. One feels that the student understands the question and the breadth of its importance. Also helpful to the argument is the way the student draws on an historical point that is germane to the illustration selected.

SAMPLE ESSAY 2

We are technologically literate. Some might argue that we have forgotten "the nature of things" in achieving this status. The ingenious among us have advanced industry, both for the production of the necessities of life and for the efficient use of resources. Both of these motives appear innocent enough. After all, they represent the best of "the American Way"! Efficiency, however, has often meant the disregard of the disposal of waste materials. It has also often meant the violation of human dignity because the work that was once honorable has become dangerous, repetitive, and unrewarding. American ingenuity is the curious creator and benefactor of the resulting environmental consequences. Consequences such as pollution, death to wildlife, and disease are the result of a lack of conscience and a refusal to recognize the negative results of the so-called progress of the American way of life. For most of us, these negative results are regarded as too far into the future to be concerned about now. Making the Earth do what we want in the name of progress shows that we do not understand the law of entropy and how it is closing in on us.

It would be possible, I suppose, to see the positive contributions of technology by looking at the small picture. Home life is more efficient; entertainment is conveniently at our fingertips; space is being conquered; military tactics are more complex and, paradoxically, more accurate in locating and defeating the enemy. Progress, power, and the quality of life are enhanced by the control of the environment made possible by technology. This argument is prevalent among those who also favor free enterprise in big business. Corporations, real estate developers, and profitable scientific ventures all benefit from this way of thinking.

It would be easy to believe that the choice of one or the other of these positions is the legacy we are forced to leave to the next generation. Actually, both choices are too extreme. The Earth should be both nurtured and nurturing; humanity can use and respectfully replenish the Earth. For every progressive effort, there must be a cautious limit or protection. For every tree cut, one must be planted; for every human being displaced, there must be a new job created. It is not an either/or proposition; it is an "all or nothing" proposition.

While pessimism about the human race is justified at this time in our history, despair is premature. With small voices, groups are creating an environment that is forcing legislators and communities to respond to the needs of nature by recycling, using biodegradable products, and, in general, becoming aware of the enormous task before us.

EXPLANATION OF ESSAY 2

The first paragraph lends assistance to the author's point of view by providing a rationale for what might prompt the author to make such a declaration. The second paragraph offers the counter-position and defends the use of technology and the progress that results from that use. Finally, the student specifically suggests the nominal but real efforts underway to foster a new consciousness, thereby alleviating some of the ultimate "gloom and doom" of the author.

Writing an essay that is a response to a value judgment creates a very specific task for the student. It demands that the student clarify the meaning of the position, understand its implications, and then respond with a counter–value statement. As simply and as much to the point as possible, the essay attends to the reader's sense of judgment and provides sufficient information that allows the reader to acknowledge the value orientation of the essay.

The essay provides a coherent and clear answer that responds to the statement without pretense. Straightforward sentences express the perspective advocated by the writer in response to the three tasks.

SECTION 4
Biological Sciences

PASSAGE I (QUESTIONS 93–95)

93. **C.** The 5′ and 3′ notations refer to two specific carbon atoms in the ring forms of the pentose sugars deoxyribose and ribose. The inorganic phosphate molecule that is part of each DNA and RNA nucleotide is covalently bonded to the 5′ carbon of the pentose. Therefore, the end of a nucleic acid molecule that has a "free" phosphate is referred to as the 5′ end. Adenine and guanine, answer choices A and C, respectively, are purine bases found in both DNA and RNA and have nothing to do with polarity of the molecules. The pentose sugar end of a nucleic acid molecule has nothing bonded to the 3′ position and is, therefore, described as the 3′ end of the molecule. You should notice in Figure 1 that each of the two strands of DNA has a 5′ end and a 3′ end, but that the two strands run in opposite directions with respect to this polarity.

94. **A.** Adenine and guanine are the two nitrogenous nucleic acid bases resembling the organic molecule purine, which has a double-ring structure, and are given that generic name; they are found in both DNA and RNA. The other three nitrogenous bases (cytosine, thymine, and uracil) found in DNA and RNA are similar to the molecule pyrimidine, which has a single-ring structure and, as a result, are described as pyrimidines. Cytosine is found in both DNA and RNA nucleotides. However, thymine is unique to DNA, while uracil is unique to RNA and, in a sense, "replaces" thymine in RNA. Among the four answer choices for this item, the only one where *both* bases are purines is answer choice A.

95. **B.** Looking at Figure 1, or simply recalling knowledge of base-pairs in double-stranded DNA, you should be able to determine that purines base-pair with pyrimidines. Answer choice B gives the only correct pairing of a purine (guanine) and a pyrimidine (cytosine). Because each molecule of guanine in a given double-stranded molecule of DNA would be paired with a molecule of cytosine, the total amounts of each are equal. (The observation that DNA always contains equal amounts of guanine and cytosine, as well as equal amounts of adenine and thymine, was made by Erwin Chargaff prior to the Watson-Crick model.) Answer choices A, C, and D offer impossible pairings between two purines or two pyrimidines and are incorrect.

PASSAGE II (QUESTIONS 96–100)

96. **D.** The fusion of an egg and sperm sets into motion the events of embryonic development beginning with a rapid change in egg membrane potential that prevents fusion with additional sperm. Unlike mammals, where there is no apparent polarity of the embryo until the blastocyst stage, embryonic axes are already determined in the zygotes of amphibians. The point of sperm penetration will be the anterior end of the developing embryo, so answer choice D is correct. The gray crescent, which forms opposite the penetration point of the sperm,

marks the site of the future blastopore and, eventually, the anus. The first cleavage is parallel to the dorsiventral axis, bisecting the gray crescent and thus dividing the two-celled embryo into left and right halves.

97. **D.** Following fertilization of the egg, the major developmental stages of an amphibian embryo, in correct sequence, are morula, blastula, gastrula, neural plate, neural groove (or fold), neural tube, tail bud, and tadpole. The only answer choice that presents a correct sequence of stages is D; other choices have stages out of proper sequence. You will need to be familiar with this sequence and the major developmental events that occur in embryology of vertebrates to answer other questions about animal development.

98. **A.** To answer this question, you must be familiar with the adult tissue and organ derivatives of the primary germ layers. Answer choice A correctly identifies ectoderm as the germ layer precursor of the nervous system, including the spinal cord and brain. The other choices are incorrect because the spinal cord is derived from ectoderm (as the embryonic neural groove or primitive streak) exclusively.

99. **C.** The question also tests your knowledge of adult derivatives of the primary germ layers, in this case the derivatives of ectoderm. Answer choice C correctly identifies the vertebrae as not being ectodermally derived. All other choices present tissues and structures that are developed from ectoderm. The vertebrae (along with the notochord, circulatory system, skeletal muscles, excretory and reproductive systems, and the lining of the coelom) are among the adult tissues derived from mesoderm.

100. **A.** Dorsal ectoderm is induced into forming the neural tube by the underlying notochord and is one example of the general phenomenon of induction. The answer choice that correctly identifies this term is A. The other choices give incorrect terms for this question, although you should be familiar with their definitions: determination refers to the fates of each cell in a developing embryo (the potential developmental fates of these cells become increasingly restricted); biologically, transformation refers to the incorporation of extrinsic genetic material into a cell's genome, especially as it occurs in bacteria; differentiation describes the progressive specialization in the form and/or function of cells and tissues throughout development.

PASSAGE III (QUESTIONS 101–104)

101. **D.** Meso compounds contain chiral centers, but they are optically inactive because of some symmetry element in the molecule. Both ribose and xylose will give diacids that have a plane of symmetry when reacted with HNO_3. Answer A is only partially correct; answers B and C are incorrect because neither lyxose nor arabinose will give meso diacids.

102. **B.** Because the Ruff degradation destroys the chiral center at the number 2 carbon (by converting it to an aldehyde), the configuration of the remaining chiral centers determines which new aldose will form. The configurations of carbons 3 and 4 of arabinose match the configuration of erythrose. None of the other answers is reasonable.

103. **A.** Because the Kiliani-Fischer synthesis adds a new chiral center non-stereoselectively, two new aldoses will form, differing only in the configuration at the new chiral center. Both gulose and idose are identical to xylose at carbons 3, 4, and 5. None of the other pairs meets this criterion.

104. **A.** To see the rotation needed to change this projection to the conventional form, it is probably easiest to rewrite it using dashed lines and wedges to indicate stereochemistry.

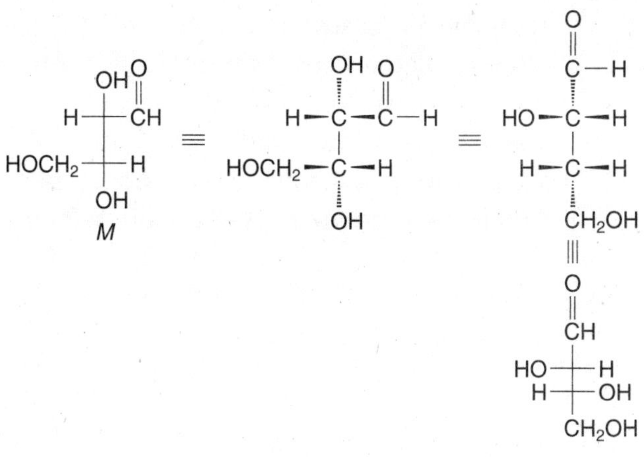

The other answers are various perturbations of incorrect rotations around the chiral centers.

PASSAGE IV (QUESTIONS 105–108)

105. **C.** To answer this question, you must apply Dalton's Law. The total pressure of a gas is the sum of the pressures that the individual gases in the mixture would exert independently (Dalton's Law). Accordingly, atmospheric pressure is the sum of the pressures of its constituent gases. Atmospheric pressure at sea level (i.e., one atmosphere) is 760 mm Hg. Because our atmosphere is approximately 21% oxygen, the partial pressure of oxygen (i.e., that part of atmospheric pressure contributed by oxygen) equals 760mm × .21, or 159 mm Hg. The correct choice is C. The actual partial pressure of oxygen entering the lungs is reduced to about 150 mm Hg because of the fact that the inspired air is saturated with water vapor (which has a partial pressure of about 47 mm Hg at body temperature).

106. **D.** This question deals with the terms used to describe various capacities of pulmonary function. That part of the total lung capacity that can be forcefully expired after a maximum inspiration is known as the vital capacity of the lungs (answer choice D). Note from reading the spirogram in Figure 2 that a certain amount of gas remains, the residual volume that cannot be expired. As a result, the lungs cannot be normally emptied of gas. The other choices are incorrect: inspiratory reserve volume is the amount of air that can be inspired after a tidal inspiration, tidal volume is the amount of air expired during each cycle of quiet breathing, and vital capacity of the lungs is the maximum amount of air that can be expired after a maximum inspiration (i.e., the maximum volume of air that can be exchanged with the environment, as can be seen from the spirogram).

107. **B.** About 70% of the carbon dioxide in mammalian blood is in the form of bicarbonate anions, so answer choice B is correct. When carbon dioxide dissolves in aqueous solution, it forms carbonic acid, which quickly dissociates into hydrogen ions and bicarbonate ions. The hydrogen ions (protons) combine with deoxyhemoglobin of red blood cells and their acidic influence is effectively buffered out. This bicarbonate buffering system is important in maintaining normal blood pH of 7.4, in addition to transporting carbon dioxide. The other choices are incorrect: carboxyhemoglobin is the combination of hemoglobin and carbon monoxide; dissolved carbon dioxide gas comprises only about 10% of the carbon dioxide carried by the blood; and carbonic anhydrase is the enzyme that catalyzes the conversion of carbonic acid to carbon dioxide and water in the pulmonary capillaries.

108. **C.** By reading the spirogram in Figure 2 and knowing that the amount of air exchanged during quiet breathing is known as the tidal volume, you can determine that this patient's tidal volume is about 500cc. The other answer choices are incorrect: 6000cc is the total lung capacity as read from the spirogram, 4800cc is the approximate vital capacity of this individual, and

3500cc is the sum of the tidal and inspiratory reserve volumes.

109. **C.** The SH^- ion would displace the bromine atom from the backside of the carbon in a nucleophilic displacement reaction (S_N2), leading to a product with inverted configuration at that carbon. Answer choice A would be formed if the reaction proceeded with retention of configuration. Answer choices B and D are not chemically feasible reactions.

110. **D.** The partial pressures of oxygen and carbon dioxide are the main determinants of whether oxygen will be picked up or released by hemoglobin. When there is a large amount of oxygen (a high partial pressure) and a low partial pressure of carbon dioxide, hemoglobin picks up oxygen. This is the case in the alveoli of the lungs. Oxyhemoglobin dissociates oxygen when the partial pressure of carbon dioxide is high and that of oxygen is low. This occurs in the tissues that are serviced by the systemic circulation.

111. **A.** The disintegration of the zona pellucida begins when the sperm penetrates the egg. The zona pellucida is one of the membranous layers that surround the unfertilized egg, which must be totally disintegrated by the time the zygote reaches the uterus. Its disintegration frees the trophoblast layer of cells, which then adheres to the uterine wall.

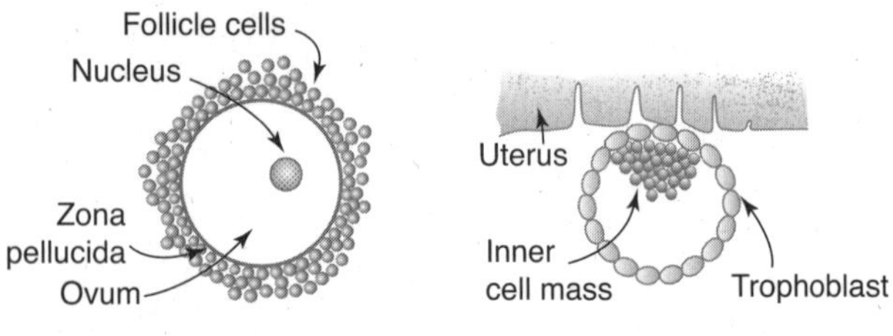

Fig. (a) Ovum before ovulation and fertilization (b) After fertilization and implantation

112. **B.** The sino-atrial (S-A) node is a small strip of specialized muscle in the wall of the heart's right atrium. This node has the contractile properties of muscle and can transmit impulses like a nerve. The S-A node generates the rhythmic self-excitatory impulse that causes a wave of contraction across the walls of the atria. This wave reaches a second mass of nodal tissue, the atrio-ventricular (A-V) node, which is then stimulated to contract. This contraction is transmitted to all parts of the ventricles, causing them to contract as a unit.

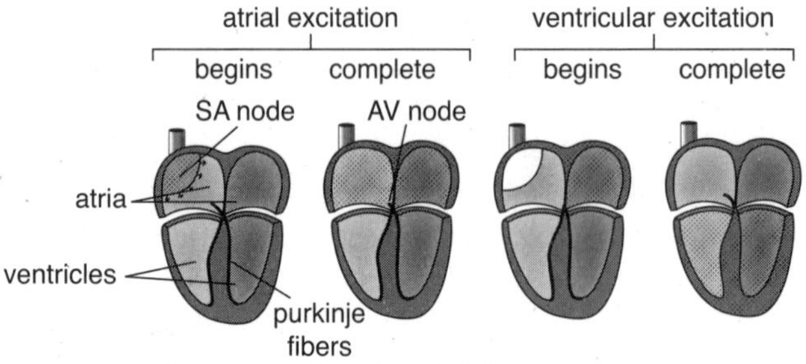

Sequence of cardiac excitation.

PASSAGE V (QUESTIONS 113–117)

113. **D.** When lactose is present as the sole energy source, the enzymes for lactose metabolism are produced. The regulatory gene is not inactivated (answer choice B). It continues to produce repressor proteins, but not at an increased rate (answer choice C). The repressor proteins do not bind to the operator (answer choice A) because of the change in their shape.

114. **C.** Recall that the control via the operon is at the level of transcription. In this case, it is the production of mRNA from DNA, which is initiated by RNA polymerase. Dehydrogenase synthetase (answer choice B) is a type of enzyme. Translation (answer choice A) is the synthesis of proteins and occurs after transcription. Replication (answer choice D) is frequently associated with the production of new DNA.

115. **C.** The operon is on the DNA. The dominant form of the structural genes must be on the same DNA strand. The three genes

must be copied together and act together. Because they must be on the same DNA strand, they are cis. Because they must be copied and work together, they are polygenic. Therefore, they are polycistonic.

116. **D.** Expression of structural genes is inhibited when lactose is absent. Lactose is the inducer. The promoter (answer choice A) and operator (answer choice B) are always present in the operon, and the RNA polymerase (answer choice C) is always present in the cell.

117. **A.** The three enzymes are always produced together and in sequence, so that the first is required for the second and the second is required for the third. When gene 1 is inhibited, no enzymes are produced. When gene 2 is inhibited, only the enzyme from gene 1, β-galactosidase, is produced. When gene 3 is inhibited, only the enzyme from gene 3, transacetylase, is inhibited. Therefore, the sequence of enzymes is β-galactosidase, permease, and transacetylase.

PASSAGE VI (QUESTIONS 118–122)

118. **D.** Answer choice D correctly identifies the location of the ion pumps in the nephron. The ion pumps located in the ascending limb of the loop of Henle are directly involved in establishing an increasingly high osmolality from renal cortex to renal medulla. Active transport of Na^+ and/or Cl^- across the epithelial walls of the ascending limb seems to be occurring. In the process, the filtrate within the tubule becomes hypotonic to the surrounding fluid. There is reabsorption of Na^+, Cl^-, amino acids, and glucose across the proximal convoluted tubule (answer A) and distal tubule walls (answer B), but in both cases the solute uptake is back into the blood and is not involved in the countercurrent multiplier system. The wall of the collecting tubule (answer C) is permeable to water but not to salt. As filtrate passes through the collecting tubule, it becomes increasingly concentrated in urea and other remaining solutes. Some of the urea diffuses into the surrounding tissue and helps account for the steep osmotic gradient encountered as the collecting tubule passes farther into the medulla.

119. **C.** By referring to Figure 1, you should be able to identify answer choice C as the only correct sequence of structures through which glomerular filtrate flows. Each of the other three choices has a portion of nephron listed that is out of sequence.

120. **B.** The ultrafiltration of blood should force fluid and small solute molecules from glomerular capillaries into the nephron. No large molecules, like blood proteins, or cellular components should enter the lumen of the nephron. Answer choice B is correct because it identifies a blood component that is too large to pass through the capillary pores of the glomerulus under normal circumstances. Answer choices A, C, and D identify molecules that are small enough to pass through the pores and are normally found in glomerular filtrate.

121. **D.** The question requires that you understand that water movement across the walls of the collecting tubule is by osmosis and does not involve active transport. Answer choice D correctly identifies this passive process. Both reabsorption (answer choices A and B) and tubular secretion (answer choice C) are ATP-dependent, active transport processes.

122. **A.** To correctly answer this question, you must know that: (1) urea is the principal nitrogenous waste produced by humans, (2) urea is produced in the liver, and (3) urea is removed from the blood by ultrafiltration in the kidney. Answer choice A includes the correct information on all three points. The

other three choices have incorrect information regarding at least one of the three points.

PASSAGE VII (QUESTIONS 123–126)

123. **B.** This question requires that you expand the binomial $(p + q)^2$ and then solve for $2pq$, which is the frequency of heterozygotes. If p represents the frequency of the dominant allele in a population and q represents the recessive, then in this item p equals 70%, or 0.7. Because $p + q = 1$, then $q = 1 - .7 = .3$. Substituting these values in the expanded binomial expression $p^2 + 2pq + q^2 = 1$, you should find that the value for $2pq$ is .42, or 42%. Therefore, the correct answer choice for this question is B. The other choices present values that represent other frequencies in this problem, so you need to be careful: the frequency of the recessive gene q in the population is 30%; the frequency of homozygous dominant individuals (p^2) is 49%; and the given frequency of the dominant allele is 70%, obviously not the same as the frequency of heterozygotes.

124. **A.** This question asks you to do a simple manipulation of the Hardy-Weinberg formula $p^2 + 2p + q^2 = 1$. Solving for p^2 yields $1 - 2pq - q^2$, so answer choice A is correct.

125. **D.** This question requires you to expand the binomial $(p + q)^2$ and then solve for p^2, which represents the frequency of homozygous dominant individuals. That value can be derived by taking the square root of .36 (or q^2, the given value for the frequency of homozygous recessive individuals). This yields .6, or q. Because $p + q = 1$, then $p = 1 - q$, or .4. Squaring .4 yields .16 (or p^2). The correct answer is found in answer choice D.

126. **D.** For this item, you must be able to work the classic Mendelian dihybrid cross. The information given in the question tells you the dominant phenotypes — tall and red — for two different genes. You don't need to know the recessive phenotypes, but you may recall that they were short and white, respectively, in Mendel's original work. The conventional ratio of 9:3:3:1 must be correctly understood to mean 9 dominant/dominant: 3 dominant/recessive: 3 recessive/dominant: 1 recessive/recessive with respect to the two characteristics. Knowing this, you can easily see that there will be $9 + 3 = 12$ dominant (red) phenotypes for *every* sixteen offspring. Answer choice D is correct; the others offer numbers that can be obtained from the numbers in the ratio, but none of these are correct.

127. **C.** The nitrogenous bases found in DNA are adenine, guanine, cytosine, and thymine. The nitrogenous bases present in RNA are adenine, guanine, cytosine, and uracil. So the pyrimidine base uracil is found in RNA instead of the pyrimidine base thymine found in DNA.

128. **D.** Many enzymes are involved in the breakdown of foods into the macromolecular components needed by the body. Of the enzymes listed, all are involved in digestion except for ligase. Ligase is the enzyme that seals nicks in DNA.

129. **B.** There is no chiral center as part of the peptide bond, so resonance delocalization does not affect optical activity. All of the other answers are properties that can be attributed to the electron delocalization in the peptide bond.

130. **C.** The axon usually, but not always, conducts impulses from the cell body. Axons can send impulses to other cells. In some neurons, they may be several feet long. In vertebrate cells, axons are usually ensheathed by Schwann cells, which provide nutrition to the axon. These Schwann cells may then be enveloped by myelin.

PASSAGE VIII (QUESTIONS 131–133)

131. **A.** Solving this problem requires you to recognize which signals in the nmr spectrum are due to the p-toluenesulfonyl moiety, subtract these from the spectrum, and deduce the structure from the remaining signals. The parasubstituted ring is responsible for the peaks in the aromatic region centered at 7.5, while the singlet at 2.5 can be attributed only to the methyl group attached to the ring. This leaves the characteristic peaks for an ethyl group at 1.1 and 3.1 and a 1 H singlet at 5.0. The only compound shown that would react with tosyl chloride to give these nmr signals is ethylamine (answer choice A).

132. **C.** The passage shows reaction with primary and secondary amines, so to answer this question, you must know only the difference between the classes of amines and that tertiary amines have the structure R_3N.

133. **B.** A proton reacting with NaOH must be adjacent to a strongly electron-withdrawing group, which will stabilize the negative charge on the product anion. The SO_2 group is very electron-withdrawing, and so the proton attached to the nitrogen is acidic.

PASSAGE IX (QUESTIONS 134–137)

134. **B.** An anticodon is a three-base sequence that is complementary to a specific codon. The translation part of protein synthesis uses this complementarity to "match" codons on mRNA with their respective anticodons on tRNA, thereby ensuring that the appropriate amino acid is inserted in the primary structure of the polypeptide being constructed. With respect to the three incorrect answer choices (A, C, and D), there is no term to describe the three-base sequence on DNA from which a codon is transcribed; the nucleotides of rRNA carry no specific information regarding the amino acid sequence in a polypeptide; mRNA contains codons, as already described.

135. **A.** Of the sixty-four possible triplets in the genetic code, sixty-one code for amino acids (from one to six amino acids for each codon) and three are nonsense triplets that do not code for amino acids but appear to function as punctuation in the translation (again, using the language metaphor). Therefore, each codon has a function in protein synthesis. The remaining answer choices incorrectly describe the code: every possible codon does not code for an amino acid because three are punctuation codons, and most amino acids have more than one codon (in fact, only methionine and tryptophan have single codons).

136. **C.** Transcription moves from the 3′ end of DNA to the 5′ end of the molecule and synthesizes a strand of mRNA having the opposite polarity (i.e., 5′ to 3′). Therefore, the complementary bases must be read in an antiparallel fashion. That is, the base at the 5′ end of the DNA molecule sequence will be the complement of the base at the 3′ end of the mRNA molecule. By carefully proceeding from the 3′ end of the hypothetical sequence of DNA presented in this item and remembering that thymine replaces uracil in DNA, the appropriate mRNA sequence can be constructed. Answer choice A is identical to the mRNA sequence given and is not possible because it contains uracil, among other reasons; answer choice B contains the correct sequence of complementary bases, but it is constructed in a parallel, not antiparallel, fashion; and answer choice

D is antiparallel, but only with respect to *entire codons,* not individual bases.

137. **D.** George Beadle and Edward Tatum's classic work with the mold *Neurospora crassa* showed that specific mutant colonies of the mold were deficient in a single enzyme and that the mutation could be inherited through a single gene. Enzymes are made of or contain proteins, while genes (in the biochemical sense) consist of a specific sequence of DNA bases. However, because it is also known that many proteins consist of two or more polypeptides, the modern interpretation of the "one gene, one enzyme" principle is correctly stated in answer choice D. The remaining choices are incorrect because one codon does not code for an enzyme or a polypeptide, only one amino acid; a nucleic acid base is only part of a nucleotide; a nucleotide is only one "letter" in a codon.

PASSAGE X (QUESTIONS 138–140)

138. **D.** Because linoleic acid has the lowest melting point of the fatty acids mentioned, answer choice D, which has two of these and one oleic acid, will have the lowest melting point of the fats shown. Answer choice A is the next lowest because it has three of the monounsaturated oleate groups. Answer choices B and C contain only saturated acids, which have higher melting points.

139. **A.** The correct answer to this question requires you to know that free radicals are stabilized by adjacent double bonds (cf., allyl- and benzyl-free radicals). The free radical intermediate that is the product of the reaction of dioxygen with linoleic acid can be stabilized by two adjacent double bonds.

R—CH=CH—CH—CH=CH—R

Oleic acid (answer choice C) and palmitoleic (answer choice B) are also susceptible to oxidation, but less so than linoleic. Answer choice D, stearic acid, will be least reactive with dioxygen.

140. **C.** The region around $3300cm^{-1}$ in the infrared is where the OH group absorbs. The only one of the fatty acids that contains an OH group is ricinolcic.

PASSAGE XI (QUESTIONS 141–143)

141. **B.** This question tests your knowledge of the types and distribution of epithelial tissues. Answer choice B correctly identifies the epithelial tissue unique to the luminal surfaces of the urinary bladder (and ureters) as transitional. Transitional epithelium is a type of stratified epithelium, and its multiple layers of rounded cells allow for considerable distension. The other three answer choices identify types of simple epithelia found as coverings elsewhere in the body.

142. **C.** Connective tissue proper is characterized by three types of fibers that are produced by fibroblasts: elastic, reticular, and collagenous fibers. Answer choice C is correct because projection fibers are actually part of the nervous system and transmit impulses from the cerebrum to other parts of the brain; therefore, they are not part of connective tissue at all.

143. **A.** Areolar (loose) connective tissue functions primarily as binding and packing for skin, muscle, and blood vessels. The areolar tissue surrounding blood vessels contains mast cells that are specialized for the production of the anticoagulant heparin, which prevents blood from clotting within the vessels. Answer choice A correctly identifies the location of these unique cells.

144. **C.** The electron transport system yields 6 ATPs, and the Krebs cycle yields 9 ATPs, for a total of 15 ATPs.

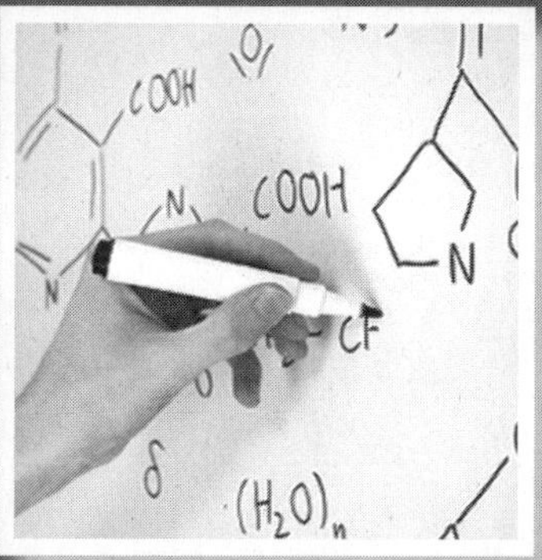

MCAT

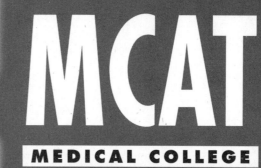

MEDICAL COLLEGE ADMISSION TEST

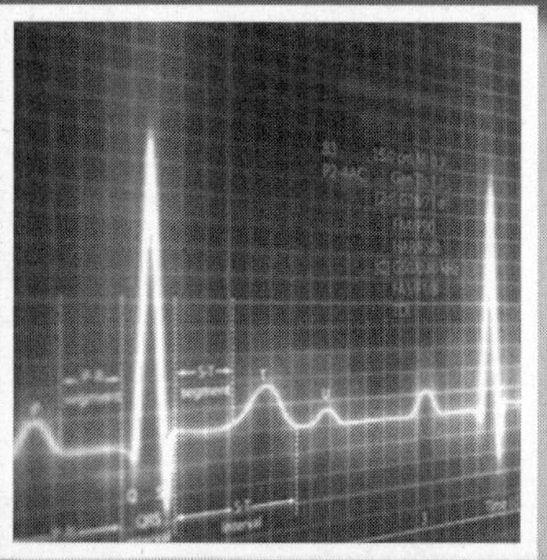

Test 4

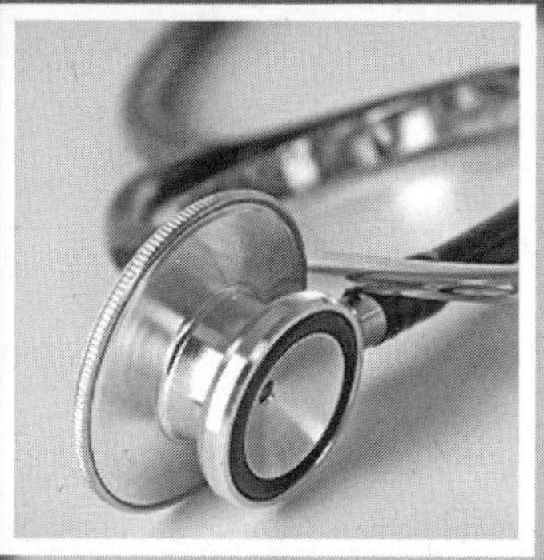

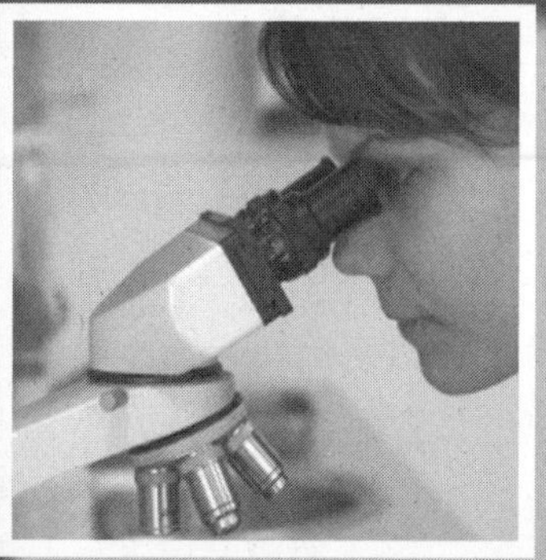

Test 4 ■ Answer Sheet

SECTION 1:
Physical Sciences

1. Ⓐ Ⓑ Ⓒ Ⓓ
2. Ⓐ Ⓑ Ⓒ Ⓓ
3. Ⓐ Ⓑ Ⓒ Ⓓ
4. Ⓐ Ⓑ Ⓒ Ⓓ
5. Ⓐ Ⓑ Ⓒ Ⓓ
6. Ⓐ Ⓑ Ⓒ Ⓓ
7. Ⓐ Ⓑ Ⓒ Ⓓ
8. Ⓐ Ⓑ Ⓒ Ⓓ
9. Ⓐ Ⓑ Ⓒ Ⓓ
10. Ⓐ Ⓑ Ⓒ Ⓓ
11. Ⓐ Ⓑ Ⓒ Ⓓ
12. Ⓐ Ⓑ Ⓒ Ⓓ
13. Ⓐ Ⓑ Ⓒ Ⓓ
14. Ⓐ Ⓑ Ⓒ Ⓓ
15. Ⓐ Ⓑ Ⓒ Ⓓ
16. Ⓐ Ⓑ Ⓒ Ⓓ
17. Ⓐ Ⓑ Ⓒ Ⓓ
18. Ⓐ Ⓑ Ⓒ Ⓓ
19. Ⓐ Ⓑ Ⓒ Ⓓ
20. Ⓐ Ⓑ Ⓒ Ⓓ
21. Ⓐ Ⓑ Ⓒ Ⓓ
22. Ⓐ Ⓑ Ⓒ Ⓓ
23. Ⓐ Ⓑ Ⓒ Ⓓ
24. Ⓐ Ⓑ Ⓒ Ⓓ
25. Ⓐ Ⓑ Ⓒ Ⓓ
26. Ⓐ Ⓑ Ⓒ Ⓓ
27. Ⓐ Ⓑ Ⓒ Ⓓ
28. Ⓐ Ⓑ Ⓒ Ⓓ
29. Ⓐ Ⓑ Ⓒ Ⓓ
30. Ⓐ Ⓑ Ⓒ Ⓓ
31. Ⓐ Ⓑ Ⓒ Ⓓ
32. Ⓐ Ⓑ Ⓒ Ⓓ
33. Ⓐ Ⓑ Ⓒ Ⓓ
34. Ⓐ Ⓑ Ⓒ Ⓓ
35. Ⓐ Ⓑ Ⓒ Ⓓ
36. Ⓐ Ⓑ Ⓒ Ⓓ
37. Ⓐ Ⓑ Ⓒ Ⓓ
38. Ⓐ Ⓑ Ⓒ Ⓓ
39. Ⓐ Ⓑ Ⓒ Ⓓ
40. Ⓐ Ⓑ Ⓒ Ⓓ
41. Ⓐ Ⓑ Ⓒ Ⓓ
42. Ⓐ Ⓑ Ⓒ Ⓓ
43. Ⓐ Ⓑ Ⓒ Ⓓ
44. Ⓐ Ⓑ Ⓒ Ⓓ
45. Ⓐ Ⓑ Ⓒ Ⓓ
46. Ⓐ Ⓑ Ⓒ Ⓓ
47. Ⓐ Ⓑ Ⓒ Ⓓ
48. Ⓐ Ⓑ Ⓒ Ⓓ
49. Ⓐ Ⓑ Ⓒ Ⓓ
50. Ⓐ Ⓑ Ⓒ Ⓓ
51. Ⓐ Ⓑ Ⓒ Ⓓ
52. Ⓐ Ⓑ Ⓒ Ⓓ

SECTION 2:
Verbal Reasoning

53. Ⓐ Ⓑ Ⓒ Ⓓ
54. Ⓐ Ⓑ Ⓒ Ⓓ
55. Ⓐ Ⓑ Ⓒ Ⓓ
56. Ⓐ Ⓑ Ⓒ Ⓓ
57. Ⓐ Ⓑ Ⓒ Ⓓ
58. Ⓐ Ⓑ Ⓒ Ⓓ
59. Ⓐ Ⓑ Ⓒ Ⓓ
60. Ⓐ Ⓑ Ⓒ Ⓓ
61. Ⓐ Ⓑ Ⓒ Ⓓ
62. Ⓐ Ⓑ Ⓒ Ⓓ
63. Ⓐ Ⓑ Ⓒ Ⓓ
64. Ⓐ Ⓑ Ⓒ Ⓓ
65. Ⓐ Ⓑ Ⓒ Ⓓ
66. Ⓐ Ⓑ Ⓒ Ⓓ
67. Ⓐ Ⓑ Ⓒ Ⓓ
68. Ⓐ Ⓑ Ⓒ Ⓓ
69. Ⓐ Ⓑ Ⓒ Ⓓ
70. Ⓐ Ⓑ Ⓒ Ⓓ
71. Ⓐ Ⓑ Ⓒ Ⓓ
72. Ⓐ Ⓑ Ⓒ Ⓓ
73. Ⓐ Ⓑ Ⓒ Ⓓ
74. Ⓐ Ⓑ Ⓒ Ⓓ
75. Ⓐ Ⓑ Ⓒ Ⓓ
76. Ⓐ Ⓑ Ⓒ Ⓓ
77. Ⓐ Ⓑ Ⓒ Ⓓ
78. Ⓐ Ⓑ Ⓒ Ⓓ
79. Ⓐ Ⓑ Ⓒ Ⓓ
80. Ⓐ Ⓑ Ⓒ Ⓓ
81. Ⓐ Ⓑ Ⓒ Ⓓ
82. Ⓐ Ⓑ Ⓒ Ⓓ
83. Ⓐ Ⓑ Ⓒ Ⓓ
84. Ⓐ Ⓑ Ⓒ Ⓓ
85. Ⓐ Ⓑ Ⓒ Ⓓ
86. Ⓐ Ⓑ Ⓒ Ⓓ
87. Ⓐ Ⓑ Ⓒ Ⓓ
88. Ⓐ Ⓑ Ⓒ Ⓓ
89. Ⓐ Ⓑ Ⓒ Ⓓ
90. Ⓐ Ⓑ Ⓒ Ⓓ
91. Ⓐ Ⓑ Ⓒ Ⓓ
92. Ⓐ Ⓑ Ⓒ Ⓓ

SECTION 4:
Biological Sciences

93. Ⓐ Ⓑ Ⓒ Ⓓ
94. Ⓐ Ⓑ Ⓒ Ⓓ
95. Ⓐ Ⓑ Ⓒ Ⓓ
96. Ⓐ Ⓑ Ⓒ Ⓓ
97. Ⓐ Ⓑ Ⓒ Ⓓ

98. Ⓐ Ⓑ Ⓒ Ⓓ
99. Ⓐ Ⓑ Ⓒ Ⓓ
100. Ⓐ Ⓑ Ⓒ Ⓓ
101. Ⓐ Ⓑ Ⓒ Ⓓ
102. Ⓐ Ⓑ Ⓒ Ⓓ
103. Ⓐ Ⓑ Ⓒ Ⓓ
104. Ⓐ Ⓑ Ⓒ Ⓓ
105. Ⓐ Ⓑ Ⓒ Ⓓ
106. Ⓐ Ⓑ Ⓒ Ⓓ
107. Ⓐ Ⓑ Ⓒ Ⓓ
108. Ⓐ Ⓑ Ⓒ Ⓓ
109. Ⓐ Ⓑ Ⓒ Ⓓ
100. Ⓐ Ⓑ Ⓒ Ⓓ
111. Ⓐ Ⓑ Ⓒ Ⓓ
112. Ⓐ Ⓑ Ⓒ Ⓓ
113. Ⓐ Ⓑ Ⓒ Ⓓ
114. Ⓐ Ⓑ Ⓒ Ⓓ
115. Ⓐ Ⓑ Ⓒ Ⓓ
116. Ⓐ Ⓑ Ⓒ Ⓓ
117. Ⓐ Ⓑ Ⓒ Ⓓ
118. Ⓐ Ⓑ Ⓒ Ⓓ
119. Ⓐ Ⓑ Ⓒ Ⓓ
120. Ⓐ Ⓑ Ⓒ Ⓓ
121. Ⓐ Ⓑ Ⓒ Ⓓ
122. Ⓐ Ⓑ Ⓒ Ⓓ
123. Ⓐ Ⓑ Ⓒ Ⓓ
124. Ⓐ Ⓑ Ⓒ Ⓓ
125. Ⓐ Ⓑ Ⓒ Ⓓ
126. Ⓐ Ⓑ Ⓒ Ⓓ
127. Ⓐ Ⓑ Ⓒ Ⓓ
128. Ⓐ Ⓑ Ⓒ Ⓓ
129. Ⓐ Ⓑ Ⓒ Ⓓ
130. Ⓐ Ⓑ Ⓒ Ⓓ
131. Ⓐ Ⓑ Ⓒ Ⓓ
132. Ⓐ Ⓑ Ⓒ Ⓓ
133. Ⓐ Ⓑ Ⓒ Ⓓ
134. Ⓐ Ⓑ Ⓒ Ⓓ
135. Ⓐ Ⓑ Ⓒ Ⓓ
136. Ⓐ Ⓑ Ⓒ Ⓓ
137. Ⓐ Ⓑ Ⓒ Ⓓ
138. Ⓐ Ⓑ Ⓒ Ⓓ
139. Ⓐ Ⓑ Ⓒ Ⓓ
140. Ⓐ Ⓑ Ⓒ Ⓓ
141. Ⓐ Ⓑ Ⓒ Ⓓ
142. Ⓐ Ⓑ Ⓒ Ⓓ
143. Ⓐ Ⓑ Ⓒ Ⓓ
144. Ⓐ Ⓑ Ⓒ Ⓓ

SECTION 1
Physical Sciences

TIME: 70 Minutes

QUESTIONS: 1–52

DIRECTIONS: Most of the questions in this section are arranged in groups, each corresponding to a descriptive passage. Based on the information given in a passage, choose the one best answer to each question in the group. Some questions are independent of a descriptive passage and of each other. Choose the one best answer to each of these questions. If you are not sure of an answer, eliminate those choices that you know are incorrect and choose an answer from among those remaining. Fill in the corresponding circle on the answer sheet to indicate your answer. You may refer to the periodic table at any time.

PASSAGE I (QUESTIONS 1–4)

A chemist determines the solubility of KNO_3 in water at a given temperature by measuring the mass of a saturated solution at that temperature and then measuring the mass of solute that remains after all the water has been removed. After determining the solubility at a variety of temperatures, the chemist plotted the solubility as a function of temperature, as shown below:

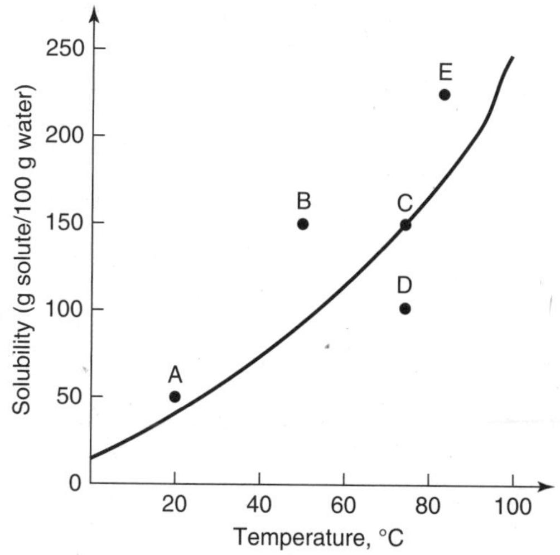

Points A, B, C, D, and E represent various aqueous solutions of KNO_3.

1. Which solution(s) is (are) unsaturated?
   A. A, B, and E
   B. A, B, C, and E
   C. C only
   D. D only

2. Addition of a tiny crystal of KNO_3 can initiate crystallization in solution(s)
   A. A, B, and E.
   B. A, B, C, and E.
   C. C only.
   D. D only.

3. At 80°C, a solution contains 100g of KNO_3 in 100g of water. This solution is
   A. unsaturated.
   B. saturated.
   C. supersaturated.
   D. either unsaturated or saturated.

4. Estimate the mass (g) of water required to dissolve 85g of KNO_3 at 80°C.
   A. 13 B. 22
   C. 50 D. 77

PASSAGE II (QUESTIONS 5–9)

A chemist studies the response of solid, liquid, and vapor phases of CO_2 to pressure and temperature changes by measuring the sublimation, freezing, and boiling temperatures of CO_2 at various pressures. The chemist also determines the temperature above which CO_2 vapor cannot matter how much pressure is applied.

These data are plotted on the curve shown below.

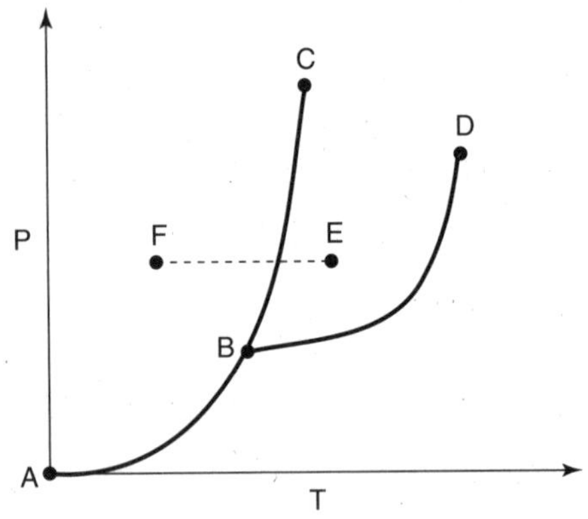

Points A, B, C, D, E, and F represent CO_2 at various conditions of pressure and temperature.

5. At all temperatures along the line connecting points A and B, the rate at which a
   A. liquid boils to form a vapor equals the rate at which vapor condenses to form a liquid.
   B. solid melts to form a liquid equals the rate at which liquid freezes to form a solid.
   C. solid melts to form a liquid exceeds the rate at which liquid freezes to form a solid.
   D. solid sublimes to form a vapor equals the rate at which vapor condenses to form a solid.

6. How many variables (degrees of freedom) must be specified to define point E?
   A. 0 B. 1
   C. 2 D. 3

7. If the chemist heats CO_2 starting at point F until point E is reached and at a constant pressure, what phase change will occur?
   A. Melting B. Boiling
   C. Sublimation D. Condensation

8. The triple point for CO_2 occurs at 5.11atm and 216.6K. When CO_2 solid is heated at 1.00atm, it
   A. melts. B. boils.
   C. sublimes. D. freezes.

9. The slope of line BC indicates that the melting point of CO_2
   A. increases with increasing pressure.
   B. increases with decreasing pressure.
   C. is not affected by changes in pressure.
   D. decreases with increasing pressure.

PASSAGE III (QUESTIONS 10–12)

"Fixed" nitrogen is nitrogen that has been combined chemically with other elements. In the Haber process, atmospheric nitrogen is fixed by allowing it to react with hydrogen to form ammonia:

$$N_2\,(g) + 3H_2\,(g) \rightleftharpoons 2\,NH_3\,(g)$$

The enthalpy change, $\Delta H°$, for this reaction is – 92 kJ.

In a quantitative study of this process, a chemist mixes the two reactants together so that the initial concentrations of nitrogen and hydrogen inside a container are 0.500M and 0.800M, respectively. When the mixture reaches equilibrium, the concentration of ammonia becomes 0.150M.

10. Calculate the concentration of N_2 in the equilibrium mixture.
    A. 0 B. 0.725M
    C. 0.425M D. 0.500M

11. The equilibrium constant for this reaction is expressed as
    A. $\frac{[N2][3H2]^3}{[NH3]^2}$ B. $\frac{[N2][H2]^3}{[NH3]^2}$

C. $\frac{[2NH_3]^2}{[N_2][3H_2]^3}$ D. $\frac{[NH_3]^2}{[N_2][H_2]^3}$

12. An increase in pressure caused by decreasing the volume of this system at equilibrium would result in a(n)
    A. increase in the number of N_2 molecules.
    B. increase in the number of H_2 molecules.
    C. decrease in the number of NH_3 molecules.
    D. increase in the concentration of NH_3.

QUESTIONS 13–16 are NOT based on a descriptive passage.

13. In an elastic collision, all of the following quantities are conserved EXCEPT
    A. momentum.
    B. velocity.
    C. kinetic energy.
    D. potential energy.

14. Isotopes of the same element have the same atomic number and a different mass number. Which statement is true?
    A. Isotopes have more protons and electrons than their element.
    B. Isotopes have fewer protons and electrons than their element.
    C. Isotopes have a different number of neutrons.
    D. Isotopes have a different number of neutrons and protons.

15. The density of a steel alloy is 7.8gm/cm^3. What would be the mass of a 2 meter × 3 meter × 5 meter block constructed out of this alloy?
    A. 2.34gm B. 2.34×10^8gm
    C. 234gm D. 3900gm

16. What does X represent in the following radioactive decay?
    $${}^{238}_{92}Y \rightarrow {}^{238}_{93}Z + X$$
    A. A proton B. An electron
    C. A neutron D. An α-particle

PASSAGE IV (QUESTIONS 17–19)

Gasoline is the name for aliphatic hydrocarbons, which are carbon chains with seven to eleven carbon atoms and sixteen to twenty-two hydrogen atoms. In ideal combustion with oxygen, gasoline would produce only water and carbon dioxide. However, the combustion engine is not perfect, and gasoline is rarely pure. Gasoline manufacturers have added lead and other additives to improve the performance of gasoline. Because the Clean Air Act of 1990 basically banned lead additives, the additive of choice has been MTBE (methyl tertiary butyl ether), a simple molecule based on methanol ($C_5H_{12}O$).

17. Calculate the ratio of oxygen molecules to octane molecules needed for ideal octane combustion.
    A. 25:2 B. 16:2
    C. 18:2 D. 7:2

18. Which of these is the correct equation for heptane's combustion?
    A. $2C_7H_{16} + 15O_2 \rightarrow 8H_2O + 7CO_2$
    B. $2C_7H_{16} + 22O_2 \rightarrow 8H_2O + 7CO_2$
    C. $C_7H_{16} + 15O_2 \rightarrow 8H_2O + 7CO_2$
    D. $C_7H_{16} + 22O_2 \rightarrow 8H_2O + 7CO_2$

19. One gallon of gasoline ideally contains 132×10^6J of chemical energy. What number of watt-hours is this equal to?
    A. 1.32×10^4W hrs
    B. 3.7×10^4W hrs
    C. 1.32×10^2W hrs
    D. 3.7×10^2W hrs

PASSAGE V (QUESTIONS 20–24)

To evaluate the thermodynamic aspects of the reaction between methane gas, CH_4, and excess oxygen at 25°C,

$$CH_4\,(g) + 2O_2\,(g) \rightarrow CO_2\,(g) + 2H_2O\,(l),$$

a chemist uses a Table of Heats of Formation to calculate the enthalpy change, $\Delta H°$, and a Table of Standard Entropies to calculate the entropy change, $\Delta S°$. Using these values in the Gibbs-Helmholtz equation, the chemist calculates the free energy change, $\Delta G°$. These values are:

$\Delta H° = -890.3$ kJ

$\Delta S° = -0.2428$ kJ/K

$\Delta G° = -817.9$ kJ

The molar masses of reactants and products are:

$CH_4 = 16$, $O_2 = 32$, $CO_2 = 44$, and $H_2O = 18$.

20. The value of $\Delta S°$ indicates that the
    A. entropy of the products is less than the entropy of the reactants.
    B. entropy of the reactants is less than the entropy of the products.
    C. reaction is rapid.
    D. reaction is slow.

21. The value of $\Delta G°$ indicates that the reaction is
    A. rapid.
    B. slow.
    C. spontaneous.
    D. nonspontaneous.

22. Because both the sign of $\Delta H°$ and the sign of $\Delta S°$ for this reaction are negative, this reaction is
    A. spontaneous only at high temperatures.
    B. spontaneous only at low temperatures.
    C. always spontaneous.
    D. never spontaneous.

23. Calculate $\Delta H°$ for the formation of eight moles of H_2O.
    A. −3561.2 kJ   B. −7122.4 kJ
    C. −222.6 kJ   D. +3721.1 kJ

24. Calculate $\Delta H°$ for the reaction
    $CO_2\,(g) + 2H_2O\,(l) \rightarrow CH_4\,(g) + 2O_2\,(g)$.
    A. −890.3 kJ   B. −732.6 kJ
    C. +732.6 kJ   D. +890.3 kJ

QUESTIONS 25–27 are NOT based on a descriptive passage.

25. If a 50kg object is raised 2 meters, what is the work that is being done?
    A. 490 J   B. 980 J
    C. 1970 J   D. 1350 J

26. The phenomenon that occurs when a wave spreads into the region behind an obstruction is known as
    A. refraction.   B. diffraction.
    C. dispersion.   D. superposition.

27. If the expression *W* in the First Law of Thermodynamics is negative, it implies all of the following EXCEPT
    A. work has been done by the system.
    B. the total internal energy has decreased.
    C. a negative amount of work has been done to the system.
    D. the system has lost heat.

PASSAGE VI (QUESTIONS 28–32)

A chemist adds a piece of tin metal to an aqueous solution containing silver ions. The chemist observes the formation of crystalline silver in the solution. The equation for this reaction is

$$Sn + 2Ag^+ \rightarrow Sn^{2+} + 2Ag$$

The chemist is able to design a voltaic cell where this reaction is used to produce electrical energy. Standard reduction potentials at 25°C are

$Sn^{2+} + 2e^- \rightarrow Sn$; E° = −0.14 V

$Ag^+ + e^- \rightarrow Ag$; E° = 0.80 V

28. Which species is the oxidizing agent in this cell?
    A. Sn   B. Ag^+
    C. Sn^{2+} D. Ag

29. What is the half-reaction that takes place at the anode?
A. $Sn \rightarrow Sn^{2+}$ B. $Sn^{2+} \rightarrow Sn$
C. $Ag^+ \rightarrow Ag$ D. $2Ag^+ \rightarrow 2Ag$

30. Calculate E° for the cell.
A. 0.66 V B. –0.66 V
C. 0.28 V D. 0.94 V

31. The cell can be abbreviated
A. $Sn/2\,Ag^+ \,||\, Sn^{2+}/2Ag$
B. $Sn/Ag^+ \,||\, Sn^{2+}/Ag$
C. $Ag^+/Ag \,||\, Sn/Sn^{2+}$
D. $Sn/Sn^{2+} \,||\, Ag^+/Ag$

32. In this cell, the electron flow between electrodes is from
A. Sn to Ag. B. Sn^{2+} to Sn.
C. Ag^+ to Ag. D. Ag to Ag^+.

PASSAGE VII (QUESTIONS 33–37)

In a study of the conditions for static equilibrium in a body acted upon by concurrent forces, a physicist suspends a 50kg ball using two ropes, as shown in the figure below (sin 30° = 0.500; cos 30° = 0.866).

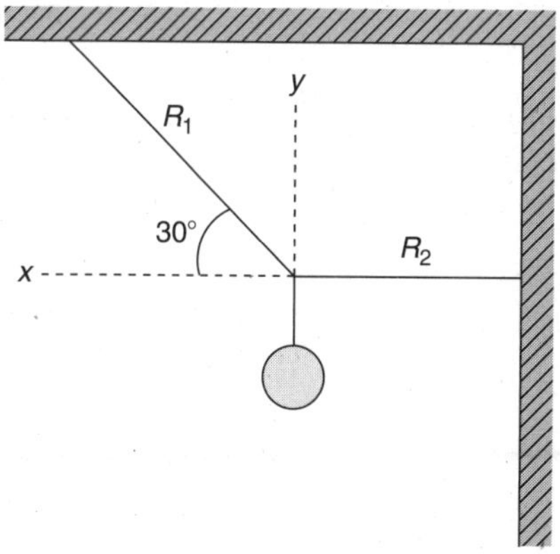

The physicist is able to calculate the various forces acting on the ball. These values are then determined experimentally using spring balances inserted along the ropes.

33. The gravitational force on the ball is
A. 50 kg up. B. 50 kg down.
C. 100 kg up. D. 100 kg down.

34. The sum of the forces exerted in the y direction by ropes R_1 and R_2 at the junction is equal to
A. 0 kg. B. 50 kg up.
C. 50 kg down. D. 100 kg up.

35. The sum of all the forces acting in the x direction is equal to
A. 0 kg. B. 50 kg up.
C. 50 kg down. D. 100 kg up.

36. The force exerted in the y direction by ropes R_1 and R_2 is
A. $R_1 \sin 30° + R_2$. B. $R_1 \cos 30° + R_2$.
C. $R_1 \sin 30°$. D. $R_1 \cos 30°$.

37. The force exerted on the ball by rope R_1 is
A. 100 kg. B. 25 kg.
C. 50 kg. D. 87 kg.

PASSAGE VIII (QUESTIONS 38–41)

In a study of Ohm's Law as applied to circuit components, a physicist sets up an electrical circuit that contains several resistors in series, a pair of resistors in parallel, and a single voltage source. A diagram of the circuit is shown below:

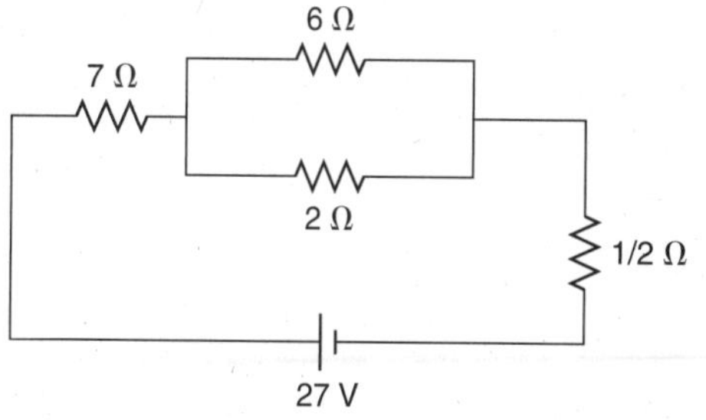

Amperages and voltages across the resistors are calculated using Ohm's Law. These values are then determined experimentally using an ammeter and a voltmeter.

38. Calculate the equivalent resistance of the 6Ω and 2Ω resistors.
    A. 1/8Ω B. 3/2Ω
    C. 2Ω D. 3Ω

39. Calculate the total resistance of the entire network of resistors
    A. 3Ω B. 5Ω
    C. 7Ω D. 9Ω

40. Calculate the current through the 7Ω resistor.
    A. 1 amp B. 3 amp
    C. 5 amp D. 7 amp

41. Calculate the voltage drop across the 7Ω resistor.
    A. 3 volts B. 7 volts
    C. 21 volts D. 24 volts

PASSAGE IX (QUESTIONS 42–45)

To study some of the properties of spherical mirrors, a physicist inserts a convex mirror having a radius of curvature of 50 cm in a mirror holder and places it at the 0-cm mark of an optical bench. The physicist makes sure that the convex surface of the mirror faces the object to be placed on the optical bench. A 60-cm-tall lamp is placed at the 100-cm mark on the optical bench. The physicist makes sure that the axes of the lamp and mirror are aligned.

42. Calculate the focal length of the mirror.
    A. 10 cm B. 20 cm
    C. 25 cm D. 40 cm

43. Calculate the distance from the mirror to the image of the lamp.
    A. 55 cm behind the mirror
    B. 40 cm behind the mirror
    C. 40 cm in front of the mirror
    D. 20 cm behind the mirror

44. How tall is the image of the lamp?
    A. 24 cm B. 28 cm
    C. 16 cm D. 12 cm

45. Which one of the following statements about convex mirrors is false?
    A. The focal length is negative.
    B. The image is always erect.
    C. The image is always virtual.
    D. The image is always in front of the mirror.

PASSAGE X (QUESTIONS 46–49)

To determine the characteristics of simple harmonic waves in stretched strings, a physicist studies various guitar strings. One of these strings is stretched (tuned) so that when it is plucked, the transverse wave produced corresponded to a note of A at a frequency of 110 Hz. This note is played at a loudness of 20 decibels (dB). The note made by this instrument interferes with a note of A made by a second instrument. The beat frequency was 5 beats per second.

The speed of these sounds in air can be calculated from the formula

$$v = 331 + 0.6\,T,$$

in which T is in °C and v in meters/second.

46. What is the frequency of this note when played one octave higher?
    A. 55 Hz B. 110 Hz
    C. 111 Hz D. 220 Hz

47. The energy of this sound is _____ times the loudness of the softest audible sound.
    A. 0.20 B. 100
    C. 200 D. 220

48. What are the possible frequencies of the note made by the second instrument?

A. 105 Hz

B. 115 Hz

C. 110 Hz or 115 Hz

D. 105 Hz or 115 Hz

49. Calculate the speed of this sound in air at 10°C.

A. 110 m/s B. 220 m/s

C. 330 m/s D. 337 m/s

QUESTIONS 50–52 are NOT based on a descriptive passage.

50. A 55-year-old woman has a near point of 100 cm. What lens should be used to see clearly an object at the normal near point of 25 cm? (Find the focal length of the required lens.)

A. 20.0 cm B. –33.3 cm

C. 33.3 cm D. –25.0 cm

51. The resistance of a piece of copper wire is 10 ohms. The resistance, in ohms, of a piece of copper wire of the same diameter but twice as long is

A. 5 Ω. B. 10 Ω.

C. 20 Ω. D. 80 Ω.

52. In the photoelectric effect, electromagnetic radiation is incident upon the surface of a metal. Which of the following is NOT a true statement about the photoelectric effect?

A. The stopping potential V_0 is proportional to v^2.

B. v_0 is characteristic of the cathode material.

C. The stopping potential is independent of the intensity.

D. There is no photocurrent unless $v > v_0$.

STOP! If time still remains, you may review work only in this section. When the time allotted is up, you may go on to the next section. STOP!

SECTION 2
Verbal Reasoning

TIME: 60 Minutes

QUESTIONS: 53–92

DIRECTIONS: The verbal reasoning section contains nine passages, each followed by a series of questions. Based on the information given in a passage, choose the one best answer to each question.

PASSAGE I (QUESTIONS 53–57)

John Hancock, born in 1737 at Braintree (presently Quincy), Massachusetts, lost his father, a Congregational pastor, at the age of seven. He spent the next six years with his grandparents at Lexington before joining his guardian, Thomas Hancock, a childless uncle and one of the richest merchant-shippers in Boston. After studying at Boston Latin School and graduating from Harvard College in 1754, John began working as a clerk in his uncle's business and learned it rapidly. In 1760–1761, while visiting London to observe the English side of the business, he attended the funeral of George II and the coronation of George III, who apparently granted him an audience. In 1763, he became a partner in his uncle's business. The uncle died the following year and willed him the firm, a fortune that was probably the greatest in New England, and a luxurious house on Beacon Street.

Hancock allied with other merchants in protesting the Stamp Act (1765), and the next year inaugurated a long legislative career; but he did not strongly identify with the patriots until two years later. At that time, British customs officials, their courage bolstered by the arrival of a British warship in Boston Harbor, charged him with smuggling and seized one of his ships. During the ensuing riots, the terrified customs officials fled to an island in the harbor. A few months later, the first major contingent of British troops sailed into port and created a tense situation that resulted in the Boston Massacre (1770). John Adams ably defended Hancock in court until the British dropped the smuggling charge, but the episode made him a hero throughout the colonies.

Other factors tied Hancock to the patriots. Samuel and John Adams, shrewdly perceiving the advantages of a rich and well-known affiliate, welcomed him into their ranks, encouraged his idolatry by the populace, and pushed him upward in the Revolutionary hierarchy. When the first provincial congress met at Salem and Concord in 1774, he acted as president as well as chairman of the vital council of safety. The second provincial congress, convening the next year at Cambridge and Concord, elected him to the Continental Congress.

On April 18, only three days after the provincial congress adjourned, British troops marched from Boston to seize rebel stores at Concord. Warned of their approach during the night by Paul Revere, Hancock and Samuel Adams, who were visiting at nearby Lexington, escaped. But the British-American clashes at Lexington and Concord marked the outbreak of war.

From 1775 until 1777, Hancock presided over the Continental Congress. The very first year, his egotism, which regularly aroused the antipathy of many members, created personal embitterment as well. Blind to his own limitations, particularly his lack of military experience, he unrealistically entertained the hope that he, instead of Washington, would be appointed as commander-in-chief of the Continental Army.

Only Hancock and Charles Thompson, the president and secretary of Congress, signed the broadside copy of the Declaration, printed the night of its adoption, July 4, 1776, and disseminated to the public the following day. At the formal signing of the parchment copy on August 2, tradition holds that Hancock wrote his name in large letters so that the king would not need spectacles to recognize him as a "traitor." After resigning as presiding officer in 1777, he remained a member of Congress until 1780, though he spent much of his time in Boston, and for the rest of his life solidified his political position in Massachusetts. In 1788, as a major general in the militia, he commanded an expedition that failed to recapture Newport, Rhode Island, from the British. He made a more tangible contribution to the war by accepting Continental currency from his debtors, even though his fortune had already been dented by wartime-induced reverses.

In 1780, the same year Hancock gave up his seat in Congress and attended his Commonwealth's constitutional convention, he was overwhelmingly elected as first governor (1780–1785). He won reelection in 1787–1793. In the interim (1785–1786), he once again sat in Congress. In 1788, he chaired the Massachusetts convention that ratified the U.S. Constitution, which he favored.

While still governor, in 1793 at the age of 56, Hancock died in Boston. His funeral, one of the most impressive ever held in New England, culminated in burial at Old Granary Burying Ground.

53. Which of the following factors is not given as associating Hancock with the patriots?
    - A. His wealth
    - B. His being charged with smuggling
    - C. His status as a hero
    - D. His acquaintance with King George

54. The passage supports the view that John Hancock
    - A. greatly profited financially from the Revolutionary War.
    - B. was a strong egotistical person.
    - C. was a smuggler.
    - D. was a reclusive personality.

55. The passage on John Hancock gives evidence primarily based on
    - A. public historical records.
    - B. eyewitness accounts.
    - C. private letters.
    - D. autobiographical revelations.

56. From this passage, it is reasonable to assume that the Boston Massacre could have been prevented if
    - A. Hancock had supported the Stamp Act.
    - B. John Adams had not defended Hancock in court.
    - C. the British had not seized one of Hancock's ships.
    - D. Hancock had not smuggled goods.

57. For the last thirteen years of his life, John Hancock
    - A. concentrated on his political position in Massachusetts.
    - B. concentrated on his business.
    - C. served in Congress.
    - D. served as governor of Massachusetts.

PASSAGE II (QUESTIONS 58–62)

John Adams and Thomas Jefferson were the first two occupants of the White House, the official residence of our nation's presidents since 1800. It is a national shrine that symbolizes the honor and dignity of the highest office in the land, and it has been the scene of many historic events and brilliant social affairs. Like the nation itself, it bears the influence of successive chief executives. Although rebuilt and modernized, it retains the simplicity and charm of its original appearance.

President George Washington approved the plans for the White House, drawn by Irish-born James Hoban, winner of a prize competition. Major Pierre Charles L'Enfant, the French artist-engineer, located the mansion in his plan of the Federal City, where the White House and the Capitol were the first public buildings erected. The cornerstone was laid on October 13, 1792. Workmen used light gray sandstone from the Aquia Creek Quarries, in Virginia, for the exterior walls. During the course of construction or soon thereafter, they were painted white. As a result, the building was unofficially termed the "White House" from an early date, but for many years it was usually referred to as the "President's House" or the "President's Palace."

In the Palladian style of architecture, the main façade resembles the Duke of Leinster's mansion in Dublin. Hoban probably derived the details of the other faces and the interior arrangement from other contemporary European mansions. He supervised the original construction, the rebuilding after the burning by British forces in 1814, and the erection of the north and south porticoes some years later. Over time, however, various architects modified Hoban's original plans, notably Benjamin H. Latrobe during and after the Jefferson administration.

President and Mrs. John Adams were the first occupants, in November 1800, when the government moved from Philadelphia to Washington. The interior had not yet been completed, and Mrs. Adams used the unfinished East Room to dry the family's wash. During Jefferson's administration the east and west terraces, or pavilions, were built. Jefferson, who practiced democratic simplicity in his social life, opened the mansion each morning to all arrivals.

During the War of 1812, British forces captured the city and set the torch to the White House, the Capitol, and other government buildings in retaliation for the destruction of some public buildings in Canada by U.S. troops. Only the partially damaged exterior walls and interior brickwork of the White House remained in the spring of 1815 when reconstruction began. In 1817, the recently elected President James Monroe was able to occupy the structure. In 1824, builders erected the south portico, and in 1829, the large north portico over the entrance and driveway. The west wing, including the president's Oval Office, was added during the first decade of the twentieth century. The east wing was built in 1942.

Over the years, the White House proper has been extensively renovated and modernized on various occasions. The old sandstone walls have been retained, however. The aim has been to keep the historical atmosphere while providing a more livable home for the president and his family.

Located on the first floor of the main building are the East Room, Green Room, Blue Room, Red Room, State Dining Room, and Family Dining Room. These richly furnished rooms are open to the public on a special schedule. The ground and second floors are restricted to the use of the presidential family and guests. On the ground floor are the Diplomatic Reception Room, Curator's Office, Vermeil Room, China Room, and Library. The second floor contains the Lincoln Bedroom, Lincoln Sitting Room, Queen's Bedroom (Rose Guest Room), Treaty Room, Yellow Oval Room, and Empire Guest Room. Neither of the wings, reserved for the president and his staff, is ordinarily accessible to the public.

The simple dignity of the White House is enhanced by the natural beauty of its informal, but carefully landscaped grounds.

58. The passage states that the White House, in its first few years of existence, was
    A. actually gray in color.
    B. fully furnished with many spare rooms.
    C. first occupied by President John Adams and his wife.
    D. located in Philadelphia.

59. The passage suggests that the original plans for the White House reflect the influence of which of the following countries?
    I. Ireland
    II. England
    III. France
    A. I only
    B. II only
    C. I and III
    D. II and III

60. Throughout the history of the White House, the building has
    A. been fully reconstructed twice.
    B. retained its original sandstone walls.
    C. undergone moderate renovation.
    D. been noted for its intricate architecture.

61. According to the author, the White House is a symbol of
    I. the power of the United States.
    II. the wealth and youth of the United States.
    III. the honor and dignity of the presidency.
    A. I only B. II only
    C. III only D. I and III

62. Which of the following is NOT a repercussion of the U.S. troops' destruction of some public buildings in Canada?
    A. British troops captured the city of Washington.
    B. The French helped remodel the burned White House in the fashion of those buildings destroyed.
    C. Only the walls and some brickwork of the White House remained after foreign troops set fire to it.
    D. The White House couldn't be occupied until 1817.

PASSAGE III (QUESTIONS 63–66)

Alcohols are members of a group of chemicals identified by their unique combination of carbon, hydrogen, and oxygen atoms. Alcohols range from methanol, which has only one carbon atom; to ethanol, with two; to the higher alcohols, with progressive additions of carbon atoms.

Because alcohols can be burned with oxygen to give off large amounts of heat, they have significant potential value as liquid fuels. In general, the higher alcohols, those with the most carbon atoms, have the highest heating value. This is because more carbon-hydrogen bonds can be broken to form carbon dioxide and water, releasing more energy. However, it is more difficult and expensive to produce the higher alcohols. Therefore, the simpler alcohols — methanol and ethanol — are favored for use as alcohol fuels.

Methanol, the simplest alcohol, has a chemical formula of CH_3OH. It is most commonly produced by gasification of coal, a nonrenewable resource. Methanol-production techniques that are acceptable in terms of environmental standards and resource availability are not cost-effective at this time. However, methanol can also be produced from environmentally safe biomass feedstocks, and much research is focused on this area.

Because ethanol, also called grain alcohol, is the intoxicant in alcoholic beverages, its production, use, distribution, and marketing are regulated by the Bureau of Alcohol, Tobacco, and Firearms of the U.S. Department of the Treasury.

Ethanol is legally measured in proof gallons. Each number of proof represents the ethanol content in increments of one-half percent by volume. Therefore, a mixture of 50 percent ethanol by volume is referred to as 100 proof, while pure ethanol, which is anhydrous, or water-free, is 200 proof.

Methanol and ethanol can be used alone as fuels for spark-ignited internal combustion engines. However, because methanol has less than half the heat content of gasoline, and ethanol has less than two-thirds, engine modifications must be made in order to achieve satisfactory performance. On the other hand, blends up to about 10 percent of either of these two alcohols with gasoline have been successfully used in vehicles without engine modifications, although other components such as fuel lines may require exchanging.

The term *gasohol* was coined and registered as a trademark in 1973 by the Nebraska Agricultural Products Industrial Utilization Committee. By its definition, gasohol is a blend of 10 percent anhydrous, agriculturally derived ethanol, and 90 percent unleaded gasoline. Through popular usage, it has become the generic term for all ethanol or methanol and gasoline blends. For the sake of accuracy, however, it is best to identify other ethanol-gasoline blends with a number identifying the percentage of ethanol used, as in fuel blend E20. Similarly, for methanol-gasoline blends, fuel blend M10 identifies a 10 percent mix in methanol gasoline. Gasohol made from its component, fermentation ethanol, is the most widely used alcohol fuel in the United States today.

63. Methanol and ethanol are favored over the higher alcohols for use as alcohol fuels because they
    - A. have fewer carbon atoms.
    - B. release more energy.
    - C. are more common.
    - D. are simpler and cheaper to produce.

64. Researchers focus on methanol as a fuel because
    - A. coal, the major source of methanol, is an ample resource.
    - B. it is a complex fuel that meets environmental standards.
    - C. it can be produced from biomass feedstocks that are safe for the environment.
    - D. coal, the major source of methanol, is cost-efficient.

65. The main point of this passage is that
    - A. ethanol and methanol are just two types of simple alcohol fuels that scientists believe will soon become common, cost-efficient, environmentally safe fuels.
    - B. alcohols are measured chemically by their additions of carbon atoms; because ethanol and methanol have a low measurement, they are unable to supply power to fuel engines.
    - C. methanol and ethanol are gasoline substitutes.
    - D. gasohol, a blend of alcohol fuels, is the fuel of the future.

66. Which of the following is a reason that alcohols have a significant potential value as liquid fuels?
    - A. They are cheap to produce.
    - B. They can be produced from renewable resources.
    - C. They can be burned to give off large amounts of heat.
    - D. They are nonpolluting.

PASSAGE IV (QUESTIONS 67–72)

A long-standing problem of philosophical theology is the problem of evil. The problem may be stated as follows:

(1) Either God cannot prevent evil or God will not prevent evil.

(2) If God cannot prevent evil, then God is not all-powerful.

(3) If God will not prevent evil, then God is not all-loving.

(4) Therefore, either God is not all-powerful or God is not all-loving.

The response to this problem has taken many forms. One response has been to claim that (2) is false. The argument here is that God has endowed human beings with a free will, a will to choose freely between good and evil. Therefore, God could not give human beings the ability to freely choose between good and evil and then intervene to make the choice of evil impossible. That would have been a negation of the gift of free will. When we talk about God's ultimate power, we mean God's ability to do any logically possible thing, but it would not be a logically possible thing for God to give genuine free will to humans and then so arrange things that this freedom could not be exercised in the choice between good and evil.

A second response has been to deny the truth of (3). The argument here is that there are some virtues that require the prior existence of evil in order to be exercised, such as sympathy or compassion. We see only a very small part of the total picture, and so we do not see the roles that evil plays in the grand scheme of things. If we did, we might understand that those evils that God allows make for a better world than there would be if those evils did not exist. Those evils may make possible the existence of virtues.

Still another response to the problem has been to point out that an underlying assumption of the problem is that there is such a thing as evil, and this has been called into question. Certainly there is what to us appears to be evil, but our perspective is only that of the very limited part of existence that we inhabit; evil is, like beauty, in the eye of the beholder, and who are we to say that evil exists from the perspective of God? All of God's creation is good, even if some parts of it from our limited perspective appear problematical. These problematical parts we deem "evil." However, if we had the perspective of the whole creation before us, we would see, as does God, that the whole of creation is perfectly good, and evil is nowhere to be found in it. What we call "evil" is really just a perceived lack of goodness, and everything that exists is good.

Finally, there have been those who found the initial argument persuasive and concluded that either God's power or God's goodness is limited. Of these two options, most have tended to infer that it is God's power that is limited. It has even been argued that this limitation of God's power invests us with a purposeful moral responsibility for the way things are. We cannot just sit back and leave it all to God, for the nature of things depends on us and our actions.

67. Based on this passage, the problem of evil shows that there is a problem with
    A. our conception of God.
    B. how to eliminate evil.
    C. whether evil exists.
    D. freedom of the will.

68. One response to the problem of evil has been to affirm that
    A. God intervenes in human affairs.
    B. evil does not exist.
    C. God can do any logically possible thing.
    D. if God will not prevent evil, then God is not all-loving.

69. According to the passage, those who deny that evil exists hold that
    A. we think evil exists because of our limited perspective.
    B. God's power is limited.
    C. evil is necessary for goodness.
    D. evil is really goodness.

70. The problem of evil claims to show that
    A. God does not exist.
    B. an all-powerful God does not exist.
    C. an all-good God does not exist.
    D. an all-good and all-powerful God does not exist.

71. One response to the problem has involved the claim that
    A. human beings have a free will.
    B. God could not choose between good and evil.
    C. good will overcome evil.
    D. human beings are evil.

72. Which of the following would be a satisfactory response to the problem of evil?
    A. To resolve to do good
    B. To have faith in God
    C. To actively participate in doing God's work
    D. To show that evil is an illusion

PASSAGE V (QUESTIONS 73–78)

There are some properties that things have as inherent or necessary parts of their very make-up, properties that we might call primary or necessary properties. This means that some properties or qualities are necessary for the thing to be what it is. There are other properties that things may have but that are not primary properties. These are properties they may or may not have without affecting their essential nature. These we may call secondary or contingent properties. For example, the property of "having three sides" is a primary property of a triangle, while the property of "being inscribed in a circle" is not. For a basketball, properties of circumference and weight are primary, while those of color are secondary.

This distinction between primary and secondary properties underlies one of the most ancient arguments for the existence of God, the so-called ontological argument.

One version of this argument notes that the term *God* signifies a supremely perfect being. The question is whether such a being exists in actuality or only as a figment of our imaginations. There can be no doubt that we have a conception of God; there is only the question as to whether or not there is anything in reality corresponding to our conception.

Now if the concept of God is that of a perfect being, then we must assume that in conceiving of God, we are conceiving of God with whatever properties a perfect being would have as primary properties, meaning that they are essential to its nature. Surely existence is just such a property, for a being that was perfect but lacked existence would be "less perfect" than a being that had those same properties and also had existence as well. But this would then mean that such a being that lacked existence would not be the most perfect being possible because another being could be conceived as "more perfect" than it. Therefore, this most perfect conceivable being would have to have as one of its essential properties the property of existence. This means that the property of existence could not be separated from the nature of that being.

There may seem to be an element of magic about this, even a kind of sophistry. Why may we not just make the same argument for any object? The answer is that this argument holds only for a being described as "a supremely perfect being" or "a being more perfect than any other." Only of such a being may it be affirmed that the property of existence is one of its primary or essential properties.

73. The ontological argument claims that
    A. whatever we conceive exists in the actual world.
    B. whatever we conceive we must conceive as having whatever primary properties it has.
    C. whatever we conceive must have whatever secondary properties it has.
    D. attempting to prove existence is futile.

74. Primary properties are properties that things
    A. must have.
    B. must have if they exist.
    C. are known to have.
    D. may or may not have as part of their nature.

75. The essential nature of a thing is determined by its
    A. secondary properties.
    B. primary properties.
    C. tertiary properties.
    D. tangible properties.

76. The reason the ontological argument does not hold for things other than God is that
    A. existence is a necessary property of God.
    B. existence is a necessary property only of a supremely perfect being.
    C. existence is a secondary property.
    D. God is omniscient.

77. If two objects had the same primary properties in common, then
    A. they would be identical.
    B. they would have the same secondary properties in common.
    C. they would be ontologically unstable.
    D. separately, they would each be the object in question.

78. According to the ontological argument,
  A. if God exists, then God exists.
  B. it is necessarily true that God exists.
  C. whatever we conceive of exists.
  D. a being even more perfect than God exists.

PASSAGE VI (QUESTIONS 79–83)

Music's power to affect moods and stir emotions has been well known for as long as music has existed. Stories about the music of ancient Greece tell of its healing powers. Leopold Mozart, the father of Wolfgang, wrote that if the Greeks' music could heal the sick, then the music of his time should be able to bring the dead back to life. Unfortunately, today's music cannot do quite that much.

The healing power of music, taken for granted by ancient man and by many primitive societies, is only recently becoming accepted by medical professionals as a new way of healing the emotionally ill.

Using musical activities involving patients, the music therapist seeks to restore mental and physical health. Music therapists usually work with emotionally disturbed patients as part of a team of therapists and doctors. Music therapists work together with physicians, psychiatrists, psychologists, physical therapists, nurses, teachers, recreation leaders, and the families of patients.

The therapy that a music therapist gives to patients can be in the form of listening, performing, lessons on an instrument, or even composing. A therapist may help a patient regain lost coordination by teaching the patient how to play an instrument. Speech defects can sometimes be helped by singing activities. Some patients need the social awareness of group activities, but others may need individual attention to build self-confidence. The music therapist must discern the type of activities that are best for each patient.

In addition to working with patients, the music therapist attends meetings with other therapists and doctors who work with the same patients to discuss progress and plan new activities. Written reports to doctors about patients' responses to treatment are another facet of the music therapist's work.

Hospitals, schools, retirement homes, and community agencies and clinics are some of the sites where music therapists work. Some music therapists work in private studies with patients sent to them by medical doctors, psychologists, and psychiatrists. Music therapy can be done in studios, recreation rooms, hospital wards, or classrooms depending on the type of activity and needs of the patients.

Qualified music therapists have followed a four-year course with a major emphasis in music plus courses in biological science, anthropology, sociology, psychology, and music therapy. General studies in English, history, speech, and government complete the requirements for a bachelor of music therapy. After college training, a music therapist must participate in a six-month training internship under the guidance of a registered music therapist.

Students who have completed college courses and have demonstrated their ability during the six-month internship can become registered music therapists by applying to the National Association for Music Therapy, Inc. New methods and techniques of music therapy are always being developed, so the trained therapist must continue to study new articles, books, and reports throughout his or her career.

79. Which statement best summarizes the central idea of this passage?
  A. Music therapy is a multifaceted area of professional life.
  B. The healing power of music therapy is extensive and intensive.
  C. Music therapy is complex and always involves the teaching of songs and instruments.
  D. A music therapist is a medical person.

80. The qualifications for becoming a licensed music therapist consist of all of the following EXCEPT
  A. working with a registered therapist.
  B. training on one's own.

C. a sustained internship.
D. the ability to utilize current therapeutic techniques.

81. Self-confidence can be rebuilt through music. Which of the following reasons supports this statement?
    I. A skill can strengthen the will to succeed.
    II. All persons have musical ability.
    III. All persons may enjoy music.
    A. I only B. II only
    C. I and III D. II and III

82. In this essay, the term *patient* specifically refers to a person
    A. in need of the services of medical personnel.
    B. in need of resocialization.
    C. in psychoanalysis.
    D. disabled by loss of coordination, hearing, or speech.

83. On the basis of the essay, the relationship of healing to music therapy is one of
    A. cause and effect.
    B. symptom and treatment.
    C. process and consequence.
    D. health and disease.

PASSAGE VII (QUESTIONS 84–87)

The official birth date of American naval aviation (sometimes referred to as the U.S. Navy's air arm) has been set as May 8, 1911. This is the date when the United States Navy bought its first aircraft. This flimsy little craft, offered for sale to the Navy by Glenn Curtis, cost the Navy $5,500. Despite the simple and fragile construction and the relatively high unit cost of this little craft, the date of the sale was an important one because it marked the birth of what has become the greatest and most effective naval air arm of any nation.

In 1890, Captain A. T. Mahan, USN, pointed out in his writings that the nation that controls the seas also controls the lands and thereby wins the wars. Despite the advancement of naval aviation, his doctrine is still very much in effect. However, a qualification to this doctrine must be added today — to control the seas, one must first control the air over the seas. To control the seas and the air over them, the Navy's air, surface, and undersea forces work as a team to accomplish this task.

The U.S. Navy has never separated its aviation branch from the other forces. This is due mainly to the foresight of those senior officers in positions of great responsibility over the past sixty years or more. Great Britain tried such a separation of its air and surface forces after World War I. This experiment did not work. As a result, the air arm was brought back into the Royal Navy only a short time before World War II. The British Admiral of the Fleet, Lord Keys, stated in 1944 that the success of the U.S. Navy in the Battle of the Philippines was made possible only because the United States Navy had been free to develop its own naval aviation. He stated further that in the complex business of waging war on the seas, no one factor or force can win alone. All forces must work together as a team. Fortunately, the U.S. Navy tends its air, surface, and undersea forces with motherly devotion and fairness, thereby creating a unified force that is unparalleled in history.

The mission of the U.S. Navy is to ensure open sea lanes in the oceans of the world in time of war and to deny their use to the enemy. The continuous appearance of new and modern sophisticated weapons changes the techniques of naval aviation. This also adds to the U.S. Navy's capabilities. However, the command of the seas is still the primary mission of the navy. Naval aviation, regardless of the sophistication of its present arms and of those to come, still has as its primary function close coordination with other forces of the navy to maintain command of the seas.

84. It can be inferred from this passage that the U.S. Navy
    I. is the oldest of the armed forces.
    II. shares its command of the seas.

III. highly parallels the thought and development of the British Navy.

A. I only B. II only
C. III only D. I and III

85. According to this passage, the U.S. Navy is
 A. the seafaring arm of the armed forces.
 B. the undersea, air, and seafaring arm of U.S. defense.
 C. comparable to the navy of Great Britain.
 D. the idea of Captain A. T. Mahan.

86. From the facts in this passage, it may be concluded that
 A. the navy has not changed its techniques since 1911.
 B. the navy commands the seas without assistance.
 C. command of the navy reflects the maternal care of the U.S. government.
 D. the future is in the hands of those leaders who have vision in matters of defense.

87. It can be reasonably inferred from this passage that war is
 I. a complex effort.
 II. necessary for peace.
 III. a necessary evil.

 A. I only B. III only
 C. I and II D. II and III

PASSAGE VIII (QUESTIONS 88–90)

Apprehension over the development and implementation of nuclear plants was confirmed in the minds of critics when the media announced the fuel meltdown at Three Mile Island near Harrisburg, Pennsylvania, in 1979 and again reinforced with the accident at the nuclear plant at Chernobyl in 1986. Environmentalists who had raised serious questions preceding and following the two catastrophes continue to press for research and development of solar energy and other non-fossil sources, such as wind and geothermal.

The federal courts entered the process in the 1970s, when an interest group charged the Atomic Regulatory Commission with unfair and inadequate procedures during a licensing process. Although the interest group convinced the United States Circuit Court of Appeals that closer judicial monitoring of the licensing process was within constitutional protections, it lost its case in the United States Supreme Court in *Vermont Yankee Nuclear Power Corporation v. Natural Resources Defense Counsel, Inc.* in 1978. The Supreme Court held that the agency's informal rule-making was based upon technical data, and the courts should not become "Monday morning quarterbacks." Other activities of interest groups, such as Public Concern, the National Audubon Society, and Worldwatch Institute, led to the demise of construction of nuclear plants with no new orders by 1978. More recent concern of interest groups and many citizens is radioactive waste disposal.

For many years, nuclear scientists have had great influence on industrial and political leaders, university administrator policymakers, and major professional groups. As early as the 1950s, the slogan "atomic energy for peace" led to full-scale plans for research and development, which was supposed to provide safe, cheap, and unlimited sources of electricity. The bandwagon gained momentum, and the nuclear reactor program became the buzzword of the 1950s and 1960s. Enthusiasts promised that atomic energy would provide the solution for combating the greenhouse effect and for promoting industrial growth.

Problems developed when industry failed to meet its promises. Construction costs were higher than predicted. Construction was complex and plagued by errors. The amount of time between initiation of construction and authorization by government to begin electrical generation far exceeded all expectations. Adding to the cost of construction and maintenance was the fact that plant constructions were unique, with variation from plant to plant. Cancellations of nuclear reactors by utility companies became prevalent during this period of time. Today, three large plants have not begun operation, and only 103 commercial nuclear plants currently generate electricity.

Pro-nuclear activists have gone back to the drawing board in search of new ideas that will again generate enthusiasm for nuclear energy and funds for industrial and university research projects. The high cost of nuclear energy remains the major factor in the decision-making process of managers of utilities. Over the years, stockholders have become disillusioned with investment in utilities with nuclear-powered plants, and management has responded accordingly.

88. Which phrase best describes the main idea in the passage?
    A. The pluralistic nature of the American society
    B. Stockholders' desire to invest in a single utility operated by the national government
    C. A need for congressional investigation of interest group infiltration into industrial research laboratories and construction sites
    D. The hopelessness of pursuing the use of nuclear power

89. Which statement summarizes the implication that can be drawn from the author's narrative?
    A. Industrial giants place philosophical and humanitarian priorities over profits.
    B. Nuclear energy is a dead issue in the United States.
    C. In our capitalist system of government, pressure exerted by ordinary citizens may eventually have an impact on major industrial development.
    D. Utility companies have abandoned General Electric and Westinghouse production goals and have become active proponents of interest groups' support of solar energy.

90. Which statement puts into perspective the current conditions in our country?
    A. The safest, most economical, and least controversial policy for development of energy alternatives to coal and oil is yet to be resolved by leaders in industry, universities, and interest groups due to the complexity of the issue.
    B. The uncertainty of decision-making by utility companies is rectified by the fact that these companies have safety and public service as the number one priority.
    C. Historically, interest groups are composed of an odd assortment of people who manufacture issues in order to bond members to the organizations.
    D. Technically, conditions for a bandwagon in support of nuclear energy that prevailed in the 1950s and 1960s are the same today, with the sole exception of the Chernobyl and Three Mile Island accidents.

PASSAGE IX (QUESTIONS 91–92)

Although February 18, 2000, marked the seventieth anniversary of the discovery of Pluto, the ninth planet in the solar system has guarded its secrets well. This frigid world is so small and distant that it appears as a featureless blob even through the largest Earth-based telescopes. It is also the only planet that has not yet been visited by a scientific spacecraft.

Despite these difficulties, a new picture of Pluto has begun to emerge during the past decade. Dedicated observational efforts using a variety of modern instruments, aided by some fortuitous celestial alignments, have produced a number of surprises. Pluto has a satellite, Charon, so large that the two objects can virtually be considered a double planet. The planet has bright polar caps and a darker, mottled equatorial region. A layer of methane ice covers most of its surface. Pluto even possesses a thin atmosphere; when the planet is farthest from the sun, all or part of the atmosphere may freeze and fall to the surface as snow. Charon's surface, which appears to be quite different from Pluto's, may be a great expanse of water ice.

Pluto's size and density are much like those of Triton, the large satellite of Neptune that was recently visited by the *Voyager 2* probe. These and other similarities suggest that both bodies may be leftover planetesimals, relics from the early days of the solar system that managed not to be swept up by the giant outer planets. In this scenario, Triton was captured by Neptune, whereas Pluto was able to survive as a bona fide planet in an independent orbit about the sun.

Clyde W. Tombugh first glimpsed Pluto in 1930 as part of a methodical photographic survey inspired by Percival Lowell, a wealthy Bostonian with a passionate interest in finding a possible trans-Neptunian planet. It was immediately evident that Pluto is an oddball in many ways. The other outer planets orbit the sun in roughly circular paths, but Pluto's highly elliptical orbit carries it from 30 to 50 times the Earth's distance from the sun and, at times, brings it closer to the sun than Neptune. This has been the case between 1979 and 1999. Pluto's orbit also is inclined 17 degrees to the plane in which the Earth revolves around the sun, far more than that of any other planets.

New insight into Pluto's complex nature has renewed interest for a spacecraft mission to this distant world. Sending a pair of spacecraft increases the likelihood that at least one encounter will be successful and, because of economies of scale, the cost would be only slightly more than for a single spacecraft. If both were successful, it would be possible to investigate timedependent phenomena on Pluto (such as changes in its atmosphere) and to image both hemispheres of Pluto and Charon at high resolution.

A mission to Pluto would complete the human endeavor to perform a preliminary reconnaissance of all the major bodies in the solar system. As each planet has shed some of its secrets, the beautiful, bewildering diversity of nature has grown ever clearer.

91. The primary purpose of this passage is to
    A. describe atmospheric conditions on Pluto.
    B. argue for additional exploration of Pluto.
    C. detail the history of Pluto's discovery,
    D. explain Lowell's scientific contribution

92. According to the author, which of the following was farthest from the sun in 1990
    A. Charon
    B. Earth
    C. Neptune
    D. Pluto

STOP! If time still remains, you may review work only in this section. When the time allotted is up, you may go on to the next section. STOP!

SECTION 3
Writing Sample

TIME: 60 minutes

2 essays, separately timed

30 minutes each

DIRECTIONS: This section tests your writing skills by asking you to write two essays. You will have 30 minutes to write each one.

During the first 30 minutes, work only on the first essay. If you finish it in less than 30 minutes, you may review what you have written, but do not begin the second essay. During the second 30 minutes, work only on the second essay. If you finish it in less than 30 minutes, you may review what you have written for that essay only. Do not go back to the first essay.

Read each assigned topic carefully. Make sure your essays respond to the topics as they are assigned.

Make sure your essays are written in complete sentences and paragraphs, and are as clear as you can make them. Make any corrections or additions between the lines of your essays. Do not write in the margins.

On the day of the test, you are given three pages to write each essay. You are not required to use all of the space provided, but do not skip lines so you will not waste space. Illegible essays cannot be scored.

PART 1

Consider this statement:

> *Layer upon layer, past times preserve themselves in the city until life itself is finally threatened with suffocation; then, in sheer defense, modern man invents the museum.*
>
> Lewis Mumford

Write a comprehensive essay in which you accomplish the following objectives: Explain what you think the statement means. Describe specifically in what ways the city encourages rather than stultifies life. Discuss the place of the city in the life of modern humans.

PART 2

Consider this statement:

> *A nation built on the idea that all men are of equal worth and equal rights summons every one of its citizens to a life-long commitment to put that idea into practical effect.*
>
> Bruce Catton

Write a comprehensive essay in which you accomplish the following objectives: Explain what you think the statement means. Describe specific situations that set up an opposition to the statement. Discuss how citizens might work toward "equal worth and equal rights."

SECTION 4
Biological Sciences

TIME: 70 Minutes

QUESTIONS: 93–144

DIRECTIONS: Most of the questions in this section are arranged in groups, each corresponding to a descriptive passage. Based on the information given in a passage, choose the one best answer to each question in the group. Some questions are independent of a descriptive passage and of each other. Choose the one best answer to each of these questions. If you are not sure of an answer, eliminate those choices that you know are incorrect and choose an answer from among those remaining. Fill in the corresponding circle on the answer sheet to indicate your answer. You may refer to the periodic table at any time.

PASSAGE I (QUESTIONS 93–96)

Figure 1

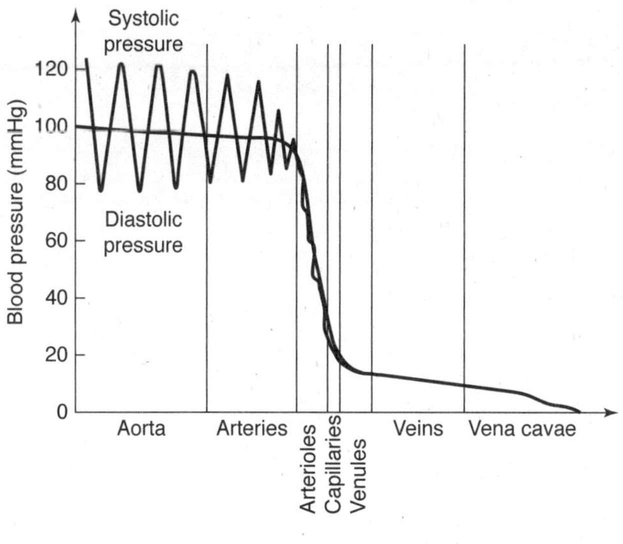

Mammalian circulatory systems are closed systems where blood is pumped by a four-chambered heart. It is often described as a double circulatory system because of the pulmonary and systemic circuits. Because cardiac muscle typically contracts as a unit, blood is driven through the vessels of the body by pulses of pressure. As blood moves farther away from the heart, the overall pressure in the system decreases. The difference in pressure caused by contraction and relaxation of the heart also decreases.

Rates of blood flow fluctuate according to changes in heart rate, stroke volume, and cross-sectional area of the vessels through which blood flows. Water is forced out of blood by hydrostatic pressure as the blood enters capillary beds from arterioles and is taken back into venules by osmotic pressure as blood leaves capillary beds. Most (about 99 percent) of this water is thus reabsorbed, but a small amount of fluid remains in the tissues of the capillary bed. This fluid is ultimately returned to the blood circulatory system through lymphatics, capillaries, and veins.

Use the information given in this passage, your general knowledge of the circulatory system, and the graph of systemic circulation that appears as Figure 1, to answer the following questions.

93. In a mammal, blood pressure is lowest in the

A. aorta.

B. vena cavae.

C. capillaries of the arm.

D. veins of the leg.

94. Lymph is returned to the blood circulatory system through large lymph ducts that empty into the

A. subclavian veins.

B. hepatic portal system.

C. abdominal aorta.

D. inferior vena cava.

95. The connection between the aorta and the pulmonary artery of a mammalian fetus is known as the
    A. foramen ovale.
    B. foramen magnum.
    C. ductus arteriosus.
    D. ligamentum arteriosum.

96. All of the following statements about the mammalian circulatory system are correct EXCEPT
    A. blood pressure is lower in a capillary bed than in the arteriole leading to it.
    B. water content of blood is regulated by concentration of blood protein.
    C. osmotic pressure across capillary walls is regulated by active transport of water.
    D. blood flows faster in the arteriole than in the capillary bed.

PASSAGE II (QUESTIONS 97–99)

The nucleotide base sequence of a section of DNA can be determined by using the Sanger Method. This involves four main steps. First, double-stranded DNA is separated into two strands. Second, a radioactively labeled primer, to which nucleotides can be added, is attached to one end of the single strands of DNA. This is shown below.

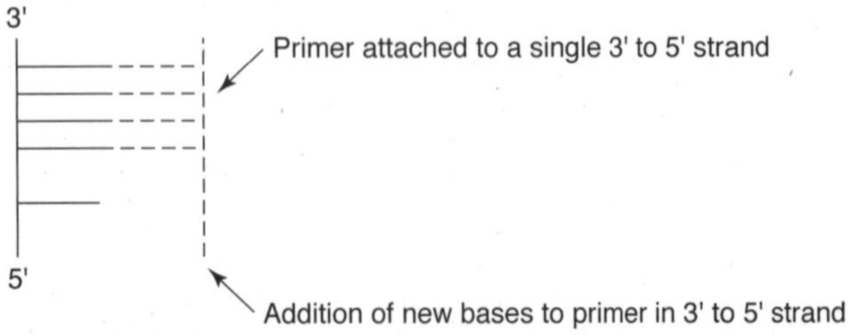

Third, the single DNA strands with the attached primer are added to four different test tubes. Each test tube contains the added material and DNA polymerase, the four nucleotide precursors, and a small amount of one special nucleotide. There are four special nucleotides: one for adenine (ddA), one for cytosine (ddC), one for guanine (ddG), and one for thymine (ddT). These special forms, called dideo-oxy-nucleotides, are shaped so that, once they are incorporated into the growing DNA, no more nucleotides are added to the chain. The DNA chains synthesized in the test tubes all start with the same labeled primer and all contain the same sequence of bases. However, they differ in length depending on where the special form of the nucleotide was added.

The final step is to analyze the new DNA using gel electrophoresis. In electrophoresis, the smaller particles move the furthest. Therefore, the shorter the DNA chains, the further they move during electrophoresis. To determine the length of the chains, the material from each test tube is added to separate gels and after a set period of time, the position of the chains along the gel is determined.

ANALYSIS OF GEL

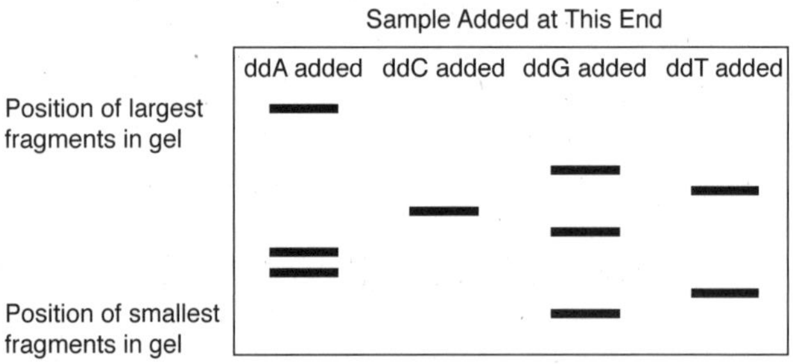

97. The sequence of nucleotide bases is the sequence of gel positions from smallest to largest fragments. Which of the following represents the DNA chain produced in the given gel analysis?
    A. A G T C G A A T G
    B. T C A G C T T A G
    C. C A T T C G A C T
    D. G T A A G C T G A

98. If the special nucleotide for adenine is shown as an asterisk (A*), which of the following could be a section of DNA chain in the gel?
    A. G T A A
    B. G T A A*
    C. G T A*A
    D. G T A* A*

99. What would be the result if all of the special nucleotides were added to each test tube, and it was not possible to distinguish among the four different special nucleotides?
   A. The results would be the same as the given results, but the spots on the gel would be thicker.
   B. There would be one spot showing the smallest fragment on each of the four gels.
   C. There would be a series of identical spots on each of the four gels.
   D. There would be one spot showing the largest fragment on each of the four gels.

PASSAGE III (QUESTIONS 100–102)

Endochondral bone formation is essentially a process of replacing a cartilaginous model with osseous tissue. The developing bone, which is highly vascularized, is formed by deposition of calcium salts of phosphate and carbonate within the intercellular matrix already defined by the chondrocytes of the cartilaginous model. Hypertrophication of chondrocytes in the shaft of the bone occurs as the model grows and calcification follows as minerals are deposited within the matrix.

Because calcification causes chondrocytes to die due to nutrient starvation, selected cells of the perichondrium are giving rise to osteoblasts. An uncalcified bone matrix known as osteoid is produced by the osteoblasts. Calcification of the perichondrium follows to form the periosteal bone collar. In the center of the developing bond, a primary ossification center is formed as cartilage is invaded by osteoblasts and vascular tissue. Two secondary ossification centers are similarly formed at the ends of the bone.

Elongation of the bone is now essentially a function of chondrocyte production in the epiphyseal plates, which are located between the primary ossification activity in the middle of the bone and the two secondary centers at each end. As long as cell division continues in the epiphyseal plates, bone growth will proceed. Eventually, the epiphyseal plates ossify and the bone will no longer increase in length.

Remodeling of bone tissue already formed occurs throughout the life of a vertebrate. Osteoblasts in the periosteum secrete osteoid as the bone is physically stressed and additional bone is deposited. Simultaneously, bone cells next to the medullary cavity are reabsorbed by osteoclasts, thereby keeping the size of the cavity proportional to the size of the bone.

Use the information given in this passage and your knowledge of the bone structure to answer the following questions.

100. The proximal epiphyseal plate of a human humerus would be closest to which of the following?
   A. The ulna
   B. The insertion of the triceps brachii
   C. The scapula
   D. The insertion of the biceps brachii

101. Knee and elbow joints arc cxamples of bone articulations known as
   A. synarthroses.
   B. synchondroses.
   C. amphiarthroses.
   D. diarthroses.

102. The shaft of a long bone is properly known as the
   A. diaphysis.
   B. epiphysis.
   C. amphiarthrosis.
   D. symphysis.

QUESTIONS 103–104 are NOT based on a descriptive passage.

103. The correct name, using the Cahn-Ingold-Prelog designation of absolute configuration, for the compound below is

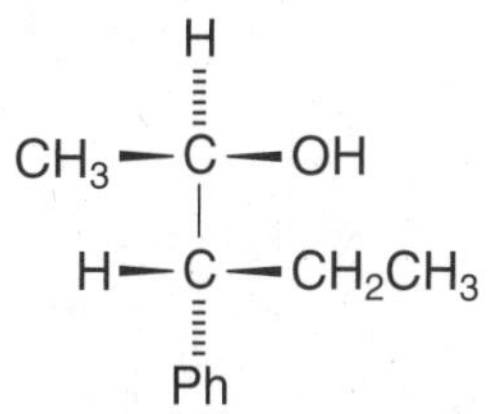

A. (2R, 3S)-3-Phenyl-2-pentanol.
B. (2R, 3R)-3-Phenyl-2-pentanol.
C. (2S, 3S)-3-Phenyl-2-pentanol.
D. (2S, 3R)-3-Phenyl-2-pentanol.

104. The correct IUPAC name for the compound shown below is

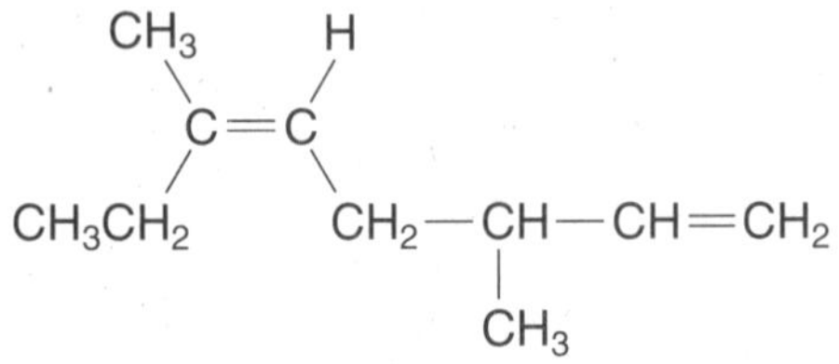

A. (E)-3, 6-dimethyl-1, 5-octadiene.
B. (Z)-3, 6-dimethyl-1, 5-octadiene.
C. (Z)-3, 6–dimethyl-3, 7-octadiene.
D. (E)-3, 6–dimethyl-3, 7-octadiene.

PASSAGE IV (QUESTIONS 105–108)

Enzymes are highly specialized proteinaceous, organic catalysts that, like all catalysts, lower the energy of activation necessary for a chemical reaction to occur. The molecule that an enzyme acts upon is known as a substrate. An enzyme greatly speeds up the specific reaction it catalyzes to the extent that one enzyme molecule can cause thousands of substrate molecules to be converted into product each second. Some enzymes contain a nonprotein component that is essential to the activity of the enzyme; others require a brief, loose bonding with metal ions or nonproteinaceous organic compounds called cofactors to catalyze the reaction.

Like inorganic catalysts, enzymes are not themselves changed during the reaction and can function repeatedly. The specificity of enzyme activity depends on steric compatibility between the substrate and the surface of the enzyme, or, more precisely, certain areas on the surface of the enzyme known as active sites. The activity of an enzyme requires that the conformation of the active site fits, or can be induced to fit, the shape of the substrate molecule. Anything that disrupts this precise fit will reduce enzyme activity or inhibit it entirely.

Suppose an enzyme catalyzes the conversion of molecule *X* to molecule *Y*. A third molecule *A*, which has no steric resemblance to *X*, binds with the surface of the enzyme at some distance from the active site and has the effect of increasing the reaction rate. A fourth molecule, *B*, which is quite similar to *X*, binds with the enzyme at the active site and has the effect of reducing the reaction rate. Adding more of molecule *X* to the reaction mixture reverses the effect of molecule *B* and the reaction rate again increases.

Figure 1 plots the rate of this enzyme-catalyzed reaction against temperature. You will have to refer to this plot and the information given above, and draw on your knowledge of enzymes in general to answer the questions in this passage.

Figure 1. Hand-drawn curve: rate versus temperature

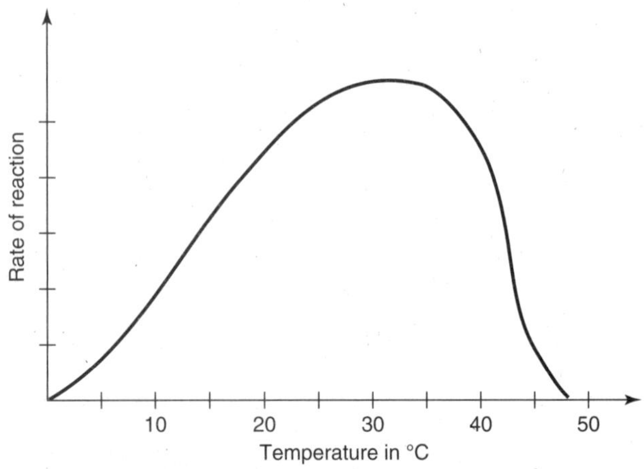

105. In this reaction, molecule *A* is
A. the substrate.
B. a competitive inhibitor.
C. a cofactor.
D. an allosteric modulator.

106. In this reaction, molecule *B* is a(n)
A. cofactor.
B. allosteric modulator.

C. noncompetitive inhibitor.
D. competitive inhibitor.

107. The optimum temperature for the reaction plotted in Figure 1 is approximately _____°C.
A. 5 B. 25
C. 35 D. 45

108. A nonprotein component part of an enzyme, as described in this passage, is known as a(n)
A. allosteric modulator.
B. prosthetic group.
C. coenzyme.
D. secondary structure.

PASSAGE V (QUESTIONS 109–111)

Steroids are defined as derivatives of perhydrocyclopentano-phenanthrene.

The most common steroid, cholesterol, is also a precursor of many other steroids that greatly influence biological activity. Shown here are several important steroids.

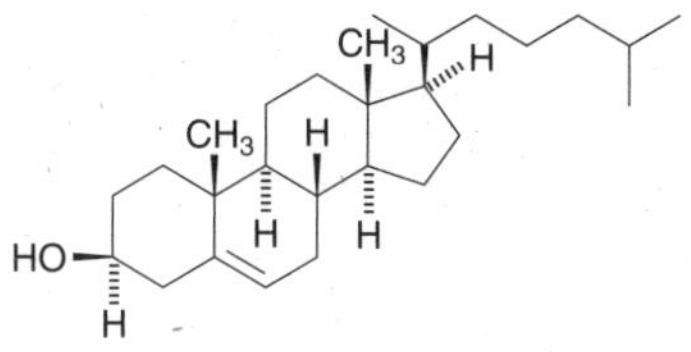

Cholesterol

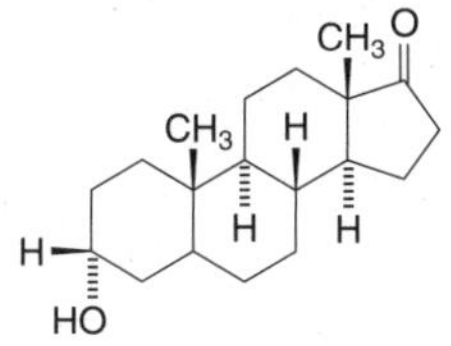

Androsterone (male sex hormone)

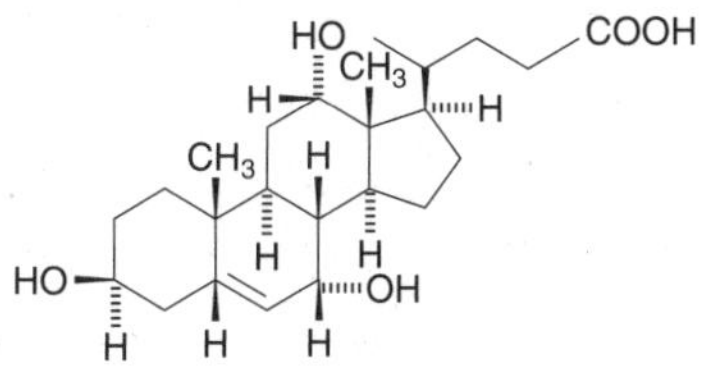

Cholic acid

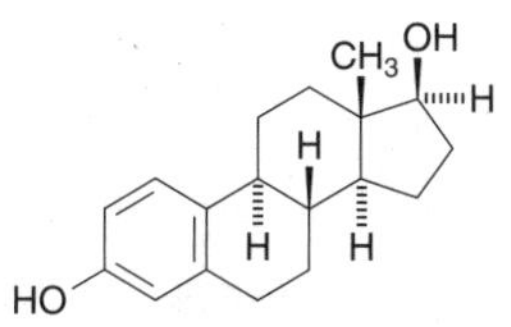

Estradiol (female sex hormone)

109. The most water soluble of the steroids shown is
A. androsterone. B. estradiol.
C. cholic acid. D. cholesterol.

110. The number of chiral centers in androsterone is
A. 1. B. 3.
C. 5. D. 7.

111. The only one of these compounds that will show absorption in the 6.5–7.5 d region of the NMR spectrum is
A. estradiol. B. androsterone.
C. cholic acid. D. cholesterol.

QUESTIONS 112–115 are NOT based on a descriptive passage.

112. The placenta originates from
A. embryonic cells.
B. maternal cells.
C. paternal cells.
D. both A and B.

113. The Golgi apparatus primarily functions in
A. packaging protein for secretion.
B. synthesizing protein for secretion.
C. packaging protein for hydrolysis.
D. synthesizing protein for hydrolysis.

114. For the protons in methyl propanoate, what is the order of *increasing* distance downfield from TMS in the NMR spectrum?

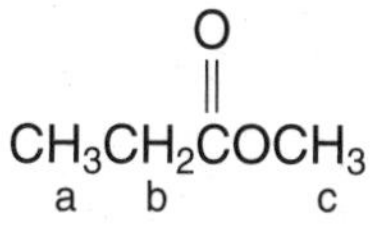

A. c, a, b B. a, b, c
C. b, c, a D. a, c, b

115. What is the major product of the following sequence of reactions?

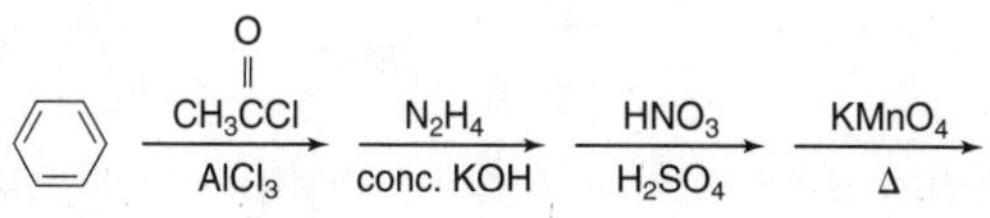

A. 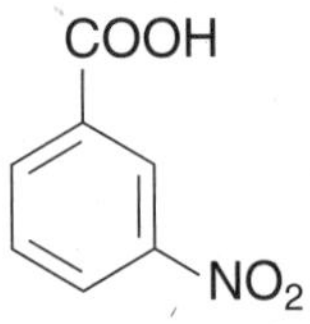

B. 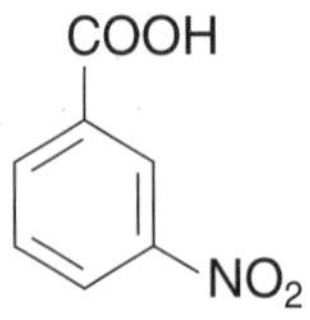

C. 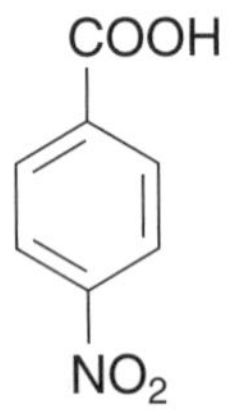

D. 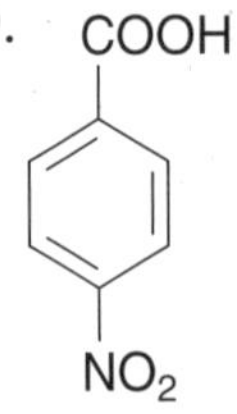

PASSAGE VI (QUESTIONS 116–118)

Regardless of the organism or tissues involved, the liberation of energy from carbohydrates involves the same fundamental biochemical reactions at the cellular level. The reactions can be divided into three basic groups — glycolysis, the Krebs (or citric acid) cycle, and the electron transport chain. Each occurs in a specific region or structure within the cell, and each consists of numerous reactions. Collectively, these three groups of reactions can be referred to as cellular respiration.

Glycolysis is essentially an anaerobic process that breaks glucose into pyruvic acid, producing some ATP and reduced coenzymes (specifically, NADH). Under certain conditions, some cells are capable of converting pyruvic acid into ethanol and carbon dioxide or into lactic acid. In these cases, the overall process is known as fermentation, and the entire breakdown of glucose to these products occurs without requiring oxygen. Under appropriate conditions, the pyruvic acid is then converted into acetyl-Coenzyme A by oxidative decarboxylation in preparation for the Krebs cycle.

The Krebs cycle is a complex series of coupled reactions that yields carbon dioxide, reduced coenzymes, and some GTP (the energy of which can then be used to synthesize ATP). The electrons carried by these reduced coenzymes are shunted to the electron transport chain, where the majority of the ATP from cellular respiration is produced by chemiosmotic synthesis. Ultimately, at their lowest energy level, these electrons are donated to oxygen and, with the addition of hydrogen ions, leave respiration as water.

116. Glycolysis takes place in the
   A. ribosome.
   B. nucleus.
   C. mitochondrion.
   D. cytosol.

117. It is generally accepted that the number of ATP molecules that can be synthesized by fermentation of one glucose molecule is
   A. 2.
   B. 18.
   C. 36.
   D. 42.

118. In eukaryotes, the electron transport chain is located in the
   A. cytosol.
   B. outer compartment of the mitochondrion.
   C. inner membrane of the mitochondrion.
   D. plasma membrane.

PASSAGE VII (QUESTIONS 119–122)

In 1931, Erich Hückel applied the principles of molecular orbital theory to aromatic compounds. He formulated the $4n + 2$ rule, which states that *planar, cyclic fully conjugated polyenes possessing* $4n + 2\pi$ *electrons will have special aromatic stability* (n is 0 or an integer). This stability leads to decreased heats of combustion and reduced reactivity with many reagents, among other properties. Hückel also recognized that certain cyclic charged intermediates could have aromatic properties and that nonbonding electrons on heterocyclic atoms could be conjugated with the π electrons in a ring.

Consider the following structures and answer questions 119–122.

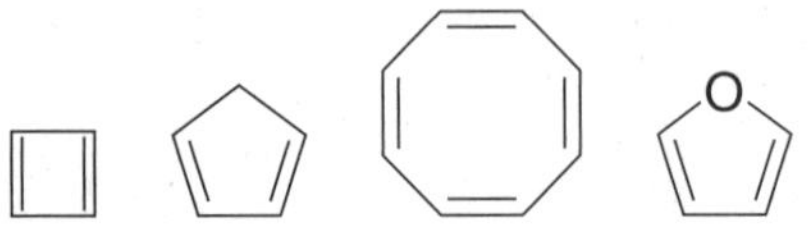

(1) (2) (3) (4)

119. Which of these compounds is aromatic?
A. 1 B. 2
C. 3 D. 4

120. Which compound can form an aromatic entity by reacting with the strong base $NaNH_2$?
A. 1 B. 2
C. 3 D. 4

121. Which of these compounds would show absorption peaks 6–8 ppm downfield from TMS in the NMR spectrum?
A. 1 B. 2
C. 3 D. 4

122. Which of the following compounds would react most readily with (aq) $AgNO_3$?

A. 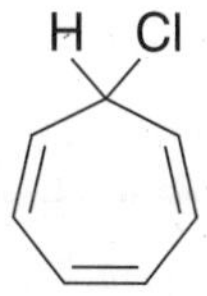

B. 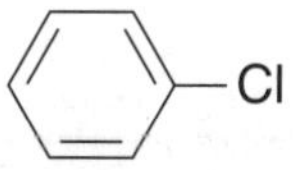

C. 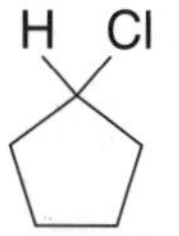

D. 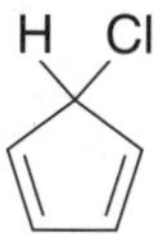

PASSAGE VIII (QUESTIONS 123–126)

One of the unifying principles of modern biology is the concept of evolutionary change. Evidence for evolutionary change existed before Darwin, but he was the first to present evidence that natural selection was the agent for such change. Among the observations that Darwin made to support the role of natural selection were morphological similarities among adults of related species. Comparative anatomy of the limbs of vertebrates suggested common origins of many of these structures, leading to the contemporary concepts of evolutionary homology and evolutionary analogy.

Additional evidence for evolutionary change was seen in comparative embryology of both invertebrate and vertebrate animals. Haeckel's conclusion of ontogenic recapitulation of phylogeny, while not literally correct, provided an intellectual framework for interpreting the developmental similarities among related taxonomic groups of organisms.

The well-known ability of plant and animal breeders to make changes in characteristics of domesticated species was interpreted by Darwin as further confirmation that variation could be selected and retained. He perceived that the only difference between natural selection and this artificial selection was that humans were acting as the agents of selection. Given the geological time frame involved in natural changes of species, he reasoned that the same mechanisms were clearly involved. The only differences were, therefore, the intensity of the selective pressures and the concomitant modification in the rate of change.

123. All of the following are homologous structures EXCEPT
A. the foreleg of a horse and the wing of a bat.
B. the wing of an insect and the wing of a bird.
C. the arm of a human and the flipper of a seal.
D. the wing of a penguin and the foreleg of a turtle.

124. Genetic variation is acted upon by natural selection to cause evolutionary change. Which of the following conditions would NOT be susceptible to natural selection?
A. A recessive allele in the homozygous condition
B. A dominant allele in the heterozygous condition
C. A recessive allele in the heterozygous condition
D. A dominant allele in the homozygous condition

125. Which of the following intrinsic isolation mechanisms would act to prevent production of interspecific hybrids *after* mating of the parents?
A. Behavioral isolation
B. Mechanical isolation

C. Ecogeographic isolation
D. Developmental isolation

126. Which of the following is NOT a general characteristic of chordates?
A. Pharyngeal gill slits
B. Vertebral column
C. Dorsal hollow nerve cord
D. Notochord

QUESTIONS 127–128 are NOT based on a descriptive passage.

127. The aldol condensation of two molecules of acetaldehyde gives the product

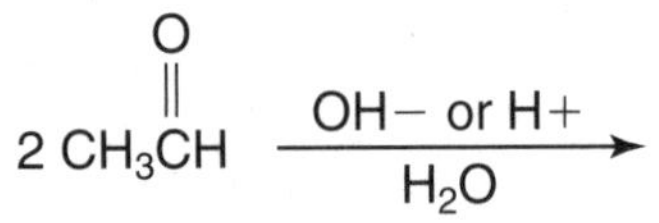

A. 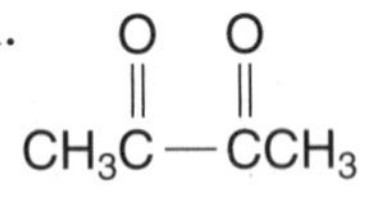

B. 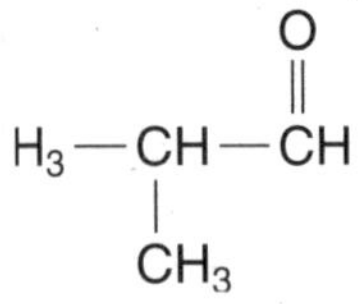

C. 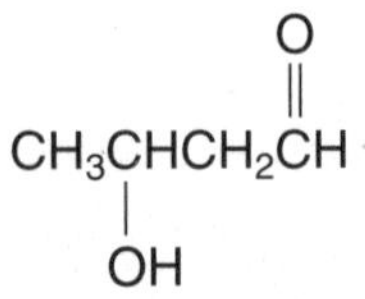

D. 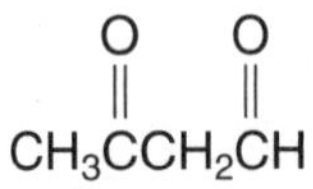

128. The interconversion of glyceraldehyde (1) and dihydroxyacetone (2) involves the intermediate

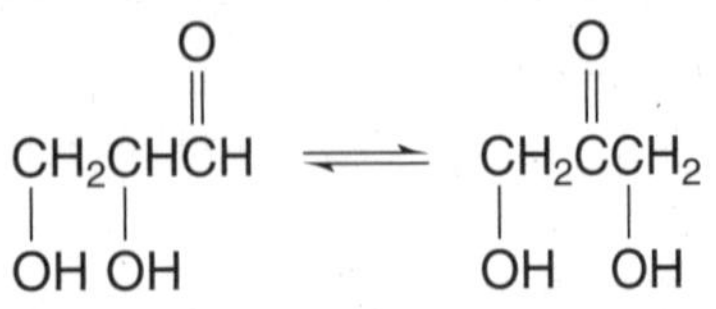

A. 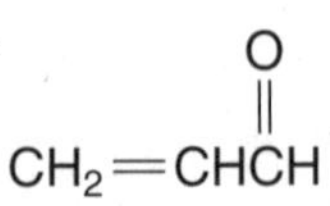

B. 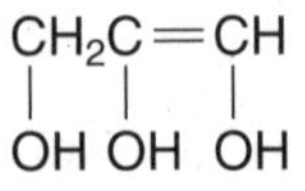

C. 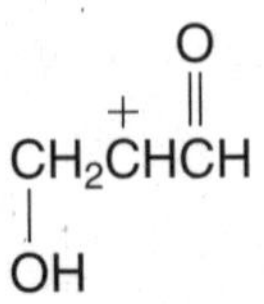

D. 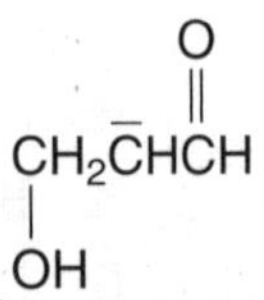

PASSAGE IX (QUESTIONS 129–134)

There are generally considered to be four major tissue types in vertebrates — epithelial, connective, muscle, and nerve. Within each category can be found subcategories with specialized cell types and/or intercellular matrices.

While many cells have some contractile properties, muscle tissues exhibit the characteristic to a much greater extent. The three principal types of muscle tissue are known as skeletal, smooth, and cardiac. The ability to generate and propagate electrochemical membrane potentials is critical to the function of these tissues. The functional unit of skeletal and cardiac muscle is known as a sarcomere and is visible using electron microscopy. A diagram of a sarcomere is given in Figure 1.

Figure 1

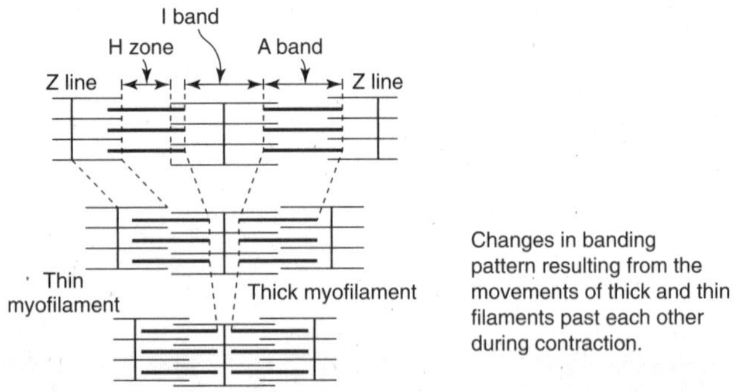

Nerve cells are specialized for response to a variety of stimuli and for the rapid transmission of changes in electrochemical membrane potentials (i.e., action potentials or nerve impulses). The extensions of nerve cells, known as fibers, can be quite long, thereby distinguishing certain neurons as the longest cells in the body. A drawing of a myelinated motor neuron is given in Figure 2.

Figure 2

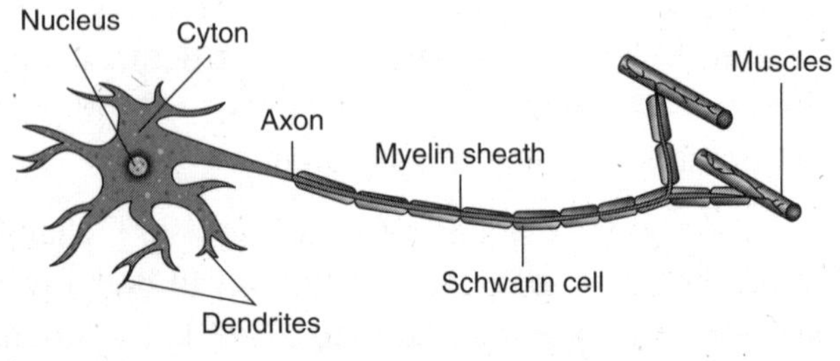

The structure of a neuron.

The establishment of an initial (resting) electrostatic potential depends largely on a differential "leakage" of potassium and, to a lesser extent, sodium ions across the membrane of the neuron. Propagation of a nerve impulse is accomplished by a series of momentary ion-specific changes in membrane permeability that first allows sodium ions to rush into the cell and then allow potassium ions to rush out of the cell, thereby reversing polarity of the membrane briefly. The resting potential is regenerated by local diffusion of ions away from the membrane surface while a sodium-potassium pump aids in maintaining the sodium and potassium ion concentration gradients across the membrane. Transmission of an impulse between neurons or between a neuron and an effector occurs at synapses. These synapses may involve a direct coupling of cells (through gap junctions) or, more commonly, a narrow space known as a synaptic cleft. Where synaptic clefts are involved, transmission depends on chemical neurotransmitters released by the presynaptic membrane that diffuse across the cleft. The neurotransmitters may have an excitatory or inhibitory effect on the postsynaptic membrane.

129. Which of the following statements correctly describes a fully contracted sarcomere compared to one that is relaxed?
   A. The A-band remains the same length.
   B. The H-zone remains the same length.
   C. The I-bands remain the same length.
   D. The Z-lines remain equidistant from each other.

130. Striations and multiple nuclei are characteristic of _____ muscle.
   A. smooth
   B. skeletal
   C. cardiac
   D. skeletal and cardiac

131. The normal resting potential of a neuron is about _____ millivolts.
   A. 120 B. 12
   C. –45 D. –70

132. When an action potential moves along skeletal muscle fibers, calcium ions are released from the sarcoplasmic reticulum. The calcium ions bind with what molecular component of the thin filaments?
   A. Actin
   B. Troponin complex
   C. Myosin
   D. Tropomyosin

133. Many neurons outside the central nervous system are enveloped by neuroglial cells called Schwann cells, which give rise to myelin sheaths. Compared to the speed of other nerve impulses, those moving along axons with myelinated sheaths travel
   A. much faster.
   B. slightly faster.
   C. slightly slower.
   D. much slower.

134. As the sodium-potassium pump functions in a neuron membrane, _____ Na^+ is(are) pumped out for every _____ k^+ pumped in.
   A. 1; 2 B. 2; 3
   C. 3; 2 D. 2; 1

PASSAGE X (QUESTIONS 135–138)

Nucleophilic substitution reactions involve the displacement of a leaving group by a nucleophile.

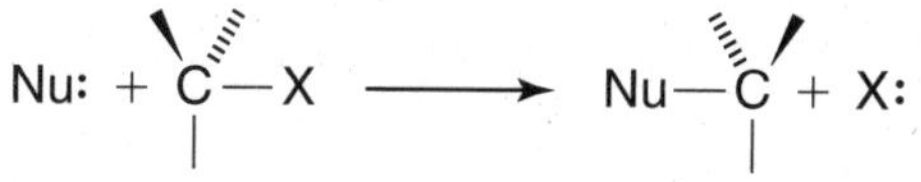

If this occurs in a one-step reaction, it is called an S_N2 mechanism. S_N2 reactions proceed with inversion of configuration at chiral centers and exhibit second-order kinetics:

Rate = k[Nu][R – X]

A one-step reaction, S_N1, involves a reactive intermediate, (1), and exhibits first-order kinetics:

Rate = k[R – X]

Because the intermediate can react with the nucleophile to give both enantiomers, a racemate is formed.

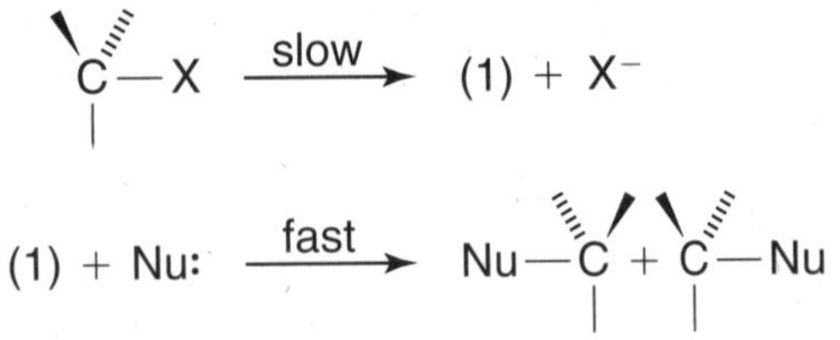

135. What kind of intermediate is (1)?
   A. A carbanion
   B. A carbocation
   C. An enolate
   D. A free radical

136. For the reaction

$$\underset{(2)}{NaOC_2H_5} + \underset{(3)}{(R)\text{—}PhCH(CH_3)Br} \xrightarrow{C_2H_5OH} PhCH(CH_3)OC_2H_5 + NaBr$$

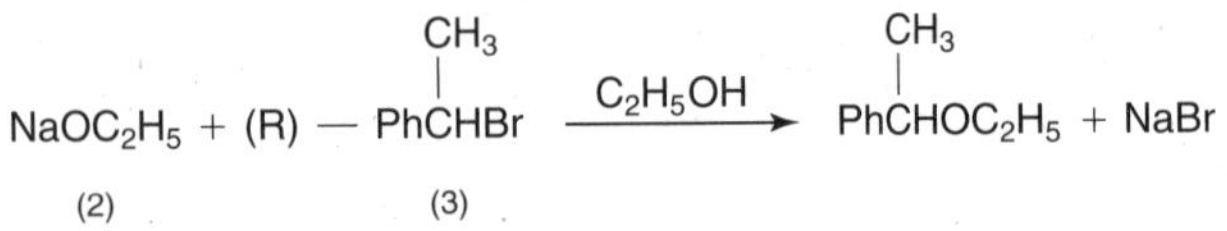

   what is the mechanism and expected rate equation if the product is found to be devoid of optical activity?
   A. S_N2, Rate = k[2][3]
   B. S_N2, Rate = k[3]
   C. S_N1, Rate = k[2]
   D. S_N1, Rate = k[3]

137. Elimination reactions compete with substitution reactions. What is the major elimination product of the following reaction?

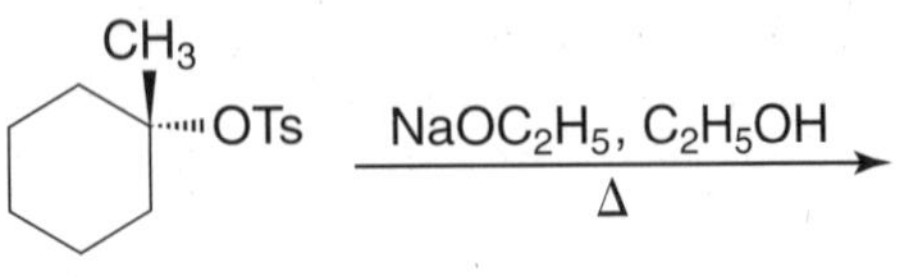

A.

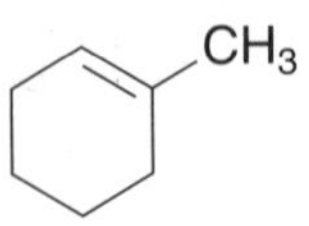

B. 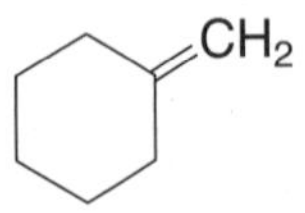

C.

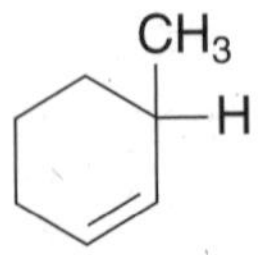

D. 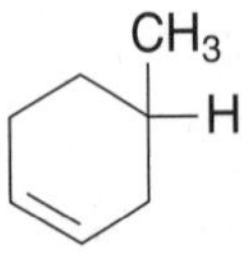

138. Acid-catalyzed elimination of alcohols an produce alkenes with rearranged carbon atoms, for example,

$$Ph\text{—}CH(CH_3)\text{—}CH_2OH \xrightarrow[\Delta]{H+} Ph\text{—}C(CH_3){=}CH_2 + Ph\text{—}CH{=}CH\text{—}CH_3$$

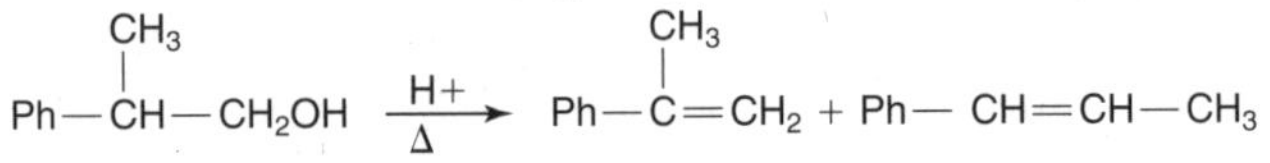

   Which of the following alcohols will NOT produce rearranged product when heated with acid?

   A. $CH_3CH_2\text{—}CH(OH)\text{—}CH(CH_3)\text{—}CH_3$ 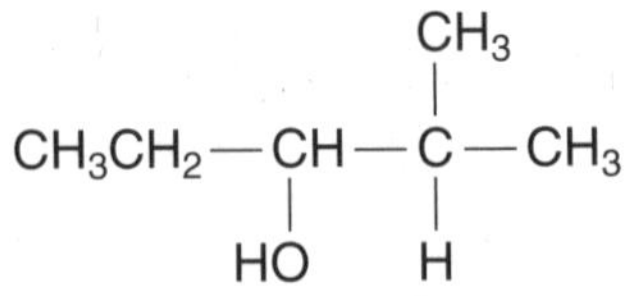

   B. $(CH_3)_3COH$

   C. $CH_3CH_2CH_2CH_2OH$

   D. $(CH_3)_3CH\text{—}CH(OH)\text{—}CH_3$ 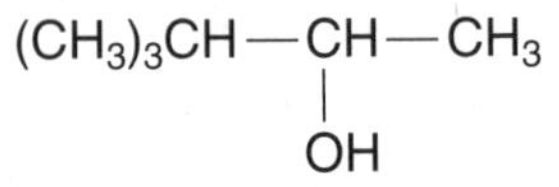

PASSAGE XI (QUESTIONS 139–141)

Many diseases are the result of pathogenic microorganisms that have become sufficiently numerous in an animal to directly affect its normal metabolism and bodily functions. Following the acceptance of Pasteur's Germ Theory of Disease in the late 1800s, many such pathogens were identified and found to be the cause of common diseases. Bacteria and viruses, as well as some eucaryotic microorganisms, were among the pathogens discovered.

Experiment 1. An animal was brought into a diagnostic laboratory suffering fro m an unknown ailment and was placed in an isolation area. Because the body temperature of the sick animal was elevated, the diagnostician suspected a pathogen, but the symptoms did not match those caused by any known microorganism. Blood work in the pathology lab indicated that a bacillus bacterium was present, and that this bacillus was also present in blood samples of other afflicted animals from the same population.

Experiment 2. After trying a variety of culture protocols and growth media, technicians found they could aerobically maintain a pure culture of the bacillus on blood agar at 37°C. Sufficient cultures of the presumed pathogenic bacillus were produced to test its virulence on laboratory animals.

Experiment 3. Healthy animals that had never shown characteristics similar to the ailments of the original animal were inoculated with pure cultures of the bacillus. They developed the same symptoms as the original animal that had been brought into the lab. They were also placed in isolation. The disease progressed in these test animals just as it had in the one first brought into the lab.

Experiment 4. Subsequent blood work showed an identical bacillus was widespread in the systems of the test animals. When this bacillus was cultured by the same protocol, it showed the same morphological and metabolic characteristics as the bacterial bacillus isolate.

139. The diagnosticians concluded that the bacterial bacillus isolate they had initially found was indeed the cause of the animal's disease. They could draw this conclusion from the results of
    - A. Experiment 1 only
    - B. Experiments 1 and 2
    - C. Experiments 1, 2, and 3
    - D. The results of all four experiments were necessary for this conclusion.

140. Which of the following cytological structures are NOT found in any bacteria?
    - A. Polysaccharide cell wall
    - B. Ribosomes
    - C. Mitochondria
    - D. Cell membrane

141. A particular bacterium requires about 45 minutes to divide by fission into two cells. If 10 bacteria are originally inoculated into a fresh culture medium and you assume all cells survive, approximately how many bacteria will exist after 12 hours of culture?
    - A. 75,000
    - B. 225,000
    - C. 475,000
    - D. 650,000

QUESTIONS 142–144 are NOT based on a descriptive passage.

142. The autonomic nervous system is involved when you
    - A. sight a deer and turn your head to see it more clearly.
    - B. run to catch the bus and develop a rapid heart rate, an increase in respiration rate, and an increase in blood pressure.
    - C. are hit by a hammer on your knee and your knee jerks.
    - D. walk barefoot, step on a thorn, and immediately raise your foot.

143. When two long-winged flies are mated, their progeny consist of 77 flies with long wings and 24 flies with short wings. The parental genotypes are
    - A. Ll × Ll.
    - B. LL × LL.
    - C. ll × ll.
    - D. LL × Ll.

144. The somatic nervous system controls
    - A. heart (cardiac) muscle.
    - B. smooth muscle.
    - C. skeletal (striated) muscle.
    - D. the erector pili.

STOP! If time still remains, you may review work only in this section. STOP!

Test 4 ■ Answer Key

1. D
2. A
3. A
4. C
5. D
6. C
7. A
8. C
9. A
10. C
11. D
12. D
13. B
14. C
15. B
16. B
17. A
18. D
19. B
20. A
21. C
22. B
23. A
24. D
25. B
26. B
27. B
28. B
29. A
30. D
31. D
32. A
33. B
34. B
35. A
36. C
37. A
38. B
39. D
40. B
41. C
42. C
43. D
44. D
45. D
46. D
47. B
48. D
49. D
50. C
51. C
52. A
53. D
54. B
55. A
56. C
57. A
58. C
59. A
60. B
61. C
62. B
63. D
64. C
65. A
66. C
67. A
68. B
69. A
70. D
71. A
72. D
73. B
74. B
75. B
76. B
77. D
78. B
79. A
80. B
81. C
82. D
83. C
84. B
85. B
86. D
87. A
88. A
89. C
90. A
91. B
92. C
93. B
94. A
95. C
96. C
97. D
98. B
99. C
100. C
101. D
102. A
103. B
104. B
105. D
106. D
107. C
108. B
109. C
110. D
111. A
112. D
113. A
114. B
115. C
116. D
117. A
118. C
119. D
120. B
121. D
122. A
123. B
124. C
125. D
126. B
127. C
128. B
129. A
130. B
131. D
132. B
133. A
134. C
135. B
136. D
137. A
138. B
139. D
140. C
141. D
142. B
143. A
144. C

SECTION 1
Physical Sciences

PASSAGE I (QUESTIONS 1–4)

1. **D.** Solution D is the only one that has a concentration lower than that of a saturated solution at the same temperature. Solution C is saturated (and at the same temperature as solution D); solutions A, B, and E are supersaturated.

2. **A.** Supersaturated solutions A, B, and E contain more solute than allowed by equilibrium considerations; they are unstable to addition of solute. Answers B and C are incorrect because solution C is saturated. Answer D is incorrect because solution D is unsaturated.

3. **A.** This solution contains less solute than that required for saturation at 80°C (170 g KNO_3/100 g water); therefore, it must be unsaturated. Answers B and D are incorrect because the solution does not contain enough solute to be saturated. Answer C is incorrect because the solution does not contain a higher concentration of solute than that required for saturation.

4. **C.** The solubility of KNO_3 at 80°C is about 170 g KNO_3/100 g water.

$$? \text{ g water} = 85 \text{ g KNO3} \times \frac{100 \text{ g water}}{170 \text{ g KNO3}}$$

$$= 50 \text{ g water}$$

Incorrect answers can result from misreading the solubility and/or setting up an equation where the units do not cancel each other to produce units of g of water.

PASSAGE II (QUESTIONS 5–9)

5. **D.** The region to the left of line *AB* is the solid region. The region to the right is the vapor region. All points along the line represent temperatures and pressures where the solid is in equilibrium with the vapor.

6. **C.** The two variables that must be specified are temperature and pressure.

7. **A.** Point F is in the solid region. Point E is in the liquid region. The phase change occurs when a solid changes to liquid, or it is melting. Answer B is incorrect because boiling is a change from liquid to vapor. Answer C is incorrect because sublimation is a change from solid to vapor. Answer D is incorrect because condensation is a change from vapor to liquid.

8. **C.** Because the pressure at the triple point, the point at which solid, liquid, and vapor coexist in equilibrium, is greater than 1.00 atm, CO_2 solid will not melt. Instead, it is converted directly into a vapor; that is, it sublimes.

9. **A.** Line *BC* is the melting point curve. For CO_2, as for most substances, this line has a positive slope. The higher the pressure along this curve, the higher the corresponding melting point.

PASSAGE III (QUESTIONS 10–12)

10. **C.** The quantity of N_2 required to produce the NH_3 is calculated from knowledge of the stoichiometric coefficients of the balanced equation:

$$? \frac{mole\ N_2}{L} = 0.150 \frac{molNH_3}{L} x \frac{1molN_2}{2molNH_3}$$
$$= 0.075 \frac{\text{mol } N_2}{L}$$

Subtracting this quantity from the initial N_2 concentration gives the remaining N_2 concentration:

$$[N_2] = 0.500\ M - 0.075\ M = 0.425\ M$$

Answer A is incorrect because some N_2 must remain at equilibrium. Answer B is incorrect because the N_2 concentration must decrease rather than increase. Answer D is incorrect because the N_2 concentration must decrease from its initial value.

11. **D.** The equilibrium constant is equal to the product of the molar concentrations at equilibrium of the products, each raised to the stoichiometric coefficient in the balanced equation, divided by the product of the molar concentrations at equilibrium of the reactants, each raised to the stoichiometric coefficient in the balanced equation. Answer choices A and B are incorrect because they show reactant concentrations in the numerator and product concentrations in the denominator. Answer choice C is incorrect because the molar concentrations should not be multiplied by the stoichiometric coefficients.

12. **D.** When the volume is decreased, the concentration of each substance is increased. Answer choices A and B are incorrect because the equilibrium would shift to the right, resulting in fewer H_2 and N_2 molecules. Answer choice C is incorrect because the equilibrium shift to the right would result in more NH_3 molecules.

13. **B.** Elastic collisions conserve energy and momentum, not velocity.

14. **C.** Although all the atoms of a given element have exactly the same chemical properties (the same atomic number, Z), they do not always have the same mass. Atoms that are chemically alike but that differ in mass are called isotopes. All isotopes of a given element have the same number of electrons and protons but have different numbers of neutrons.

15. **B.** Using the equation

$$\text{Density} = \frac{\text{Mass}}{\text{Volume}}$$

we obtain

$$\text{Mass} = (\text{Density})(\text{Volume})$$

Because density is in gm/cm^3, let us use the CGS system. Therefore, we must convert the measurements of the block into centimeters.

2 meters = 200 centimeters
3 meters = 300 centimeters
5 meters = 500 centimeters

Now, finding the volume of the block

$$V = 1 \times w \times h = 200 \times 300 \times 500$$

Finally, we can find the mass:

$$\text{Mass} = (7.8\ \text{gm/cm}^3)(3.0 \times 10^7\ \text{cm}^3)$$
$$\text{Mass} = 2.34 \times 10^8\ \text{gm}$$

16. **B.** Balancing the reaction we obtain

$$^{238}_{92}Y \rightarrow {}^{238}_{93}Z + {}^{0}_{-1}X.$$

Because there is no change in mass number, and the charge on the emitted particle is -1, X must be an electron. In this case, a neutron has been split, producing a proton and an electron. The electron is emitted, and the proton is retained, resulting in an increase of nuclear charge with no loss of nuclear mass.

PASSAGE IV (QUESTIONS 17-19)

17. **A.** The correct combustion equation is

$$2C_8H_{18} + 25O_2 \rightarrow 18H_2O + 16CO_2$$

The coefficients octane and oxygen are 2 and 25, respectively. Therefore, the ratio of oxygen to octane must be 25:2.

18. **D.**

$$C_7H_{16} + 22O_2 \rightarrow 8H_2O + 7CO_2$$

19. **B.**

$$?W \times hrs = 132 \times 10^6 J\left(\frac{Wxs}{J}\right)\left(\frac{hrs}{3.6 \times 10^2 s}\right)$$

$$= 37 \times 10^3 W \times hrs$$

PASSAGE V (QUESTIONS 20-24)

20. **A.**

$$\Delta S = S_{products} - S_{reactants}$$

Because the value $\Delta S°$ for this reaction is negative, this difference must result from subtracting a larger reactant entropy from a smaller product entropy. Answer choice B is incorrect because subtracting a smaller reactant entropy from a larger entropy results in a positive value of $\Delta S°$. Answers C and D are incorrect because the value of $\Delta S°$ gives no indication of the rate of reaction.

21. **C.** $\Delta G°$ has a negative value in this reaction. If $\Delta G°$ is negative, the reaction is spontaneous. Answer choice D is incorrect because a reaction is nonspontaneous only if $\Delta G°$ is positive. Answers A and B are incorrect because the value of $\Delta G°$ gives no indication of the rate of reaction.

22. **B.**

$$\Delta G° = \Delta H° - T\Delta S°$$

The reaction will be spontaneous when $\Delta G°$ is negative. Because $\Delta H°$ is negative, this term will tend to make $\Delta G°$ negative. Because $\Delta S°$ is negative, the $-T\Delta S°$ term is positive and will tend to make $\Delta G°$ positive. If T is small enough (at low temperatures), the positive $T\Delta S°$ term will be smaller than the negative $\Delta H°$ term, and the resulting $\Delta G°$ will be negative.

23. **A.**

$$?\ kJ = 8 \text{ mol } H_2O \times \frac{-890.3 kJ}{2 \text{ mol } H_2O}$$

$$= -3561.2 kJ$$

Incorrect answers can result from setting up an equation so that the units do not cancel each other to produce units of kJ.

24. **D.** $\Delta H°$ for a reaction is equal in magnitude but opposite in sign to $\Delta H°$ for the reverse reaction. The reaction given in this equation is the reverse of the reaction for the data given.

$$\Delta H°_{reverse} = -(\Delta H°_{forward})$$
$$= -(-890.3 \text{ kJ})$$
$$= +890.3 \text{ kJ}$$

25. **B.** Work is the change in potential energy

W = $PE_f - PE_i$; PE_i = zero.
W = m h g
W = (50 kg)(2 m)(9.8 m/s^2) = (100)(9.8) J
W = 980 J

26. **B.** Diffraction is the tendency of a wave to spread into a region behind an obstruction. This also includes the tendency of a wave to spread out when passing through a small aperture.

27. **B.** The First Law of Thermodynamics is $U = Q + W$. If W is negative, work has been done by the system on the outside world, and this has caused a decrease in the internal energy of the system. Nothing can be said about the heat of the system unless more information is given about U and Q.

PASSAGE VI (QUESTIONS 28–32)

28. **B.** An oxidizing agent causes the oxidation of another species. In the process, the oxidizing agent is reduced. Reduction is the gain of electrons. In this reaction, Ag^+ gains electrons and is the oxidizing agent. Answer choice D is incorrect because Ag is the end product of the reduction. Answer A is incorrect because Sn is the reducing agent. Answer C is incorrect because Sn^{2+} is the end product of the oxidation of Sn.

29. **A.** The anode is the electrode where oxidation takes place. Oxidation is the loss of electrons. At the anode:

$$Sn \rightarrow Sn^{2+} + 2e^-.$$

Answer choices B, C, and D are incorrect because they are reduction half-reactions.

30. **D.** Reversing the equation for the standard reduction potential changes the sign of E°:

$$Sn \rightarrow Sn^{2+} + 2e^-; E°_{ox} = +0.14 \text{ V}$$

Doubling each quantity in the standard reduction potential does not affect E°:

$$2e^- + 2\,Ag^+ \rightarrow 2\,Ag; E°_{red} = +0.80 \text{ V}$$

Adding the two half-reactions

$$Sn \rightarrow Sn^{2+} + 2e^-; E°_{ox} = +0.14 \text{ V}$$
$$2e^- + 2\,Ag^+ \rightarrow 2\,Ag; E°_{red} = +0.80 \text{ V}$$
$$Sn + 2\,Ag^+ \rightarrow Sn^{2+} + 2\,Ag; E°_{tot} = +0.94 \text{ V}$$

31. **D.** In this notation, the anode reactant and product are shown on the left side of the double line; the cathode reactant and product are shown on the right side of the double line; the double line represents a salt bridge. Answer choices A and B are incorrect because they show oxidizing and reducing agents together at the anode. Answer choice C is incorrect because the anode and cathode half-reactions are each on the wrong side of the double lines.

32. **A.** At the anode (Sn) electrons are produced:

$$Sn \rightarrow Sn^{2+} + 2e^-$$

These electrons travel to the cathode (Ag), where they are picked up by the Ag^+ ions:

$$e^- + At^+ \rightarrow Ag$$

Answer choices B, C, and D are incorrect because they indicate electron flow between forms of the same element.

PASSAGE VII (QUESTIONS 33–37)

33. **B.** The gravitational force is just the weight.

34. **B.** The upward forces exerted by the ropes must equal the downward force exerted by the ball, i.e., 50 kg.

35. **A.** Because the ball does not move, the sum of the forces must be zero.

36. **C.** $R_1 \sin 30°$ is the *y*-axis component of the force exerted by rope 1. Rope 2 does not exert a force in the *y* direction because the force exerted by rope 2 is normal to the *y* direction.

37. **A.** The upward force exerted in the *y* direction by rope R_1, sin 30°, must equal the downward force exerted by the ball, i.e., 50 kg.

$$R_1 \sin 30° = 50 \text{ Kg}$$
$$R_1 = \frac{50 \text{ Kg}}{0.5} = 100 \text{ Kg}$$

PASSAGE VIII (QUESTIONS 38–41)

38. **B.** For the resistors in parallel:

$$\frac{1}{R_{parallel}} = \frac{1}{R_1} + \frac{1}{R_2} = \frac{1}{6} + \frac{1}{2}$$
$$\frac{1}{R_{parallel}} = \frac{3}{2}\,\Omega$$

39. **D.** For the resistors in series:

$$R_{total} = R_3 + R_p + R_5$$
$$= 7 + \frac{3}{2} + \frac{1}{2} = 9\Omega$$

40. **B.** Current is the same throughout a series network. Therefore, the current through the 7Ω resistor is the same as the current through the total of the resistors in series given in Question 84.

$$I = \frac{V}{R} = \frac{27}{9} = 3 \text{ amps}$$

41. **C.** Now that the current is known, the voltage drop is just found by Ohm's Law.

$$V = IR = 3 \times 7 = 21 \text{ volts}$$

PASSAGE IX (QUESTIONS 42–45)

42. **C.** The focal length is half the radius of curvature:

½ × 50 cm = 25 cm.

43. **D.** The image distance obeys the rule

$$\frac{1}{f} = \frac{1}{D_o} + \frac{1}{D_i}$$

where f is the focal length (which is negative in a convex mirror), D_0 is the object distance, and D_i is the image distance.

$$\frac{1}{-25cm} = \frac{1}{100cm} + \frac{1}{D_i}$$
$$\frac{1}{D_i} = \frac{-25cm - 100cm}{(25cm)(100cm)}$$
$$D_i = -20cm$$

The negative sign indicates that the image is behind the mirror.

44. **D.** The sizes of the object S_0 and the image S_i are in the same ratio as their respective distances.

$$\frac{S_i}{S_o} = \frac{D_i}{D_o}$$
$$S_i = S_o\left(\frac{D_i}{D_o}\right) = 60cm\left(\frac{-20cm}{100cm}\right) = -12cm$$

45. **D.** In convex mirrors, the image is always behind the mirror.

PASSAGE X (QUESTIONS 46–49)

46. **D.** An increase of one octave represents doubling the frequency:

2 × 110 Hz = 220 Hz.

47. **B.** Because each 10 decibels have 10 times the energy of the softest audible sound, this sound has 10 × 10, or 100 times the loudness of the softest audible sound.

48. **D.** Beats result from alternating constructive and destructive interference. The beat frequency is the difference between the frequencies of the two notes; therefore, frequency of the second note is 110 ± 5 Hz.

49. **D.** Using the formula given in the problem:

$$v = 331 + 0.6(10) = 337 \text{ m/s}.$$

50. **C.** We would like a lens that brings objects from 25 cm to 100 cm. Note that s' is negative because the image is supposed to be located on the same side of the lens as the object.

$$s = +25 \text{ cm}, s' = -100 \text{ cm}$$
$$\frac{1}{f} = \frac{1}{s} + \frac{1}{s'} = \frac{1}{25} = \frac{1}{100}$$
$$f = 33.3cm$$

51. **C.** When the length of a conductor is increased, the number of collisions between free electrons and vibrating atoms increases. Doubling the length of a conductor doubles the average number of collisions. In general, the resistance is directly proportional

to the length of the conductor. Therefore, if a piece of wire is doubled in length, then its resistance is doubled.

52. **A.**

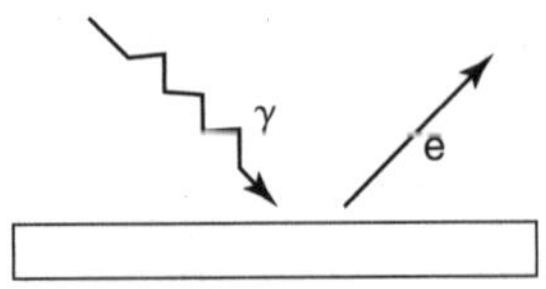

In the photoelectric effect, by conservation of energy,

$$h\upsilon = \tfrac{1}{2} mv^2 + \phi$$

where ϕ is the work function of the metal. Furthermore,

$$eV_0 = \tfrac{1}{2}mv^2.$$

As a result, the stopping potential V_o is directly proportional to the incident light frequency υ:

$$eV_o = h \; - \qquad \text{or } V_o = \frac{h}{e} \; - \; \frac{}{e}$$

In fact, this is one way of determining Planck's constant.

SECTION 2
Verbal Reasoning

PASSAGE I (QUESTIONS 53–57)

53. **D.** In the second paragraph, Answer choices B and C are listed as factors identifying Hancock with the patriots. Answer choice A is given as an additional factor at the start of the third paragraph. Answer choice D is not given as a factor that tied Hancock to the patriots.

54. **B.** In the fifth paragraph, mention is made of Hancock's egotism, which "regularly aroused the antipathy of many members." The passage states that Hancock's fortune was dented by wartime financial reverses; he did not profit from the war (answer choice A). Answer choice C is false; though Hancock was accused of smuggling by the British, the charges were dropped. His political activity and egotism show that answer choice D is false.

55. **A.** The narrative reports matters of public record and does not purport to give elements from the other kinds of sources listed.

56. **C.** British customs officials, bolstered by the presence of a warship in the Boston harbor, seized one of Hancock's ships after accusing him of smuggling. Repercussions of this action resulted in the Boston Massacre. Hancock *did* support the Stamp Act (answer choice A), and was falsely accused of smuggling (answer choice D). Adams successfully defended Hancock in court *after* the Boston Massacre (answer choice B).

57. **A.** In the sixth paragraph, we learn that Hancock remained a member of Congress until 1780, and for the rest of his life (thirteen years) "solidified his political position in Massachusetts." During this period, he did serve in Congress for a time and he did serve as governor for a time, but he did neither for the whole thirteen-year period; therefore, answer choices C and D are not entirely correct. There is no evidence for answer B.

PASSAGE II (QUESTIONS 58–62)

58. **C.** President Adams and his wife were the first occupants of the White House in November 1800. This was right after the government moved to Washington (answer choice D). The interior had not yet been completed (answer choice B). The passage also states that during construction or very soon after, the White House was painted white; therefore, answer choice A is incorrect because the gray color was immediately painted over, not left unpainted for the first years of the building's existence, like the question poses.

59. **A.** The original architect of the White House, James Hoban, was Irish and most likely fashioned the White House after a duke's mansion in Dublin. French architects *later* helped design additions (II), and the British had no part in the building's construction (III).

60. **B.** During the War of 1812, when the British captured the city and burned the White House, only the building's exterior walls and interior brickwork remained. The White House was rebuilt only once after this 1812 fire, not twice (answer choice A). It has undergone extensive renovations, however, making answer choice C incor-

rect. The building has nevertheless retained its simple design, making answer choice D also incorrect.

61. **C.** This point is made in the opening paragraph, and no claim is made about the elements listed in the other choices.

62. **B.** When U.S. troops destroyed some Canadian buildings, the British captured Washington in retaliation (answer choice A) and burned the White House, leaving only walls and brickwork unharmed (answer choice C). Reconstruction of the building caused it to be unfit and unfinished for living until 1817, when President Monroe moved in (answer choice D). The French did not offer any assistance in reconstructing the White House, although two French architects, L'Enfant and Latrobe, worked on designs for additions for the buildings before and after the 1812 reconstruction. Therefore, B is not true.

PASSAGE III (QUESTIONS 63–66)

63. **D.** This point is made at the end of the second paragraph. Notice that they are not favored fuels because they are more common, as answer C claims; if they are more common, it is because they are favored and are simpler and cheaper to produce.

64. **C.** Methanol is the simplest, not the most complex alcohol (answer choice D). It is most commonly produced by coal, a nonrenewable source *not* in ample supply (answer A) and that is costly to use (answer B). Research focuses on environmentally safe production of methanol (answer C).

65. **A.** More research is needed, but ethanol and methanol are simple, cost-efficient, environmentally positive fuels that can be blended to power engines. Answer choice D is incorrect because gasohol is a blend of alcohol fuels and gasoline. Answer B is incorrect because ethanol and methanol can be used alone to ignite some engines, not all, making answer C incorrect.

66. **C.** This reason is given at the start of the second paragraph. Notice that not all alcohol fuels are cheap to produce and not all come from renewable resources. Nothing is said about pollution being a factor in making alcohols valuable fuels.

PASSAGE IV (QUESTIONS 67–72)

67. **A.** The second paragraph explains the problem as one of how we define God's attributes. Answers B, C, and D are associated with other responses to the problem of how we conceive God.

68. **B.** This is explained in the fourth paragraph. Answer choices A and C are not suggested as responses to the problems, and answer D is simply one of the premises of the problem, not a response to the problem.

69. **A.** This position is mentioned in the fourth paragraph. Both answer choices B and C are suggested as being part of different responses to the problem than that which denies the existence of evil. Answer D is incorrect because if the existence of evil is denied, it therefore cannot be goodness.

70. **D.** See statement (4). The problem presented is not that God does not exist (answer choice A), and neither answer choice B nor C, taken singly, is correct. The problem is that God is not both all-good and all-powerful, which is answer D.

71. **A.** This is explained in the second paragraph. The other choices are not discussed in the passages as parts of a proposed solution.

72. **D.** This is explained in the fourth paragraph. The other choices would represent

responses to how we should deal with the existence of evil, but these would not be responses to the problem of evil.

PASSAGE V (QUESTIONS 73–78)

73. **B.** This is explained in the first paragraph. Answer choices A, C, and D are not affirmed in the passage.

74. **B.** This is explained in the first two sentences. Answer choice A is incorrect because, if a thing does not exist, it will not have any properties, including primary properties. Answer C is incorrect because primary properties do not depend on their being known, and answer D is incorrect because an object cannot exist as what it is without primary properties.

75. **B.** This is explained in the second sentence. The first paragraph rules out answer choice A, and answers C and D are never mentioned as possibilities in the passage.

76. **B.** This is explained in the fourth paragraph. Answer choice A gives no answer to the question of why the argument would not apply to other things, and answer C is denied by the argument made in the fourth paragraph. Answer choice D is not mentioned in the text.

77. **D.** Individual human beings have, as humans, the same primary properties, but they are not identical, so answer choice A is false, and they do not have the same secondary properties, so answer choice B is false. Answer choice C is not mentioned in the passage.

78. **B.** This is explained in the fourth paragraph. Answer choice A is true but it is not what the ontological argument claims, and answer C is also not the claim of the argument. The argument does not support answer choice D.

PASSAGE VI (QUESTIONS 79–83)

79. **A.** Answer choice A is correct because it includes the broad spectrum of the discussion of music therapy in the passage. Answer choice B is too narrow in its response. Answer choice C contains an error in isolating teaching from a variety of options. Answer choice D is plainly untrue because it is too vague to be true without qualification.

80. **B.** The passage mentions that answer choices A, C, and D are needed for a person to qualify as a music therapist. Answer choice B refers to self-training, while the passage indicates training under supervision.

81. **C.** Because a person's will to succeed may vary as much as a person's enjoyment of music, options I and III have the potential to rebuild self-confidence. Therefore, answer choice C is correct. Answer choice A represents only option I. Answer choices B and D represent option II, which states that all people have musical ability; this is false.

82. **D.** D is the only answer that clarifies the fact that music therapists relate to persons with disabilities, rather than to persons either under the care of medical personnel (answer choice A), a social worker (answer choice B), or a psychoanalyst (answer choice C).

83. **C.** This answer requires you to be aware of the simple logic in relating the process of music therapy to the consequences of healing while not inferring any more than this from the passage. Cause and effect might be a logical choice, but that implies a completed fact. In most cases, it is not known that music therapy will indeed heal. It is known that a probable consequence of music therapy is healing. Answer choice B indicates a relationship between symptom and treatment, and answer choice D indicates a rela-

tionship between disease and health. In both cases, a medical model is implied. Both B and D are too medically specific.

PASSAGE VII (QUESTIONS 84–87)

84. **B.** An important aspect of the U.S. Navy fleet is its kinship to its air force, which allows the fleet to protect the skies and seas at the same time; therefore option II is correct. There is not enough information in the passage to know if the U.S. Navy is the oldest of the armed forces, so answer choices A and D are incorrect because they offer option I. Option III suggests that the U.S. Navy is similar to the British Navy when, in fact, the failure of the early British Navy was due to the lack of development between the Navy and its air force—a key aspect of the U.S. Navy; therefore, answer choice C is incorrect because option III is presented.

85. **B.** This answer is correct because it is the most thorough and complete answer. Answer choice A is exclusive. Answer choice C is incorrect because there is not enough information in this passage to determine whether the two navies are comparable. Though the idea of a navy was important to Captain Mahan, it cannot be concluded that the navy was the idea of one individual; therefore, answer choice D is incorrect.

86. **D.** Answer choice A is a negative statement refuted by the essay. Answer choice B undermines the joint efforts of the air force and army. Answer choice C is restrictive in its focus and leaves "maternal care" unclear. Answer choice D focuses on the theme of the essay and captures the essence of it; therefore, it is correct.

87. **A.** Because the passage emphasizes the complexity of need for development and cooperation among the many facets of the armed forces, option I is correct. Options II and III are incorrect because peace is never mentioned in the article, and no judgments are made as to the ramifications of having a navy. Because answer choice A offers only option I, it is correct. Answer choices B, C, and D offer options II and III, so they are incorrect.

PASSAGE VIII (QUESTIONS 88–92)

88. **A.** The author identifies several competing segments of our pluralistic society. Different groups of people vie for power in the policy-making arena. In this analysis, the author describes legislators, government executives, interest groups, university faculty, and industry and business leaders with competing ideas and different operating centers of power. Answer choice B is incorrect. Stockholders are private citizens and groups who have independently chosen to invest in utilities that function in a capitalist system of government. The author does not imply that stockholders are interested in a socialist system of government. Answer choice C is incorrect. Although the author aptly describes a highly emotional environment created by conflicting views, the analysis does not lead the reader to conclude that members of interest groups have gained power in the atomic energy industry. Answer choice D is incorrect. The reader has misinterpreted the chronological analysis of events described by the author. Rather than propose that nuclear power is at best hopeless and should be abandoned, the author tends to be sympathetic toward the problems that have beset the development of atomic energy.

89. **C.** The essay vividly portrays how ordinary citizens can change the course of industrial development if they organize in interest groups and as stockholders. Consider the facts that the author has presented, and it becomes clear that these people have been

partly responsible for slowing the bandwagon of earlier years. Lack of orders and reduction in funds for research and development are the end product. Answer choice A is incorrect. The author does not imply that the bottom line of industry has changed from profits to higher ideals. However, he does imply that, once major problems are eliminated, atomic energy can improve the environment and provide a better quality of life. Answer choice B is incorrect. The fact that arguments are still prevalent and funds are still allocated for new research has kept nuclear energy a lively issue in the private and public sectors of our country and elsewhere. Answer choice D is incorrect. While utility companies have quit ordering atomic reactors and constructing new plants, their major concern appears to be strictly a matter of business investment that will attract and keep investors. The author does not infer that solar energy has attracted serious attention of utility companies.

90. A. The overall theme of the author is the difficulty of finding a solution for supplying energy when alternatives are controversial and scientific developments are complex. The author, in his short analysis, makes a balanced presentation because he considers the various views of leaders in industry, universities, and interest groups. Answer choice B is incorrect. Actually, the author has described the certainty of utility management as it responds to stockholders' concerns. Utility policy-makers know that safety and good service should be important factors that investors consider, but dividends paid to stockholders are of major importance in any business. Answer choice C is incorrect. The author does not let us know his personal feelings about interest groups, but he does carefully describe major concerns of interest groups who have organized to fight the development of nuclear energy. The purpose of the essay is not to perform a psychological analysis of members of interest groups or any other group described in the study. Answer choice D is wrong. The author's comparison of the bandwagon effect in the 1950s and the 1960s does not support the thesis that conditions are the same with the exception of two unfortunate accidents. Rather, the author has systematically described events that have dulled the enthusiasm for large public and private expenditures on research and construction of atomic plants. Although interest has revived somewhat, promoters of atomic energy today speak to an entirely different audience whose members have either experienced or witnessed failures and unexpected costs.

PASSAGE IX (QUESTIONS 91–92)

91. **B.** The author begins the passage by telling us that, although Pluto was discovered many years ago, we know little about it. In the next few paragraphs, the author briefly mentions what little we do know about Pluto was discovered. In the final two paragraphs, the author returns to the argument that further exploration is needed. To some extent, answer choices A, C, are mentioned in the passage. Nevertheless, each is there only to add to the overall argument in favor of additional exploration. Thus, anser choices A, C, and are all incorrect because they are not the main focus ot the passage.

92. **C.** In the first sentence, the author describes Pluto as the "ninth planet," but we do not know whether this refers to distance or discovery. Later in the passage, we are given more information and can deduce that at the time Pluto was discovered, it mant both. We are also told in the fourth paragraph that Pluto's highly elliptical orbit at times brings it closer to the sun than Neptune. In the next sentence, the author directly states that between 1979 and 1999 Pluto had been closer to the sun than Neptune.

Therefore, answer choice D is invorrect. Answer chioce B is wrong because the author tells us in the fourth paragraph that Pluto's orbit is 30 to 50 times farther from the sun than the Earth. As a satellite of Pluto. Charon is necessarily very close to Pluto. We are not told exactly how close, but it is reasonable to assume close enough that Charon is not farther from the sun than Neptune at the same time Pluto is closer than Neptune. If this assumption was not the case, and keeping in mind that the author has told us Pluto had been closer to the sun than Neptune in 1990, it would be necessary to know exactly where Charon was in its orbit around Pluto at the time of answering this question to answer it correctly—certainly an unreasonable requirement.

SECTION 3
Writing Sample

SAMPLE ESSAY 1

Commuters trapped in their cars on a jammed freeway, or those wedged into crammed buses or trains entering or leaving a city, would agree with the statement that in the city "life itself is finally threatened with suffocation." Outsiders who have fought the masses and pollution to reach the city find themselves overwhelmed in vast tracts of glass-faced skyscrapers that honor money and greed. Workers, like drones, live out an existence of depressing sameness, scurrying from appointment to appointment, driven by machines meant to serve them but that often appear to enslave them. Once people have returned to the suburbs — real estate costing so much in cities that few can afford to live there — the cities become desolate wastelands of crime and disease. The homeless and poor sleep on the warm air vents in the doorways of skyscrapers or on station benches where commuters will once again stream by heedlessly the following morning.

Cities, built for humankind's ease, entertainment, safety, and business, have become unlivable, Mumford suggests, because of the accretion of layers of the past. When the Industrial Revolution herded people into cities, there was no forethought and little planning as to how such cities could accommodate the millions of people that would eventually attempt city life. As a result, the "city" is built upon the errors of the past and is doomed to repeat them. For example, the water and sewage systems very often belong to the nineteenth century; to repair or replace them would not only bankrupt the city but also disrupt its business life. The mass transport systems designed to carry the labor force into the city are either totally dismantled because of obsolescence, with no funds to resurrect them, or operate on antiquated methods that waste rather than save time and money. The judicial system and police force are strained to the limit, laboring in buildings that belong to another century, or in streets that form a warren where criminals can escape or turn back upon the enforcer. The very infrastructure of the city seems tottering, ready to fall with the next crime-wave.

No wonder modern humans, "in sheer defense," invent the museum. How much easier to gaze longingly at the past achievements of humans in the Smithsonian than to contemplate the soaring murder rate in the city of Washington, D.C.! Mumford's statement suggests that we cannot survive in the city, but we can erect monuments to it.

The museum then becomes a testament to the fact that people once did live in cities and led lives both full and satisfying. Modern humans invent the museum as a haven of rest and peace from the modern city life; people in Florence escape the screech of traffic to wonder at medieval art, and people in New York escape pressure and marvel at the ruins of ancient Egypt. Modern humans mull over the past life of the "city" and perhaps yearn for those places so carefully chosen by our ancestors.

Admittedly, Mumford's view is gloomy, seeing only one side of the darkened city. After a period of "urban blight" in the seventies, cities have begun to recapture the magic, if not the calm, of past city life. Areas that were architecturally stunning but have fallen into neglect have been resurrected into art galleries or antique malls, bringing more commerce to flagging city coffers. Cynics may scoff at the quality of life in such areas, but the city will come to life again if the projects are well conceived. One such project, Faneuil Hall in Boston, exemplifies the aims of a city (which itself was turning into a museum) determined to revitalize its existence.

Similarly, New York, for all its rapidly decaying infrastructure, managed to revive the Seaport area that brings more acclaim with each new development of the project. "The city that never sleeps" offers the best in drama, ballet, and music for those who can afford it. If, like Boston, New York would serve the people with improved travel and housing, the city could live again as the civilized metropolis it once was.

In other words, city life can be resurrected. The seemingly out-of-grasp civility of past eras can be relived outside the museum. There is a place for the city in the life of modern humanity — we simply have to be more careful and thoughtful about the *quality* of life we choose for the city. Culture should be available for everyone. Parks should be safe for joggers at midnight. Riverfronts should be populated by thriving businesses. The displaced poor must be offered humane living conditions. We should preserve the life of the city within the city and not simply within the museum.

EXPLANATION OF ESSAY 1

The essay deals with all three tasks fully, paying particular attention to the key words of the tasks: *explain*, *describe* and *discuss*. Paragraphs one through four explain thoroughly each part of the statement: the suffocating life of the modern city; the reason being the accretions of the past; the invention of the museum as a defense. The opening paragraph involves the reader in the explanation because most people have suffered city commutes. It also introduces the notion of city dwellers as drones, an idea which plays as a useful motif.

Paragraph two deals with the "layer upon layer of past times," showing how the past has caused problems in the present, using specific examples from the life of the city. Paragraphs three and four extend the explanation into the concept of the museum becoming a monument to the city, a testament that people could once survive happily within a city.

Paragraph five sets up an argument against the statement that cities are indeed livable for the modern human, giving specific examples of cities that have revitalized themselves. Paragraph six then discusses the place of the modern city, picking up details from the previous paragraphs to bring the essay to a satisfying, wrapped-up ending.

Each paragraph is clearly structured with a topic sentence, limiting sentence, and evidence to back up the topic. For example, paragraph two sets up the topic sentence about cities being unlivable. Two limiting sentences focus on past lack of planning and present living with errors. The next sentence gives examples to "prove" the central point. The last sentence gives a dramatic conclusion suggesting that cities are about to crumble. The entire paragraph reads like a miniature essay, as it should.

Each sentence in each paragraph relates to another, often by giving very simple signals to the reader. Time links or transitions like "*Once* people have returned to the suburbs . . ." (paragraph one), introductory phrases such as "*For example* . . ." (paragraph two), and comparison links such as "*Similarly* . . ." (paragraph three) are several examples. All such linking devices make for unity within the paragraph and push the meaning forward.

Besides sentence links within the paragraphs, strong links or transitions *between* the paragraphs hold the essay together: "No wonder modern humans . . ." (paragraph two into three) simply picks up on all the negatives of the previous paragraph and moves to the point of the museum smoothly. "As a result" would also have worked but is not so forceful. "The museum *then* becomes a testament . . ." (paragraph three into four) is both a time transition and a consequence transition. Thus, it would have also worked but is more formal than the voice of the essay requires. "In other words, city life can be resurrected" (last paragraph) gathers together all the previous points and moves the reader to the conclusion.

Overall, the writing is clear and to the point. The sentence structure is varied, mixing long sentences with multiple subordinate clauses: "Outsiders who have fought the masses" (paragraph one), with short simple sentences:

"Culture should be available for everyone . . ." (last paragraph). Vocabulary is apt "Commuters *trapped . . . wedged . . . crammed . . .*" (paragraph one). The mechanics of the paper (spelling, punctuation, syntax) are sound. Together they provide an unimpeded piece of prose for the reader.

SAMPLE ESSAY 2

Ideally, in the "best of all possible worlds," the concept of all men being created equal, with "equal worth and equal rights" should indeed work. No matter what race, gender, class, or religion people are born into, they should have equality if the nation where they are born has committed to such a belief. It should not matter what color people are because all colors should be equal, one not having more positive connotation over the others. When a nation like America committed itself to equality, a certain idealism was at play. The men making the commitment of belief, signing the belief into law, were automatically superior to those for whom they were making the commitment: the masses, many illiterate, many incapable of signing, never mind reading, the document pledging equality. However, having made such a pledge, every member of the nation should set aside personal ambition and preferences to promote equal worth and equal rights. All people should be entitled to housing and the safety of the family home. All people should live in neighborhoods where it is safe to walk after dark. Jobs and education should be available to all, each person receiving equal, not elitist, treatment. Expert health care should be available for everyone at the same cost, at the same level of excellence. Last, each person within the nation should be accorded equal worth, human dignity, owning a name and identity that all respect equally. There should be race harmony within a nation made up of a "salad bowl" of peoples; there should be no class system because class suggests a caste system of "higher" and "lower"; and there should be a melding of different religions because no one religious choice is "better" than another.

Of course, in the real world, George Orwell's statement holds more validity than Catton's: "All {men} are born equal but some are more equal than others." A child born into the "Nob Hill" area of a city in America will definitely be "more equal" than one born in an inner-city ghetto. A Nob Hill child will be entitled to have a safe home and environment; the ghetto child may not have a permanent home, and the environment will be dangerous. The Nob Hill child will automatically inherit an education pattern: private school with first-class teachers and state-of-the-art equipment, followed by Ivy League universities. If the child is a girl, she may encounter problems with certain schools not welcoming her in certain disciplines and certain jobs not in her province, but money and status can usually overcome such barriers. The ghetto child meanwhile inherits no pattern of education; he or she is not "entitled" to private schools and universities, nor a choice of equal jobs. The ghetto girl can look forward to a life on welfare or menial jobs where she will not be paid equally for the same job performed by males. Inequality in health will have already demonstrated itself, even before the birth of each child, in prenatal care; the birth itself in totally different hospitals (if indeed the ghetto birth takes place in a hospital) will underline the inequality. Finally, human dignity will not be afforded the ghetto child even if she or he makes it out of the ghetto and makes it into the life on Nob Hill — the gap lessens, but the identity remains, the label cannot be removed.

Within such structures how can every citizen make a life-long commitment to put equality into practice? Given that absolute equality is impossible — we are all different in all kinds of ways from birth — citizens must make a conscious effort to practice the original concept of our forefathers. There must be made available the means for all people to achieve equality. Education is the obvious means to raise everyone to a suitable standard of living, affording the poorest of its citizens the highest level of learning. No nation committed to equality should lower its standards to the lowest common denominator. The upheaval in communist countries proves that abject equality is not the answer (and within such equality some definitely were "more equal" than others, as the leaders of Romania demonstrated). A structure should exist, however, where all people have access to forms of education to help those who so wish to move across race, gender, religion, class, and color barriers.

EXPLANATION OF ESSAY 2

The essay immediately sets up the thesis that equality is possible only in an ideal world. It explains the concept behind the statement in terms of what should happen in a nation built on the belief of equality for all people. The first two paragraphs set up the pattern for the rest of the essay, within the explanation of the statement. The next long paragraph takes each one of the points in the previous paragraph as an argument against the statement that, in America, equal worth and equal rights are not feasible because of an entrenched hierarchical society. The last paragraph deals with the possible solution for an "acceptable equality" — one that everyone can agree on and work toward, based on improved education levels.

The essay fulfills the tasks demanded by tapping into the notion of the founding fathers, as well as Orwell's statement on "equality," and the events in communist countries. The essay is structured on a contrast basis using the two classes of children as examples. Each point in the first two paragraphs is dealt with in the next, with a repetition in the conclusion of the categories used in the opening lines (race, gender, religion, and color), bringing the essay full circle and providing cohesion.

The paragraphs develop from a clearly stated topic sentence, limiting sentences, and examples. Simple sentences cue the reader to the structure of the paragraph: "Last" (paragraph one); "Finally" (paragraph two). A rhetorical question starts the last paragraph; the following text then attempts to answer that question.

Each paragraph flows smoothly into the next with the use of simple transitional phrases or words: "Of course, in the real world . . ." (paragraph one into two, pushing the readers forward yet reminding them of the contrast between the "ideal" and "real"); "Within such structures . . . " (paragraph two into three, pulling together the ideas of the last paragraph but pushing forward to an answer for the problem).

The sentences are suitably varied and often rely on parallel structure or repetition to stress certain points: "All people should be entitled . . . "; "All people should live in neighborhoods . . ." The use of punctuation is appropriate, as is the vocabulary. Words to be stressed are often "lifted" into quotation marks: "salad bowl," "entitled." The awkwardness of using the "he or she" construction has been avoided through the use of the plural or "the child." Overall the language skills and techniques work well, never impeding or making the reader stumble over clumsy sentences, poor spelling, or weak punctuation.

SECTION 4
Biological Sciences

PASSAGE I (QUESTIONS 93–96)

93. **B.** As can be seen from the graph of blood pressure in a human circulatory system (Figure 1), the lowest blood pressure exists just before blood is returned to the heart from systemic circulation. Pressure is highest in the aorta and then decreases through arterial, capillary, and venous circulation.

94. **A.** There are two principal ducts that return lymph to the circulatory system: the thoracic duct and the right lymphatic duct. The thoracic duct is the larger of the two and empties into the left subclavian vein, while the right lymphatic duct empties into the right subclavian vein. None of the other choices describe vessels that participate in the return of lymph to the circulatory system.

95. **C.** This item tests your understanding of fetal circulation in mammals. Answer choice C gives the correct name of the connection between the aorta and the pulmonary artery. Answer choice A is the name of the opening between the atria of a fetal heart, while answer choice D gives the name of the adult derivative of the ductus arteriosus. Answer choice B is the name of the large opening in the occipital bone of the cranium through which the spinal cord passes.

96. **C.** Osmotic pressure of any solution is determined by the concentration of solute. Active transport of water does not occur, either across the walls of capillaries or through any other membranes; only solute can be actively transported. The other statements in this item correctly state facts regarding mammalian circulation.

PASSAGE II (QUESTIONS 97–99)

97. **D.** The smallest fragment is G, and the largest fragment is A. The nucleotide bases between the smallest and largest are those given in answer choice D and can be read from the bottom to the top of the gel. The base sequence in answer choice A is from the largest fragment to the smallest. The base sequences in answer choices B and C are the complimentary bases of answer choices A and D, respectively. The base sequence given in answer C would be on the 3′ to 5′ strand, where the first base cytosine is given.

98. **B.** The special nucleotide is in the final position of the section of chain because no nucleotides can be added after the special nucleotide. Therefore, the section of chain is G T A A*, with the special nucleotide A* being added last. In A, there is no special nucleotide. This cannot be a section of DNA chain because nucleotides would continue to be added. In answer choices C and D, nucleotides are added after the special nucleotide. This does not occur.

99. **C.** As long as there was no way to distinguish among the different special nucleotides, all of the possible chain lengths would be present in each test tube. Therefore, there would be a series of identical spots on each of the four gels (answer choice C). One small fragment (answer

choice B) suggests that only one special nucleotide was added; thus no further nucleotide bases were incorporated. One large fragment (answer choice D) suggests that the special nucleotide was added only in the last position in all four test tubes. The results would not be the same because the four special nucleotides are in different test tubes and, as a result, are distinguishable.

PASSAGE III (QUESTIONS 100–102)

100. **C.** This question requires knowledge of skeletal anatomy and the directional terminology used in anatomy. The term *proximal* means "toward the main mass of the body" (as opposed to distal) so the proximal epiphyseal plate of the humerus would be in the head of that bone. Among the choices given, answer choice C is correct because the scapula is closest to the head of humerus. The other choices are incorrect because they all identify anatomical features found near the distal end of the humerus.

101. **D.** The classification of articulations, based on degree of movement permitted, recognizes three types: synarthroses (immovable), amphiarthroses (slightly movable), and diarthroses (freely movable). The knee and elbow joints are classic examples of diarthroses, so answer choice D is correct. You should be familiar with other examples of diarthroses — shoulder and hip joints, intercarpal and intertarsal joints, etc. You may also need to be familiar with examples of synarthroses (answer choice A) and amphiarthroses (answer choice C). Answer choice B, which is incorrect for this question, gives the term *synchondrosis*, which refers to the epiphyseal plates of long bones, a subtype of synarthrotic joint.

102. **A.** This question is another test of your knowledge of bone nomenclature. The proper name for the shaft of a long bone is "diaphysis," so answer choice A is correct. An epiphysis (answer choice B) is the end segment of a long bone, which during growth of the individual was separated from the diaphysis by the epiphyseal plate. Answer choice C is incorrect because it gives the term used to refer to the type of bone joint that is slightly movable (i.e., an amphiarthrosis). A symphysis (answer choice D) is a type of amphiarthrosis, examples of which are seen in intervertebral and in the sacroiliac joints.

103. **B.** The Cahn-Ingold-Prelog system of nomenclature uses priorities to establish the R or S designation. With the lowest priority group oriented away from the observer, the R designation is given if movement from the highest to next highest priority is clockwise. If it is counterclockwise, the atom is designated S. Manipulation of the structure shown will allow easy designation of the absolute configuration, if you know how to assign priorities.

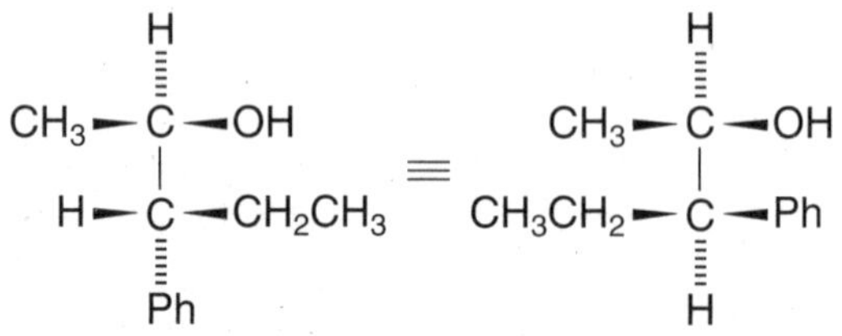

104. **B.** The 1, 5-octadiene describes the longest chain containing the diene, using the lowest possible numbers to locate the double bonds (following the 1 and 5 carbons). Once these numbers are assigned, the 3, 6-dimethyl follows. Assignment of stereochemistry at the 5, 6 double bond is made by assigning priorities to the groups attached to each carbon of the double bond. Because the higher priority groups are on the same side of the double bond, the Z (zusammen) designation is given. E (entgegen) indicates that the higher priority groups are on opposite sides of the double bond. The 1, 2 double bond has

no stereochemistry (two hydrogens are on one carbon), so no designation is necessary. Answer choice C would allow you to draw the correct structure for the molecule, but it is incorrect nomenclature because the numbers are larger. Answer choices A and B have the wrong stereochemistry for the double bond.

PASSAGE IV (QUESTIONS 105–108)

105. **D.** This question requires that you know about enzyme kinetics. Because molecule *A* affects the rate of enzyme activity and does so by binding with the enzyme at a site physically distinct from the active site, it must be an allosteric modulator, or regulator. Therefore, answer choice D is correct. It should be noted that allosteric inhibitors may themselves be products of a series of enzyme reactions that regulate one of the previous enzymes (often the first of the series) through feedback inhibition. The other answer choices are incorrect: molecule *A* is obviously not the substrate because it is not changed by the reaction; a competitive inhibitor reduces enzyme activity by binding with the enzyme at the active site; and a cofactor is usually a small inorganic or metal ion that is required for catalytic activity.

106. **D.** Because molecule *B* reduces the rate of this reaction by binding at the active site, it is acting as a competitive inhibitor of the enzyme, and answer choice D is correct. The effect of competitive inhibitors is reversible by increasing the substrate concentration. The other answer choices are incorrect because cofactors bind with the enzyme loosely, if at all, and do not inhibit the reaction (actually, they may be required for activity); allosteric modulators can inhibit enzyme reactions (e.g., through feedback inhibition), but they do not bind at the active site; and noncompetitive inhibitors are reversible inhibitors of enzyme activity that bind away from the active site.

107. **C.** By simply reading the plot seen in Figure 1, you can determine that the optimum temperature (i.e., the one at which the reaction proceeds fastest) is about 35°C (C). At 5° and 25°C, the reaction is occurring, but more slowly than at 35°C. At 45°C, the reaction has almost entirely ceased most likely because the enzyme has been denatured.

108. **B.** The nonprotein structural component described in the passage is called a prosthetic group, correctly given by answer choice B. An allosteric modulator (answer choice A) is a molecule, often a product of a subsequent enzyme reaction in a series that regulates enzyme activity by binding with the enzyme away from the active site. Coenzymes (answer choice C) are often required for enzyme activity, but they are separate, usually organic molecules and are not part of the structure of enzymes.

PASSAGE V (QUESTIONS 109–111)

109. **C.** Cholic acid, which emulsifies dietary fats in the small intestine, has three OH groups and one COOH group. These are polar hydrogen-bonding groups that enhance water solubility. None of the other three would exhibit any water solubility because they are largely nonpolar and hydrophobic.

110. **D.** Chiral centers have four different groups bound to a carbon atom. Androsterone has seven such carbons.

111. **A.** The 6.5–7.5 δ area of the NMR spectrum is where aromatic protons appear. The only one of the steroids with an aromatic ring, ring A, is estradiol.

112. **D.** The placenta is a region where a portion of the embryonic chorion and the maternal

uterine wall join. It functions in the exchange of nutrients, wastes, and gases between the mother and the fetus. (See the figure below.)

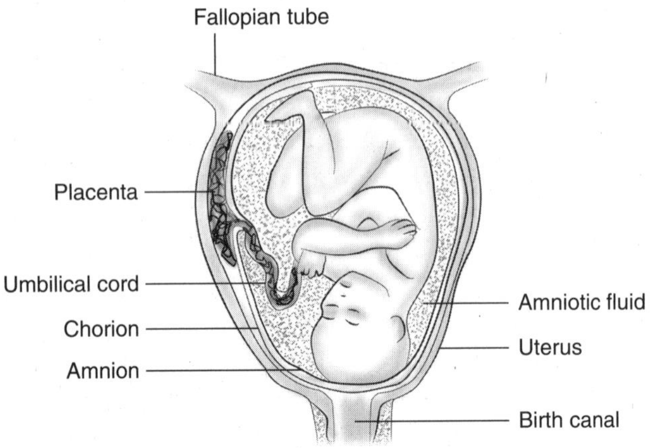

113. **A.** The Golgi apparatus is an organelle that is responsible only for the packaging of protein for secretion.

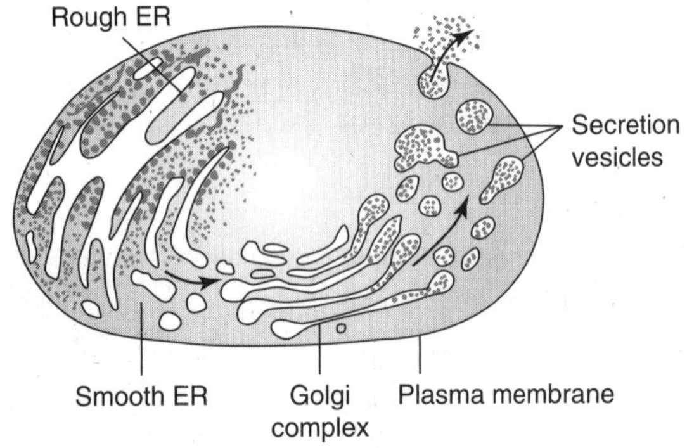

Schematic representation of the secretion of a protein in a typical animal cell. The large arrows represent the probable route of secreted proteins.

114. **B.** This question requires knowledge of NMR chemical shifts. Alkyl protons, *a*, are not deshielded and appear close to TMS (about 1.0 δ). Protons on a carbon adjacent to a carbonyl group can be found in the 2.0–2.5 δ region. Protons on a carbon attached to an oxygen usually occur in the 3.5–4.0 δ region. The other answers are perturbations of the correct answer.

115. **C.** Your knowledge of several chemical reactions is tested by this question. The reactions would yield the following products:

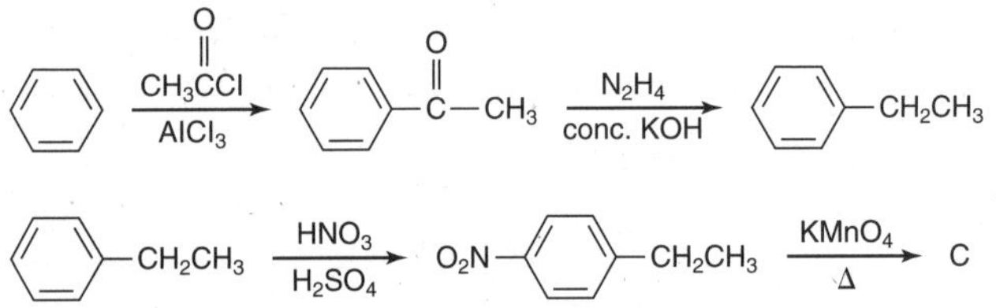

The first reaction is a Friedel-Crafts acylation. It is followed by a Wolff-Kishner reduction, which produces an ortho-para directing ethyl group. Nitration then produces para-nitroethylbenzene (and some ortho), which can be oxidized to *p*-nitrobensoic acid (answer choice C). Answer choice A would be the product if the ethyl group was meta direction. Answer choice B would be the product if no oxidation of the ethyl group took place. Answer choice D is not a feasible answer because no reaction shown would lead to the vinyl group.

PASSAGE VI (QUESTIONS 116–118)

116. **D.** The enzymes that catalyze the reactions known as glycolysis are soluble proteins found in the cytosol, or cytoplasm. The end result of this process is pyruvic acid, ATP, and NADH+H^+. Ribosomes are the site of protein synthesis (i.e., translation of mRNA) and the nucleus contains chromosomal DNA and is the site of transcription. Mitochondria have catabolic enzymes, specifically those of the Krebs cycle and the electron transport chain, but they are not involved in glycolysis.

117. **A.** Fermentation of glucose is an anaerobic process that produces either lactic acid (as in skeletal muscle) or ethanol and carbon dioxide (as in yeast cells). There is a direct yield of two molecules of ATP per glucose molecule fermented in this process, so answer choice A is correct. Complete aerobic metabolism of one glucose molecule yields thirty-six molecules of ATP, the number given in answer choice C. (It yields thirty-eight in procaryotes.) Answer choices B and D do not reflect the number of ATP molecules produced by

either aerobic or anaerobic breakdown of glucose and are therefore incorrect.

118. **C.** The carrier molecules (Co-enzyme Q, cytochromes, and other proteinaceous molecules acting as enzymes) of the electron transport chain are located within the inner membrane of mitochondria; therefore, answer choice C is correct. The other choices are incorrect: the cytosol is the location of the enzymes of glycolysis, the outer compartment of the mitochondrion is the site of the electrochemical gradient established by H+ pumped out of the inner compartment, and the plasma membrane contains no enzymes directly related to intermediary metabolism.

PASSAGE VII (QUESTIONS 119–122)

119. **D.** To answer this and succeeding questions, you must know that each carbon-carbon bond has two π electrons that can be delocalized if they are conjugated with other double bonds.

120. **B.** Sodium amide, $NaNH_2$, will react with acidic protons in a neutralization reaction.

$$NaNH_2 + RH \text{ S } NH_3 + Na^+R^-$$

Ordinary hydrocarbons are not acidic; they are cyclopentadiene (answer choice B) and will react to form an aromatic entity where the electrons of the carbonion conjugate with the four π electrons of the double bonds. None of the other compounds can react with a base to form an aromatic entity.

121. **D.** This question tests your knowledge of NMR spectrometry. The area described is the aromatic region of the spectrum; therefore, only the aromatic compound 4 will show peaks there. The other compounds will absorb in the alkene region.

122. **A.** Silver nitrate reacts with halides to give a precipitate of silver halide. Ordinarily, one must destroy the organic molecule by a sodium fusion reaction to yield Na*X* before getting a reaction with silver nitrate. Answer choice A, however, will react readily with silver nitrate to yield a trophylium cation.

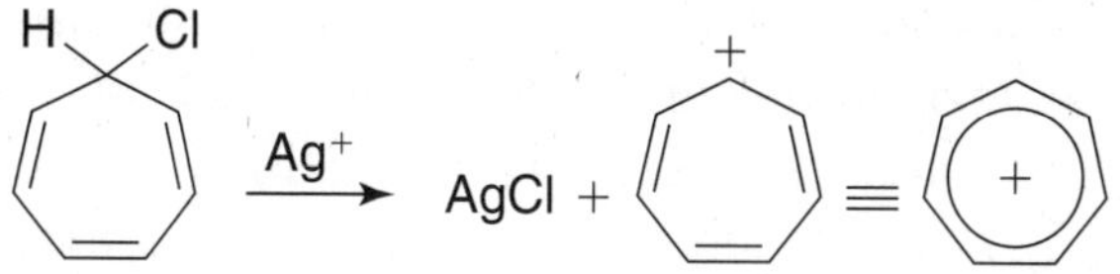

The tropylium ion has 6 π electrons, and these can form different resonance structures by delocalization of the positive charge and π electrons. The stability of this aromatic species enhances the reactivity of its precursor. Answer choice B is an aromatic compound, and the C—Cl bond is very strong. Breaking the bond would actually disrupt an aromatic species. Answer choice D would yield a cation where delocalization is theoretically possible, but the 4 π electrons would not be aromatic. Answer choice C is an ordinary alkyl halide, which would not be reactive.

PASSAGE VIII (QUESTIONS 123–126)

123. **B.** This item tests your understanding of homologous and analogous structures. Homologous structures have evolved from a common ancestral form. Of the answer choices presented, all but answer choice B represent structures that are homologous as vertebrate forelimbs because they have common bone structures. The wing of an insect is *analogous* to the wing of a bird because it has a common function, but because it evolved independently from the bird wing, it is not homologous.

124. **C.** For an allele to be subject to selective pressures, it must be expressed (i.e., there must be a phenotype). A heterozygote expresses the dominant phenotype, while the recessive allele is masked from selective pressure. Answer choice C describes this

situation; the other three answer choices all indicate alleles that would be expressed and therefore would be susceptible to positive and negative selective pressures.

125. **D.** All four answer choices in this item identify mechanisms that act to prevent interspecific hybridization. However, answer choices A, B, and C describe mechanisms that act to *prevent* mating between species. In those cases where interspecific mating can occur, developmental isolation (as well as gametic isolation) prevents the formation of viable offspring. Answer choice D correctly identifies this situation. In some instances, viable hybrid offspring can develop, but they may be subject to other isolating mechanisms such as hybrid sterility (e.g., a mule).

126. **B.** The classic characteristics of the phylum Chordata are the occurrence of pharyngeal gill slits, a notochord, and a dorsal hollow nerve cord at some time in the animal's development. A cartilaginous or bony vertebral column is found only in the subphylum Vertebrata and therefore is *not* a general phylum characteristic.

127. **C.** The aldol condensation is a reaction between an enolate ion and an uncharged aldehyde. The product is an aldehyde with an alcohol functional group (aldol). Answer choice D would require the displacement of a hydride ion. Answer choices A and B are not feasible products of an aldol condensation.

128. **B.** The interconversion occurs through a symmetrical ene-diol intermediate that involves keto-enol tautomerism. None of the other possibilities is feasible.

PASSAGE IX (QUESTIONS 129–134)

129. **A.** This item tests your knowledge of the sliding-filament theory of skeletal and cardiac muscle contraction. The functional unit of a muscle known as a sarcomere is diagrammed in Figure 1 near the beginning of this passage. The sarcomere contracts as the thick myosin slide by the thin actin filaments. This is accomplished as cross bridges from the myosin "pull" the actin filaments. During the contraction of a sarcomere, the Z lines move closer to each other, the I bands of each sarcomere shorten, and the H zone gradually disappears. The A band remains virtually the same length because it corresponds to the length of the myosin filaments. Answer choice A is a correct description of this fact.

130. **B.** Smooth muscle has no cross striations, but both cardiac and skeletal muscle show striations due to the arrangement of actin and myosin into sarcomeres. Unlike cardiac muscle, however, skeletal muscle is multinucleate. Answer choice B correctly identifies skeletal muscle as the only striated, multinucleate muscle.

131. **D.** The inside of a neuron is about 70 millivolts negative compared to the outside (the actual value may range from –65mv to –85mv in neurons and muscle cells). This potential difference is referred to as the resting membrane potential, or simply resting potential, of the neuron. The only correct value for a neuron resting potential is given in answer choice D.

132. **B.** In this item, your understanding of the complex process of muscle fiber contraction is tested. As an action potential moves along a muscle cell, calcium ions released from the sarcoplasmic reticulum bind with one of two regulatory proteins found as part of the thin filaments. The protein with which calcium binds is known as the troponin complex, so the correct answer choice is B. This binding causes a slight conformational change in the other regulatory protein known as tropomyosin. Because of this change, the myosin cross bridges can then attach to specific sites on the actin, and the contraction process can proceed.

133. **A.** Neurons that are enveloped by Schwann cells have action potentials only at the nodes of Ranvier (see Figure 2 in the middle of the passage). These neurons, therefore, transmit impulses by the jumping of action potentials from node to node. The type of conduction is known as saltatory conduction and is much more rapid than conduction in neurons without Schwann cells, so the correct answer choice for this item is A.

134. **C.** The sodium-potassium pump moves sodium ions from the inside of a cell to the outside, and it moves potassium ions from the outside to the inside. The "pump" is actually a protein embedded in the cell membrane that resembles a rocker switch as it changes from one conformation to another. These conformational changes (or at least one of them) require energy in the form of ATP and result in sodium ions being pumped out and potassium ions being pumped into the cell in a ratio of approximately 3:2 during each cycle. This ratio is correctly given in answer choice C.

PASSAGE X (QUESTIONS 135–138)

135. **B.** The step leading to (1) involves heterolysis of the C–X bond. Because X^- is formed, the carbon is left with a positive charge. A free radical (answer choice D) would form if bond homolysis occurred. Answer choice A or C would be formed if an acid-base reaction removed a proton.

136. **D.** Loss of optical activity means that an S_N1 reaction is the likely mechanism; because ionization of the alkyl halide is the rate-determining (slow) step, the rate is dependent on the concentration of alkyl halide. Answer choice C would imply that sodium ethoxide was involved in the rate-determining step; it is not. The loss of optical activity rules out answer choices A and B.

137. **A.** Reaction of the base with a hydrogen beta to the leaving group (OTs) is required for elimination. Only answer choices A and B show products of such a reaction. Answer choice B is not correct because it is a less substituted alkene than A (Saytzeff's rule).

138. **B.** t-Butyl alcohol will react via a tertiary carbocation that will not rearrange.

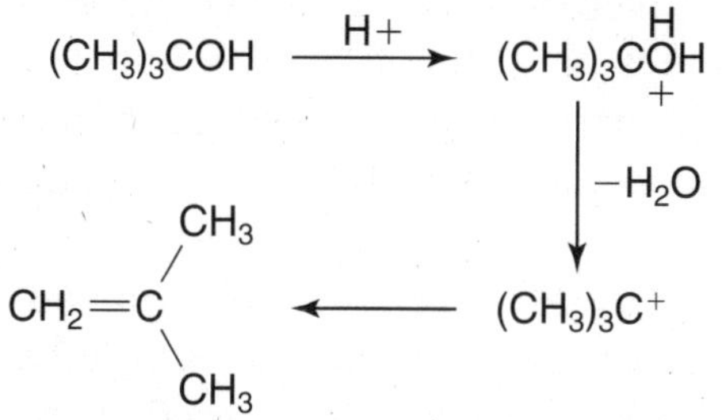

Protonation and dehydration of answer choices A and D will yield secondary cations that can rearrange by a hydride shift to a more stable tertiary cation. Answer choice C will yield a primary cation that can rearrange to a more stable secondary cation.

PASSAGE XI (QUESTIONS 139–141)

139. **D.** The four "experiments" described in the passage are actually descriptions of the application of the rules of procedure known as Koch's Postulates. Only after successfully completing all four steps, as described in the passage or in analogous situations, can it be concluded that a suspected pathogen is actually the cause of a disease.

140. **C.** In this item you must recall the components of a bacterial cell. Bacteria have cell walls, not made of cellulose like plant cell walls, but of a related polysaccharide. While bacteria are prokaryotic, they do have ribosomes, which are not membrane-bound organelles. Bacterial ribosomes are different, however, from those of eukaryotes in several aspects. All bacterial cells are enclosed in a cell membrane that exists just inside the cell

wall. Given this information, answer choice C is the only one possible. You should also be able to make this selection by recalling that only eukaryotes have mitochondria and they are not found in bacteria.

141. **D.** This item requires you to calculate the approximate number of bacterial cells that will be produced after a given time period. Given the replication time of forty-five minutes, you should be able to determine that a single bacterium will go through sixteen divisions in twelve hours to produce 2^{16}, or approximately 65,000, cells. Because there were ten bacterial cells initially placed inoculated into the medium, there will be approximately $10 \times 65{,}000 = 650{,}000$ cells at the end of twelve hours.

142. **B.** The autonomic nervous system innervates the heart, some glands, the smooth muscles of the digestive tract, the respiratory system, the reproductive system, and the blood vessels. Only answer choice B describes processes innervated by the autonomic pathways. The other choices are all parts of the somatic pathways of the nervous system that usually innervate skeletal muscle.

143. **A.** By dividing one group of progeny by the other, 77/24, the Mendelian ratio of approximately 3:1 is obtained. This suggests that the long-winged phenotype is dominant to the short-winged phenotype. This in turn implies that neither of the parents were homozygous because that situation would not have produced any short-winged flies:

LL × LL	LL × *ll*
↓	↓
All LL	All L*l*
↓	↓
Long-winged	Long-winged

Because some recessive flies are the result of the cross, both parents must have had a recessive, *l*, and allele. Constructing a Punnet Square, we find:

	L	*l*
L	LL	L*l*
l	L*l*	*ll*

75% – phenotypically long
25% – phenotypically short

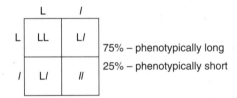

144. **C.** The somatic nervous system innervates skeletal muscles, which are under voluntary control. The other muscles are controlled by the autonomic nervous system.

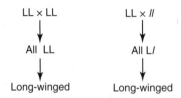

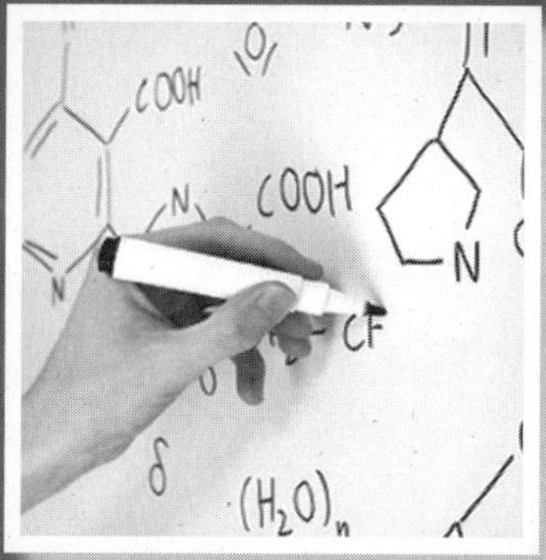

MCAT

MEDICAL COLLEGE

ADMISSION TEST

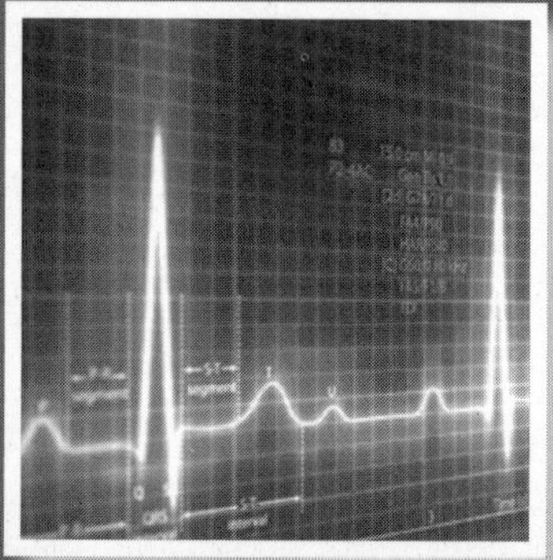

Test 5

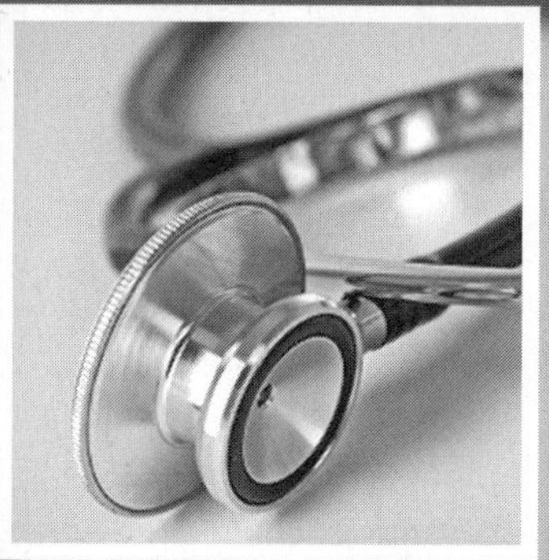

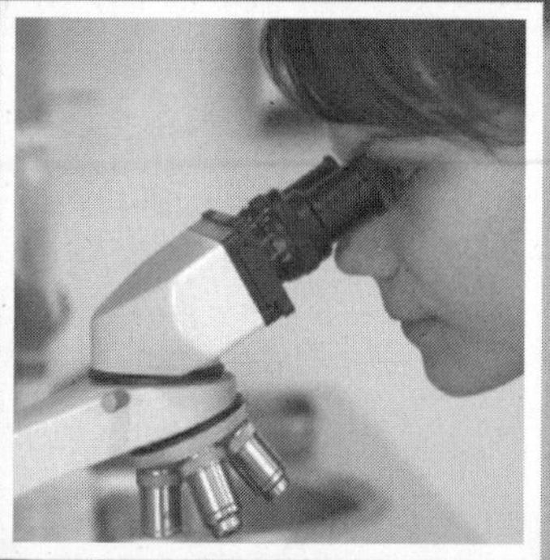

Test 5 ■ Answer Sheet

SECTION 1: Physical Sciences

1. Ⓐ Ⓑ Ⓒ Ⓓ
2. Ⓐ Ⓑ Ⓒ Ⓓ
3. Ⓐ Ⓑ Ⓒ Ⓓ
4. Ⓐ Ⓑ Ⓒ Ⓓ
5. Ⓐ Ⓑ Ⓒ Ⓓ
6. Ⓐ Ⓑ Ⓒ Ⓓ
7. Ⓐ Ⓑ Ⓒ Ⓓ
8. Ⓐ Ⓑ Ⓒ Ⓓ
9. Ⓐ Ⓑ Ⓒ Ⓓ
10. Ⓐ Ⓑ Ⓒ Ⓓ
11. Ⓐ Ⓑ Ⓒ Ⓓ
12. Ⓐ Ⓑ Ⓒ Ⓓ
13. Ⓐ Ⓑ Ⓒ Ⓓ
14. Ⓐ Ⓑ Ⓒ Ⓓ
15. Ⓐ Ⓑ Ⓒ Ⓓ
16. Ⓐ Ⓑ Ⓒ Ⓓ
17. Ⓐ Ⓑ Ⓒ Ⓓ
18. Ⓐ Ⓑ Ⓒ Ⓓ
19. Ⓐ Ⓑ Ⓒ Ⓓ
20. Ⓐ Ⓑ Ⓒ Ⓓ
21. Ⓐ Ⓑ Ⓒ Ⓓ
22. Ⓐ Ⓑ Ⓒ Ⓓ
23. Ⓐ Ⓑ Ⓒ Ⓓ
24. Ⓐ Ⓑ Ⓒ Ⓓ
25. Ⓐ Ⓑ Ⓒ Ⓓ
26. Ⓐ Ⓑ Ⓒ Ⓓ
27. Ⓐ Ⓑ Ⓒ Ⓓ
28. Ⓐ Ⓑ Ⓒ Ⓓ
29. Ⓐ Ⓑ Ⓒ Ⓓ
30. Ⓐ Ⓑ Ⓒ Ⓓ
31. Ⓐ Ⓑ Ⓒ Ⓓ
32. Ⓐ Ⓑ Ⓒ Ⓓ
33. Ⓐ Ⓑ Ⓒ Ⓓ
34. Ⓐ Ⓑ Ⓒ Ⓓ
35. Ⓐ Ⓑ Ⓒ Ⓓ
36. Ⓐ Ⓑ Ⓒ Ⓓ
37. Ⓐ Ⓑ Ⓒ Ⓓ
38. Ⓐ Ⓑ Ⓒ Ⓓ
39. Ⓐ Ⓑ Ⓒ Ⓓ
40. Ⓐ Ⓑ Ⓒ Ⓓ
41. Ⓐ Ⓑ Ⓒ Ⓓ
42. Ⓐ Ⓑ Ⓒ Ⓓ
43. Ⓐ Ⓑ Ⓒ Ⓓ
44. Ⓐ Ⓑ Ⓒ Ⓓ
45. Ⓐ Ⓑ Ⓒ Ⓓ
46. Ⓐ Ⓑ Ⓒ Ⓓ
47. Ⓐ Ⓑ Ⓒ Ⓓ
48. Ⓐ Ⓑ Ⓒ Ⓓ
49. Ⓐ Ⓑ Ⓒ Ⓓ
50. Ⓐ Ⓑ Ⓒ Ⓓ
51. Ⓐ Ⓑ Ⓒ Ⓓ
52. Ⓐ Ⓑ Ⓒ Ⓓ

SECTION 2: Verbal Reasoning

53. Ⓐ Ⓑ Ⓒ Ⓓ
54. Ⓐ Ⓑ Ⓒ Ⓓ
55. Ⓐ Ⓑ Ⓒ Ⓓ
56. Ⓐ Ⓑ Ⓒ Ⓓ
57. Ⓐ Ⓑ Ⓒ Ⓓ
58. Ⓐ Ⓑ Ⓒ Ⓓ
59. Ⓐ Ⓑ Ⓒ Ⓓ
60. Ⓐ Ⓑ Ⓒ Ⓓ
61. Ⓐ Ⓑ Ⓒ Ⓓ
62. Ⓐ Ⓑ Ⓒ Ⓓ
63. Ⓐ Ⓑ Ⓒ Ⓓ
64. Ⓐ Ⓑ Ⓒ Ⓓ
65. Ⓐ Ⓑ Ⓒ Ⓓ
66. Ⓐ Ⓑ Ⓒ Ⓓ
67. Ⓐ Ⓑ Ⓒ Ⓓ
68. Ⓐ Ⓑ Ⓒ Ⓓ
69. Ⓐ Ⓑ Ⓒ Ⓓ
70. Ⓐ Ⓑ Ⓒ Ⓓ
71. Ⓐ Ⓑ Ⓒ Ⓓ
72. Ⓐ Ⓑ Ⓒ Ⓓ
73. Ⓐ Ⓑ Ⓒ Ⓓ
74. Ⓐ Ⓑ Ⓒ Ⓓ
75. Ⓐ Ⓑ Ⓒ Ⓓ
76. Ⓐ Ⓑ Ⓒ Ⓓ
77. Ⓐ Ⓑ Ⓒ Ⓓ
78. Ⓐ Ⓑ Ⓒ Ⓓ
79. Ⓐ Ⓑ Ⓒ Ⓓ
80. Ⓐ Ⓑ Ⓒ Ⓓ
81. Ⓐ Ⓑ Ⓒ Ⓓ
82. Ⓐ Ⓑ Ⓒ Ⓓ
83. Ⓐ Ⓑ Ⓒ Ⓓ
84. Ⓐ Ⓑ Ⓒ Ⓓ
85. Ⓐ Ⓑ Ⓒ Ⓓ
86. Ⓐ Ⓑ Ⓒ Ⓓ
87. Ⓐ Ⓑ Ⓒ Ⓓ
88. Ⓐ Ⓑ Ⓒ Ⓓ
89. Ⓐ Ⓑ Ⓒ Ⓓ
90. Ⓐ Ⓑ Ⓒ Ⓓ
91. Ⓐ Ⓑ Ⓒ Ⓓ
92. Ⓐ Ⓑ Ⓒ Ⓓ

SECTION 4: Biological Sciences

93. Ⓐ Ⓑ Ⓒ Ⓓ
94. Ⓐ Ⓑ Ⓒ Ⓓ
95. Ⓐ Ⓑ Ⓒ Ⓓ
96. Ⓐ Ⓑ Ⓒ Ⓓ
97. Ⓐ Ⓑ Ⓒ Ⓓ

98. Ⓐ Ⓑ Ⓒ Ⓓ
99. Ⓐ Ⓑ Ⓒ Ⓓ
100. Ⓐ Ⓑ Ⓒ Ⓓ
101. Ⓐ Ⓑ Ⓒ Ⓓ
102. Ⓐ Ⓑ Ⓒ Ⓓ
103. Ⓐ Ⓑ Ⓒ Ⓓ
104. Ⓐ Ⓑ Ⓒ Ⓓ
105. Ⓐ Ⓑ Ⓒ Ⓓ
106. Ⓐ Ⓑ Ⓒ Ⓓ
107. Ⓐ Ⓑ Ⓒ Ⓓ
108. Ⓐ Ⓑ Ⓒ Ⓓ
109. Ⓐ Ⓑ Ⓒ Ⓓ
110. Ⓐ Ⓑ Ⓒ Ⓓ
111. Ⓐ Ⓑ Ⓒ Ⓓ
112. Ⓐ Ⓑ Ⓒ Ⓓ
113. Ⓐ Ⓑ Ⓒ Ⓓ
114. Ⓐ Ⓑ Ⓒ Ⓓ
115. Ⓐ Ⓑ Ⓒ Ⓓ
116. Ⓐ Ⓑ Ⓒ Ⓓ
117. Ⓐ Ⓑ Ⓒ Ⓓ
118. Ⓐ Ⓑ Ⓒ Ⓓ
119. Ⓐ Ⓑ Ⓒ Ⓓ
120. Ⓐ Ⓑ Ⓒ Ⓓ
121. Ⓐ Ⓑ Ⓒ Ⓓ
122. Ⓐ Ⓑ Ⓒ Ⓓ
123. Ⓐ Ⓑ Ⓒ Ⓓ
124. Ⓐ Ⓑ Ⓒ Ⓓ
125. Ⓐ Ⓑ Ⓒ Ⓓ
126. Ⓐ Ⓑ Ⓒ Ⓓ
127. Ⓐ Ⓑ Ⓒ Ⓓ
128. Ⓐ Ⓑ Ⓒ Ⓓ
129. Ⓐ Ⓑ Ⓒ Ⓓ
130. Ⓐ Ⓑ Ⓒ Ⓓ
131. Ⓐ Ⓑ Ⓒ Ⓓ
132. Ⓐ Ⓑ Ⓒ Ⓓ
133. Ⓐ Ⓑ Ⓒ Ⓓ
134. Ⓐ Ⓑ Ⓒ Ⓓ
135. Ⓐ Ⓑ Ⓒ Ⓓ
136. Ⓐ Ⓑ Ⓒ Ⓓ
137. Ⓐ Ⓑ Ⓒ Ⓓ
138. Ⓐ Ⓑ Ⓒ Ⓓ
139. Ⓐ Ⓑ Ⓒ Ⓓ
140. Ⓐ Ⓑ Ⓒ Ⓓ
141. Ⓐ Ⓑ Ⓒ Ⓓ
142. Ⓐ Ⓑ Ⓒ Ⓓ
143. Ⓐ Ⓑ Ⓒ Ⓓ
144. Ⓐ Ⓑ Ⓒ Ⓓ

SECTION 1
Physical Sciences

TIME: 70 Minutes

QUESTIONS: 1–52

DIRECTIONS: Most of the questions in this section are arranged in groups, each corresponding to a descriptive passage. Based on the information given in a passage, choose the one best answer to each question in the group. Some questions are independent of a descriptive passage and of each other. Choose the one best answer to each of these questions. If you are not sure of an answer, eliminate those choices that you know are incorrect and choose an answer from among those remaining. Fill in the corresponding circle on the answer sheet to indicate your answer. You may refer to the periodic table at any time.

PASSAGE I (QUESTIONS 1–5)

A bullet of mass $m_1 = 0.01$ kg is fired with a muzzle speed of 100 m/sec to the RIGHT along the horizontal. The gun recoils with a speed of 1 m/sec. The bullet encounters an approximately constant force of air resistance equal to its weight as it heads toward a block of mass $m_2 = 1$ kg, which is initially at rest on a rough horizontal surface a distance of 10 m from where the bullet was fired. The bullet imbeds itself in the block, a process that takes 0.01 sec from the initial time of contact. The combination bullet-in-block then slides 2 m before coming to rest. Use $g = 10$ m/sec^2.

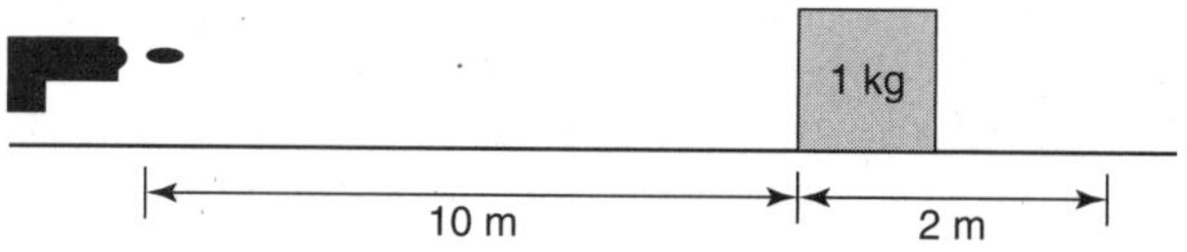

1. The mass of the gun is
   A. 1 g.
   B. 100 g.
   C. 0.01 kg.
   D. 1 kg.

2. The speed of the bullet as it impacted the block was
   A. 100 m/s.
   B. 101 m/s.
   C. 99 m/s.
   D. 0 m/s.

3. The impulse received by the earth during the bullet's flight was
   A. 0.01 kgm/s LEFT.
   B. 0.01 kgm/s RIGHT.
   C. 1 kgm/s RIGHT.
   D. 1 kgm/s LEFT.

4. The average force experienced by the bullet during impact was
   A. 10,000 N.
   B. 9800 N.
   C. 9900 N.
   D. 98 N.

5. The acceleration of the combination over the 2 m slide was
   A. 0.24 m/s^2 LEFT.
   B. 9.8 m/s^2 LEFT.
   C. 49 m/s^2 RIGHT.
   D. 1 m/s^2 LEFT.

PASSAGE II (QUESTIONS 6–8)

Carbon dioxide is soluble in water and is used to carbonate soft drinks. Tommy's favorite part of drinking pop is the fizz. He discovered, to his mother's annoyance, that he can create more fizz by adding teaspoons of sugar to his drink. The solubility of CO_2 in pure water is 1.45g of CO_2/1L at 298K. After his initial discovery, Tommy begins experimenting with other solutes.

6. If he adds equal molar amounts of NaCl and sucrose to adjacent glasses of pop, how would the volume of CO_2 evolved from the glass containing salt compare with that evolved from the glass with added sugar?
   A. The soda with salt added would produce half the volume produced from adding sugar.
   B. Both glasses would produce the same volume of CO_2 because equal molar amounts of NaCl and sucrose were added.
   C. The soda with salt added would produce twice as much volume as the soda with added sugar.
   D. Adding NaCl would not cause any CO_2 gas to be evolved.

7. Aspartame is an artificial sweetener found in many diet sodas. It has a formula weight of 294.31 g/mole. Sucrose has a formula weight of 342.30 g/mole. What would you expect if equal masses of sucrose and aspartame were added to two adjacent glasses of soda?
   A. The glass containing sucrose would release more CO_2.
   B. The glass containing aspartame would release more CO_2.
   C. Both glasses would release the same amount of CO_2.
   D. Adding aspartame would not cause any CO_2 gas to be evolved.

8. While eating at a diner, Tommy's father, a chemistry professor, asks the waitress for low-sodium salt. The waitress brings him two unlabeled saltshakers. One contains pure NaCl, and the other contains the low-sodium variety. The low-sodium variety is a mixture of NaCl and KCl. Using his knowledge of colligative properties, Tommy's father pours equal masses of each into separate glasses of seltzer water to determine which one was the KCl/NaCl mixture. How can he determine which shaker contains the low-sodium salt?
   A. The NaCl/KCl mixture should cause twice as much CO_2 to be evolved.
   B. The NaCl/KCl mixture should cause half as much CO_2 to be evolved.
   C. The NaCl/KCl mixture should cause less CO_2 to be evolved.
   D. The NaCl/KCl mixture should cause more CO_2 to be evolved.

PASSAGE III (QUESTIONS 9–12)

In a bungee fall (also known as a bungee jump), the bungee cord is tied around the person's ankle, the person falls head first, and (hopefully) doesn't hit the ground when the cord is fully stretched, just before the person springs back upward. There are various ways to model the physics of a bungee fall. In the simplest model, the bungee cord is considered to obey Hooke's Law exactly; that is, it performs like a perfect massless spring where the force is proportional to the stretch length and the proportionality constant is known as the spring constant. The stretch length refers to the length that the spring is stretched beyond its equilibrium (unstretched) length. Also, the energy of the perfect spring is purely mechanical; no energy is transferred to thermal energy, so it behaves as if there were no damping forces that would attenuate the oscillation amplitude.

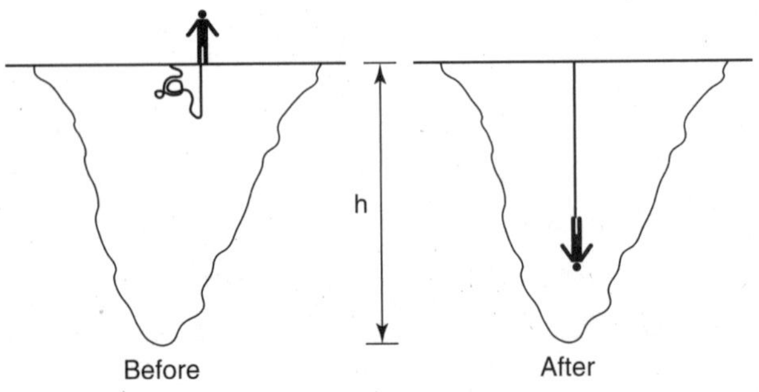

In a more accurate model, the real elastic properties of a bungee cord are measured and used to determine the stretch length of the cord in an actual fall. A sample curve for the force applied on a bungee cord as a function of stretch length is shown below.

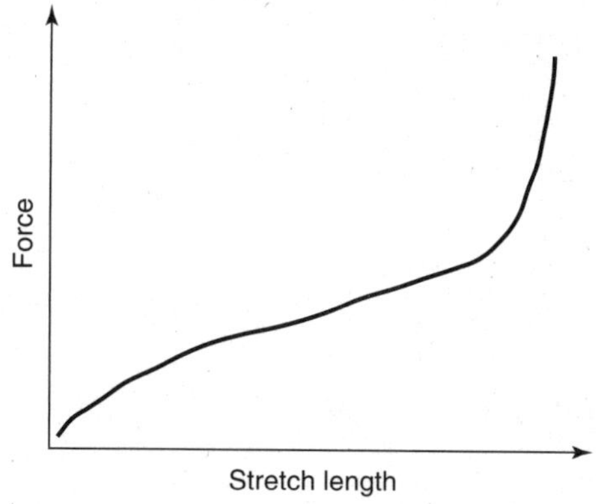

One obtains a more accurate approximation of a real bungee cord by including the conversion of mechanical energy into thermal energy as the cord is stretched. This conversion of energy results in damped oscillations for the person following the bungee fall. As time progresses, they oscillate with successively smaller and smaller amplitude. The amplitude, A, follows a negative exponential as a function of time according to the equation, $A = A_o e^{-\lambda t}$. The decay constant, λ, determines how quickly the oscillations attenuate. Sample data for the natural log of the amplitude of oscillation of a man on a bungee cord as a function of time are shown below.

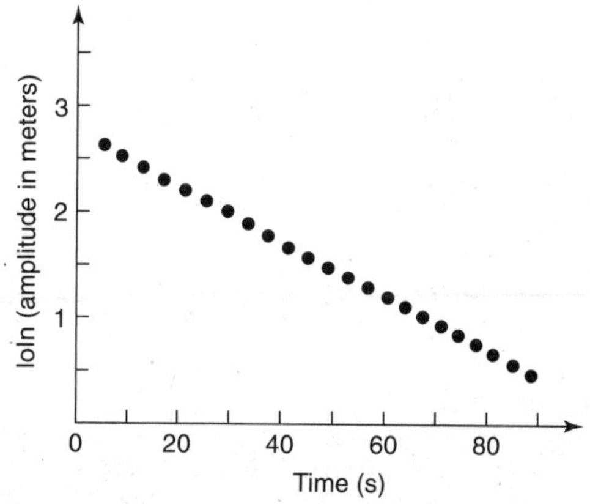

For the following questions, neglect air resistance.

9. An 80-kg man performs a bungee fall. When the man is at the bottom of the fall, the cord is stretched an additional 30 m from its unstretched length. At the bottom of the fall, the man is located 90 m below the point from which he fell. Assuming that this bungee cord behaves like a perfect massless spring, determine its spring constant.
   A. 650 kg/s^2
   B. 360 kg/s^2
   C. 240 kg/s^2
   D. 160 kg/s^2

10. What is the approximate oscillation frequency of the 80-kg man as he moves up and down following the fall? Again, assume that the bungee cord behaves like a perfect massless spring with a spring constant of 300 kg/s^2.
    A. 4 Hz
    B. 1 Hz
    C. 0.3 Hz
    D. 0.08 Hz

11. From the graph of the force versus stretch length, at what length is the bungee cord most elastic? That is, where does a given force change produce the greatest change in length?
    A. When the cord is short before it has been stretched
    B. When the cord is long after it has been significantly stretched
    C. When the cord has been stretched by a moderate amount
    D. The elasticity is the same no matter what the length of the cord.

12. From the graph of attenuating amplitude with time, determine the approximate value of the decay constant for attenuation.
    A. 0.02 s^{-1}
    B. 0.4 s^{-1}
    C. 4 s^{-1}
    D. 100 s^{-1}

QUESTIONS 13–16 are NOT based on a descriptive passage.

13. What is the total resistance of the circuit below?
    A. 12 Ω
    B. 4.7 Ω
    C. 8/3 Ω
    D. 2 Ω

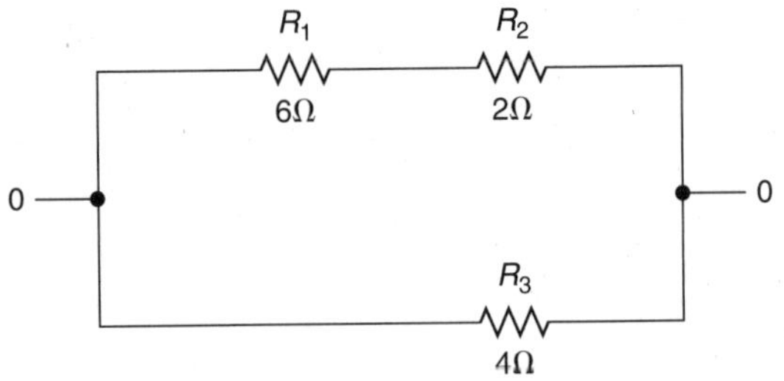

14. Two forces of 10 newtons and 6 newtons act on an object. In order to produce a resultant force of 4 newtons, how many degrees apart must they be oriented with respect to each other?
    A. 45°
    B. 60°
    C. 90°
    D. 180°

15. A 25-lb cannonball is shot from a cannon horizontally situated 3 ft above the ground. The muzzle velocity is 550 ft/sec. At the same time, an identical 25-lb cannonball is dropped from the same 3 ft height. Assuming ideal conditions, the dropped cannonball will strike the ground
    A. before the one that was shot.
    B. with a lesser vertical velocity than the shot cannonball.
    C. with greater vertical velocity than the shot cannonball.
    D. at the same time as the one that was shot.

16. A 100-gram marble strikes a 25-gram marble lying on a smooth horizontal surface squarely. In the impact, the speed of the larger marble is reduced from 100 cm/sec to 60 cm/sec. What is the speed of the smaller marble immediately after impact?
    A. 60 cm/sec
    B. 100 cm/sec
    C. 40 cm/sec
    D. 160 cm/sec

PASSAGE IV (QUESTIONS 17–26)

The laws of thermodynamics are especially relevant in today's society, considering the problems that we face in supplying the nation with energy. Are we really running out of energy? How long will it take? What are the consequences of using various types of energy? These questions involve many of the principles of thermodynamics. You should be familiar with terms such as state function, energy, entropy, enthalpy and free energy, and the equations associated with the laws. The following is some useful information for working problems in this section.

Bond Energies (kcal/mole)

H – H	104	C – O	83
H – F	135	C = O	178
H – O	111	O = O	118
H – Cl	103	Cl – Cl	58
C – Cl	79	C = C	146
H – C	87	C – C	83

Heats of Formation (kcal/mole)

CO (g)	–26.4	Fe_3O_4 (s)	–267
CO_2 (g)	–94.1	FeO (s)	–63.7
Fe_2O_3 (s)	–197	SO_2 (g)	–71.0

Free Energy of Reaction (kJ/mole)

CO (g) $\frac{1}{2}O_2$ (g) $\rightarrow$ CO_2 (g) –257.2

	$G°_f$ (kJ/mo)	$H°_f$ (kJ/mol)	$S°_f$ (J/mol K)
Fe_3O_4 (s)	–1018	–1121	145.3
FeO (s)	NA	–272.0	60.75
Fe_2O_3 (s)	–743.6	–825.5	87.40
CH_3CH_2OH (l)	–174.8	–277.6	161
CH_3CHO (g)	–133.7	–166	266
H_2O (g)		–242	188.7
H_2O (l)		–286	–

Experiment 1

This experiment was designed to study the vaporization of water.

$$H_2O\ (l) \longleftrightarrow H_2O\ (g)$$

Experiment 2

In this experiment, the change in entropy involved in the vaporization of one mole of Freon, CCl_2F_2 (coolant used in refrigeration and air conditioning), at 25° was found to be

57.7 J/(mol K). These chloro-floro-hydrocarbons are believed to be responsible for the depletion occurring in the ozone layer above the earth.

Experiment 3

It has been found that alkenes undergo addition reactions in the presence of halogens rather than the substitution reactions observed with alkanes (catalyst needed for alkanes). The following is an example of an addition reaction using ethene (ethylene):

$$C_2H_4 + Cl_2 \longrightarrow C_2H_4Cl_2$$

Experiment 4

The most desirable iron ores contain hematite, Fe_2O_3, or magnetite, Fe_3O_4. The oxide is reduced in blast furnaces by carbon monoxide:

$$Fe_2O_3\ (s) + 3CO\ (g) \longrightarrow 2Fe\ (s) + 3CO_2\ (g)$$

Most of the oxide is reduced to molten iron by the carbon monoxide, although some is reduced directly by coke (carbon):

$$Fe_2O_3\ (s) + 3C\ (s) \longrightarrow 2Fe\ (l) + 3CO\ (g)$$

Experiment 5

In another oxidation-reduction reaction, iron is oxidized to form magnetite, while the carbon in carbon dioxide is reduced to form carbon monoxide:

$$3FeO\ (s) + CO_2\ (g) \longrightarrow Fe_3O_4\ (s) + CO\ (g)$$

Experiment 6

The first reaction is simply a condensation reaction:

$$H_2O\ (g) \longrightarrow H_2O\ (l) \qquad (1)$$

The following reaction is a decomposition reaction involving limestone:

$$CaCO_3\ (s) \longrightarrow CaO\ (s) + CO_2\ (g) \qquad (2)$$

In the blast furnace used in Experiment 5, coke is mixed with limestone, and crushed iron ore is admitted at the top of the furnace as the "charge." A blast of hot air from the bottom burns the coke to carbon monoxide with the evolution of more heat:

$$2C\ (s) + O_2\ (g) \longrightarrow 2CO\ (g) + \text{heat}$$

The limestone, called a flux, is added to react with the silica gangue in the ore to form a molten slag of calcium silicate.

$$CaO\ (s) + SiO_2\ (s)\ (\text{gangue}) \longrightarrow \underset{(\text{slag})}{CaSiO_3}\ (l)$$

Experiment 7

Ethanol, or ethyl alcohol, was first prepared by fermentation a long time ago—the most ancient literature contains references to beverages that were obviously alcoholic! The fermentation of blackstrap molasses, the residue from the purification of cane sugar, sucrose, is one important source of ethanol:

$$C_{12}H_{22}O_{11} + H_2O \xrightarrow{\text{yeast}} 4CH_3CH_2OH + 4CO_2$$

In one experiment, the oxidation of ethanol results in the formation of acetaldehyde and hydrogen. Many different reagents can be used to oxidize ethanol.

$$CH_3CH_2OH\ (l) \longrightarrow CH_3CHO\ (g) + H_2\ (g)$$

Experiment 8

The internal energy, E, of a specific amount of a substance represents all the energy contained within the substance. It includes all kinds of energy. The difference between the internal energy of the products and the internal energy of the reactants of a chemical reaction of physical change is related to the heat lost or gained and the work done on or by the system.

In this experiment, a gas is heated up and gains 65 J of heat from the surroundings. As the gas heats up, it does work on the surroundings equal to 22 J.

Experiment 9

The following reaction involves the oxidation of iron in ferrous oxide to form hematite, Fe_2O_3, but it can also be classified as a combination reaction:

$$4FeO\ (s) + O_2\ (g) \longrightarrow 2Fe_2O_3\ (s)$$

17. Consider the reaction in Experiment 1. What is the energy needed to change two moles of liquid water into water vapor?
A. 484 kJ B. 572 kJ
C. 377.4 kJ D. 88 kJ

18. Use the data in Experiment 2 to determine the heat that will be evolved when 100 grams of liquid Freon vaporizes at 25°C.
A. −14.2 kJ B. 14.2 kJ
C. −17.2 kJ D. 17.2 kJ

19. Given the bond energies in the passage and the reaction studied in Experiment 3, calculate the energy change in the reaction that resulted.
A. 42 B. −37
C. +37 D. 47

20. Find the heat (enthalpy) of reaction for the reduction of hematite with carbon monoxide as discussed in Experiment 4.
A. −28 B. 28
C. 486.4 D. −486.4

21. Determine the heat (enthalpy) of reaction for the equation under study in Experiment 5.
A. −8.2 B. 8.2
C. 136.5 D. −135.6

22. Consider the reactions under study in Experiment 6. Increasing the temperature in these reactions would make
A. both more spontaneous.
B. both less spontaneous.
C. (1) more spontaneous and (2) less spontaneous.
D. (2) more spontaneous and (1) less spontaneous.

23. In Experiment 7, suppose that 100 gm of ethanol are oxidized. Approximately how many moles of hydrogen gas are produced?
A. 0.5 moles B. 1 mole
C. 2 moles D. 4 moles

24. What are q, w, and the change in internal energy for the conditions described in Experiment 8?
A. $q = +65$; $w = +22$; E = +43
B. $q = +65$; $w = -22$; E = +87
C. $q = -65$; $w = -22$; E = +87
D. $q = -65$; $w = +22$; E = −87

25. Consider the reaction discussed in Experiment 9. Which of the following sets of answers will be the correct signs for each of the quantities?
A. $H = +$; $S = +$; $G = ?$
B. $H = -$; $S = -$; $G = ?$
C. $H = +$; $S = -$; $G = +$
D. $H = -$; $S = +$; $G = -$

26. Consider the following phase diagram. Point *B* on this diagram represents

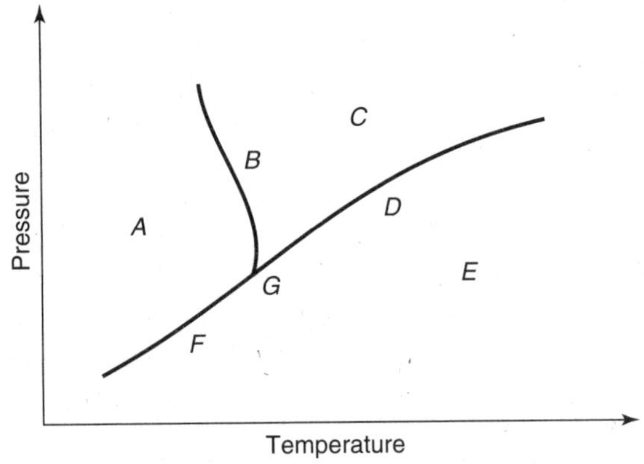

A. solid, liquid, and equilibrium
B. liquid, gas, and equilibrium
C. solid, gas, and equilibrium
D. solid, liquid, gas, and equilibrium

PASSAGE V (QUESTIONS 27–30)

The solenoid that is connected to the starter in your automobile may look something like the one pictured below. S is your ignition switch, which allows the solenoid to draw current from your 12-volt battery. This energizes the solenoid, which then produces a magnetic field in opposition to that of the permanent magnet in its core. As a result, the permanent magnet is pushed upward, closing the contact of a spring switch that connects the starter to your battery and allowing it to draw sufficient current to start your car. The solenoid has resistance $R = 3\Omega$ and is wound about a core with a permeability of $\mu = 25 \times 10^{-7}$ H/m. When the ignition switch is closed, the magnetic field (B) at the center of the solenoid is measured to be 0.1 T.

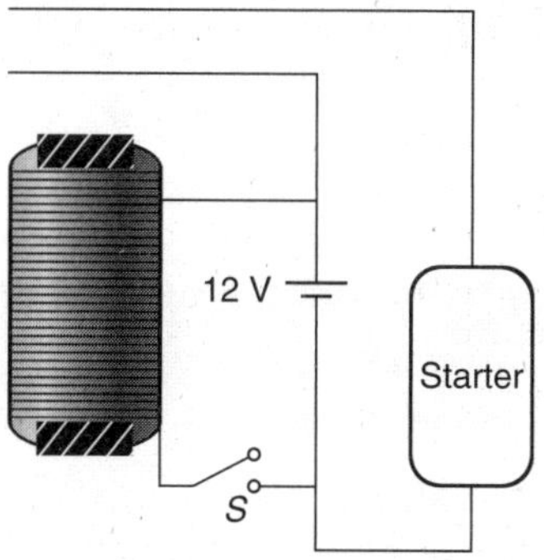

27. What current will flow in the solenoid when the ignition switch is closed?
    A. 0.25 A B. 4 A
    C. 36 A D. 120 A

28. What is the number of turns per unit length of coil that comprises this solenoid?
    A. 10,000 B. 160,000
    C. 1,100 D. 500

29. The quantity that is computed as the product of the magnetic field strength (B) times the cross-sectional area (A) of the solenoid is called
    A. magnetic flux.
    B. the magnetic field.
    C. electromagnetic radiation.
    D. a Faraday.

30. The process by which the permanent magnet reacts by being pushed upward from the solenoid is called magnetic
    A. induction.
    B. deduction.
    C. invasion.
    D. repulsion.

PASSAGE VI (QUESTIONS 31–33)

A truck driver in Minnesota pulls into a warehouse in the middle of winter. The temperature outside is −10°F, and the temperature inside is 50°F. After the truck is unloaded, it can no longer fit through the garage door. The shock absorbers, without the load, have expanded and made the truck taller. The truck driver releases air from the tires until the truck can fit out the door. He then drives to the nearest gas station to refill his tires. The tires, when filled to capacity, have a volume of 30 *L*. Overfilling the tires will only increase the pressure but not the volume in the tires. The trucker then drives home and parks in his garage.

31. The pressure inside the tires before the trucker pulls into the warehouse is 30 psi. What is the pressure inside the tires when they come to thermal equilibrium with the inside of the warehouse? (Assume that the mass of the truck and its load have no effect on the pressure, and that there is no change in volume.)
    A. 12.9 psi B. 26.5 psi
    C. 34.0 psi D. 50 psi

32. What volume would the air occupy if the truck driver released all of the air from 1 tire inside the warehouse?
    A. 14.7 L B. 61.2 L
    C. 69.4 L D. 122.4 L

33. If the air in the tire is composed of 80% N_2 and 20% O_2 by mass, what is the partial pressure exerted by the N_2 gas in the tire when the truck is inside the warehouse?
    A. 24.0 psi B. 24.6 psi
    C. 28.6 psi D. 1.8 atm

PASSAGE VII (QUESTIONS 34–37)

A robot used to deliver parts along an assembly line is programmed so that its time at each station is minimized and correlated with the work being done on the line. Its motion has been modeled with the use of simple linear fitting so that its accelerations are assumed constant over different time intervals. A portion of this modeling over an eight-second interval is shown in the graph below.

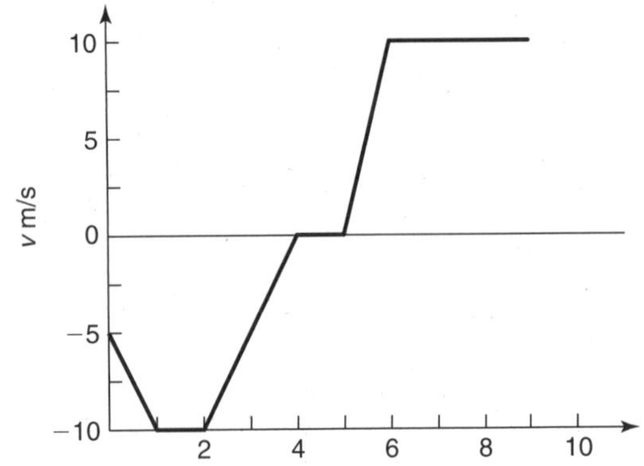

34. What is the robot's speed at $t = 1.5$ seconds?

A. 0 m/s B. 10 m/s

C. 5 m/s D. 10 m/sec^2

35. What is the robot's average speed between $t = 2$ and $t = 4$ seconds?

A. 0 m/s B. 5 m/s

C. 3.33 m/s D. 10 m/s

36. The robot is at rest at

A. 4.5 s. B. 1.5 s.

C. 6.5 sec. D. 7 sec.

37. What is the robot's average acceleration between $t = 4$ and $t = 7$ seconds?

A. 0 m/s^2 B. 5 m/s^2

C. 10 m/s^2 D. 3.33 m/s^2

QUESTIONS 38–40 are NOT based on a descriptive passage.

38. How many coulombs of charge are required to plate out 127 g of Cu^{2+} (molecular weight of Cu = 63.5 g/mole)?

A. 2 C B. 3 C

C. 4 C D. 5 C

39. If the average adult inhales 300 L of air a day, how much oxygen will be inhaled in that length of time? (Air is composed of 78% N_2, 20% O_2, and 2% other elements.)

A. 60 L B. 15 L

C. 600 L D. 6 L

40. Compound X has an atomic number of 25. It forms an ion with the electronic configuration,

$1s^2\ 2s^2\ 2p^6\ 3s^2\ 3p^6\ 3d^5$.

What is the proper ionic symbol for X?

A. X^+ B. X^{2+}

C. X^{3+} D. X^{4+}

PASSAGE VIII (QUESTIONS 41–44)

Carbon has 4 valence electrons. The electron configuration for carbon is $[He]2s^22p^2$. The s atomic orbital lies closer to the nucleus than the p orbitals and is therefore lower in energy. All three p orbitals are equivalent in energy and are orthoganol (90°) to one another. Covalent bond formation occurs through the overlap of atomic orbitals.

Methane (CH_4), a greenhouse gas, is composed of one carbon covalently bonded to 4 hydrogens. The covalent bonds in methane form the overlap of 1s orbitals of the hydrogen atoms with the atomic orbitals on carbon. If you were to construct methane in this way and combined the hydrogen 1s orbitals with the orbitals on carbon, you would get a strange result. The structure you would obtain would have one short bond (from the overlap of the C 2s orbital and a hydrogen 1s orbital) and three longer bonds of equal length that are 90° apart (from the overlap of three 2p orbitals with 1s orbitals on three hydrogens). Experimental evidence proves this structure to be wrong. Methane is tetrahedral, with all of its bond lengths (110pm) and bond angles (~109°) being equivalent.

To get a structure for methane that more closely approximates reality, we must use the concept of orbital hybridization. Orbital hybridization allows us to "mix" atomic orbitals to yield

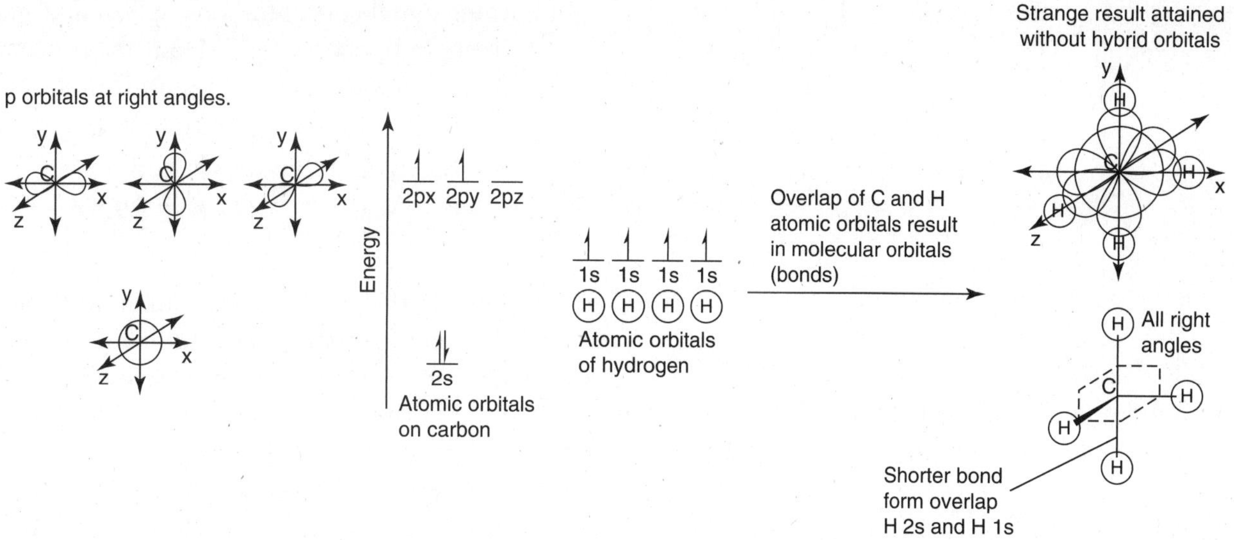

new hybrid atomic orbitals. To get the structure of methane, we need 4 equivalent atomic orbitals on carbon. This can be accomplished by hybridizing the 2s and three 2p orbitals. This results in four new sp^3 hybrid atomic orbitals. Each new sp^3 orbital is identical in energy and shape and oriented 109° relative to each other. Overlap of these sp^3 hybrid orbitals with the 1s orbitals on the hydrogens provides a more accurate picture of methane, which has 4 equivalent bonds and has a tetrahedral geometry.

41. Which energy diagram best represents the hybrid orbitals of carbon in methane?

A.

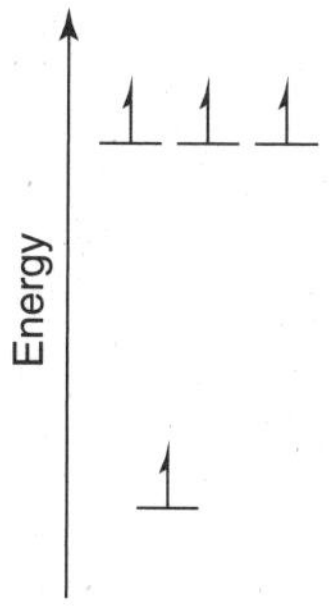

B.

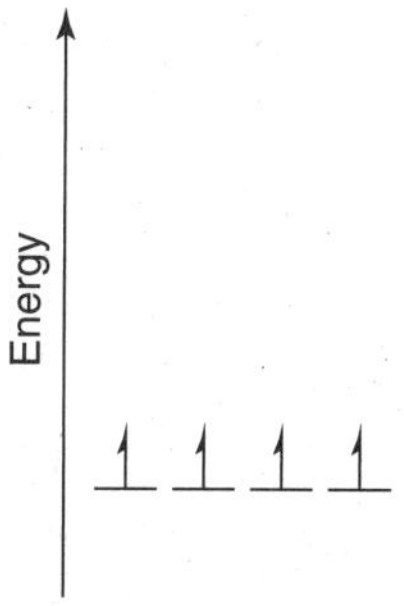

C.

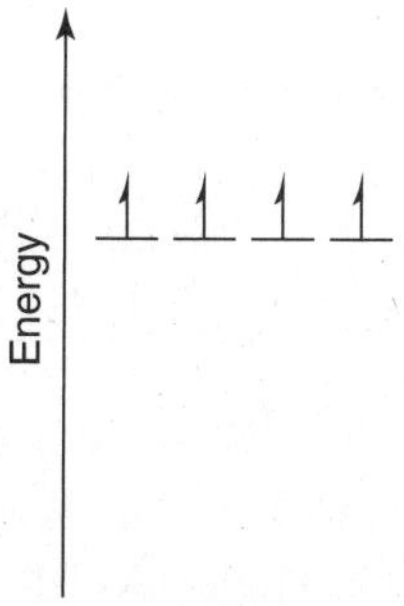

D.

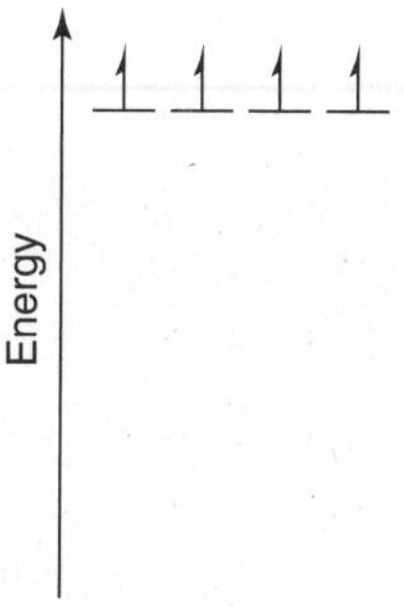

42. How many molecular orbitals are produced in the formation of methane by the overlap of 1s orbitals of four hydrogen and the four sp^3 orbitals on carbon?

A. 4 B. 8

C. 16 D. 6

43. Ethylene contains a carbon-carbon double bond. The carbons involved in this bond are both sp^2 hybridized. The double bond consists of one sigma and one pi bond. The sigma bond results from the overlap of two sp^2 hybrid atomic orbitals. The pi bond results from the overlap of unhybridized p atomic orbitals. What is the correct energy diagram for an sp^2 hybridized carbon in ethylene?

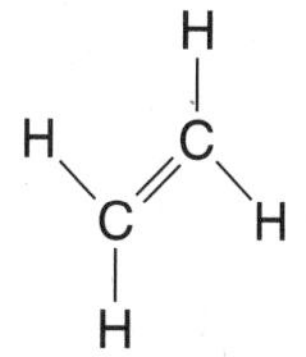

A.

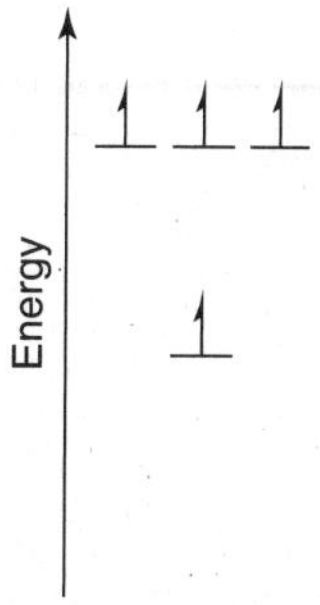

B.

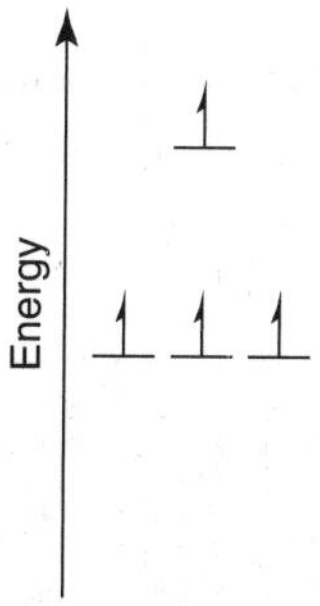

C.

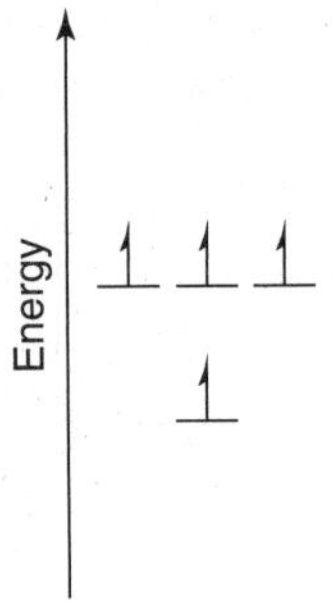

D.

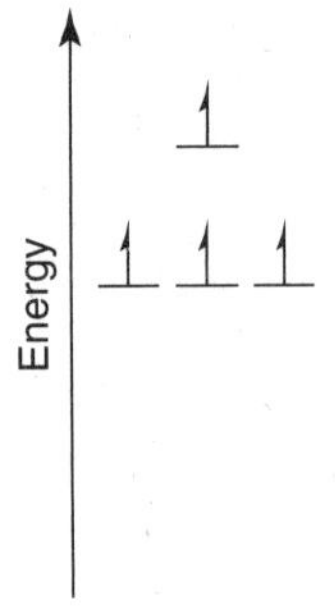

44. What is the hybridization of phosphorous in each step of the following reaction?

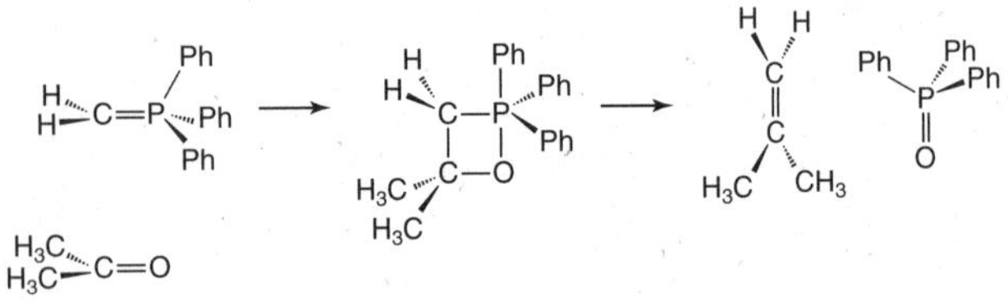

A. sp^3, sp^3d, sp^3 B. sp^3d, sp^3d, sp^3d
C. sp^3, sp^3, sp^3 D. sp^2, sp^3d, sp^2

PASSAGE IX (QUESTIONS 45–48)

Aqueous bromine solutions react with alkenes to form bromohydrins. Bromohydrins are useful starting materials in organic synthesis. The net reaction for the reaction of bromine with 2-methyl propene, as well as its proposed mechanism, is shown below.

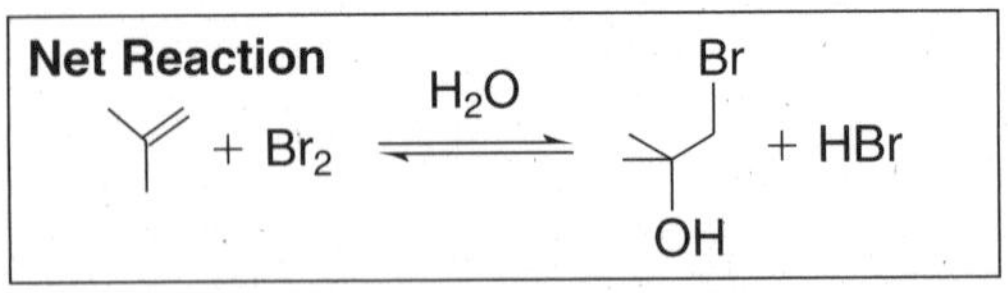

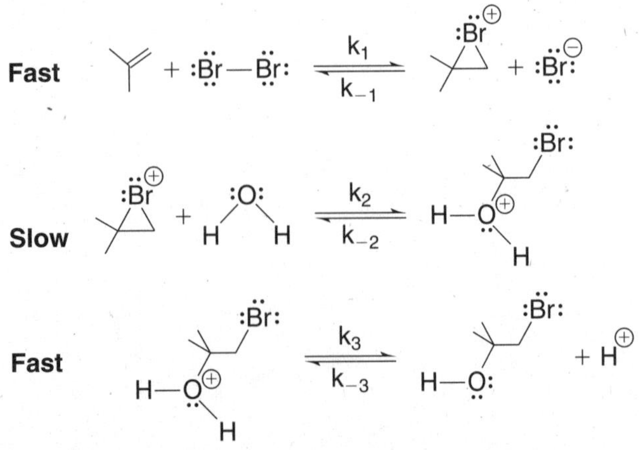

45. If the initial concentrations of bromine and 3-methylpropene are 0.25M, and the concentration of product at equilibrium is 0.1M, what is the value of the equilibrium constant?

A. K = 0.444 B. K = 3.33
C. K = 4.44 D. K = 29.6

46. During the reaction, the concentrations of 3-methylpropene, bromine, and bromohydrin were found to be 0.08M, 0.6M, and 0.82M, respectively. If the equilibrium constant is K = 15.0, what is the reaction quotient, and in which direction must the reaction proceed to reach equilibrium?

A. Q = 14.0; the reaction will proceed to the right.
B. Q = 14.0; the reaction will proceed to the left.
C. Q = 17.1; the reaction will proceed to the right.
D. Q = 17.1; the reaction will proceed to the left.

47. What is the rate law for the reaction?

A. $k[H_2O][Br_2][C_4H_8]$; $k = k_2\,(k_1/k_{-1})$
B. $k[C_4H_8][Br_2]$; $k = (k_1k_2/k_{-1}k_{-2})$
C. $k[C_4H_8][Br_2]$; $k = k_2(k_1/k_{-1})$
D. $k([C_4H_8][Br_2])^{1/2}$; $k = k_2\,(k_1/k_{-1})^{1/2}$

48. If the amount of water were doubled, what effect would it have on the rate of the reaction?

A. The rate of reaction would be halved.
B. Water does not appear in the rate law, so doubling the amount of water would have no effect on the rate.
C. The rate of reaction would double.
D. The rate of the reaction would be quadrupled.

PASSAGE X (QUESTIONS 49–52)

Defibrillators are devices designed to deliver a large electric current to the chest to stop heart fibrillations that occur during a heart attack. The potential difference between the terminals of a battery is first transferred to a capacitor. A special circuit then repeatedly steps up this potential difference until the potential between the two capacitor plates is in the thousands of volts. A paddle is then connected to each capacitor plate, and the paddles are placed on the chest. The voltage across the capacitor plates is transferred to the chest cavity for a very short amount of time. A large current flows to stimulate the heart back to its normal rhythm.

Typical defibrillators have a parallel plate capacitor with a capacitance equal to 100 mF and operate at 5000 volts. Between the locations of the paddles on the chest, the resistance of the chest can be modeled as three resistors in parallel, one for higher-resistance tissues (for example, bone), moderate-resistance tissues (for example, muscle), and low-resistance tissues (for example, blood). For an average chest, these tissues would have resistances of 6000, 2000, and 1000 ohms, respectively.

49. If all of thc energy stored in the capacitor is transferred to the chest, how much energy is transferred to the chest?

A. 100 J B. 625 J
C. 1250 J D. 2500 J

50. How much current is delivered to the average chest when a typical defibrillator is used?

A. 40 A B. 24 A
C. 15 A D. 8.3 A

51. If the capacitor in the defibrillator device consists of two parallel plates separated by a distance of 2 mm and no dielectric is used, what is the electric field between these plates?

A. 500,000 N/C
B. 2,500,000 N/C
C. 800,000 N/C
D. 1,650,000 N/C

52. Suppose that the parallel plate capacitor in the defibrillator is charged to 5000 volts and then isolated from the electric circuit. The parallel plate capacitor is then connected in parallel to another identical parallel plate capacitor so that the charges distribute equally between the two capacitors. What is the ratio of energy stored in this parallel combination to the energy stored in the original single capacitor?

A. 1/2 B. 2/1
C. 1/4 D. 1/1

STOP!

If time still remains, you may review work only in this section. When the time allotted is up, you may go on to the next section.

STOP!

SECTION 2
Verbal Reasoning

TIME: 60 Minutes

QUESTIONS: 53–92

DIRECTIONS: The verbal reasoning section contains nine passages, each followed by a series of questions. Based on the information given in a passage, choose the one best answer to each question.

PASSAGE I (QUESTIONS 53-57)

Granting that computer literacy consists in knowing what sorts of skills and what levels of skills can and should be taught using computers, where should the literate educator stand on the question?

Computers are marvelous tools that, when used as electronic blackboards, interactive simulators, and conjecture testers, greatly improve sociality and intuition in the classroom. Provided one does not narrow one's goal to forcing the student to think procedurally like a computerized problem-solver, there is no limit to the level of skill that imaginative new learning environments may be able to foster. Computers are also useful as rule-following, literal-minded tutees, as long as one limits oneself to teaching elementary math and programming, as most LOGO users now do.

But the outlook for the computer as tutor is less bright. If one accepts our skill model, one is forced to conclude that the level of skill appropriately taught using the computer is quite limited. At the beginning level, the computer can be useful for drill and practice in subjects requiring nothing more than the memorization of facts, rules, and procedures such as spelling and subtraction. In restricted areas, where trained competence, not educated expertise, is the goal, computers and interactive media like videodisks may indeed prove useful. However, one should not attempt to tutor any higher level of skill, for that would require giving logic machines skills that have proven to be beyond their capacities.

We have seen that the advocates of computers as tutors and tutees think, like Socrates and Plato, that we cannot teach what we do not understand and that we only understand what we can formulate in the sorts of rules and procedures used by a logic machine. If that were true, teachers could be gradually replaced by computers. But teachers are no doubt aware, and parents must become aware, that expertise in teaching does not consist in knowing complicated rules about their discipline and about coaching — what tips to give, when to keep silent, when to intervene — although teachers may have learned such rules in graduate school. What an expert teacher gains from experience is not more facts about some field plus rules of coaching of the sort he or she once explicitly followed as a beginner; rather, the teacher learns intuitively and spontaneously to draw on the commonsense knowledge and experience he or she shares with the student in order to provide the tips and examples needed by the advanced beginner. The teacher also learns how to motivate the involved practice by which a student gains experience in any domain.

From Hubert L. Dreyfus and Stuart E. Dreyfus, *Mind over Machine,* 1986.

53. The primary subject of the passage is
    A. what constitutes computer literacy.
    B. the qualities good teachers must have.

C. appropriate uses of computers in education.

D. limitations of computers as educational tools.

54. The authors believe that computers as educational tools can be effective in developing

I. logical skills.

II. procedural problem-solving skills.

III. classroom sociality.

A. I only

B. I and II

C. II and III

D. I, II, and III

55. One can infer from the passage that the authors believe that the acquisition of expertise derives chiefly from

A. experience and intuition.

B. mastery of the facts in a given discipline.

C. careful coaching and problem-solving.

D. logic combined with informed advice.

56. With which of the following statements would the authors most likely agree?

A. One can teach what one does not understand.

B. Expert teachers derive their expertise largely from rules learned in graduate school.

C. Teachers can be replaced by computers.

D. We only understand what we can formulate in logical rules and procedures.

57. Which of the following statements best summarizes the authors' view of the use of computers in education?

A. Their uses are virtually unlimited.

B. They can be very useful educational tools as long as their limitations are recognized.

C. They can be valuable but are generally abused because people fail to realize that they can be used only as tools, not as tutors or tutees.

D. They are greatly overrated and should seldom be used.

PASSAGE II (QUESTIONS 58–63)

In both oral and typographic cultures, information derives its importance from the possibilities of action. Of course, in any communication environment, input (what one is informed about) always exceeds output (the possibilities of action based on information). But the situation created by telegraphy, and then exacerbated by later technologies, made the relationship between information and action both abstract and remote. For the first time in human history, people were faced with the problem of information glut, which means that simultaneously they were faced with the problem of a diminished social and political potency.

You may get a sense of what this means by asking yourself another series of questions: What steps do you plan to take to reduce the conflict in the Middle East; or the rates of inflation, crime and unemployment? I shall take the liberty of answering for you: You plan to do nothing about them. You may, of course, cast a ballot for someone who claims to have some plans, as well as the power to act. But this you can do only once every two or four years by giving one hour of your time, hardly a satisfying means of expressing the broad range of opinions you hold. Voting, we might say, is next to the last refuge of the politically impotent. The last refuge is, of course, giving your opinion to a pollster, who will get a version of it through a desiccated question, and then will submerge it in a Niagara of similar opinions, and convert them into — what else? — another piece of news. As a result, we have here a great loop of impotence: The news elicits from you a variety of opinions about which you can do nothing except to offer opinions as more news, about which you can equally do nothing.

Prior to the age of telegraphy, the information-action ratio was sufficiently close so that most people had a sense of being able to control some of the contingencies in their lives. What people knew about had action-value. In the information world created by telegraphy, this sense of potency was lost, precisely because the whole world became the context for news. Everything became everyone's business. For the first time, we were sent information that answered no question we had asked, and that, in any case, did not permit the right to reply.

We may say then that the contribution of the telegraph to public discourse was to dignify irrelevance and amplify impotence. But this was not all: Telegraphy also made public discourse essentially incoherent. It created a world "of broken time and broken attention," to use Lewis Mumford's phrase. The principal strength of the telegraph lay in its capacity to move information, not collect it, explain it, or analyze it. In this respect, telegraphy was the exact opposite of typography. Books, for example, are an excellent container for the accumulation, quiet scrutiny, and organized analysis of information and ideas. A book is an attempt to make thought permanent and to contribute to the great conversation conducted by authors of the past. Therefore, civilized people everywhere consider the burning of a book a vile form of anti-intellectualism. But the telegraph demands that we burn its contents. The value of telegraphy is undermined by applying the tests of permanence, continuity, or coherence. The telegraph is suited only to the flashing of messages, each to be quickly replaced by a more up-to-date message.

Adapted from Neil Postman, *Amusing Ourselves to Death*, 1985.

58. The author regards voting chiefly as
    A. a satisfying way of expressing an individual's various political beliefs.
    B. a way of directly contributing to the solution of important national and international problems.
    C. the crucial act upon which democracy depends.
    D. a relatively ineffective expression of powerlessness.

59. From the passage, it is clear that the author regards polls chiefly as
    A. a means of manufacturing news.
    B. an effective way of influencing public opinion.
    C. an attempt to shape foreign and domestic policy.
    D. part of a system of political checks and balances.

60. "Information-action ratio" refers to
    A. the relationship between accurate information and government policies based on accurate information.
    B. the degree to which people can take meaningful action on the basis of information they receive.
    C. the individual's need to have global and not merely local news.
    D. the relationship between historical facts and current events.

61. According to the author, people in pre-telegraphic cultures had a greater sense of being able to control some of the contingencies in their lives than people in telegraphic cultures because
    A. the context of their news was less global.
    B. they derived their news chiefly from oral sources.
    C. their news had less action-value.
    D. there was greater personal contact between individuals.

62. According to the author, telegraphy has
    I. made public discourse more incoherent.
    II. increased the flow of irrelevant information.

III. given individuals a greater sense of social responsibility.

A. I only

B. I and II

C. I and III

D. I, II, and III

63. The author's statement that the "telegraph is suited only to the flashing of messages" is designed to support his contention that telegraphy

A. dignifies irrelevance.

B. increases the individual's sense of political impotence.

C. created a world of broken time and broken attention.

D. makes the relationship between information and action abstract.

PASSAGE III (QUESTIONS 64–69)

We base our expectations of the future on what we have observed about the past, both in our daily lives and in our professions. It was the great philosopher David Hume who called to our attention the problem we face as we do this.

Hume pointed out that no matter how many observations we have made of a correlation between events, we can never be sure that this correlation will be repeated in the future. There is no way for us to know whether the future will resemble the past that we have observed. Furthermore, there is no observation we can make about any particular object or event that will necessarily reveal to us its future nature, or how it will be related to other objects or events in the future, or even if there will be a future at all. An examination of the present and past, no matter how detailed and complete, will not suffice as proof that the future will be one way rather than another.

It might be thought that, although we cannot know the future with certainty, we can at least have some assurance of probability about the resemblance of the future to the past. But even here, Hume raised questions about the validity of this assumption. How can we say that the past makes a particular future more likely, except by appealing to the fact that this is the way things have always been, so that we project this expectation into the future? The projection of either probability or certainty into the future, however, is the very point at issue.

As a result, there is a critical problem involving the conceptual basis on which we conduct our lives, the justification for the extrapolation of past observations to future expectations. This is a problem for which we have as yet no satisfactory solution. Still, we continue to shape and fashion our lives as if this problem did not exist.

Hume observed that this disposition to fashion expectations of the future based on the past is a part of our human nature. He did not urge us to try to reshape our human nature as we form these expectations. What must be considered is not what we do but rather the nature of our justification for what we do.

64. The main problem considered in the passage concerns the

A. truth of our judgments about the future.

B. justification of our judgments about the future.

C. probability of our judgments about the future.

D. existence of the future.

65. Based on this passage, we should conclude that

A. the future will not resemble the past.

B. the future may not resemble the past.

C. the future will probably not resemble the past.

D. there are no grounds for saying what might or will happen in the future.

66. According to the passage, the philosopher David Hume would be most likely to say that

A. we should live only for today and take no care for tomorrow.

B. we should predict the future in terms of probability rather than certainty.
C. we should be aware that our knowledge of the future rests on an uncertain foundation.
D. we should not make predictions about the future.

67. According to the passage, our assurance about how the future will be
A. rests on no foundation at all.
B. rests on no justified foundation at all.
C. rests on no justified foundation that we can prove.
D. is guaranteed by the sources of past predictions.

68. The problem identified in the passage could be
A. solved by gathering more data.
B. solved by being more precise in analyzing our data.
C. solved by both gathering more data and being more precise in analyzing the data.
D. in how we justify the relevance of this data to our prognostications.

69. Hume would say that judgments of probability are no better than judgments of certainty because
A. either one of them may turn out to be false.
B. each requires a presumption of the relevance of past information to future expectations.
C. each requires a presumption of the effect of the past on the future.
D. our human nature is such that no knowledge is possible for us.

PASSAGE IV (QUESTIONS 70–73)

The literature on elderly drug use indicates that the elderly are at high risk for drug misuse, and that they may also be at considerable risk for drug abuse involving legal drugs. In addition, a small group of elderly opiate addicts exists. There are findings that some addicts do mature out of their addiction, but the majority adapts and conceals their habit by using other drugs, such as hydromorphone hydrochloride; by decreasing their daily usage; and by substituting more legally available substances such as alcohol or barbiturates. The abusive use of drugs by the elderly may be associated with coping problems related to retirement, physical problems, loss of family and friends, dependence, and feelings of depression and low self-esteem.

Elderly alcohol abuse is a more widely acknowledged and more thoroughly researched problem than elderly drug abuse. One-third of alcoholics developed their problems after entering their elderly years. Their drinking seems to be related more to attempts to cope with the stresses and problems of old age than to more deeply rooted psychological difficulties. Elderly alcohol abusers are likely to drink more often but in smaller quantities than younger alcohol abusers. Elderly alcohol abusers also have fewer severe and obvious social or physical problems or impairments than do younger alcohol abusers. Hiding, denial, or lack of awareness of the problem is common among the elderly. As the environmental stresses of the growing elderly population increases and as increasing proportions of the elderly become non-abstainers, the number of elderly alcoholics may increase dramatically over the next ten to fifteen years.

Drug abuse among the elderly may follow a pattern comparable to that for alcohol abuse. Neither elderly alcohol abusers nor elderly drug abusers seem to mature out to the extent previously believed. An aging of both abuser populations is likely, along with reductions, adaptations, and concealment of abuse as old age is reached. Both forms of abuse may either begin or recur during old age. Elderly alcoholism and elderly drug abuse appear mainly to involve small but frequent doses of legal substances. For many elderly persons, alcohol abuse and other drug abuse may be part of a single pattern.

Adolescence and old age have many similarities that may relate to drug abuse. Both involve uncertain and changing roles and self-concepts, lower social status, disadvantages with respect to employment and income, shifting and uncertain social supports, and other characteristics. Both groups are limited in their ability to become self-reliant and assert their independence and have limited resources for coping. Both groups find drugs readily available, although they come from different sources. This, and the elderly's regard for lawfulness and social conformity, results primarily in illicit drug use among adolescents and licit drug use among the elderly.

The stepping-stone theory, in which initial use of alcohol and tobacco is said to lead gradually to marijuana use and then to hard drug use among adolescents, may have a parallel in the use of licit drugs by the elderly. Psychological characteristics of the aged, including reduced intellectual and problem-solving abilities, may also increase the tendency among some elderly persons to return to the use of more primitive defense mechanisms such as somatization and, so, to drug use. In addition, psychoactive drug use may reflect the more passive copying styles of many older adults.

70. The passage predicts that the number of elderly alcoholics may increase dramatically in the near future due to
    A. the longer life expectancy that will be achieved during this time.
    B. greater environmental stresses on a larger elderly population.
    C. the decreasing availability of illicit drugs.
    D. the increasing expense of licit drugs.

71. According to information contained in the passage, it can be concluded that
    A. one-third of all alcoholics are elderly.
    B. one-third of all elderly alcoholics had not developed their problems before entering their elderly years.
    C. one-third of persons entering their elderly years have become alcoholics.
    D. most elderly people are depressed.

72. According to the stepping-stone theory, which of the following would be most likely to occur?
    A. An adolescent who uses cocaine later becomes an alcoholic.
    B. An adolescent who drinks begins to smoke cigarettes.
    C. An adolescent who is a cocaine addict becomes an opium addict when elderly.
    D. An elderly person who abuses over-the-counter sleeping medication becomes dependent on barbiturates.

73. The passage suggests that the elderly's regard for lawfulness and social conformity
    A. helps to explain the low incidence of drug abuse among the elderly.
    B. helps to explain which substances are most likely to be abused by the elderly.
    C. decreases once the elderly person begins to abuse drugs.
    D. stands in the way of solutions.

PASSAGE V (QUESTIONS 74–78)

The submarine first became a major component in naval warfare during World War I, when Germany demonstrated its full potential. Wholesale sinking of Allied shipping by the German U-boats almost swung the war in favor of the Central Powers. Then, as now, the submarine's greatest advantage was that it could operate beneath the ocean surface where detection was difficult. Sinking a submarine was comparatively easy once it was found — but finding it before it could attack was another matter.

During the closing months of World War I, the Allied Submarine Devices Investigation Committee was formed to obtain more effective underwater detection equipment from science and technology. The committee developed a reasonably accurate device for locating a submerged submarine. This device was a trainable hydrophone, which was attached to the bottom of the ASW ship, and used to detect screw noises and other sounds that came from a submarine. Although the committee disbanded after World War I, the British made improvements on the locating device between that time and World War II and named the device after the committee.

American scientists further improved on the device, calling it sonar, a name derived from the underlined initials of the words <u>so</u>und <u>na</u>vigation and <u>r</u>anging.

At the end of World War II, the United States improved the snorkel (a device for bringing air to the crew and engines when operating on submerged diesels) and developed the Guppy (short for "greater underwater propulsion power"), a conversion of the fleet-type submarine of World War II fame. The superstructure was changed by reducing the surface area, streamlining every protruding object, and enclosing the periscope shears in a streamlined metal fairing. Performance increased greatly with improved electronic equipment, additional battery capacity, and the addition of the snorkel.

Since World War II, the submerged endurance of the submarine has improved sufficiently to make submarine detection difficult. The problem increases as the submarine goes faster and deeper and stays down longer. To cope with the modern submarine, we now have better detection devices, more modern weapons, and newer ships, but the battle for supremacy is a never-ending one.

During World War II, submarines sent millions of tons of shipping to the bottom. Early in the war, England's lifelines were nearly strangled by German submarines. American submarines played a large role in the defeat of Japan by sinking nearly all her merchant marine. Obviously, the submarine is a potent weapon, requiring equally effective countermeasures. The United States and Great Britain were successful in developing equipment, weapons, and tactics that enabled the destruction of the German submarine force. Japan was never able to develop an effective defense against our submarines.

74. The purpose of this passage is to
    A. explain why the Allies won World War II.
    B. identify the major improvements in submarine technology since World War I.
    C. explain why submarines will not be important in future wars.
    D. compare Allied and German submarine technology.

75. The greatest difficulty in anti-submarine warfare is
    A. finding the enemy submarine.
    B. sinking the enemy submarine once it is found.
    C. drawing the enemy submarine to the surface.
    D. escaping the enemy submarine once contact is made.

76. During World War II, the primary means of submarine detection was based on
    A. surface sightings.
    B. intelligence reports.
    C. satellite surveillance.
    D. sound reports.

77. Which of the following countries did *not* participate in the development of the submarine detection device that was eventually known as sonar?
    A. Germany
    B. Great Britain
    C. The United States
    D. France

78. The author of the passage says that, in the early part of World War II,
    A. American submarines almost destroyed Japanese shipping.
    B. German submarines almost destroyed shipping to England.
    C. English submarines almost destroyed shipping to Germany.
    D. Japanese submarines almost destroyed American shipping.

PASSAGE VI (QUESTIONS 79–83)

Americans know of Hebrew as the language of the Old Testament. Hebrew had been a living language; that is, it was spoken as a native language by a community of people, at least until the first century, B.C., and possibly for several centuries after that. But even though it has ceased to be a living language in this sense, a large and important body of literature has remained in constant daily use for prayer and study.

During the Middle Ages and into the Renaissance, Hebrew served as a *lingua franca* for Jews throughout the world, and the literature was expanded by scholars and poets. As a result, Hebrew remained familiar, and in the last century successful efforts were begun to revive it as a modern language.

Today, Hebrew is the official language of the state of Israel. It is taught to immigrants who speak a wide variety of native languages, with the goal of having all of Israel's inhabitants able to speak it.

To be sure, modern Hebrew is different from the Biblical languages. The phonology (sound system) has been simplified, and new syntactic patterns and vocabulary have been developed to express concepts not dreamed of two thousand years ago. But the modern language is unmistakably the descendant of the language of the Psalms and the prophets.

Modern Hebrew is a living language, and as such, it is changing daily. Slang expression, coinages, variant pronunciations, and grammatical innovations are characteristic of any living language. Furthermore, Hebrew is spoken and written in a variety of styles. These vary from highly formal to highly informal.

Formal spoken style is very similar to the literary style and is more like the traditional Hebrew that is taught. Formal style is used, as the name implies, for public speaking, official meetings, radio news broadcasts, or on other occasions where the speaker would use deferential or deliberate speech.

Informal spoken style is that used by native speakers in ordinary, relaxed conversation. It is often more rapid than the formal style and is the speech which seems most "natural" to native Israelis.

There is a highly informal style that contains much slang, contractions, and dropping of sounds, and is fairly rapid. The student should not attempt to learn it until he or she is fairly fluent in the ordinary informal style.

The goal of studying a language is performance. One "knows" Hebrew in the same sense that one "knows" how to drive a car. It is not necessary to be an automotive engineer or to know the technical terms for the parts of a car in order to be a good driver. Many excellent drivers even have wrong notions about the mechanical aspects of an automobile. Similarly, it is not necessary to be able to discuss accurately and comprehensively the grammar of a language in order to speak it fluently and correctly. Intensive drilling will produce the proper habits. When one is able to participate in conversation easily and fluently with a minimum of either "accent" or conscious effort, then one has achieved the goal of studying a language.

79. Modern Hebrew and Biblical Hebrew are identical in
    A. phonology.
    B. syntax.
    C. vocabulary.
    D. no precise way.

80. A living language is identified as one that
    A. has a long history.
    B. is richly expressive.
    C. is spoken as a native language by a community of people.
    D. has both written and oral forms.

81. The passage represents the goal of studying a language as
    A. knowing the grammar of the language.
    B. conversational ease in using the language.
    C. broadening one's cultural heritage.
    D. learning the vocabulary of the language.

82. The passage states that the state of Israel has the goal of having all its inhabitants
   A. learn to speak Hebrew.
   B. speak only Hebrew.
   C. learn Biblical Hebrew.
   D. learn both Biblical and modern Hebrew.

83. The passage represents knowing a language as
   A. knowing how to do something.
   B. knowing why something is the way it is.
   C. being able to explain how something works.
   D. being able to read.

PASSAGE VII (QUESTIONS 84–87)

Perhaps the most remarkable trauma seen by the paleopathologist is trephination or the surgical removal of a portion of the skull. The earliest written accounts of trephination are found in the Hippocratic writings (460–377 B.C.). However, the evidence of trephining goes back at least to the Neolithic period (10,000 B.C.).

It is clear that the identification of the cause of holes in the skull cannot always be made. However, there are some criteria that will be important in any analysis. The first question to be resolved is whether the hole is the result of mechanical intervention. Evidence for curing or scraping may still exist even if healing has taken place. The next problem to be clarified is if the cutting was done before or after death. The significant question here is whether we are seeing the product of a surgical procedure or the result of some postmortem ritual. Any evidence of healing or inflammatory reaction to the cutting is indicative of trephination. However, it is possible that a patient can die during the trephination or so soon after it that no reaction takes place. Such a situation in an archaeological example of trephination may be indistinguishable from postmortem ritual removal. In such situations the demonstration of unambiguous trephination in the same geographical area would certainly be significant in interpreting the equivocal cases. Another important criterion is the presence of fracture in association with evidence of cutting. Many, if not most, trephinations occur in association with skull fracture. As with most other problems in paleopathology, careful observation combined with a comprehensive knowledge of the options is the most important prerequisite in determining the presence of trephination.

In trephination, four basic responses can occur. First, in those cases where trauma preceded the trephination procedure, death may be due to the initial trauma. Second, the surgical procedure itself may cause death. Third, the surgical procedure may not directly cause death but may introduce disease organisms that cause infection and possibly death. Fourth, there may be no complications resulting from surgery, in which case the individual survives with varying degrees of repair to the surgically induced defect. If there is no healing, as evidenced by the lack of remodeling of the cut edges or fill in of exposed spaces, the reasonable assumption is that death occurred at the time of, or shortly after, surgery. A zone of porous, reactive bond surrounding the surgical area suggests survival for some time after surgery, but with the possibility of infection complicating the healing process and causing death. Partial to complete refill of the surgical defect is indicative of recovery and long-term survival after surgery.

84. Trephination is a surgical procedure involving the removal of a portion of the skull in
   A. a living patient.
   B. a corpse.
   C. either a living patient or a corpse.
   D. a postmortem ritual.

85. The passages specifies that many trephinations
   A. cause skull fractures.
   B. result from skull fractures.
   C. are associated with skull fractures.
   D. leave scars.

86. In this passage, the word *trauma* should be taken to mean a
    A. painful emotional response to something.
    B. frightful or fearful condition.
    C. bodily wound, injury, or shock.
    D. dream state.

87. Which of the following would be the best evidence for long-term survival after trephination?
    A. Partial refilling of the damaged skull
    B. Exposed spaces in the skull
    C. Signs of an inflammatory reaction
    D. Absence of reshaping or the cut edges of the skull

PASSAGE VIII (QUESTIONS 88–91)

Restoring the seceded states to the Union was the central issue in American politics from 1865–1869. This was preeminently a constitutional question involving the distribution of power between the states and the federal government. Considered from a strictly legal standpoint, reunification presented perplexing difficulties. Social and economic turmoil resulting from the destruction of slavery vastly complicated the problem, if it did not make a peaceful solution virtually impossible. Behind the rhetoric of states' rights and federal supremacy, the core elements in the Reconstruction problem were the status and rights of the former Confederates on the one hand, and the status and rights of the emancipated slaves on the other. The task of postwar Union policy was to reconcile the demands of these conflicting groups while restoring the federal system according to Northern republican principles.

Reconstruction as a problem in constitutional politics began with the disruption of the Union in the months before Sumter and continued throughout the war. The first ideas on the subject to be given practical expression were those advanced by President Lincoln at the beginning of the war. In his message to Congress in July 1861, and in a series of executive actions in subsequent months, Lincoln held that secession was null and void, and that the so-called seceded states were, therefore, still in the Union. He admitted that the Southern states were out of their normal relationship to the other states and the federal government because they had no loyal governments and were controlled by persons in rebellion against federal authority. But the states, as political entities distinguished from their governments, still were in the Union. So all that was necessary for Reconstruction was the suppression of actual military rebellion, the creation of loyal state governments by loyal citizens, and the resumption of normal relations with the federal government.

Lincoln assumed that it was the duty of the federal government to assist the states in Reconstruction. The justification for this assumption he found in Article IV, Section 4, of the Constitution, by which the United States guaranteed every state a republican form of government. All subsequent Reconstruction schemes drew upon this constitutional provision as justification for federal controls.

Finally, Lincoln assumed that the president had authority to carry through a competent Reconstruction program with little congressional assistance. A principal step in the plan was the suppression of rebellion, already being accomplished under the president's war powers. Lincoln admitted that in practice Congress would have final authority to pass upon presidential Reconstruction because it could seat delegates from Southern states at its discretion.

Lincoln's plan had two great virtues. It was consistent, for it rested upon the same premise of the nullity of secession upon which the administration had prosecuted the war. And it was simple in execution and promised a rapid restoration of a normally functioning constitutional system. Its great practical weakness was that Congress could destroy it merely by refusing to seat delegates from the reconstructed states.

88. The primary purpose of this passage is to
    A. criticize Congress for refusing Southern delegates.
    B. describe Lincoln's Reconstruction plan.

C. explain the failure of Reconstruction.

D. highlight the causes of the Civil War.

89. According to the author, one of the most important parts of the Reconstruction problem involved

A. the rights of former slaves.

B. states' rights advocates.

C. suppression of military rebellion.

D. congressional support.

90. The author tells us Lincoln believed the federal government should

A. leave Reconstruction to Congress.

B. let the states develop a Reconstruction plan.

C. stay out of Reconstruction.

D. assist states in Reconstruction.

91. Lincoln justified his plan based on

A. congressional authority.

B. a constitutional provision.

C. federal supremacy.

D. administrative expertise.

PASSAGE IX (QUESTION 92)

The intensely hot conditions that prevailed at the universe's birth probably lie forever beyond the reach of even the largest particle accelerators. Investigators of low-temperature physics, however, have long surpassed nature. In the 15 billion years since the Big Bang, no point in the universe at large has reached a temperature cooler than three kelvins (the temperature of the cosmic microwave background). In laboratories, however, temperatures measured in nanokelvins and picokelvins are being achieved. The phenomena being studied at such temperatures are not only new to physicists, they have never occurred before in the history of the cosmos.

Of all the unusual phenomena that ultralow temperatures elicit, perhaps the most spectacular are superfluidity — the frictionless flow of a fluid — and its electronic analogue, superconductivity. Superfluidity in liquid ^{4}He, the common isotope of helium, has been known since 1938. In 1972, Douglas D. Osheroff, Robert C. Richardson, and David M. Lee of Cornell University found that the rare isotope ^{3}He could also become superfluid. Exploration of the properties of this new kind of matter has been a central project of ultralow-temperature physics for the past decade and a half.

The behavior of superfluid ^{3}He can be very intricate even though its structure is that of a simple liquid, composed of identical, chemically inactive, rare gas atoms. In addition to being worthy of study for its own sake, this combination of the simple and the complex makes superfluid ^{3}He an ideal substance in which to study many other condensed-matter problems, ranging from the properties of neutron stars to those of high-temperature superconductors.

Laboratory studies of the behavior of superfluid ^{3}He may eventually yield insight about forms of matter found nowhere on the earth. It is conjectured, for example, that the neutron matter (neutronium) in rapidly rotating pulsars is superfluid, even though the temperature in neutron stars is about 100 million kelvins. Neutron matter clearly cannot be studied in the laboratory, but it may be possible to mimic its behavior by means of rotating superfluid ^{3}He or ^{4}He. Neutrons, like ^{3}He atoms, are fermions, and it is believed that neutronium becomes superfluid by the same Cooper-pair mechanism operating in ^{3}He. Only detailed theoretical calculations can tell whether the correspondence between superfluid ^{3}He and neutronium is sufficiently close for such models to yield useful results. If so, experiments will be performed on ^{3}He with neutron stars in mind.

The experimental verification of such a possibility may lie far in the future because such a transition may take place only at temperatures well below those to which liquid helium can be cooled at present. Nevertheless, there is little doubt that those temperatures will eventually be reached.

92. The primary purpose of the passage is to
    A. discuss properties of neutron stars.
    B. identify isotopes of helium.
    C. explain the value of ultralow-temperature experiments.
    D. describe how superfluids are formed.

STOP!

If time still remains, you may review work only in this section. When the time allotted is up, you may go on to the next section.

STOP!

SECTION 3
Writing Sample

TIME: 60 minutes

2 essays, separately timed

30 minutes each

DIRECTIONS: This section tests your writing skills by asking you to write two essays. You will have 30 minutes to write each one.

During the first 30 minutes, work only on the first essay. If you finish it in less than 30 minutes, you may review what you have written, but do not begin the second essay. During the second 30 minutes, work only on the second essay. If you finish it in less than 30 minutes, you may review what you have written for that essay only. Do not go back to the first essay.

Read each assigned topic carefully. Make sure your essays respond to the topics as they are assigned.

Make sure your essays are written in complete sentences and paragraphs, and are as clear as you can make them. Make any corrections or additions between the lines of your essays. Do not write in the margins.

On the day of the test, you are given three pages to write each essay. You are not required to use all of the space provided, but do not skip lines so you will not waste space. Illegible essays cannot be scored.

PART 1

Consider this statement:

"The tree of humanity forgets the labour of the silent gardeners who sheltered it from the cold, watered it in time of drought, shielded it against wild animals; but preserves faithfully the names mercilessly cut into its bark."

Heine, *The Romantic School, 1833*

Write a comprehensive essay where you accomplish the following objectives. Explain what you think the statement means. Discuss what you think Heine meant by "silent gardeners." Whose names do you think are "mercilessly cut" on the tree? Be sure to include examples.

PART 2

Consider this statement:

"As soon as any part of a person's conduct affects prejudicially the interests of others, society has jurisdiction over it, and the question whether the general welfare will or will not be promoted by interfering with it, becomes open to discussion. But there is no room for entertaining any such question when a person's conduct affects the interests of no persons besides himself...."

John Stuart Mill, *On Liberty*

Write a comprehensive essay where you accomplish the following objectives. Explain the meaning of Mill's statement. Consider Mill's idea in relation to a specific situation that might contradict or limit this idea. Discuss the possibility of resolving this contradiction.

STOP! If time still remains, you may review work only in this section. When the time allotted is up, you may go on to the next section. STOP!

SECTION 4
Biological Sciences

TIME: 70 Minutes

QUESTIONS: 93–144

DIRECTIONS: Most of the questions in this section are arranged in groups, each corresponding to a descriptive passage. Based on the information given in a passage, choose the one best answer to each question in the group. Some questions are independent of a descriptive passage and of each other. Choose the one best answer to each of these questions. If you are not sure of an answer, eliminate those choices that you know are incorrect and choose an answer from among those remaining. Fill in the corresponding circle on the answer sheet to indicate your answer. You may refer to the periodic table at any time.

PASSAGE I (QUESTIONS 93–95)

A diagram of a "typical" animal cell is presented in Figure 1. In reality, there are many kinds, sizes, and shapes of animal cells depending on their position and function within body tissues. However, the basic roles of the organelles depicted in Figure 1 remain the same regardless of tissue type. The presence of a membrane-bound organelle distinguishes eukaryotic from prokaryotic cells.

FIGURE 1

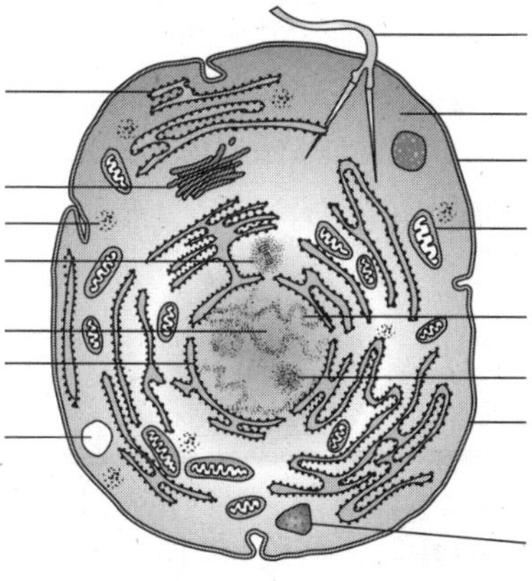

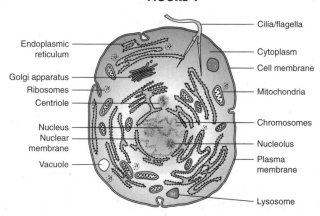

The plasma membrane that delimits a cell from its surrounding medium is basically a bilayer of phospholipids into which are inserted a variety of extrinsic and intrinsic proteins. Movement of substances through the plasma membrane and within the cell can occur passively or actively. The membrane contains a variety of channels and pumps to regulate this movement, although it remains subject to external factors such as the osmotic pressure of the surrounding fluids.

Nuclear division (karyokinesis) is usually followed by cell division (cytokinesis) in animal cells. Somatic cells of animals undergo a type of karyokinesis known as mitosis, which proceeds in a series of stages as part of an overall cell cycle. This cycle usually approximates a twenty-four-hour period but may occur in less than an hour or take several days to complete.

93. The following stages of the cell cycle occur directly after mitosis:
    A. S, G_1, G_2.
    B. G_1, G_2, S.
    C. G_1, S, G_2.
    D. S, G_2, G_1.

94. The stage of mitosis where separation of chromatids at the centromere occurs is
    A. metaphase.
    B. anaphase.
    C. telophase.
    D. prophase.

95. Celery sticks that are left in a dish of freshwater for several hours become stiff and hard. Celery sticks left in a salt solution become limp and soft. From this, we can deduce that the cells of the celery sticks are
    A. hypotonic to both freshwater and the salt solution.
    B. hypertonic to both freshwater and the salt solution.
    C. hypertonic to freshwater but hypotonic to the salt solution.
    D. hypotonic to freshwater but hypertonic to the salt solution.

PASSAGE II (QUESTIONS 96–99)

The external sex organs of male and female mammals are homologous structures, having developed from an embryonic bisexual primordium called the genital tubercle. Differentiation of human genitalia occurs during the eighth week of development. Production of testosterone and a polysaccharide called mullerian inhibitory factor (MIF) by the newly differentiated testes causes masculinization of the genital tubercle and associated structures. In the absence of MIF and testosterone, these structures develop into female genitalia.

Gametogenesis in mammals, as in other animals, is by meiosis. Both spermatogenesis and oogenesis are initiated during embryonic development and both are arrested in the first meiotic division, not to resume until puberty. Germ cells that migrate from the yolk sac early in embryological development are the source of the spermatogonia and oogonia from which sperm and eggs develop. Spermatogonia reproduce themselves mitotically so that sperm production is continuous throughout the adult life of males, while the number of oogonia remains fixed after embryogenesis.

Spermatogenesis produces four functional spermatozoa, but the unequal cleavages of oogenesis result in only one functional ovum. Furthermore, the second meiotic division of oogenesis occurs only if the secondary oocyte is fertilized. Because of unequal cleavages, virtually all of the cytoplasm of the oogonium is preserved in the ovum and, therefore, the zygote. The other products of oogenesis, the polar bodies, degenerate and have no known function in reproduction.

A further difference between male and female gamete production in mammals can be seen in the cyclic nature of ovulation. While sperm are produced continuously by males, females release an egg or eggs periodically during menstrual cycles (in humans and some other primates) or estrous cycles. These cyclic ovulations are under complex hormonal control and cease during the middle to late stages of adult life. In humans, this phenomenon is known as menopause and usually occurs between the ages of forty and fifty years.

96. Which of the following is a correct, but not necessarily complete, sequence of four cells formed during spermatogenesis in animals?
    A. Primary spermatocyte, secondary spermatocyte, spermatogonium
    B. Secondary spermatocyte, spermatid, spermatozoan
    C. Spermatogonium, spermatid, primary spermatocyte
    D. Spermatozoan, spermatid, secondary spermatocyte

97. The structure in which oogenesis occurs in mammalian ovaries is known as a(n)
    A. follicle.
    B. oocyte.
    C. corpus luteum.
    D. endometrium.

98. Spermatogenesis occurs in the ____ of mammals.
    A. epididymis
    B. prostate gland
    C. seminiferous tubules
    D. vas deferens

99. The external female genital structure that is homologous to (i.e., arose from the same embryonic tissue as) the penis is the
   A. vagina.
   B. cervix.
   C. labia majora.
   D. clitoris.

PASSAGE III (QUESTIONS 100–104)

Collection of the mechanical, thermal, chemical, electromagnetic, or other forms of stimulus energy from the environment and converting it into the electrochemical energy of nerve impulses is the function of various sensory receptors found in animals. These receptors differ in complexity, from single-neuron mechanoreceptors of the skin to the large, multi-receptor eyes and ears of vertebrates.

The process of converting stimulus energy into nerve impulses is known as transduction. The senses of vision and hearing represent two different mechanisms of transduction, each with varying degrees of integration.

In the vertebrate eye, transduction of light energy involves cis-trans isomerization of photosensitive molecules located in receptor cells of the retina. The light-induced conformational changes ultimately lead to action potentials in sensory neurons of the retina through changes in permeability of the neuron membranes. The original photosensitive form of the receptor molecules is reestablished by an enzymatic, energy-dependent conversion. Qualitative and quantitative differences in light are perceived by integration of the action potentials of the two kinds of photoreceptor cells, the rods and cones. In this way, humans and certain other vertebrates can detect changes in wavelength and light intensity as color and brightness.

Hearing involves the transduction of pressure waves in the atmosphere into action potentials. This process involves mechanical movements of membranes and the ossicles of the middle ear that then induce pressure waves in the fluids of the cochlea. Displacement of the cilia of sensory hair cells located on the basilar membrane of the organ of Corti cause action potentials to form in sensory neurons of the cochlear nerve. Different frequency sounds cause different portions of the basilar membrane to vibrate, and the hair cells of those portions are thereby stimulated. The cochlear nerve carries impulses from different parts of the basilar membrane to correspondingly different parts of the cerebral cortex. The brain then perceives differences in volume and pitch of sound, respectively, by the number of action potentials received and the particular region of the cerebral cortex that receives them. High-amplitude sound causes more sensory neurons to fire, and the cerebral cortex is mapped to recognize impulses from specific regions of the basilar membrane.

Use the information presented in this passage and your general knowledge of vision and hearing in mammals to answer the following questions.

100. The following is a correct, but not necessarily complete, sequence of structures through which sound waves act in mammalian hearing.
   A. Malleus, stapes, round window, vestibular canal
   B. Stapes, oval windows, round window, tympanic canal
   C. Tympanic membrane, malleus, round window, vestibular canal
   D. Oval window, vestibular canal, tympanic canal, round window

101. Compared to the cones of a human eye, rods are
   A. less sensitive to light intensity.
   B. more numerous.
   C. concentrated in the center of the retina.
   D. capable of detecting color.

102. The cilia of sensory hairs on the basilar membrane are embedded in the
   A. round window.
   B. tectorial membrane.
   C. oval window.
   D. vestibular canal.

103. There is a certain region of the vertebrate eye known as the blind spot. This region is actually the
   A. edge of the lens.
   B. fovea centralis.
   C. exit point of the optic nerve.
   D. macula lutea.

104. The inner ear of mammals also contains the apparatus for balance and equilibrium. Changes in the position of the head with respect to gravity, as in bending forward, are detected by hair cells in chambers known as the
   A. semicircular canals.
   B. vestibular canal.
   C. statocyst.
   D. utricle and saccule.

QUESTIONS 105–109 are NOT based on a descriptive passage.

105. A molecule passing from the nucleus to the cytoplasm must pass through two membranes. Which other organelle has a double membrane?
   A. Mitochondrion
   B. Golgi apparatus
   C. Ribosome
   D. Endoplasmic reticulum

106. Secretory proteins that are synthesized on the _____ are destined for packaging in the _____ before they are released by exocytosis.
   A. rough endoplasmic reticulum; nucleus
   B. rough endoplasmic reticulum; Golgi apparatus
   C. smooth endoplasmic reticulum; rough endoplasmic reticulum
   D. Golgi apparatus; rough endoplasmic reticulum

107. Colchicine inhibits the formation of microtubules. Which cellular process would be disrupted by colchicine?
   A. Growth
   B. Respiration
   C. Cytokinesis
   D. Meiosis

108. The developmental homologue (homologues) to the front flipper of the seal is (are)
   A. a bird's wing.
   B. a cat's paw.
   C. a butterfly's wing.
   D. both a bird's wing and a cat's paw.

109. Alleles
   A. are always expressed
   B. can cross over.
   C. are variations of genes on homologous chromosomes.
   D. are always sex-linked.

PASSAGE IV (QUESTIONS 110–113)

FIGURE 1. Characteristics of Red, Intermediate, and White Muscle Fibers

	Red (Type I)	**Intermediate (Type IIA)**	**White (Type IIB)**
Diameter	Small	Intermediate	Large
Z-line thickness	Wide	Intermediate	Narrow
Glycogen content	Low	Intermediate	High
Resistance to fatigue	High	Intermediate	Low
Capillaries	Many	Many	Few
Myoglobin content	High	High	Low
Respiration type	Aerobic	Aerobic	Anaerobic
Twitch rate	Slow	Fast	Fast
Myosin ATPase content	Low	High	High

The muscle fibers of skeletal muscles can be categorized into two fundamental groups based on the time required to reach maximum tension following stimulation. These two muscle fiber types are known as slow-twitch and fast-twitch; muscles containing a predominance of slow-twitch fibers may require as much as 100 msec to reach maximum tension, while a muscle made up primarily of fast-twitch fibers may reach maximum tension in as little as 10 msec. Because of differences in myoglobin content, these fibers are also identified as red (slow-twitch) and white (fast-twitch) fibers.

As can be seen from Figure 1, fast-twitch and slow-twitch fibers differ in a variety of ways. Figure 1 also characterizes a special type of fast-twitch fiber, an intermediate form, that has a greater capacity for aerobic production of ATP than the classic fast-twitch type.

Use the information from Figure 1 and your knowledge of muscle fiber characteristics in general to answer the questions following this passage.

110. Muscles involved in maintaining posture would be expected to contain predominantly
   A. white muscle fibers.
   B. red muscle fibers.
   C. intermediate muscle fibers.
   D. anaerobically respiring muscle fibers.

111. From the information in Figure 1, it can be deduced that the muscle fiber type(s) with large numbers of mitochondria is (are)
   A. type I.
   B. type IIA.
   C. type IIB.
   D. both type I and type IIA.

112. The three muscle fiber types described in this passage are all found in skeletal muscle. Skeletal muscle fibers are similar to smooth muscle fibers in which of the following ways?
   A. Both are multinucleate.
   B. Both have sarcomeres.
   C. Both have electrical synapses.
   D. Both contract in response to Ca^{++}.

113. The most common neurotransmitter of vertebrate neuromuscular synapses is
   A. epinephrine. B. acetycholine.
   C. norepinephrine. D. serotonin.

PASSAGE V (QUESTIONS 114–117)

Quite unlike the way it was perceived before the development of electron microscopy, a eukaryotic cell is now known to have an internal supporting meshwork called the cytoskeleton (see Figure 1). The fibers making up the cytoskeleton (microfilaments, microtubules, and intermediate filaments)

FIGURE 1

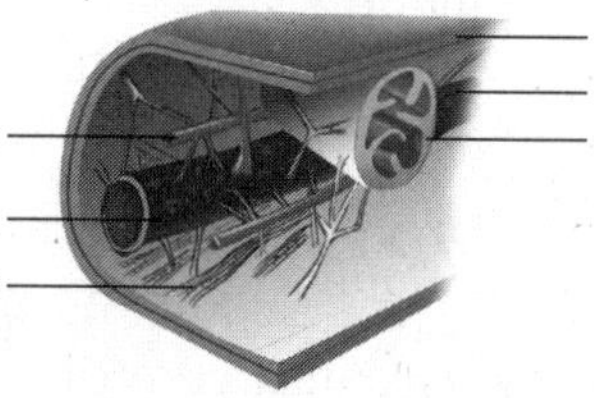

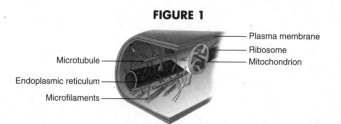

may be assembled and reassembled in a variety of ways, thus enabling a cell to change morphology. These fibers are also associated with a cell's ability to move, by their involvement with muscle cell contraction, activity of flagella and cilia, and formation of pseudopodia during amoeboid movement. Materials are transported within a cell by moving along pathways determined by the arrangement of these fibers. Cellular import and export of materials can involve vacuole formation by cytoskeleton-induced changes in the cell membrane. There are many methods of cellular import/export of materials. Cytoskeleton-induced changes do account for vacuole formation.

Microtubules are particularly important in the structure and motion of flagella and cilia. The arrangement of paired tubules and the mechanism of movement seen in cross-sections of flagella and cilia is identical for all eukaryotes. The proteins in these paired tubules slide past one another in a way that is similar to the sliding-filament contraction of skeletal muscle.

In a similar comparison, centrioles and the basal bodies to which flagella and cilia are anchored have common structures involving microtubules. Basal bodies serve as the template from which cilia and flagella are initially patterned. Centrioles are virtually identical to basal bodies, and they seem to have a role in the organization of microtubule structure during cell growth. Centrioles are not present in cells of vascular plants (with the exception of flagellated gametes).

114. The type of intercellular junction that connects cardiac muscle fibers and allows for direct, electrical synapsing is known as a
 A. tight junction.
 B. desmosome.
 C. plasmodesmata.
 D. gap junction.

115. As seen with electron microscopy, a cross section of a eukaryotic cilium or flagellum consists of _____ pairs of microtubules surrounding a central core of _____ pair(s) of microtubules.
 A. 6; 1
 B. 7; 2
 C. 9; 2
 D. 9; 3

116. The spindle fibers that appear during prophase of mitosis consist of
 A. microfilaments.
 B. kinetochores.
 C intermediate filaments.
 D. microtubules.

117. Which of the following events of cytokinesis is most likely to involve microfilaments?
 A. Centripetal cell wall formation in fungi
 B. Centrifugal cell wall formation in plants
 C. Cleavage furrow formation in animals
 D. Cell plate formation in plants

PASSAGE VI (QUESTIONS 118–121)

The numerous enzymatic processes involved in all of the different aspects of cellular metabolism are regulated in a variety of ways. One of the most common regulatory mechanisms is that of feedback inhibition. This occurs when an end product of the enzymatic process accumulates in a sufficiently high enough concentration to inhibit a crucial enzyme, which is usually involved in the beginning of the pathway. The flow of substances through the enzymatic pathway is prevented and, as a result, there is no further end-product formation.

For example, the amino acid isoleucine is produced in the following manner:

$$\text{threonine} \xrightarrow{\text{threonine deaminase}} \alpha\text{-ketobutyrate} \rightarrow \rightarrow \rightarrow \rightarrow \text{isoleucine}$$

As isoleucine accumulates, it will inhibit the enzyme threonine deaminase that will prevent the further production of isoleucine. Conversely, as the concentration of isoleucine decreases, threonine deaminase will become active once again, and the production of isoleucine will increase. In this way, the amount of end product generated by an enzymatic pathway can be matched precisely to the metabolic need for that product.

118. In a metabolic pathway regulated by feedback inhibition, the rate of the entire reaction is determined by
 A. the activity of the last enzyme in the pathway.
 B. end-product concentration.
 C. substrate concentration.
 D. activator concentration.

119. Feedback inhibition serves a useful purpose in cellular metabolism because it
 A. speeds up the rate at which enzymatic reactions occur.
 B. reduces the availability of substrates.
 C. regulates the flux through an enzymatic pathway, matching product supply to demand.
 D. provides a means for genetic regulation of metabolic processes.

120. The opposite of feedback inhibition is
 A. positive feedback, in which an increase in end product increases enzyme activity.
 B. negative feedback, in which an increase in end product decreases enzyme activity.
 C. competitive inhibition, in which a molecule similar in structure to the

substrate blocks the active site of the enzyme.

D. positive modulation, in which a decrease in substrate increases enzyme activity.

121. When a high concentration of isoleucine is present, what effect would increasing the threonine concentration have on threonine deaminase activity?

A. Enzyme activity would increase, resulting in the production of isoleucine.

B. Enzyme activity would decrease due to a threonine-induced conformational change in the enzyme's structure.

C. There would be no effect on enzyme activity because the high concentration of isoleucine would inhabit threonine deaminase.

D. There would be no effect on enzyme activity because the high concentration of threonine would inhibit threonine deaminase.

QUESTIONS 122–123 are NOT based on a descriptive passage.

122. Nitrous acid converts cytosine to uracil by deamination. This type of conversion in one DNA strand would lead to a change in the complementary base in the other strand to

A. adenine.

B. cytosine.

C. thymine.

D. guanine.

123. Messenger RNA does not contain

A. adenine.

B. uracil.

C. guanine.

D. thymine.

PASSAGE VII (QUESTIONS 124–129)

Carboxylic acids can be modified to form several useful derivatives, shown below:

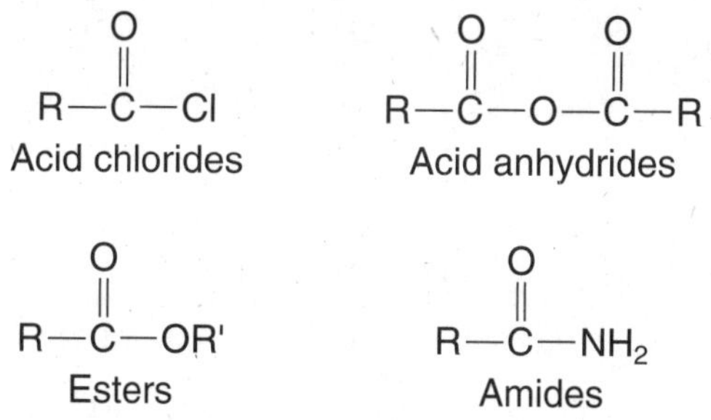

All of these may be hydrolyzed by an aqueous acid or base. Acid chlorides and anhydrides may be reactive enough to be hydrolyzed by water alone. Amides are the most stable of the derivatives toward hydrolysis. The mechanism of hydrolysis may be written as follows:

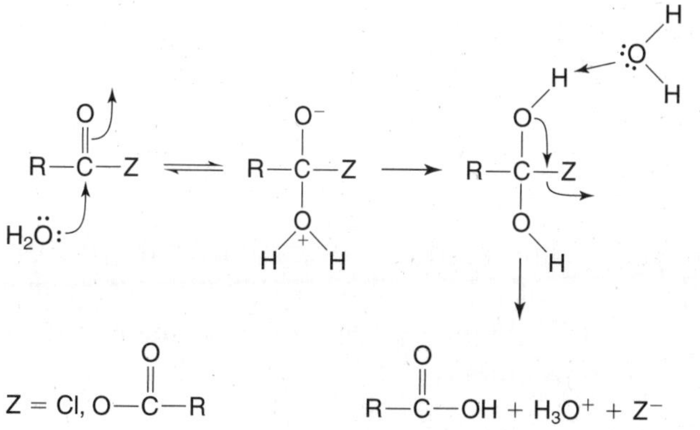

124. Acid added to the water increases the rate of hydrolysis because it

A. protonates the carbonyl oxygen.

B. protonates the carbonyl carbon.

C. protonates the leaving group.

D. stabilizes the product.

125. The hydrochloric acid hydrolysis of ethyl benzoate in water labeled with oxygen-18 yields the following labeled product:

A. benzoic acid.

B. benzoyl chloride.

C. benzoic anhydride.

D. ethanol.

126. Which of the following reactions is suitable for preparing benzamide?

A. $PhC(=O)Cl + NH_3$

B. 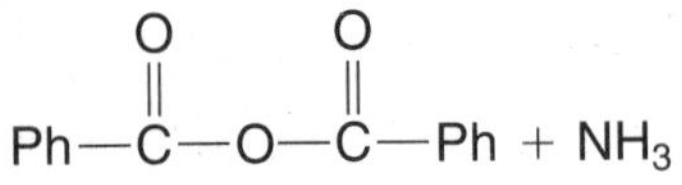

C. 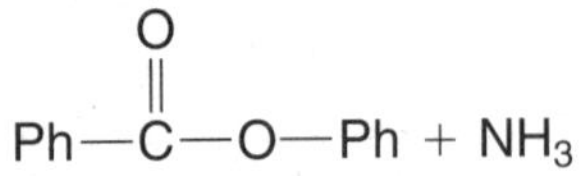

D. All of the above.

127. Biological reactions frequently involve the phosphate ion as a leaving group; 1,3-bisphosphoglycerate has the following structure:

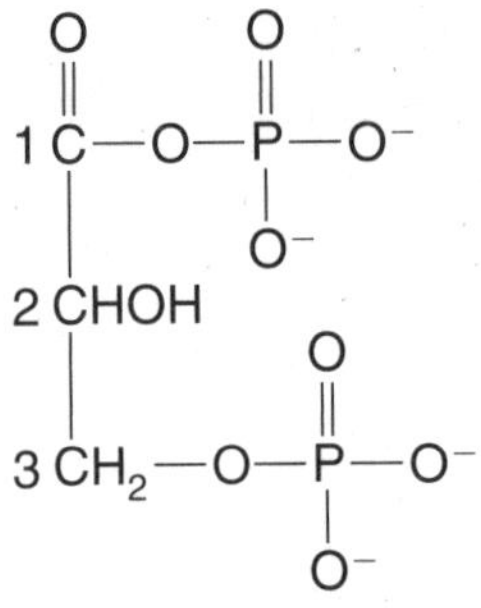

Which product will result from the hydrolysis of 1,3-bisphosphoglycerate under conditions that remove only *one* of the phosphate groups?

A. 2-phosphoglycerate
B. 1-phosphoglycerate
C. 3-phosphoglycerate
D. 4-phosphoglycerate

128. Which of the following amines will be *least* reactive toward an acid chloride or acid anhydride?

A. 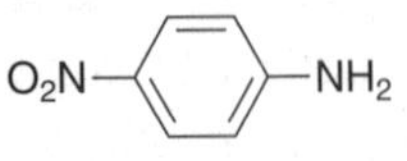

B. 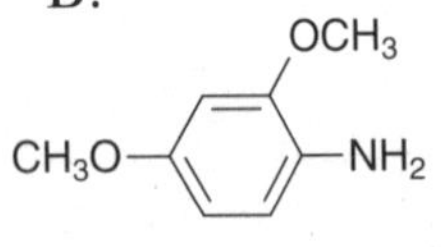

C. 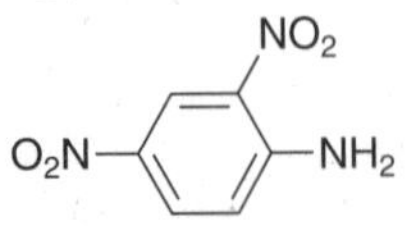

D. 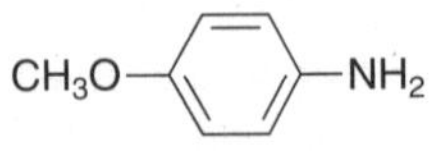

129. The following sequence of reactions would produce which product?

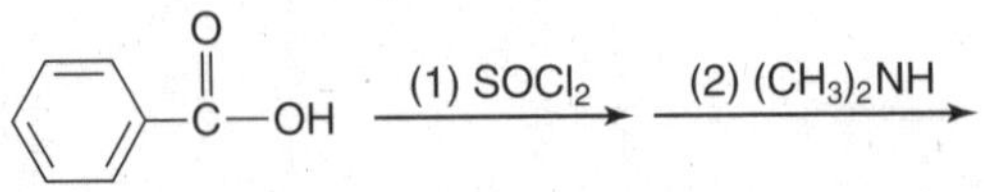

A. 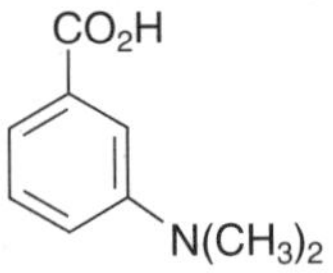

B. 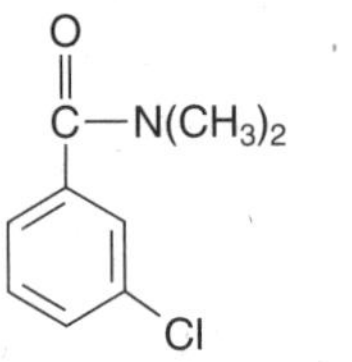

C. 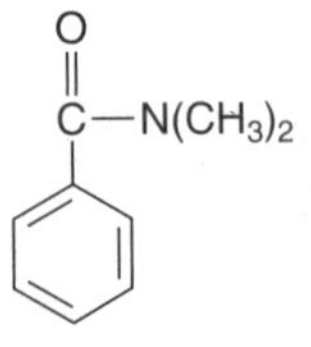

D. 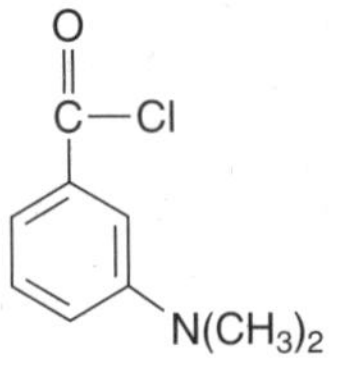

PASSAGE VIII (QUESTIONS 130–133)

Vertebrates, like all other heterotrophic organisms, must obtain their energy-rich molecules from food sources outside their bodies. This food is taken into a two-ended digestive tract that allows one-way transport and processing of these ingested substances. The fundamental processes that occur in the vertebrate digestive system are ingestion, digestion, absorption, and elimination (defecation) of indigestible materials. The organic molecules ingested are usually in the form of large polymers that are mechanically and chemically broken down into the monomeric constituents at various points within the system.

Digestion begins in the buccal cavity and involves both mechanical and enzymatic activity. The majority of digestive activity, however, occurs in the stomach and small intestine. The gastric juice produced by the stomach consists of hydrochloric acid and digestive enzymes, produced in the form of inactive precursors known as zymogens. After leaving the stomach, the partially digested food is acted upon by a variety of other enzymes secreted into the lumen of the digestive tract by the pancreas, liver, and the wall of the small intestine itself. Most absorption of the digested food molecules occurs in the small intestine. The large intestine functions primarily in the reabsorption of water from the digestive tract, the excretion of certain salts from the circulatory system, and the reabsorption of bile salts for return to the liver.

Once food has entered the esophagus, its movement is accomplished by peristaltic contractions of the digestive tract. At certain points along the tract, rings of muscle called sphincters regulate the movement of the material within the tract. Not all food molecules ingested can be broken down by the action of the human digestive tract. Cellulose, for example, cannot be enzymatically digested and is passed through the tract essentially untouched. Such undigestible material is considered necessary to provide bulk for the stimulation of peristalsis.

130. All of the following enzymes are produced by the pancreas *except*
    A. trypsin.
    B. lipase.
    C. chymotrypsin.
    D. pepsin.

131. Villi and microvilli are found lining the inside of a mammal's
    A. small intestine.
    B. stomach.
    C. esophagus.
    D. large intestine.

132. The movement of the tongue during chewing forms food in the buccal cavity into a mass known as a
    A. chyme.
    B. pylorus.
    C. bolus.
    D. caecum.

133. Enzymes to digest starch are produced by both the
    A. salivary glands and stomach.
    B. pancreas and salivary glands.
    C. stomach and small intestine.
    D. small intestine and pancreas.

PASSAGE IX (QUESTIONS 134–136)

Cystic fibrosis is an autosomal recessive genetic disease. It is due to one of several mutations on the long part of chromosome 7 and results in the production of a defective cystic fibrosis regulatory protein. The normal cystic fibrosis regulatory protein is similar to a group of proteins that are important in active transport of materials across membranes.

There are about 250,000 nucleotide base pairs in the gene for the cystic fibrosis regulatory protein. The nucleotide sequence of a small section of DNA, the resulting mRNA code, and the amino acid composition of the protein for the corresponding section are given below. Also given is the mRNA and amino acid sequence for the same short section in individuals with one form of cystic fibrosis.

Normal Individual

DNA

5′	A	T	T	A	A	A	G	A	A	A	A	T	A	T	C	A	T	C
3′	T	A	A	T	T	T	C	T	T	T	T	A	T	A	G	T	A	G

T	T	T	G	G	T	3′
A	A	A	C	C	A	5′

mRNA

5′	A	U	U	A	A	A	G	A	A	A	A	U	A	U	C	A	U	C

U	U	U	G	G	U	3′

Amino acids

Ile	Lys	Glu	Asn	Ile	Ile	Phe	Gly

Individual with Cystic Fibrosis

mRNA

5′	A	U	U	A	A	A	G	A	A	A	A	U	A	U

C	A	U	C	G	G	U	3′

Amino acids

Ile	Lys	Glu	Asn	Ile	Ile	Gly

134. The mRNA code is mostly degenerate. This means that two or more codons occur for one amino acid. Which of the given codons show the degeneracy of the code?

A. TAA and GGT
B. ATT and ATC
C. ATT and AUU
D. AUU and AUC

135. Which of the following best describes the cystic fibrosis regulatory protein found in individuals with a severe form of cystic fibrosis?

A. It is missing the amino acid Phe.
B. The mRNA is missing nucleotide base pairs.
C. It has seven amino acids instead of eight.
D. It is only a small part of the protein found in normal individuals.

136. What is the most probable explanation of this result?

A. The codon UAA is a nonsense codon that stops the addition of amino acids.
B. The individual does not have sufficient energy to continue producing proteins.
C. The DNA contains many Okazaki fragments, one of which gives the two amino acids.
D. The nucleotides bound together on the tailing (right) end of the mRNA prevent proper reading of the mRNA.

QUESTIONS 137–140 are NOT based on a descriptive passage.

137. The hybridization of carbons a, b, and c in the following compound is

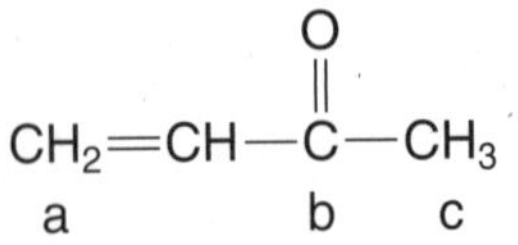

A. a = sp^2 b = sp c = sp^3
B. a = sp b = sp c = sp^3
C. a = sp^2 b = sp^2 c = sp
D. a = sp^2 b = sp^2 c = sp^3

138. All of the following are reasonable resonance contributors to the structure of N, N-dimethyl formamide *except*

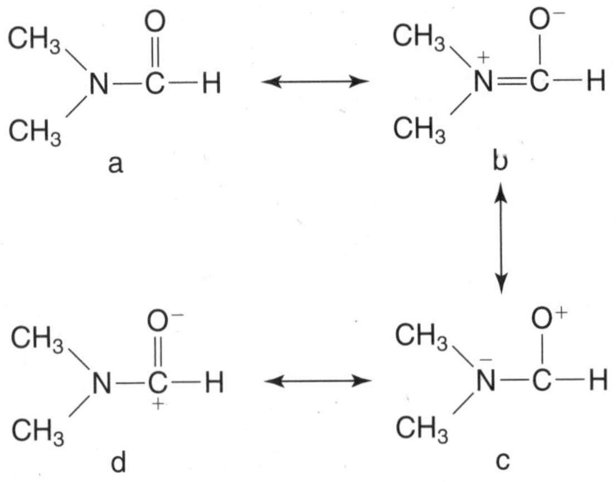

A. a
B. b
C. c
D. d

139. What sequence of reactions would be used to carry out the following synthesis?

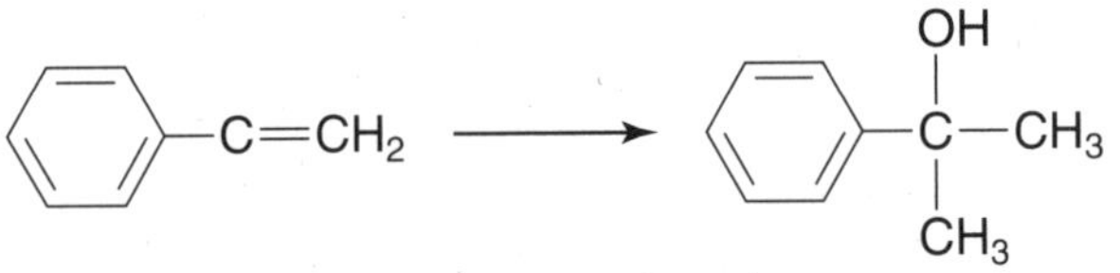

A. 1) CH_3MgI 2) Cr_2O_3 3) H_3O+, Δ
B. 1) Br_2/CCl_4 2) KOH/CH_3CH_2OH 3) CH_3MgI 4) H_3O+
C. 1) H_2O, H+ 2) Cr_2O_3 3) CH_3MgI 4) H_3O+
D. 1) CH_3MgI 2) Cr_2O_3 3) $LiAlH_4$

140. Which will be the shortest carbon-carbon bond in the structure shown?

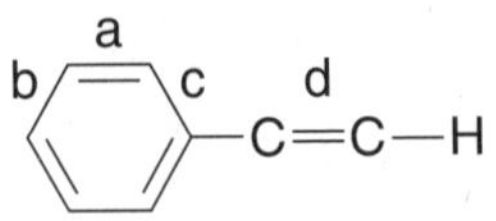

A. a
B. b
C. c
D. d

PASSAGE X (QUESTIONS 141–143)

Newman projections are a convenient way of indicating spatial arrangements and interactions for many compounds. Shown below are Newman representations of conformational states of ethane, C_2H_6, viewed along the C-C bond.

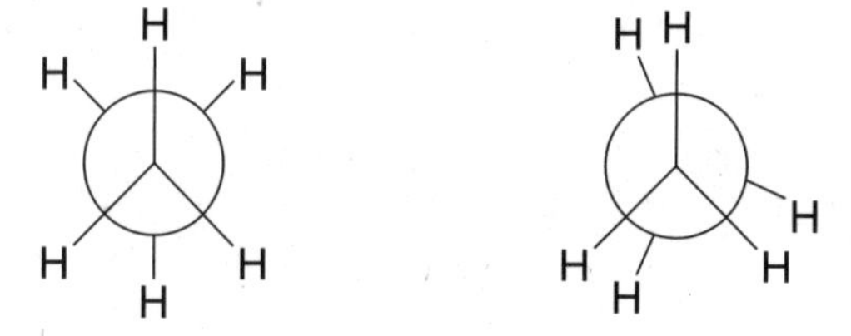

Staggered Eclipsed

The conformation states of n-butane, C_4H_{10}, viewed along the C_2-C_3 bond, may be represented as

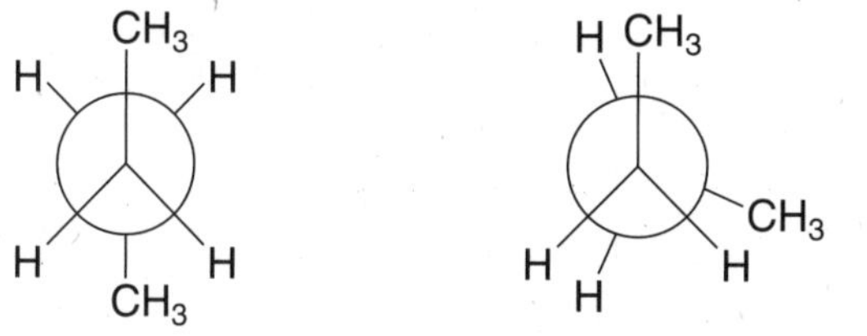

Anti Eclipsed-1

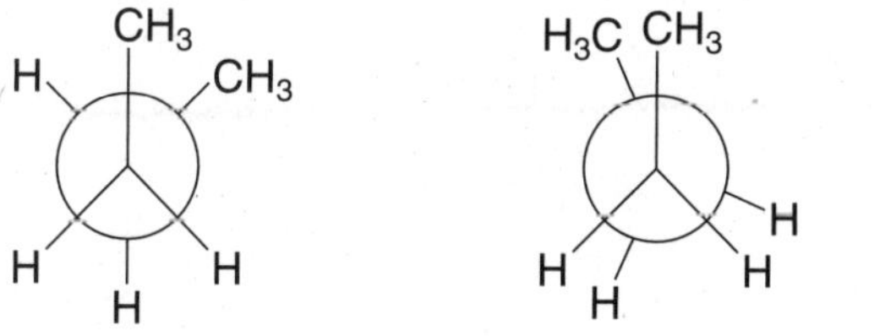

Gauche Eclipsed-2

Successive rotations of 60° around the C_2-C_3 bond give the plot of potential energy versus conformational states of n-butane:

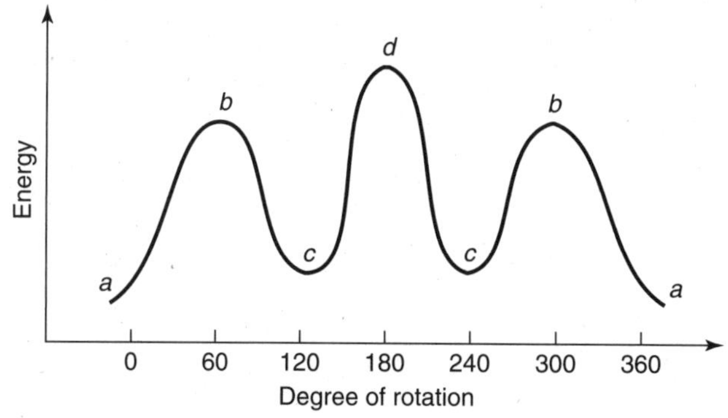

For Questions 141–143, match the position on the energy diagram that corresponds to the conformation shown above.

141. Anti
   A. a B. b
   C. c D. d

142. Gauche
   A. a B. b
   C. c D. d

143. Eclipsed-2
   A. a B. b
   C. c D. d

PASSAGE XI (QUESTION 144)

Carboxylate ions are formed by the reaction of carboxylic acids with bases.

$$RCO_2H + B^- \rightarrow RCO_2^- + BH$$

Phenolate ions are formed by the reaction of phenols with bases.

$$ArOH + B^- \rightarrow ArO^- + BH$$

In general, carboxylic acids will react with aqueous $NaHCO_3$, while the stronger base NaOH must be used for reaction with phenols. Phenols such as 2,4-dinitrophenol, however, will react with $NaHCO_3$.

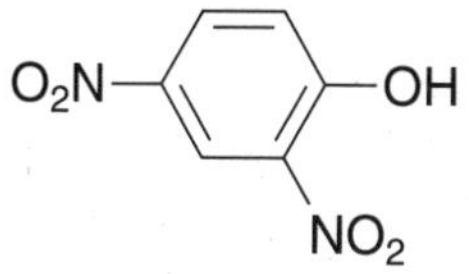

144. 2,4-Dinitrophenol is very acidic because the
   A. electron-withdrawing nitro groups stabilize the phenolate ion.
   B. electron-donating nitro groups stabilize the phenolate ion.
   C. nitro groups increase the melting point of the compound.
   D. nitro groups change the conformation of the ring.

STOP! If time still remains, you may review work only in this section. STOP!

Test 5 ■ Answer Key

1. D
2. C
3. B
4. D
5. A
6. C
7. B
8. C
9. D
10. C
11. C
12. A
13. C
14. D
15. D
16. D
17. D
18. B
19. B
20. A
21. A
22. D
23. C
24. A
25. D
26. A
27. B
28. A
29. A
30. D
31. C
32. C
33. B
34. B
35. B
36. A
37. D
38. C
39. A
40. B
41. C
42. B
43. D
44. A
45. A
46. A
47. D
48. A
49. C
50. D
51. B
52. A
53. C
54. D
55. A
56. A
57. B
58. D
59. A
60. B
61. A
62. B
63. C
64. B
65. D
66. C
67. C
68. D
69. B
70. B
71. B
72. D
73. B
74. B
75. A
76. D
77. A
78. B
79. D
80. C
81. B
82. A
83. A
84. A
85. C
86. C
87. A
88. B
89. A
90. D
91. B
92. C
93. C
94. B
95. C
96. B
97. A
98. C
99. D
100. D
101. B
102. B
103. C
104. D
105. A
106. B
107. D
108. D
109. C
110. B
111. D
112. D
113. B
114. D
115. C
116. D
117. C
118. B
119. C
120. A
121. C
122. A
123. D
124. A
125. A
126. D
127. C
128. C
129. C
130. D
131. A
132. C
133. B
134. D
135. A
136. A
137. D
138. C
139. C
140. D
141. A
142. C
143. D
144. A

SECTION 1
Physical Sciences

PASSAGE I (QUESTIONS 1–5)

1. **D.** By the conservation of momentum, the product of the mass of the bullet times its speed must equal the product of the mass of the gun times its recoil speed, or

$$m_b v_b = m_g v_g$$
$$(0.01 \text{ kg})(100 \text{ m/s}) = m_g(1 \text{ m/s})$$
$$1 \text{ kg} = m_g$$

2. **C.** Using the kinematic formula for constant acceleration, we obtain the following:

$$v^2 = 2ad\ v_0^2$$
$$v^2 = 2(-10 \text{ m/s}^2)(10 \text{ m}) + (100 \text{ m/s})^2$$
$$v^2 = 9800$$
$$v = 99 \text{ m/s}$$

Even without having calculated the acceleration above, one should realize that all other answers are unreasonable in this question.

3. **B.** An impulse is defined as the change in the momentum of an object. As a result, the bullet experiences an impulse, having slowed down due to the air resistance. The impulse is

$$I = \Delta p = p_f - p_i = m(v_f - v_i)$$
$$= (0.01 \text{ kg})(99 \text{ m/s} - 100 \text{ m/s})$$
$$= -0.01 \text{ kgm/s}$$

But, by the conservation of momentum, the earth must experience an equal but opposite impulse. So the correct response is to the RIGHT, or the NEGATIVE of the impulse experienced by the bullet.

4. **D.** The other definition of impulse is through Newton's Second Law as the product of the average force experienced by the object times the amount of time the force acts on the object, or

$$I = F\Delta t$$
$$F = I/\Delta t$$
$$= (0.98 \text{ kgm/s})/(0.01 \text{ sec})$$
$$= 98 \text{ N}$$

5. **A.** We use the same kinematic equation as earlier, but this time we'll find the acceleration given the initial and final speeds of the combination and the distance over which it travels:

$$\frac{v^2 - v0^2}{2d} = a$$

$$(0^2 - (0.98 \text{ m/s})^2)/(2(2)) = a = -0.24 \text{ m/s}^2$$

The NEGATIVE sign, once again, reminds us of the direction of the acceleration as it slows the combination down along the rough surface.

PASSAGE II (QUESTIONS 6–8)

To understand Questions 6 – 8, you must understand stoichiometric relationships, gas laws, and basic acid base definitions and normality.

6. **C.** The solubility of CO_2 will be decreased by the addition of another solute. The solubility of CO_2 is a colligative property and depends on the number of solute molecules dissolved. One mole of NaCl dissociates and provides two moles of solute

so it causes twice as much CO_2 evolution compared to sucrose.

7. **B.** The solubility of CO_2 decreases as the moles of added solute increases. Because aspartame has a lower molar mass, a given mass of aspartame provides more moles of solute than sucrose. For example,

1.0g aspartame × (1 mole aspartame/294.31g aspartame) = 3.4×10^{-3} mole "solute"

versus

1.0g sucrose × (1mole sucrose/342.30g sucrose) = 2.9×10^{-3} mole "solute"

8. **C.** Potassium has a higher atomic mass than sodium. The average molar mass of the KCl/NaCl mixture will be higher than pure NaCl. As a result, an equal mass of KCl/NaCl mixture will provide fewer moles of solute compared to pure NaCl. Thus, the low-sodium salt should result in less CO_2 gas being evolved.

PASSAGE III (QUESTIONS 9–12)

9. **D.** Using conservation of energy, the man's initial gravitational potential energy (mgh) when he starts to fall must equal the final spring energy ($kx^2/2$) when he is at the end of the fall. Equating these two formulas, we get $kx^2/2 = mgh$, so

$$k = 2mgh/x^2 = 2(80kg)(9.8m/s^2)(90m)/(30m)^2 \sim 2(80kg)(10m/s^2)(90m)/(900m^2)$$

$$= 60kg/s^2.$$

10. **C.** The oscillation frequency is given by

$$f = \frac{1}{2\pi}\sqrt{\frac{k}{m}} = \frac{1}{2\pi}\sqrt{\frac{300kg/s^2}{80kg}} \sim \frac{1}{6}\sqrt{4s^{-2}} \sim 0.3s^{-1} = 0.3\text{Hz}$$

11. **C.** The slope of the graph $\Delta F/\Delta x$ determines the elasticity of the cord. When the cord stretches easily, Δx is large, and the slope is small. This occurs in the middle of the graph when the cord has been stretched by a moderate amount.

12. **A.** The graph is represented by the equation $A = A_0e^{-\lambda t}$. Taking the natural log of both sides of this equation yields

$$\ln(A) = \ln(A_0) + \ln(e^{-\lambda t})$$
$$= \ln(A_0) - \lambda t.$$

This equation has the form $y = mx + b$, which is the equation for a straight line. The y coordinate is represented by ln(A), and the x coordinate is represented by t. The slope is $-\lambda$. The slope of the graph is approximately $-2/100$ s $= -0.02$ s^{-1}. Therefore, the decay constant, λ, is 0.02 s^{-1}. Note that there are no units for the natural log of the amplitude.

13. **C.** Resistances R_1 and R_2 are in series, so we can use the following formula to combine them.

$$R_{\text{Total}} = R_1 + R_2 + R_3 + \ldots + R_n$$

Therefore,

$$8\,\Omega = 6\,\Omega + 2\,\Omega$$

Now, we have simplified the circuit to

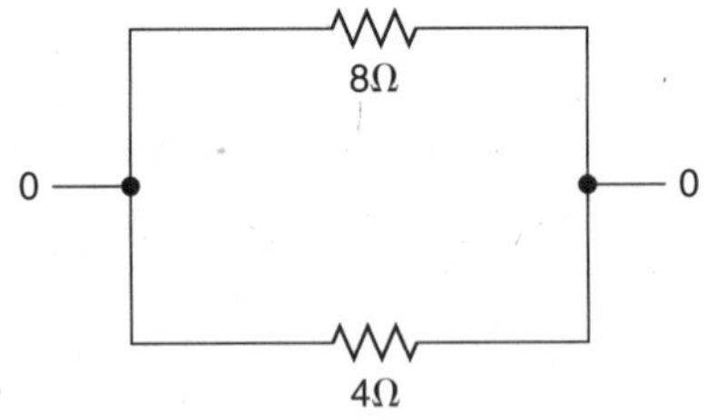

which has two resistors connected in parallel. We then use the following:

$$\frac{1}{R_{Total}} = \frac{1}{R_1} + \frac{1}{R_2} + \frac{1}{R_3} + \ldots + = \frac{1}{R_n}$$

Therefore,

$$\frac{1}{R_{Total}} = \frac{1}{8\Omega} + \frac{1}{4\Omega} = \frac{3}{8}\Omega;\ \text{and}\ R_{Total} = \frac{8}{3}\Omega$$

14. **D.** Because the resultant force is the difference between the two forces, the forces must be oriented exactly opposite to each other.

15. **D.** Gravitational acceleration on a body is unaffected by the horizontal velocity if ideal conditions are assumed, that is, if there is no wind resistance. The two cannonballs, therefore, strike the ground simultaneously.

16. **D.** The law of conservation of momentum is applicable here, as it is in all collision problems. Therefore,

 Momentum after impact = Momentum before impact.

 Momentum after impact = $M_{B1} \times V_{B1}$ = 100 gm × 100 cm/sec = 10,000 gm × cm/sec

 Momentum after impact = $M_{A1} \times V_{A1} + M_{A2} \times V_{A2}$ = 100 gm × 60 cm/sec + 25 gm × V_{A2} cm/sec

 Then, 10,000 gm-cm/sec = 6000gm-cm/sec + 25 g × V_{A2}.

 V_{A2} = 160 cm/sec.

PASSAGE IV (QUESTIONS 17–26)

Questions 17–26 require an understanding of the laws of thermodynamics. Also, knowledge of various phases (phase diagrams) is required.

17. **D.** From the table, the energy given off in forming one mole of H_2O (g) is 242 kJ, while the energy given off in forming one mole of H_2O (l) is 286 kJ. The difference, 286 kJ − 242 kJ = 44 kJ, is the energy needed to change one mole of liquid water into water vapor. Therefore, 2(44 kJ) = 88 kJ are needed to convert two moles.

18. **B.** The equation needed for working this problem is $\Delta G° = \Delta H° - T\Delta S°$, which gives the relationship among free energy, enthalpy, and entropy. The change in free energy is a measure of the spontaneity of the reaction. If the change in free energy is negative, the reaction is spontaneous; if it is positive, the reaction is nonspontaneous; and if it is zero, the reaction is at equilibrium. In this case, the reaction is at equilibrium — true for any phase occurring at the boiling point, melting point, or sublimation point.

 $0 = \Delta H° - T\Delta S°$

 $0 = \Delta H° - 298\ \text{K}\ (57.7\ \text{J/mole K})$

 $\Delta H° = 1.72 \times 10^4\ \text{J/mole} = 17.2\ \text{kJ/mol} \times 1\ \text{mole}/121\ \text{g} \times 100\text{g}$

 $= 14.2\ \text{kJ}$

 This is the amount of heat required for 100 grams, which is less than 1 mole.

19. **B.** Energy is released when a bond is broken, so the sign is negative. On the other hand, energy is absorbed when a bond is broken, so the sign is positive. To calculate the change in energy for the reaction, we only need to add the energy of the bonds formed (−) and subtract from the energy required for the bonds broken.

 4 C-H bonds + 1 C=C bond + 1 Cl−Cl bond Reactants

 4(87) + 1(146) + 1(58) = 552

 4 C-H bonds + 1 C−C bond + 2 Cl−Cl bonds Products

 4(87) + 1(83) + 2(79) = −589

 Change in energy = 552 − 589 = −37.

20. **A.** The heat of formation of Fe_2O_3 (s) is given, so you may write the equation for the formation of a compound from its elements.

 $2Fe\ (s) + 3/2O_2\ (g) \rightarrow Fe_2O_3\ (s)\ H°$ − 743.6

 This equation must be reversed so that Fe_2O_3 appears on the left-hand side of the equation because that is where it appears in the equation that we are evaluating. When you reverse an equation, you must also change the sign of the enthalpy change. Use this equation with the one given in the passage to find the equation you want.

Fe_2O_3 (s) → 2Fe (s) + 3/2O_2 (g) + 743.6

3CO (g) + 3(1/2)O_2 (g) → 3CO_2 (g)
3(−257.2)

The second equation must be multiplied by 3 to eliminate the oxygen and also because there are 3 CO and 3 CO_2 in the equation required. When an equation is multiplied by a number, the change in enthalpy must also be multiplied by the same number.

Adding the two equations together cancels the oxygen and gives the required equation:

Fe_2O_3 (s) + 3CO (g) → 2Fe (s) + 3CO_2 (g) − 28 kJ

21. **A.** You must use Hess's Law. Look up the heats of formation for all of the reactants and products. If a reactant or product has a coefficient, multiply the enthalpy by the coefficient. Add the enthalpies for all of the products and the enthalpies for the reactants. Subtract the sum of the enthalpies of the reactants from the sum of the enthalpies for the products. This is the change in enthalpy for the reaction or the heat of reaction.

$$\Delta H = [1(-267) + 1(-26.4)] - [3(-63.7) + 1(-94.1)]$$

$$\Delta H = -8.2 \text{ kJ/mole}$$

You get answer choice B if you subtracted reactants from products, answer choice C if you didn't multiply the enthalpy for FeO by three, and answer choice D if you didn't multiply by three and subtracted products from reactants.

22. **D.** Use the equation

$$\Delta G = \Delta H - T\Delta S.$$

If ΔH is + and ΔS is +, increasing the temperature will make the reaction more spontaneous. However, if ΔH is − and ΔS is −, increasing the temperature will make the reaction less spontaneous.

ΔH = − and ΔS = − Equation (1)

ΔH = + and ΔS = + Equation (2)

Therefore, answer choice D is correct.

23. **C.** The number of moles of ethanol (CH_3CH_2OH) that correspond to 100gm is determined by dividing the number of grams by the atomic weight. The atomic weight is 2(12gm/mole) for C + (16gm/mole) for O + 6(1gm/mole) for H = 46gm/mole. Therefore, 100gm represents approximately 2 moles. From the reaction, 1 mole of ethanol produces 1 mole of H_2, so there will be 2 moles of hydrogen gas produced.

24. **A.** Any process where heat is absorbed has a positive q. (Endothermic process: q = +, exothermic process: q = −.) When the system does work, it loses energy, so w = +. If work is done on the system, the system gains energy, so w = −. Use the equation

$$\Delta E = q - w$$

Therefore, if q = + and w = +, then ΔE = 65 − (22) = 43.

25. **D.** First, find the change in enthalpy for the reaction:

$$\Delta H = 2(-1121) - 4(-272.0) = -1154 \text{ kJ/mole}$$

Then, find the change in entropy for the reaction:

$$\Delta S = 2(145.3) - 4(60.75) = 47.6 \text{ J/mole K}$$

Because ΔH is negative and ΔS is positive, the change in free energy will always be negative, and the reaction is spontaneous at any temperature.

You get answer choice A if you obtained the wrong sign for ΔH, answer choice B if you obtained the wrong sign for ΔS, and answer choice C if you obtained the wrong sign for ΔH *and* ΔS.

26. **A.** In the phase diagram A = solid, C = liquid, and E = gas:

    B = equilibrium between solid and liquid – melting point

    D = equilibrium between liquid and gas – boiling point

    F = equilibrium between solid and gas – sublimation point

    G = equilibrium between all three – triple point

PASSAGE V (QUESTIONS 27-30)

27. **B.** Ohm's Law gives the relationship among the voltage V, the resistance R, and current I as

    $V = IR$ or $I = V/R = (12\ V)/(3\Omega) = 4A.$

    Answer choice A is the mathematical inverse sometimes achieved by incorrect algebra, while answer choice C is the product of V times R, an incorrect statement of Ohm's Law.

28. **A.** The relationship for the magnetic field (B) at the center of a long solenoid is:

    $B = \mu nI$

    where n is the number of turns per unit length of core, and I is the current in the windings. Thus,

    $n = B/\mu I = (0.1\ T) / (25 \times 10^{-7}\ \text{H/m})(4\ \text{A})$

    $n = 10{,}000$

29. **A.** Magnetic flux through a solenoid is found to be the product of the constant field times the cross-sectional area. Electromagnetic radiation (answer choice C) results from oscillatory fields, not steady fields, while the Faraday (answer choice D) is the unit of capacitance, not magnetic flux.

30. **D.** The repulsive nature of like magnetic poles is the cause of the motion of the permanent magnet here. Answer choice A involves changing magnetic fields through secondary coils, not the interaction between fields and magnets.

PASSAGE VI (QUESTIONS 31-33)

Questions 31–33 require an understanding of the polarity of molecules in determining the attractive forces between molecules. You must know that the strongest attractive forces exist between ions. These attractive forces decrease as the polarity of the molecule decreases. In general, the stronger the attractive forces between the molecules, the lower the vapor pressure and the higher the boiling point. Increasing the attractive forces in the solution will therefore lower the vapor pressure and increase the boiling point of the solution. If the attractive forces are all alike, then the molecular weight will control the vapor pressure and boiling point.

31. **C.** This is a Gay-Lussac's Law problem. There is no change in volume.

    $P_1/T_1 = P_2/T_2$

    $P_2 = (P_{1X}\ T_2)/T_1$

    $P_1 = 30\text{psi}$ $\qquad P_2 = ?$

    $T_1 = -10°F$ $\qquad T_2 = 50°F$

    $°C = 5/9(-10°F - 32°F)$

    $°C = 5/9(50°F - 32°F)$

    $T_1 = -23.3°C$ $\qquad T_1 = 10°C$

    $T_1 = -23.3 + 273 = 249.7K$

    $T_1 = 10 + 273 = 283K$

    $T_1 = 249.7K$ $\qquad T_2 = 283K$

    $P_2 = (30\text{psi} \times 283K)/(249.7K)$

    $P_2 = 34\ \text{psi}$

32. **C.** This is a Boyle's Law problem. There is no change in temperature. The initial

pressure is the tire pressure inside the garage (see the answer explanation for Question 31). We don't have to convert psi to another unit (atm, Torr, mm Hg) because the psi units will cancel each other in the equation.

$P_1V_1 = P_2V_2$

$V_2 = P_1V_1/P_2$

$P_1 = 34$ psi $\quad P_2$ 1 atm $= 14.7$ psi

$V_1 = 30L \quad V_2 = ?$

$V_2 = (34\text{psi} \times 30\text{L})/14.7$ psi

$V_2 = 69.41$

33. **B.** This problem involves Dalton's Law for partial pressures. The total pressure exerted by a mixture of gases is the sum of the partial pressures. The partial pressure for a component in a mixture of gases is equal to the total pressure multiplied by the mole fraction of the component. To find the partial pressure of N_2 (ρ_{N2}), we first have to calculate the mole fraction (x_{N2}) of N_2 in air. Air = 80% N_2 by mass. If we assume that we have 100g of air, then we have 80g N_2 and 20g of O_{2-}.

Mole N_2 = 80g $N_2 \times$ (1mol N_2/28g N_2) 2.86 mol N_2

Mole O_{2-} = 20g $O_{2-} \times$ (1 mole O_{2-}/ 32g O_{2-}) 0.625 mol O_{2-}

Total mole = 3.485 mol

X_{N2} = 2.86mol N_2/3.485 mol = 0.82

$P_{N2} = P_{tot} X_{N2} = 34\text{psi} \times 0.82$

P_{N2} = 24.6 psi.

PASSAGE VII (QUESTIONS 34–37)

34. **B.** The speed or, more precisely, the instantaneous speed of an object is determined from the graph on the *v*-axis as the magnitude of the velocity. At 1.5 s, the velocity is shown to be –10 m/s, so that the speed must be 10 m/s. Answer choice A is the value of the slope of the graph at that point and is the acceleration, not the speed of the object. The units are incorrect in answer choice D.

35. **B.** The average speed of an object is found as the mathematical average of half the sum of the initial and final values and is:

$$s = ½(s_i + s_f) = ½(10 \text{ m/s} + 0) = 5 \text{ m/s}$$

36. **A.** To be at rest is to have zero speed. When an object has zero velocity, it has zero speed. This occurs throughout the time interval between 4 s and 5 s, so answer choice A is the only answer that fits within this range. All other answers are within range where the slopes are zero and the accelerations are zero, not necessarily the speeds.

37. **D.** The average acceleration of an object is defined as the ratio of the change in the velocity to the time interval over which it changes. Therefore, it is

$$a = \frac{v_f - v_i}{t} = \frac{(10m/s) - (0m/s)}{(3s)} = 3.33m/s$$

38. **C.** This question deals with the phenomenon of electrolysis. When an electric current is applied to a solution containing ions, the ions will either be reduced or oxidized to their electronically neutral state.

To answer this question, you must realize that Cu^{2+} ions exist in solution. To plate out copper, 2 electrons must be added to obtain the copper atom, Cu. Because the Cu^{2+} must gain electrons, it must be reduced. The amount of electricity that produces a specific amount of reduction (or oxidation) is related by $q = nF$ (Faraday's Law), where q = the quantity of electricity in coulombs, n = number of equivalents oxidized or reduced, and F = Faradays. The number of equivalents equals the weight of material oxidized or reduced (m) divided by the gram-equivalent weight of the material (M_{eq}); that is,

$$N = \frac{M}{M_{eq}}.$$

A Faraday = 96,490 coulombs or one mole of electrons.

Because copper ion requires two electrons for reduction, the gram-equivalent weight is one half of the atomic weight or 31.75g-equiv. Therefore, you have

$$q = \frac{127}{31.75} F = 4F$$

39. **A.** If a person inhales 300L of air a day, which contains 20% O_2, he or she would inhale

$20\% \times 300L$

of oxygen per day. This is equal to

$0.20 \times 300L = 60L.$

40. **B.** The ionic symbol of an atom is equal to the charge on the atom. This charge is determined by comparing the atomic number Z to the number of electrons, as shown in the electronic configuration. The atomic number corresponds to the net positive charge on the nucleus, and the number of electrons indicates the magnitude of the negative charge of the electron cloud.

The electronic configuration of hydrogen is written as $1s^1$; "1s" indicates the atomic orbital, and the superscript 1 indicates that there is one electron in the orbital. You can determine the number of electrons present by taking the sum of the superscripts. The net charge of an atom is found by adding the net negative charge (the sum of the electrons) and the net positive charge (the atomic number, which is equal to the number of protons). For hydrogen, ($Z = 1$) $1s^1$, the net negative charge is -1 and the net positive charge is +1. Thus, the atom is neutral; no ionic symbol is used. This method is used to find the ionic symbols for the atoms described in the problem.

PASSAGE VIII (QUESTIONS 41–44)

41. **C.** Mixing four atomic orbitals will produce four equivalent hybrid orbitals. The energy of each orbital is identical. The energy of the new atomic orbitals will lie somewhere between the 2s and 2p atomic orbitals.

42. **B.** The number of orbitals is conserved. In hybrid orbitals, the mixing of four atomic orbitals produces four hybrid atomic orbitals (four sp^3 orbitals). Mixing three atomic orbitals produces three hybrid atomic orbitals (3 sp^2 orbitals), mixing two atomic orbitals produces two hybrid atomic orbitals, etc. The same is true for the overlap of atomic orbitals to form bonds (molecular orbitals). If four sp^3 orbitals on the carbon combine with four 1s orbitals on hydrogen, then eight molecular orbitals are formed. In the case of methane, four molecular orbitals are bonding orbitals and four are antibonding orbitals.

43. **D.** An sp^2 hybridized carbon results from the mixing of the 2s orbital with two 2p orbitals to produce three sp^2 hybridized orbitals of equal energy. The energy of these orbitals will lie somewhere between the energy of the 2s and 2p unhybridized orbitals. There is also one 2p orbital that was not mixed with the others. This remains unaffected and has the same energy as a normal 2p orbital.

44. **A.** The electronic geometry of an atom is a good indication of its hybridization.

Linear sp

Trigonal planar/bent (120°) sp^2

Tetrahedral/trigonal pyramide/bent (109°) sp^3

Trigonal bipyramide/"seesaw"/T-shaped sp^3d

Octehedral/square planar sp^3d^2

PASSAGE IX (QUESTIONS 45–48)

45. **A.** We need to find the equilibrium concentrations of the products and reactants and plug them into the expression:

$$K = [C_4H_8BrOH][HBr]/[Br_2][C_4H_8]$$

The equilibrium concentration of C_4H_8BrOH is given (0.1 M). According to the balanced equation, the concentration of Br– will be the same as the C_4H_8BrOH. Also, for every mole of C_4H_8BrOH produced, 1 mole of C_4H_8 and Br_2 is consumed. Therefore, the concentration of reactants can be found by subtracting the equilibrium concentration of the products from the reactants:

Br_2	$+ C_4H_8$	C_4H_8BrOH	HBr
0.25	0.25	0	0
−0.1	−0.1	+0.1	+0.1
0.15	0.15	0.1	0.1

$K = [0.1] [0.1]/[0.15] [0.15]$

$K = 0.444$

46. **A.** The expression for the equilibrium constant is

$K = [C_4H_8BrOH][HBr]/[C_4H_8][Br_2]$

$[C_4H_8BrOH] = [HBr]$

Substituting:

$K = [C_4H_8BrOH]^2/[C_4H_8][Br_2]$

$Q = [0.82]^2/[0 .08][0.6]$

$Q = 14.0$

The reaction quotient is less than K. The reaction will proceed until Q = K. The concentration of products must increase, and the concentration of reactants must decrease for this to occur, so the reaction proceeds toward the right.

47. **D.** The rate of reaction is determined by the slowest elementary step in the mechanism. In this case, it is the second step:

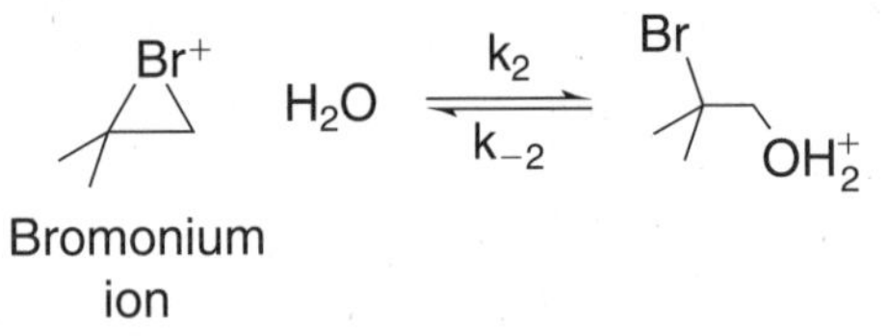

Rate = δ[bromonium ion]/ δt = k_2 [bromonium ion]

H_2O doesn't appear in the rate law because it is the solvent and its concentration is essentially constant. We cannot measure the concentration of the bromonium ion, so we must express it in terms of some species we can measure.

The first reaction is a dynamic equilibrium (the rate of the forward and reverse reactions is equal):

k_1 $[C_4H_8]$ $[Br_2]$ k_{-1} $[Br^-]$ [bromonium ion]

and $[Br^-]$ = [bromonium ion]

So,

k_1 $[C_4H_8]$ $[Br_2]$ = k_{-1} [bromonium ion]^2

We can then rearrange to get an expression for the [bromonium ion]:

[bromonium ion]^2 = $k_1/k_{-1}[C_4H_8]$ $[Br_2]$

[bromonium ion] = $(k_1/k_{-1}[C_4H_8]\ [Br_2])^{1/2}$

We then substitute this expression into our initial rate law:

RATE = k $([C_4H_8]\ [Br_2])^{1/2}$ where $k = k_2\ (k_1/k_{-1})^{1/2}$.

48. **A.** The rate of the reaction would be halved. It is true that water does not appear in the rate law because its concentration is effectively constant, but doubling the amount of water would effectively half the concentration of the other reactants. (See the answer explanation for Question 47 for the rate law).

For example,

Rate = k $([C_4H_8]\ [Br_2])^{1/2}$

Original amount of H_2O:

Rate = k $([1.0][1.0])^{1/2}$ = 1.0

Doubling amount of H_2O:

Rate = k$([0.5][0.5])^{1/2}$ = 0.5

PASSAGE X (QUESTIONS 49–52)

49. **C.** The electrical energy, U, stored in a capacitor is given by the equation, $U = CV^2/2$. We have $U = (100 \times 10^{-6}\ F)(5 \times 10^3\ V)^2/2 = 2500/2\ J = 1250\ J$. Note that if you use MKS units (Farads and volts), the solution will be in MKS units (Joules).

50. **D.** From Ohm's Law, voltage = (current) (resistance), so current = voltage/resistance. We have three resistors in parallel with a parallel resistance that is determined by the equation $1/R = 1/R_1 + 1/R_2 + 1/R_3$. We have

$$1/R = 1/6000 + 1/2000 + 1/1000$$
$$= 1/6000 + 3/6000 + 6/6000$$
$$= 10/6000.$$

So $R = 6000/10 = 600$ ohms and current = 5000 volts/600 ohms = 8.3 amps.

51. **B.** For a parallel plate capacitor, the electric field, E, between the plates is determined from the distance, d, between the plates by the equation $V = Ed$, so that $E = V/d$. We have, $E = 5000$ volts/2 mm = 5000 volts/2×10^{-3} m = 2500×10^3 V/m = 2,500,000 V/m = 2,500,000 N/C. Note that MKS units for electric field are V/m or N/C.

52. **A.** The charge has distributed equally on each capacitor plate, so each capacitor has one-half the charge of the original capacitor. The voltage is related to the charge, q, and capacitance by $V = q/C$. Therefore, if the charge on each capacitor has dropped by a factor of 2, the voltage on each capacitor has also dropped by a factor of 2. The total energy of the two-capacitor system is therefore $U = C(V/2)^2/2 + C(V/2)^2/2 = CV^2/4$. This value is exactly one-half the energy stored, $CV^2/2$, of the original capacitor. There is no violation of conservation of energy because the energy has been converted into thermal energy in the connecting wires between the two capacitors.

SECTION 2
Verbal Reasoning

PASSAGE I (QUESTIONS 53–57)

53. **C.** The passage is concerned chiefly with the proper uses of computers in education, that is, what they can and cannot do, and what some of the potential dangers are in using them. Answer choices A, B, and D are included in the passage, but they do not constitute its chief subject matter.

54. **D.** Paragraph two asserts that computers as educational tools can foster logical skills, classroom sociality, and procedural problem-solving skills. The authors also warn against making logical skills and procedural problem-solving skills the only goals of computer use in education.

55. **A.** Although mastery of facts (answer choice B), careful coaching (answer choice C), and logic (answer choice D) are important in early stages, expertise derives from intuition and experience (see paragraph four).

56. **A.** Rules learned in graduate school are a first step in teaching, but expertise derives from intuition and experience (so not answer choice B). Because computers do not function on the basis of experience and intuition, they cannot replace teachers (so not answer choice C). The authors disagree with the assumptions made by advocates of computers as tutors that we cannot teach what we do not understand, and that we understand only what we can formulate in logical rules and procedures (so not answer choice D).

57. **B.** The authors believe computers can teach a wide range of skills and can be used as tools, tutors, and tutees, but they cannot teach educated expertise (that is, their uses as tutors are quite limited).Therefore, answer choice B best summarizes the authors' view of the use of computers in education.

PASSAGE II (QUESTIONS 58–63)

58. **D.** Postman says that the last refuge of the politically impotent is to give one's opinion to a pollster. Next to the last refuge is voting, so answer choice D is the correct choice. Answer choices A and B are in conflict with the author's main thesis; the author does not discuss voting as a crucial democratic act.

59. **A.** The second paragraph makes clear that the author regards polls chiefly as instruments for gathering opinions, which are then compiled and presented as news, thus completing a "loop of impotence" (i.e., information about which the public can do nothing). Polls may or may not influence foreign policy and public opinion and may or may not play a role in a system of checks and balances, but the author's interest is in polls as part of a telegraphic information system that contributes to the public's sense of helplessness.

60. **B.** The information-action ratio involves input (what one is informed about) and output (the possibilities of action based on information). The possibility of meaningful action based on received information was relatively high in pre-telegraphic cultures, but technological advances have made the relationship abstract and remote. The ratio

does not involve accuracy of information or the relationship between history and current events. Local news may be more relevant for meaningful action than global news, but the ratio refers to all forms of news.

61. **A.** Because the context of news for people in pre-telegraphic cultures was more local than global, they received more relevant news (i.e., news that could result in meaningful action). Some pre-telegraphic cultures were oral, but some were not (so not answer choice A). The author does not discuss degrees of personal contact among individuals in various types of culture (so not answer choice D). News, of course, had more, not less, action-value (not answer choice C).

62. **B.** Telegraphy has made public discourse more incoherent (see paragraph four) and has provided information upon which no meaningful action can be based. However, it has not increased the public sense of social responsibility, even though it has provided more information (see paragraph two).

63. **C.** The author's statement occurs in the context of his discussion of the ways in which telegraphy has made public discourse essentially incoherent. Telegraphy had indeed dignified irrelevance (answer choice A), increased a sense of political impotence (answer choice B), and made the information-action relationship more abstract (answer choice D), but the particular statement made in answer choice C supports his argument in paragraph four about incoherent public discourse (Mumford's "broken time and broken attention").

PASSAGE III (QUESTIONS 64–69)

64. **B.** This problem, discussed throughout the passage, is summarized in the fourth paragraph.

65. **D.** Based on the points made in the third paragraph of this passage, there are no grounds for saying what might or will happen in the future.

66. **C.** Nothing in the passage relates to an acceptance of answer choice A. According to paragraph three, projections of probable future events are no more justified than projections of certainty, so answer choice B is also not a good choice. The final paragraph gives reasons for rejecting answer choice D. This leaves answer choice C, which is supported by the cautions made in the first and fourth paragraphs.

67. **C.** We do have a foundation (our observations of the past and present), so answer choice A is false, and we do not claim to know that our foundation is not justified, so answer choice B is false. The problem is that we cannot prove the justification of our foundation. Answer choice D is not a factor mentioned in the passage.

68. **D.** The second paragraph indicates that none of the procedures mentioned in answer choices A, B, and C would solve the problem because the problem is not in the amount of data or our analysis of this data, but in how we justify the relevance of this data to our judgments about the future.

69. **B.** Paragraphs two and three consider this issue. Becauase Hume's concern is with belief and not actuality — in particular, with the basis for our belief, not the truth of our belief — answer choice A is irrelevant. The effect of the past on the future (answer choice C) is also not Hume's concern. There is no claim in this passage to support answer choice D.

PASSAGE IV (QUESTIONS 70–73)

70. **B.** The final sentence of paragraph two gives these reasons for the predicted increase in the number of elderly

alcoholics. No mention is made of changes in the life expectancy, the availability of illicit drugs, or the expense of licit drugs, so answer choices A, C, and D are incorrect.

71. **B.** Because paragraph two states that one-third of alcoholics developed their problems after entering their elderly years, it can be concluded that this population had not developed their problems before entering their elderly years. No information is given in this passage about the percentage of the alcoholic population that is elderly or about the percentage of the elderly population that is alcoholic, so both answer choices A and C are incorrect. Answer choice D is not stated explicitly as a general explanation.

72. **D.** The trend among adolescents, described in the last paragraph, begins with both alcohol and cigarettes and leads first to marijuana and then to hard drugs, so both answer choices A and B are incorrect. Answer choice C is not relevant to the theory. Because the trend outlined by the theory is from "weaker" to "stronger" drugs, answer D is the best choice.

73. **B.** This connection is suggested in paragraph four. The relative incidence of drug abuse among the elderly is not discussed in this passage, so answer choice A is incorrect. In the first paragraph, the desire among elderly addicts to conceal their habits is mentioned, so answer choice C is also incorrect. Answer choice D is never mentioned.

PASSAGE V (QUESTIONS 74–78)

74. **B.** The passage considers only the naval aspect of World War II, not its overall outcome, so answer choice A is incorrect. The final paragraph mentions the continuing competition between ship and submarine technology, which suggests that submarines will continue to be important, so answer choice C is incorrect. German submarine technology is not compared to Allied technology, so answer choice D is also incorrect.

75. **A.** This point is made in the first paragraph.

76. **D.** The passage describes the development of asdic and sonar technologies for the detection of submarines, and both were based on detecting the sound from submarines. The other elements were not described as methods for locating submarines in this passage.

77. **A.** Paragraphs two and three describe the development of the hydrophone by the Allies, its improvement and renaming as asdic by the British, and its further refinement and renaming as sonar by the Americans. The only possible correct answers are Germany and France, and because Germany was not a member of the Allied Powers (as paragraph one indicates), it is the correct choice.

78. **B.** This claim is made in the fourth paragraph. Notice that answer choice A is not correct because, while American submarines nearly destroyed the Japanese merchant marine, this is not mentioned as occurring early in the war.

PASSAGE VI (QUESTIONS 79–83)

79. **D.** In the fourth paragraph, modern Hebrew is said to be unmistakably the descendent of Biblical Hebrew, but in none of these ways are the two identical.

80. **C.** This point is made in the opening paragraph.

81. **B.** This point is discussed in the last paragraph of the passage.

82. **A.** This point is made in the third paragraph. The author does not claim that the state of Israel is attempting to have only Hebrew spoken, so answer choice B is false.

83. **A.** In the last paragraph, the comparison is made between knowing a language and knowing how to drive a car. The stress is on performance (knowing how) rather than explanation (knowing why).

PASSAGE VII (QUESTIONS 84–87)

84. **A.** In the second paragraph, evidence is described that differentiates between cutting of a skull before death (during trephination of a living patient) and after death (as part of a postmortem ritual).

85. **C.** In the second paragraph, we are told that "many, if not most, trephinations occur in association with skull fracture." We cannot draw from this any conclusion about whether the surgical procedure causes or results from fracture, and so neither answer choice A nor answer choice B is a valid assumption; answer choice D is not explicitly mentioned.

86. **C.** The passage does not deal with trauma as a psychological condition, and the first and third paragraphs refer to the physical trauma associated with trephination.

87. **A.** The final paragraph mentions this as an indication of long-term survival. This paragraph also mentions answer choices B and D as evidence for death during or shortly after surgery because no healing has had time to occur. Answer choice C may be associated with short-term or long-term survival because the inflammatory reaction indicates that death was not immediate, but this does not eliminate infection as a complicating factor that might have prevented a complete recovery.

PASSAGE VIII (QUESTIONS 88–91)

88. **B.** The passage begins with a description of the Reconstruction problem, then tells us of Lincoln's plan and how he justified it, and concludes by explaining the plan's virtues. Answer choice A is incorrect because the author does not say Congress *did* refuse to seat Southern delegates; he only informs us this was a weakness of the plan that was *possible* to occur. Answer choice C is incorrect because Reconstruction did not fail (the Southern states once again became a functioning part of the Union), and there is nothing in the passage to suggest otherwise. Answer choice D is incorrect because the author does not attempt to highlight or otherwise consider what *caused* the Civil War. Instead, he is concerned with what happened *after* the war.

89. **A.** The author tells us this in the first paragraph when he uses the words *core elements* and then lists the status and rights of emancipated (i.e., former) slaves. In this same sentence, the author suggests that the discussion of states' rights and federal supremacy is rhetoric. In this sense, the author is using *rhetoric* with a slightly negative connotation, meaning they are not the important parts of the Reconstruction problem. Therefore, answer choice B is incorrect. Answer choice C is incorrect because this was part of Lincoln's plan. Certainly, the suppression of military rebellion is important, but the author mentions it only in passing and does not indicate it has particular significance. Answer choice D is incorrect because congressional support would be for the Reconstruction *plan* and not part of the *problem* for which the plan is being developed.

90. **D.** This point is made in the first sentence of the third paragraph. Answer choice A is

clearly incorrect because the author tells us of Lincoln's plan for Reconstruction and notes that the plan could be destroyed by Congress. For the same reasons, answer choice B is also incorrect. If Lincoln believed Reconstruction should be left to either Congress or the states, he would not have bothered to formulate his own plan. This same reasoning also makes answer choice C incorrect.

91. **B.** In the third paragraph, we are specifically told Lincoln justified his plan under Article IV, Section 4 of the Constitution. Congressional authority, in particular the ability to seat Southern delegates, certainly could affect the plan, but it was not a *justification* for the plan, making answer choice A incorrect. Along the same lines, federal supremacy is an issue to be considered, but it is not a justification for the plan. So answer choice C is incorrect. Answer choice D is incorrect because there is no mention in the passage of administrative *expertise*. The only direct mention of the administration is when the author tells us Lincoln's plan was consistent with the way the administration prosecuted the war.

PASSAGE IX (QUESTION 92)

92. **C.** After giving some background information in the first three paragraphs, the authors tell of the value of ultralow-temperature experiments in the fourth. In particular, such experiments will provide further information on condensed-matter problems such as the properties of neutron stars. Answer choice A is incorrect because the passage suggests we do not know the properties of neutron stars. In fact, this is the information that researchers hope to gain by ultralow-temperature experiments. Two isotopes of helium are mentioned in the passage: ^{3}He and ^{4}He. Nevertheless, the authors give no indication that their discovery was either made recently or as the result of these experiments. These particular two isotopes are mentioned simply because they form superfluids at ultralow temperatures. Thus, answer choice B is incorrect. Despite discussing superfluids throughout the passage, we are not told *how* superfluids are formed in experiments, except that they require ultralow temperatures. So answer choice D cannot be the primary purpose of the passage.

SECTION 3
Writing Sample

SAMPLE ESSAY 1

History is a form of social memory. Just as individuals remember some experiences and forget others, so the human race selects some events and records these events in history books. In this way, a few events are considered important and a few individuals are considered famous, while most of human experience and those who experienced it are forgotten.

Heine makes a clear distinction between those who are forgotten by history and those who are remembered. Who are the "silent gardeners" who, according to Heine, are forgotten? The phrase is a metaphor. It implies that humanity lives and grows like a plant or tree in a garden. It implies that some individuals are nurturing like gardeners. They help to meet the needs of fellow humans just as a gardener provides care for the plants in a garden. They help to protect fellow humans just as a gardener protects plants from the cold and from wild animals. According to Heine, these gardeners are "silent." They do not call attention to themselves. Their achievements are not recorded in history books, and they are forgotten.

Many different people might serve as examples. Parents who spend time with their children and raise them into good adults would be examples of nurturers who are not famous. A teacher whose efforts go unheralded might also be an example. In fact, anyone who simply does a good job and thereby provides for the needs of others might be tending to at least a part of the garden. Perhaps one reason the "silent gardeners" are forgotten is that they are just doing what we expect everyone to do ideally.

In contrast to these "silent gardeners" are those whose names are "mercilessly cut" in the bark of humanity. Now the image is that of a tree. The action is a violent one. The metaphor implies that to be remembered in history, an individual must do something to hurt others. There are many obvious examples. History books are full of outrageous dictators, from Nero to Hitler, who are famous for their cruelty.

One might argue with Heine that some of the nurturers are in fact remembered. One could point to such famous examples as Gandhi, Socrates, Martin Luther King, and Mother Theresa. A more basic argument, however, could be directed at the metaphor itself. While humans tame animals and raise crops, humans themselves are not raised to serve the needs of some other species. Heine's metaphor separates the nurturers from the nurtured. At this point, the metaphor breaks down. If humans are viewed as animals in nature just like other wild animals, then the destructive humans may be a part of nature. As much as we might detest these violent individuals when they threaten us personally, they may have a role in the scheme of things. Heine may misrepresent the human condition as tame, separating it from the natural context of other wildlife.

EXPLANATION OF ESSAY 1

The essay explains what Heine means by "silent gardeners." It is essential that the essay accomplish the specific tasks assigned in the directions. In the first paragraph, the writer sets up an intellectual framework for how the quote will be interpreted. In this framework, history is viewed as "social memory." The general assignment, to explain what the whole statement means, is broken down into several more manageable tasks. The first of these is to explain what Heine means by "silent gardeners." The writer explains the term by the method of expansive paraphrase. The terms are put in his or her own words, expanding upon the phrase in order to explore all of its implications. First considerations go to the implications of "gardeners" as a metaphor because the noun establishes the underlying meaning of the noun phrase. The writer then discusses the implications of "silent" because the adjective modifies the meaning of the noun. By paraphrasing Heine's phrase, an understanding of the quote is demonstrated.

The essay explains whose names are "mercilessly cut" on the tree. In the fourth paragraph, the writer tackles the second of the assigned tasks. Because Heine's statement makes a distinction, the sides of that distinction must, to a certain extent, be defined in terms of each other. The writer shows an awareness of this relationship by beginning the fourth paragraph, "In contrast to these 'silent gardeners' . . ." This opening phrase serves as a signpost, guiding the reader from one paragraph to the next. Signposts of this sort are essential to expressing the logical structure of the essay.

The essay includes specific examples of both of the above groups. The directions conclude with the explicit admonition: "Be sure to include examples." When directions are so explicit, it is imperative to follow them in order to do well on the assignment. Those evaluating the essays are sure to look for specific examples in determining whether the writer has accomplished the assigned tasks. After explaining in the second paragraph what Heine means by "silent gardeners," the writer immediately illustrates this explanation with specific examples: parents, teachers, and others. After explaining in the fourth paragraph what Heine means by those whose names are "mercilessly cut" on the tree, the writer points out specific examples: Nero and Hitler. In choosing appropriate examples, the writer demonstrates an ability to move intellectually from the general to the specific, to understand the general in terms of the specific and the specific in terms of the general. Perhaps most important, however, by providing specific examples, the writer demonstrates the ability to follow directions and accomplish the assigned task.

Note that the assigned tasks need not be accomplished in the essay in exactly the same order they are presented in the directions. Different strategies may all be successful. The important thing is not following a particular sequence, but rather making sure that *all* of the assigned tasks have been accomplished. If the directions had explicitly requested a sequence, then the writer should follow that sequence. In general, however, a variety of setups may be successful as long as every assigned task is accomplished.

The essay not only demonstrates an understanding of the quote, but goes beyond this to a criticism of Heine's point of view. The directions ask the writer to "discuss what you think Heine meant by 'silent gardeners.'" The phrase, "Discuss what you think," opens the essay up for some interpretation. The directions do not specifically ask, however, for any discussion of the issues beyond this interpretation of what Heine meant. Therefore, before the writer launches into a discussion of personal views on the topic, it is essential that the writer should have already accomplished all of the tasks assigned in the directions. In this case, this means giving an interpretation of the quote (specifically, the two sides of the distinction) and citing examples to illustrate that interpretation. This having been accomplished, the writer may still enhance the essay by going beyond the limitations of a paraphrase.

The grammar is correct according to accepted standards. The sentences are well constructed. The paragraphs are unified and coherent. There are no sentence fragments. There are no run-on sentences. There are no errors in subject-verb agreement, parallel syntax, pronoun case, or verb inflection. The syntax is clear and unambiguous. The language is not wordy or repetitious. Each paragraph addresses a particular topic. Within each paragraph, the sentences move easily and naturally through the logic of the discussion. There are no abrupt transitions, and punctuation and style conform to accepted standards.

SAMPLE ESSAY 2

Mill makes a distinction between those actions that harm another person and those actions that have no effect on anyone else. According to Mill, only actions of the first type should be subject to legal regulations.

Examples of the first type of action are obvious enough. It is generally assumed that there should be laws to protect the individual from the harmful actions of others. Murder, rape, and robbery are all punishable because they are actions against members of society.

It is not so obvious however, to determine when, in Mill's words, "a person's conduct affects the interests of no persons besides himself." The law forbids suicide, for example, but apparently Mill would argue that society is not warranted in interfering with suicide because the harmful action is not directed at someone else. By the same token, the law should not interfere with risky activities such as tightrope walking, mountain climbing, or skydiving. The same argument might be extended to narcotics addiction and gambling.

One difficulty with this sort of argument is that the consequences of an action are seldom limited enough to affect no one else. A suicide, a drug addict, or a gambler may hurt his or her immediate family. Even if there is no immediate family, there are neighbors and others in the vicinity who suffer because of the suicide's action. No one lives in total independence of everyone else. Every individual is necessarily a part of society. A drug addict, for example, becomes a problem for society because he or she causes a drain on the health and law enforcement resources of the community.

What Mill sees as the proper concern of law might be more applicable to civil law. In civil law, one individual can sue another for an amount equal to damages or harm incurred as a result of the actions of the other individual. In criminal law, on the other hand, it is not actually the harmed individual who is a party to the case, but the state. A criminal is arrested, tried, and punished by society — the state, as a whole. Criminal law might then be said not merely to protect one individual from another, but to enforce the moral values of society. The criminal has transgressed, not necessarily against an individual but against society. In the case of civil law, a transgression against moral values that cannot be properly deemed as the values of society could not be considered a valid legal argument.

EXPLANATION OF ESSAY 2

The first sentence is about the main topic: the distinction made by Mill. The writer does not discuss the essay itself or writing the essay. The writer does not refer to him- or herself. Instead, the writer directs the reader's attention to the topic.

The writer follows the directions for writing the essay and demonstrates an understanding of the quote. The writer does this by explaining the distinction that Mill has made. The writer demonstrates understanding by *paraphrasing* the quotation, restating Mill's idea in his or her own words. For example, Mill's reference to an individual's conduct that "affects prejudicially the interests of others" is paraphrased as "actions that harm another person." Similarly, Mill's reference to an individual's conduct that "affects the interests of no persons besides himself" is paraphrased as "actions that have no effect on anyone else." By putting Mill's ideas in his or her own words, the writer demonstrates an understanding of those ideas.

The writer also follows the directions for writing the essay and demonstrates an understanding of the quote by choosing appropriate examples. As examples of "actions that harm another person," the writer lists "murder, rape, and robbery." As examples of actions that might be considered to "have no effect on anyone else," the writer discusses suicide, tightrope walking, mountain climbing, drug addiction, and gambling. The writer recognizes that some of these actions might in fact be harmful to others. The writer shows understanding by exploring the issue in relation to these concrete examples. By choosing appropriate examples, the writer demonstrates an understanding of the abstract terms in Mill's statement.

In the last two paragraphs, the writer extends the discussion beyond a simple restatement of Mill's idea. The point is not whether Mill is right or wrong. Nor is the point whether you agree with the writer's opinion or not. Judge the essay solely on how well the writer argues his or her point, whatever that point may be. The writer could just as well agree or disagree with Mill, but he or she follows the directions for writing the essay by presenting an example that contradicts or limits Mill's thesis and by considering how this contradiction might be resolved.

The essay is organized in a series of unified and coherent paragraphs. Each paragraph has a particular function in the development of the argument. The first paragraph is an introduction. The second and third paragraphs present the two sides of Mill's distinction. The fourth and fifth paragraphs extend the discussion beyond this restatement and explanation of Mill's idea. The unity, coherence, and logical sequence of the paragraphs give the essay the appearance of being carefully planned. In this way, the writer presents him- or herself as someone who has considered the topic in some detail and is not just writing down whatever he or she happens to think of next.

A consistent style is maintained; it is neither so casual as to seem careless nor so formal as to seem pretentious. The writer avoids clichés. In this way, the style does not become a distinction but instead directs the attention of the reader to the topic.

The writer uses correct spelling, grammar, and standard idioms. The writer observes the generally accepted grammar rules concerning subject verb agreement, verb forms, and sentence punctuation. The writer avoids constructions with ambiguous modifiers or ambiguous pronouns. In this way, the writing does not call attention to itself but rather allows the reader to focus on the topic.

SECTION 4
Biological Sciences

PASSAGE I (QUESTIONS 93–95)

93. **C.** This item tests your ability to identify the stages of the cell cycle. Answer choice C gives the correct sequence of stages that immediately follow mitosis (and cytokinesis, in most cases).

94. **B.** The four stages of mitosis are presented as possible choices for this item, which tests your knowledge of the events of these stages. Pairs of sister chromatids (the "diad") appear during mitosis, line up independently at the cells' equatorial plate during metaphase, and separate at the centromeres during anaphase. Telophase features thc uncoiling of chromatids and the appearance of new nuclear membranes, and usually marks the time of cytokinesis. Based on this information, answer choice B is correct.

95. **C.** In this item, you are asked to recall osmotic relationships that exist between the cytoplasm of living cells and certain solutions. Osmosis is the diffusion of water across cell (or other differentially permeable) membranes in response to concentration gradients. A solution that is hypertonic to a reference solution will tend to gain water across a membrane; one that is hypotonic will tend to lose water. Answer choice C correctly identifies the relationships between the living cells and the two solutions where they were placed.

PASSAGE II (QUESTIONS 96–99)

96. **B.** To answer this question, you must recall the events of spermatogenesis in animals. Spermatogonia, located in the outer region of seminiferous tubules, develop from primordial germ cells that migrate to this region during the fourth week of embryonic development. The spermatogonia undergo mitotic and cytokinetic divisions to form a primary spermatocyte and another spermatogonium, thereby perpetuating themselves. Meiosis begins with the primary spermatocyte and produces secondary spermatocytes, and then haploid spermatids. The spermatids mature into spermatozoa (with the help of Sertoli, or nurse cells). Answer choice B offers the only correct sequence of cells formed during spermatogenesis. You should also be familiar with the corresponding, but significantly different, process of oogenesis.

97. **A.** Oogonia begin meiosis in ovarian structures called primordial follicles. Primordial follicles then become primary and secondary follicles as meiosis proceeds. By the time it is ready for ovulation, the structure is known as a vesicular ovarian, or graafian, follicle and contains a secondary oocyte. Answer choice A gives the correct term for this structure. The other choices are incorrect: an oocyte — primary and then secondary (answer choices B and C) — follows the oogonium in the sequence of cells produced during oogenesis; the endometrium (answer choice D) is the highly vascularized inner lining of the uterus.

98. **C.** In mammals, spermatogenesis occurs in the seminiferous tubules of the testes. Answer choice C correctly identifies the location of spermatogenesis. In the epididymis (answer choice A), spermatozoa acquire

motility and are stored prior to ejaculation. The prostate gland (answer choice B) surrounds the urethra of the male and adds an alkaline secretion to the semen during ejaculation. The vas deferens (answer choice D) is the tube that carries sperm from the epididymis to the ejaculatory duct.

99. **D.** As described in the passage, male and female genitalia are homologous; the female homologue of the penis is the clitoris, having also developed from a genital tubercle. Answer choice D correctly identifies this structure. The other answer choices are incorrect: the vagina (A), which is not part of the external female genitalia, is the tubular opening between the uterus and the vestibule of the female reproductive tract; the cervix (B), also not part of the external genitalia, is the opening of the uterus into the vagina; the labia majora (C), which are external genitalia, develop from the labioscrotal folds (they are homologous to the scrotum of male genitalia).

PASSAGE III (QUESTIONS 100–104)

100. **D.** To answer this question, you must recall the structures of the outer, middle, and inner ear in the sequence of their involvement in detecting sound. Sound waves collected by the external ear (pinna) cause small vibrations of the tympanic membrane. These vibrations, in turn, cause movement in the following structures or fluids in sequence: malleus, incus, stapes, oval window, fluid of vestibular canal, fluid of tympanic canal, and the round window. The malleus, incus, and stapes are bones (ossicles) of the middle ear, while the remaining structures are part of the cochlea of the inner ear. Given this information, the only correct answer choice is D.

101. **B.** Rods and cones differ in several ways; you need to recall those differences to answer this question. Answer choice B correctly indicates that rods are more numerous than cones. Answer choice A is incorrect because rods are actually more sensitive to light, not less. Rods are most numerous at the periphery of the retina, not in the center (the fovea centralis has none), and so answer choice C is incorrect. Answer choice D is also incorrect: rods are not color-sensitive; they only provide quantitative information about light. In addition to these differences, you should know that cones provide greater visual acuity, principally because ganglion cells receive information from individual cones in the fovea (the ratio of rods-to-ganglia in the periphery of the retina is much higher).

102. **B.** The cilia of sensory hair cells located on the basilar membrane of the cochlea are embedded in the tectorial membrane, so answer choice B is correct. Distortion of these sensory hairs causes nerve impulses to be sent to specific regions of the cerebral cortex where they are interpreted as sound of a particular frequency. The structures indicated by the other three answer choices for this question are involved in hearing but are not in direct contact with the sensory hair cilia.

103. **C.** To answer this question correctly, you must be familiar with the anatomy of the retina of the vertebrate eye. The axons of the ganglion neurons transmitting information from photoreceptor cells (i.e., rods and cones) are in the vitreous chamber and exit the eye through the retina. The area where they come together to form the optic nerve as they leave the vitreous chamber is known as the optic disc, or blind spot (because there are no photoreceptors in this region). Answer choice C correctly identifies the blind spot as the optic nerve's exit point. The other answer choices are incorrect: the edge of the lens (A) is rich in rods and very sensitive to dim light; the fovea centralis

(B) is the area of sharpest vision, with a dense population of cones, near the center of the retina; and the macula lutea (D), also rich in cones, is the area immediately surrounding the fovea.

104. **D.** Of the three areas of the inner ear — vestibule, semicircular canals, and cochlea (also known as labyrinth) — the vestibule has two interconnected sacs called the utricle and saccule. These sacs have receptors that are sensitive to straight-line movements of the head and to gravity. Answer choice D correctly identifies these chambers. The other three answer choices are incorrect: the three semicircular canals (A) are also located in the labyrinth, but they respond to rotational movements of the head; the vestibular canal (B), or scala vestibuli, is the fluid-filled upper chamber in the cochlea, separated from the lower chamber (scala tympani) except for a narrow connection at the apex called the helicotrema; and a statocyst (C) is a mechanoreceptor of invertebrates, containing sand or other granular substances, that functions as an organ of equilibrium.

105. **A.** Mitochondria generate energy in the form of ATP. They are enclosed by two membranes: the outer membrane is a continuous covering, while the inner membrane is thrown into many folds that extend to the interior of the organelle. These folds, called cristae, greatly increase the surface area of the inner membrane. This increases the metabolic efficiency of the confined space of the mitochrondia because it allows for many more enzymes of the respiratory process to be inserted.

106. **B.** The protein to be secreted is synthesized on the rough endoplasmic reticulum. Vesicles containing small quantities of the synthesized protein bud off from the endoplasmic reticulum. These vesicles carry the proteins to the Golgi apparatus. There, the protein is concentrated by the removal of water, and it is released in the form of secretory granules. These granules containing the protein are separated from the cytoplasm by a membrane that can fuse with the plasma membrane. When the secretory granule fuses with the plasma membrane, its contents are expelled from the cell by exocytosis.

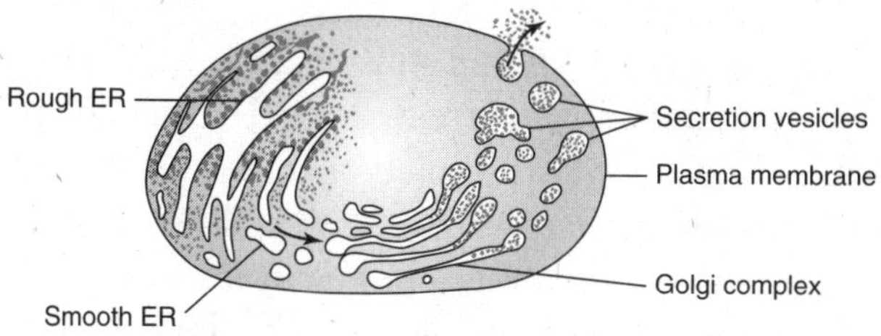

107. **D.** Centrioles are made by microtubules. As a result, their activity will be blocked by colchicine because they participate in the formation of spindle fibers. If spindle formation is blocked, meiosis (and mitosis) will not proceed beyond metaphase.

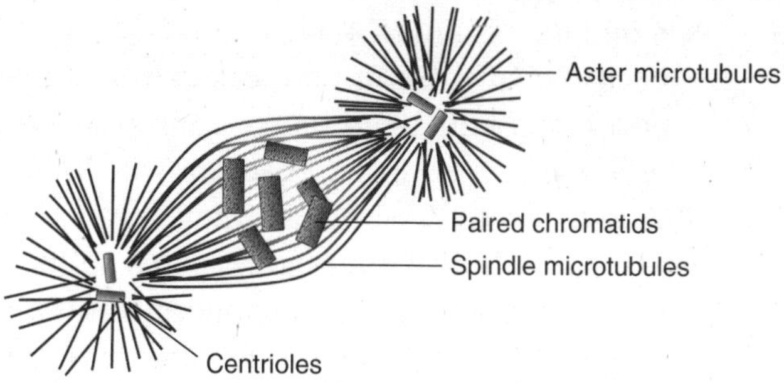

108. **D.** Homologous structures have similar evolutionary origins. They may have diverged in their functions and phenotypic appearance, but their relationships to adjacent structures and embryonic development are essentially the same. The bonds of seal flippers, bird wings, and cat paws are very similar; this reveals their common ancestry.

109. **C.** Alleles are variations of genes. They occupy the same loci on homologous chromosomes, and they are responsible for the variety that appears in the phenotypes of all organisms.

PASSAGE IV (QUESTIONS 110–113)

110. **B.** Because postural muscles are skeletal muscles that must sustain contractions over long periods of time, it would be advantageous for them to have the characteristics of red muscle fibers listed in Figure 1. These muscles, in fact, have a predominance of type I, or red muscle, fibers, so answer choice B is correct. Type IIB, white muscle fibers, with anaerobically adapted fast-twitch characteristics, would not be found in great numbers in postural muscles. Nor would intermediate type IIA fibers be found in postural muscles, despite their increased capacity for aerobic respiration. Anaerobically respiring muscle fibers (i.e., type IIB) would not be expected in postural muscles for reasons already presented. Therefore, answer choices A, C, and D are incorrect.

111. **D.** High aerobic capacity implies large numbers of mitochondria because of the need for utilization of the electron transport chain contained there. Therefore both type me and type IIA (also known as fast-twitch red fibers because they have a lot of myoglobin) would be expected to have large numbers of mitochondria. Answer choice D correctly identifies this information and is the best answer. Type IIB fibers, which are adapted for anaerobic production of ATP, have significantly fewer mitochondria, so answer choice C is obviously incorrect.

112. **D.** In this question, you must be aware of similarities and differences between skeletal and smooth muscle fibers. One of the similarities is that contraction in cardiac, skeletal, and smooth muscle fibers is induced by calcium ions. In the case of cardiac and skeletal muscle fibers, the calcium comes from the sarcoplasmic reticulum; for smooth muscle fibers, calcium comes from extracellular fluids. However, both skeletal and smooth fibers contract in response to calcium, so answer choice D is correct. The other answer choices are incorrect: skeletal muscle fibers are multinucleate, but smooth fibers are uninucleate; smooth muscle fibers do not have sarcomeres; and neither skeletal nor smooth muscle fibers have electrical synapses. (However, cardiac muscle does have electrical synapses.)

113. **B.** All of the choices listed for this question identify known neurotransmitters. Acetylcholine is used at parasympathetic nerve endings, some neurons of the central nervous system, and at the neuromuscular junction (synapse) of somatic motor neurons. Therefore, the correct answer choice is B. Epinephrine (answer choice A), norepinephrine (answer choice C) (both are catecholamines), and serotonin (answer choice D) all serve as neurotransmitters in the peripheral and/or the central nervous systems. However, the predominant neurotransmitter at neuromuscular junctions is acetylcholine.

PASSAGE V (QUESTIONS 114–117)

114. **D.** This question requires knowledge of intercellular junctions. Gap junctions (answer choice D) are circular interconnections between adjacent cells large enough to allow small molecules to move from cell to cell. They also allow action potentials to pass directly from one cell to another as in the so-called electrical synapses of cardiac muscle (intercalated discs are essentially gap junctions), so answer choice D is correct. Tight junctions (answer choice A) and desmosomes (answer choice B) are two other intercellular junctions of animal cells; plasmodesmata (answer choice C) are membrane-lined channels through cell walls of adjacent plant cells.

115. **C.** All cilia and flagella of eukaryotic cells have the same cross-sectional ultrastructure that consists of two central pairs of microtubules surrounded by nine additional pairs, so answer choice C is correct. This structure runs the length of the cilium or flagellum and connects with a basal body having a ring of nine triplets of microtubules (the same structure as a centriole). Adjacent pairs of microtubules slide past one another due to dynein cross-arms attaching and reattaching.

116. **D.** Microtubules have a variety of functions, among them is the separation of chromatids in mitosis and meiosis where they form the spindle fibers; therefore, answer choice D is correct. Answer choices A and C identify two other fibers found as part of the structure of the cytoskeleton, but microfilaments and intermediate filaments are not involved in spindle fiber architecture. Answer choice B identifies the region of the centromere of a chromatid to which spindle fibers attach, but it is incorrect because it is part of the chromatic, not the spindle, fiber.

117. **C.** This question requires that you can distinguish among the three principal types of cytokinesis. Answaer choice C is correct because cleavage (of animal cells) involves a contractile ring of actin microfilaments that pinch off the cytoplasm into two units (myosin is probably involved also, although it has not been directly seen). Cytokinesis in plants and fungi (and some protists) involves the formation of new cell walls, either from the center outward in plants (answer choice B), or from the periphery inward in fungi (answer choice A). The cell plate (answer choice D), or phragmoplast, is the precursor of the centrifugally formed cell wall of plants.

PASSAGE VI (QUESTIONS 118–121)

118. **B.** This question requires an understanding of the process of feedback inhibition in which the concentration of end product determines the degree of enzyme inhibition and thus determines the overall rate of reaction. Answer choice A is incorrect because the activity of the last enzyme of a pathway depends on the amount of substrate reaching it, which in turn depends on the activity of the enzymes preceding it. Answer choice C is incorrect because substrate concentration has little effect on reaction rate if enzyme inhibition is present. Answer choice D is incorrect because the rate is determined by inhibitor, not activator, concentration.

119. **C.** Feedback inhibition is important in metabolic processes because it offers a mechanism whereby the production of a substance can be matched precisely to the demand that exists for that substance, minimizing the waste of both materials and energy. Answer choice A is incorrect because feedback inhibition slows down enzymatic reactions. Answer choice B is incorrect because the availability of substrate is unaffected by enzyme inhibition. Answer choice D is incorrect because feedback inhibition is not a form of genetic regulation.

120. **A.** The opposite of feedback inhibition occurs when an increase in end-product concentration increases enzyme activity instead of decreasing it. Answer choice B is incorrect because negative feedback is the same as feedback inhibition. Answer choice C is incorrect because competitive inhibition will also decrease enzyme activity. Answer choice D is incorrect because a change in substrate concentration is not involved in positive modulation.

121. **C.** Because feedback inhibition by isoleucine decreases threonine deaminase activity, increasing the availability of substrate would have little, if any, effect on enzyme activity. Answer choice A is incorrect

because enzyme activity would remain depressed. Answer choice B is incorrect because isoleucine, not threonine, induces the conformational change leading to decreased enzyme activity. Answer choice D is incorrect because threonine does not inhibit the enzyme.

122. **A.** Cytosine normally binds to guanine, and uracil normally binds to adenine. A conversion of cytosine to uracil would lead to a conversion of guanine to adenine in the complementary strand. Thus, a CG to AU (or AT) event has occurred.

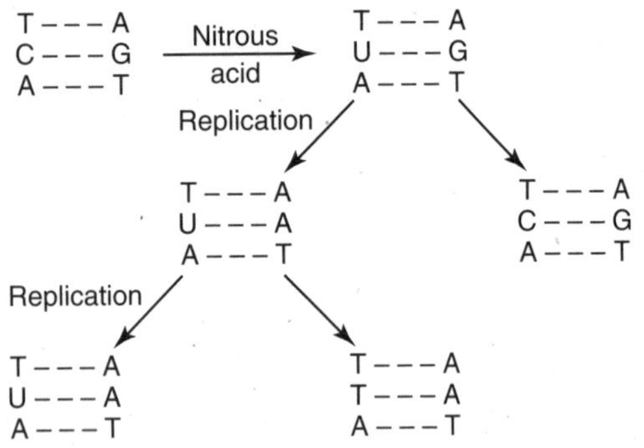

123. **D.** RNA contains uracil; DNA contains thymine. Uracil is the base partner of adenine in RNA. One way of distinguishing between RNA and DNA is to check for the presence of uracil.

PASSAGE VII (QUESTIONS 124–129)

124. **A.** To answer this question, you must recognize that the nonbinding electron-pairs of oxygen will be protonated by acid. Protonation of the carbonyl oxygen greatly diminishes the electron density on the carbonyl carbon.

$$\ddot{O}: \quad \overset{+}{:O}-H \quad :\ddot{O}-H$$
$$R-\overset{\parallel}{C}-Z \xrightarrow{H^+} R-\overset{\parallel}{C}-Z \rightleftharpoons R-\overset{\parallel}{\underset{+}{C}}-Z$$

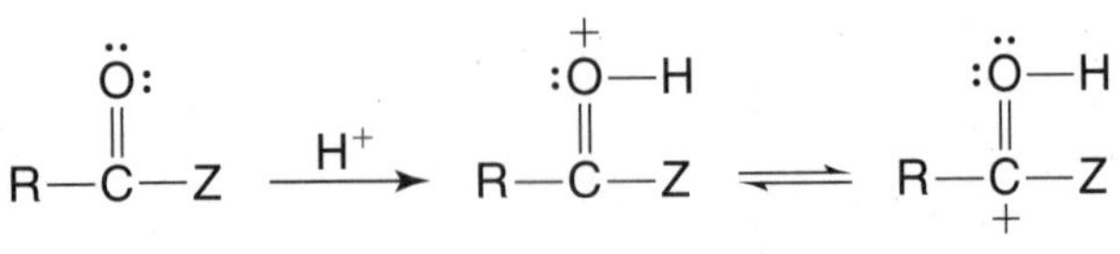

Answer choice A is not correct because the proton will not be attracted to the elec-

tron-deficient carbon atom. Neither answer choice C nor answer choice D can account for the enhanced reactivity.

125. **A.** References to the mechanism show that the oxygen of the attacking water becomes incorporated into the product acid.

$$Ph-\overset{O}{\overset{\parallel}{C}}-OEt \xrightarrow[H_2O]{HCl \atop 18} Ph-\overset{O}{\overset{\parallel}{C}}-\overset{18}{O}H + EtOH$$

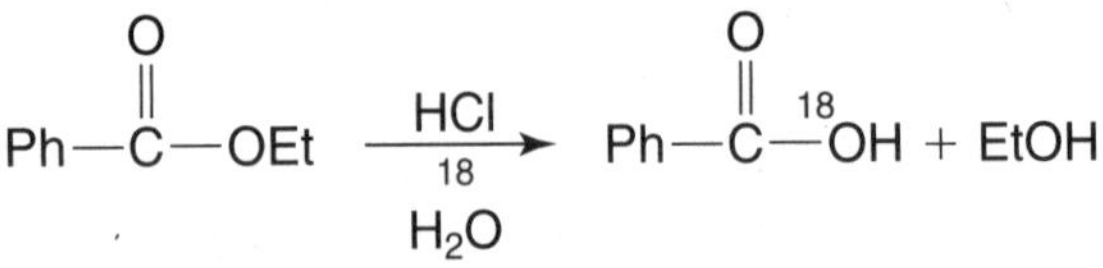

Ethanol (answer choice D) will contain the oxygen to which it was attached in the ester. Benzoyl chloride (answer choice B) and benzoic anhydride (answer choice C) are not products of the reaction.

126. **D.** The product of all of these reactions is a stable amide.

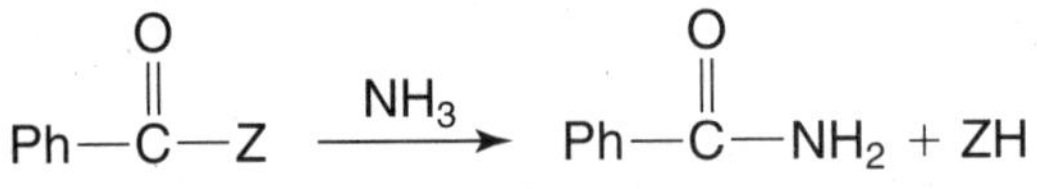

$$Ph-\overset{O}{\overset{\parallel}{C}}-Z \xrightarrow{NH_3} Ph-\overset{O}{\overset{\parallel}{C}}-NH_2 + ZH$$
$$Z = Cl, OOCPh, OPh$$

The acid chloride will react most readily, but the anhydride and ester can also be used in the preparation.

127. **C.** Because we are looking for the *product* of the reaction, we must realize that the most easily removed phosphate is on carbon 1. This is an anhydride; carbon 3 has a phosphate ester. Because anhydrides are more labile than esters, the anhydride will be hydrolyzed, leaving the ester on carbon 3.

128. **C.** Any of these will theoretically react with an acid chloride or anhydride in the manner of NH₃, except that a substituted amide will be formed. Because the reaction depends on nucleophilic attack of the carbonyl group by the unshared pair of electrons on the nitrogen atom, any substituents that are electron-withdrawing will slow the reaction. The methoxy groups are electron-donating; therefore neither answer choice B nor answer choice D is correct. The nitro group is electron-withdrawing; because the

amine shown in answer choice A has *two* nitro groups, it will react slower than the amine shown in answer choice C.

129. **C.** The reaction with thionyl chloride, $SOCl_2$, will produce the acid chloride. This will react with the amine to give N,N-dimethylbenzamide. The other answers involve reaction with the ring, which would not occur.

PASSAGE VIII (QUESTIONS 130–133)

130. **D.** This item tests your knowledge of the enzymes secreted into the digestive tract. The pancreas is one of two principal sources of enzymes, the other being the glands of the small intestine. Trypsin, lipase, and chymotrypsin (in addition to amylase) are produced by the pancreas. Pepsin is produced as pepsinogen by the stomach, *not* by the pancreas, and is the correct choice.

131. **A.** Villi and microvilli are found in the small intestine. While villi are small but visible projections of the mucosa, microvilli can be visualized only with an electron microscope. Along with larger foldings of the intestine, these structures serve to increase the surface area of the intestinal lining.

132. **C.** The ovoid mass of food that enters the esophagus from the mouth is called a bolus, so answer choice C is correct. The term *chyme* (answer choice A) refers to the semiliquid material that enters the duodenum from the stomach, pylorus (answer choice B) refers to the *opening* through which chyme enters the duodenum, and the caecum (answer choice D) is a blind pouch at the point where the small intestine meets the large intestine.

133. **B.** There are two sources of amylase — the salivary glands and the pancreas. Answer choice B correctly identifies these glands. The stomach and small intestine both produce enzymes, but neither produces amylase.

PASSAGE IX (QUESTIONS 134–136)

134. **D.** Both AUU and AUC are mRNA codons that code for the amino acid Ile (answer choice D). It is the mRNA, not the DNA, that has the codon. Therefore, answer choices B and C are incorrect. In answer choice B, ATT and ATC are the 5′ to 3′ DNA nucleotide bases that give mRNA codons for Ile. In answer choice C, ATT and AUU are nucleotide sequences of DNA and the resulting mRNA for Ile. The two nucleotides in answer choice A, TAA and GGT, are at either end of the 5′ to 3′ DNA.

135. **A.** Phe, which requires the codon UUU, is missing in answer choice A. The mRNA is missing nucleotide base pairs, and this results in the defective protein; it does not describe the protein. There are seven amino acids instead of eight (answer choice C) in the given section, but the whole protein is much larger. The mutation is a change on only a small part of the protein in the individual with cystic fibrosis, but the rest of the protein is the same (answer choice D). A second type of mutation is found in some individuals with a cystic fibrosis. It occurs within the same section of DNA as above. This mutation gives the following mRNA and amino acid sequence.

mRNA

5′	A	U	U	A	A	A	U	A	A	A	U

A	U	C	A	U	C	G	G	U	3′

Amino acids

Ile	Lys

136. **A.** Three codons mean stop; one of them is UAA. This mutation is inherited, so the

energy level of the individual (answer choice B) would not be a factor. During DNA replication, there are Okazali fragments but they are tied together. Also, the mRNA was correctly copied, so these fragments cannot be the cause of production of only two amino acids (answer choice C). In some cases, the nucleotides on a single strand of mRNA can bind together. However, there is no obvious complementary sequence of nucleotides on the tailing (right) end of the mRNA (answer choice D).

137. **D.** This question tests your knowledge of bond hybridization. Carbons that form double bonds, whether to each other or to other atoms, are sp^2. Carbons that form single bonds to four other atoms are sp^3.

138. **C.** A resonance form with only six electrons on electronegative oxygen is very unlikely. Nitrogen has too many electrons, also. Answer choice A is the uncharged, conventionally written form. Answer choices B and D are reasonable resonance contributors.

139. **C.** To solve synthetic problems, one usually works backward. Comparing the product to starting material, you can see that a methyl group has been added and a tertiary alcohol formed. This can be the product of a Grignard reagent and a ketone. A ketone can result from oxidation of a secondary alcohol, which can be formed by adding H^3O^+ to an alkene. This sequence is found in answer choice C, with the fourth step being hydrolysis of the Grignard adduct. Answer choice A is not feasible because a Grignard does not add to an alkene. The first two steps of answer choice B would lead right back to the alkene. Answer choice D has the same limitation as answer choice A.

140. **D.** Multiple bonds are generally shorter than single bonds because the increased overlap of orbitals brings the nuclei closer together. For the same reason, triple bonds are shorter than double bonds. Therefore, the acetylene bond, d, will be the shortest bond in this molecule; c is a single bond; and a and b are actually equivalent because of electron delocalization within the aromatic ring. Their length is intermediate between single and double bonds.

PASSAGE X (QUESTIONS 141–143)

141. **A.** The anti-conformation has the two methyl groups, which are larger than hydrogens and farthest apart, so it will have the lowest potential energy.

142. **C.** The gauche conformation has the methyl groups close to each other, but not with the direct overlap of the eclipsed forms; it is more stable than they are, but less stable than the anti-conformation.

143. **D.** The direct methyl-methyl interaction makes eclipsed-2 the least stable conformation.

PASSAGE XI (QUESTION 144)

144. **A.** The negative charge on a phenolate ion can be delocalized onto the ring to some extent, but the delocalization is not as effective as if it were onto two equivalent oxygen atoms, as in a carboxylate ion. Nevertheless, strongly electron-withdrawing groups on the ring can stabilize the phenolate ion to the point that it is as stable as some carboxylate ions. Answer choice B is incorrect on two counts: the nitro groups are not electron-donating, and they would not stabilize the negative charge if they were. Answer choices C and D have nothing to do with acidity. In no case is answer choice D a true statement.

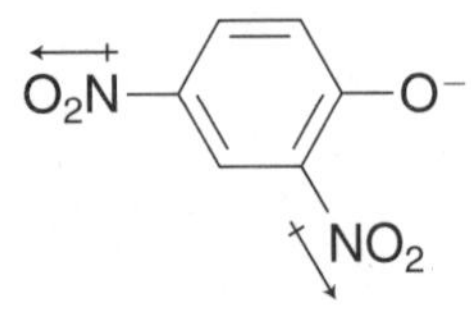

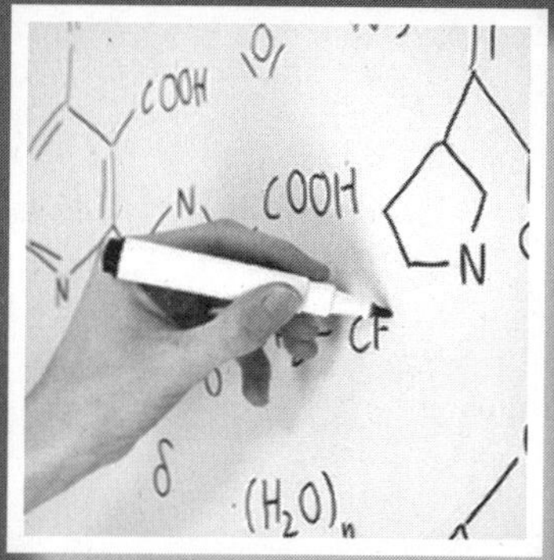

MCAT

MEDICAL COLLEGE ADMISSION TEST

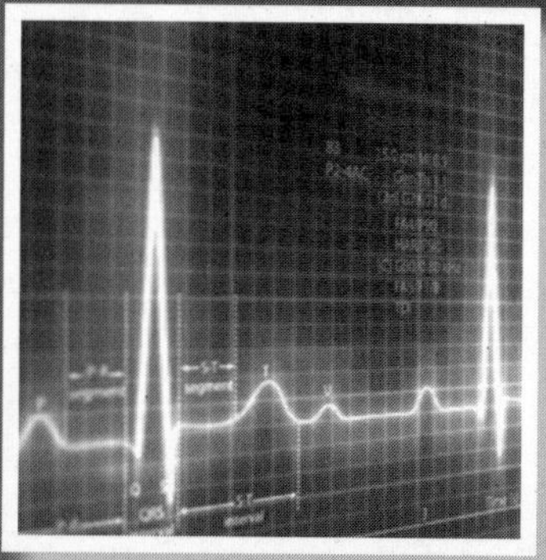

Test 6

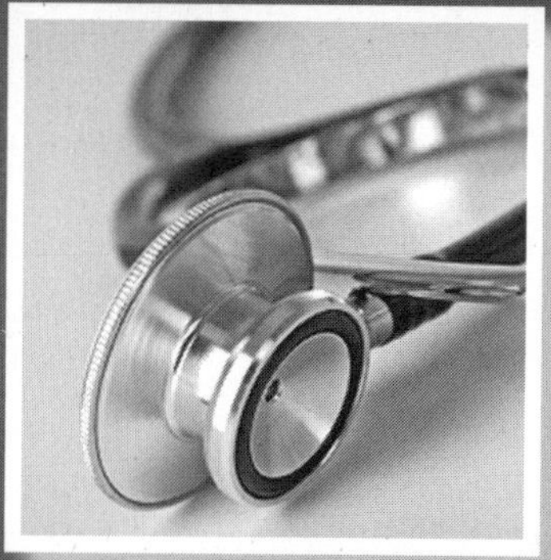

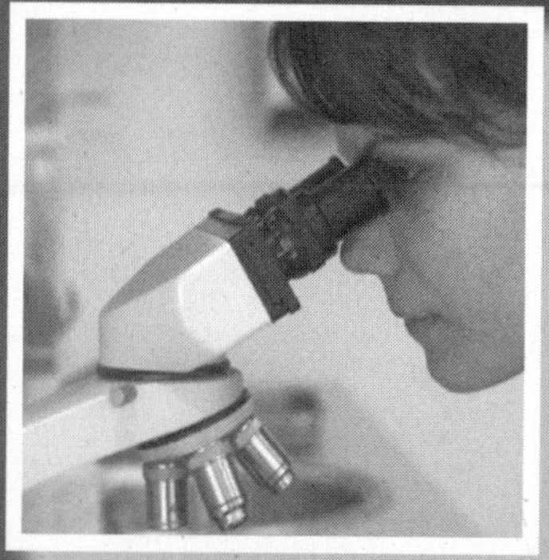

Test 6 ■ Answer Sheet

SECTION 1: Physical Sciences

1. Ⓐ Ⓑ Ⓒ Ⓓ
2. Ⓐ Ⓑ Ⓒ Ⓓ
3. Ⓐ Ⓑ Ⓒ Ⓓ
4. Ⓐ Ⓑ Ⓒ Ⓓ
5. Ⓐ Ⓑ Ⓒ Ⓓ
6. Ⓐ Ⓑ Ⓒ Ⓓ
7. Ⓐ Ⓑ Ⓒ Ⓓ
8. Ⓐ Ⓑ Ⓒ Ⓓ
9. Ⓐ Ⓑ Ⓒ Ⓓ
10. Ⓐ Ⓑ Ⓒ Ⓓ
11. Ⓐ Ⓑ Ⓒ Ⓓ
12. Ⓐ Ⓑ Ⓒ Ⓓ
13. Ⓐ Ⓑ Ⓒ Ⓓ
14. Ⓐ Ⓑ Ⓒ Ⓓ
15. Ⓐ Ⓑ Ⓒ Ⓓ
16. Ⓐ Ⓑ Ⓒ Ⓓ
17. Ⓐ Ⓑ Ⓒ Ⓓ
18. Ⓐ Ⓑ Ⓒ Ⓓ
19. Ⓐ Ⓑ Ⓒ Ⓓ
20. Ⓐ Ⓑ Ⓒ Ⓓ
21. Ⓐ Ⓑ Ⓒ Ⓓ
22. Ⓐ Ⓑ Ⓒ Ⓓ
23. Ⓐ Ⓑ Ⓒ Ⓓ
24. Ⓐ Ⓑ Ⓒ Ⓓ
25. Ⓐ Ⓑ Ⓒ Ⓓ
26. Ⓐ Ⓑ Ⓒ Ⓓ
27. Ⓐ Ⓑ Ⓒ Ⓓ
28. Ⓐ Ⓑ Ⓒ Ⓓ
29. Ⓐ Ⓑ Ⓒ Ⓓ
30. Ⓐ Ⓑ Ⓒ Ⓓ
31. Ⓐ Ⓑ Ⓒ Ⓓ
32. Ⓐ Ⓑ Ⓒ Ⓓ
33. Ⓐ Ⓑ Ⓒ Ⓓ
34. Ⓐ Ⓑ Ⓒ Ⓓ
35. Ⓐ Ⓑ Ⓒ Ⓓ
36. Ⓐ Ⓑ Ⓒ Ⓓ
37. Ⓐ Ⓑ Ⓒ Ⓓ
38. Ⓐ Ⓑ Ⓒ Ⓓ
39. Ⓐ Ⓑ Ⓒ Ⓓ
40. Ⓐ Ⓑ Ⓒ Ⓓ
41. Ⓐ Ⓑ Ⓒ Ⓓ
42. Ⓐ Ⓑ Ⓒ Ⓓ
43. Ⓐ Ⓑ Ⓒ Ⓓ
44. Ⓐ Ⓑ Ⓒ Ⓓ
45. Ⓐ Ⓑ Ⓒ Ⓓ
46. Ⓐ Ⓑ Ⓒ Ⓓ
47. Ⓐ Ⓑ Ⓒ Ⓓ
48. Ⓐ Ⓑ Ⓒ Ⓓ
49. Ⓐ Ⓑ Ⓒ Ⓓ
50. Ⓐ Ⓑ Ⓒ Ⓓ
51. Ⓐ Ⓑ Ⓒ Ⓓ
52. Ⓐ Ⓑ Ⓒ Ⓓ

SECTION 2: Verbal Reasoning

53. Ⓐ Ⓑ Ⓒ Ⓓ
54. Ⓐ Ⓑ Ⓒ Ⓓ
55. Ⓐ Ⓑ Ⓒ Ⓓ
56. Ⓐ Ⓑ Ⓒ Ⓓ
57. Ⓐ Ⓑ Ⓒ Ⓓ
58. Ⓐ Ⓑ Ⓒ Ⓓ
59. Ⓐ Ⓑ Ⓒ Ⓓ
60. Ⓐ Ⓑ Ⓒ Ⓓ
61. Ⓐ Ⓑ Ⓒ Ⓓ
62. Ⓐ Ⓑ Ⓒ Ⓓ
63. Ⓐ Ⓑ Ⓒ Ⓓ
64. Ⓐ Ⓑ Ⓒ Ⓓ
65. Ⓐ Ⓑ Ⓒ Ⓓ
66. Ⓐ Ⓑ Ⓒ Ⓓ
67. Ⓐ Ⓑ Ⓒ Ⓓ
68. Ⓐ Ⓑ Ⓒ Ⓓ
69. Ⓐ Ⓑ Ⓒ Ⓓ
70. Ⓐ Ⓑ Ⓒ Ⓓ
71. Ⓐ Ⓑ Ⓒ Ⓓ
72. Ⓐ Ⓑ Ⓒ Ⓓ
73. Ⓐ Ⓑ Ⓒ Ⓓ
74. Ⓐ Ⓑ Ⓒ Ⓓ
75. Ⓐ Ⓑ Ⓒ Ⓓ
76. Ⓐ Ⓑ Ⓒ Ⓓ
77. Ⓐ Ⓑ Ⓒ Ⓓ
78. Ⓐ Ⓑ Ⓒ Ⓓ
79. Ⓐ Ⓑ Ⓒ Ⓓ
80. Ⓐ Ⓑ Ⓒ Ⓓ
81. Ⓐ Ⓑ Ⓒ Ⓓ
82. Ⓐ Ⓑ Ⓒ Ⓓ
83. Ⓐ Ⓑ Ⓒ Ⓓ
84. Ⓐ Ⓑ Ⓒ Ⓓ
85. Ⓐ Ⓑ Ⓒ Ⓓ
86. Ⓐ Ⓑ Ⓒ Ⓓ
87. Ⓐ Ⓑ Ⓒ Ⓓ
88. Ⓐ Ⓑ Ⓒ Ⓓ
89. Ⓐ Ⓑ Ⓒ Ⓓ
90. Ⓐ Ⓑ Ⓒ Ⓓ
91. Ⓐ Ⓑ Ⓒ Ⓓ
92. Ⓐ Ⓑ Ⓒ Ⓓ

SECTION 4: Biological Sciences

93. Ⓐ Ⓑ Ⓒ Ⓓ
94. Ⓐ Ⓑ Ⓒ Ⓓ
95. Ⓐ Ⓑ Ⓒ Ⓓ
96. Ⓐ Ⓑ Ⓒ Ⓓ
97. Ⓐ Ⓑ Ⓒ Ⓓ

98. Ⓐ Ⓑ Ⓒ Ⓓ
99. Ⓐ Ⓑ Ⓒ Ⓓ
100. Ⓐ Ⓑ Ⓒ Ⓓ
101. Ⓐ Ⓑ Ⓒ Ⓓ
102. Ⓐ Ⓑ Ⓒ Ⓓ
103. Ⓐ Ⓑ Ⓒ Ⓓ
104. Ⓐ Ⓑ Ⓒ Ⓓ
105. Ⓐ Ⓑ Ⓒ Ⓓ
106. Ⓐ Ⓑ Ⓒ Ⓓ
107. Ⓐ Ⓑ Ⓒ Ⓓ
108. Ⓐ Ⓑ Ⓒ Ⓓ
109. Ⓐ Ⓑ Ⓒ Ⓓ
110. Ⓐ Ⓑ Ⓒ Ⓓ
111. Ⓐ Ⓑ Ⓒ Ⓓ
112. Ⓐ Ⓑ Ⓒ Ⓓ
113. Ⓐ Ⓑ Ⓒ Ⓓ
114. Ⓐ Ⓑ Ⓒ Ⓓ
115. Ⓐ Ⓑ Ⓒ Ⓓ
116. Ⓐ Ⓑ Ⓒ Ⓓ
117. Ⓐ Ⓑ Ⓒ Ⓓ
118. Ⓐ Ⓑ Ⓒ Ⓓ
119. Ⓐ Ⓑ Ⓒ Ⓓ
120. Ⓐ Ⓑ Ⓒ Ⓓ
121. Ⓐ Ⓑ Ⓒ Ⓓ
122. Ⓐ Ⓑ Ⓒ Ⓓ
123. Ⓐ Ⓑ Ⓒ Ⓓ
124. Ⓐ Ⓑ Ⓒ Ⓓ
125. Ⓐ Ⓑ Ⓒ Ⓓ
126. Ⓐ Ⓑ Ⓒ Ⓓ
127. Ⓐ Ⓑ Ⓒ Ⓓ
128. Ⓐ Ⓑ Ⓒ Ⓓ
129. Ⓐ Ⓑ Ⓒ Ⓓ
130. Ⓐ Ⓑ Ⓒ Ⓓ
131. Ⓐ Ⓑ Ⓒ Ⓓ
132. Ⓐ Ⓑ Ⓒ Ⓓ
133. Ⓐ Ⓑ Ⓒ Ⓓ
134. Ⓐ Ⓑ Ⓒ Ⓓ
135. Ⓐ Ⓑ Ⓒ Ⓓ
136. Ⓐ Ⓑ Ⓒ Ⓓ
137. Ⓐ Ⓑ Ⓒ Ⓓ
138. Ⓐ Ⓑ Ⓒ Ⓓ
139. Ⓐ Ⓑ Ⓒ Ⓓ
140. Ⓐ Ⓑ Ⓒ Ⓓ
141. Ⓐ Ⓑ Ⓒ Ⓓ
142. Ⓐ Ⓑ Ⓒ Ⓓ
143. Ⓐ Ⓑ Ⓒ Ⓓ
144. Ⓐ Ⓑ Ⓒ Ⓓ

SECTION 1
Physical Sciences

TIME: 70 Minutes

QUESTIONS: 1–52

DIRECTIONS: Most of the questions in this section are arranged in groups, each corresponding to a descriptive passage. Based on the information given in a passage, choose the one best answer to each question in the group. Some questions are independent of a descriptive passage and of each other. Choose the one best answer to each of these questions. If you are not sure of an answer, eliminate those choices that you know are incorrect and choose an answer from among those remaining. Fill in the corresponding circle on the answer sheet to indicate your answer. You may refer to the periodic table at any time.

PASSAGE I (QUESTIONS 1–4)

A man pulls a 25-kg crate at a constant speed of 2 m/s up a hill using a rope inclined at 25° with respect to the 30° incline. The force of friction between the crate and the slope is f = 53.33 N and is assumed to be constant over the entire 20-m long slope. The rope does not stretch as it is pulled, and the tension in the rope is maintained constant. Use the value of $g = 10 \text{m/s}^2$.

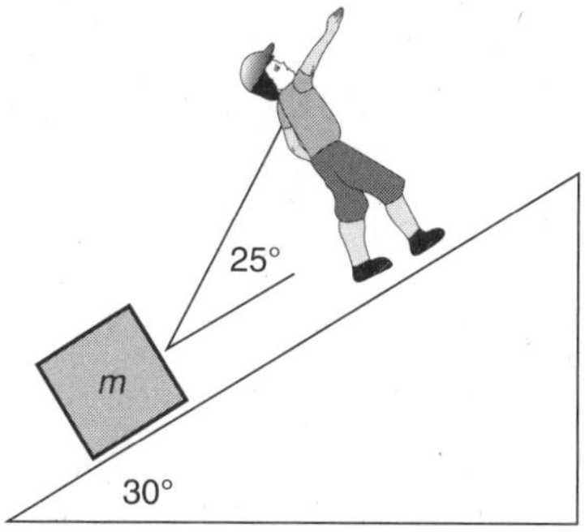

1. How much work is done by gravity in moving the crate up the slope?
   A. −5,000 J B. −4,330 J
   C. −2,500 J D. −2,868 J

2. How much work is done by the frictional force in moving the crate up the slope?
   A. −1,067 J B. −4,330 J
   C. −2,500 J D. −1,570 J

3. How much work is done by the contact force (often called the NORMAL force) between the crate and the slope in moving the crate up the slope?
   A. 0 J B. 5,000 J
   C. 2,500 J D. −1,067 J

4. How much work is done by the man in moving the crate up the slope?
   A. 1,067 J B. 4,330 J
   C. 5,000 J D. 3,567 J

PASSAGE II (QUESTIONS 5–7)

A 2-kg mass attached to an ideal Hookean spring is constrained to oscillate along one dimension on a horizontal frictionless surface. A mark has been placed at an arbitrary location on the table to designate the $x = 0$ position for this motion. As the mass oscillates without loss of energy, it traces the path shown on the graph below.

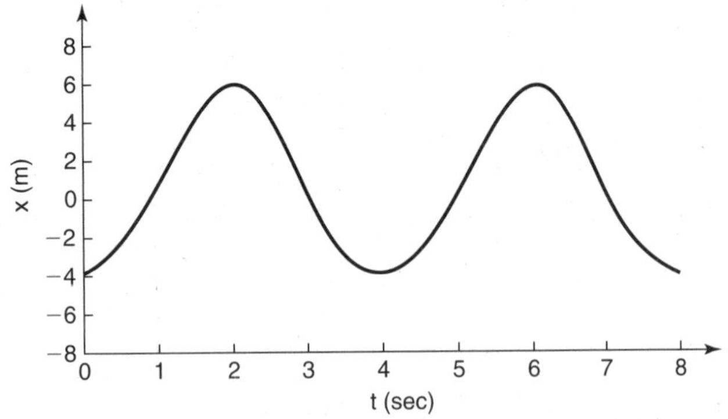

5. What is the amplitude of the motion for this oscillator?
   A. 6 m
   B. −4 m
   C. 5 m
   D. 2 m

6. What is the period of the oscillator?
   A. 2 s
   B. 4 s
   C. 6 s
   D. 8 s

7. When is the mass moving the slowest?
   A. At t = 1 s
   B. At t = 2.5 s
   C. At t = 5 s
   D. At t = 6 s

PASSAGE III (QUESTIONS 8–12)

Atom A located in Group V in the second row of the periodic table combines with atom B, which is located in Group VII in the third row of the periodic table.

Various laboratory experiments indicate that each atom in the periodic table has a different ability to attract the electrons in a covalent bond, resulting in a bond polarity. The difference in their electronegativities leads to varying degrees of ionic or covalent bonding. Measurement of the dipole moment of the molecule in the laboratory indicates the degree of polarity.

Atom C whose electronic configuration is

$1s^2 2s^2 2p^6 3s^2 3p_x^{\,1} 3p_y^{\,1} 3p_z^{\,1}$

also combines with atom B. However, atom C forms two different compounds with atom B. When more than one compound can be formed between two elements, the molecular geometry (arrangement of atoms around the central atom) is different in each case. This difference in arrangement can be detected by measuring bond angles, bond lengths, and dipole moments.

Valence shell electron pair repulsion theory and hybridization are the two theoretical explanations offered to explain the experimentally determined bond angles and molecular geometries.

8. The compound formed between atom A and atom B has the formula _____, would be classified as _____, and contains bonds but is a _____ because it has a _____ molecular geometry.
   A. NCl_3; ionic; polar covalent; nonpolar; pyramidal
   B. NCl_3; covalent; polar covalent; polar; pyramidal
   C. NCl_3; ionic; polar covalent; polar; trigonal planar
   D. NCl_3; covalent; polar covalent; nonpolar; trigonal planar

9. The compound formed between atom B and atom C, which is not formed by atom A and atom B, has the formula _____ and exhibits _____ hybridization and a _____ molecular geometry.
   A. PCl_3; sp^3; tetrahedral
   B. PCl_5; sp^3d; trigonal bipyramidal
   C. PCl_5; sp^2d^2; pentagon
   D. PCl_5; sp^3d; square

10. Which of the following is NOT a valid set of quantum numbers for an electron in element C (as described in Passage III)?
    A. $n = 3; l = 0; m_l = 1; m_s = +\frac{1}{2}$
    B. $n = 3; l = 1; m_l = 1; m_s = +\frac{1}{2}$
    C. $n = 3; l = 1; m_l = 1; m_s = -\frac{1}{2}$
    D. $n = 3; l = 1; m_l = 0; m_s = -\frac{1}{2}$

11. Element B contains ___ protons, ___ electrons, and ___ neutrons and will form a

___ ion whose radius will be ___ the radius of the parent atom.

A. 17; 17; 17; −1; <
B. 17; 17; 18; −1; <
C. 17; 17; 18; −1; >
D. 17; 18; 18; +1; <

12. The molecular orbital diagram for the molecule formed between two atoms of element A indicates that the molecule is _____, with _____ electrons in the bonding molecular orbitals and _____ electrons in the antibonding molecular orbitals, which results in a bond order of _____.

A. diamagnetic; 8; 4; 2
B. paramagnetic; 8; 2; 3
C. paramagnetic; 7; 4; 2
D. diamagnetic; 8; 2; 3

PASSAGE IV (QUESTIONS 13–16)

A meter stick, whose center of gravity is found to be at exactly its midpoint, is pivoted at $x = 0$ cm by a frictionless pivot. It is maintained horizontal with the use of a spring balance that is attached to the stick at $x = 20$ cm. The angle (θ) between the stick and the direction of the applied force on the balance is permitted to vary between 90° and 150°, while the meter stick is kept horizontal, during which time the force registered by the balance changes. A 2 N weight is hung at $x = 95$ cm on the stick so that its weight is vertically downward at that point. The table and figure below record the above information, as well as some values of the spring force versus the angle.

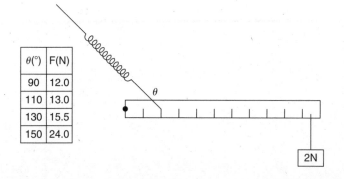

θ(°)	F(N)
90	12.0
110	13.0
130	15.5
150	24.0

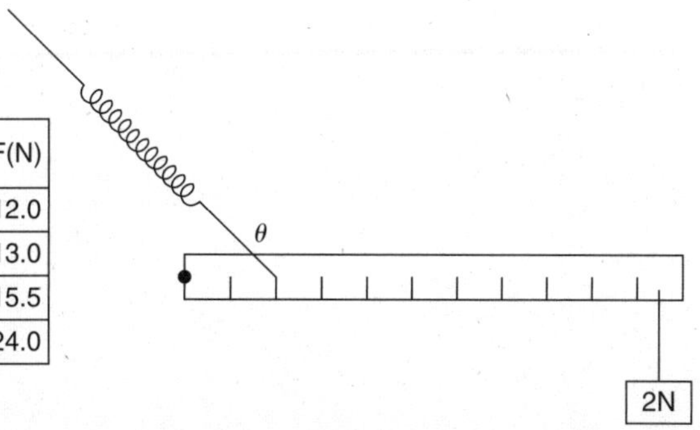

13. Compute the torque on the stick about its pivot created by the 2 N mass.

A. 1 Nm
B. 1.5 Nm
C. 2 Nm
D. 1.9 Nm

14. Compute the torque on the stick about its pivot created by the spring balance when it is at 90°.

A. 0 Nm
B. 2.4 Nm
C. 3.6 Nm
D. 5 Nm

15. If the meter stick were held below the horizontal, the

A. torque due to the 2 N weight would not change.
B. angle between the spring balance and the stick could not be 90°.
C. angle would be exactly 90°.
D. torque due to the weight of the meter stick would change.

16. Which diagram below best illustrates the direction of the force exerted by the pivot on the stick when the angle of the spring balance is 150°?

A.
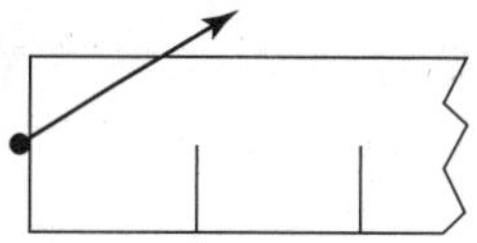

B.
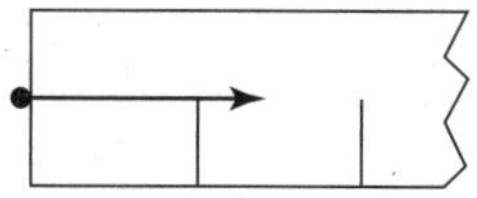

C.
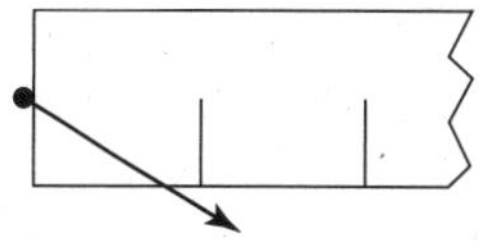

D.
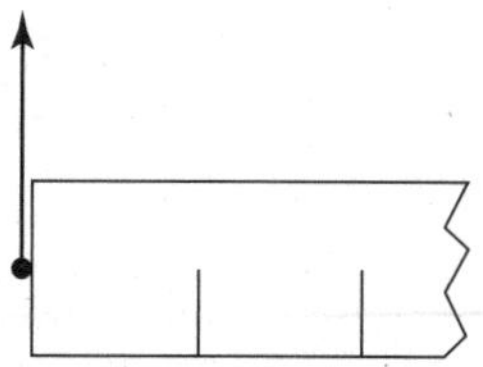

PASSAGE V (QUESTIONS 17–20)

A thermodynamic system comprised of a non-ideal gas is taken through the cycle shown below as a $P - V$ diagram. The process from state c to state a is adiabatic and requires that 500 J of work be done on the gas. Getting to state a from state b, however, requires that 750 J of work be done on the gas along the isothermal path shown, during which time 300 J of heat flows out of the gas. The process from state b to state c takes place at constant volume.

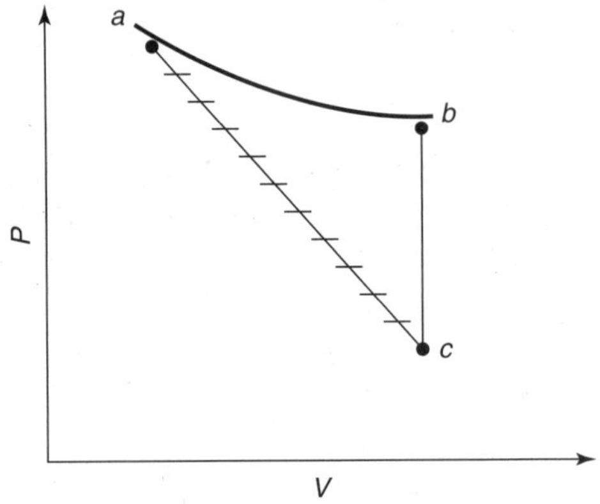

17. How much work is done by the gas during one complete cycle traversed counterclockwise?

    A. 0 J B. 250 J
    C. −250 J D. −1,250 J

18. What is the change in the internal energy of the gas during the process from state a to state b?

    A. 0 J B. 1050 J
    C. 450 J D. −450 J

19. How much heat is absorbed by the gas during the process from state c to state a?

    A. 500 J B. 250 J
    C. 0 J D. −250 J

20. How much heat flows out of the gas during the process from state b to state c?

    A. 300 J B. 50 J
    C. 0 J D. 250 J

QUESTIONS 21–25 are NOT based on a descriptive passage.

21. A concave makeup mirror is placed 2.0 cm from a nose. The image of the nose is located 5.0 cm behind the mirror. What is the focal length of the mirror?

    A. 1.4 cm B. 2.0 cm
    C. 2.5 cm D. 3.3 cm

22. Equipotential lines for a certain region of space are semicircles, as shown in the diagram below. Each line is labeled in units of volts. From this diagram, determine the approximate value of the electric field at point P. A length scale is shown at the bottom right of the diagram.

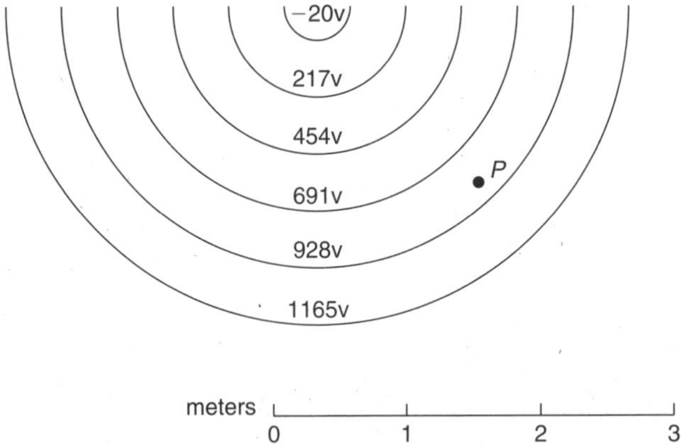

    A. 320 N/C B. 470 N/C
    C. 640 N/C D. 850 N/C

23. A U-shaped section of wire is located in a 0.8-Tesla magnetic field that points into the page, as shown below. A 3-amp current flows in the wire in the indicated direction. Determine the direction of the *net* force on the entire U-shaped section of wire. The length of sections A, B, and C are 2 cm, 5 cm, and 2 cm, respectively.

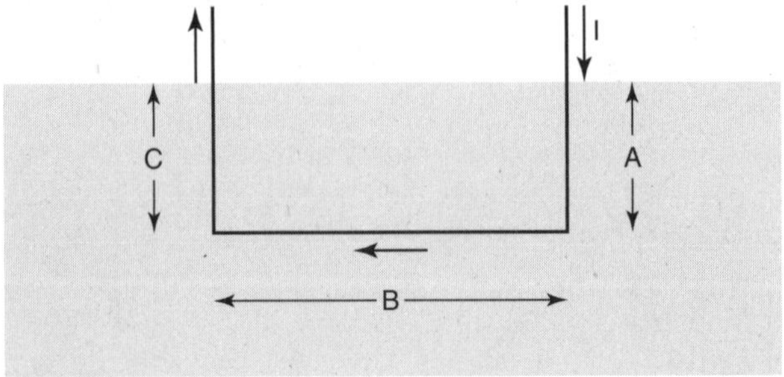

A. Into the page
B. Out of the page
C. Up
D. Down

24. Which of the following is *not* a characteristic of an exothermic reaction?
 A. The potential energy of the products is lower than the potential energy of the reactants.
 B. There is a negative ΔH.
 C. There is energy of activation.
 D. There is a positive ΔH.

25. Liquid helium tanks have pressure relief valves that allow high-pressure gas to escape. Assume that 5 kg of helium are held in a container of volume 1.50 m^3. If no pressure relief valve were used, determine the approximate pressure exerted by the gas on the walls of the container when the helium is at room temperature. You may treat the helium as an ideal gas.
 A. 2.1×10^6 N/m^2
 B. 3.5×10^6 N/m^2
 C. 4.2×10^6 N/m^2
 D. 6.4×10^6 N/m^2

PASSAGE VI (QUESTIONS 26–30)

EXPERIMENT 1

The following data was obtained when the reaction below was studied:

$$2A + B + 3C \rightleftharpoons \rightarrow \text{Products}$$

Initial Rate	[A]	[B]	[C]
3	1	1	1
6	2	1	1
27	1	1	3
3	1	4	1

EXPERIMENT 2

The concentrations of B and C were kept constant and the concentration of A was observed over time.

Time, min	[A]
0	0.400
10	0.300
20	0.200
30	0.150
40	0.100
50	0.075
60	0.500

EXPERIMENT 3

A given set of concentrations of A, B, and C was used to determine the rate of the reaction at various temperatures.

Temperature (°C)	k(L mol^{-1}s^{-1})
283	1.2×10^{-4}
302	3.5×10^{-4}
355	6.8×10^{-3}
393	1.8×10^{-2}
430	1.7×10^{-1}

26. The rate of disappearance of A should be _____ the rate of disappearance of B, while the disappearance of C should be _____ the rate of disappearance of B.
 A. twice; twice
 B. twice; triple
 C. one-half; one-third
 D. one-half; one-half

27. Tripling the concentration of C _____ the initial rate of the reaction by a factor of _____.
 A. increases; 3
 B. increases; 9
 C. increases; 2
 D. There is no obvious relationship.

28. Combine the answers to the previous two questions with the effect of increasing the concentration of B by a factor of 4 to determine the rate law for this reaction. The rate law is
 A. rate = $k[A][B][C]^2$
 B. rate = $k[A]^2[C]$
 C. rate = $k[A][C]^2$
 D. rate = $k[A]^2[B][C]^3$

29. The overall order of this reaction is
    A. 6. B. 4.
    C. 5. D. 3.

30. How much faster will a reaction be at 65°C compared to the same reaction at 25°C?
    A. 4 times B. 8 times
    C. 16 times D. 2 times

PASSAGE VII (QUESTIONS 31–34)

A 1.5-V dry cell battery with internal resistance (r) is connected in series with an external resistor (R) and an ammeter, as shown in the figure below. A current of 0.15 A is measured. A voltmeter is also attached at the terminals of the battery, as shown. With the circuit connected, it records a value of 1.40 V. When the circuit is broken — i.e., when the resistor is disconnected from the battery — the voltmeter records a value of 1.50 V.

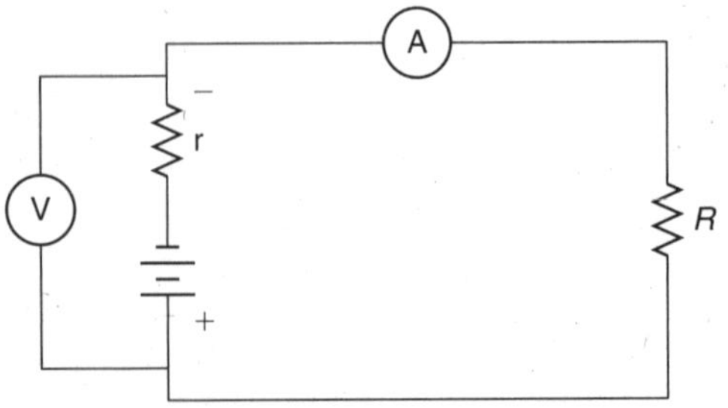

31. The voltage reading of 1.5 V recorded when the circuit is broken is called the _____ of the battery.
    A. energy B. electromotive force
    C. power D. equipotential

32. The value of the external resistance is
    A. 10 Ω. B. 8.50 Ω.
    C. 0.21 Ω. D. 9.33 Ω.

33. The value of the internal resistance of the battery is
    A. 9.33 Ω. B. 0.67 Ω.
    C. 1.50 Ω. D. 10 Ω.

34. If the mass of the external resistor is 2 grams and its specific heat capacity is 0.5 J/(g°C), approximately how much time will it take to increase in temperature by 10°C? Assume that the loss of heat to the surroundings is negligible.
    A. 10 s B. 25 s
    C. 50 s D. 120 s

PASSAGE VIII (QUESTIONS 35–39)

A converging lens of focal length $f_1 = +20$ cm is located 10 cm to the left of a diverging lens of focal length $f_2 = -15$ cm. A 10-cm tall object is placed 40 cm to the left of the converging lens. The image produced by the converging lens (as if it were alone) will act as the object for the diverging lens.

35. If the diverging lens were not there, the image would be located _____ the converging lens.
    A. 40 cm to the left of
    B. 20 cm to the right of
    C. 40 cm to the right of
    D. at infinity to the right of

36. If the diverging lens were not there, the image would be
    A. inverted and smaller than the object.
    B. inverted and the same size as the object.
    C. upright and larger than the object.
    D. not visible at all.

37. The diverging lens acts to
    A. confine the region for viewing the object.
    B. magnify the object.
    C. intensify the object.
    D. produce a virtual image of the object.

38. The final image produced by the combined system is located
    A. 20 cm to the left of the converging lens.
    B. 30 cm to the right of the diverging lens.

C. 10 cm to the right of the diverging lens.
D. at infinity to the left of the diverging lens.

39. The total magnification of the system is

A. $-\frac{1}{3}$ B. $+\frac{2}{3}$
C. -1 D. $+1$

PASSAGE IX (QUESTIONS 40–42)

Alkenes are organic molecules that can be prepared by the dehydration of alcohols under acidic conditions. The first steps in the mechanism of these reactions are the protonation of the alcohol, followed by removal of water to produce a positively charged reactive intermediate. A number of reaction pathways are available to this reactive intermediate, which results in a complex mixture of alkene products. As a result, the acid-catalyzed dehydration of alcohols is rarely used as a synthetic method for the preparation for alkenes. One of many mechanistic pathways for the formation of an alkene product is shown below:

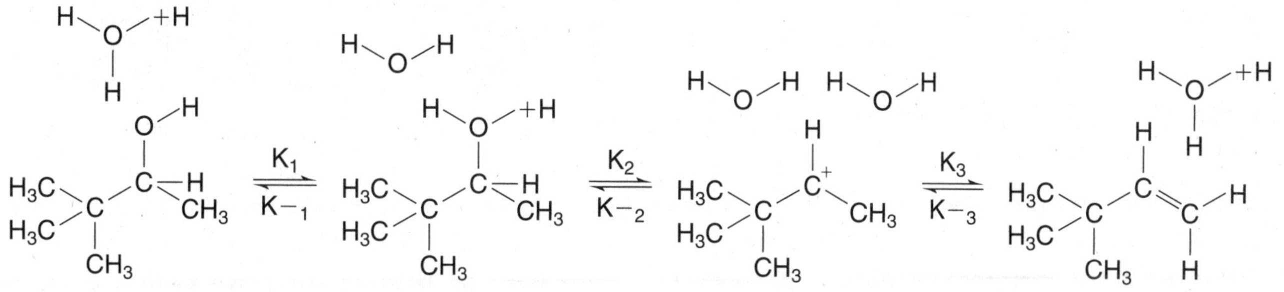

A B C D
Reactive Intermediate Product

The formation of **C** is the rate-determining step. Reactive intermediate **C** cannot be isolated and reacts further to produce alkene **D** by the loss of an H^+.

40. What is the rate law for the formation of B from A?
A. $\delta B/\delta t = (k_1/k_{-1})[A][^+H_3O]/[B]$
B. $\delta B/\delta t = k_1[A][^+H_3O]$
C. $\delta B/\delta t = k_1[A]$
D. $\delta B/\delta t = (k_1/k_{-1})[A][^+H_3O]/[B]$

41. What is the expression for the equilibrium constant for the reaction of A going to B?
A. $K = (k_1/k_{-1})[A][^+H_3O]/[B]$
B. $K = (k_{-1}/k_1)[B]/[^+H_3O][A]$
C. $K = k_1/k_{-1}$
D. $K = k_{-1}/k_1$

42. What is the rate law for the overall reaction?
A. $\delta D/\delta t = k_3[C]$
B. $\delta D/\delta t = (k_3/k_{-3})[D]/[C]$
C. $\delta D/\delta t = k_2[B]$
D. $\delta D/\delta t = (k_2k_1/k_{-1})[A]$

PASSAGE X (QUESTIONS 43–46)

In the book *The Little Prince* by Antoine de Saint-Exupéry and Richard Howard, the little prince lives on a small planet. The planet's size and rate of rotation allows the prince to watch sunsets continuously by simply moving his chair after each setting. The authors would like us to believe that the little prince liked to watch sunsets. A more likely reason the little prince chases the sun is that his planet has no water to regulate its temperature. As a result, the sunny side of the planet must be exceedingly hot, and the shady side must be exceedingly cold. To maintain a livable temperature, the little prince needs to maintain a position that is continuously at dusk.

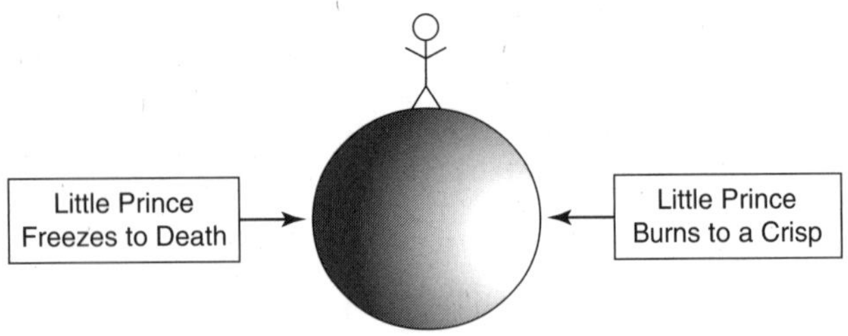

Suppose the little prince moves to another planet that is composed entirely of water to regulate the temperature. Water has a heat of vaporization of λH_{vap} = 40.7kJ/mol and a heat of fusion of LH_{fus} = 6.0kJ/mol. During the day, some of the sun's energy is used in the evaporation of water. This energy is released at night by the condensation of water. If the planet has ice caps, these too would help regulate the temperature by their melting and freezing. The high heat capacity (C = 4.18J/g°C) of water also makes the planet resistant to large changes in temperature.

The little prince's new water planet has a mass of 1.0×10^6kg. During the day, the sun supplies 1.0×10^8 kJ of energy to the planet. This amount of energy is enough to liquefy two metric tons of iron.

43. If the planet is composed entirely of liquid water, what is the planet's change in temperature after it absorbs this 1.0×10^8 kJ of heat energy?

A. $\Delta T = +24°C$ B. $\Delta T = +43°C$
C. $\Delta T = -43°C$ D. $\Delta T = +0.024°C$

44. If some of the sun's energy is used to evaporate 20,000kg of water during the day, how much of the sun's energy is left to heat the liquid water on the planet? What is the change in temperature of the liquid water?

A. $q = 4.52 \times 10^7$ kJ; $\Delta T = -11°C$
B. $q = 4.52 \times 10^7$ kJ; $\Delta T = +11°C$
C. $q = 5.48 \times 10^7$ kJ; $\Delta T = +13°C$
D. $q = 5.48 \times 10^7$ kJ; $\Delta T = -13°C$

45. At night, 20,000kg of water vapor condense and are returned to the planet surface. What is the temperature change of the planet?

A. $\Delta T = +11°C$ B. $\Delta T = -11°C$
C. $\Delta T = +13°C$ D. $\Delta T = -13°C$

46. During the day, the little prince sits on an iceberg. Eventually, the iceberg melts and the little prince has to go swimming. The iceberg has a mass of 100,000kg and is in equilibrium with the liquid water on the planet. What is the temperature of the water when the little prince goes for a swim?

A. $T = +8°C$ B. $T = -8°C$
C. $T = -16°C$ D. $T = +16°C$

PASSAGE XI (QUESTIONS 47–49)

Hydrogen has 1 valence electron in a 1s atomic orbital (AO). The s orbital is spherically shaped. Two hydrogen atoms may combine to form an H_2 molecule. The process of bond formation involves the overlap (or mixing) of the 1s AO of the hydrogen atoms. This process produces two new orbitals referred to as molecular orbitals (MO). Each new MO can hold two electrons. One MO is lower in energy than an unbonded 1s AO and is called a bonding orbital. The other MO produced is higher in energy than a 1s AO and is called an antibonding orbital.

Electrons occupying the bonding MO are stabilized by both hydrogen nuclei. As a result, the electrons in this MO are lower in energy than electrons in the uncombined H 1s AO. Adding an electron to the bonding MO results in the release of energy. This is why hydrogen atoms can combine to form H_2 molecules.

Electrons in antibonding MOs are destabilized relative to electrons in an H 1s AO. An energy input is required to place electrons in these MOs. The energy needed to place electrons in an antibonding MO is greater than the amount of energy released from putting an electron in a bonding MO.

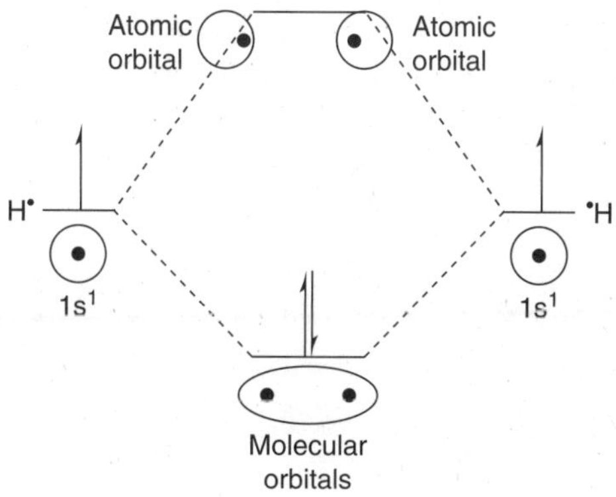

47. If H^+ and H• were combined to form a molecule, how would its bond length and bond strength compare to a normal H_2 molecule composed of 2H• atoms?
    A. Same bond length, same bond strength
    B. Shorter bond length, greater bond strength
    C. Longer bond length, weaker bond strength
    D. No bond would form.

48. If H^+ and $H{:}^-$ were combined to form a molecule, how would its bond length and bond strength compare to a normal H_2 molecule composed of 2H• atoms?
    A. Same bond length, same bond strength
    B. Shorter bond length, greater bond strength
    C. Longer bond length, weaker bond strength
    D. No bond would form.

49. If $H{:}^-$ and H• were combined to form a molecule, how would its bond length and bond strength compare to a normal H_2 molecule composed of 2H• atoms?
    A. Same bond length, same bond strength
    B. Shorter bond length, greater bond strength
    C. Longer bond length, weaker bond strength
    D. No bond would form.

QUESTIONS 50–52 are NOT based on a descriptive passage.

50. H_2(g) reacts with I_2(g) to give HI(g) at 700°K. However, when *X* is introduced to the system, it is observed that the reaction now occurs at the same rate at 400°K. *X* is a(n)
    A. substitution agent.
    B. linking agent.
    C. enzyme.
    D. catalyst.

51. The salt produced by the equimolar reaction of acetic acid with sodium hydroxide is
    A. neutral. B. acidic.
    C. alkaline. D. aprotic.

52. In a certain experiment, a constant 100-N horizontal force is applied to two blocks resting on a horizontal frictionless surface. The block on the left has a mass of 8 kg and the block on the right has a mass of 12 kg.

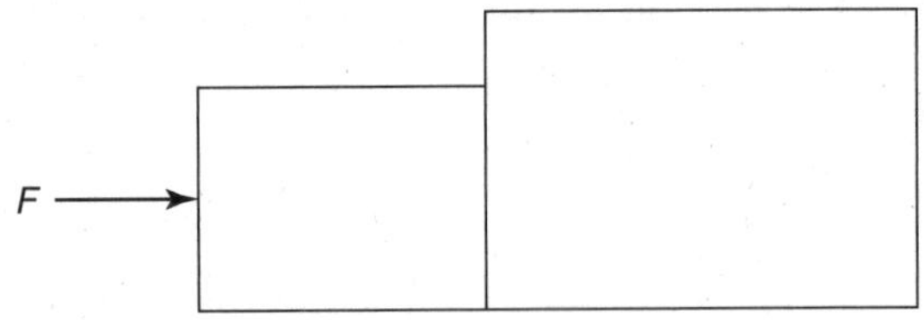

Determine the contact force between the two blocks.

A. 100 N B. 80 N
C. 60 N D. 0 N

STOP!

If time still remains, you may review work only in this section. When the time allotted is up, you may go on to the next section.

STOP!

SECTION 2
Verbal Reasoning

TIME: 60 Minutes

QUESTIONS: 53–92

DIRECTIONS: The verbal reasoning section contains nine passages, each followed by a series of questions. Based on the information given in a passage, choose the one best answer to each question.

PASSAGE I (QUESTIONS 53–57)

In his classic book *Ethics*, G. E. Moore presented an ethical theory and defended it by offering a detailed critique of a number of alternative theories.

One of the important distinctions Moore brought out was the reasons that may lead us to think an action is right or wrong and the reasons that actually constitute an action's being right or wrong. This is a plausible distinction, but one that we are apt to overlook. The difference Moore was calling to our attention here is between the considerations that may be effective in causing us to understand or believe that an action is right and the very different matter of what makes the action right. In another context, we might see this distinction in the mechanism by which we determine or come to believe that someone is a girl and not a boy. Normally, we rely on such facts as the name or the attire of the person, when in fact we know that these clues are entirely incidental to the person's actual gender. A person being named "Mary" is a good reason for our belief that the person so named is a girl, but it is no reason at all for why the person actually is a girl.

Applying this point to the rightness of actions, Moore urged that we carefully determine whether such things as our own or others' approval of an action is merely a reason for our belief in the rightness of an action or the sort of thing that actually makes an action right.

In challenging the idea that approval of some sort is what actually makes an action right, Moore noted that there are several difficulties with this view. For example, consider the case where two people are disagreeing about whether or not a certain action is right. If the rightness of the act were constituted only by the individual's approval of it — if "right" simply means "approved of" — then these two people could not, in fact, disagree with one another at all. Their statements that the act in question is or is not right are not in conflict because they are actually talking about two different things: their separate feelings of approval.

If it is said, instead, that the approval that is relevant here is general approval (the approval of most people in a society), then a moral reformer's assertion, "I know that most people approve of this action but I believe that this action is wrong," would be self-contradictory because it means, "I know that most people approve of this action but I believe that this action is what most people do not approve of." If general approval determines rightness, then the individual moral reformer's belief would not be sufficient for reclassifying as wrong an act that is approved of by most members of the society.

Moore argued that we should not confuse our approval of an action with the reasons for it being true that the action is right. It may be true that the reason why we think an action is right is that we approve of it, but this is a very different thing from the reason why the action is, in fact, right.

53. According to this passage, Moore considered our own or others' approval of an action to be an invalid reason for
   A. our believing the action is right.
   B. the action being right.
   C. our performing the action.
   D. not doing the action.

54. According to the passage, if everyone agrees that an action is right,
   A. the action is right.
   B. it is true that the action is right.
   C. it is possible that the action is not right.
   D. it should be abided.

55. Suppose someone was raised to believe that stealing is all right. Moore would accept this as an explanation for
   A. why this person would believe that stealing is right.
   B. why stealing would be right.
   C. why stealing would be right for this person.
   D. why stealing is immoral.

56. In this passage, it is argued that
   A. what is right is the same as what a person approves of.
   B. people do not disagree about what is right.
   C. approval is not what makes an action right.
   D. majority consensus determines what is right.

57. If we were to apply Moore's principles of reasoning, we would regard the fuel gauge on an automobile as
   A. a reason for our believing how much fuel is in the automobile.
   B. a reason for how much fuel is in the automobile.
   C. irrelevant to how much gas we put in the car.
   D. unreliable.

PASSAGE II (QUESTIONS 58–62)

Since life began eons ago, thousands of creatures have come and gone like the dinosaur — sometimes rendered extinct by naturally changing ecological conditions, but more recently by humans and their activities.

If extinction is part of the natural order, some people ask: "Why save endangered species? What makes a relatively few animals and plants so special that effort and money should be expended to preserve them?"

Congress addressed these questions in the preamble to the Endangered Species Act of 1973, holding that endangered and threatened species of fish, wildlife, and plants "are of esthetic, ecological, educational, historical, recreational, and scientific value to the Nation and its people." In making this statement, Congress was summarizing a number of convincing arguments advanced by thoughtful scientists, conservationalists, and others who are greatly concerned by the disappearance of wildlife.

Sadly, we can no longer attribute the increasing decline in our wild animals and plants to "natural" processes. Many are declining because of exploitation, habitat alteration or destruction, pollution, or the introduction of new species of plants and animals to an area. As mandated by Congress, protecting endangered species and restoring them to the point at which their existence is no longer jeopardized is the primary objective of the U.S. Fish and Wildlife Service's Endangered Species Program.

Passage of the Endangered Species Act of 1973 gave the United States one of the most far-reaching laws ever enacted by any country to prevent the extinction of imperiled animals and plants. The act created a national program that today involves the federal government, the states, conservation organizations, individual citizens, business and industry, and foreign governments in a cooperative effort to conserve endangered wildlife throughout the world. Under the law, the secretary of the interior (acting through the U.S. Fish and Wildlife Service) has broad powers to protect and conserve all forms of wildlife and plants that he or she finds in serious jeopardy. The secretary of commerce, acting through the National Marine Fisheries Service, has similar authority for protecting and conserving most marine life.

As of August 1984, more than 300 native mammals, birds, reptiles, crustaceans, plants, and other life forms were officially protected on the U.S. List of Endangered and Threatened Wildlife and Plants. In addition, more than 500 foreign species have been listed.

Habitat destruction is the most serious worldwide threat to wildlife and plants, followed by overexploitation for commercial, sporting, or other purposes. Disease, predation, inadequate conservation laws, and other natural or human-made factors may also contribute to a species' decline — making it a candidate for listing as endangered or threatened. The act defines an "endangered" species as one that is in danger of extinction throughout all or a significant portion of its range. A "threatened" species is defined as one that is likely to become endangered within the foreseeable future.

The Fish and Wildlife Service follows a formal "rule-making" procedure in determining which species should be placed on the U.S. List of Endangered and Threatened Wildlife and Plants.

A "rule-making" is the process used by federal agencies (and many states) to propose and later adopt regulations that have the effect of law and apply to all U.S. residents. The proposed rule-making is published in the *Federal Register*, a daily government publication, and after a suitable period for public comment and possible revision, it is published again as a final rule. Endangered or threatened species are placed on the list, reclassified, or deleted through this process.

58. The passage implies that it is possible for the public to influence the government's decisions regarding endangered species by
   A. mentioning that the rule-making proposals become final rules only after a period of public access allowing for commentary.
   B. indicating the need for popular vote to pass the Endangered Species Act of 1973.
   C. citing statistics that were based on public feedback.
   D. stating the law that requires public majority to pass the *Federal Register*.

59. Which of the following best represents the main idea of the passage?
   A. The Endangered Species Act of 1973 was an important development in the preservation of endangered wildlife.
   B. The federal government's current involvement in conservation of endangered plants and animals was bolstered by public involvement in the late 1960s.
   C. Human-made factors have had negative effects on wildlife, forcing the intervention of the secretaries of commerce and the interior to work in conjunction with the public to create legitimate conservation laws for the nation.
   D. Modern human existence has negatively altered natural habitats, prompting the installment of the Endangered Species Act that promotes the conservation of endangered species worldwide.

60. What is the author's purpose in mentioning dinosaurs in the beginning of the passage?
   A. To develop similarities between the plight of one animal to another animal described later in the passage
   B. To contrast ancient and modern attitudes toward wildlife
   C. To express the need for government control of wildlife
   D. To present a well-known example to later contrast the difference between natural and human-made extinction

61. As opposed to "threatened" wildlife, an "endangered" species has which of the following criteria?
    I. Overexploitation for commercial purposes
    II. Danger of extinction throughout most of its life range
    III. The likelihood of extinction in the near future

    A. II only
    B. I and II
    C. I and III
    D. II and III

62. According to the passage, all of the following apply to the "rule-making" procedure EXCEPT for which one?
    A. The procedure is used by federal and state agencies to propose and adopt regulations.
    B. Public access to and commentary on the documented rule-making procedure may prompt the reevaluation of the endangered species list and the proposals.
    C. The procedure produces regulations that act as laws and apply to all U.S. citizens.
    D. The proposals are made into final rules only after a period of time during which the secretaries of commerce and the interior approve all revisions and pass them to Congress.

PASSAGE III (QUESTIONS 63–67)

It is a matter for public concern that American universities begin 1989 in serious difficulty explaining what they are, what they should teach, and by what right they teach.

The universities' crisis is related to a profound problem of the twentieth century, a cause of war in our times, which is the problem of truth — an intellectual problem, obviously, but a political one as well. If truth doesn't exist or cannot be determined, why do we do what we do? If it does exist and can be determined, and I possess the truth while you are in error, why should I not send you to prison or Siberia in order to eliminate error from society?

The Western civilization that produced the ferocious modern politico-ideological "truth" systems of Marxism-Leninism, mutating into Stalinism and Nazism-Fascism, is the same civilization that has most effectively resisted the ideologizing of knowledge. It has defended free thought and created, in the course of its history, the democratic political system that actually asks people to decide a nation's course. It has done this on a continuing assumption of the possibility of discovering the truth about things through reason.

The values of this civilization, "the West," are now questioned, directly or indirectly, in the course of the university controversy. First there is debate about cultural relativism, which was most publicized at Stanford University. People ask why the thought and art of the West should be taught in the American university, rather than the thought and art of China and India.

People ask why the oral literature of Africa or the preliterate cultures of the North American Indian should be shunted off onto the margins of what is considered civilization. Women note that few women are among the "great" figures taught in the university and challenge that this should be so.

A political explanation is proposed, which says European or European-descended white men have always controlled Western universities and dominated Western cultural life, imposing what suited them.

This obviously is true but it is just as obviously reductionist. To say that Western society is Eurocentric is to repeat oneself. To say that its culture has been dominated by men is to state an historical fact, not only about this civilization but all others as well. Yet self-interest, plot, and power-brokerage are not satisfactory explanations. To claim that they are is to deny implicitly those values or standards exist outside the play of power, or that judgments have been or can be made which are not those of power-in-action.

Behind the cultural relativism of the controversy is the influence of "postmodernism," which says that universal principles and values and the Western liberal, rationalist effort to discover general truths are no longer credible.

The founding assumption of the Western university is that reality is perceived through reason. Postmodern thought holds to the contrary that reason has become "pluralized" and relativized, and reality is indeterminate. Knowledge exists only as "regimes" of knowledge, which is to say political systems (an academic department or intellectual school, for example) dictate that certain things are so and use power, pain, and reward to make this accepted.

The civilization we live in would be incomprehensible and unworkable if we abandoned the beliefs that reason can arbitrate the moral claims of society and that truth exists and is ascertainable. Philosopher Alastair MacIntyre argues that our moral identity and civilization are integrally related, and if we abandon a belief in truth for a cultural relativism, we are giving up all possibility of moral judgment.

From William Pfaff, "American Universities, Moral Reasoning and the Greeks." © 1989 by Los Angeles Times Syndicate.

63. According to the author, the two conflicting modes of thought in the crisis he describes are
    - A. those of preliterate and postliterate cultures.
    - B. Marxism and Nazism.
    - C. postmodernism and liberal rationalism.
    - D. Fascism and postmodernism.

64. Which of the following statements most accurately states the author's view of Western civilization's response to the problem of truth?
    - A. The West has refused to deal with the problem.
    - B. The West has abandoned rationalism in favor of repressive politico-ideological "truth" systems.
    - C. The West has used "truth" systems as an excuse for war and for exploiting non-Western cultures.
    - D. The West has both produced repressive "truth" systems and preserved free thought and open inquiry.

65. The author's discussion of the problem of truth is intended chiefly to
    - A. demonstrate the decline of moral responsibility in Western civilization.
    - B. indicate that universities are powerless to cope with large historical movements.
    - C. illustrate the harmful effects of "truth" systems.
    - D. place the current crisis in universities in a broad intellectual and political context.

66. According to the author, all of the following beliefs of Western civilization are threatened by postmodernism EXCEPT the belief that
    - A. truth can be discovered through reason.
    - B. reality is indeterminate.
    - C. reason can arbitrate society's moral claims.
    - D. general truths transcend political systems.

67. Based on the author's discussion, it can be inferred that postmodern thought contains all of the following ideas EXCEPT that
    - A. universal values do not exist.
    - B. knowledge exists only as a political system.
    - C. objective inquiry is the best means of discovering truth.
    - D. "reality" cannot be discovered through reason.

PASSAGE IV (QUESTIONS 68–72)

The relationship of a king toward his people is rightly compared to that of a father to his children, and to a head of a body composed of diverse members. For it was as fathers that the good princes and magistrates of the people of God acknowledged themselves to their subjects. And for all other well-ruled commonwealths, the style of *pater patriae* (father of his country) was ever and is commonly used with kings. The proper office of a king toward his subjects agrees very well with the office of the head toward the body and all members thereof. For from the head, being the seat of judgment, proceedeth the care and foresight of guiding and preventing all evil that may come to the body or any part thereof. The head cares for the body; so doth the king for his people. As the discourse and direction flows from the head, and the execution according thereunto belongs to the rest of the members, everyone according to their office: so is it betwixt a wise prince and his people. As the judgment coming from the head may not only employ the members, every one in its own office, as long as they are able for it; but, likewise, in case any of them affected with any infirmity must care and provide for their remedy, in case it be curable, and if otherwise has someone cut them off for fear of infecting the rest: even so is it betwixt the prince and his people. And as there is ever hope of curing any diseased member by the direction of the head, as long as it is whole; but by the contrary, if it be troubled, all the members are partakers of that pain, so is it betwixt the prince and his people.

And now to speak first of the father's part, consider what duty his children owe to him, and whether upon any pretext whatever it will not be thought monstrous and unnatural for his sons to rise up against him, to control him at their appetite, and when they think good to slay him, or to cut him off, and adopt to themselves any other they please in his room. Can any pretense of wickedness or rigor on his part be a just excuse for his children to put hand to him? In case it were true that the father hated and wronged the children never so much, will any man endowed with the least spark of reason think it lawful for them to meet him with the line? Yea, suppose the father were furiously following his sons with a drawn sword, is it lawful for them to turn and strike again, or make any resistance but by flight? I think surely if there were no more but the example of brute beasts and unreasonable creatures, it may serve well enough to qualify and prove my argument. We read often the piety that the storks have to their old and decayed parents: and generally we know that there are many sorts of beasts and fowls that with violence and many bloody strokes will beat and banish their young ones from them, how soon they perceive them to be able to fend for themselves; but we never read nor heard of any resistance on their part, except among vipers; which proves such persons as ought to be reasonable creatures, and yet unnaturally follow this example, to be endued with their viperous nature.

And for the similitude of the head and the body, it may very well fall out that the head will be forced to cut off some rotten member to keep the rest of the body in integrity: but what state the body can be in, if the head for any infirmity that can fall to it be cut off, I leave it to the reader's judgment.

To conclude, if the children may upon any pretext that can be imagined lawfully rise up against their father, cut him off, and choose any other whom they please in his room; and if the body for the well of it may for an infirmity that may be in the head strike it off, then I cannot deny that the people may rebel, control, and displace, or cut off their king, at their own pleasure, and upon respects moving them.

Adapted from James Stuart, *The True Law of Free Monarchies*. (1598).

68. Which of the following statements most accurately describes the organization of the passage?
    A. It takes the form of a syllogism (a major premise, minor premise, and conclusion).

B. It takes the form of an "if X, then Y" proposition.
C. It takes the form of argument by analogy (two controlling metaphors).
D. It uses inductive logic, proceeding from particulars to a generalization.

69. The author alludes to "beasts and fowls" chiefly to support his argument that
A. the king's subjects should not resist his irrational, violent behavior.
B. the king serves as protector for even his most unworthy subjects.
C. civil obedience protects humankind from the chaos of the natural order.
D. a benign monarchy is analogous to natural law.

70. Which of the following statements most accurately summarizes the relationships among the four paragraphs?
A. The first two present one argument, and the last two present a second argument.
B. The first introduces two metaphors, the second and third each develop one, and the fourth deals with both.
C. Each of the first three has a different controlling metaphor, and the fourth presents a conclusion.
D. The first, third, and fourth draw their controlling metaphors from man, and the second derives its controlling metaphor from nature.

71. The author believes that
A. subjects may rebel only with ample cause.
B. monarchs should be replaced only when an overwhelming majority of their subjects desires change.
C. violent revolution is sometimes justified.
D. monarchs may never be lawfully replaced.

72. The weakest arguments in the passage result from
A. a failure to define terms.
B. introducing examples (such as the viper) that contradict other examples.
C. the failure to provide historical background.
D. taking metaphors literally, as in the head/body metaphor.

PASSAGE V (QUESTIONS 73–76)

Genius is supposed to be a power of producing excellencies that are out of the reach of rules of art, a power that no precepts can teach and no industry can acquire.

This opinion of the impossibility of acquiring those beauties that stamp the work with the character of Genius, supposes that it is something more fixed than it is in reality; and that we always do, and always did agree in opinion, with respect to what should be considered as the characteristic of genius. But the truth is, the degree of excellence that proclaims Genius is different in different times and places; and what shows it to be so is that mankind has often changed its opinion upon this matter.

When the arts were in their infancy, the power of merely drawing the likeness of any object was considered one of their greatest efforts. But when it was found that every man could be taught to do this and a great deal more merely by the observance of certain precepts, the word Genius shifted application and was given only to him who added the peculiar character of the object he represented; to him who had invention, expression, grace, or dignity; in short, to him who possessed those qualities, or excellencies, the power of producing that could not then be taught by any known and promulgated rules.

What we now call Genius begins, not where rules abstractly end, but where known vulgar and trite rules no longer hold any place. Even works of Genius, like every other effect, as they must have their cause, must likewise have their rules. It cannot be by chance that excellencies are produced with any constancy or certainty, for this is not the nature of chance. Yet the rules by which men of extraordinary parts work, are either such that they discover by their own peculiar observations, or a nice texture as not easily to admit being expressed in words; especially as artists are not very frequently skillful in that mode of communicating ideas. Unsubstantial, however, as these rules may seem and as difficult as it may be to convey them in writing, they are still seen and felt in the mind of the artist; and he works from them with as much certainty, as if they were embodied, as I may say, upon paper. It is true that these refined principles cannot always be made palpable, like the more gross rules of art. Yet it does not follow that the mind may be put in such a train that it shall perceive, by a kind of scientific sense, that propriety which words, particularly words of unpracticed writers such as we are, can but very feebly suggest.

Invention is one of the great marks of Genius, but if we consult experience, we shall find that it is by being conversant with the inventions of others that we learn to invent; as by reading the thoughts of others we learn to think.

73. Which of the following statements best describes the function of the first paragraph?
    A. It offers historical background for the author's topic.
    B. It states a position that the author will attempt to refute.
    C. It states the first of the author's two-part argument.
    D. It states the main thesis of the essay, which is developed in subsequent paragraphs.

74. Based on the passage, with which of the following statements would the author disagree most strongly?
    A. Genius is innate and can never be taught.
    B. Standards of Genius rise as more is learned of the rules of art.
    C. Works of Genius follow certain rules, even if those rules are hidden from common view.
    D. Men of Genius may discover rules of art through their own acute observations.

75. Which of the following ideas in the essay is an unsupported claim, based neither on an appeal to history nor on experience?
    I. Artistic rules in works of Genius are seen and felt in the mind of the artist.
    II. Artists can learn invention.
    III. The degree of excellence that is called Genius differs in various times and locales.
    A. I only
    B. II only
    C. I and III
    D. I, II, and III

76. The primary purpose of the passage is to
    A. analyze the differences between genuine and supposed works of Genius.
    B. trace the history of different conceptions of Genius.
    C. distinguish between works of Genius and works of invention.
    D. argue that Genius is not out of the reach of the rules of art.

PASSAGE VI (QUESTIONS 77–80)

Three months ago, we wrote about the costly retreat from the humanities on all the levels of American education. It has become apparent to us that one of the biggest problems confronting American education today is the increasing vocationalization of our colleges and universities. Schools are under pressure to become job-training centers and employment agencies.

The pressure comes mainly from two sources. One is the growing determination of many citizens to reduce taxes, which is understandable but irresponsible when connected to the reduction of vital public services. The second source of pressure comes from parents and students who scorn courses that do not teach people how to become attractive to employers in a tightening job market.

It is absurd to believe that development of skills does not also require systematic development of the human mind. Education is being measured more by the size of the benefits the individual can extract from society than by the extent to which the individual can come into possession of his or her full powers. The result is that the life-giving juices are in danger of being drained out of education.

Instead of trying to shrink the liberal arts, Americans ought to pressure colleges and universities to increase the ratio of the humanities to the sciences.

The irony of the emphasis being placed on careers is that nothing is more valuable for anyone who has had a professional or vocational education than to be able to deal with abstractions or complexities, or to feel comfortable with subtleties of thought and language. The doctor who knows only about disease is at a disadvantage alongside the doctor who knows at least as much about people as about pathological organisms. The lawyer who argues in court from a narrow legal base is no match for the lawyer who can connect legal precedents to historical experience. The business executive whose competence in general management is bolstered by an artistic ability to deal with people is of prime value to his company. For the technologist, the engineering of consent can be as important as the engineering of moving parts. Just in terms of career preparation, therefore, a student is shortchanged by shortcutting the humanities.

But even if it could be demonstrated that the humanities contribute nothing directly to a job, they would still be an essential part of the educational equipment of any person who wants to come to terms with life. The humanities would be expendable only if human beings didn't have to make decisions that affected their lives and the lives of others; if the human past never existed or had nothing to tell us about the present; if human relations were random aspects of life; and if no special demands arose from the accident of being born a human being instead of a hen or a hog.

Finally, there would be good reason to eliminate the humanities if a free society were not absolutely dependent on a functioning citizenry. If the main purpose of a university is job training, then the underlying philosophy of our government has little meaning. The debates that went into the making of American society concerned not just institutions or governing principles but the capacity of humans to sustain those institutions. The fundamental question sensed by everyone at the American Constitutional Convention was whether the people themselves would understand what it meant to hold the ultimate power of society, and whether they had enough of a sense of history and destiny to know where they had been and where they ought to be going.

Jefferson was prouder of having been the founder of the University of Virginia than of having been president of the United States. He knew that the educated and developed mind was the best assurance that a political system could be made to work — a system based on the informed consent of the governed. If this idea fails, then all the saved tax dollars in the world will not be enough to prevent the nation from turning on itself.

Adapted from Norman Cousins, "How to Make People Smaller Than They Are," © *The Saturday Review* (December 1978).

77. The primary purpose of the passage is to
    A. argue that the liberal arts are more vocationally useful than professional education.
    B. lament the passing of a golden era in American higher education.
    C. argue that the humanities are the most important part of the curriculum.
    D. argue that too much money is being spent on vocational and professional education.

78. Which of the following reasons does the author offer to support his contention that Americans ought to pressure universities to

increase the ratio of the humanities to the sciences?

I. The humanities are useful for people who have had professional or vocational educations.

II. Free societies depend absolutely on citizens educated in the humanities.

III. The humanities are essential in helping people understand and cope with their lives as human beings.

A. I only
B. I and II
C. II and III
D. I, II, and III

79. The author's discussion of doctors, lawyers, and business executives is designed chiefly to

A. provide evidence to support his claim that the humanities provide valuable job-related skills.
B. point out the weaknesses of vocational education.
C. illustrate his argument that the humanities are important for anyone wishing to come to terms with life.
D. argue that the "life-giving juices" are being drained out of education.

80. Judging from this passage, which of the following best expresses the author's conception of the proper primary function of education?

A. It ought to develop a broad range of job-related skills.
B. It should fulfill the emotional and psychological needs of the individual.
C. It ought to develop systematically the full mental capacities of the individual.
D. It should be tailored to the special interests and life objectives of each individual.

PASSAGE VII (QUESTIONS 81–86)

The right of nature, which writers commonly call *jus naturale*, is the liberty each man has to use his own power as he wills himself for the preservation of his own nature, that is to say, of his own life; and consequently of doing anything which in his own judgment and reason he shall conceive to be the aptest means thereunto.

By Liberty is understood, according to the proper signification of the word, the absence of external impediments, which impediments may oft take away part of a man's power to do what he would, but cannot hinder him from using the power left him according as his judgment and reason shall dictate to him.

A law of nature (*lex naturalis*) is a precept or general rule found out by reason, by which a man is forbidden to do that which is destructive to his life or taketh away the means of preserving the same; and to omit that by which he thinketh it may be best preserved. Those that speak of this subject confuse *Jus* and *Lex*, Right and Law; yet these ought to be distinguished because Right consisteth in liberty to do or to forbear, whereas Law determineth and bindeth to one of them: Law and Right differ as much as obligation and liberty, which in one and the same matter are inconsistent.

And because the condition of man . . . is a condition of war of everyone against everyone, in which case everyone is governed by his own reason, and there is nothing he can make of us that may not be a help unto him in preserving his life against his enemies: it followeth that in such a condition every man has a right to every thing, even to one another's body. And therefore as long as this natural right of every man to every thing endureth, there can be no security to any man (how strong or wise soever he be) of living out the time which nature ordinarily alloweth men to live. And consequently, it is a precept or general rule of reason that every man ought to endeavor peace as far as he has hope of obtaining it; and when he cannot obtain it, that he may seek and use all helps and advantages of war. The first branch of which containeth the first and fundamental law of nature, which is to seek peace and follow it. The second, the sum of the right of nature, which is to use all means we can to defend ourselves. From this fundamental law of nature, by which men are commanded to endeavor peace, is derived this second law: that a man be willing, when others are so too, insofar as for peace and defence of himself he shall think necessary, to lay down this right to all things, and be contented with so much liberty against other men as he would allow other men against himself. For as long as any man holdeth this right of doing anything he liketh, so long are all men in the condition of war. But if other men will not lay down their right, as well as he, then there is no reason for anyone to divest himself of his. For that he were to expose himself to pray (to which no man is bound) rather than dispose himself to peace. This is that law of the Gospel: Whatsoever you require that others should do to you, that do ye to them.

From Thomas Hobbes, *Leviathan* (1651).

81. According to the author, the right of nature and a law of nature
    A. spring from the same desire for peace.
    B. are naturally compatible.
    C. have been clearly delineated by previous writers.
    D. are in conflict with one another.

82. The author derives his first law of nature from
    A. reason.
    B. observation of nature.
    C. Biblical authority.
    D. history.

83. One can infer from the passage that the author believes
    A. in absolute monarchy.
    B. that effective government depends on the consent of the governed.
    C. that liberty is best achieved in a democratic society.
    D. that only rugged individualists can lead satisfying lives.

84. According to the author, the first and second laws of nature spring from man's
    A. desire for self-preservation.
    B. need for social institutions.
    C. desire for liberty.
    D. essentially benign constitution.

85. The author suggests that man need not follow the second law of nature
    A. when it conflicts with the first law of nature.
    B. if other men refuse to relinquish their rights of nature.
    C. when it infringes on his personal identity.
    D. when it conflicts with Biblical teachings.

86. Which of the following statements is most accurate?
    A. The right of nature and the two laws of nature derive from the same impulse for self-preservation; they differ chiefly insofar as the former considers man as an individual and the latter considers man as a social being.
    B. The right of nature deals with man's liberty whereas the two laws of nature deal with man's desire for peace and the right to defend himself.
    C. The author believes that the laws of nature ought to take precedence over the right of nature, but that men always give priority to the right of nature when the two are in conflict.
    D. The right of nature and the two laws of nature both derive from reason, but only the former deals with self-preservation, while the latter deal only with peace and prosperity.

PASSAGE VIII (QUESTIONS 87–90)

Incrementalism is a strategy used to reduce the enormous problems of decision-making and calculation arising during the budgetary process. Incrementalism assumes that the calculation of each year's budget uses some base as a starting point, such as last year's budget, and focuses attention on the marginal changes. In a broad sense, this base can be zero, as in zero base budgeting. The usual case, however, is to use the previous year's budget as the base, with the expectation that the next budget will be an expansion of it.

The first test of incrementalism considers the continuity of the organization requesting the budget. Many organizations continue their activities from year to year without a great deal of fluctuation. Their requirements for funding are relatively stable, and their ongoing programs are continued as long as constituency needs are being met. Such organizations do not need to consider alternatives beyond those required to maintain their services. Only when the organization is not meeting its constituency's needs is it necessary to adapt procedures and strategies and consider new alternatives.

When new alternatives are proposed, they usually come in the form of new programs or an expansion of old programs. For the organization making a budgetary decision, the additional or expanded programs are those that will receive the greatest attention since they are the items that have not been previously discussed. The other items appearing in the request have been discussed and settled, and unless there are specific reasons for doing so, they need not be considered again. This strategy benefits those who must process large amounts of information by substantially reducing the items needing consideration. The information necessary to adequately consider even one or two programs can be enormous. Reconsideration of the entire budget on a yearly basis would make the task impossible.

The behavioral approach helps to explain why budgeting is done incrementally. The first problem facing a consideration of the entire budget is the nonintegration of the organizational goals. Each subunit of an organization can have its own goals that may not always be in line with the goals of the organization as a whole. Thus, the organization at times pursues conflicting goals. Rather than attempting to resolve this situation all at once, the goals are dealt with one at a time. This approach limits the number of decisions that must be made at a given time.

Second, in problem-solving there is a tendency to look in one's own backyard first, i.e., trying something similar to what has been done previously, but different enough to solve the problem. This looks at the problem in small increments in an attempt to keep costs down. The search is not for the best solution to the problem, only an adequate one. Thus, the chances are better that small changes will adequately solve the problem at less cost than a complete reconsideration of the problem to find the best solution.

87. The primary purpose of the passage is to
   A. describe the federal budgetary process.
   B. highlight alternative budgetary systems.
   C. show why incrementalism is used.
   D. examine the shortcomings of zero base budgeting.

88. According to the author, stable organizations that continue their operations from year to year are
   A. more likely to use incrementalism.
   B. not involved in problem-solving.
   C. more likely to have consistent sets of goals.
   D. more likely to examine their entire budget on a yearly basis.

89. From the passage, it can be deduced that zero-base budgeting is
   A. another form of incrementalism.
   B. a problem-solving strategy.
   C. a strategy used to reduce the enormous problems of decision-making and calculations.
   D. an unacceptable way of budgeting when compared with incrementalism.

90. The author would most likely agree that
   A. zero-base budgeting is preferred to incrementalism.

B. under incrementalism, both old and new programs receive careful scrutiny.
C. extensive problem searches are more economical.
D. incrementalism may not be perfect, but it is understandable.

PASSAGE IX (QUESTIONS 91–92)

The Reverend Jerry Falwell, founder of the Moral Majority, said in a television interview: "Homosexuality is immoral. The so-called 'gay rights' are not rights at all because immorality is not right. God hates homosexuality, and so do we. But we do not hate the homosexual; we want to help him by helping him overcome his sin."

Falwell speaks for a large number of Americans who feel that there is something deeply objectionable about homosexuality. In other societies, of course, people have other views. The rulers of present-day Iran agree with Falwell and take his view to an extreme: there, homosexuals may be castrated or killed or both. In England, on the other hand, a more tolerant attitude is taken, and all legal penalties were removed over three decades ago. What attitude are we to take? One possibility is that we might agree with Falwell and say that homosexuality is in fact immoral. Or we might disagree and say that in fact homosexuality is *not* immoral. But there is a third alternative. We might say something like this:

Falwell is expressing his own personal opinion, and many may agree with him. But others may have different opinions. Where morality is concerned, there are no "facts," and no one is "right." He has his opinion; others have their opinions; and that's the end of it.

This is the basic thought behind *Ethical Subjectivism*. Ethical subjectivism is the idea that our moral opinions are based on our feelings, and nothing more. In this view, there is no such thing as "objective" right or wrong. It is a fact that some people are homosexual, and some are heterosexual; but it is not a fact that one is good and the other bad. So when someone such as Falwell says that homosexuality is wrong, he is not stating a fact about homosexuality. Instead, he is merely saying something about his feelings toward it.

Of course, ethical subjectivism is not simply an idea about the evaluation of homosexuality. Exactly the same applies to any moral judgment whatever.

We should be clear about what *kind* of theory this is. Ethical subjectivism is not a theory about what things are good and what things are bad. It does not try to tell us how we should live or what moral opinions we should accept. It is not that sort of theory. Instead, it is a theory about *the nature of moral judgments*. It says that no matter what moral judgments we make, we are only expressing our personal feelings, and nothing more. People who accept this theory will still have moral opinions, of course — they might be in favor of gay rights or opposed to them. But whatever stance they choose, they will not believe their choice represents the "truth." They will recognize that their opinions merely represent their own personal feelings.

91. The primary purpose of the passage is to
    A. explain the theory of ethical subjectivism.
    B. offer an explanation for homosexuality.
    C. criticize Falwell's views.
    D. defend objective determinations of right and wrong.

92. From the passage, according to Falwell,
    A. there is no objective right and wrong.
    B. absolute moral rules cannot be maintained.
    C. homosexuality breeds intolerance.
    D. it is the act not the actor that must be corrected.

STOP! If time still remains, you may review work only in this section. When the time allotted is up, you may go on to the next section. STOP!

SECTION 3
Writing Sample

TIME: 60 minutes

2 essays, separately timed

30 minutes each

DIRECTIONS: This section tests your writing skills by asking you to write two essays. You will have 30 minutes to write each one.

During the first 30 minutes, work only on the first essay. If you finish it in less than 30 minutes, you may review what you have written, but do not begin the second essay. During the second 30 minutes, work only on the second essay. If you finish it in less than 30 minutes, you may review what you have written for that essay only. Do not go back to the first essay.

Read each assigned topic carefully. Make sure your essays respond to the topics as they are assigned.

Make sure your essays are written in complete sentences and paragraphs, and are as clear as you can make them. Make any corrections or additions between the lines of your essays. Do not write in the margins.

On the day of the test, you are given three pages to write each essay. You are not required to use all of the space provided, but do not skip lines so you will not waste space. Illegible essays cannot be scored.

PART 1

Consider this statement:

> *"Pens are most dangerous tools, more sharp by odds*
>
> *Than swords, and cut more keen than whips or rods."*
>
> John Taylor (1580–1653)

Write a unified essay in which you perform the following tasks: (1) Explain what you think the above statement means. (2) Describe a specific situation where pens are *not* as powerful as swords. (3) Discuss what you think determines whether or not the pen is mightier than the sword.

PART 2

Consider this statement:

> *"Patience is the strongest of strong drinks, for it kills the giant Despair."*
>
> Douglas Jerrold (1803–1857)

Write a unified essay in which you perform the following tasks: (1) Explain what you think the above statement means. (2) Describe a specific situation where patience may *not* overcome despair. (3) Discuss what you think determines whether or not patience is the best means of fighting despair.

STOP! If time still remains, you may review work only in this section. When the time allotted is up, you may go on to the next section. STOP!

SECTION 4
Biological Sciences

TIME: 70 Minutes

QUESTIONS: 93–144

DIRECTIONS: Most of the questions in this section are arranged in groups, each corresponding to a descriptive passage. Based on the information given in a passage, choose the one best answer to each question in the group. Some questions are independent of a descriptive passage and of each other. Choose the one best answer to each of these questions. If you are not sure of an answer, eliminate those choices that you know are incorrect and choose an answer from among those remaining. Fill in the corresponding circle on the answer sheet to indicate your answer. You may refer to the periodic table at any time.

PASSAGE I (QUESTIONS 93–95)

Human pedigrees are used in genetics to study inherited traits. Circles represent females; squares represent males. Parents are joined by a horizontal line between their symbols; sibling offspring are suspended below their parents from a horizontal line. The symbols of individuals affected by a specific genetic trait are darkened in, as shown below.

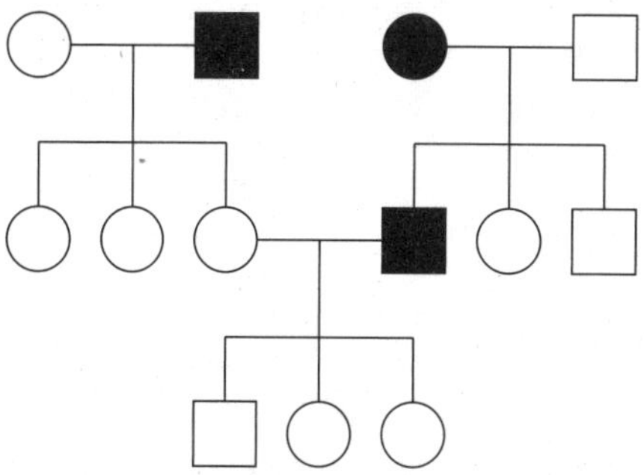

Pedigree A

93. *Could* the trait indicated in pedigree A be caused by a sex-linked gene?
   A. No, this trait could not be sex-linked.
   B. Yes, this trait could be due to a sex-linked dominant gene.
   C. Yes, this trait could be due to a sex-linked recessive gene.
   D. Yes, this trait appears to be due to a holandric sex-linked gene.

94. If the trait concerned in pedigree B is caused by an autosomal recessive gene, what is the probability that the couple indicated by the arrows will have an affected child? (They plan to have just one child.)
   A. Zero
   B. $\frac{1}{4}$
   C. $\left(\frac{1}{3}\right)^3$ or $\frac{1}{8}$
   D. $\frac{1}{4} \times \frac{1}{4}$ or $\frac{1}{16}$

95. If the trait concerned in pedigree C is caused by a sex-linked recessive gene, what is the chance that the couple, indicated by the arrows, would have an affected child?
   A. $\left(\frac{1}{2}\right)^2$
   B. $\left(\frac{1}{2}\right)^3$
   C. $\left(\frac{1}{2}\right)^4$
   D. $\left(\frac{1}{2}\right)^5$

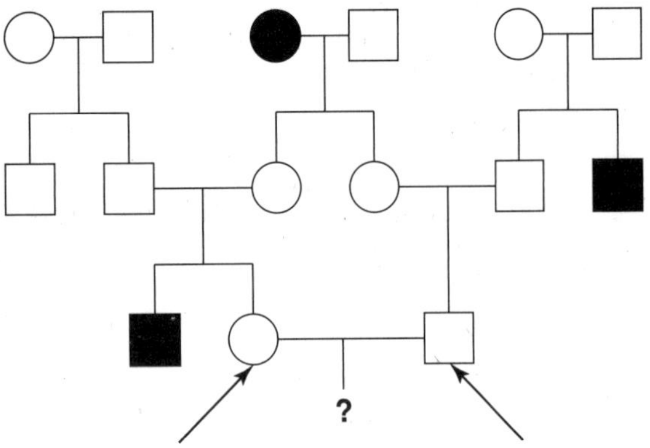

Pedigree C

PASSAGE II (QUESTIONS 96–98)

Male animals produce gametes by a process called spermatogenesis, which involves two meiotic divisions and a maturation process. The overall result is the production of haploid sperm from a diploid organism. Humans have a diploid chromosomal number of 46.

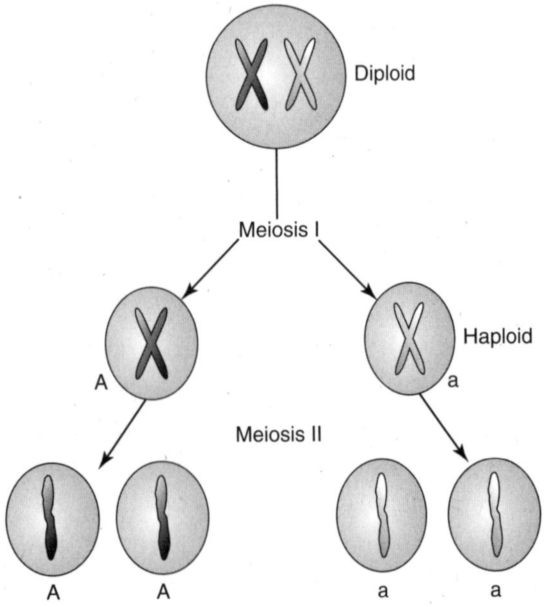

Overview of Meiosis
(Spematogenesis in a hypothetical animal with 2N = 2)

96. In the human male, how many chromosomes would be present in a primary spermatocyte at Prophase I?
    A. 23
    B. 46
    C. 92
    D. No chromosomes would be present; only chromatids would be.

97. In the human male, how many chromosomes would be present in a primary spermatocyte at Anaphase I?
    A. 23
    B. 46
    C. 92
    D. No chromosomes would be present; only chromatids would be.

98. In the human male, the following cells are haploid:
    A. spermatids, sperm.
    B. primary spermatocytes after Metaphase I.
    C. secondary spermatocytes.
    D. only spermatids.

PASSAGE III (QUESTIONS 99–101)

The cell membranes of living systems maintain an internal environment that is distinct from the external environment. The tubes below have selectively permeable membranes at their bottoms. The test tubes initially contain 10 ml of:

Test Tube	Solution
A	Distilled water
B	0.5% glucose in water
C	1.0% glucose in water

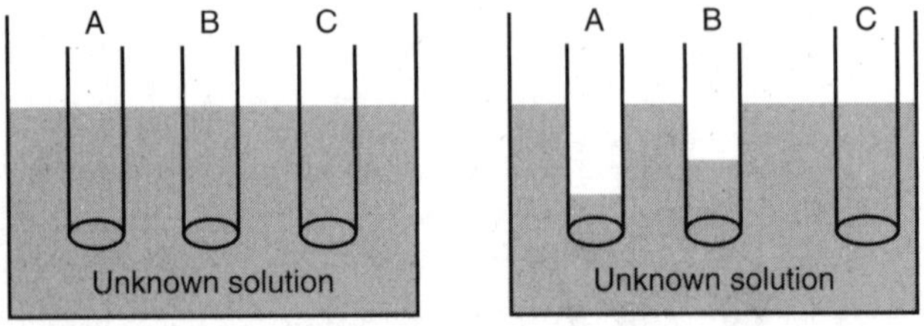

At start of experiment **After two hours**

The results after two hours are shown in the figure. Refer to this figure to answer the following questions.

99. What is the concentration of the unknown solution?
   A. 100% water
   B. 99.5% water
   C. 99.0% water
   D. It cannot be determined from the information provided.

100. If a red blood cell is placed in a hypertonic solution, the cell will
   A. shrink as water moves out.
   B. swell as water moves inward.
   C. maintain its shape by osmosis.
   D. maintain its shape, but its organelles will collapse inward.

101. Without expending energy, molecules can move into or out of cells by
   I. passing though pores formed by pore proteins in the plasma membrane.
   II. binding to a carrier protein in the plasma membrane.
   III. diffusing though the lipid phase of the plasma membrane.
   A. I only
   B. II and III
   C. III only
   D. I, II, and III

PASSAGE IV (QUESTIONS 102–105)

Gel electrophoresis of proteins has shown a surprising amount of diversity at the molecular level. The majority of proteins that exhibit polymorphism have only two alleles, one whose "fast" allozyme migrates rapidly compared to the other "slow" allozyme. These allozymes (variant forms of an enzyme) are often not known to confer different degrees of fitness. A population of fruit flies was examined, and "fast" and "slow" esterases were subsequently found. A representative gel electrophoretogram of six individuals' esterases is shown.

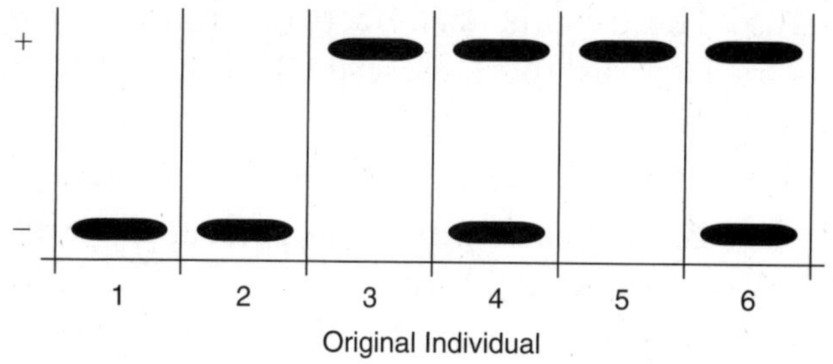

102. From the electrophoretogram shown above, it can be concluded that
   A. individual 4 is heterozygous for different versions of this enzyme (allozymes).
   B. individuals 1 and 2 have only the slow allozyme and are therefore less fit.
   C. the most adaptive phenotype would be shown by individuals 3 and 5.
   D. individual #6 appears to be homozygous.

103. The relationship between different allozymes is that they
   A. are the products of different alleles.
   B. catalyze the same reaction.
   C. are products of different alleles *and* catalyze the same reaction.
   D. don't catalyze the same reaction.

104. If the "slow" allozyme could function only within the lower part of the range of normal temperatures, and the "fast" allozyme functioned throughout this temperature range, the
   A. "slow" allozyme homozygote would be considered to be the most "fit" phenotype.
   B. "fast" allozyme homozygote would be considered to be the most "fit" phenotype.
   C. heterozygote would be the least "fit" phenotype.
   D. allozyme constitution of an individual would not be related to fitness.

105. The results of electrophoretic studies such as those described above indicate that
   A. genotypes are not relevant to fitness.
   B. Darwinian fitness does not apply at the molecular level.
   C. genetic variability at the molecular level is commonly found in biological populations.
   D. all proteins that exhibit polymorphism have four alleles.

QUESTIONS 106–109 are NOT based on a descriptive passage.

106. Following fertilization, the zygote undergoes a series of rapid mitotic divisions. The stage at which a solid ball of cells is formed is called the
   A. morula.
   B. blastula.
   C. gastrula.
   D. fetus.

107. The area of the brain responsible for coordinating voluntary muscle movement is the
   A. cerebrum.
   B. cerebellum.
   C. thalamus.
   D. hypothalamus.

108. Pepsin requires _____ for proper activity.
   A. vitamin C
   B. enzymes
   C. acidity
   D. basicity

109. One of the simplest kinds of behavior is the knee jerk, in which a tap below the knee causes the leg to jerk up. This behavior requires as a minimum which of the following combination of structures?
   A. A motor neuron and a muscle
   B. A receptor and at least two segments of the spinal chord
   C. A receptor neuron, a motor neuron, and a muscle
   D. An intact spinal cord and a brain

PASSAGE V (QUESTIONS 110–112)

Evolution is a central concept in biology. Understanding biology requires the study of genes in populations and the mechanisms that may result in genetic diversity, speciation, or extinction. In Hardy-Weinberg genetic equilibrium, gene and genotypic frequencies remain constant over many generations. If there were two different alleles for a particular locus, the frequency of the dominant allele "A" would be termed "p," and that of the recessive allele "a" would be called "q."

The diploid generation would be distributed with the frequencies p^2 for AA, 2pq for Aa, and q^2 for aa. These frequencies would remain the same generation after generation, as long as there were no forces that disturbed this equilibrium. Disturbance could come from random events in small populations, genetic changes, assortative mating, and natural selection. Evolution would never occur if populations remained in genetic equilibrium. Darwin's "Theory of Natural Selection" is the principal, unifying concept that provides the framework for ongoing biological studies today. The theory could be summarized as "differential reproduction of genetic variants results in evolutionary change."

Although many gene frequency changes may be due to genetic drift, selection is a significant factor in effecting evolutionary changes. Darwin provided the theoretical basis for the development of population genetics. Molecular biologists as well as naturalists actively study evolutionary biology today.

110. Darwin's theory of natural selection, the "survival of the fittest," as it is understood today,
   A. is generally understood to refer to the progressive evolution of larger, stronger organisms.
   B. refers to the relative ability of individuals with different genotypes to have different reproductive success.

C. has been replaced by the concept of punctuated equilibrium.
D. None of the above

111. Random fluctuations in gene frequencies due to small population size are called
A. genetic equilibrium.
B. heterosis.
C. genetic drift.
D. natural selection.

112. Selection acts upon
A. populations.
B. individual phenotypes.
C. species.
D. genes.

PASSAGE VI (QUESTIONS 113–117)

If an organism is to grow, mature, and replace injured or worn-out parts, cellular division must occur. The process of nuclear division that results in two identical daughter nuclei is called mitosis. Cytokinesis refers to the division of the cytoplasm. These complex components of cell division usually occur simultaneously, but they can occur independently. Both processes are controlled by intricate interactions among genes, their products, and environmental factors. The following questions concern mitosis and cytokinesis.

113. The constricted area at which two identical chromatids are joined is called the
A. centriole.
B. centrosome.
C. centromere.
D. centrochore.

114. If the somatic chromosome number of a species is 46, how many chromosomes would be present in a cell during anaphase?
A. 23 B. 46
C. 92 D. 12

115. The stage during which chromosomes replicate is
A. prophase. B. metaphase.
C. anaphase. D. interphase.

116. The protein structure to which spindle microtubules attach is the
A. centromere. B. centriole.
C. centrosome. D. kinetochore.

117. Animal cells usually undergo cytokinesis by
A. a contractile ring of actin filaments, which cleaves one cell into two.
B. the phragmoplast forming a telophase furrow.
C. the formation of a cell plate across the equator.
D. binary fission.

PASSAGE VII (QUESTIONS 118–122)

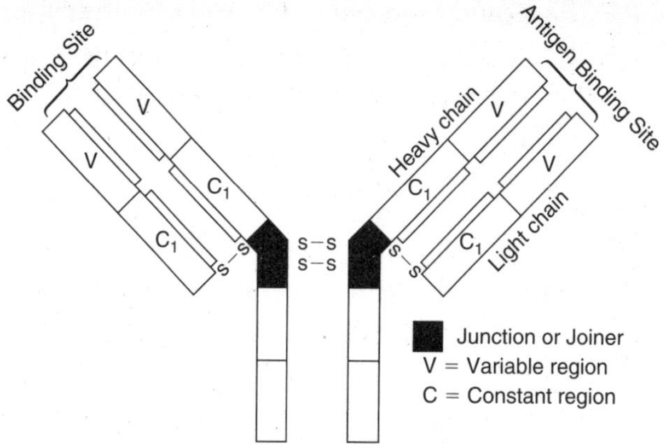

An Antibody Molecule

Organisms have evolved mechanisms to defend themselves against foreign invaders. Vertebrates have a variety of types of white blood cells that respond to foreign molecules. These cells come from stem cells in the bone marrow. Any specific immune cell can make only *one* kind of antibody. Mammals have immune cells that can produce antibodies that specifically react with virtually any foreign substance — the potential to form billions of different antibodies, more types of antibodies than the total number of genes in the organism. An illustration of an antibody molecule is shown above.

118. The vertebrate immune response involves the following different types of cells that respond in a highly specific manner.
  A. Erythrocytes and phagocytes
  B. T cells and B cells
  C. Reticulocytes and phagocytes
  D. Phagocytes only

119. The Y-shaped antibody molecule is produced by
  A. infected cells.
  B. T cells.
  C. B cells.
  D. phagocytes.

120. The Y-shaped antibody molecule consists of how many different types of polypeptides?
  A. 1
  B. 2
  C. 3
  D. 4

121. The antibody molecule illustrated
  A. could bind two different kinds of antigens.
  B. could bind only one kind of antigen.
  C. is a dimer, which could bind one particular type of antigen at two different sites.
  D. Both B and C

122. Using your knowledge of the variability of immunoglobulin structure, select the variants that are present in all members of a species.
  A. Allotypes
  B. Idiotypes
  C. Isotypes
  D. Phenotypes

PASSAGE VIII (QUESTIONS 123–125)

Early microscopists discovered that every animal and plant tissue consisted of small units called cells. All living organisms are composed of one or more cells, the basic units of biological structure and function. Various structures and organelles have evolved to support the life processes of cells. To understand how an organism lives and interacts with its environment, one must understand the cell.

123. There are many different kinds of cells, but all share the following features:
  A. mitochondria and nuclei.
  B. endoplasmic reticulum and centrioles.
  C. a plasma membrane and DNA genetic information.
  D. protein coat.

124. The function of the nucleous is to
  A. produce ribosomal subunits.
  B. orient the cellular poles during cytokinesis.
  C. store messenger RNA before transport to the endoplasmic reticulum.
  D. process, package, and store lipids and proteins for the nuclear membrane.

125. The mitochondria is the organelle that
  I. has the enzymes and cofactors for the process known as respiration.
  II. is descended from other mitochondria.
  III. breaks down organic molecules, coupling these catabolic reactions with energy-capturing reactions, which store this energy in other molecules to be used for other cellular processes.
  A. I, II, and III
  B. I and II
  C. I and III
  D. II and III

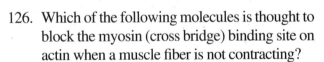

QUESTIONS 126–128 are NOT based on a descriptive passage.

126. Which of the following molecules is thought to block the myosin (cross bridge) binding site on actin when a muscle fiber is not contracting?
  A. Calcium
  B. Troponin
  C. Tropomyosin
  D. ATP

127. During development, the stage in which there is a hollow ball of cells is called
  A. gastrulation.
  B. blastulation.

C. morulation.
D. the isolecithal stage.

128. A harmless animal that represents another species that is dangerous to a predator is an example of
A. Mullerian mimicry.
B. Batesian mimicry.
C. cryptic appearance.
D. mutualism.

PASSAGE IX (QUESTIONS 129–133)

In organisms that reproduce asexually, nuclear division is accomplished by mitosis and each of the daughter cells receives an exact copy of the parental genetic material. All of the offspring of asexual reproduction are essentially genetically identical, resulting in little if any genetic variability among different generations.

Sexually reproducing species, however, exhibit a high degree of genetic variability. This variability is due mainly to the process of meiosis, during which gamete formation occurs. Meiosis differs from mitosis because the daughter cells contain only half the number of chromosomes of the parental cells. This is necessary to ensure that the chromosome number of a species remains constant because sexual reproduction involves the union of two gametes. The zygote formed in this manner will then have the full complement of chromosomes.

Human cells contain two copies of each chromosome type (1 maternal and 1 paternal), each of which contains slight variants of the same genes. There are 46 total chromosomes, or 23 pairs of chromosomes, in each cell. During the first meiotic division, the pairs of homologous chromosomes segregate randomly into daughter cells. Each daughter cell therefore contains some chromosomes of maternal origin and some of paternal origin. During the second meiotic division, the two chromatids that make up each chromosome separate and assort randomly into daughter cells. The number of possible chromosomal combinations that can result simply because of random assortment of chromosomes and chromatics is 2^n, where n is the number of pairs of chromosomes. In humans, the number of possible combinations is 2^{23}, or 8,388,608. The number of possible chromosomal combinations that can result when two gametes unite to form a zygote is $(2^n)^2$. Thus, it can be seen how the events that occur during meiosis increase the number of different genetic combinations and hence contribute to the potentially high genetic variability in a sexually reproducing species.

129. A clone, which is a group of genetically identical organisms derived from a single parent, is a result of which type of division?
A. Cytokinesis
B. Meiosis
C. Reduction
D. Mitosis

130. Which of the following statements best describes one of the major benefits of sexual reproduction?
A. The genetic variability associated with sexual reproduction allows a species to adapt readily to a changing environment.
B. The genetic variability associated with sexual reproduction is of great importance in an unchanging environment for species continuity.
C. Chromosome number remains constant, unlike asexual reproduction, in which chromosome number doubles with each generation.
D. All of the progeny of sexual reproduction will be genetically identical.

131. In a cell containing 3 pairs of chromosomes, how many possible chromosomal combinations exist for each daughter cell?
A. 64
B. 8
C. 16
D. 3

132. One of the important events that occurs during meiosis, but not in mitosis, is
   A. replication of the chromosomal material.
   B. a doubling of the chromosome number.
   C. a reduction by half of the chromosome number.
   D. nuclear division.

133. During prophase of the first meiotic division, chromatids of homologous chromosomes often exchange parts, a process known as crossing over. How does this affect genetic variability?
   A. It increases genetic variability to a greater extent than random assortment alone.
   B. It decreases genetic variability by producing daughter cells that are very similar to each other.
   C. It does not affect genetic variability because homologous chromosomes are exactly alike.
   D. It decreases genetic variability by reducing the possible number of chromosomal combinations.

PASSAGE X (QUESTIONS 134–137)

Ten grams of iodine (I_2) were added to 10 grams of acetone in a 500-cc flask; 1.6 molar sodium hydroxide was added slowly to the flask with thorough mixing. The reaction was kept cool and proceeded until the brown color of the iodine was gone. All that remained was a yellow solution and a yellow precipitate.

134. The yellow precipitate is most likely
   A. sodium iodide.
   B. iodoform.
   C. sodium acetate.
   D. hydrogen iodide.

135. If radioactive iodine were used in the reaction, where in the products would the radioactivity be found?
   A. Precipitate
   B. Supernatant
   C. Precipitate *and* supernatant
   D. It cannot be determined.

136. If radioactive sodium (in the form of sodium hydroxide) were used in the reaction, where in the products would the radioactivity be found?
   A. Precipitate
   B. Supernatant
   C. Precipitate *and* supernatant
   D. It cannot be determined.

137. Which of the following will NOT react with the precipitate to produce I_2 gas?
   A. F_2
   B. Cl_2
   C. Br_2
   D. CO_2

PASSAGE XI (QUESTIONS 138–142)

(−) 2–bromo octane is reacted with sodium hydroxide.

138. The main product is
   A. (−) 2-octanol.
   B. (+) 2-octanol.
   C. (±) 2-octanol.
   D. some optically *inactive* product.

139. This type of reaction is classified as
   A. E1.
   B. E2.
   C. S_N1.
   D. S_N2.

140. Which of the following will react in this manner slower than the 2-bromo octane?
   A. $CH_3(CH_2)_6CH_2Br$
   B. $CH_3(CH_2)_4CHBrCH_2CH_3$
   C. $CH_3(CH_2)_4CBr(CH_3)_2$
   D. $CH_3(CH_2)_3CHBr(CH_2)_2CH_3$

141. Which of the following is true of the above reaction?
   A. It involves second-order kinetics.
   B. It involves an elimination.
   C. Both of the above
   D. None of the above

142. What will the major product be if (+) 2-bromo octane is used?
   A. (+) 2-bromo octanol
   B. (−) 2-bromo octanol
   C. (−) 2-octanol
   D. (+) 2-bromo octane

QUESTIONS 143–144 ARE NOT based on a descriptive passage.

143. Which reagents should be used to prepare ethers by the Williamson method?
   A. Primary alcohol, butyl chloride, sodium metal
   B. Primary alcohol, sodium, HCl
   C. Sodium borohydride, butyl chloride
   D. Sodium borohydride, butylchloride, HCl

144. A Barr body is a highly condensed and genetically inactive X chromosome. The following table summarizes the genotype of the sex chromosomes, the sex and phenotype of the individual, and the number of Barr bodies present.

Genotype of Sex Chromosomes	Phenotype	Number of Barr Bodies
XX	Normal female	1
XY	Normal male	0
X	Turner syndrome female	0
XXX	Triplo-X female	2
XXY	Klinefelter syndrome male	1
XXXY	Klinefelter syndrome male	2
XYY	XYY syndrome male	0

Which of the following best explains the number of Barr bodies?
   A. The number of X chromosomes minus one
   B. The number of X and Y chromosomes minus two
   C. The number of X and Y chromosomes divided by two
   D. The number of X chromosomes minus the number of Y chromosomes

STOP! If time still remains, you may review work only in this section. STOP!

Test 6 ■ Answer Key

1.	C	37.	D	73.	B	109.	C
2.	A	38.	A	74.	A	110.	B
3.	A	39.	D	75.	A	111.	C
4.	D	40.	B	76.	D	112.	B
5.	C	41.	C	77.	C	113.	C
6.	B	42.	D	78.	D	114.	C
7.	D	43.	A	79.	A	115.	D
8.	B	44.	C	80.	C	116.	D
9.	B	45.	A	81.	D	117.	A
10.	A	46.	D	82.	A	118.	B
11.	C	47.	C	83.	B	119.	C
12.	D	48.	A	84.	A	120.	B
13.	D	49.	C	85.	B	121.	D
14.	B	50.	D	86.	A	122.	C
15.	D	51.	C	87.	C	123.	C
16.	C	52.	C	88.	A	124.	A
17.	C	53.	B	89.	A	125.	A
18.	D	54.	C	90.	D	126.	C
19.	C	55.	A	91.	A	127.	B
20.	B	56.	C	92.	D	128.	B
21.	D	57.	A	93.	A	129.	D
22.	B	58.	A	94.	C	130.	A
23.	D	59.	D	95.	B	131.	B
24.	D	60.	D	96.	B	132.	C
25.	A	61.	B	97.	B	133.	A
26.	B	62.	D	98.	C	134.	B
27.	B	63.	C	99.	C	135.	C
28.	C	64.	D	100.	B	136.	B
29.	D	65.	D	101.	D	137.	D
30.	C	66.	B	102.	A	138.	B
31.	B	67.	C	103.	C	139.	D
32.	D	68.	C	104.	B	140.	C
33.	B	69.	A	105.	C	141.	A
34.	C	70.	B	106.	A	142.	C
35.	C	71.	C	107.	B	143.	A
36.	B	72.	D	108.	C	144.	A

SECTION 1
Physical Sciences

PASSAGE I (QUESTIONS 1–4)

1. **C.** Work is defined through the combination of the force F on an object (mg downward) over a displacement D (along the slope) times the cosine of the angle θ between these two vectors:

$$W_g = mgD\cos\theta = (25\text{ kg})(10\text{ m/s}^2)(20\text{ m})\cos(120°)$$
$$W_g = -2500\text{ J}$$

Answer choice A is obtained by neglecting the relationship with the angle; answer choice B is obtained by using the angle of the slope (30°) instead of the angle between the vectors; and answer choice D is obtained by using the angle $\theta = 55°$, the sum of the two angles given.

2. **A.** The frictional force f is given in the problem and the same relationship should be used:

$$W_f = fD\cos\theta = (53.33\text{ N})(20\text{ m})\cos(180°)$$
$$W_f = -1067\text{ J}$$

Answer choices B and C are inserted as in the previous question to imply that the work done by friction might be identical to the work done by the gravitational field.

3. **A.** Once again, we rely on the same relationship to compute the work done by the contact force as:

$$W_c = ND\cos\theta = N(20\text{ m})\cos(90°)$$
$$W_c = 0$$

The work is zero because there is no component of the contact force along the direction of motion. As a result, it is not necessary to compute the actual force N. Answer choice B is the opposite of the simple (weight) × (distance) that many believe to be the work done in opposition to gravity. Answer choice C comes from the incorrect notion that the contact force simply opposes that of gravity.

4. **D.** The simplest approach here is to recognize that there is no net force on the crate (zero acceleration) and thus *no net work is done*. Therefore, the sum of the work by each of the four forces is *zero*, the last force being the effort of the man through the tension in the rope. Therefore:

$$W_m = -(W_g + W_f + W_c)$$
$$W_m = -(-2500\text{ J} - 1067\text{ J} + 0)$$
$$W_m = +3567\text{ J}$$

PASSAGE II (QUESTIONS 5–7)

5. **C.** The amplitude A of a simple harmonic oscillator is defined as ½ the difference between the minimum and maximum displacement. In this case, we have a maximum value of +6 m, a minimum value of −4 m, so:

$$A = ½((6\text{ m}) - (-4\text{ m})) = 5\text{ m}$$

Answer choices A and B are both attempts to assume that the oscillator is symmetric when it is not.

6. **B.** The period T of the oscillator is defined as the time for one complete oscillation. Because the points at the center are deceptive, we rely on the turning points to determine this. Two consecutive maximum displacements occur at $t = 2$ and $t = 6$ seconds, so

$$T = 6\text{ s} - 2\text{ s} = 4\text{ s}.$$

7. **D.** The velocity of an object is found by taking the slope of the displacement versus time graph. When the slope is *zero*, the mass has the slowest speed. This occurs at $t = 0$, $t = 2$, $t = 4$, and $t = 6$ seconds on our graph. Answer choices A and C present situations where the mass moves the fastest.

PASSAGE III (QUESTIONS 8–12)

The passage requires an understanding of electronic configuration, bonding, hybridization, molecular geometries, and their effect on the polarity of molecules.

8. **B.** Nitrogen is atom A and chlorine is atom B. Nitrogen will form only one compound with chlorine. No expanded octet is possible because the nitrogen atom is too small to accommodate more than 8 electrons around the central atom. The bonding is covalent because nitrogen and chlorine are both nonmetal atoms. Metals and nonmetals form ionic bonds; however, nonmetals form polar covalent bonds with other nonmetals. A nonmetal will also form a nonpolar covalent bond with itself.

   Nitrogen, the central atom, possesses 5 valence electrons. The unpaired electrons in the p subshell bond to the unpaired electron in each of 3 different chlorine atoms to give 8 valence electrons around nitrogen. Eight valence electrons form 4 pairs of electrons — 3 bonding pairs and 1 lone (nonbonding) pair of electrons. To minimize the repulsion between the pairs of electrons, the four pairs are arranged in a tetrahedral. However, because the lone pair of electrons occupies one of the positions in the tetrahedral, the molecular geometry will no longer be a symmetrical tetrahedral but will resemble a pyramid with N at the apex.

   The covalent bond between N and Cl is polar because the two atoms have different electronegativities, which is the ability to attract the electrons in a covalent bond. The greater the difference in the electronegativity, the more polar the bond. Because the pyramidal molecule is not symmetrical, there is no way for the polarities of the bonds to cancel each other, and the resulting molecule must be polar.

9. **B.** Phosphorus is a larger atom than nitrogen; therefore, P will form both PCl_3 and PCl_5. The bonding in PCl_3 exhibits sp^3 hybridization, with the lone pair of electrons occupying one of the tetrahedrally arranged orbitals. However, the bonding in PCl_5 is described as sp d because one of the original 3s electrons is promoted to an empty 3d orbital, and hybridization results in five equivalent orbitals made from one s, three p, and one d orbital — sp^3d. The resulting molecule has ten valence electrons around the central atom and is said to possess an expanded octet.

   Five pairs of electrons can be arranged in two different ways — a square with one pair up or down (square pyramidal) or a triangle with one pair up and one pair down (trigonal bipyramidal). The number of 90° angles must be made as small as possible to minimize the repulsion between the electron pairs. In the square pyramidal shape, there would be eight 90° repulsions; whereas in the trigonal pyramidal, there would be six 90° repulsions. Consequently, there will be six 90° and three 120° bond angles in the trigonal bipyramidal molecule.

   All of the bonds in this molecule will be polar because the electronegativities of P and Cl are different. However, because this is a symmetrical molecule, the bond polarities will cancel each other, resulting in a nonpolar molecule.

10. **A.** The principal quantum number, n, can have an integral value excluding zero. The azimuthal quantum number, l, can be 0 to $n - 1$. The magnetic quantum number, m_1, can have values from $-l$ to $+l$. The spin quantum number, m_s, can have values of

+½ or −½. Answer choice A is not a valid set: if $l = 0$, m_l must be 0 because the absolute value of m_l must not be greater than the absolute value of l.

11. **C.** Element B is chlorine, which has an atomic number of 17; that means it has 17 protons and 17 electrons if it is a neutral atom. There are 18 neutrons in this atom if we assume that it is the atom of chlorine with a mass number of 35 (35 − 17 = 18). Chlorine forms a negative one ion because it needs only one electron to complete its outer shell of electrons. This negative one ion is larger than the parent atom because of electronic repulsion between the added electron and the other electrons in this region of space.

12. **D.** Bond order = (bonding electron − antibonding electrons)/2
$$= (8 - 2)/2 = 3$$
All the electrons are paired so the molecule is diamagnetic. (See figure below.)

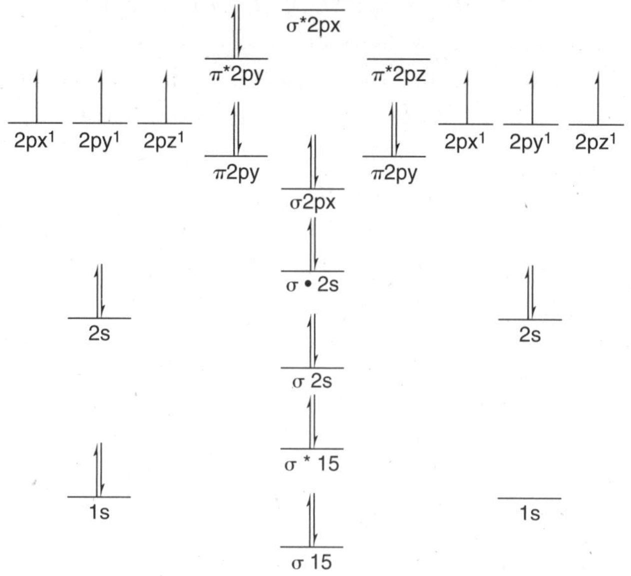

PASSAGE IV (QUESTIONS 13–16)

13. **D.** Torque τ is determined by the product of the force F times the moment arm d from the pivot point.

$$\tau = dF = (0.95\text{ m})(2\text{ N}) = 1.90\text{ Nm}$$

14. **B.** Torque is also found as the product of the distance r from the pivot times the force F times the sin θ (θ being the angle between the directions of r and F). Thus

$$\tau = rF \sin\theta = (0.2\text{ m})(12\text{N}) \sin(90°) = 2.4\text{ Nm}$$

15. **D.** Because the torque sensitivity depends on the angle between the directions of r and F, any nonhorizontal placement of the stick would yield a different value of the torque due to the weight of the stick, which appears at the 50-cm mark and is directed vertically downward. Answer choice A is incorrect because this weight also points vertically downward under all conditions. Answer choices B and C are incorrect because this angle can be freely adjusted by moving the spring independent of the stick.

16. **C.** For static equilibrium to be achieved, the sum of the torques and the sum of the forces must be zero. In the diagram below, the forces are shown on the meter stick, with the length of each vector representing the approximate magnitude of each force. The exact value for the weight of the meter stick is not needed. In addition to the forces shown, for the net force to sum to zero on the meter stick, it is clear that the pivot must supply a force downward and to the right. Therefore, answer choice C is the only possible choice.

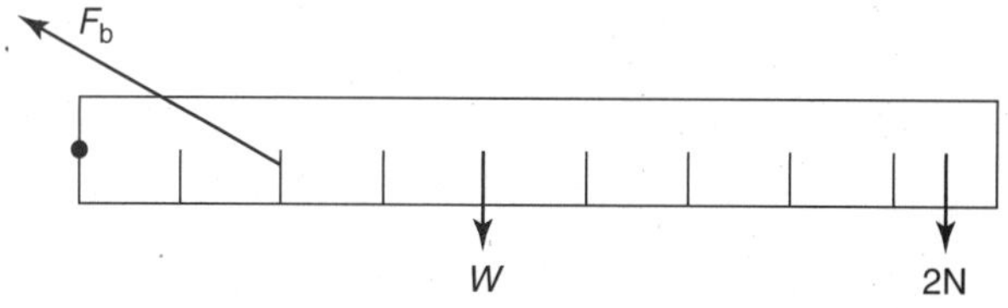

PASSAGE V (QUESTIONS 17–20)

17. **C.** Because *zero* work is done during the constant volume process ($dW = PdV$), the total work is just the sum of the two given, accounting for the correct directions:

$$W_{ba} = -750\text{ J, while } W_{ac} = +500\text{ J}$$

as defined by positive work being done *by* the gas. As a result, a net work of –250 J is found. Answer choice D accounts only for magnitudes and not the different directions, while answer choice B is correct only for a *clockwise* traversal of the cycle.

18. **D.** The first law of thermodynamics can be stated as

$$\Delta U = Q - W,$$

with U being the internal energy of the gas and Q the heat gained by the gas. Because the process from $a - b$ is just the reverse of the process from $b - a$, we have

$$Q_{ab} = +300 \text{ J},$$
$$W_{ab} = +750 \text{ J},$$

and therefore

$$\Delta U_{ab} = (300 \text{ J}) - (750 \text{ J}) = -450 \text{ J}$$

19. **C.** The process $c - a$ is adiabatic, and thus, by definition, no heat flows into or out of the gas during this process.

20. **B.** To compute the heat flow in or out of the gas, we rearrange the first law as

$$Q = \Delta U + W.$$

We must know ΔU_{bc} to determine Q_{bc}. We obtain this by recognizing that the internal energy change over the entire cycle is *zero*. Thus, the sum of the answers to questions 18 and 19 must be negated in the process from $b - c$

$$\Delta U_{bc} = -(\Delta U_{ab} + \Delta U_{ca}) = -((-450 \text{ J}) + (500 \text{ J})) = -50 \text{ J}$$

Because no work is done during the constant volume process,

$$Q_{bc} = \Delta U_{bc} + W_{bc} = -50 \text{ J} + 0 = -50 \text{ J}$$

21. **D.** The formula to determine the focal length, f, from the object distance, d_o, and image distance, d_i, is $1/f = 1/d_o + 1/d_i$. It is important to remember that when an image is behind a mirror, the image must be virtual because no light rays can emanate from that image. The image distance is then negative, so

$$1/f = 1/(2.0 \text{ cm}) + 1/(-5.0 \text{ cm}) = 5/10 - 2/10 = 3/10$$

and $f = 10/3 \sim 3.3$ cm.

To find the secondary focal length, set $s_0 = -\infty$.

22. **B.** The electric field is equal to the gradient of the electric potential or the change in the electric potential per unit length. The length is measured perpendicular to the equipotential lines. Subtracting adjacent equipotential lines yields 237 volts. Adjacent lines are separated by about 0.5 m. Therefore, $E = \Delta V/\Delta x = 237$ volts/0.5 meters ~ 470 V/m. It is also important to realize that the units, volts per meter (V/m), are equivalent to newtons per coulomb (N/C).

23. **D.** The direction of the force on a current in a magnetic field is determined from the equation $F = IL \times B$. The cross product of the length, L, and the magnetic field, B, is determined by the fact that the length vector is in the direction of the current. Using the right-hand rule, for section A, the fingers of the right hand go in the direction of the current (down), and these are crossed in the direction of the magnetic field (into the page). The direction of the thumb (and therefore the force) is to the right. For section C, similar application of the right-hand rule yields a force to the left. Because A and C sections have the same length, the forces are equal and opposite. The net force is determined by section B, which yields a direction down using the right-hand rule.

24. **D.** All reactions, exothermic or endothermic, that involve any type of bond breaking will have an energy of activation, though it may be very low. An exothermic reaction has a negative ΔH (change in enthalpy). Because heat is being liberated, it is only logical that the potential energy of the products should be lower than the potential energy of the reactants. This is summarized in the diagram shown.

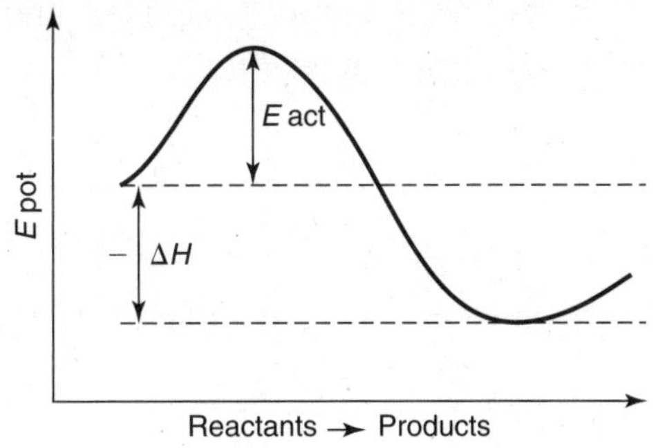

25. **A.** From the periodic table, there are 4 g of helium per mole, and room temperature is about 25°C or 25 + 273 ~ 300 K. Using the ideal gas equation, PV = nRT, we obtain

$$P = \frac{nRT}{V} \sim \frac{(500g)\frac{mole}{4g}8.3\frac{J}{moleK}(300K)}{1.5m^3}$$
$$= \frac{(5000)(8.3)(300)}{6}\frac{J}{m^3}$$
$$= (5000)(8.3)(50)\frac{J}{m^3}$$
$$= (5 \times 10^3)(4.15 \times 10^2)\frac{N}{m^2} \sim 21 \times 10^5\frac{N}{m^2}$$
$$= 2.1 \times 10^6\frac{N}{m^2}$$

Note that J/m^3 is the same as N/m^2. Another name for these units is Pascals.

PASSAGE VI (QUESTIONS 26–30)

The passage requires an understanding of the interpretation of experimental rate data, rates of reactions, rate laws, and the mathematical relationships among these.

26. **B.** Using the coefficients in the stoichiometric equation shows that 2 molecules of A would disappear for each B, and 3 molecules of C would disappear with each molecule of B. Consequently, the rate of disappearance of A would be twice the rate of disappearance of B, and the rate of disappearance of C would be three times the rate of disappearance of B.

The same kind of relationships would hold for the appearance of products on the right-hand side of the equation.

27. **B.** Using row 1 and row 3 in experiment 1 shows that the concentration of A and B remains constant while the concentration of C triples (1 M to 3 M). The initial rate increases from 3 to 27, so the rate must increase by a factor of 9 (27/3 = 9):

$$\text{rate} = k[C]^2$$

28. **C.** We already know that

$$\text{rate} = k[A][C]^2$$

Using row 1 and row 4 of experiment 1 reveals that quadrupling the concentration of B has no effect on the initial rate of the reaction. This means that B cannot be involved in the rate-determining step in the reaction and therefore cannot be in the rate law expression.

29. **D.** The order of the reaction can be obtained by simply adding the superscripts in the rate equation:

$$1 + 2 = 3$$

30. **C.** In general, increasing the temperature by 10° doubles the reaction rate. Because the temperature increases by four multiples of ten, the reaction rate will double four times: 2^4, or 16 times. The rate will be 16 times faster at 65°C.

PASSAGE VII (QUESTIONS 31–34)

31. **B.** The term *electromotive force (EMF)* is historical in nature. The battery is often called a "seat of EMF." Because the EMF is actually a potential difference that drives electrical charges to higher potential, it cannot be considered equipotential (answer choice D). Answer choices A and C are dimensionally incorrect.

32. **D.** Ohm's Law gives us the relationship between the potential difference *V* across

any resistor R and the current I through the resistor as

$$V = IR$$

or

$$R = V/I = (1.40\text{ V})/(0.15\text{ A}) = 9.33\ \Omega.$$

Answer choice A is obtained by using the EMF of the battery instead of the terminal voltage (V_t) recorded while the resistor is connected.

33. **B.** We must realize that the difference between the EMF, which can be likened to the maximum possible ability for the battery to move charges, and the terminal voltage is through the internal resistance of the battery and is given by

$$V_t = \text{EMF} - Ir$$
$$V_t + Ir = \text{EMF}$$
$$Ir = \text{EMF} - V_t$$
$$r = (\text{EMF} - V_t)/I = ((1.5\text{ V}) - (1.4\text{ V}))/(0.15\text{ A})$$
$$r = 0.67\ \Omega$$

Note that the sum of $R + r = 10\ \Omega$ as expected. The battery and the external resistor share the total EMF. Answer choice A is provided again for those who neglect to account for the fact that the battery is the supply of the voltage.

34. **C.** The thermal energy is related to the power by E = Pt, where t is the time. The specific heat capacity, c, is related to the thermal energy; the change in temperature, ΔT; and the mass, m, by E = cm ΔT. Therefore, Pt = cm ΔT and t = cm. ΔT/P = (0.5 J/(g°C))(2 g)(10°C)/(.21 J/s) ~ 50 s.

PASSAGE VIII (QUESTIONS 35–39)

35. **C.** The relationship between the distance from the object to the lens, *o*; the distance from the image to the lens, *i*; and the focal length of the lens, *f* is:

$$\frac{1}{o} + \frac{1}{i} = \frac{1}{f}$$

because $o = 40$ cm and $f = +20$ cm:

$$\frac{1}{i} = \frac{1}{f} - \frac{1}{o} = \frac{1}{(20\text{ cm})} - \frac{1}{(40\text{ cm})} = \frac{1}{40\text{ cm}}$$

that yields the answer $i = +40$ cm. The + signifies that the image is *real* and thus is located where the light actually goes—through the lens—which is to the *right* of the lens.

36. **B.** The magnification m relationships yield both the size and orientation of the image relative to the object:

$$m = -\frac{i}{o};|m| = \frac{h_1}{h_o}$$

where h_i and h_o are the heights of the image and object, respectively. Therefore, the results for this case are:

$$m = -(40\text{ cm})/(40\text{ cm}) = -1$$
$$|m| = 1$$

This says that the image is the same size as the object but *inverted*, due to the *negative* result for *m*.

37. **D.** A diverging lens spreads light away from the optical axis, not allowing it to converge as in the formation of a real image. The image is then said to be *virtual*. Diverging lenses can only produce images smaller than the object, so answer choice B is incorrect. The light intensity is a measure of power per unit area. So answer choice C is not correct for a diverging lens, which cannot intensify a beam due to its spreading effects.

38. **A.** Using the formula established earlier,

$$\frac{1}{o} + \frac{1}{i} = \frac{1}{f}$$

with o = –30 cm (the negative sign required for virtual) and f = –15 cm

$$\frac{1}{i} = \frac{1}{f} - \frac{1}{o} = \frac{1}{(-15\text{ cm})} - \frac{1}{(-30\text{ cm})} = \frac{1}{-30\text{ cm}}$$

This gives i = –30 cm, or 30 cm to the *left* of the diverging lens. Because the diverging lens is 10 cm to the *right* of the converging lens, this final image must be located 20 cm to the *left* of the *converging* lens. Answer choice C would be the result had the object distance been taken as *positive* instead of negative.

39. **D.** As before, the magnification for the diverging lens is

$$m = -\frac{i}{o}; |m| = \frac{h_1}{h_o}$$

so that

m = – (–30 cm)/(–30 cm) = –1

This says that the *inverted* object is *re-inverted* but kept the same size. Therefore, the *total* magnification (m_T) is just the products of the two individual magnifications and is

$$m_T = (-1)(-1) = +1$$

It is interesting to note that this particular optical system has simply brought a real object closer to the lens system without changing its size or orientation. Answer choices A and B would be correct only if demagnification occurred, which it has not. Answer choice C is the magnification of each lens separately, not the combined effect.

PASSAGE IX (QUESTIONS 40-42)

40. **B.** The rate of formation of B is the rate constant times k_1 multiplied by the reactants raised to their stoichiometric coefficients. Note that even though ^+H_3O acts as a catalyst and does not appear in the net equation, it does appear in the rate law for the elementary step of A going to B.

41. **C.** The equilibrium constant for A to B is K=[B]/[A]. At equilibrium, the rate of formation of B is equal to k_1[A] and the rate of formation of A is k_{-1}[B]. At equilibrium, the rate of the forward and back reactions is equal:

$k_{-1}[B] = k_1[A]$ this rearranges to $[B]/[A] = k_{-1}/k_1$

therefore, $K = k_{-1}/k_1$

42. **D.** The rate law for the reaction is determined by the rate-determining step (B to C). The rate law for this step is rate = k_2[B]. The concentration of [B] is not known. The elementary steps that occur before the rate-determining step can be assumed to be at equilibrium. This fact allows us to find an equivalent expression for [B] that we can substitute into the rate law.

At equilibrium: $k_{-1}[B] = k_1[A]$ and $[B] = k_1/k_{-1}[A]$.

Substituting this equality for [B] gives:

Rate = $(k_2k_1/k_{-1})[A]$

PASSAGE X (QUESTIONS 43-46)

43. **A.** The temperature change is calculated using the expression

q = m × specific heat × ΔT.

This rearranges to:

ΔT = q/(m × specific heat).

Plugging in the values q = 1×10^{11}J, m = 1×10^9g; SH = 4.18J/g°C, we get:

1.0×10^{11}J/(4.18J/g°C × 1.0×10^9 g) = 23.92°C ~ 24°C

44. **C.** The process of evaporation requires energy. As a result, there is less energy to heat the liquid water on the planet's surface. The amount of energy lost is equal to the energy required to vaporize the 20,000kg of water.

(heat entering planet) = (energy used to heat $H_2O_{(l)}$) + (energy used to vaporize $H_2O_{(l)}$)

To find the energy available to heat the liquid water, we must first find the energy used to vaporize $H_2O_{(l)}$. Subtract this from the total energy. The energy that is left is used to calculate the temperature change of the liquid water.

(heat entering planet) – (energy used to vaporize $H_2O_{(l)}$) = (energy used to heat $H_2O_{(l)}$)

$(1 \times 10^{11}J)$ – (moles H_2O vaporized) H_{vap} = (energy used to heat $H_2O_{(l)}$)

moles H_2O vaporized $= 2.0 \times 10^7 g\ H_2O \times (1 mole\ H_2O/18g) = 1.11 \times 10^6 mole$

$H_{vap} = 40.7 kJ/mole$

(energy used to heat $H_2O_{(l)}$)$= (1 \times 10^8 kJ) - [(1.11 \times 10^6 mole) \times (40.7 kJ/mole)]$

$= (1 \times 10^8\ kJ) - (4.52 \times 10^7 kJ)$

$= 5.48 \times 10^7 kJ$

The temperature change of the water is calculated using the energy above and the expression:

$\Delta T = q/(mass \times SH)$

We use the values $q = 5.48 \times 10^7 kJ$ or $5.48 \times 10^{10} J$,

mass = total mass H_2O – mass H_2O_{vap},

$SH = 4.18 J/g^oC$

$\Delta T = (5.48 \times 10^{10} J)/[(1.0 \times 10^9 g - 2.0 \times 10^7 g) \times 4.18 J/g^oC]$

$\Delta T = +13.4^oC \sim +13^oC$

45. **A.** When the H_2O vapor condenses, the energy it absorbed in the vaporization process is released (–q). This energy enters the H_2O liquid (+q). From the previous question, we know that

$q = 4.52 \times 10^7 kJ$ or $4.52 \times 10^{10} J$

Using the expression:

$q = m \times SH \times \Delta T \rightarrow \Delta T = q/(m \times SH)$

$\Delta T = 4.52 \times 10^{10} J/(1.0 \times 10^9 g \times 4.18 J/g^oC)$

$= 10.8 \sim 11^oC$

46. **D.** The iceberg and the liquid water are at equilibrium, so the water is at 0°C. The temperature of the water will not increase until the iceberg is completely melted. To find the temperature that the water is raised to, we first need to calculate the amount of energy needed to melt the iceberg. The energy remaining after this phase change can be used to heat the water.

The amount of heat needed to melt the iceberg is

$q = (moles\ H_2O) \times H_{fus}$

moles $H_2O = 1.0 \times 10^8 g \times (1$ moles $H_2O/18g) = 5.56 \times 10^6$ mole

$H_{fus} = 6.0 kJ/mol$

$q = (5.56 \times 10^6\ mol) \times (6.0 kJ/mol)$

$q = 3.33 \times 10^7 kJ$

The temperature that the water is raised to can be found using:

$\Delta T = q/(m \times SH)$

We use the values $q = (1.0 \times 10^8 kJ - 3.33 \times 10^7 kJ) = 6.67 \times 10^7 kJ$ or $6.67 \times 10^{10} J$

$m = 1.0 \times 10^9 g$

$SH = 4.18 J/g°C$

$\Delta T = 6.67 \times 10^{10} J/[(1.0 \times 10^9 g) \times (4.18 J/g°C)]$

$\Delta T = 15.9°C \sim 16°C$

PASSAGE XI (QUESTIONS 47–49)

47. **C.** Bond formation occurs because the electron in the bonding MO is lower in energy than it would be if it remained in the H1s AO. Adding an electron to this MO would result in the release of energy. The

amount of energy released from adding one electron to the bonding MO is less than the energy that would be released from adding two electrons. Therefore, the bond is weaker and longer than a bond formed from 2H• atoms.

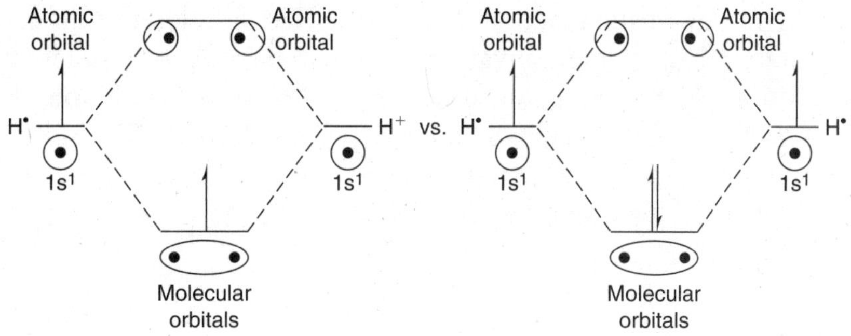

48. **A.** Bond formation occurs because the electrons in the bonding MO are lower in energy than they would be if they remained in the H1s AO. The molecule would be identical to a H_2 formed from 2H• atoms. Therefore, the bond has the same bond length and bond strength.

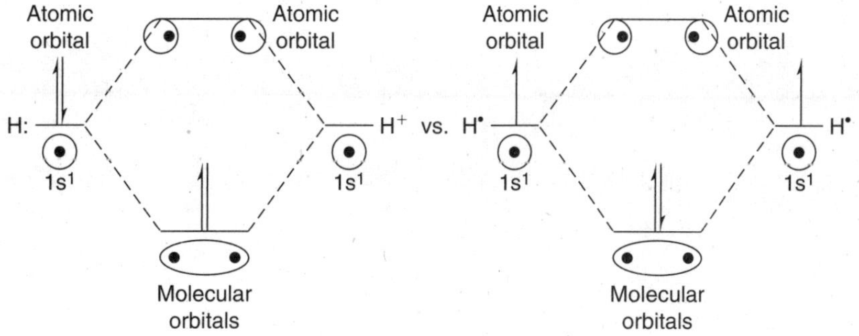

49. **C.** The bond would be longer and weaker than a bond formed from 2H• atoms. The electron in the antibonding MO represents repulsive interactions between electrons. Adding electrons to this MO requires an input of energy. This input of energy is greater than the amount of energy released from putting an electron in the bonding MO. In effect, the presence of an electron in the antibonding MO more than cancels the stabilization from one electron in the bonding MO. So the bond is longer and weaker than a bond formed from 2H• atoms.

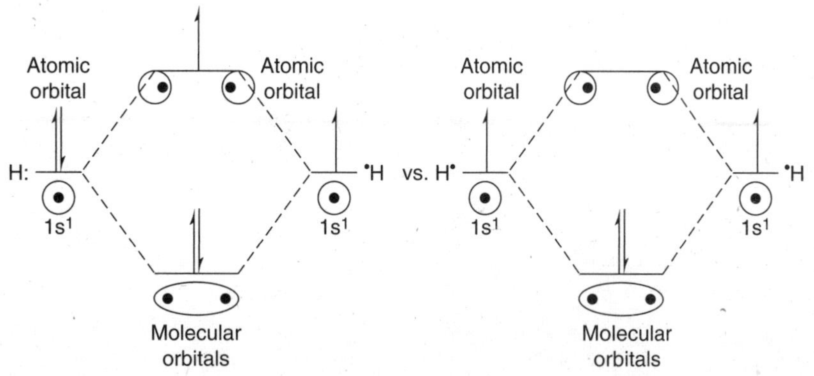

50. **D.** In this reaction, *X* serves to reduce the temperature required for product formation to occur. This lowering of the required reaction temperature is analogous to a decrease in the activation energy of the reaction. By definition, a catalyst lowers the activation energy of a reaction. So *X* is determined to be a catalyst. An enzyme is defined as a biochemical catalyst and is inapplicable in this case because the reaction in question is not biochemical in nature.

51. **C.**

HOAc + NaOH	$\rightarrow$	NaOAc + H_2O
acetic acid		sodium acetate

The reaction of equimolar quantities of a weak acid and a strong base produces a basic (alkaline) salt and water.

52. **C.** The acceleration of both blocks can be determined by F = ma, where F is the net external force on the system (100 N) and m is the total mass of the two blocks (20 kg). The acceleration of each block is therefore 5 m/s^2. A force diagram for the block on the left is shown below. Using Newton's Second Law for this block, we obtain $F_{net} = F - F_c = m_1a$, so F_c, the contact force, is

$$F_c = F - m_1a = 100\text{ N} - (8\text{ kg})(5\text{ m/s}^2) = 60\text{ N}.$$

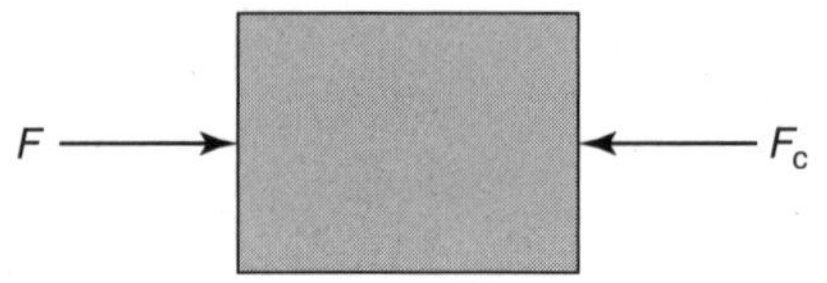

SECTION 2
Verbal Reasoning

PASSAGE I (QUESTIONS 53–57)

53. **B.** The concluding paragraph of this passage makes this clear and also shows why answer choice A is incorrect. This passage does not consider Moore's views on reasons for acting (answer choice C). Answer choice D is not relevant.

54. **C.** Agreement is no guarantee that an action is right, only that everyone believes it to be right. As a result, answer choices A and B are incorrect. As paragraphs three and five imply, it is possible that everyone will agree that an action is right, while the action is wrong, so answer choice C is the best one. Answer choice D is not a valid option.

55. **A.** The facts of a person's upbringing would serve to explain why this person believed as he or she did, but would not explain the truth of the person's belief, so both answer choices B and C should be rejected. Answer choice D is beside the point.

56. **C.** The fourth and fifth paragraphs show that people can disagree about what is right and that their individual or collective approval does not ensure an action's rightness. Therefore, answer choices A and B should be rejected. Answer choice D contradicts the passage.

57. **A.** The fuel gauge is the normal reason we have for holding the belief about how much fuel we have. The fuel gauge, however, is not the cause of how much fuel we have, so answer choice B is false. Answer choice C contradicts the passage, and answer choice D is not supported by the information we have.

PASSAGE II (QUESTIONS 58–62)

58. **A.** The passage does not mention popular vote (answer choice B), and it offers simple statistics that require no public response (answer choice C). While the public may have a chance to comment on the *Federal Register*, it is not a document that needs to be "passed," especially by public vote (answer choice D). The passage does mention the accessibility of the *Federal Register* to the public for commentary; therefore, answer choice A is correct.

59. **D.** While it is important to acknowledge the impact of the Endangered Species Act of 1973, answer choice A merely names the act and does not include an explanation of its application. Answer choice B is incorrect because it mentions "public involvement," a topic not covered in this passage. Answer choice C is incorrect not only because it again presents this false public interaction, but also because it focuses on the United States (the "Nation") and omits the connection with other countries that also honor conservation laws. Answer choice D embodies the topics of why species are endangered, what has been done about it, and by whom it was done, making choice D the most complete answer of the four choices.

60. **D.** The passage states that habitat destruction, a human-made force, is the most serious threat to wildlife and plants. To demonstrate the importance and consequence of environment, the author uses the dinosaur to show what natural extinction is compared to the human-made habitat-

altering extinction of today. Answer choice A is incorrect because the passage does not focus solely on one particular animal. Answer choice B is incorrect because ancient attitudes are not actually presented in the passage. Answer choice C is incorrect because the government in no way affected the life of the dinosaur.

61. **B.** Option III is the definition of a "threatened" species; therefore, any answer with that option is incorrect. Option I applies to both "endangered" and "threatened" species. Option II defines an "endangered" species according to the passage. Answer choice B offers both Options I and II.

62. **D.** The Fish and Wildlife Service works with the *Federal Register*; there is no involvement of either secretaries or Congress in the placement of a species on the published endangered list.

PASSAGE III (QUESTIONS 63–67)

63. **C.** The two modes of thought involved in the "identity crisis" discussed by the author are that of liberal rationalism, which maintains that truth can be discovered through reason, and that of postmodernism, which maintains that knowledge exists only as political systems, that reality is indeterminate, and that reason has become "pluralized." Fascism, Marxism, and Nazism are "truth" systems produced by modern Western civilization, but not the modes of thought involved in the current university crisis (consequently, not answer choice D or answer choice B). Both modes are those of literate cultures (and so not answer choice A).

64. **D.** In paragraph three, the author asserts that Western civilization has produced such politico-ideological "truth" systems as Nazism and Marxism, but it has also been the civilization that has most effectively resisted the ideologizing of knowledge, thereby preserving free thought and open inquiry. Consequently, it has not ignored the problem of truth (not answer choice A) or abandoned rationalism (not answer choice B). It has used "truth" systems as a basis for war, but that is only one aspect of the problem of truth in the twentieth century (hence not answer choice C).

65. **D.** The author conceives the current university crisis as part of the larger twentieth-century intellectual and political problem of truth. He seeks to define that problem in paragraphs two and three before addressing the university crisis in the remainder of the passage. What the author perceives to be the possible decline of moral responsibility has not yet happened, but may if postmodern thought prevails (and so not answer choice A). As the remainder of the passage makes clear, the author believes that intellectual crises in universities have far-reaching consequences (not answer choice B). The author discusses the harmful effects of "truth" systems, but that is not the primary function of his discussion of truth (not answer choice C).

66. **B.** One of the beliefs of postmodern thought is that reality is indeterminate; therefore, that belief is not threatened by postmodernism. Other postmodern beliefs are that truth or knowledge exist only as political systems (not answer choice D), and that there is no such thing as universal truth and that reason has been "pluralized" (not answer choice A). The author says that our civilization would be unworkable if we abandon our belief that reason can arbitrate the moral claims of society, that is, if we capitulate to postmodernism, which does not share that belief (not answer choice C).

67. **C.** Postmodernism asserts that the effort to discover truth through reason is no longer credible (not answer choice D), that knowledge exists only as political "regimes" (not answer choice B), and that universal values do not exist because truth is relative (not answer choice A). The tradition of liberal

rationalism maintains that objective inquiry is the best means of discovering truth.

PASSAGE IV (QUESTIONS 68–72)

68. **C.** The passage presents its argument by means of analogy, specifically, two metaphors that are introduced at the beginning and then developed throughout the passage (the king as a father and the king as the head of a physical body). The other three answer choices are inaccurate.

69. **A.** The author uses examples drawn from the natural world to support his argument that the king's behavior, even at its most violent and irrational, ought not to be resisted by his subjects. Beasts and fowls, he says, do not resist when they are beaten and banished by their parents; by analogy, neither should subjects resist the king, their father, when he behaves in a similar fashion. The king and his subjects are analogous to the natural order, but the king depicted in this instance is not benign.

70. **B.** The metaphors of the king as father and as head are introduced in the first paragraph. The second paragraph develops the metaphor of king as father, while the third paragraph develops the king-as-head metaphor. The fourth paragraph uses both metaphors in stating the conclusion to what is a single argument throughout the passage.

71. **C.** The last paragraph makes it clear that the author believes that the king may never be lawfully replaced (they may not "choose any other whom they please in his room"). In the author's view, there is never ample cause for rebellion, and violent revolution is never justified.

72. **D.** The author's metaphor comparing the king to the head of a physical body suggests that the king is the seat of wisdom and power, but the metaphor does not effectively support his argument that a king can never be replaced when the metaphor is taken literally. Cutting the head off a physical body obviously destroys the whole, but replacing a ruler does not necessarily destroy a country. There are no key terms that the author leaves undefined (not answer choice A). The author's example of the viper is an exception that the author believes proves the "natural law" he discusses (not answer choice B).

PASSAGE V (QUESTIONS 73–76)

73. **B.** The first paragraph states that it is generally believed that Genius cannot be taught through rules or acquired by hard work, a position that the author attempts to refute in the remainder of the passage. It does not offer historical background, nor is it part of the author's argument or his thesis.

74. **A.** The entire passage is designed to argue that Genius can be taught. The other three statements are all ones with which the author would agree (and which are in fact present in the passage in similar forms).

75. **A.** Option I is a simple assertion, Option II is based on an appeal to experience, and Option III is based on an appeal to history.

76. **D.** All of the passage is designed to refute the idea in paragraph one that Genius is beyond the reach of rules. The other choices are either mistaken (answer choices A and C) or partial explanations (answer choice B) of the passage's main purpose.

PASSAGE VI (QUESTIONS 77–80)

77. **C.** The author argues that the humanities are not only neglected, but that they ought to be at the center of higher education. Although liberal arts can be vocationally useful, that is not the chief thrust of the author's argument, nor is he primarily concerned with amounts of money spent on

different kinds of education or with lamenting the loss of a less vocationally oriented past.

78. **D.** The author offers three reasons why the ratio of the humanities to the sciences should be increased: Option I is the chief subject of paragraph five, Option II is the chief subject of paragraphs seven and eight, and Option III is the chief subject of paragraph six.

79. **A.** The author argues that doctors, lawyers, and business executives who are liberally educated have an advantage over those who are not, even when the only consideration is career preparation. Answer choice B is a plausible answer when vocational education is compared with liberal education, but that is not the chief point of the author's discussion of doctors, lawyers, and executives in paragraph five. The author discusses answer choices C and D, but not specifically in relation to these professionals.

80. **C.** In paragraph three, the author suggests that the proper objective of education is to enable the individual to come into possession of his or her full powers, an idea that is repeated in the final paragraph in the author's assertion that Jefferson believed that the educated and developed mind is of paramount importance if free society is to be preserved. For the author, the primary function of education is not connected to vocational concerns (not answer choice A) or personal emotional needs (not answer choice B), nor is it to cater to the individual's special interests, which may be merely vocational.

PASSAGE VII (QUESTIONS 81–86)

81. **D.** The author says that law and right differ as much as obligation and liberty, which are inconsistent (paragraph three). They do spring from the same desire, but it is the desire for self-preservation (not answer choice A). They are naturally incompatible, not compatible (not answer choice B). The author's task is to define and analyze these concepts, not to rely on discussions of previous writers (not answer choice C).

82. **A.** The first law of nature (seek peace and follow it) derives from the "general rule of reason" that "every man ought to endeavor peace as far as he has hope of obtaining it; and when he cannot obtain it, that he may seek and use all helps and advantages of war" (paragraph four). The author analyzes man's natural state, but derives his laws from a reasoning process (not answer choice B). Neither Biblical authority nor history is the source of his laws, although they may be in agreement with both Biblical authority and human history.

83. **B.** The author believes that man must form social contracts based on mutual obligations if he is to achieve self-preservation in society. Such contracts depend on consent if they are to work; lack of consent on either side leads to chaos and war. Therefore, the correct answer choice is B. Absolute monarchy is not based on mutual consent. Rugged individualists probably cannot lead satisfactory lives unless they are willing to give up significant portions of personal liberty. Absolute liberty, in fact, cannot be achieved in any society, democratic or otherwise, nor does the author discuss the relative merits of democracy.

84. **A.** All natural laws derive ultimately from man's desire for self-preservation. Man needs social institutions, but that need springs from his desire for self-preservation (not answer choice B). The right of nature, not the law of nature, is based on the desire for liberty (not answer choice C). The author's discussion of man's natural state makes clear it is a condition of constant warfare, not one that suggests that man's nature is essentially benign (not answer choice D).

85. **B.** Toward the end of the last paragraph, the author says that man is not obligated to follow the second law of nature (to lay down his right of nature) if other men refuse to give up their right of nature. The first and second laws of nature are compatible (not answer choice A). The second law of nature is also compatible with the "law of the Gospel" (not answer choice D). The right of nature always conflicts with personal freedom, but purely personal considerations must be subordinated to social considerations if the laws of nature are to work (not answer choice C).

86. **A.** The right of nature and the laws of nature do derive ultimately from the same impulse (self-preservation); the former considers the rights of man as an individual, whereas the latter seeks to establish laws that enable man to survive when interacting with other men. Answer choice B is incorrect because the two laws of nature do not deal with man's right to defend himself; instead, they focus on man's obligation to give up certain forms of liberty in order to achieve peace. The right of nature and the law of nature do conflict, but the author does not suggest that man invariably chooses the right of nature when the two conflict (not answer choice C). The right of nature and the laws of nature both derive from reason, but they also deal with self-preservation (hence not answer choice D).

PASSAGE VIII (QUESTIONS 87–90)

87. **C.** Answer choice C is correct because the author begins with an explanation of incrementalism, provides a test for incrementalism, then explains why it is used. Answer choice A is incorrect primarily because it is too broad. Although incrementalism is part of the federal budgetary process, it is only one aspect of it, and this passage does not describe, or even outline, the entire budgetary process. Similarly, answer choice B is incorrect because the author is not concerned with alternative budgetary systems. Zero-base budgeting is mentioned only in the first paragraph and only as a means of defining incrementalism, so answer choice D is also incorrect.

88. **A.** The purpose of the second paragraph is to present a test of incrementalism. The test involves the stability of the organization. Given the definition of incrementalism in the first paragraph, the reader can conclude stable organizations are more likely to use incrementalism. This conclusion also makes answer choice D incorrect. The third paragraph's discussion of how stable organizations consider new alternatives like problem solving makes answer choice B incorrect. The author does not make a connection between stable organizations and the consistency of organizational goals. These two topics are considered separately and, given the information contained in the passage, the reader should not link the two.

89. **A.** If one asked the author whether zero could be the base in incrementalism, he would respond, "In a broad sense this can be zero, as in zero-base budgeting. Please read the first paragraph of my passage." Answer choice B is incorrect because from the first paragraph we can conclude ZBB is a budgetary system—not a method of problem solving. Answer choice C is an incorrect answer because it is actually a definition of incrementalism. Answer choice D is not the best answer because a zero base does not necessarily mean that ZBB is more comprehensive than incrementalism. There is no direct indication in the passage whether ZBB is accepted. We are told only that it exists.

90. **D.** Answer choice D is correct because the author devotes a good portion of the passage to describing why incrementalism is used. Although the author does not specifically indicate any problems with incrementalism, the tone of the passage is resigned. The author seems to suggest incrementalism is

forced on the budgetary process. There are some good points to it, but its shortcomings are not mentioned. Answer choice A is incorrect because of the author's statement at the end of the third paragraph and his generally favorable description of incrementalism throughout the passage. Given the author's definition of incrementalism in the first paragraph, answer choice B is also incorrect. Answer choice C is incorrect because the point of the fifth paragraph is to describe how to keep costs down by looking at the problem incrementally.

PASSAGE IX (QUESTIONS 91–92)

91. **A.** The author uses attitudes toward homosexuality to illustrate and present the theory of ethical subjectivism. In the fifth paragraph, the author specifically states that ethical subjectivism is not just about evaluations of homosexuality, but applies to any moral judgment. Although used as an example, the author makes no attempt to *explain* homosexuality (answer choice B). Similarly, the author is not *criticizing* Falwell's views. To do so would be contrary to ethical subjectivism. The author may object to Falwell's statements to the extent they suggest homosexuality is objectively immoral, but the statements are used only as an example and are not the primary purpose of the passage (answer choice C). Answer choice D is incorrect because the focus of the passage is ethical subjectivism, which holds that moral judgments are only expressions of personal feelings and not objective determinations of right and wrong. In addition, the author does not imply that ethical subjectivism is any better or worse than any other moral philosophy. (To do so, of course, would be contrary to ethical subjectivism.)

92. **D.** This is made clear from the last sentence of the first paragraph in which Falwell says that he does not hate the homosexual, but rather the act of homosexuality. Given Falwell's statements and the author's use of them as an example of a person holding a moral judgment out as an objective determination of something that is wrong, it should be clear Falwell *does* believe in objective right and wrong, making answer choice A incorrect. For the same reasons, answer choice B is incorrect because Falwell *does* believe homosexuality to be absolutely immoral. Answer choice C is incorrect because the author does not suggest a connection between homosexuality and intolerance. In addition, the author notes England's tolerant attitude toward homosexuality.

SECTION 3
Writing Sample

SAMPLE ESSAY 1

John Taylor remarks upon the strength of written words by suggesting that they are even more powerful than tangible steel. No doubt, words carved by a writer's pen may do crippling harm to humans and surpass the longevity of a simple physical laceration. Taylor begins his observation regarding written words and the pens that produce them with a metaphor, likening the pens to "dangerous tools." Just as tools may be used to construct or demolish, so pens, too, may be used to enhance; but more important, Taylor stresses the pen's potential to destroy as implied by his choice of "painful" word pairs: sharp/swords, cut/keen, whips/rods. Like a parent cautions a young child about a knife or scissors, so Taylor reminds the reader of the harm that words can inflict.

A common response to Taylor's remark that would contradict his belief in the power of the written word can be found echoing in the playgrounds and schoolyards of all of our childhoods: "Sticks and stones may break my bones but words will never hurt me." This chant proclaims the immediate and painful results of abuse by physical objects, while attempting to combat the threat posed by words. Although visible damage will most certainly not be seen when hurling words rather than rocks, this lyric works to deny the internal psychological and emotional suffering that can be caused by disdainful words or unchecked verbal emotion. A physical wound caused by swords, whips, and rods, or sticks and stones, for that matter, may soon heal; but the mental wound caused by the sharper wit of pens is often much deeper and lasting. Not only is the recorded word there for the victim to see and feel, it is there for contemporaries as well as future generations to ponder.

If one is to learn from history, one must remember that words — whether spoken or written — must be chosen carefully, for their might has been demonstrated throughout the ages. The imperishable effect of the written word as compared to the timely pain of physical abuse can be summed up when one considers the teeming amount of published accounts of modern and ancient opinion available in our libraries. Compare their accessibility to the chances of viewing the scars of a deep wound on any body. Long after the body has passed into oblivion, the opinion of that person may remain among the living but more ominously, it may be entombed on the bookshelves.

EXPLANATION OF ESSAY 1

The essay addresses all three tasks: (1) Taylor's view of the might or power of the pen is explained and interpreted. (2) The essay contains a paragraph that contests Taylor's opinion with a childhood taunt that claims that words are unable to cause pain. (3) The essay compares the lasting effects of the written word versus the ephemeral pain of physical injury and makes a historically proven conclusion about each in relation to the other.

The grammar, spelling, and punctuation conform to suggested standards. Organization, depth of thought, control of vocabulary, and variation of sentence structure are evident.

SAMPLE ESSAY 2

Douglas Jerrold extols the positive effects of patience as he compares it to a "strong drink," suggesting results through its usage similar to those of an alcoholic beverage. Because this metaphor seems favorable in that patience — like a drink — can slay an emotion as undesirable as despair, it can be inferred that the repercussions of patience are also propitious. These characteristics are needed to overcome such a dire state of consciousness as despair. However, by using personification and by ascribing such power to Patience, the message becomes clear that if one can partake of this strongest of strong drinks, one will not be inclined to surrender to despondency and the giant Despair will be slain.

It is important to note, however, that people must be careful that they do not become complacent by relying too heavily on patience. Some literature of the past, particularly fairy tales, has presented women, for instance, with role models of overly patient females. These characters are so patient; in fact, they become passive and do not work to better their situation. For example, some of the women passively wait or sleep, like Sleeping Beauty; or instead of relying on their own abilities, they hope for rescue, like Cinderella as she prays for a fairy godmother, or Rapunzel as she wishes for a prince.

Although Douglas Jerrold advocates imbibing the strong drink of Patience to conquer Despair, it seems that overreliance on patience and passivity can induce the same ill-effects of the alcohol to which it is compared: a blurring of vision creating the inability to see what and when action must be taken. Just as it is difficult to rise from the depths of a drunken existence that is as firmly rooted in despair as it can be caused by it, it is equally laborious to stir one's own soul to action having been made dormant by the excessive patience it practiced — in moderation at one time — for its own good.

EXPLANATION OF ESSAY 2

The essay addresses all three tasks: (1) Jerrold's idea of Patience is defined and explained in relation to the metaphor and the object of Despair. (2) A conflicting view, presenting the disadvantages of patience, is presented using examples. (3) A resolution of moderation is offered.

The essay uses relevant examples and clearly, concisely, and logically presents the argument. The grammar, spelling, and punctuation conform to suggested standards. Organization, depth of thought, and control of vocabulary and sentence structure are evident.

SECTION 4
Biological Sciences

PASSAGE I (QUESTIONS 93–95)

This passage requires a basic understanding of Mendelian inheritance and sex linkage, and the ability to apply the basic rules of probability of independent events.

93. **A.** This pedigree could not represent a sex-linked trait. A sex-linked recessive trait would have to be exhibited by all sons if it is exhibited by the mother. A holandric trait is carried on the Y chromosome and would not be exhibited by females. A father who showed a sex-linked dominant trait would have to pass that trait on to all of his daughters.

94. **C.** The male is heterozygous because his mother exhibits the trait. The probability of his sperm carrying the recessive allele is therefore ½. The female's mother is heterozygous because her mother exhibits the trait. The probability that the female received the recessive allele is ½. If the female is heterozygous, ½ of her eggs would carry the allele. Because all three events must occur to have a homozygous recessive child, the probability of having an affected child would be the product of these three probabilities, $\frac{1}{2} \times \frac{1}{2} \times \frac{1}{2}$.

95. **B.** The female could be heterozygous for the trait in question; the chance that she is heterozygous is ½ because her mother showed herself to be a heterozygote by having an affected son. If the female in question is heterozygous, half (½) of her eggs would carry the recessive gene. All daughters of this couple would receive their father's X chromosome with its dominant gene. Therefore, only sons could be affected. Half (½) of the offspring are expected to be male: those that are fertilized by a Y-bearing sperm. All three events must occur (heterozygous female, recessive X egg, X-bearing sperm) to have an affected child. The chance of the occurrence is the product of the probabilities of these independent events: $\frac{1}{2} \times \frac{1}{2} \times \frac{1}{2}$.

PASSAGE II (QUESTIONS 96–98)

This passage involves meiosis, specifically spermatogenesis. To respond correctly to the questions in this section, one must know the stages of meiosis and the chromosomal constitution at each of these stages.

96. **B.** The diploid number of chromosomes is present at Prophase I. These chromosomes replicate and synapse during this phase of meiosis. A replicated chromosome, two identical chromatids joined by a common centromere, is considered to be one chromosome.

97. **B.** At Anaphase I, homologous chromosomes (each chromosome consists of identical chromatids joined at the centromere) travel to opposite poles. All of the chromosomes that were present before Prophase I are present in the cell as well. The chromatids will not separate until the second meiotic division.

98. **C.** The two secondary spermatocytes produced after the completion of Meiosis I are haploid. They have one replicated chromosome of each type, 23 chromosomes in all. Meiosis II is similar to a mitotic division;

the identical sister chromatids separate and travel to opposite poles at Anaphase II. The products of Meiosis II are haploid spermatids, which develop into haploid sperm. The primary spermatocyte is diploid.

PASSAGE III (QUESTIONS 99–101)

Understanding this passage requires a basic knowledge of osmosis, the diffusion of water across a selectively permeable membrane. The net movement of water will be from the side with a higher concentration of water to the side with a lower concentration.

99. **C.** Because tube C does not change fluid levels, the unknown solution must have the same concentration of water as tube C. Tube C is 1.0% glucose, and therefore 99.0% water.

100. **B.** The red blood cell would swell as water moved inward. Water will move across a selectively permeable membrane from a hypotonic solution (less solute, more water) to a hypertonic solution (more solute, less water). The process of water moving across a semipermeable membrane is called osmosis.

101. **D.** Molecules may move into or out of cells in several ways. Molecules such as ions and water molecules will move by diffusion through plasma membrane pores from a region of higher concentration to a region of lower concentration. Lipid-soluble molecules can diffuse directly through the lipid phase of the membrane. Carrier-facilitated diffusion involves carrier proteins, often called permeases, which interact with the molecule and ease diffusion through the membrane.

PASSAGE IV (QUESTIONS 102–105)

Underlying this passage is an understanding of the relationship between genes and proteins. The representative electrophoretogram reveals that the enzyme in question exists in two forms that are separable by electrophoresis. Individuals may show one or both forms.

102. **A.** To answer this question, one must interpret the electrophoretic results and understand the meaning of the term *allele*. Alleles are genes that code for different versions of the same product, in this case, an enzyme. Individuals 4 and 6 show both allozymes and therefore appear to be heterozygous for this gene. Individuals 1 and 2 are homozygous for the "slow" allele, but there is no evidence given concerning relative fitness of this allele. Likewise, there is no evidence that the "fast" allele in 3 and 5 is more adaptive.

103. **C.** This question requires the understanding that alleles code for a different molecular version of a product that serves a particular function. In this case, the alleles code for different versions of an enzyme (allozymes) whose function is to catalyze the same reaction.

104. **B.** This question assigns a differential range of function for the two allozymes. If one allozyme (in this case, the "fast" allele product) functions throughout the normal temperature range, and the other "slow" allozyme has restricted function within this range, homozygotes for the broad-range allele would be most fit.

105. **C.** The introductory passage states that gel electrophoresis revealed a surprising amount of diversity at the molecular level, indicating that genetic variability at the molecular level is a widespread phenomenon. The information in this section does not address fitness.

106. **A.** The mitotic divisions of the zygote lead to a solid ball of cells called the morula. As the cells of the morula divide further, a fluid-filled cavity forms. This hollow ball of cells is the blastula. When the cells of the blastula differentiate into three layers, the mass is known as a gastrula. The developing organism is called a fetus.

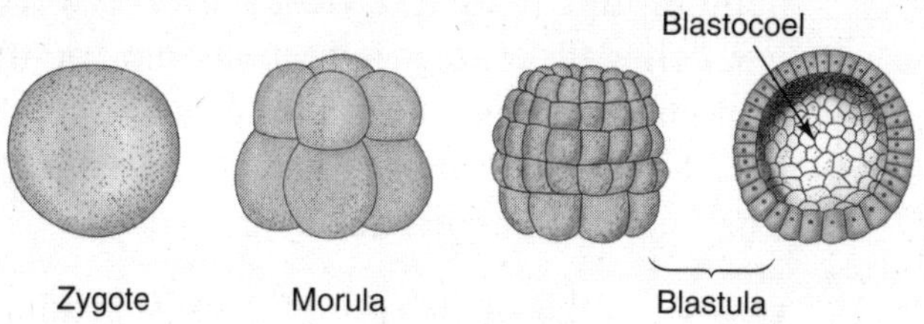

107. **B.** The cerebellum regulates and coordinates muscle contractions. Its size in different animals corresponds roughly with the amount of muscular activity of the animal. Removal of the cerebellum results in the loss of the ability to coordinate voluntary muscle movement.

108. **C.** Pepsin is one of the few enzymes whose optimum pH is not 7. Pepsin requires a low pH of 1.5 to 2.5 for proper activity. The acidity of the stomach is maintained for optimal activity of the protease pepsin.

109. **C.** Highly developed animals can react extremely quickly to certain types of stimuli. This can be important when the animal comes into contact with harmful stimuli, such as fire or sharp objects piercing the skin. The faster the animal responds, the less damage is done.

These kinds of responses do not involve the brain because conscious input is unnecessary and would slow the response. Instead, the impulse is carried from the receptor neuron directly to the spinal cord and then back out through a motor neuron to the appropriate muscle. Thus, the receptor neuron, the motor neuron, and the muscle are the only structures necessary for the reflex action to occur.

PASSAGE V (QUESTIONS 110–112)

This section involves the basic conc epts of evolution and population genetics. To answer these questions, one must understand natural selection and the conditions under which Hardy-Weinberg genetic equilibrium prevails.

110. **B.** Natural selection results in a differential in reproductive success between individuals of different genotypes. In the game of evolution, the winners are genotypes that succeed in passing on more genes to the next generation than other genotypes.

111. **C.** For Hardy-Weinberg equilibrium, the population must be large enough for the laws of probability to prevail. In small populations, events unrelated to fitness can cause wide fluctuations in gene frequencies, or genetic drift.

112. **B.** Individual phenotypes have different success at contributing their genes to the next generation. Those phenotypes that have relatively fewer descendants have been selected against. Selection acts on the individual phenotypes with the best adaptive traits to select for survival those organisms that can respond best to certain conditions.

PASSAGE VI (QUESTIONS 113–117)

Cell and nuclear division are studied in elementary biology courses, but these cellular events are truly complex. Timing, chromosomal structure, and cell structure are important to these processes. The questions in this section require an understanding of the sequence of events in and the basic structures of mitosis and cytokinesis.

113. **C.** The centromere is also called the primary construction. It is the point where sister chromatids are joined. Because this region is relatively uncondensed, it appears to be very narrow or even indiscernible under the microscope. The spindle fibers attach in this region on the kinetochore structures located at the centromere.

114. **C.** At prophase and metaphase, 23 pairs, or 46 chromosomes, are replicated. Each chromosome has identical sister chromatids

joined at the centromere. At anaphase, the replicated chromosomes travel to opposite poles, doubling the number of chromosomes in the cell at that time to 92.

115. **D.** Replication of chromosomes occurs during the "S" stage of the cell cycle when the DNA content in the nucleus doubles. The "S" stands for "synthesis," specifically, DNA synthesis. The "S" stage is in mid-interphase.

116. **D.** The kinetochore is the actual structure to which spindle microtubules attach. The replicated chromosome consists of two identical chromatics joined at the centromere region. Two kinetochores per chromosome develop in late prophase, one pointed toward each pole. The microtubules of the spindle attach to the kinetochores. The centriole is a self-reproducing organelle associated with nuclear division. The centrosome is the differentiated region of the cytoplasm that contains the centriole.

117. **A.** Animal cells undergo cytokinesis by means of a contractile ring of actin filaments that divide the cell into two. Pragmoplasts and cell plates are characteristic of plant cells. Binary fission is an amitotic, asexual division process of prokaryotes.

PASSAGE VII (QUESTIONS 118–122)

Although the vertebrate immune response is complex, these questions concern basic elements of that response. One needs to know the nature of cell-mediated and humoral immunity and the principal organs, cells, and molecules involved.

118. **B.** T and B lymphocytes respond to specific invading organisms. Cells that also respond but are not listed here are natural killer (NK) cells that respond to viruses and nonself tissues. Erythrocytes are red blood cells that contain oxygen-transporting hemoglobin. Phagocytes are scavenger cells; they are not responsible for the immune response. Reticulocytes are young red blood cells just after loss of their nuclei. They mature into erythrocytes.

119. **C.** B cells or B lymphocytes produce antibodies after stimulation by a specific antigen. T cells or T lymphocytes (answer choice B) directly attack foreign cells or substances in the cell-mediated immune response. Phagocytes (answer choice D) are scavenger cells.

120. **B.** The Y-shaped antibody molecule consists of two identical "heavy" and two identical "light" polypeptide chains held together by disulfide bridges. Therefore, just two different types of polypeptides exist in an antibody molecule: the "heavy" chain and the "light" chain.

121. **D.** As described in the passage, antibodies are specific for one particular type of antigen. The antibody molecule illustrated has two binding sites and therefore could bind this type of antigen at both active sites.

122. **C.** Isotypes are variants present in all members of a species. Examples of isotypic variants are the different antibody classes and subclasses. Allotypes, however, are variants that are due to intraspecies genetic differences. Each individual has a specific allotype at each of its immunoglobulin gene loci, which often differ from those present in other individuals. Idiotypes are variants due to a large amount of structural heterogeneity in the immunoglobulin V regions. This is related to the production of a wide variety of different V regions to bind diverse antigens. Finally, phenotypes are the physical appearances of an individual; some phenotypes, such as blood groups, are completely determined by heredity, while others, such as stature, are readily altered by environmental agents.

PASSAGE VIII (QUESTIONS 123–125)

This section is concerned with the basics of cell architecture. The specific structure of a cell is directly related to its function. Some features are common to all cells; others vary according to the cell's origin and/or function.

123. **C.** All cells have a plasma membrane and DNA as genetic information. Prokaryotic cells do not have mitochondria, nuclei, endoplasmic reticulum, or centrioles. Viruses are considered to be noncellular particles; they have a protein coat but no plasma membrane. RNA or DNA may serve as viral genetic information.

124. **A.** The nucleolus is the region of ribosomal rRNA synthesis and the assembly of ribosomal subunits. It is formed around the nucleolar organizing region on a particular chromosome, the region of DNA that codes for rRNA.

125. **A.** The inner membrane of the mitochondrion contains cofactors for electron transport, and the mitochondrial matrix has the enzymes of the Krebs or citric acid cycle. Thus, the process of respiration occurs within the mitochondrion. This process involves breaking down the acetyl group on acetyl coenzyme A, passing the hydrogen atoms down electron carriers via the electron transport chain where coupled reactions form energy-rich ATP molecules from ADP. Mitochondria are descended from mitochondria; they duplicate by a binary fission process.

126. **C.** Tropomyosin, a linear protein, attaches to actin and covers the myosin-binding sites when the muscle is not contracting.

127. **B.** A developing embryo undergoes three drastically different stages in its early development. These states are temporally continuous but have been given separate names. The single zygote divides many times and becomes a ball of cells called the morula. A fluid-filled cavity is formed in the center of the morula, changing it into a hollow ball of cells called the blastula. Blastulation is followed by gastrulation, where the three germ layers differentiate. The gastrula period extends until the early forms of all of the major structures are laid down in neurulation. After this, the developing organism is referred to as a fetus.

128. **B.** Cryptic appearance, Mullerian mimicry, and Batesian mimicry are ways that organisms can avoid becoming the victims of predators. The cryptic appearance of some organisms enables them to blend into their surroundings, becoming invisible to their potential attackers. Mullerian mimicry involves the evolution of two or more inedible or unpleasant-tasting species so that they resemble one another. Batesian mimicry, however, involves the resemblance of an unprotected, harmless species to a dangerous species. This makes it difficult for the predator to distinguish between the two forms. Once the predator has tasted the noxious species, it tends to stay away from both species.

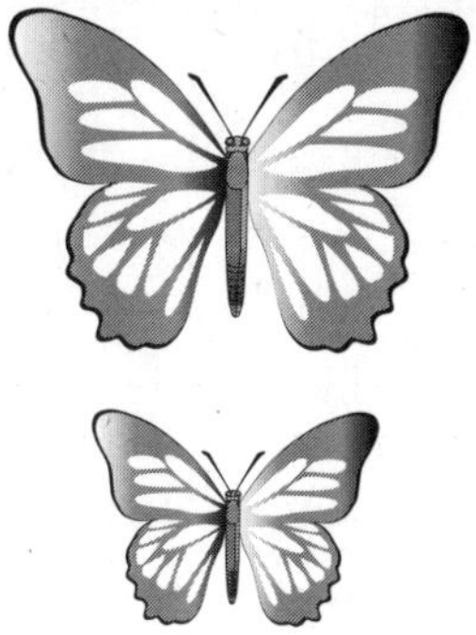

An Example of Batesian Mimicry.

Top: The Monarch butterfly, a distasteful species. Bottom: The Viceroy, a species that mimics the Monarch. Species in the group to which the Viceroy belongs ordinarily have a quite different appearance.

PASSAGE IX (QUESTIONS 129–133)

129. **D.** Mitosis gives rise to daughter cells that are identical to the parent cell; it is the only

type of nuclear division that could result in clone formation. Answer choice A is incorrect because cytokinesis is the division of cytoplasm that occurs in both mitosis and meiosis. Answer choices B and C are incorrect because they refer to the same type of division that results in genetically variable daughter cells.

130. **A.** Sexual reproduction introduces a great deal of genetic variability into a population. If the environment changes, the traits necessary to survive in the new environment may also change. When there are many variations of traits available, it is likely that some individuals will possess the traits best suited to the new environment and will be able to survive and reproduce. Answer choice B is incorrect because genetic variability is not as important in an unchanging environment. Answer choice C is incorrect because the chromosome number remains constant in both sexual and asexual reproduction. Answer choice D is incorrect because the offspring of sexual reproduction are genetically different from each other.

131. **B.** If a cell contains three pairs of chromosomes, the number of possible combinations is 2^3, or 8 different combinations. For example, if a cell contains the chromosome pairs Aa, Bb, and Cc, the possible chromosome combinations are:

ABC	ABc	Abc	AbC
aBC	aBc	abC	abc

132. **C.** During meiosis, the chromosome number is reduced by half, so that when two gametes unite to form a new individual, the chromosome number is once again restored to normal. Answer choices A and D are incorrect because these events occur in both meiosis and mitosis. Answer choice B is incorrect because the chromosome number is reduced by half during meiosis.

133. **A.** When individual chromatids exchange parts, genetic variability is increased to an even greater extent than with random assortment alone. Following crossover, each homologous chromosome contains one original chromatid and one altered chromatid. In this case, meiosis would result in four genetically different daughter cells. Answer choice B is incorrect because the daughter cells will be genetically different. Answer choice C is incorrect because homologous chromosomes contain slight variations of the same genes and are not identical. Answer choice D is incorrect because the number of chromosomal combinations is not reduced.

PASSAGE X (QUESTIONS 134–137)

134. **B.** The reaction occurs in two steps. Iodine will react with acetone to form hydrogen iodide and triiodoacetone, which is readily reversible:

$$3I_2 + CH_3COCH_3 \rightarrow 3HI + I_3CCOCH_3.$$

However, the hydrogen iodide will react irreversibly with sodium hydroxide to form sodium iodide and water:

$$3NaOH + 3HI \rightarrow 3NaI + 3H_2O.$$

The triiodoacetone also reacts with the sodium hydroxide to form sodium acetate and iodoform:

$$Cl_3COCH_3 + NaOH \rightarrow CH_3COOH + CHI_3.$$

Because iodoform is quite insoluble in water, it is the precipitate.

135. **C.** Remember, iodine will be in the precipitate as iodoform and in the supernatant as sodium iodide.

136. **B.** The only compound the sodium ends up in is sodium acetate, which is quite soluble in water and, as a result, in the supernatant as well.

137. **D.** Remember, electronegativity *decreases* as one moves down the periodic table. Because all of the listed halogens are above iodine, they can all displace it. An example using fluorine would be:

$$F_2 + 2CHI_3 \rightarrow 2CHI_2F + I_2 \uparrow.$$

The other halogens would react the same way.

PASSAGE XI (QUESTIONS 138–142)

138. **B.** This is an S_N2 reaction. The OH^- replaces the Br, and the optical activity is reversed. See the illustration below.

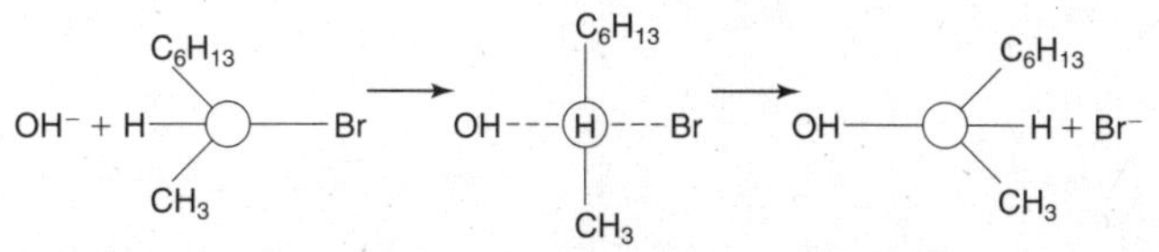

An Example of an S_N2 Reaction.

Note that the optical activity of the product has been reversed. Also note the intermediate form in the middle.

139. **D.** It involves substitution (answer choices A and B are elimination), and the optical activity of the product is reversed.

140. **C.** The bromine in this compound is on a 3° carbon.

141. **A.** S_N2 stands for substitution, second-order kinetics. The rate law for this states:

$$\text{Rate} = k[CH_3(CH_2)_5CHBrCH_3]\,[OH^-],$$

where k is the reaction rate constant.

142. **C.** An S_N2 reaction will still occur, and the optical activity will be reversed.

143. **A.** The Williamson synthesis of ethers is important because of its versatility in the laboratory. This method of synthesis can be used to make asymmetrical ethers as well as symmetrical ethers. In the Williamson synthesis, an alkyl halide is allowed to react with a sodium alkoxide (or sodium phenoxide),

$$\underset{\text{Alkyl halide}}{R—X} + \underset{\text{Sodium alkoxide}}{R'—O^-\,Na^+} \rightarrow$$

$$\underset{\text{Ether}}{R—O—R'} + Na^+X^-,$$

where R represents an alkyl group and X a halide (Cl, Br, I, or F). [The yield from RX is: $CH_3 > 1° > 2° (> 3°)$.]

The sodium alkoxide is made by direct action of sodium metal on dry alcohols:

$$R—OH + Na \rightarrow R—O^-\,Na^+ + {}^1\!/_2\,H_2\uparrow$$

144. **A.** The Barr bodies mask an X chromosome, so that only one X chromosome is active in each somatic cell of females. As a result, the X chromosome's expression is the same in males and females. For the given answer choices, only answer choice A is consistent with the number of Barr bodies observed.

MCAT

MEDICAL COLLEGE ADMISSION TEST

Subject Index

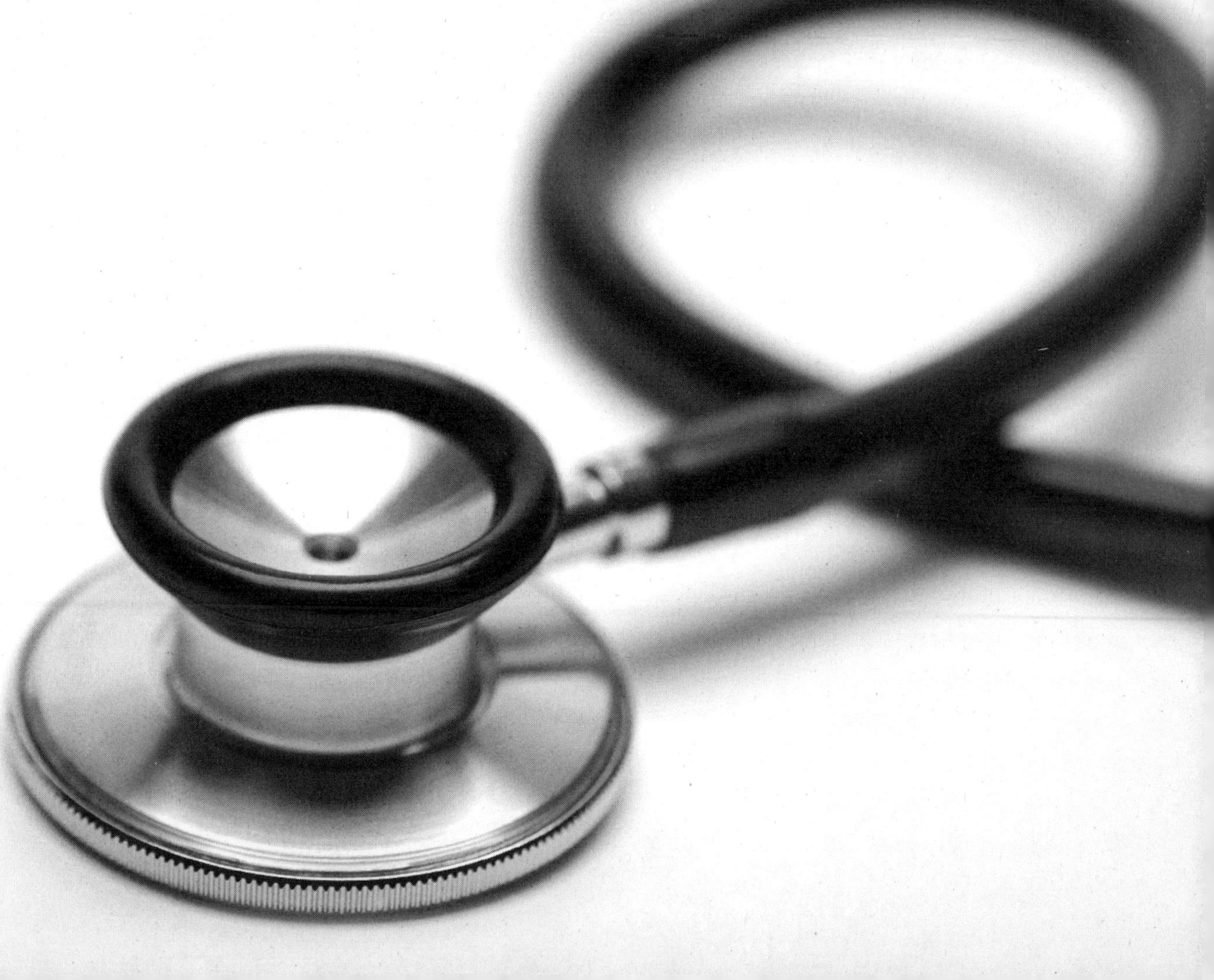

Index

A

D

E

F

J

K

L

M

N

Q

R

V

W

X

Y

Z

MCAT

MEDICAL COLLEGE
ADMISSION TEST

Appendix

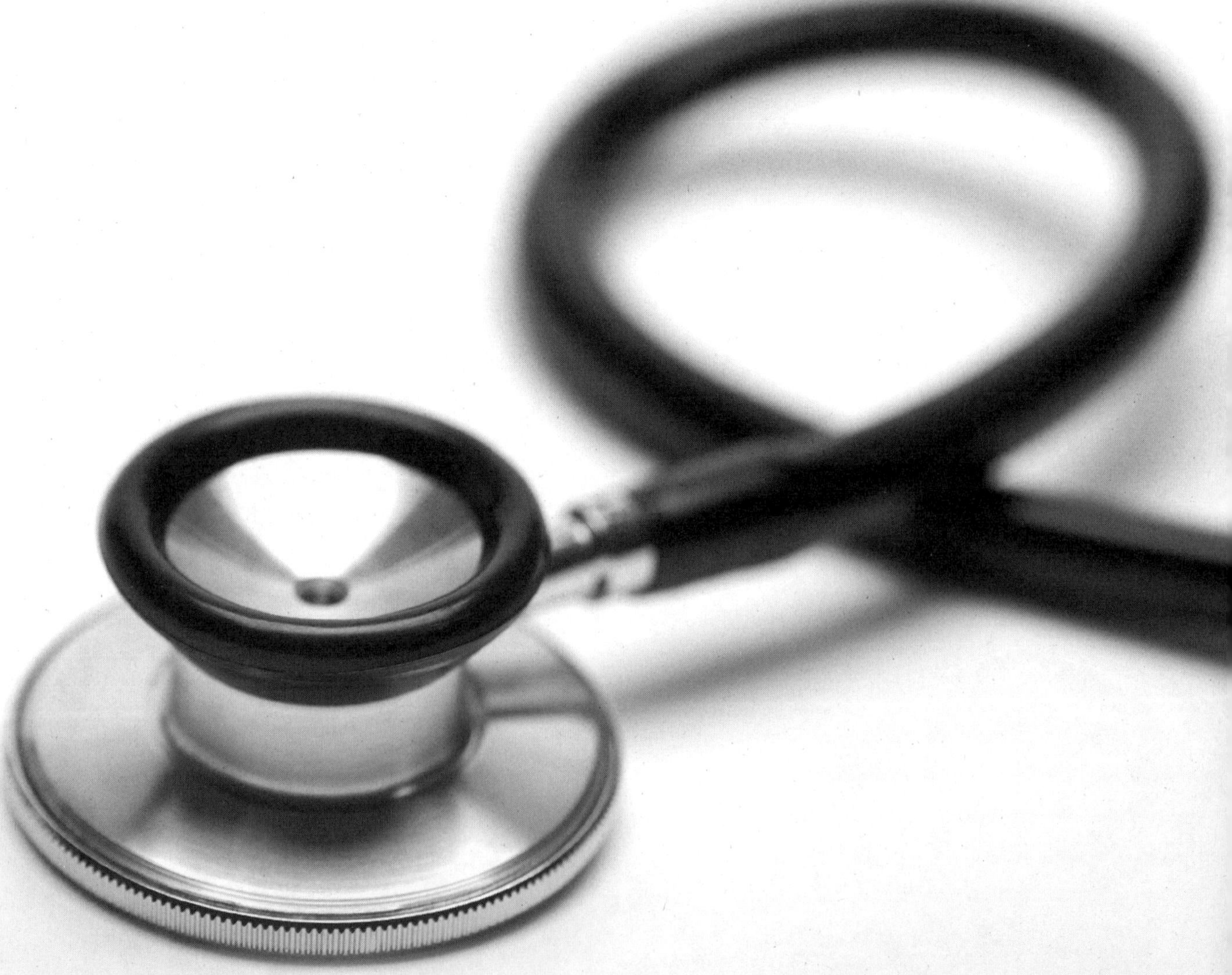

LIST OF UNITS AND MEASUREMENTS

	Dimension	Units
	Length	meter
	Time	second
	Mass	kilogram
Derived Dimensions	Acceleration	m/s^2
	Velocity	m/s
	Force	kg ◊ m/s^2
	Momentum	kg ◊ m/s
	Torque	kg ◊ m^2/s^2
	Angular Momentum	kg ◊ m^2/s^2
	*Electrostatic Charge	coulomb (C)
	Energy/Work	Joule (kg ◊ m^2/s^2)
	Power	Watt (kg ◊ m^2/s^3)
	Potential Difference	Volt (kg ◊ m^2/c ◊ s^3)
	Current	Ampere (c/s)

KEY

Example cell: 22 Ti, Titanium: 47.88, A1/B1, 4.5, $[Ar]3d^24s^2$, 1,670°, 1.54, 3,289°, hcp, 3, **4**, 6.82 (group 4, IVA, IVB)

- Atomic Number
- Atomic Weight; ( ) indicates most stable or best known isotope
- Density (g/cm^3; for gases: g/L at 0°C, 1 atm)
- Melting Point, °C
- Boiling Point, °C
- Oxidation State(s) (bold indicates most stable state)
- Group Classification
- Symbol
- Name
- Acidity/Basicity
- Electronic Configuration
- Electronegativity
- Crystal Structure
- First Ionization Potential

Metal / Metalloid / Non-Metal

Alkali Metals (group 1) · Alkaline Earth Metals (group 2) · Halogens (group 17) · Noble Gases (group 18)

Group	1	2	3	4	5	6	7	8	9	10	11	12	13	14	15	16	17	18
	IA	IIA	IIIA	IVA	VA	VIA	VIIA	VIIIA	VIIIA	VIIIA	IB	IIB	IIIB	IVB	VB	VIB	VIIB	VIII
	IA	IIA	IIIB	IVB	VB	VIB	VIIB	VIII	VIII	VIII	IB	IIB	IIIA	IVA	VA	VIA	VIIA	0

No.	Symbol	Name	Atomic Weight	Acidity/Basicity	Density	Electronic Configuration	Melting Point, °C	Electronegativity	Boiling Point, °C	Crystal Structure	Oxidation State(s)	First Ionization Potential
1	H	Hydrogen	1.00794	A1/B1	0.0899	$1s^1$	-259.34°^{TP}	2.20	-252.88°	hcp	**1**	13.598
2	He	Helium	4.002602	—	0.1785	$1s^2$	-272.375° (25 atm)	—	-268.93°	hcp	—	24.587
3	Li	Lithium	6.941	B3	0.97	$[He]2s^1$	180.5°	0.98	1,342°	bcc	**1**	5.392
4	Be	Beryllium	9.012182	A1/B1	1.8477	$[He]2s^2$	1,287°	1.57	2,471°	hcp	**2**	9.322
5	B	Boron	10.811	A2	2.31	$[He]2s^2p^1$	2,075°	2.04	2,550°	tet	**3**	8.298
6	C	Carbon	12.011	A2	2.25	$[He]2s^2p^2$	4,492°^{TP}	2.55	3,825°^{SP}	hex	2,±**4**	11.26
7	N	Nitrogen	14.00674	A3	1.25046	$[He]2s^2p^3$	-210.0°	3.04	-195.79°	hex	2,±**3**,4,5	14.534
8	O	Oxygen	15.9994	—	1.429	$[He]2s^2p^4$	-218.79°	3.44	-182.95°	cub	**-2**	13.618
9	F	Fluorine	18.9984032	—	1.69	$[He]2s^2p^5$	-219.62°	3.98	-188.12°	mon	**-1**	17.422
10	Ne	Neon	20.1797	—	0.9002	$[He]2s^2p^6$	-248.59°	—	-246.08°	fcc	—	21.564
11	Na	Sodium	22.989768	B3	0.97	$[Ne]3s^1$	97.72°	0.93	883°	bcc	**1**	5.139
12	Mg	Magnesium	24.3050	B3	1.74	$[Ne]3s^2$	650°	1.31	1,090°	hcp	**2**	7.646
13	Al	Aluminum	26.981539	A1/B1	2.702	$[Ne]3s^2p^1$	660.32°	1.61	2,519°	fcc	**3**	5.986
14	Si	Silicon	28.0855	A1/B1	2.33	$[Ne]3s^2p^2$	1,414°	1.90	3,265°	fcc	**4**	8.151
15	P	Phosphorus	30.973762	A2	1.82	$[Ne]3s^2p^3$	44.15°	2.19	277°	cub	±3,4,**5**	10.486
16	S	Sulfur	32.066	A3	2.07	$[Ne]3s^2p^4$	115.21°	2.58	444.6°	orh	±2,4,**6**	10.36
17	Cl	Chlorine	35.4527	A3	3.214	$[Ne]3s^2p^5$	-101.5°	3.16	-34.04°	tet	±**1**,3,5,7	12.967
18	Ar	Argon	39.948	—	1.784	$[Ne]3s^2p^6$	-189.35°	—	-185.85°	fcc	—	15.759
19	K	Potassium	39.0983	B3	0.86	$[Ar]4s^1$	63.38°	0.82	759°	bcc	**1**	4.341
20	Ca	Calcium	40.078	B3	1.54	$[Ar]4s^2$	842°	1.00	1,484°	fcc	**2**	6.113
21	Sc	Scandium	44.95591	B1	2.989	$[Ar]3d^14s^2$	1,541°	1.36	2,830°	hcp	**3**	6.54
22	Ti	Titanium	47.88	A1/B1	4.5	$[Ar]3d^24s^2$	1,670°	1.54	3,289°	hcp	3,**4**	6.82
23	V	Vanadium	50.9415	A1/B1	5.96	$[Ar]3d^34s^2$	1,910°	1.63	3,407°	bcc	2,3,4,**5**	6.74
24	Cr	Chromium	51.9961	A3	7.2	$[Ar]3d^54s^1$	1,907°	1.66	2,671°	bcc	2,**3**,6	6.766
25	Mn	Manganese	54.93805	A3	7.47	$[Ar]3d^54s^2$	1,246°	1.55	2,061°	cub	**2**,3,4,6,7	7.435
26	Fe	Iron	55.847	A1/B1	7.86	$[Ar]3d^64s^2$	1,538°	1.83	2,861°	bcc	2,**3**	7.870
27	Co	Cobalt	58.9332	A1/B1	8.92	$[Ar]3d^74s^2$	1,495°	1.88	2,927°	fcc	**2**,3	7.86
28	Ni	Nickel	58.6934	B2	8.9	$[Ar]3d^84s^2$	1,455°	1.91	2,913°	fcc	**2**,3	7.635
29	Cu	Copper	63.546	B2	8.94	$[Ar]3d^{10}4s^1$	1,084.62°	1.9	2,562°	fcc	1,**2**	7.726
30	Zn	Zinc	65.39	A1/B1	7.14	$[Ar]3d^{10}4s^2$	419.58°	1.65	907°	hcp	**2**	9.394
31	Ga	Gallium	69.723	A1/B1	6.095	$[Ar]3d^{10}4s^2p^1$	29.76°	1.81	2,204°	orh	**3**	5.999
32	Ge	Germanium	72.61	A1/B1	5.35	$[Ar]3d^{10}4s^2p^2$	938.25°	2.01	2,833°	fcc	**4**	7.899
33	As	Arsenic	74.92159	A2	5.72	$[Ar]3d^{10}4s^2p^3$	817°^{TP}	2.18	614°^{SP}	rhm	±**3**,5	9.81
34	Se	Selenium	78.96	A3	4.81	$[Ar]3d^{10}4s^2p^4$	221°	2.55	685°	hex	-2,**4**,6	9.752
35	Br	Bromine	79.904	A3	3.119	$[Ar]3d^{10}4s^2p^5$	-7.2°	2.96	58.8°	orh	±**1**,5	11.814
36	Kr	Krypton	83.8	—	3.74	$[Ar]3d^{10}4s^2p^6$	-157.36°	—	-153.22°	fcc	—	13.999
37	Rb	Rubidium	85.4678	B3	1.532	$[Kr]5s^1$	39.31°	0.82	688°	bcc	**1**	4.177
38	Sr	Strontium	87.62	B3	2.6	$[Kr]5s^2$	769°	0.95	1,382°	fcc	**2**	5.695
39	Y	Yttrium	88.90585	B1	4.469	$[Kr]4d^15s^2$	1,526°	1.22	3,336°	hcp	**3**	6.38
40	Zr	Zirconium	91.224	A1/B1	6.49	$[Kr]4d^25s^2$	1,855°	1.33	4,409°	hcp	**4**	6.84
41	Nb	Niobium	92.90638	A2	8.57	$[Kr]4d^45s^1$	2,477°	1.6	4,744°	bcc	3,**5**	6.9
42	Mo	Molybdenum	95.94	A3	10.2	$[Kr]4d^55s^1$	2,623°	2.16	4,639°	bcc	2,3,4,5,**6**	7.099
43	Tc	Technetium	(97.9072)	A3	11.5	$[Kr]4d^55s^2$	2,157°	1.9	4,265°	hcp	**7**	7.28
44	Ru	Ruthenium	101.07	A2	12.3	$[Kr]4d^75s^1$	2,334°	2.2	4,150°	hcp	2,3,**4**,6,8	7.37
45	Rh	Rhodium	102.9055	A1/B1	12.4	$[Kr]4d^85s^1$	1,964°	1.28	3,695°	fcc	2,**3**,4	7.46
46	Pd	Palladium	106.4	B2	12.02	$[Kr]4d^{10}$	1,554.9°	2.2	2,963°	fcc	**2**,4	8.34
47	Ag	Silver	107.8682	A1/B2	10.5	$[Kr]4d^{10}5s^1$	961.78°	1.93	2,162°	fcc	**1**	7.576
48	Cd	Cadmium	112.411	B2	8.642	$[Kr]4d^{10}5s^2$	321.07°	1.69	767°	hcp	**2**	8.993
49	In	Indium	114.818	A1/B2	7.3	$[Kr]4d^{10}5s^2p^1$	156.6°	1.78	2,072°	tet	**3**	5.786
50	Sn	Tin	118.710	A1/B1	7.28	$[Kr]4d^{10}5s^2p^2$	231.93°	1.96	2,602°	fcc	2,**4**	7.344
51	Sb	Antimony	121.757	A2	6.618	$[Kr]4d^{10}5s^2p^3$	630.63°	2.05	1,587°	rhm	±**3**,5	8.641
52	Te	Tellurium	127.60	A2	6.25	$[Kr]4d^{10}5s^2p^4$	449.51°	2.1	988°	hcp	-2,**4**,6	9.009
53	I	Iodine	126.90447	A3	4.93	$[Kr]4d^{10}5s^2p^5$	113.7°	2.66	184.4°	orh	±**1**,5,7	10.451
54	Xe	Xenon	131.29	—	5.89	$[Kr]4d^{10}5s^2p^6$	-111.75°	—	-108.04°	fcc	—	12.13
55	Cs	Cesium	132.90543	B3	1.879	$[Xe]6s^1$	28.44°	0.79	671°	bcc	**1**	3.894
56	Ba	Barium	137.327	B3	3.594	$[Xe]6s^2$	727°	0.89	1,897°	bcc	**2**	5.212
57	La	Lanthanum	138.9055	B3	6.146	$[Xe]5d^16s^2$	920°	1.10	3,455°	hex	**3**	5.577
58	Ce	Cerium	140.115	B2	6.77	$[Xe]4f^15d^16s^2$	799°	1.12	3,424°	fcc	**3**,4	5.466
59	Pr	Praseodymium	140.90765	B2	6.773	$[Xe]4f^36s^2$	931°	1.13	3,510°	hex	**3**,4	5.422
60	Nd	Neodymium	144.24	B2	7.0	$[Xe]4f^46s^2$	1,016°	1.14	3,066°	hex	**3**	5.489
61	Pm	Promethium	(144.9127)	B2	7.264	$[Xe]4f^56s^2$	1,042°	1.13	3,000°	dcp	**3**	5.554
62	Sm	Samarium	150.36	B2	7.536	$[Xe]4f^66s^2$	1,072°	1.17	1,790°	rhm	2,**3**	5.631
63	Eu	Europium	151.965	B2	5.244	$[Xe]4f^76s^2$	822°	1.2	1,596°	bcc	2,**3**	5.666
64	Gd	Gadolinium	157.25	B2	7.901	$[Xe]4f^75d^16s^2$	1,314°	1.2	3,264°	hcp	**3**	6.141
65	Tb	Terbium	158.92534	B1	8.23	$[Xe]4f^96s^2$	1,359°	1.2	3,221°	hcp	**3**,4	5.842
66	Dy	Dysprosium	162.50	B1	8.551	$[Xe]4f^{10}6s^2$	1,411°	1.22	2,561°	hcp	**3**	5.927
67	Ho	Holmium	164.93032	B1	8.8	$[Xe]4f^{11}6s^2$	1,472°	1.23	2,694°	hcp	**3**	6.018
68	Er	Erbium	167.26	B1	9.066	$[Xe]4f^{12}6s^2$	1,529°	1.24	2,862°	hcp	**3**	6.101
69	Tm	Thulium	168.93421	B1	9.321	$[Xe]4f^{13}6s^2$	1,545°	1.25	1,946°	hcp	2,**3**	6.18436
70	Yb	Ytterbium	173.04	B1	6.966	$[Xe]4f^{14}6s^2$	824°	1.1	1,194°	fcc	2,**3**	6.25394
71	Lu	Lutetium	174.967	B1	9.84	$[Xe]4f^{14}5d^16s^2$	1,663°	1.27	3,393°	hcp	**3**	5.42589
72	Hf	Hafnium	178.49	A1/B1	13.31	$[Xe]4f^{14}5d^26s^2$	2,233°	1.3	4,603°	hcp	**4**	7.0
73	Ta	Tantalum	180.9479	A2	16.6	$[Xe]4f^{14}5d^36s^2$	3,017°	1.5	5,458°	bcc	**5**	7.89
74	W	Tungsten	183.84	A2	1.935	$[Xe]4f^{14}5d^46s^2$	3,422°	2.36	5,555°	bcc	2,3,4,5,**6**	7.98
75	Re	Rhenium	186.207	A2	20.5	$[Xe]4f^{14}5d^56s^2$	3,186°	1.9	5,596°	hcp	-1,2,4,6,**7**	7.88
76	Os	Osmium	190.23	A2	22.61	$[Xe]4f^{14}5d^66s^2$	3,033°	2.2	5,012°	hcp	2,3,**4**,6,8	8.7
77	Ir	Iridium	192.22	B2	22.65	$[Xe]4f^{14}5d^76s^2$	2,446°	2.20	4,428°	fcc	2,3,**4**,6	9.1
78	Pt	Platinum	195.08	B2	21.45	$[Xe]4f^{14}5d^96s^1$	1,768.4°	2.28	3,825°	fcc	2,**4**	9.0
79	Au	Gold	196.96654	A1/B1	19.31	$[Xe]4f^{14}5d^{10}6s^1$	1,064.18°	2.54	2,856°	fcc	1,**3**	9.225
80	Hg	Mercury	200.59	B2	13.546	$[Xe]4f^{14}5d^{10}6s^2$	-38.83°	2.0	356.73°	rhm	1,**2**	10.437
81	Tl	Thallium	204.3833	B2	11.85	$[Xe]4f^{14}5d^{10}6s^2p^1$	304°	2.04	1,473°	hcp	**1**,3	6.108
82	Pb	Lead	207.2	A1/B1	11.34	$[Xe]4f^{14}5d^{10}6s^2p^2$	327.46°	2.33	1,749°	fcc	**2**,4	7.416
83	Bi	Bismuth	208.98037	A2	9.78	$[Xe]4f^{14}5d^{10}6s^2p^3$	271.4°	2.02	1,564°	rhm	**3**,5	7.289
84	Po	Polonium	(208.9824)	A1/B1	9.196	$[Xe]4f^{14}5d^{10}6s^2p^4$	254°	2.0	962°	cub	2,**4**	8.42
85	At	Astatine	(209.9824)	—	—	$[Xe]4f^{14}5d^{10}6s^2p^5$	302°	2.2	337°	—	±**1**,3,5,7	—
86	Rn	Radon	(222.0176)	—	9.73	$[Xe]4f^{14}5d^{10}6s^2p^6$	-71°	—	-61.7°	—	—	10.748
87	Fr	Francium	(223.0197)	B3	—	$[Rn]7s^1$	27°	0.7	677°	bcc	**1**	—
88	Ra	Radium	(226.0254)	B3	5.8	$[Rn]7s^2$	700°	0.9	1,536°	bcc	**2**	5.279
89	Ac	Actinium	(227.0278)	[illegible]	10.07	$[Rn]6d^17s^2$	1,051°	1.1	3,198°	fcc	**3**	6.9
90	Th	Thorium	232.0381	B1	11.72	$[Rn]6d^27s^2$	1,750°	1.3	4,788°	fcc	**4**	6.08
91	Pa	Protactinium	231.03588	B1	15.37	$[Rn]5f^26d^17s^2$	1,572°	1.5	—	bct	4,**5**	5.89
92	U	Uranium	238.0289	A1/B1	19.07	$[Rn]5f^36d^17s^2$	1,135°	1.38	3,818°	bcc	3,4,5,**6**	6.05
93	Np	Neptunium	(237.0482)	A1/B1	20.45	$[Rn]5f^46d^17s^2$	644°	1.36	—	orh	3,4,**5**,6	6.19
94	Pu	Plutonium	(244.0642)	A1/B1	19.816	$[Rn]5f^67s^2$	640°	1.28	3,228°	mcl	3,**4**,5,6	5.8
95	Am	Americium	(243.0614)	A1/B1	13.67	$[Rn]5f^77s^2$	1,176°	1.3	2,607°	hcp	**3**,4,5,6	5.993
96	Cm	Curium	(247.0703)	A1/B1	13.51	$[Rn]5f^76d^17s^2$	1,345°	1.3	—	dcp	**3**	6.02
97	Bk	Berkelium	(247.0703)	—	14.78	$[Rn]5f^97s^2$	1,050°	1.3	—	dcp	**3**,4	6.23
98	Cf	Californium	(251.0796)	—	—	$[Rn]5f^{10}7s^2$	900°	1.3	—	—	**3**	6.3
99	Es	Einsteinium	(252.083)	—	—	$[Rn]5f^{11}7s^2$	860°	1.3	—	—	**3**	6.42
100	Fm	Fermium	(257.0951)	—	—	$[Rn]5f^{12}7s^2$	1,527°	1.3	—	—	**3**	6.5
101	Md	Mendelevium	(258.1)	—	—	$[Rn]5f^{13}7s^2$	827°	1.3	—	—	2,3	6.58
102	No	Nobelium	(259.1009)	—	—	$[Rn]5f^{14}7s^2$	827°	1.3	—	—	2,3	6.65
103	Lr	Lawrencium	(262.11)	—	—	$[Rn]5f^{14}6d^17s^2$	1,627°	—	—	—	**3**	—
104	Rf	Rutherfordium	(261.108)	—	—	$[Rn]5f^{14}6d^27s^2$	—	—	—	—	—	—
105	Db	Dubnium	(262.114)	—	—	$[Rn]5f^{14}6d^37s^2$	—	—	—	—	—	—
106	Sg	Seaborgium	(266.121)	—	—	$[Rn]5f^{14}6d^47s^2$	—	—	—	—	—	—
107	Bh	Bohrium	(264.124)	—	—	$[Rn]5f^{14}6d^57s^2$	—	—	—	—	—	—
108	Hs	Hassium	(269.134)	—	—	$[Rn]5f^{14}6d^67s^2$	—	—	—	—	—	—
109	Mt	Meitnerium	(268.138)	—	—	$[Rn]5f^{14}6d^77s^2$	—	—	—	—	—	—
110	Uun	Ununnilium	(271.146)	—	—	—	—	—	—	—	—	—
111	Uuu	Unununium	(272.153)	—	—	—	—	—	—	—	—	—
112	Uub	Ununbium	(277)	—	—	—	—	—	—	—	—	—
114	Uuq	Ununquadium	(289)	—	—	—	—	—	—	—	—	—
116	Uuh	Ununhexium	(289)	—	—	—	—	—	—	—	—	—

LANTHANIDE SERIES: 58–71 · ACTINIDE SERIES: 90–103

MEDICAL COLLEGE ADMISSION TEST

Additional ANSWER SHEETS

SECTION 1: Physical Sciences

1. Ⓐ Ⓑ Ⓒ Ⓓ
2. Ⓐ Ⓑ Ⓒ Ⓓ
3. Ⓐ Ⓑ Ⓒ Ⓓ
4. Ⓐ Ⓑ Ⓒ Ⓓ
5. Ⓐ Ⓑ Ⓒ Ⓓ
6. Ⓐ Ⓑ Ⓒ Ⓓ
7. Ⓐ Ⓑ Ⓒ Ⓓ
8. Ⓐ Ⓑ Ⓒ Ⓓ
9. Ⓐ Ⓑ Ⓒ Ⓓ
10. Ⓐ Ⓑ Ⓒ Ⓓ
11. Ⓐ Ⓑ Ⓒ Ⓓ
12. Ⓐ Ⓑ Ⓒ Ⓓ
13. Ⓐ Ⓑ Ⓒ Ⓓ
14. Ⓐ Ⓑ Ⓒ Ⓓ
15. Ⓐ Ⓑ Ⓒ Ⓓ
16. Ⓐ Ⓑ Ⓒ Ⓓ
17. Ⓐ Ⓑ Ⓒ Ⓓ
18. Ⓐ Ⓑ Ⓒ Ⓓ
19. Ⓐ Ⓑ Ⓒ Ⓓ
20. Ⓐ Ⓑ Ⓒ Ⓓ
21. Ⓐ Ⓑ Ⓒ Ⓓ
22. Ⓐ Ⓑ Ⓒ Ⓓ
23. Ⓐ Ⓑ Ⓒ Ⓓ
24. Ⓐ Ⓑ Ⓒ Ⓓ
25. Ⓐ Ⓑ Ⓒ Ⓓ
26. Ⓐ Ⓑ Ⓒ Ⓓ
27. Ⓐ Ⓑ Ⓒ Ⓓ
28. Ⓐ Ⓑ Ⓒ Ⓓ
29. Ⓐ Ⓑ Ⓒ Ⓓ
30. Ⓐ Ⓑ Ⓒ Ⓓ
31. Ⓐ Ⓑ Ⓒ Ⓓ
32. Ⓐ Ⓑ Ⓒ Ⓓ
33. Ⓐ Ⓑ Ⓒ Ⓓ
34. Ⓐ Ⓑ Ⓒ Ⓓ
35. Ⓐ Ⓑ Ⓒ Ⓓ
36. Ⓐ Ⓑ Ⓒ Ⓓ
37. Ⓐ Ⓑ Ⓒ Ⓓ
38. Ⓐ Ⓑ Ⓒ Ⓓ
39. Ⓐ Ⓑ Ⓒ Ⓓ
40. Ⓐ Ⓑ Ⓒ Ⓓ
41. Ⓐ Ⓑ Ⓒ Ⓓ
42. Ⓐ Ⓑ Ⓒ Ⓓ
43. Ⓐ Ⓑ Ⓒ Ⓓ
44. Ⓐ Ⓑ Ⓒ Ⓓ
45. Ⓐ Ⓑ Ⓒ Ⓓ
46. Ⓐ Ⓑ Ⓒ Ⓓ
47. Ⓐ Ⓑ Ⓒ Ⓓ
48. Ⓐ Ⓑ Ⓒ Ⓓ
49. Ⓐ Ⓑ Ⓒ Ⓓ
50. Ⓐ Ⓑ Ⓒ Ⓓ
51. Ⓐ Ⓑ Ⓒ Ⓓ
52. Ⓐ Ⓑ Ⓒ Ⓓ

SECTION 2: Verbal Reasoning

53. Ⓐ Ⓑ Ⓒ Ⓓ
54. Ⓐ Ⓑ Ⓒ Ⓓ
55. Ⓐ Ⓑ Ⓒ Ⓓ
56. Ⓐ Ⓑ Ⓒ Ⓓ
57. Ⓐ Ⓑ Ⓒ Ⓓ
58. Ⓐ Ⓑ Ⓒ Ⓓ
59. Ⓐ Ⓑ Ⓒ Ⓓ
60. Ⓐ Ⓑ Ⓒ Ⓓ
61. Ⓐ Ⓑ Ⓒ Ⓓ
62. Ⓐ Ⓑ Ⓒ Ⓓ
63. Ⓐ Ⓑ Ⓒ Ⓓ
64. Ⓐ Ⓑ Ⓒ Ⓓ
65. Ⓐ Ⓑ Ⓒ Ⓓ
66. Ⓐ Ⓑ Ⓒ Ⓓ
67. Ⓐ Ⓑ Ⓒ Ⓓ
68. Ⓐ Ⓑ Ⓒ Ⓓ
69. Ⓐ Ⓑ Ⓒ Ⓓ
70. Ⓐ Ⓑ Ⓒ Ⓓ
71. Ⓐ Ⓑ Ⓒ Ⓓ
72. Ⓐ Ⓑ Ⓒ Ⓓ
73. Ⓐ Ⓑ Ⓒ Ⓓ
74. Ⓐ Ⓑ Ⓒ Ⓓ
75. Ⓐ Ⓑ Ⓒ Ⓓ
76. Ⓐ Ⓑ Ⓒ Ⓓ
77. Ⓐ Ⓑ Ⓒ Ⓓ
78. Ⓐ Ⓑ Ⓒ Ⓓ
79. Ⓐ Ⓑ Ⓒ Ⓓ
80. Ⓐ Ⓑ Ⓒ Ⓓ
81. Ⓐ Ⓑ Ⓒ Ⓓ
82. Ⓐ Ⓑ Ⓒ Ⓓ
83. Ⓐ Ⓑ Ⓒ Ⓓ
84. Ⓐ Ⓑ Ⓒ Ⓓ
85. Ⓐ Ⓑ Ⓒ Ⓓ
86. Ⓐ Ⓑ Ⓒ Ⓓ
87. Ⓐ Ⓑ Ⓒ Ⓓ
88. Ⓐ Ⓑ Ⓒ Ⓓ
89. Ⓐ Ⓑ Ⓒ Ⓓ
90. Ⓐ Ⓑ Ⓒ Ⓓ
91. Ⓐ Ⓑ Ⓒ Ⓓ
92. Ⓐ Ⓑ Ⓒ Ⓓ

SECTION 4: Biological Sciences

93. Ⓐ Ⓑ Ⓒ Ⓓ
94. Ⓐ Ⓑ Ⓒ Ⓓ
95. Ⓐ Ⓑ Ⓒ Ⓓ
96. Ⓐ Ⓑ Ⓒ Ⓓ
97. Ⓐ Ⓑ Ⓒ Ⓓ
98. Ⓐ Ⓑ Ⓒ Ⓓ
99. Ⓐ Ⓑ Ⓒ Ⓓ
100. Ⓐ Ⓑ Ⓒ Ⓓ
101. Ⓐ Ⓑ Ⓒ Ⓓ
102. Ⓐ Ⓑ Ⓒ Ⓓ
103. Ⓐ Ⓑ Ⓒ Ⓓ

104. Ⓐ Ⓑ Ⓒ Ⓓ
105. Ⓐ Ⓑ Ⓒ Ⓓ
106. Ⓐ Ⓑ Ⓒ Ⓓ
107. Ⓐ Ⓑ Ⓒ Ⓓ
108. Ⓐ Ⓑ Ⓒ Ⓓ
109. Ⓐ Ⓑ Ⓒ Ⓓ
110. Ⓐ Ⓑ Ⓒ Ⓓ
111. Ⓐ Ⓑ Ⓒ Ⓓ
112. Ⓐ Ⓑ Ⓒ Ⓓ
113. Ⓐ Ⓑ Ⓒ Ⓓ
114. Ⓐ Ⓑ Ⓒ Ⓓ
115. Ⓐ Ⓑ Ⓒ Ⓓ
116. Ⓐ Ⓑ Ⓒ Ⓓ
117. Ⓐ Ⓑ Ⓒ Ⓓ
118. Ⓐ Ⓑ Ⓒ Ⓓ
119. Ⓐ Ⓑ Ⓒ Ⓓ
120. Ⓐ Ⓑ Ⓒ Ⓓ
121. Ⓐ Ⓑ Ⓒ Ⓓ
122. Ⓐ Ⓑ Ⓒ Ⓓ
123. Ⓐ Ⓑ Ⓒ Ⓓ
124. Ⓐ Ⓑ Ⓒ Ⓓ
125. Ⓐ Ⓑ Ⓒ Ⓓ
126. Ⓐ Ⓑ Ⓒ Ⓓ
127. Ⓐ Ⓑ Ⓒ Ⓓ
128. Ⓐ Ⓑ Ⓒ Ⓓ
129. Ⓐ Ⓑ Ⓒ Ⓓ
130. Ⓐ Ⓑ Ⓒ Ⓓ
131. Ⓐ Ⓑ Ⓒ Ⓓ
132. Ⓐ Ⓑ Ⓒ Ⓓ
133. Ⓐ Ⓑ Ⓒ Ⓓ
134. Ⓐ Ⓑ Ⓒ Ⓓ
135. Ⓐ Ⓑ Ⓒ Ⓓ
136. Ⓐ Ⓑ Ⓒ Ⓓ
137. Ⓐ Ⓑ Ⓒ Ⓓ
138. Ⓐ Ⓑ Ⓒ Ⓓ
139. Ⓐ Ⓑ Ⓒ Ⓓ
140. Ⓐ Ⓑ Ⓒ Ⓓ
141. Ⓐ Ⓑ Ⓒ Ⓓ
142. Ⓐ Ⓑ Ⓒ Ⓓ
143. Ⓐ Ⓑ Ⓒ Ⓓ
144. Ⓐ Ⓑ Ⓒ Ⓓ

MEDICAL COLLEGE ADMISSION TEST

Additional ANSWER SHEETS

SECTION 1: Physical Sciences

1. (A) (B) (C) (D)
2. (A) (B) (C) (D)
3. (A) (B) (C) (D)
4. (A) (B) (C) (D)
5. (A) (B) (C) (D)
6. (A) (B) (C) (D)
7. (A) (B) (C) (D)
8. (A) (B) (C) (D)
9. (A) (B) (C) (D)
10. (A) (B) (C) (D)
11. (A) (B) (C) (D)
12. (A) (B) (C) (D)
13. (A) (B) (C) (D)
14. (A) (B) (C) (D)
15. (A) (B) (C) (D)
16. (A) (B) (C) (D)
17. (A) (B) (C) (D)
18. (A) (B) (C) (D)
19. (A) (B) (C) (D)
20. (A) (B) (C) (D)
21. (A) (B) (C) (D)
22. (A) (B) (C) (D)
23. (A) (B) (C) (D)
24. (A) (B) (C) (D)
25. (A) (B) (C) (D)
26. (A) (B) (C) (D)
27. (A) (B) (C) (D)
28. (A) (B) (C) (D)
29. (A) (B) (C) (D)
30. (A) (B) (C) (D)
31. (A) (B) (C) (D)
32. (A) (B) (C) (D)
33. (A) (B) (C) (D)
34. (A) (B) (C) (D)
35. (A) (B) (C) (D)
36. (A) (B) (C) (D)
37. (A) (B) (C) (D)
38. (A) (B) (C) (D)
39. (A) (B) (C) (D)
40. (A) (B) (C) (D)
41. (A) (B) (C) (D)
42. (A) (B) (C) (D)
43. (A) (B) (C) (D)
44. (A) (B) (C) (D)
45. (A) (B) (C) (D)
46. (A) (B) (C) (D)
47. (A) (B) (C) (D)
48. (A) (B) (C) (D)
49. (A) (B) (C) (D)
50. (A) (B) (C) (D)
51. (A) (B) (C) (D)
52. (A) (B) (C) (D)

SECTION 2: Verbal Reasoning

53. (A) (B) (C) (D)
54. (A) (B) (C) (D)
55. (A) (B) (C) (D)
56. (A) (B) (C) (D)
57. (A) (B) (C) (D)
58. (A) (B) (C) (D)
59. (A) (B) (C) (D)
60. (A) (B) (C) (D)
61. (A) (B) (C) (D)
62. (A) (B) (C) (D)
63. (A) (B) (C) (D)
64. (A) (B) (C) (D)
65. (A) (B) (C) (D)
66. (A) (B) (C) (D)
67. (A) (B) (C) (D)
68. (A) (B) (C) (D)
69. (A) (B) (C) (D)
70. (A) (B) (C) (D)
71. (A) (B) (C) (D)
72. (A) (B) (C) (D)
73. (A) (B) (C) (D)
74. (A) (B) (C) (D)
75. (A) (B) (C) (D)
76. (A) (B) (C) (D)
77. (A) (B) (C) (D)
78. (A) (B) (C) (D)
79. (A) (B) (C) (D)
80. (A) (B) (C) (D)
81. (A) (B) (C) (D)
82. (A) (B) (C) (D)
83. (A) (B) (C) (D)
84. (A) (B) (C) (D)
85. (A) (B) (C) (D)
86. (A) (B) (C) (D)
87. (A) (B) (C) (D)
88. (A) (B) (C) (D)
89. (A) (B) (C) (D)
90. (A) (B) (C) (D)
91. (A) (B) (C) (D)
92. (A) (B) (C) (D)

SECTION 4: Biological Sciences

93. (A) (B) (C) (D)
94. (A) (B) (C) (D)
95. (A) (B) (C) (D)
96. (A) (B) (C) (D)
97. (A) (B) (C) (D)
98. (A) (B) (C) (D)
99. (A) (B) (C) (D)
100. (A) (B) (C) (D)

101. Ⓐ Ⓑ Ⓒ Ⓓ
102. Ⓐ Ⓑ Ⓒ Ⓓ
103. Ⓐ Ⓑ Ⓒ Ⓓ
104. Ⓐ Ⓑ Ⓒ Ⓓ
105. Ⓐ Ⓑ Ⓒ Ⓓ
106. Ⓐ Ⓑ Ⓒ Ⓓ
107. Ⓐ Ⓑ Ⓒ Ⓓ
108. Ⓐ Ⓑ Ⓒ Ⓓ
109. Ⓐ Ⓑ Ⓒ Ⓓ
110. Ⓐ Ⓑ Ⓒ Ⓓ
111. Ⓐ Ⓑ Ⓒ Ⓓ
112. Ⓐ Ⓑ Ⓒ Ⓓ
113. Ⓐ Ⓑ Ⓒ Ⓓ
114. Ⓐ Ⓑ Ⓒ Ⓓ
115. Ⓐ Ⓑ Ⓒ Ⓓ
116. Ⓐ Ⓑ Ⓒ Ⓓ
117. Ⓐ Ⓑ Ⓒ Ⓓ
118. Ⓐ Ⓑ Ⓒ Ⓓ
119. Ⓐ Ⓑ Ⓒ Ⓓ
120. Ⓐ Ⓑ Ⓒ Ⓓ
121. Ⓐ Ⓑ Ⓒ Ⓓ
122. Ⓐ Ⓑ Ⓒ Ⓓ
123. Ⓐ Ⓑ Ⓒ Ⓓ
124. Ⓐ Ⓑ Ⓒ Ⓓ
125. Ⓐ Ⓑ Ⓒ Ⓓ
126. Ⓐ Ⓑ Ⓒ Ⓓ
127. Ⓐ Ⓑ Ⓒ Ⓓ
128. Ⓐ Ⓑ Ⓒ Ⓓ
129. Ⓐ Ⓑ Ⓒ Ⓓ
130. Ⓐ Ⓑ Ⓒ Ⓓ
131. Ⓐ Ⓑ Ⓒ Ⓓ
132. Ⓐ Ⓑ Ⓒ Ⓓ
133. Ⓐ Ⓑ Ⓒ Ⓓ
134. Ⓐ Ⓑ Ⓒ Ⓓ
135. Ⓐ Ⓑ Ⓒ Ⓓ
136. Ⓐ Ⓑ Ⓒ Ⓓ
137. Ⓐ Ⓑ Ⓒ Ⓓ
138. Ⓐ Ⓑ Ⓒ Ⓓ
139. Ⓐ Ⓑ Ⓒ Ⓓ
140. Ⓐ Ⓑ Ⓒ Ⓓ
141. Ⓐ Ⓑ Ⓒ Ⓓ
142. Ⓐ Ⓑ Ⓒ Ⓓ
143. Ⓐ Ⓑ Ⓒ Ⓓ
144. Ⓐ Ⓑ Ⓒ Ⓓ